DE RE MEDICA

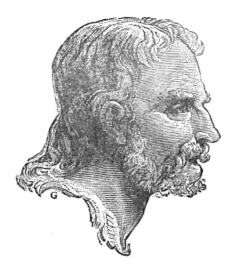

CELSUS, Aurelius Cornelius

30 B.C. — A.D. 38

DE RE MEDICA

Editio Tertia

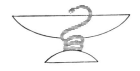

INDIANAPOLIS, INDIANA, U.S.A.

ELI LILLY AND COMPANY

1951

TO THE MEDICAL PROFESSION

In offering this publication to the medical profession,

Eli Lilly and Company emulates

the purpose and title of the original classic work of Celsus,

DE RE MEDICA *(the first treatise for medical reference),*

first published in Florence in 1478.

This book is a presentation of therapeutic suggestions

in common diseases.

Contents

SECTION 1 PAGE 1   *Common Diseases — Suggested Treatment*

SECTION 2 PAGE 281   *Drugs — Actions and Uses*

SECTION 3 ———   *Colored Plates*

SECTION 4 PAGE 517   *Laboratory Tests*

SECTION 5 PAGE 551   *Poisons and Antidotes*

SECTION 6 PAGE 563   *Useful Tables*

SECTION 7 PAGE 591   *Selected List of Lilly Products*

SECTION 8 PAGE 627   *Index*

Common Diseases

Suggested Treatment

INFECTIOUS DISEASES *

BACTERIAL DISEASES

ABSCESS

An abscess is a circumscribed collection of pus in a cavity formed by necrosis and disintegration of tissues. It is usually surrounded by a wall of inflammatory tissue. Sterile abscesses may be due to local deposits of irritant drugs or toxins. Usually abscesses are due to infection. The so-called "cold abscess," without active inflammation, is usually due to tuberculosis. The acute or warm abscess is typically caused by *Staphylococcus aureus* but may be due to any micro-organism. In the case of furuncles and carbuncles (p. 232) the agent gains access through hair follicles. In abscesses of deep organs the agent is usually carried in the blood, either in the course of bacteremia or in an infected embolus.

An acute abscess may cause three types of symptoms: (1) local inflammation, with redness, swelling, increased heat, tenderness, and, later, fluctuation; (2) pressure on adjacent structures; and (3) constitutional symptoms of infection.

Diagnosis of a superficial abscess is usually simple. Deep-seated abscesses may present difficulty because of the overlapping of symptoms of the infection to which the abscess may be secondary.

Abscesses extend from their starting points along avenues of least mechanical and immunological resistance. They may reach surfaces (point) and evacuate themselves spontaneously.

Treatment—The first principle of treatment of acute abscesses is drainage. If there are constitutional symptoms or the abscess is spreading rapidly, the patient should receive systemic anti-infective therapy (p. 286). As a general rule, an abscess should not be incised for drainage until it has localized; that is, until pus is present and is surrounded by a definite wall of inflammatory tissue. Maintenance of free drainage is of the utmost importance. Local anti-infective therapy may have value.

Tuberculous (cold) abscesses should be protected as much as possible from movement. Treatment is directed to the primary disease. If a cold abscess is increasing rapidly in size, if it is pointing and threatening to break, or if it is interfering with the patient's health, it should be aspirated. Open drainage should be avoided except in the presence of mixed infection.

ANTHRAX

Anthrax is an acute, contagious, infectious disease caused by *Bacillus anthracis*, a gram-positive club-shaped rod. The disease is primarily one of animals, especially cattle and sheep. It is transmitted secondarily to man by contact with infected animals or with the hair, hides, wool, meat, or feces of such animals and is thus largely an occupational disease of tannery, textile, slaughterhouse, farm,

---

* Infections involving principally a single organ or tissue are discussed under the organ concerned (see Index).

1

and veterinary workers. The organism usually enters the body through the skin but occasionally may do so through the lungs or gastro-intestinal tract. The mortality rate with modern therapy approximates 8 percent.

Following an incubation period of one to seven days, the cutaneous type of the disease manifests itself by the development of a painless papule which occurs most frequently on an exposed part of the body. The lesion may itch as it progresses in twelve to twenty-four hours to a vesicle with a dark hemorrhagic center which is later surrounded by brawny edema. A serous or hemorrhagic fluid is discharged, and a hard, depressed, dark-colored eschar forms which lasts for a week or two. The regional lymphatics and lymph nodes are swollen and tender. The pulmonary type of the disease occurs less frequently, usually begins gradually, and resembles a severe pneumonia. The gastro-intestinal type is rare.

Diagnosis of the three types may be made by finding the encapsulated organisms in gram-stained smears or cultures of the cutaneous lesion, sputum, or vomitus. It should be confirmed by animal inoculation. Blood cultures are sometimes positive early in the disease and are not necessarily a bad prognostic sign.

In the differential diagnosis, one must consider carbuncle (p. 232), early chancre (p. 10), impetigo (p. 236), and sycosis vulgaris (p. 237).

Treatment—The drug of choice is penicillin (for dosage, see p. 289). Treatment also includes bed rest, immobilization of the affected extremity, and dressings of penicillin or 5 percent sulfonamide ointment. Some authors report favorable results utilizing sulfonamides systemically (p. 293).

Prophylaxis is directed at the prevention of human contact with infected animals and materials. Infected animals should be cremated or buried deeply. Individuals subject to exposure should wear protective clothing, gloves, and respirators. Proper ventilation is important.

BRUCELLOSIS

Brucellosis (undulant fever) is an acute or chronic, specific septicemic infection of man and animals caused by *Brucella melitensis* (goat type), *Br. abortus* (bovine type), or *Br. suis* (swine type). The bovine type is usually the mildest infection. The mortality is from 2 to 5 percent.

The incubation period varies from five to thirty days but averages fourteen days. In the most common form, the onset is gradual, with generalized aching, headache, anorexia, chilliness, insomnia, backache, and stiffness or pain in the neck and various joints. The temperature rises to 104° to 105°F., with exacerbation of symptoms and extreme weakness. Constipation is common. There may be a progressive weight loss. The temperature increases slowly in the afternoon or evening, accompanied by chilly sensations and followed by drenching sweats. The temperature returns to only slightly elevated levels by morning. The febrile phase lasts from six days to three weeks, recurring after a very few days of normal temperature.

There are many clinical variations of the disease. Spontaneous recovery may occur in a few weeks, or the disease may persist for years. A malignant form is characterized by sudden onset, acute course, sustained high fever, and high fatality rate. A short-duration infection occurs, with fever for one week but with weakness and irritability for many weeks. A very mild form with recurrent mild symptoms may require intensive study for diagnosis.

Diagnosis depends upon recovery of the organism from the blood by culture or guinea-pig inoculation; repeated positive agglutination reactions in a titer of at least 1:50; or positive skin test to Brucellergen, 0.1 cc. of a 1:1,000 solution given intracutaneously in one arm with a normal saline control in the other. The reaction read at twenty-four and forty-eight hours is positive only in the presence of erythema, edema, and induration of greater diameter than 1 cm.

The protean symptomatology makes the differential diagnosis difficult, but typhoid fever (p. 14), the typhoidal type of tularemia (p. 13), tuberculosis (p. 12), rheumatic fever (p. 46), and malaria (p. 34) must be considered. Abdominal pain and tenderness may lead to confusion with acute appendicitis and cholecystitis. Long-enduring cases may be mistaken for functional emotional or psychological disturbances.

Treatment—At present, the most effective therapy is either aureomycin (p. 291) or chloramphenicol (p. 292) alone or in combination with streptomycin (p. 289).

CHANCROID

Chancroid ("soft chancre"), a venereally acquired local bacterial infection of the genitalia caused by *Hemophilus ducreyi*, is characterized by single or multiple necrotic ulcers and often is complicated by inflammation and suppuration of the regional lymph glands. The incubation period varies from one to twenty-four days, but the average is from three to five days.

The typical lesion is a tender, circumscribed ulcer with ragged, undermined edges, the base showing purulent granulations. Multiple lesions develop by autoinoculation. Untreated lesions may heal spontaneously in days or weeks, leaving varying degrees of scarring and destruction. Prolonged, widespread, destructive ulcers may occur in some cases unless treatment is prompt and adequate.

Diagnosis is made with certainty by finding *H. ducreyi* on smear or culture. For dependable results, these procedures require skill and experience. The skin test utilizing specific antigen is useful. It becomes positive in from eight to twenty-five days after infection. However, since skin sensitivity remains for life following an attack of the disease, the test is of positive diagnostic value only when one can be certain that he is dealing with an initial infection. When smears are negative, presumptive diagnosis must depend upon clinical appearance and exclusion of syphilis (p. 10), granuloma inguinale, and lymphogranuloma venereum (p. 23). Since multiple infection with more than one venereal disease is common, particular care must be taken to rule out all such possibilities. To rule out syphilis, at least a four-month serologic follow-up is necessary.

Treatment—Sulfonamides are specific therapy; 2 to 4 Gm. daily by mouth for seven days are usually curative. Local therapy with sulfonamide powder or ointment for four to five days is a useful adjunct. Aureomycin, chloramphenicol, and streptomycin are also effective, but they are considered by some clinicians to be less desirable because they may mask coexisting syphilis.

Bed rest is required for febrile patients with acutely inflamed glands. These should never be incised; if fluctuation develops, the gland should be aspirated aseptically by means of a 20-gauge needle introduced through a small wheal of local anesthetic solution.

The complication of phimosis or paraphimosis should be treated with compresses of warm saturated solution of magnesium sulfate. Circumcision or dorsal slit is rarely necessary.

A rapidly spreading necrotic, gangrenous ulcer may occur, often because of secondary infection by anaerobic spiral organisms. It is best treated by a combination of systemic administration of penicillin and local application of hydrogen peroxide, one part in four parts of water.

DIPHTHERIA

Diphtheria is an infection, usually of the upper respiratory tract, with *Corynebacterium diphtheriae*. It is transmitted directly by contact with a case or carrier and indirectly by articles soiled by fresh discharges. It has become relatively uncommon because of the almost complete protection afforded by immunization.

Diphtheria is a local infection, characterized by development of a distinctive membrane. The lesion itself is dangerous only when it includes the larynx, where it may occlude the respiratory passage. The other danger in diphtheria lies in the soluble exotoxin, which, after absorption, may produce myocardial inflammation or degeneration, or nerve paralysis, particularly of the third, sixth, and ninth cranial nerves. Many strains of the causative agent have been identified, some of which are nonvirulent. Virulence is determined by intracutaneous inoculation into guinea pigs.

Diagnosis of diphtheria is made by culture of the organism from the lesions. The disease may be suspected from the typical membrane, which is gray or gray-green, adherent, of a mouselike odor, and surrounded by a dull-red edematous area. The membrane usually forms on the tonsils, from which it spreads, but it may occur only in the pharynx, nasopharynx, or larynx and trachea. When it occurs only in relatively inaccessible areas, diphtheria may not be suspected until complications occur. The differential diagnosis includes acute tonsillitis (p. 9), Vincent's angina (p. 124), and infectious mononucleosis (p. 48).

Prevention is achieved by immunization. All infants should be immunized (p. 324), and a boosting dose should be administered before the child enters school.

Treatment—When diphtheria is suspected, the lesion should be cultured, and antitoxin should be given at once before the results of the culture are known. For dosage, see page 335. The usual precautions regarding sensitivity to the serum should be taken (p. 334).

Patients with diphtheria should be kept in bed and isolated until three nasal and three throat cultures taken at least twenty-four hours apart are negative. If positive cultures persist after the patient is clinically well, a virulence test should be made. Carriers can sometimes be cured by repeated topical application of penicillin powder to the tonsils or by systemic administration of the antibiotic. It has no value against the disease.

Laryngeal or tracheal obstruction should be treated by intubation or tracheotomy. Myocarditis requires absolute bed rest and the general handling of cardiac failure (p. 65). Digitalis should be given only when congestive failure is present.

BACILLARY DYSENTERY

Bacillary dysentery is an acute or chronic, infectious, inflammatory disease of the colon caused by four organisms of the genus *Shigella*. *S. dysenteriae* causes more severe symptoms than the others. *S. sonnei* infections are often resistant to treatment. Infections by *S. paradysenteriae* and *S. ambigua* are somewhat less severe. The mortality has varied widely from 0 to 70 percent, but with good management it usually will not exceed 1 percent.

The incubation period ranges from one to seven days. In the usual case the onset is abrupt, with fever developing early and rarely exceeding 104°F. Griping abdominal pains are followed shortly by diarrhea with twenty to forty stools a day. The symptoms increase in severity, and within twenty-four hours the patient is passing the typical dysenteric stool consisting of mucus, pus, and blood accompanied by tenesmus. Abdominal tenderness over the colon and the sudden onset may be mistaken for appendicitis. Headache, vomiting, malaise, or drowsiness usually occurs.

The fulminating type of the disease not uncommonly is accompanied by collapse and may be marked by chill, high fever, and vomiting, followed shortly by falling temperature, profound toxemia, and death.

The chronic form of the disease is said to exist if the dysentery persists for more than a month. The patient persistently passes loose stools containing small amounts of mucus. Commonly there are periods of exacerbation and remission, the periods of active disease being accompanied by fever and diarrhea with varying amounts of blood, mucus, and characteristic cellular exudate. Each bout results in increasing scarring and fibrosis of the colon.

Diagnosis of the disease is based upon the character of the stools and recovery of the organism on culture. The typical mucopurulent stool varies from pale pink to bright red in color. Microscopically, a cover-slip preparation reveals an abundant cellular exudate rich in polymorphonuclear white blood cells, a variable quantity of red blood cells, and a certain proportion of large cells; some of the latter are large white cells, and others are macrophages which may contain ingested red cells. Many of the

white cells appear to be undergoing necrosis or to be "ghost" cells. The white blood cell count is usually normal and rarely over 16,000. Leukopenia may occur in the most severe forms of the disease.

Complications include monoarticular or polyarticular arthritis after the acute stage is passed, myocarditis, neuritis, peripheral circulatory failure, intestinal perforation, chronic peritonitis, and renal failure. One attack may produce immunity to the attacking strain but not to other strains or species.

In the differential diagnosis, amebic dysentery (p. 33), balantidial dysentery, malarial dysentery (p. 34), cholera, intussusception, irritable colon (p. 135), ulcerative colitis (p.135), and carcinoma must be considered.

Treatment—In the acute type, the sulfonamides are the drugs of choice (for dosage, see p. 295). They should be given as early as possible and continued until the stools have been normal in number and consistency for two days. Because of the large fluid and electrolyte losses in the stools, it is doubly important to provide an adequate intake of these substances to prevent sulfonamide precipitation in the kidneys (see pp. 295 and 52). Severe toxemia may be combated by antiserum, 40 to 80 cc. diluted in 500 cc. of isotonic salt solution, administered intravenously twice daily. General measures include bed rest and an easily assimilated diet rich in protein and vitamins. Daily administration of a mild saline cathartic, such as 4 Gm. of sodium sulfate in 200 cc. of hot water, should be begun early and continued until the disease subsides.

Repeated cultures should be made for three weeks after completion of treatment to ascertain whether or not the patient has become a carrier.

Treatment of the chronic type may be difficult. Chemotherapy with the sulfonamides, often for prolonged periods, is important. The diet should be low in roughage but adequate in regard to protein and vitamins. Small amounts of saline cathartics are helpful (see above). The condition of the colon should be followed by sigmoidoscopy. Visualization of ulcers may allow direct application of 10 to 20 percent silver nitrate solution on a cotton swab. Autogenous vaccines have been of benefit in some instances.

Prophylaxis depends upon prevention of food and water contamination by feces of infected individuals, whether through food handlers, transfer by houseflies, or water contamination with feces. Since carriers are not uncommon, control of food handlers is of great importance.

ERYSIPELAS

Erysipelas is an acute inflammatory disease of the skin (infrequently of the mucous membranes) caused by *Streptococcus hemolyticus,* usually Group A. Lowering of resistance and previous attacks are predisposing factors. The organism usually gains entrance through a wound, fissure, or abrasion. Untreated, the disease usually lasts four to eight days, frequently terminating by crisis and with a mortality of 5 to 10 percent. Relapses are not uncommon.

Following an incubation period of one to three days, prodromata may appear, such as chill and fever, vomiting, malaise, headache, and anorexia. The skin lesion begins with or shortly after the prodromata as a small, red, shiny, swollen, tender area, the edge of which becomes raised, sharply demarcated, and indurated. Vesicles or blebs may form. The region first involved may clear while the infection spreads at the periphery. Extension is by continuity, frequently along the lymphatics, giving rise to tongue-shaped projections. As local healing begins, the vesicles dry to form crusts, and flaky desquamation occurs.

Ninety percent of attacks occur on the face. Frequently beginning on the nose or in the nostril, the process spreads to both cheeks to give a "butterfly" appearance followed by facial edema. In similar fashion the disease may arise and spread from surgical wounds, the umbilicus of the newborn, or the vulva after parturition. The disease may appear in the pharynx, fauces, and nose, where it is marked by intense diffuse redness and severe pain.

The principal complication is abscess formation. Superficial gangrene, suppuration in the nasal sinuses, or extension to and thrombosis of the cavernous sinus may occur. Bacteremia and pneumonia are serious complications.

Diagnosis of the facial type usually is easily made from the appearance. An increase of white blood cells, especially polymorphonuclears, is usually present. Streptococci may be recovered from the edges of the lesion.

The disease must be differentiated from erythematous eczema (p. 235) and erysipeloid. The latter resembles erysipelas locally but causes no systemic symptoms. It is due to *Erysipelothrix rhusiopathiae* (*B. erysipelatos-suis*), which is the cause of swine erysipelas. It is contracted from animals by contact and responds readily to penicillin.

Treatment—The patient should be isolated. Penicillin or sulfadiazine is usually curative (for dosage, see pp. 289 and 295, respectively). Because of the possibility of relapse, bed rest should be continued until the temperature has been normal for two or three days. The patient's comfort may be promoted by local application of emollients (p. 479).

GAS GANGRENE

Gas gangrene is an acute, fulminating infection occurring in massive lacerations and deep puncture wounds. Development of the disease is favored by heavy deposits of dirt and extensive muscle damage (such as often accompany war wounds or civilian compound fractures) and by impairment of tissue nutrition (such as may be present at the site of amputation for diabetic or arteriosclerotic gangrene). The most common causative organisms are *Clostridium perfringens, Cl. bifermentans,* and *Cl. septicum.* They are gram-positive, sporeforming, anaerobic bacilli. Muscles primarily are attacked, with the production of a virulent toxin and gas bubbles in the tissues. Severe local and systemic symptoms may appear abruptly within ten to twelve hours after the injury.

The rapid destruction of muscle tissue and the dissection of tissue layers by the gas result in severe pain and swelling. Gangrene may extend to the skin. A watery, offensive wound exudate loaded with large gram-positive bacilli is pathognomonic. Sometimes gas in the tissues is appreciated first by x-ray, and sometimes it never is detected clinically. There are also usually profound intoxication with high fever, rapid pulse, extreme apprehension, and a bronzing of the face, chest, and arms.

Treatment—Prophylactic measures consist in early radical wound débridement and the intramuscular administration of polyvalent antitoxin (combined concentrated tetanus-gas-gangrene antitoxin.) Both penicillin (p. 289) and sulfonamides (p. 295) should be given as early as possible. It is fairly well established that these drugs have little or no effect on the growth of the causative organisms. However, they should be used freely, because other susceptible organisms may be contributing support to the course of the infection.

Once the signs of the disease have developed, large doses of the antitoxin are recommended, 100,000 to 150,000 units the first twenty-four hours and then smaller doses as indicated. X-ray therapy has been recommended and may have some prophylactic value. Freshly prepared zinc peroxide solution packed loosely into the open wounds is also of value. If the systemic intoxication is severe and the swelling and gangrene are extreme, immediate guillotine amputation may be necessary. The systemic effects require careful attention to the maintenance of normal water and electrolyte balance. Frequent blood transfusions are advisable.

GLANDERS

Glanders is an infectious disease which primarily affects horses, mules, and donkeys and is only rarely transmitted to man. The disease is caused by the organism *Malleomyces mallei*, a gram-negative, nonmotile rod with rounded ends which exhibits bipolar staining with methylene blue. Glanders is rare in the United States and Canada but common in the Orient and the Balkans. It is an occupational risk in laboratory workers and in persons associated with equine animals. The portal of entry usually is a wound contaminated with the feces or discharges from the mucous membranes of infected animals. The conjunctiva and respiratory tract are less usual routes. An acute and a chronic form of the disease are recognized. The prognosis in the former is extremely grave; in the latter, a mortality of 50 to 70 percent may be expected in untreated cases.

The variable incubation period, averaging four days, is followed by a gradual onset with generalized symptoms. In the acute form of the disease the temperature rises to 104°F. The local cutaneous lesions are ulcers with irregular edges and sloughing yellow-grayish bases. Subcutaneous and intramuscular nodules (farcy buds) appear along the lymphatics and are gradually transformed into abscesses. The lesions may occur in the nose or on other mucous membranes. An exanthematous eruption indicates severe sepsis, in which case blood cultures are positive. Delirium and coma precede death in one to seven weeks.

The chronic type of the disease is remittent. An irregular fever develops in one to four weeks; subcutaneous or intramuscular abscesses or tumors appear on the extremities, head, and neck but rarely on the trunk. Bones, joints, and lungs may be involved. Emaciation develops. The disease may run a course of six weeks to fifteen years.

Diagnosis is difficult, but the disease should be suspected in any wound infection in an individual with a history of contact with infected animals. Positive complement-fixation and agglutination tests are diagnostic. The organism may be identified by smear, culture, or animal inoculation. There is disagreement regarding the value and safety of the skin test with mallein. In the differential diag-

nosis, the glanders-like melioidosis caused by *M. pseudomallei* must be considered.

Treatment—The patient should be kept in bed, isolated, and his discharges disinfected. The treatment of choice is sulfonamides given systemically (for dosage, see p. 295). In addition, 5 percent sulfonamide ointment may be applied to the ulcers.

Prevention of glanders in man depends upon suppression of the disease in animals and avoidance of contact with infected animals or contaminated materials. Laboratory personnel should be extremely cautious in handling the causative organism.

GONORRHEA

Gonorrhea is an acute infectious disease, almost always localized, due to the gram-negative organism *Neisseria gonorrhoeae*. The gonococcus has a predilection for certain parts of the body and the type of cell which is found therein. Columnar and transitional columnar cells of the urethra are particularly susceptible to invasion by these bacteria. In the male, the anterior and posterior urethra, prostate gland, seminal vesicles, vas deferens, and epididymis are common sites of attack. The uncomplicated disease is usually confined to the anterior urethra. In women, the inner surfaces of the labia minora, vestibule, urethra, paraurethral glands (Skene's), vulvovaginal glands (Bartholin's), interior of the cervix, endometrium at menstruation, fallopian tubes, ovaries, and pelvic peritoneum are susceptible. The anus and rectum are less commonly attacked. The conjunctiva of the eye is also less frequently a site of infection.

Transmission in males of all ages is by sexual contact. The minimum incubation period is forty-eight hours, but seventy-two hours to five days is the usual time. Over a week is not uncommon.

The disease in males is characterized by a mucoid urethral or serous discharge, which rapidly becomes purulent. Pain or aching on urination may be present. In very acute cases, tenesmus and hematuria are noted. Untreated cases will run a course of three to eight weeks but may enter a chronic form lasting up to six months or more. The incidence of complications is less since specific chemotherapy appeared, but acute prostatitis and epididymitis are still seen. Rectal and external palpation will usually reveal their presence. Arthritis is less common, except in untreated cases. The tendency for a single joint to be painfully swollen is characteristic. The persistence of a discharge without symptoms is noted in chronic cases of cowperitis, strictures, prostatitis, and vesicular infection. Urinary obstruction and retention are among the most serious end results. Sterility due to fibrosis of the vas deferens may occur also.

The differential diagnosis of the acute disease in the male involves various causes of nonspecific urethritis, which may be chemical, catarrhal, protozoal, pyogenic, herpetic, and traumatic. The culture and identification of the gonococcus is the only certain method of diagnosis. The chronic and other forms of the disease will involve distinction from nonspecific prostatitis, tuberculous epididymitis, rheumatic arthritis, and even bacterial endocarditis.

In the female, the urinary symptoms are less prominent because of the absence of urethral glands. When first seen, most cases present a cervicitis or infection of the endocervical glands. The factors of poor drainage and menstruation often prolong the disease and cause treatment failures. Salpingitis is common in untreated cases and occurs following menstruation. Concurrent local peritonitis often is seen. The differential diagnosis from acute ruptured appendicitis is difficult, but a careful history, positive cervical smears, evidence of bilateral involvement, and pelvic examination will usually be conclusive. When the history is unreliable, the diagnosis is difficult. Bartholin's abscess is usually due to the gonococcus, but recovery of the organism is rare. Chronic endocervicitis due to *Trichomonas*, nonspecific leukorrhea, and lacerations of childbirth often confuses the diagnosis. Chronicity of infection in the female is the rule rather than the exception, for the patient is rarely seen in the acute stage of her illness when cure would be simpler.

Gonorrheal ophthalmia in newborn infants is less common since most states require prophylactic silver nitrate drops at delivery. Prompt diagnosis and treatment with penicillin ointments (5,000 units per Gm.) will avoid the tragedy of blindness.

Vulvovaginitis in young, immature females is a common form of gonorrhea, especially in institutions. The preadolescent vaginal epithelium is particularly susceptible to the gonococcus, as is the urethra and rectum.

Treatment—Acute gonorrhea is most simply treated with a single injection of 300,000 units of procaine penicillin (p. 288). Some urologists advocate, in addition in the male, gentle irrigation of the urethra with a 1:10,000 solution of potassium permanganate three times daily for three days. Three negative smears and cultures at one-week intervals are necessary before the patient can be assumed to be free of infection. In women, it is advisable to take cervical smears and cultures at the end of each of three successive menstrual periods. If any of the cultures are positive, the patient should at once receive an injection of 600,000 units. For those few that still do not respond, a course of hyperpyrexia and aqueous penicillin (40,000 units every three hours, for a total of 320,000 units) is advised. Because there may be penicillin-fast strains of this organism, large doses of sulfadiazine, aureomycin, or streptomycin may result in remarkable recoveries when penicillin has failed.

The treatment of chronic prostatitis may require massage and the introduction of 5 percent mild silver protein solutions. Occasionally, surgical drainage is necessary to destroy an untouched focus of infection.

The treatment of the female is less successful in that drainage of foci, such as Bartholin's cysts and pelvic abscesses, may be required in addition to penicillin therapy. The dosage is similar, but more prolonged treatment is often necessary.

Vulvovaginitis in children is responsive to estrogenic hormones or sulfonamides, but recurrences and chronicity are found. Procaine penicillin, 100,000 units intramuscularly for three doses in the acute phase of this disease, usually produces excellent results. Reports of success with lower doses have been made, but relapses have also been noted in these series. Rigid culture criteria and follow-up for at least six months are necessary. Elimination of sources of adult infection in the family, institution, or foster home is equally as important as chemotherapy in these cases.

Arthritis due to gonococci may require aspiration of the joint and instillation of penicillin (20,000 units) solution in isotonic salt solution, but systemic injection should always be tried first.

Endocarditis is a serious but rare complication of this disease. Response to large doses of penicillin has been favorable.

PLAGUE

Plague is an acute infectious disease of men and rodents caused by *Pasteurella pestis* and transmitted by rat fleas and other less important biting insects. An area of endemic sylvatic (rodent) plague exists in the western portion of the United States, where the reservoirs are ground squirrels and prairie dogs.

The bubonic type has an incubation period of two to ten days, but it is usually less than five. In nonimmunized individuals the onset is abrupt, with fever of 103° F., frontal headache, and backache.

The bloated face, injected conjunctiva, swollen coated tongue, staggering gait, stumbling incoherent speech, and obvious apprehension are practically diagnostic in the early stages of a severe attack. Buboes (swellings of the lymph nodes draining the portal of entry) occur in 75 percent of cases, usually within forty-eight hours of onset of fever. Death may occur at any stage, but survival for five days is a good prognostic sign. The mortality rate is 30 percent or more. In favorable cases, general improvement starts between the third and sixth days, the buboes resolving slowly or going on to suppuration.

Pneumonic plague is a highly contagious, uniformly fatal, lobular, hemorrhagic pneumonitis. The incubation period usually is two or three days. The onset is gradual, without a distinct chill. Within twenty-four to thirty-six hours, the temperature rises to 103° to 105°F., pulse to 110 to 130, respirations to thirty to sixty, and a painless productive cough appears. The sputum becomes copious, thin, watery, stained with bright-red blood, and loaded with *Past. pestis*. Death usually occurs within five days.

Septicemic plague is uncommon. It is characterized by immediate prostration and the development of hemorrhages and skin lesions. It usually is rapidly fatal, sometimes within twenty-four hours after onset, but rarely later than three days.

Diagnosis of plague depends upon recognition of *Past. pestis* in cultures or animal inoculations of blood, sputum, or material aspirated from a bubo.

In the differential diagnosis, tularemia (p. 13), typhus (p. 17), typhoid fever (p. 14), syphilis (p. 11), and filariasis must be considered.

Prevention of the disease consists in destruction of animal reservoirs, rodent and flea control, and isolation of infected cases plus disinfection of contaminated materials.

Immunization may be accomplished with plague vaccine (first dose, 0.5 cc., followed after an interval of seven to ten days by a second dose of 1 cc.). Additional 1-cc. boosting doses may be used every four to six months.

Treatment should be initiated promptly. Streptomycin is probably the drug of choice (for dosage, see p. 289). Sulfadiazine is also effective, sulfathiazole less so; by mouth, 4 Gm. should be given every four hours day and night until the temperature is normal, followed by 0.5 Gm. every four hours for ten to fifteen days. In fulminating cases, intravenous administration should be used until oral treatment

can be initiated. Of course, with such large doses special attention must be given to keeping the urine large in volume and alkaline in reaction (p. 295). Good nursing care is essential. Morphine may be used to control restlessness and delirium.

RATBITE FEVER

Ratbite fever (sodoku) is an infectious disease transmitted to man by the bite of wild rats or, rarely, other animals, including cats, dogs, and a variety of rodents. *Spirillum minus* is the usual cause of the disease, though recently another organism, *Streptobacillus moniliformis*, has been implicated in some cases in the United States. One to three weeks after inoculation, there develop headache, chills, enlargement of regional lymph nodes, spiked fever, and a maculopapular rash. At the time of these manifestations, the original wound may become secondarily inflamed and edematous; it may eventually ulcerate. During convalescence, successive febrile paroxysms commonly recur over a period of several weeks. The mortality rate is about 10 percent.

Other conditions which closely resemble ratbite fever are tularemia (p. 13) and relapsing fever (see below). Diagnosis of ratbite fever should be considered in any patient having a febrile disturbance with a history of ratbite. It may be confirmed by intraperitoneal inoculation into white mice, rats, or guinea pigs of specimens of the patient's blood, primary lesion, or regional lymph nodes. If the disease is suspected, therapy should be undertaken without waiting for laboratory confirmation of diagnosis.

Prior to the advent of penicillin, neoarsphenamine (0.6 Gm.) or Mapharsen (0.06 Gm.) was known to be effective against *S. minus* infections. Six doses were recommended to prevent relapses. Recently, several cases of *Streptobacillus moniliformis* infection have been successfully treated with penicillin.

For prophylaxis, wounds produced by ratbites should be cauterized with fuming nitric acid.

RELAPSING FEVER

Relapsing fever is divisible into two principal types: louse-borne, transmitted from man to man, caused by the spirochete *Borrelia recurrentis;* and tick-borne, caused by *B. duttonii*, transmitted from man to man and animals to man. Both are characterized by a recurrent spirochetal septicemia. The disease is endemic in Russia, northern and tropical Africa, China, and India.

The incubation period is two to twelve days

(average seven). The onset is sudden, with chilliness or rigor, fatigue, anorexia, headache, and pain in the back or joints. The temperature may reach 104° to 105° F. and be accompanied by rapid pulse, flushed face, and frequently nausea and vomiting and abdominal pain. The spleen, and as commonly the liver, is enlarged, often tender. The high remittent fever terminates by crisis in two to seven days, with profuse sweating and sometimes collapse. Relapses occur at irregular intervals of three to ten days. In the louse-borne disease, paroxysms last four to seven days; relapses are less severe than the original attack and are usually less than four in number. The mortality varies from 2 to 50 percent. In the tick-borne disease, paroxysms last two to four days and are more severe than in the louseborne. Usually there are more than four relapses, and cerebrospinal symptoms may be more severe. The mortality is about 5 percent.

Variable manifestations include violet-red petechial rash on the shoulders and limbs; hemorrhages from the nose, gums, or gastro-intestinal tract; herpes; cough, pain in the chest, signs of bronchitis; lymphadenopathy; conjunctivitis; iritis; cranial nerve palsy; and meningitis. In some epidemics, jaundice is common.

Diagnosis depends upon recognition of the spirochetes in the blood during the febrile period, characteristic temperature curves, and the presence of the vectors.

Treatment includes good nursing, bed rest, liquid diet, and cold spongings. Although arsenicals are considered specific, they may be ineffective in some cases, particularly when infection has been tickborne. Neoarsphenamine (0.6 Gm.) or Mapharsen (0.04 to 0.06 Gm.) should be given intravenously in the early stages of the initial attack or of a relapse. One dose usually is curative, but two or three may be required. The drugs should not be given in the middle or terminal stages of an attack because of the possibility of collapse, or in the afebrile period because of the possibility of production of arsenic-resistant strains of *Borrelia*. It appears that penicillin in a total dosage of 1,560,000 to 2,800,000 units given in 40,000-unit doses every three hours may be effective. It may be given during any stage of the disease.

STREPTOCOCCUS UPPER-RESPIRATORY INFECTIONS

Under this title are included several conditions formerly regarded as distinct entities but now coming to be accepted as a group with fundamental etiological and epidemiological similarities; principally, these are scarlet fever and streptococcus sore throat (acute follicular tonsillitis). It has been demonstrated that several strains of Lancefield Group A hemolytic streptococci may cause infectious processes, the symptomatology of which depends upon the nature of the toxins thrown off by the particular strain and upon the immunological status of the individuals affected. Thus the same organism may cause scarlet fever in one individual and merely sore throat in another. The difference is due to the fact that the latter individual is resistant to the erythrogenic (rash-producing) toxin. Many persons are asymptomatic carriers of the organism, especially during epidemic periods.

Diagnosis of streptococcus sore throat may be made on clinical grounds in the majority of cases. Important signs are sudden onset, often with headache and prostration; intense redness of the palate, tonsillar region, and pharynx; edema, especially of the tonsils if they are present; exudate on the tonsils, fauces, or pharynx; and swelling and tenderness of the anterior cervical lymph glands. Not all these signs need be present. Exudate is often lacking. Laboratory evidence of the infection may be secured by culture of Group A hemolytic streptococci from the nose or throat (bearing in mind that certain individuals may be carriers) or by serologic demonstration of an increase of antistreptococcic antibodies.

Streptococcus upper-respiratory infection must be differentiated particularly from two other diseases. One is influenza (p. 22), which in general produces more severe systemic manifestations with minimal signs in the pharynx (usually redness without edema). The other is a respiratory tract infection related apparently to so-called "atypical" or virus pneumonia (p. 117), perhaps being a milder form of the same disease; its most prominent symptom is cough.

Scarlet fever may be suspected when a patient with acute sore throat has a punctate rash which blanches on pressure. It is most evident usually about the neck, chest, groin, inner thighs, and folds of the skin. Circumoral pallor may be present. In doubtful cases the Schultz-Charlton reaction may be employed; 0.2 cc. of scarlet-fever antitoxin is injected intradermally in an area of definite erythema as soon as possible after appearance of the rash. Local disappearance of the rash in four to twenty-four hours is pathognomonic; failure of disappearance does not exclude scarlet fever. The differential diagnosis also includes drug rash (p.227), serum sickness and other forms of allergy, measles (p. 24), rubella (p. 31), erysipelas (p. 5), typhus and other rickettsial fevers (p. 16), syphilis (see below), diphtheria (p. 3), exanthem subitum, and acrodynia.

Many complications may follow streptococcus respiratory infections. Early in the disease, septic complications due to direct extension or bacteremia may occur. Later, suppurative lesions may develop, the most common being otitis media (frequently followed by mastoiditis). Others include pneumonia (p. 115), empyema, meningitis, peritonsillar or retropharyngeal abscess, sinusitis, and occasionally lateral sinus thrombosis. Still other complications may occur after subsidence of the disease; the most important is glomerulonephritis (p. 218).

Treatment of the infection itself may be accomplished effectively by penicillin (for dosage, see p. 289). Sulfonamides are also of value. The patient should be isolated during the infectious period, and disinfection, both concurrent and terminal, should be practiced. A series of cultures negative for hemolytic streptococci, taken from the nose, throat, or suppurating lesions, should determine when isolation can be terminated safely.

Bed rest is essential for three weeks, whether the infection is mild or severe, and should be prolonged in the presence of complications. In scarlet fever the skin should be kept clean with nonirritating soaps. Itching may be an indication for mild antipruritic lotions (p. 480). Bland oils (p. 479) may be used to correct excessive dryness associated with desquamation.

Prompt and sufficiently prolonged administration of penicillin usually prevents complications. However, these should be watched for, and the urine should be examined periodically for a month for evidence of nephritis.

The rash of scarlet fever can be controlled by scarlet-fever antitoxin or pooled convalescent serum. It must be given early. A single intramuscular injection of 9,000 to 18,000 antitoxic units (National Institute of Health; approximately equal to 450,000 to 900,000 neutralizing units) of antitoxin or 80 to 100 cc. of convalescent serum is usually sufficient. Since severe allergic reactions from the antitoxin may occur in individuals sensitive to horse serum, preinjection precautions should be observed (p. 334).

Where there is constant possibility of exposure to streptococcus infection, as in staffs and inmates of institutions, it may in some instances be advisable to immunize actively against the rash of scarlet fever. Susceptibility to the rash is indicated by local inflammation, 1 cm. or more in diameter, which develops after intradermal injection of 0.1 cc. of diluted, standardized scarlet-fever toxin (Dick test) and persists for more than twenty-four hours. Two types of immunizing toxin are available; the tannic-acid-precipitated form is preferred. It is given at weekly intervals in five subcutaneous injections of 650, 2,500, 10,000, 30,000, and 100,000 skin-test units, respectively. Reactions are often severe. The immunity protects only against the rash and not against streptococcus infection itself.

SYPHILIS

Syphilis is a chronic contagious disease due to the *Spirochaeta pallida* (*Treponema pallidum*). It is acquired almost wholly through direct contact with open lesions, since the organism does not survive drying. The congenital form is transmitted from the mother through the placenta.

Natural History—From the beginning, syphilis is always a generalized disease. The organisms enter the blood stream within a few minutes after inoculation and spread throughout the body within twenty-four hours. There is then a primary incubation period which lasts days to months but averages something less than four weeks. At the end of this period there appears at the site of inoculation in many, but by no means all, patients a so-called "primary lesion," or chancre. Since the success of therapy varies inversely with the duration of infection and since the chancre is the first recognizable lesion, it is most important that it be seen and identified.

Although it may take various forms, the uncomplicated lesion often appears first as a papule which grows and becomes a smooth, regularly bordered ulcer that has a "punched-out" appearance. If uncomplicated, it is painless. It is usually single rather than multiple and is accompanied by enlargement of adjacent lymph nodes (the satellite bubo). Confirmation of the nature of the primary sore is sought by dark-field examination for the presence of spirochetes in serum from the untreated chancre or aspirated lymph from a satellite bubo. Extragenital chancres have been found on the lips, tongue, fingers, eyelids, skin, and other locations.

About six weeks after the appearance of the chancre there is usually an explosion of lesions throughout the body, the most obvious of which are those which involve the skin and mucous membranes. These cutaneous manifestations may take a variety of forms but are most often maculopapular. When the scalp is involved, there may be a patchy alopecia. This secondary stage may last for two years or more, during which time various manifestations may appear and regress.

During this early period of infection the lesions are ordinarily benign, leaving no permanent damage. Following it there is usually a long period of apparent quiescence varying from a few years to life. During this period of relative balance between the infectious agent and the tissues of the host, a large majority of the organisms are eliminated; those that remain become localized, often to make trouble later as the various tissues become allergic to them.

Thus, the early lesions contain many spirochetes and are dangerous to others but not to the patient, whereas the late lesions contain few spirochetes and are relatively noninfectious but are extremely dangerous to the patient because of their destructive nature.

This alteration in reaction to the syphilitic infection usually takes place about three years after infection in untreated cases, but it may vary from two years to twenty. The altered response consists typically in infiltration with plasma cells, lymphocytes, and epithelioid cells, followed by obliterative endarteritis of the surrounded blood vessels. The result is degeneration and scarring. Lesions of this kind, termed "gummata" when they form tumors, may be of any size. They do the most damage when they arise in vital structures, notably the liver, the cardiovascular system (where they may give rise to aortitis, aortic insufficiency, and aortic aneurysm), and the nervous system and its coverings. In addition, there may be parenchymatous degeneration, particularly of the nervous system. When this involves the spinal cord, it usually produces tabes dorsalis; when the cerebral cortex, paresis.

Diagnosis of syphilis varies in ease and certainty, depending on the stage of the disease and other factors. Finding of the typical spirochetes in dark-field preparations of primary and secondary lesions is pathognomonic. In the absence of such a finding, a complete physical examination, omitting absolutely no part of the body that can be seen or palpated, may disclose suggestive lesions. A history of exposure or of lesions suggesting primary or secondary syphilis may be helpful but is sometimes elicited only with difficulty.

Besides history, physical examination, and dark-field examination, serologic tests are extremely use-

ful. Of these, the complement-fixation tests have largely given way to the flocculation tests. There is also a trend toward the quantitative determinations, since they give much more useful information for diagnosis and for judging the response to treatment. The flocculation tests, which include the Kahn, Eagle, Hinton, Kline, Mazzini, cardiolipin, and others, measure the concentration in the blood serum of the globulin reagin. Normally the serum contains less than one Kahn unit of reagin per cc. After infection with syphilis the titer usually, but not always, rises so that in 35 to 50 percent of patients 12 Kahn units may be reached at the end of the second week, although sometimes six weeks or more may be required. As the infection persists, the level is ordinarily maintained at 160 Kahn units or higher, occasionally in excess of 5,000 Kahn units.

Unfortunately, certain other infections and immunizing procedures also raise the reagin level, but seldom beyond 40 Kahn units. Malaria, brucellosis, dengue, yellow fever, infectious mononucleosis, and other less common diseases may have this effect. However, serial tests in such false positives are likely to show great fluctuation in values, often above 10 Kahn units but seldom above 40. Similar false positives may follow repeated blood donations or immunization against smallpox, influenza, yellow fever, or other infections. Thus, no patient should be given a diagnosis on the basis of a single serologic test or, in the absence of positive findings in history or physical examination, on the basis of tests on a single specimen. A negative serologic test (or a series of them) is without significance, since in many cases the tests remain negative, particularly in syphilis of the nervous system or cardiovascular system.

Once the diagnosis has been confirmed, the complete co-operation of the patient must be solicited or success in treatment cannot be expected. Tact, patience, and skill in handling the initial interview can do much to assure that the patient will do his part in carrying out instructions during treatment and in reporting back to the physician at regular intervals. If the patient is helped in adjusting to the fact that syphilis is his present illness and if he is properly advised on what precautions he must take because of his infectious condition, not only will there be less chance of a lapse in treatment but such a patient becomes an effective agent in preventing spread of the disease.

Treatment—Until the advent of penicillin, treatment consisted in the administration of preparations of arsenic and bismuth, sometimes mercury, and sometimes iodides (see p. 296 *et seq.*). Neoarsphen-amine, Clorarsen, and Mapharsen were the most widely used arsenicals. When it was demonstrated that penicillin possessed a strong antitreponemal action, combined therapeutic programs were adopted in which penicillin was used in conjunction with arsenic or bismuth or both.

At the present time, penicillin alone is considered the treatment of choice in primary and secondary syphilis. The standard schedule is ten daily injections of 600,000 units (preferably of procaine penicillin). In case of serologic or clinical relapse, this course should be repeated. Infantile congenital syphilis and syphilis during pregnancy are treated in similar fashion, the dose being reduced according to age in the former case. In late syphilis, the same schedule should be repeated several times as indicated by the clinical and serologic picture presented by each case. Neurosyphilis is treated with very large doses of penicillin, often associated with either fever therapy, or arsenic and bismuth, or with both. Although no final judgment can be passed as yet, penicillin alone has appeared to be adequate therapy for these stages of syphilitic infection.

As was true with other agents used in the therapy of syphilis, penicillin may give rise to Jarisch-Herxheimer reactions in many patients. Although of no major importance in the earlier stages of the disease, they may be of serious consequence in syphilis of the cardiovascular or nervous system. Therefore, the doses should be low in the first days of treatment when these systems are involved.

The decision as to cure is to be based on both clinical and laboratory evidence. Repeated blood serologic studies and spinal-fluid examinations are basic in judging therapeutic results. It is to be emphasized that treatment must be adequate. Inadequate therapy is often worse for the patient than none.

TETANUS

Tetanus (lockjaw) is an acute infectious disease due to the toxin of *Clostridium tetani*. The spores of this organism are omnipresent and are extremely resistant to destruction. The disease may occur as the result of implantation of the spores in any wound, accidental or surgical, but it usually occurs following deep puncture wounds. Concomitant necrosis of tissue, the presence of a foreign body, or pyogenic infection is usually required for growth of the organism. The mortality from the disease, even with the best of care, may exceed 50 percent.

After an incubation period of three days to three weeks, averaging five to ten days, either generalized or localized tetanus may develop. Localized tetanus is characterized by persistent and unyielding rigidity of local muscle groups in the region of the wound. It may persist for weeks or months and disappear without residuals. It is the least likely to be fatal.

Generalized tetanus usually first presents stiffness of the jaw, sometimes accompanied and usually followed by restlessness, irritability, stiffness of the neck, and difficulty in swallowing. As the disease progresses, the muscles of the neck and back become rigid, stiffness of the jaw becomes severe (trismus), characteristic rigid smiling facies develops (risus sardonicus), abdominal muscles may become rigid, opisthotonos may occur, and painful convulsions develop. There is fever of 101° to 104°F. Cyanosis, asphyxia, and death usually result from spasm of the respiratory muscles. The prognosis is grave and is somewhat in proportion to the length of time between the initial symptoms and the occurrence of convulsions. The longer this period, the better the prognosis.

In the differential diagnosis, meningitis (p. 165), tetany (p. 195), strychnine poisoning, and impacted, infected molar teeth must be considered.

Treatment—There is growing evidence that the most important phase of the treatment of tetanus is control of the muscle spasms. Although tetanus antitoxin (p. 335) is still employed by many clinicians, the survival rate appears to be as good without it as with it. Convulsions may be controlled by paraldehyde, 10 to 40 cc. by rectum every three hours, or by intravenous barbiturates (p. 390) in doses just adequate for control. Stridor may require tracheotomy. Oxygen may be indicated. Adequate nutrition and hydration may require an indwelling gastric tube.

Active immunity can be induced by administration of tetanus toxoid (p. 326). In case of a wound or burn in a previously immunized patient, adequate prophylaxis consists in a boosting dose of toxoid (p. 326). In the absence of previous active immunization, tetanus antitoxin may be given when a patient has a wound likely to be contaminated with tetanus spores (for dosage, see p. 335).

TUBERCULOSIS

Tuberculosis is an infectious disease caused by the *Mycobacterium tuberculosis*. The agent may gain entrance to the body through inhalation or by ingestion. First contact with the organism usually results in the so-called primary or childhood type of infection, involving one or more of the following: parenchyma of the lungs, cervical lymph nodes, bronchial and hilar pulmonary lymph nodes, and mesenteric lymph nodes. These lesions, which are of the caseous type, may progress, and the infection may become disseminated; but more commonly they regress slowly, leaving fibrotic and sometimes calcified nodes containing a few live bacilli. Systemic symptoms may be trivial. As a result of the primary infection, however, most if not all of the tissues of the body become allergic to tuberculoprotein. This type of allergy involving the skin is the basis of the tuberculin test (p. 339).

In the past, a large percentage of the adult population has shown evidence of "healed" primary tuberculosis. When such an individual is reinfected or when for unknown reasons he is autoinfected by release of active bacilli from the "healed" lesions, the course of the disease in this secondary or adult type is quite different because of the allergic and immunobiologic response resulting from the primary infection.

The adult type of the disease may involve any organ or tissue but is most common in the lungs. It may be acute or chronic. The lesions are of a characteristic inflammatory nature and are termed "tubercles." The traditional signs and symptoms include fatigability, weight loss, malaise, anorexia, pallor, fever, sweats (especially at night), pain or swelling (depending on the location of the lesions), and, in the case of pulmonary tuberculosis, cough, which may vary from a slight hack to a severe, persistent type. However, in many cases the disease is active for years without obvious signs or symptoms, the person considering himself to be in good health.

Because of the silent nature of most primary and many second-type infections, the importance of examining the lung fields and adjacent areas by x-ray cannot be overemphasized. Nor can the value of case finding of contacts be minimized. Among children and adolescents the skin test with tuberculin (p. 339) or one of its derivatives is extremely valuable, although when positive it is not a criterion of activity.

Treatment will vary in individual cases, depending on the degree of advancement of the disease and the symptoms presented. Rest is the most important single item, the degree of restriction depending on the individual condition. An adequate diet is essential, with attention to adjuncts such as vita-

mins. Heliotherapy under expert supervision, and occasionally radiotherapy, may be useful.

Since the patient with tuberculosis must learn and adopt for many years a special program of living, it is often wise for him to undergo a period of sanatorium care. This is especially important when the presence of tubercle bacilli in the sputum renders him a source of infection to the members of the household.

Often other special medical and surgical measures are of value, such as collapse therapy in pulmonary tuberculosis. Recently, streptomycin and dihydrostreptomycin (p. 289) and para-aminosalicylic acid (p. 296) have shown some promise in selected cases, but much time must elapse before full evaluation is possible.

TULAREMIA

Tularemia is primarily an acute infectious disease of wild rodents. It is caused by *Pasteurella tularensis*, a gram-negative bacillus, and occurs throughout the United States and in many other parts of the world. The disease usually is transmitted to man by contact with infected animals (especially wild rabbits) and by the bites of infected deer flies or wood ticks. It may also be acquired by ingestion of undercooked infected game or contaminated water. The mortality ranges around 4 percent.

The organism can penetrate the unbroken skin or mucous membrane and requires an incubation period of two to seven days, with an average of three and one-half days. The usual history of onset is a sudden chill, rise of temperature to 103° or 104° F., prostration, headache, and severe malaise.

The disease may take one of two forms: ulceroglandular or typhoidal. The ulceroglandular type is characterized by a painful red papule, usually on the fingers or forearm, progressing to a pustule which rapidly necroses to form a shallow, punched-out ulcer with indurated borders. The regional lymph nodes enlarge and are painful. They frequently become fluctuant and rupture spontaneously. The fever runs a spiking course and in untreated cases lasts an average of thirty days. The ulcer heals with considerable scarring.

The typhoidal form does not have an external lesion; there may be local lesions in the mouth or pharynx with regional lymphadenitis. Fever may be accompanied or followed by vomiting, excruciating abdominal pains, and diarrhea. The course may be fulminant.

An oculoglandular form, usually unilateral, is seen occasionally when the patient has wiped the conjunctiva with infected materials or a contaminated hand. The inferior palpebral conjunctiva presents several small ulcers, and the regional lymph nodes are enlarged and may suppurate. Recovery in three to five weeks is the rule.

Atypical pneumonia and regional lymphadenitis without a local lesion are less frequent.

A secondary anemia is common, and a moderate leukocytosis is the rule. Occasional skin eruptions are seen and disappear within a week.

Diagnosis is dependent upon a history of contact with rabbits, ticks, or deer flies; the physical findings of an ulcer and lymphadenitis; an intracutaneous or percutaneous allergic skin test with detoxified, formalin-killed *Past. tularensis* as antigen; inoculation of blood into guinea pigs; culture and identification of the organism on cystine media from the dead animal or the local lesion; and the appearance of specific agglutinins in the blood during the second week with a rise during the third week.

Differential diagnosis includes chancre of syphilis (p. 10), influenza (p. 22), typhoid fever (see below), pneumonia (p. 115), brucellosis (p. 2), and streptococcus infections.

Treatment—The drug of choice is streptomycin administered intramuscularly in doses of 0.5 to 1 Gm. daily for six days. Prompt recovery and avoidance of complications usually follow. Aureomycin also appears to be effective in the limited number of cases treated.

Prevention is dependent upon care in handling wild rabbits and avoidance of ticks and deer flies.

TYPHOID FEVER

Typhoid fever is an acute generalized infection caused by the gram-negative organism *Eberthella typhosa*, which enters the body through the gastrointestinal tract, most commonly in infected water but frequently in contaminated food, especially milk, oysters, and other shellfish. Human carriers have been found and are dangerous as food handlers. The mortality varies from 7 to 14 percent.

The lesions of typhoid fever are widespread. They consist of submiliary granulomata. The most striking gross lesions occur in the small intestine, where there is inflammatory enlargement of the solitary lymph nodes and Peyer's patches. This usually proceeds to ulceration into the lumen of the intestine and may lead to the complications of hemorrhage and perforation. The liver and spleen contain many lesions and are usually enlarged.

The incubation period varies from five to forty days, averaging ten to fourteen days. The onset is not acute. Prodromal symptoms include chills or chilly sensations alternating with hot flashes, headache, backache, anorexia, diarrhea or constipation, epistaxis, generalized aching, and frequently bronchitis. The fever rises in a steplike fashion to reach 103° to 104° F. in seven to ten days, remains at this level ten to fourteen days, and regresses with wide daily fluctuations for seven to ten days. Sudden changes in the temperature may herald complications. The pulse is dicrotic and characteristically slow in comparison with the fever. On the seventh to tenth day a rose-colored elevated rash appears, with lesions 2 to 4 mm. in diameter which blanch on pressure. It comes in crops and is present most abundantly on the abdomen but also on the chest and back. Each crop persists two to three days and leaves a brownish stain. Delirium, listlessness, photophobia, twitching of the muscles, and somnolence are usually indications of a severe infection. The spleen is ordinarily enlarged. Acute nephritis or pyelitis may occur. Relapse is not uncommon, occurring five to ten days after the temperature has reached normal levels. It is usually mild and runs a short course.

Complications are not rare, the most important being perforation of the small bowel and intestinal hemorrhage. Others include cholecystitis, thrombosis (usually femoral and occurring after the fourth week), bronchitis, myocardial degeneration, peripheral neuritis, periostitis, and osteitis and osteomyelitis (sometimes months after clinical recovery).

Diagnosis is aided by the history of onset, especially when connected with a visit to a known typhoid area. Other important diagnostic aids are blood cultures (especially during the first week), urine and feces cultures, and the Widal reaction (usually positive in the second week). It is important to remember that previous immunization against typhoid fever can lead to a positive Widal test for several years. A leukopenia of 3,000 to 5,000 is the rule.

Many diseases simulate typhoid fever. The following most frequently give difficulty in the differential diagnosis: miliary tuberculosis, pyelitis (p. 224), typhus (p. 17), trichinosis (p. 41), brucellosis (p. 2), and meningitis (p. 165).

Treatment—Good nursing care is the most important part of treatment. A high-carbohydrate, high-caloric, soft and liquid diet is essential. Fluids should be given freely. Hemorrhage requires absolute quiet, cessation of feedings, transfusions, and an ice bag to the abdomen. Perforation requires surgery.

Chloramphenicol (p.292) appears to be of value in typhoid fever. It is given in doses of at least 0.5 Gm. every four hours for ten or twelve days. Patients should be watched closely for relapse after the drug is discontinued.

Convalescence may be slow. Bed rest is advised for seven to ten days after fever disappears, during which time the diet is increased to normal.

Strict isolation must be enforced to prevent spread. Immunization is the only effective prophylaxis (p. 329). Chloramphenicol is of little value in treating the carrier state.

WEIL'S DISEASE

Weil's disease (spirochetal jaundice, icterohemorrhagic spirochetosis) is an acute infection occasionally transmitted to man through the contamination of skin, food, or drink with the urine or feces of wild rats. These rodents are often permanent carriers and constitute the major source of infection, though occasionally mice, cats, sheep, and foxes may carry the organism, *Leptospira icterohaemorrhagiae*. Dogs are subject to a similar disease caused by *L. canicola*, which is rarely transmitted to man.

Most cases give a history of exposure to wet, rat-infested places, such as trenches, mines, sewers, fish markets, and slaughterhouses. In some areas of the world it is an occupational disease. Characteristic symptomatology, following an incubation period of four to nineteen days, includes headache, malaise, fever, prostration, conjunctival injection, nausea, jaundice, hemorrhages at various sites, and uremia. In milder cases, icterus does not occur and convalescence may be rapid. In severe cases, jaundice is noted about the fifth day. It is progressive and is accompanied by enlargement of the liver, signs of renal impairment, and a hemorrhagic tendency. Death may ensue, or convalescence may be prolonged.

Mild instances of the disease may be confused with influenza. The more serious cases resemble epidemic hepatitis and yellow fever. Diagnosis of Weil's disease usually rests upon demonstration of the organism in the blood during the first few days of the infection or in the urine from the tenth to the twentieth day. Occasionally this demonstration may be accomplished through dark-field examination; more commonly, inoculation of the specimen into young guinea pigs (leading to jaundice, hemorrhages, and death) is necessary. Recently a serologic test has proved of value.

Treatment—Even though this is a spirochetal disease, the arsenicals are completely ineffective in treatment. In-vitro experiments substantiate the value of penicillin, which should be used despite the lack of much clinical confirmation. Recommended dosage is at least 300,000 units daily until the patient has been afebrile for three days.

The importance of rodent control as a prophylactic measure is apparent. Where rats are present, food, drink, and skin should be protected from their excreta.

WHOOPING COUGH

Whooping cough is an acute infectious disease of the respiratory tract, caused by the organism *Hemophilus pertussis*. It is primarily a disease of early life. The mortality varies with the age group, decreasing from 25 percent in affected individuals under one year of age and 10 percent in those between one and two years of age to almost no fatalities in those older than five. The incubation period is usually from seven to fourteen days.

The course and clinical picture may be extremely variable. In the "typical" case, three stages of the disease, each lasting approximately two weeks, are seen. The catarrhal stage begins with a mild cough which progresses to resemble that of bronchitis. Coryza and sneezing are usually present. During the spasmodic stage the cough becomes aggravated, occurs in a series of explosive efforts, and ends with a sudden forceful inspiratory crow or whoop. Large amounts of thick, ropy, mucoid material are coughed up and swallowed or vomited. Cyanosis may occur. In the convalescent stage, the number and severity of paroxysms decrease and the symptoms gradually abate. An intercurrent infection may cause the major symptoms to reappear weeks or months after the disease subsides. Some cases may be very mild. The disease should be suspected when an individual of any age has an unexplained long-standing cough.

The most important complication is bronchopneumonia, usually of the interstitial type. Atelectasis, acute emphysema, bronchial asthma, otitis media, or convulsions may occur. Bronchiectasis may be a late sequel.

Diagnosis in the spasmodic stage can usually be made on clinical evidence. In the catarrhal stage it rests on identification of *H. pertussis* in cultures of nasal swabs (for technic, see p. 546). A characteristic leukocytosis of 15,000 to 40,000 or more, mostly lymphocytes, occurs in the late catarrhal or early spasmodic stage. Agglutinin and complement-fixation tests of the patient's serum become positive during the spasmodic stage.

Prevention depends on immunization and on protection from exposure. Specific active immunization may be carried out at any age but is best performed in the first half-year of life. Vaccination may be started as early as one month of age if alum-precipitated vaccine is used (p. 327). The exposed nonimmune infant should be given hyperimmune serum (p. 336).

Treatment—Aureomycin (p. 291) and chloramphenicol (p. 292) appear to be of value in the limited number of cases studied as of this writing. If the individual has been vaccinated previously, a boosting dose of vaccine (p. 327) should be injected during the catarrhal stage. Blood transfusions from adult immune donors, the intramuscular injection of 20 to 40 cc. of convalescent serum, or the injection of serum of hyperimmunized adults may be beneficial.

To control secondary invading organisms, if present, 0.1 Gm. of sulfadiazine per Kg. of body weight or 300,000 units of penicillin per twenty-four hours should be administered. General measures, such as fresh air, maintenance of surrounding temperature at 65° to 75°F., frequent small feedings, and a snug abdominal support, are very helpful. An x-ray of the lungs and a tuberculin test are recommended during convalescence. Mild sedatives may aid in reducing paroxysms.

YAWS

Yaws (frambesia tropica) is a spirochetal disease caused by *Treponema pertenue*. The great majority of cases occur before puberty. Infection takes place readily through abrasions of the skin, the agent being transmitted by flies or by direct contact. Yaws is essentially but not entirely limited to warm climates.

The disease ordinarily has three stages. The primary single lesion appears at the site of inoculation following an incubation period of three to four weeks which may be marked by indigestion, nocturnal headache, joint pains, and fever. It starts as a papule which grows and finally breaks the overlying skin to form a painless, fungoid, crusted, yellowish-red tubercle, 1 to 2 inches in diameter, which has been likened in appearance to a fig turned inside out. The lesion is often altered in appearance by secondary infection.

Six weeks to three months later the symptoms listed above recur, and there is usually a generalized eruption of lesions similar to the primary one. Those on the palms and soles are very painful and

are of different appearance because of the nature and thickness of the skin in these areas. Sometimes the secondary lesions are papular or licheniform. There is a generalized lymphadenopathy as in syphilis. Successive crops of lesions may come out for periods of a few months to three years.

The tertiary lesions are varied; gummatous nodules and deep ulcerations are characteristic. Bone lesions and a destructive rhinopharyngitis (gangosa) are not uncommon. Goundou, an entity marked by hornlike exostoses of the nasal and frontal bones, is believed to be a form of tertiary yaws. Late visceral (including cardiovascular) and central-nervous-system lesions are not observed. Prenatal transmission is unknown.

Although yaws is distinct from syphilis (p. 10) as a disease, no means have yet been found to distinguish the causative agents, and the serologic reactions are identical. Sometimes the differential diagnosis may be difficult. Tertiary yaws may be confused with cutaneous leishmaniasis and blastomycosis.

Treatment—In the primary and secondary stages, yaws can be cured by penicillin, aureomycin, or chloramphenicol.

RICKETTSIAL DISEASES

The rickettsiae are small gram-negative microorganisms, intermediate between bacteria and viruses, which live within the cells of their host. The only filtrable member of the group is that causing Q fever. The rickettsial diseases are transmitted to man by insects.

The organisms attack the endothelium of the arterioles and arterial capillaries, giving rise to proliferation and necrosis. There is also perivascular infiltration of round cells. The changes occur principally in the vessels of the skin, central nervous system, and myocardium. The lesions appear as microscopic swellings. They may produce thrombosis and hemorrhage.

The diseases caused by rickettsiae may be divided into four groups: typhus, spotted fever, tsutsugamushi disease, and Q fever (see Table 1). The Weil-Felix agglutination reaction, formerly employed for differentiation of the rickettsiae, has now been superseded by complement-fixation tests.

EPIDEMIC TYPHUS

Epidemic (louse-borne) typhus is an acute infectious disease caused by *Rickettsia prowazekii prowazekii*. It does not occur in the United States. Epi-

TABLE 1 — *Classification of Rickettsial Diseases*

Disease	Organism	Vector
Typhus Group		
Epidemic typhus	*R. prowazekii prowazekii*	louse
Endemic (murine) typhus	*R. prowazekii typhi*	flea
Spotted Fever Group		
Rocky Mountain spotted fever	*R. rickettsii*	tick
South American spotted fever	*R. rickettsii*	tick
Fièvre boutonneuse	*R. conorii*	tick
South African tick-bite fever	*R. conorii*	tick
Tsutsugamushi Group		
Tsutsugamushi disease (scrub typhus)	*R. tsutsugamushi*	mite
Q Fever Group		
Australian Q fever	*Coxiella burnetii*	tick
American Q fever	*Coxiella burnetii*	tick

demic typhus is transmitted by the body louse, either by the introduction of infected louse feces through the louse bite or other small abrasions or by inhalation of dust containing dry louse feces. The disease is basically a disseminated focal vasculitis and perivasculitis, with thrombosis and hemorrhage, principally of vessels in the skin, brain, heart, and kidneys. Following an incubation period of five to fifteen days, averaging ten to twelve, the disease begins fairly suddenly with chilly sensations, headache, and general malaise. The fever climbs steadily during three to four days and is accompanied by very severe headache. The nervous system is severely affected, with apathy, disorientation, stupor, incontinence, and sometimes deafness. Although early there is relative bradycardia, the pulse rate rises during the second week and becomes poor in quality, and the blood pressure may fall precipitously to as low as 70/40. Cough is an early and distressing symptom. Signs of pneumonitis appear, and a secondary bacterial pneumonia may develop. Renal failure, with oliguria and nitrogen retention, is common.

The characteristic rash occurs about the fourth to sixth day. At first rose-colored, macular, and blanching on pressure, it soon becomes petechial or hemorrhagic and changes to a brown color. It appears first on the volar aspect of the arms, spreading to the sides of the chest, abdomen, and lower extremities and rarely involving the head and neck. During the second week, the fever remains elevated and the patient is desperately ill. Recovery begins in the third week, the temperature falling to normal in one or two days. General weakness and asthenia persist for weeks. Complications include secondary bacterial bronchopneumonia, parotitis, otitis media, and gangrene of the skin. The mortality varies

from 10 to 60 percent, averaging 20 to 30 percent for adults and somewhat less for children. The prognosis becomes worse with increasing age. Death occurs usually between the fourteenth and eighteenth days, rarely before the tenth.

A leukopenia may occur during the first week. The urine findings are similar to those in other acute infectious diseases. Serologically, diagnosis may be established by complement-fixation test.

Treatment—Aureomycin (p. 291) and chloramphenicol (p. 292) are specific therapy. Good nursing care, maintenance of fluid balance and nutrition, careful attention to the skin, and symptomatic drug therapy are of great importance.

Control of lice and immunization are essential for prophylaxis. In vaccinated individuals, the disease is considerably modified; the fever lasts only a few to ten days, the exanthem frequently fails to appear, and death occurs very infrequently. Headache and depression are the prominent symptoms.

Brill's disease is believed to represent a reactivation in this country of a long-standing Old World typhus infection. There is no recent history of lousiness or bites. The symptoms are those of a mild typhus infection.

ENDEMIC TYPHUS

Endemic (murine) typhus is an acute infectious disease caused by *Rickettsia prowazekii typhi*. It is transmitted to man by the rat flea and occurs in the southern portion of the United States, Africa, Asia, and parts of South America. The disease has an incubation period of six to fourteen days. The symptoms are similar to those of epidemic typhus but are not so severe. The fever, as in epidemic typhus, lasts about fourteen days. The eruption, which appears about the fifth day, is not as hemorrhagic or extensive as in the epidemic form. The fatality rate is usually less than 5 percent. Diagnosis can be established by complement-fixation test. Treatment is the same as for epidemic typhus.

ROCKY MOUNTAIN SPOTTED FEVER

Rocky Mountain spotted fever (tick fever) is an acute infectious disease caused by *Rickettsia rickettsii*. It is transmitted by the tick Ixodidae. In the Rocky Mountain and Pacific Coast states, the wood tick is the principal vector; in the East and South, the dog tick. The disease is primarily an endangiitis, especially of the peripheral blood vessels. The mortality varies greatly but ranges around 22 percent.

The incubation period varies from two to fourteen days, being shortest in severe infections. Usually, after several days of malaise, anorexia, and chilly sensations, the disease begins suddenly, frequently with a chill. Generalized muscular and joint pains, severe headache, short dry cough, and photophobia appear rapidly and cause prostration. Following the chill, the temperature rises rapidly to 102° to 104°F., reaching a maximum of 104° to 105°F. during the second week. By the end of the second week the temperature begins to fall by lysis and is normal by the end of the third week. The pulse gradually becomes of poor quality, and its rate increases out of proportion to the fever. Respirations become rapid. Restlessness and insomnia are common, and delirium occurs in severe cases. On the third to fifth day the rash appears— usually first on the ankles, wrists, and back; later on the forehead, arms, legs, chest, and abdomen; sometimes on the mucosa of the mouth and pharynx. At first consisting of rose-colored macules 1 to 5 mm. in diameter, not elevated or palpable and disappearing on pressure, the rash gradually becomes purplish in color and confluent, then persists on pressure and becomes petechial. Rather large areas of cutaneous and subcutaneous hemorrhage may appear. The rash subsides with the temperature, but pigmented spots may remain for some time. Desquamation, usually slight except over areas of severe hemorrhage, occurs on recovery. Necrosis of the skin may appear in the third week. Pneumonia, the principal complication, occurs infrequently.

The disease must be differentiated from measles (p. 24), meningitis (p. 165), and endemic typhus (see above). The complement-fixation test is diagnostic.

Treatment—Aureomycin (p. 291) and chloramphenicol (p. 292) are specific treatment. Good nursing care is essential, with emphasis on adequate nutrition, relief of insomnia and restlessness, maintenance of fluid balance, and transfusions. Yearly immunization with Rocky Mountain spotted fever vaccine (two injections with a five-day interval) is advised in endemic areas. Recovery from the disease gives immunity for a long period of years.

Prophylaxis depends upon the reduction in number and limitation of distribution of ticks. Avoidance of exposure to ticks through use of a one-piece working garment is advisable for those working in tick-infested areas. Ticks found on the body should be removed promptly.

TSUTSUGAMUSHI DISEASE

Tsutsugamushi disease (scrub typhus, mite-borne typhus) is a specific febrile disease transmitted by a mite and caused by the organism *Rickettsia tsutsugamushi*. The mortality rate varies from 40 to 60 percent to as low as 1 to 15 percent. The disease is not known to occur in the United States.

Q FEVER

Q fever was first described in Australia but was later demonstrated in northwestern United States (nine-mile fever). The causative organism, *Coxiella burnetii*, is transmitted by several species of ticks. After a short incubation period, fever, severe headache, and prostration occur. There is no rash. A pneumonitis resembling virus pneumonia appears, and it is believed possible that the disease may be spread from man to man as an air-borne infection. Treatment is the same as for epidemic typhus (see above).

DISEASES DUE TO FILTRABLE VIRUSES

THE COMMON COLD

The common cold (acute coryza) is an ill-defined, acute, self-limited disease of the upper respiratory tract. The condition is more common than all other diseases of man combined. The etiological agent is presumed to be one or more filtrable viruses. In uncomplicated cases, the disease runs a benign course of four to seven days.

This infection is found throughout the world but is most common in temperate zones. A definite seasonal incidence has been observed, the greatest being in the months of September, October, January, February, and April, at which times abrupt changes in weather are common. Predisposing factors include crowding, poor ventilation, prolonged exposure to a combination of cold and damp, prolonged wearing of wet shoes and clothing, and allergic conditions.

Although sporadic colds are usually not communicable, the epidemic type is highly communicable, especially from several hours before to a few days after symptoms appear. Children generally are more susceptible than adults. The incubation period varies from twelve hours to four days following exposure.

The earliest symptom is usually itching or burning in some portion of the upper respiratory tract, generally in the area of the posterior nares. There may be sneezing. A watery nasal discharge appears and soon becomes almost continuous. The nasal mucosa becomes engorged and swollen, blocking the respiratory passages. The lymphoid follicles are enlarged. A nonproductive cough may appear and, when present, is frequently distressing. The patient may complain of vague aching in the back and extremities. Chilly sensations may be experienced. Headache is not uncommon. The degree of malaise and prostration varies greatly. The conjunctivae become suffused, the tongue may be dry and coated, swallowing often is difficult, the sense of smell is impaired, and the patient loses his appetite.

As the disease progresses, the nasal discharge gradually becomes thicker, yellow-gray in color, and mucoid as secondarily invading organisms become established. The external nares and angles of the mouth may become excoriated. Many individuals develop herpetiform lesions (herpes labialis, p. 21). The temperature may rise to 100° to 102°F. The disease usually subsides gradually; the discharge decreases in quantity and appetite returns, but the individual feels somewhat weakened. Relapse may occur seven to twelve days after the initial attack. The most frequent complications are bronchitis, pyogenic infection of the paranasal sinuses, otitis media, and influenza.

The differential diagnosis may be critical and complex, since most acute communicable diseases begin with upper-respiratory-tract symptoms. Allergic reactions, chemical rhinitis, mechanical irritation from foreign bodies, and nasal anatomical abnormalities also require consideration.

Treatment—There is no specific treatment. It has been shown that the initial manifestations of coryza are caused by an allergic reaction to the infecting organism. Antihistaminic drugs (p. 509) given early and in adequate doses may relieve this and thereby prevent secondary bacterial invasion. They are best given in combination with ephedrine every four hours during the day. Ephedrine is omitted at night to permit sleep. Results will be better if medication is continued at night by giving an enteric-coated tablet containing the antihistaminic drug at bedtime.

Most patients usually are more comfortable in bed, and bed rest should be imperative if the temperature rises above 100°F. The individual should be kept warm and dry and in a well-ventilated room. Analgesics, such as acetylsalicylic acid, 5 grains, may relieve aching. Since these will cause perspiration in many individuals, drafts should be avoided. Warm drinks are soothing. Inhaling steam may be beneficial, especially in the presence of bronchial involvement. Codeine, 5 to 10 mg. (1/12 to 1/6 grain) every four hours, may be used to control coughing. Vasoconstrictors (p. 376) may be used topically or by inhalation to reduce the hyperemia of the nasal mucous membranes.

The routine use of penicillin or the sulfonamides in the treatment of uncomplicated acute colds is not indicated. These drugs may be of benefit, however, if secondary infection arises or if complications occur.

Prophylaxis depends particularly upon protection from exposure. Good ventilation of working and sleeping spaces and avoidance of crowds are of greatest importance. Exposure in wet clothing or wet shoes also should be avoided.

Vaccines have been the subject of much controversy. They have no prophylactic effect against the virus infection but may be of benefit in preventing secondary infection of the respiratory tract.

CHICKENPOX

Chickenpox (varicella) is an acute infectious disease caused by a specific virus which is similar to, but apparently not identical with, that of herpes zoster (p. 21). The disease occurs almost exclusively in children. It is transmitted by contact with an affected individual, by air-borne droplets, and through articles soiled by discharges from an infected person. Chickenpox is rarely fatal. One attack usually results in permanent immunity.

After an incubation period of ten to twenty-one days (average, twelve to seventeen days), mild prodromata such as nasopharyngitis, headache, loss of appetite, mild fever, and malaise may occur, but usually the onset is sudden. An evanescent maculopapular rash develops and quickly becomes vesicular. The lesions occur mostly on the face, shoulders, and trunk, although occasional lesions are seen in the mouth or pharynx. The conjunctivae, larynx, and scalp also are affected occasionally. The vesicles are unilocular, slightly elevated, and surrounded by an erythematous area. They persist for three or four days and do not become pustular unless secondarily infected. As they dry up, they may have a depressed center. The lesions form crusts which drop off in six or seven days. New lesions appear in crops, and all stages may be seen at one time in the same area. Three or more successive crops are the rule. Occasionally, there are so few vesicles as to escape notice.

The constitutional reaction usually is mild, with little or no fever. In severe cases, which are more common in adults, there may be fever of 103° to 104°F. A leukocytosis is common, but otherwise there are no significant laboratory findings.

The most frequent complication is infection of the vesicles to form pustules. Rupture by scratching may result in ulceration and severe infection, with pockmarks as sequelae. Occasionally, hemolytic streptococci invade the lesions, causing cellulitis. Encephalitis may occur in severe cases, usually appearing toward the end of the febrile period but sometimes being delayed until the second or third week.

In the differential diagnosis, one should consider smallpox (p. 32), impetigo (p. 236), and drug eruptions (p. 227).

Treatment—There is no specific treatment. The patient should be isolated, and all articles used in the sickroom should be sterilized. Scratching should be prevented, preferably by application of a local anesthetic such as 'Surfacaine' Cream. Sulfadiazine ointment (5 percent) may be applied to control skin infections. Crusts should not be disturbed. Sedatives, such as phenobarbital (p. 392), may be helpful to control restlessness.

Quarantine frequently is not effective in controlling the transmission of the disease. For prophylaxis, 15 to 20 cc. of convalescent serum or immune globulin may be given as early as possible following exposure. This is rarely indicated and is not completely successful.

DENGUE

Dengue (breakbone fever) is an acute, rarely fatal, febrile disease caused by a specific virus which is transmitted by certain species of *Aëdes* mosquitoes. The disease occurs in the Southeastern and Gulf states, sometimes in epidemic proportions.

The usual incubation period is from five to nine days but may vary from two and one-half to fifteen days. Prodromal symptoms of malaise, muscle pains, headache, and chilliness appear six to twelve hours before the fever in about one-half of the cases. In others the onset is sudden, with muscular and severe joint pains, backache, malaise, anorexia, intense supraorbital and postorbital aching, sharp pain on moving the eyes, and pronounced mental depression. The temperature rises rapidly in a matter of hours to 102° to 105°F. It occasionally returns to normal in the middle of the febrile period, giving a "saddleback," or diphasic, type of curve. The temperature quite frequently is highest during the twenty-four hours before the crisis. Salicylates reduce fever sharply and may cause atypical spiking. The heart rate increases in proportion to the fever during the first twenty-four hours, but after this time there usually is a relative bradycardia. An absolute bradycardia may occur during convalescence.

Gastro-intestinal manifestations consist in anorexia, constipation, epigastric discomfort, colicky pain, and abdominal tenderness. Altered taste sensations are common. Prostration is pronounced. Other less frequent manifestations are photophobia, drenching sweats, sore throat, cough, epistaxis, dysuria, hyperesthesia, pain in the groins and testicles, and delirium. The face, neck, and chest may be flushed, and a punctiform rash may appear at pressure points early in the disease. Lymphadenopathy is common, particularly of the inguinal, posterior cervical, and epitrochlear glands. The spleen is usually not enlarged. Although pain in the large joints may be exquisite, no objective findings occur. True nuchal rigidity is absent.

A maculopapular or scarlatiniform rash may develop on the third to fifth day and last for three or four days. It begins on the chest, trunk, and abdomen and spreads to the extremities and face. The incidence of rash varies in different epidemics. Itching of the palms and soles is common, but desquamation occurs rarely.

It is believed that much milder infections occur, without rash and lasting only one to three days. Such attacks have been produced by inoculating heterologous strains in individuals a few months after recovery.

Convalescence may extend several weeks, during which time there is pronounced asthenia and disturbances of visual accommodation (from weakness or paralysis of the ciliary muscles). Fatalities have been reported in large foreign epidemics, but it is doubtful whether dengue is a primary cause of death in the United States. Immunity develops with recovery from an attack and persists for at least two years and probably longer. Several strains of virus have been identified, and recovery from infection with one has been shown to give partial immunity against others for at least two months.

Laboratory findings are not diagnostic except for serologic tests using specific virus antigens. The white blood cell count may be normal during the first twenty-four hours with a relative and absolute decrease in lymphocytes and an increase in immature neutrophils. Leukopenia then develops because of decrease in neutrophils. Lymphocytes increase and predominate at the end of the febrile period and early in convalescence. The blood count usually returns to normal within a week. The urine is normal. Spinal-fluid changes have been reported but have not occurred in proved infections.

Diagnosis during epidemics is not difficult but may require differentiation from influenza, typhus, measles, rheumatic fever, scarlet fever, and malaria.

Prevention is based upon eradication or control of *Aëdes* mosquitoes. There is no vaccine for immunization.

Treatment is nonspecific and supportive. Opiates may be needed to relieve pain. Antipyretics and analgesics are usually indicated. Good nursing care is important. The fluid intake should be large.

HERPES LABIALIS

Herpes labialis (fever blister, cold sore) is an acute infectious disease caused by the filtrable virus of herpes simplex. The disease may occur by itself, may accompany other infectious diseases (particularly pneumonia, meningococcic meningitis, and coryza), or may appear when the normal body economy is upset, as following fever therapy. Immunity does not follow an attack, and recurrence is common. Recovered individuals become carriers of the organism.

The virus of herpes simplex produces several disease entities, depending upon the tissue attacked. Eczema herpeticum (Kaposi's varicelliform eruption) is a serious complication of infantile eczema. Acute herpetic gingivostomatitis is a common disease of children characterized by fever, irritability, inflamed swollen gums, vesiculation of the oral mucous membranes, fetor oris, and regional lymphadenopathy. Herpetic stomatitis may recur and produce similar local lesions, but little or no systemic reaction develops.

Infection of the eye results in conjunctivitis and, more commonly, keratoconjunctivitis. The classical Parinaud's syndrome with unilateral conjunctivitis and preauricular node enlargement is caused by herpes simplex virus. Herpetic meningoencephalitis is a recognized clinical entity which cannot readily be differentiated from meningoencephalitis caused by other viruses except by special cultural or serologic methods.

The onset of herpes labialis usually is accompanied by burning and itching which continues through the course of the disease. Small painful swellings appear in the affected area. These develop rapidly into vesicles surrounded by a small erythematous area. The lesions dry to form crusts and subside in five to ten days. If the disease occurs in the buccal mucosa, discrete punched-out ulcers and erosions develop (canker sores). The disease may occur anywhere in the skin or mucous membranes but is seen most frequently at mucocutaneous junctions of the face, lips, genitalia, conjunctiva, and cornea. Corneal herpes may result in scarring. Generally, however, there is little or no constitutional reaction unless the lesions become infected secondarily. Confusion with herpes zoster (see below) may occur if the lesions have a segmental distribution.

Treatment—There appears to be no specific treatment. Aureomycin and chloramphenicol have been tried with doubtful results.

Vesicles on the skin may be dried and secondary infection prevented by application of an antiseptic tincture (p. 304). Mild astringents such as Burow's solution (p. 481), compresses, or Benzoin Tincture may be soothing. Irradiation with x-rays (75 r unfiltered) in the early stages of the disease may be helpful. As a prophylactic measure, smallpox vaccination repeated four to eight times at intervals of one to two weeks may be tried, although results are not consistently good.

HERPES ZOSTER

Herpes zoster (shingles) is an acute infectious nonepidemic disease caused by a virus similar to, but apparently not identical with, that of chickenpox (varicella). Exposure to one disease has appeared to give rise to the other in many authenticated cases. However, the general incidence is different. Herpes zoster is more common in adults; chickenpox occurs almost exclusively in children.

Herpes zoster involves the dorsal root ganglia or extramedullary ganglia of sensory nerves. Severe infections sometimes attack motor roots, resulting in temporary (rarely permanent) paralysis. Attacks may occur spontaneously, or they may be precipitated by local or general disease, trauma, or intoxication. Lesions are usually unilateral. Lasting immunity generally develops following an attack, but there is no cross protection against the varicella virus.

The incubation period is believed to be seven to fourteen days. Following a prodromal period of three or four days during which the patient is uneasy, the temperature is elevated, and varying degrees of pain and hyperesthesia are present in the cutaneous area supplied by the involved nerves. This is followed by the appearance of an erythematous and vesicular eruption along the course of the nerve. The vesicles contain a clear or slightly cloudy yellow fluid and very closely resemble those of chickenpox. Both infections cause the appearance of eosinophilic inclusion bodies in the nuclei of infected cells. Ordinarily, the vesicles in zoster do not involve the corium, but large lesions may involve all layers of the skin, in which case scarring is likely. Severe pain is encountered frequently, and neuralgic pains may persist when the disease subsides.

The infection runs a course of several weeks, during which time the temperature remains elevated and systemic symptoms occur. These are usually more severe if the attack is primary than if it has been precipitated by some other condition. Involvement of the first branch of the sensory division of the trigeminal nerve may cause corneal ulceration and result in serious damage. The major complication is secondary infection of the lesions.

The disease sometimes must be differentiated from herpes labialis (p. 21) and in its early stages from neuralgia, pleurisy, arthritic root pains, and tabetic crises. In many cases of herpes zoster, the regional lymph nodes are enlarged and tender for a day or two before the appearance of vesicles. When pain and hyperesthesia have a nerve-root distribution, the regional lymph nodes should be palpated. If they are tender without obvious cause, the diagnosis usually turns out to be herpes zoster.

Treatment—Any form of treatment is more successful if started early than if started later. Chloramphenicol (p. 292) and aureomycin (p. 291) appear to attack the virus directly and shorten the course of the disease. Immediate relief of pain and apparent shortening of the attack follow block of the affected nerves as centrally as they are accessible. Peripheral nerve block gives better results than sympathetic block. The injections should be repeated two or three times as pain returns.

Less dramatic but somewhat similar results can be achieved in early cases by injection of posterior pituitary extract. Doses of 2 or 3 U.S.P. Units are given every half hour until the patient shows circumoral pallor or a significant change in blood pressure, whichever occurs first. Suitable doses are then continued every few hours for about twenty-four hours. Posterior pituitary should not be given in the presence of pregnancy or cardiovascular disease, and the patient should be warned to avoid exertion because of the effect of the drug on coronary circulation.

Secondary infection of the lesions should be treated vigorously with penicillin (p. 288) or the sulfonamides (p. 293). Local therapy in uncomplicated cases is directed at prevention of scarring by topical application of antiseptic powders, plain shake lotions, or Lassar's paste. Greasy ointments cause maceration of the lesions and promote infection and scarring. Pain and discomfort may be relieved with demulcents (such as 'Surfacaine' Cream or Lotion) provided the lesions are not intact. Large doses of vitamin B complex started early in the disease may assist in the prevention of postherpetic neuritis. Roentgen irradiation is effective in some cases if given early.

INFLUENZA

Influenza is an acute, self-limited, highly contagious disease which occurs frequently in epidemic and rarely in pandemic outbreaks. It is characterized by symptoms which are predominantly constitutional, even though the infection itself is limited to the respiratory tract. The causative organism is a filtrable virus of the influenza group, believed to be disseminated from person to person by direct contact or droplet infection. Two groups of viruses, A and B, have been identified. Each type is represented by different strains which, though similar in many respects, differ immunologically. Little is known of the pathology of uncomplicated influenza virus infection. The clinical manifestations of infection with either type vary considerably, but, as a rule, A strains cause more fulminating and prolonged attacks.

Following an incubation period of twelve to forty-eight hours, the onset is sudden, with fever, chills or chilly sensations, malaise, generalized aching pains (particularly in the back and extremities).

headache, nausea, vomiting, and varying degrees of prostration. Fever of remittent type develops rapidly and ranges from 100° to 105°F. Coryza usually begins shortly after the onset, sore throat may develop, and a dry, irritative cough frequently occurs. Gastro-intestinal symptoms may appear but usually are severe only in children, in whom they may be the predominant findings. The respiratory symptoms (cough, substernal pain, feeling of tightness) become more severe as the disease develops. A thin, mucoid sputum is produced which later becomes mucopurulent. In uncomplicated cases, the fever persists for one to five days; it then falls rapidly and the respiratory symptoms abate. Convalescence is rapid, but there may be a prolonged period of weakness and depression.

Complications usually become manifest about the third or fourth day of the disease and are caused by associated bacteria, usually streptococci, staphylococci, or pneumococci. The cough may increase in severity, and increasing amounts of sputum may indicate the onset of bronchitis (p. 112). Sinusitis (p. 111) with severe headaches, fever, and prostration may occur. The most serious complication is pneumonia (p. 115), which may develop (1) almost concurrently with the influenza (in which case it may run a fulminating course), (2) more slowly during the course of the disease, or (3) suddenly after apparent recovery. In the last two instances, the pneumonia may present a somewhat bizarre picture because the areas of infection in the lungs may be deep-seated and isolated. Other complications include otitis media (p. 242), bronchitis (p. 112), bronchiectasis (p. 115), pulmonary abscess, simple purpura (p. 105), and epistaxis (p. 110). Although infrequent, pericarditis, endocarditis, and thrombophlebitis may occur. The recognition of complications depends upon the characteristic symptoms and physical signs of the complication in question. They should be suspected if the fever lasts more than five days.

None of the generally available laboratory tests are of diagnostic value. In research laboratories, the following procedures have proved useful: hemagglutinin inhibition, complement fixation, and virus culture in chick embryos.

Treatment—There is no specific treatment. The patient should be kept in bed from the onset of the disease until convalescence is well established; even then, activities should be restricted for seven to ten days. Large quantities of fluids by mouth are desirable during the febrile period. Symptomatic treatment with analgesics (p. 405) and codeine (p. 403) is usually indicated. Complications are treated as if they were primary diseases.

The prognosis of uncomplicated influenza is excellent; but in complicated cases, particularly during pandemics, the mortality rate may reach 20 to 40 percent. The most frequent sequelae are chronic bronchitis, chronic bronchiectasis, and pulmonary fibrosis.

Prophylaxis depends primarily on avoiding contact with known cases. Vaccines for immunization against influenza virus are available. Current preparations contain the Lee strain of type B virus and the PR8 and FM-1 strains of type A. The antigenicity of each is quite specific, and little or no protection is afforded against other strains. Immunity develops about seven days after injection of the vaccine and remains for a variable period of time, probably not exceeding six to nine months. Immunization should be performed in advance of an expected epidemic; and since sporadic and epidemic cases are more likely to appear during cold weather, the optimal time for vaccination is in the fall. Revaccination should be carried out three or four months later. Vaccination upon the appearance of an epidemic is of value, but, because of rapid dissemination of infection, many individuals will not be protected in time. For dosage and administration, see page 323. The vaccine is prepared from viruses grown in embryonated chicken eggs; therefore, individuals with egg sensitivity should be treated with caution or not at all.

LYMPHOGRANULOMA VENEREUM

Lymphogranuloma venereum (lymphogranuloma inguinale, lymphopathia venereum, fourth or sixth venereal disease, venereal bubo) is an infectious disease caused by a specific viruslike organism which is closely related to the infective agent of psittacosis (p. 30). Both organisms belong to a group that appears to be intermediate between rickettsiae and viruses.

The disease is of world-wide occurrence. It is usually transmitted by venereal contact and is characterized by acute and chronic tissue changes in the inguinal and anorectal regions and by constitutional symptoms, all of which produce a wide variety of clinical features. There is an evanescent, usually undetected, primary lesion followed by regional lymphadenitis, suppuration, fistula formation, and pronounced fibrotic changes which may give rise to stricture of the rectum and elephantiasis of the genitalia. Extragenital infections are uncommon but have been identified in the eye, mouth, and meninges. The inflammatory reaction in the lymph nodes is prolonged and consists of subacute or chronic granulomatous changes with mononuclear infiltration, small areas of necrosis, at times giant cells, and much proliferation of fibrous tissue. It closely resembles lesions of tuberculosis and syphilis.

The incubation period is usually a few days but may be several weeks. The primary lesion is a small vesicle which ruptures, leaving a shallow, nonindurated ulcer with sharply demarcated edges. The lesion is usually painless and heals in seven to ten days. It most frequently is located in men on the coronary sulcus, prepuce, or glans, and in women on the posterior vaginal wall, fourchette, or cervix. It may develop in the urethra, in the anal region, or on the female external genitalia. The initial lesion is discovered in less than one-half of cases.

Several weeks to two months after exposure to infection, or seven to fourteen days from the appearance of the vesicle, the characteristic buboes develop in the regional lymph nodes. Because of the location of the primary lesion, the inguinal nodes are commonly involved in men and the iliac and anorectal nodes in women. In temperate zones unilateral involvement is the rule, but bilateral lesions are common in the tropics. At first, the lymph glands are discrete, movable, and slightly tender. Later they become adherent to the underlying tissues to form a large, tender, inflammatory mass.

The adenitis is accompanied by constitutional symptoms of chills, fever, excessive perspiration, anorexia, vomiting, prostration, pains in the chest and muscles, stiffness of the neck, headache, epistaxis, bronchitis, and weight loss. At times the infection becomes systemic, causing generalized lymphadenopathy, splenomegaly, and hepatomegaly. Scarlatiniform rashes appear occasionally.

If the disease is untreated, the tertiary stage develops, with extension of the infection and pronounced fibrosis, which may result in proctitis, strictures, perirectal and perianal abscesses, vaginorectal and vaginovesical fistulas, and elephantiasis of the external genitalia. Secondary infections may cause death from sepsis.

Lymphogranuloma venereum must be differentiated from chancroid, pyogenic lymphadenitis, tuberculous lymphomata, gonorrhea, syphilis, granuloma inguinale, balanitis, plague (pestis minor), tularemia, carcinoma and tuberculosis of the rectum, and ulcerative colitis.

The Frei test is employed for routine diagnosis.

Intradermal injections are made of 0.1 cc. each of Frei test antigen and control material supplied with the antigen. The reaction is read in two and four days. A positive test is indicated by induration at least 6 mm. in minimum diameter at the site of antigen injection plus induration no more than 5 mm. in maximum diameter at the control injection. Since the antigen and control are prepared by use of chick embryo, the test is likely to be unsatisfactory in patients allergic to hen eggs.

The Frei test does not become positive for seven to forty days after the onset of adenitis; therefore, in suspected cases, negative tests should be repeated at intervals. False negatives may be caused by fever, tuberculosis, menstruation, and coexistent early syphilis or chancroid. Once established, a positive test remains so for life. Hence, the test is diagnostic for the current illness only if there is reasonable assurance that the patient has not previously been infected with the lymphogranuloma virus.

Antigen is also available for the complement-fixation test, which may become positive earlier than the Frei test and which becomes negative again after the infection has been eradicated. However, the antigen also gives positive complement-fixation tests in the presence of psittacosis. Tissue biopsy is of diagnostic value; stained smears of pus (Macchiavello's stain) may reveal typical cone or dumb-bell-shaped basophilic gamma bodies and chains of the smaller azurophilic elementary bodies. The organism can be cultured in embryonated chicken eggs and by intracerebral inoculation in mice. Hyperproteinemia occurs in lymphogranuloma venereum and will cause a positive formol-gel test. However, it is not specific, because it is also found in leishmaniasis, leprosy, and multiple myeloma.

Treatment—Aureomycin (p. 291) and chloramphenicol (p. 292) appear to be effective. Penicillin is of no value except possibly in the presence of secondary infection. Streptomycin has value, but resistant strains have been encountered. Sulfadiazine, if continued for long periods of time in interrupted courses of one or two weeks, is curative.

MEASLES

Measles is a specific, generalized, acute infection which is most common in children. It is characterized by acute upper-respiratory symptoms, catarrhal inflammation of mucous membranes, and a maculopapular skin eruption. Measles is the most common of all communicable diseases and occurs in all countries of the world, but it is more prevalent in temperate climates than in tropical ones. In urban areas, it is endemic but spreads to epidemic proportions about every two or three years, generally during the colder months of the year.

The etiological agent is a filtrable virus. The organism is found in the nasal secretions and in the blood stream, being most abundant twenty-four hours before the rash appears. Thus, the period of infectivity is greatest during the catarrhal stage and until the rash is maximum. After this, it decreases rapidly to zero as desquamation is established. Outside of the body, the organism is destroyed rapidly by light and air.

The incubation period is symptomless and extends from the time of infection to the first appearance of catarrhal symptoms. It averages nine to eleven days. The prodromal period, or period of invasion, begins on about the tenth day after infection. The early symptoms closely resemble those of a common cold and include mild fever, headache, malaise, increased irritability, and fatigue. Anorexia is usually profound. Vomiting often is troublesome, and diarrhea may occur. As the catarrhal inflammation increases, lacrimation and photophobia develop. The conjunctivae become red, and there is sneezing, nasal discharge, and a hard, dry cough. The swollen face, watering eyes, and puffed lips give a characteristic woebegone facial expression.

At about this time, examination of the oral mucosa may reveal Koplik's spots. These are small, slightly elevated, pin-point, white or bluish-white spots surrounded by dark-red areolae. They commonly occur on the buccal mucous membrane opposite the molar teeth and are best seen by direct daylight. The number varies from two or three at first to many, which may coalesce and involve whole areas of the mucosa. They are most numerous just before the skin rash appears.

As the Koplik's spots increase, a mottled red rash develops over the entire oral mucous membrane, particularly that of the soft palate. This enanthema sometimes precedes the Koplik's spots and at times is accompanied by a fine transitory eruption on the skin of the face.

The temperature is elevated and persists at moderate levels for one or two days; then it falls suddenly to normal or subnormal, only to rise sharply as the skin-rash, or exanthematous, stage develops. This may occur in a few hours or may be delayed as long as two or three days. The fever exceeds that of the prodromal period by one or two degrees and may be either continuous or remittent. The face becomes covered by the patchy eruption and appears swollen and edematous. The eyes are red, have a mucopurulent secretion, and are sensitive to light. A similar secretion is discharged from the partially obstructed nose. There is a persistent, dry, metallic cough. The patient is drowsy and stuporous but becomes restless and irritable when disturbed.

When the rash begins to fade, after about two days, rapid improvement occurs. The temperature may drop by lysis or crisis; the cough becomes looser; the mental symptoms subside; and the appetite returns. Photophobia often disappears rapidly; even so, the eyes remain weak, and conjunctivitis may develop if they are exposed to strong light too soon.

The exanthema begins on the head at the hair margin, usually behind the ears. Very early, it also appears between the scapulae, but at this stage it is less prominent about the mouth, cheeks, and nose and in front of the ears. Later, but during the first twenty-four hours, it spreads down the back to the iliac crests, the face becomes extensively involved (except for the cheeks), and the eruption begins to appear on the chest, abdomen, shoulders, and anterior surfaces of the arms. By the third day, the rash usually covers the head, trunk, shoulders, and anterior surfaces of the arms and thighs. The elbows and feet often remain free.

The rash is at its peak by the fifth day, but it requires only about three days to become fully developed in any one area. The lesions begin as small pink macular spots which soon become elevated papules and darken in color. These may remain discrete or, as more frequently happens, may become confluent. The individual spots feel nodular. Petechiae may appear as the result of increased capillary fragility. The skin in the vicinity of the rash is greasy from augmented activity of the sebaceous glands. Factors which affect capillary circulation influence distribution and intensity of the eruption. The effect of warm baths in hastening its appearance is a well-known example. Contrary to popular belief, there is no evidence that sparsely distributed or pale eruptions presage a less favorable prognosis.

Fading is noted on about the fifth day and proceeds in the order of appearance of the rash. A slight pigmentation may remain for two or three weeks. Desquamation usually begins with the fading and is distinguished by fine, branny scaling which is most notable on the face, neck, and thighs. The amount of desquamation is generally proportional to the severity of the rash.

Laboratory findings are not diagnostic. Blood counts give variable results, although a neutropenia with reduction in mature segmented forms is common. The blanching test, using convalescent serum intracutaneously, is of no value. Previously positive tuberculin tests may become negative.

Differential diagnosis is not difficult with typical cases after the rash has appeared. In the catarrhal stage, demonstration of Koplik's spots is the only means of positively establishing diagnosis. These are often absent in infants and in mild cases. Diseases which may be confused with measles are rubella, exanthema subitum, fourth disease, scarlet fever, variola, varicella, typhus fever, typhoid fever, cerebrospinal meningitis, serum sickness, drug rashes, and septicemia.

Measles may lower the resistance to other infections. This is exemplified by the well-known aggravating effect it has on previously acquired tuberculous infections. Many acute infections may be associated with the disease, diphtheria being one of the most serious. Secondary infection of the respiratory tract is not infrequent, especially in infants and in poorly nourished children. Pneumonia is particularly serious in these groups but may develop in any case and at any stage of the disease. Measles encephalomyelitis may develop on about the fourth to sixth day after the fever has subsided. It carries a high mortality, and many who survive develop residual abnormalities.

Prevention—Recovery from measles results in practically absolute protection, yet attempts to produce active immunity by artificial inoculation have not been uniformly successful.

Infants whose mothers have had the disease inherit passive immunity for about six months. Injection of convalescent serum or immune globulin affords similar protection but is effective only for about three weeks. This method may be used to prevent the disease in physically debilitated individuals and young infants or to stop epidemics in institutions. Injections are given intramuscularly as soon after exposure as possible and before the fourth day of incubation.

Modification of measles is the procedure of choice for normal, susceptible individuals following exposure. Convalescent serum or immune globulin is given on the sixth or seventh day after the rash has appeared in the individual from whom the infection was acquired.

When modification is successful, the incubation period is sometimes prolonged and the prodromal period almost suppressed. Koplik's spots do not develop. The eruption is mild and often fleeting and is not accompanied by constitutional symptoms or complications. Permanent immunity is almost always produced.

Treatment—Specific therapy with serum or globulin is not generally employed. It may be indicated for debilitated individuals, particularly those recovering from other diseases, or in the presence of chronic pulmonary or cardiac disease. Large doses are required. The results are equivocal.

General management includes bed rest in a well-ventilated room with constant temperature of approximately 70° F. Direct sunlight is best excluded, but the room does not need to be darkened. Sedatives and antipyretics are usually indicated. The diet should be nutritious but bland enough to avoid aggravating the tendency toward diarrhea. Mild laxatives or enemas may be employed at the onset of the infection. Ordinary cleanliness is usually sufficient for care of the skin, but antipruritic applications such as 'Surfacaine' Cream or Lotion may be necessary. Boric acid compresses and Yellow Mercuric Oxide Ointment are useful in relieving the discomfort caused by the conjunctivitis. Dark glasses or eyeshades also give considerable relief. Laryngitis and bronchitis may be severe enough to require use of a croup kettle and sedative cough mixtures (p. 379). Nasal obstruction is best relieved by inhalation of volatile vasoconstrictors or administration of aqueous solutions as drops or sprays (p. 376).

MUMPS

Mumps is an acute, infectious, and communicable systemic disease characterized by swelling and tenderness of one or more of the salivary glands and by a tendency to involve other glandular organs and the central nervous system.

The etiological agent is a filtrable virus which is transmitted by direct contact. It is surmised that transmission occurs by droplet infection through the oral cavity. The channel by which the virus finds its way to the salivary glands is not known. It is believed to be indirect, by way of the blood stream or lymphatics, and not direct by way of the duct orifices. This is supported by evidence which indicates that mumps is a systemic disease with predilection for the salivary glands, the meninges, encephalon, pancreas, and adult gonads.

Except for young infants, who may inherit immunity, infection can occur at any age but is most frequent between five and fifteen years. Sporadic cases are common in urban areas at any season, but incidence increases during the colder months and occasionally reaches epidemic proportions when opportunity for intimate exposure is present.

Individual susceptibility is believed to be low, for many completely escape the classical form of the disease. Since one attack almost always confers lasting immunity, unrecognized infections without salivary-gland involvement probably account for this seemingly low incidence. Immunity develops whether one or more than one gland is involved.

The pathological changes in the salivary glands are hyperemia and edema of the affected gland substance and surrounding tissue, with disintegration of the acinar cells and infiltration of mononuclear cells. Healing is complete and takes place by removal of the debris and regeneration of the acinar epithelium without scarring.

The period of incubation averages seventeen to twenty days. Extremes of less than a week to thirty days are reported. The contagious period begins one or two days before onset and lasts until the swelling has disappeared some twelve to fourteen days later.

Prodromal symptoms are often absent or so mild that they are unnoticed until swelling of the face appears. In certain instances, there may be noted slight fever of 99° to 100°F., malaise, chilliness, anorexia, nausea, vomiting, diarrhea, headache, dryness of the throat, neuralgic pains, and disturbed sleep. As a rule, mild to moderate constitutional symptoms are present in the prodromal stage and febrile period, although many children have so little malaise that they object to enforced bed rest. After one to three days, dull, aching pain and tenderness develop in the affected gland, and soon there follows swelling which progresses quite rapidly. Meningeal irritation is present occasionally, as evidenced by vertigo, intense headache, stiffness of the neck, fever of 102° to 104°F., and even convulsions.

The salivary glands may be infected singly, bilaterally in pairs, or in asymmetrical combinations. The parotid glands are involved in the majority of cases, and bilaterally in about 70 percent. The submaxillary glands are frequently affected and sometimes the sublinguals. It is unusual for both parotids to be involved simultaneously; more often the second gland becomes swollen two or three days after the first, or at times onset is delayed until all swelling in the first gland has disappeared. The degree and duration of the inflammation in multiple involvement are quite variable. Usually the swelling begins to subside after two or three days, at which time there is rapid subjective improvement.

Fever of 102°F. is commonly present during the first three or four days of the disease; but after this time, elevation of temperature indicates either extension to another gland or a complication. With parotid infection, the orifice of Stensen's duct (located on the buccal surface at the level of the crown of the second upper molar) is red and swollen. This sign is helpful in diagnosis but does occur in other conditions and therefore is not specific. No discharge can be produced by milking the duct. The salivary secretions may or may not be reduced in amount. In some cases, excessive dryness of the mouth may lead to stomatitis.

The pulse rate is usually slow in proportion to the amount of fever. Epistaxis, deafness, tinnitus, and abdominal pain are noted occasionally in severe cases. The spleen is often palpable at the height of illness.

The blood diastase activity is increased with salivary-gland involvement and is even higher in the presence of acute pancreatitis. The blood count may be normal, but as a rule there is an early leukopenia followed by a slight leukocytosis with a relative and often an absolute lymphocytosis. The urine may contain a trace of protein and an occasional cast when fever is present. The blood sedimentation rate is not affected in uncomplicated cases. A complement-fixation test has been described and is of value in differentiating mumps meningoencephalitis from infection with other neurotropic viruses.

Orchitis is rarely seen before puberty. It develops sometime in the second or third week, after fever and swelling of the salivary glands have subsided. In exceptional instances, the testes may be the first or even the only tissue involved. Sudden high fever and malaise appear and are soon followed by swelling and tenderness of one or, less commonly, both testicles. The swelling may be sufficient to stretch the tunica albuginea, tunica vaginalis, and scrotum, in which case pain is severe. After three to seven days, the swelling and fever slowly subside. Some temporary diminution in size of the testes may then be noted, but complete recovery is the rule. Aspermia has been reported to result from bilateral mumps orchitis, but there are extremely few authentic cases of eunuchism or impotency recorded. In the female, oöphoritis may occur but is relatively infrequent.

Neurological complications in the form of meningitis, encephalitis, or meningoencephalitis are uncommon but may develop at any stage of the disease, more often during or shortly after recovery from the salivary swelling. Manifestations vary with the type of involvement, from mild psychic changes to fever, headache, vomiting, delirium, lethargy, neck rigidity, increased deep reflexes, positive Kernig's sign, and convulsions. The spinal fluid is under increased pressure and contains globulin and an increased number of cells, predominantly lymphocytes. The cell increase does not necessarily parallel the severity of manifestations. There is some indication that pleocytosis may occur in practically all cases of mumps, even though there is no obvious evidence of central-nervous-system involvement. The spinal-fluid findings have caused diagnostic difficulty in differentiating cases of mumps occurring in the late summer and early fall from preparalytic anterior poliomyelitis and other diseases caused by neurotropic viruses. The prognosis as to recovery from neurological complications is good, although permanent deafness, blindness, spastic paralysis, idiocy, and even death have occurred.

Acute pancreatitis is not an uncommon complication of mumps. It generally begins in the first week of illness but sometimes appears later. The onset is sudden, with severe epigastric pain, tenderness, prostration, vomiting, and fever. Recovery is complete. Mumps pancreatitis is believed not to affect the islands of Langerhans or to cause permanent injury to the exocrine glands. Isolated cases of diabetes mellitus have developed soon after recovery but are considered to be examples of coincidence. Steatorrhea is equally rare.

Other glands, such as the prostate, thyroid, thymus, mammary, and lacrimal, may be involved occasionally. Nephritis, labyrinthitis, arthritis, endocarditis, pericarditis, and pleurisy are rare complications.

Prevention—Recovery from mumps, whether the classical parotitis or the more obscure systemic type of infection, produces a lasting immunity. This immunity causes specific skin hypersensitivity to the virus which may be detected by intradermal injection of mumps virus skin-test antigen (p. 338).

The test may be employed at any age for determining susceptibility to mumps. It is particularly useful during and after adolescence to identify those who should be protected against the disease and the complications which so frequently develop in this age group. Because of the relatively long incubation period of mumps, there is time to apply the test after exposure and to vaccinate individuals who require protection. As a matter of fact, the test itself produces some increase in immunity. However, active immunization with mumps virus vaccine or repeated tests do not affect the skin reaction.

Adults who are susceptible to infection, as shown by lack of circulating complement-fixing antigen or by a negative skin test, may be immunized with mumps virus vaccine (p. 323). Complement-fixation titers increase within one week. Epidemics of mumps are prone to occur in segregated populations and may be prevented or aborted by administration of the vaccine to all susceptible individuals.

Routine immunization before adolescence is not recommended for the reason that the artificially induced immunity may wane and permit infection to occur at an older age when there is greater danger from complications. It is not known whether induced immunity in infants and children can be maintained indefinitely by administration of boosting doses. Immunity to mumps is found in many individuals who have never had clinical manifestations of parotitis. It is possible that actively immunized children may develop subclinical infections and thereby acquire permanent protection. Until these points have been clarified, administration of mumps virus vaccine to infants and children should be limited to special circumstances in which the need for protection outweighs any possible disadvantages.

Individuals who are allergic to eggs may develop severe reactions and should not be immunized with the vaccine.

Treatment—Children should be isolated until swelling of the salivary glands and all complications have subsided. Fever or other constitutional reactions are indications for bed rest. In order to avoid complications, it is traditional for adults to remain in bed for two or three weeks. The diet need not be restricted unless chewing is difficult or painful, in which case soft or liquid food is desirable during the acute stage.

Hot or cold applications to the affected parts afford some relief from pain. For swelling of the salivary glands, absorbent cotton held in place by a snug bandage is often preferred. Analgesics, sedatives, and antipyretics may be used symptomatically. Oral hygiene should be encouraged unless mouthwashes and gargles increase the discomfort.

In adult men having mumps, orchitis can be prevented in almost all, if not all, by prophylactic administration of 5 mg. diethylstilbestrol daily for three or possibly four weeks beginning as soon as the diagnosis of mumps is made. Smaller doses may be ineffective. If the patient already has orchitis when first seen, the severity and duration may be reduced by diethylstilbestrol therapy in the above dosage. No side-effects have been noted.

In any case of orchitis, the scrotum should be supported by a sling or pillow. Ice bags give considerable relief but should be discontinued for one hour in every three or four. Diathermy has been recommended and is said to give prompt symptomatic relief and to hasten resolution. Severe cases may require surgical treatment consisting of multiple incisions through the tunica albuginea. Psychotherapy is generally needed to allay the patient's fear of impotence and sterility.

Central-nervous-system involvement may cause sufficient increase in spinal-fluid pressure to necessitate spinal puncture and drainage.

POLIOMYELITIS

Poliomyelitis is an acute infectious disease caused by a filtrable, neurotropic virus. It is characterized by mild, upper-respiratory or gastro-intestinal symptoms, occasionally by signs of central-nervous-system invasion, and rarely by residual, flaccid paralysis of voluntary muscles. Several immunologically different strains of virus have been isolated. In recent years the disease has occurred frequently as an epidemic. The principal mode of dissemination is not known, but human carriers are probably an important source of infection. It is most prevalent during the late spring, summer, and early fall seasons. The disease may take a very mild form or a more severe form with paralysis. Recovery from an attack is believed to produce immunity to the infecting strain of virus, but the individual may remain susceptible to other strains. Secondary attacks do occur and may produce paralysis, but it is believed that most are asymptomatic.

Symptoms of the disease become apparent after an incubation period of five to thirty-five days, averaging between nine and thirteen days. In the mild form of the disease the onset usually is sudden, with fever, malaise, headache, vomiting, restlessness, irritability, somnolence, and temperature over 100° F. Neurological symptoms usually are indefinite, and all symptoms subside in four to six days.

In the more severe cases the onset is similar, but symptoms of neurological involvement soon are manifest; muscle tenderness, stiffness of the neck and back, and pain on flexion of the neck are almost universal. Kernig's sign may be positive. On sitting, the patient may assume a tripod position with his arms propped to relieve strain on the back muscles. The fever lasts up to ten days, and the temperature may be 105° F. or higher. In about 50 percent of cases, fever may decrease several days after onset, only to reappear together with signs of neurological involvement. The symptoms of meningitis and myelitis become more pronounced toward the end of the febrile period, and flaccid paralysis is evident. The parts affected vary widely—from isolated muscle groups to apparently complete involvement of all the striated muscles. The muscles themselves are not attacked by the virus but are affected through inflammation or degeneration of the lower motor neurons. The reflexes may become erratic or hyperactive and later are diminished or absent. The disease may involve the brain, particularly the brain stem. Respiratory paralysis may result from involvement of the respiratory center or from paralysis of the thoracic or diaphragmatic musculature. Bulbar paralysis may be heralded by a nasal tone in the patient's voice followed by difficulty in swallowing. Breathing becomes difficult, and fluid accumulates in the pharynx and respiratory tree. Visual defects from involvement of the optic nerve and permanent mental changes from cortical damage do not occur. Shock and coma are not infrequent.

Diagnosis of the mild form of the disease is difficult, but it should be suspected in summer in a child with an unexplained fever greater than 101° F., particularly during an epidemic. In the more severe forms of the disease, evidence of paralysis must be watched for carefully. There are no diagnostic laboratory tests, but a lumbar puncture may reveal an increased cell count up to 150 (usually predominantly mononuclear cells) and some increase in globulin. After paralysis has appeared, the number of mononuclear cells nearly always increases but rarely exceeds 400 cells per cc. The sugar content of the spinal fluid is normal; the colloidal gold curve is not diagnostic but may be shifted to the left. The differential diagnosis includes rheumatic fever (p. 46), meningococcus infections (p. 165), tuberculous meningitis (p. 166), and virus encephalitides (p. 164).

Treatment is not specific. Adequate fluids, complete bed rest, easily assimilated diet, and careful nursing care are essential for both the mild form of the disease and the early stage of the more severe form. As the paralysis appears, care should be taken not to have bedclothes weigh on the patient's extremities. A vertical board at the foot of the bed as a footrest usually is comforting. Moist heat to the paralyzed limbs is helpful in reducing pain and spasm. Beginning in early convalescence, good supervised physical therapy is essential to re-educate muscles and improve blood supply. Splinting at any stage of the disease is inadvisable. Later, braces and physical therapy may be required to restore function of the affected parts.

In the bulbar type of the disease, as fluids begin to accumulate in the pharynx, aspiration may be necessary. Difficulty in swallowing necessitates intravenous administration of fluids. Paralysis of the respiratory centers may become so severe as to require placing the patient in a respirator. Since laryngeal spasm is common, tracheotomy should be performed on nearly every patient requiring the respirator. Frequent aspiration of fluid from the respiratory tree is essential. Administration of oxygen may be required. Dependence of the patient upon the respirator should be avoided as convalescence begins.

Prognosis at any stage of the disease should be cautious. Recovery from the mild form is the rule. In cases involving the limbs, recovery may vary widely—from no apparent residual effects to severely crippling paralysis—and the original course of the disease frequently cannot be used to predict the long-term recovery. In the bulbar form of the disease, recovery varies widely also.

Prophylaxis depends upon avoiding carriers and individuals in the acute stages of the disease. Precautions against infection should be followed in the sickroom, and isolation of cases is maintained for three weeks from date of onset. Overtiring, fatigue, overexertion, sudden chilling, crowds, surgical procedures, and unnecessary contact with ill persons are to be avoided in the presence of an epidemic. Sanitary measures, reduction of the fly population, and careful personal cleanliness may be encouraged, although there is no proof that these influence the course of an epidemic.

PSITTACOSIS

Psittacosis (ornithosis) is an acute infectious disease of the lungs caused by a filtrable virus which is transmitted to man through contact with the nasal discharges and droppings of infected birds. Parrots, parakeets, pigeons, and ducks are believed to be the principal reservoirs, but the disease is known to occur in other birds also.

Following an incubation period of seven to fifteen days, the onset of the disease may be abrupt or insidious. The initial symptoms usually are malaise, headache, anorexia, and backache. Fever begins early, may be remittent in type, remains high for a week or ten days, and declines in the second or third week by lysis. The pulse rate is slow. The presence of pulmonary disease may be difficult to detect on physical examination. Patchy areas of consolidation may be found. X-ray examination reveals hazy, irregularly distributed areas of increased density. Cough is present and is usually nonproductive, although blood-streaked sputum may be raised when secondary infection is present. Epistaxis occurs in one-fourth of cases. Occasionally, scattered rose-colored macules resembling rose spots may be seen. Relapses occur occasionally. Complications are not frequent. The disease subsides gradually, and the convalescent period is usually extended.

The disease must be differentiated from atypical pneumonia (p. 117), influenza (p. 22), typhoid fever (p. 14), and mild tuberculosis (p. 12).

The most useful laboratory test is the complement-fixation reaction with serum and psittacosis antigen. Lymphogranuloma venereum (p. 23) also will give a positive test; but titers decrease during convalescence, whereas in psittacosis titers continue to rise for several months. Complement fixation remains positive in carriers and in those constantly exposed to infected birds. The virus may be recovered from the sputum and identified. The blood count is not typical; either leukocytosis or leukopenia may be found.

Treatment—There is no known specific treatment. Bed rest, adequate fluids, and other supportive measures are required. Chloramphenicol has been found effective in experimental infections. It may be administered in an initial dose of 3 Gm. followed by 0.5 to 1 Gm. every four hours for five to ten days.

The prognosis in untreated cases varies with age, older persons being more severely affected. The mortality rate is approximately 20 percent in the absence of treatment.

Prophylaxis depends upon avoidance of birds known to carry the disease, such as parrots and pigeons, and strict isolation precautions in the case of affected persons.

RABIES

Rabies (hydrophobia) is an acute infectious disease of the central nervous system caused by a filtrable virus and transmitted to man in the saliva of an infected animal. All mammals are susceptible to the disease, but the dog is the most frequent carrier affecting man. When the virus is introduced into a wound, it becomes established in nerve tissue and migrates to the brain, where it produces a fulminating encephalitis. Once symptoms occur, the disease is inevitably fatal.

The incubation period varies from ten days to seven months or more but is rarely less than fifteen days or more than five months. It is influenced by the location and severity of the bite and, probably, by the dose of virus received. Bites on the face and head, deep bites anywhere, and bites by wolves and other wild animals result in the shortest incubation periods.

The onset of the disease is characterized by a short, prodromal period of depression, fever, headache, anorexia, nausea, sore throat, and malaise. This is followed by uncontrollable restlessness, hyperesthesia of the skin, and hypersensitivity to light and sound. Abnormal sensation at the site of infection is an early and significant sign. Agitation and anxiety succeed restlessness, saliva appears in copious quantities, deep reflexes become hyperactive, and convulsions occur as the result of very slight stimuli such as a breath of wind. Attempts to swallow result in forcible expulsion of fluids from spasmodic contraction of the muscles of deglutition and accessory muscles of respiration. This may be so violent as to cause prolonged apnea with cyanosis and gasping attempts at respiration. Dyspnea is not infrequent. Tetanic rigidity or epileptiform seizures may be seen. Death intervenes in two to three days because of dehydration and cardiac and respiratory failure (usually during a convulsion). In some cases, not all of the symptoms may occur; instead, the prodromal symptoms are followed by high fever, pains in the region of the bite, and paralysis which becomes generalized and fatal. Others may survive the stage of excitement and appear to improve, only to lapse into rapidly progressing paralysis.

Dehydration may affect the blood count, but in its absence the red cells are normal and the white cells are increased to 20,000 or more per cu.mm. The spinal-fluid pressure may be slightly increased. The fluid is clear; protein is slightly increased; and the count rarely exceeds 100, with mononuclear cells predominating.

Occasionally, hysteria may be confused with the disease but is easily differentiated. Ordinarily the diagnosis is not difficult, but without a history of exposure the disease may be confused with fulminating poliomyelitis and the encephalitides. Tetanus may develop from animal bites but usually has a short incubation period of six to fourteen days.

Trismus is rarely present in rabies, and the muscle spasticity is intermittent and usually limited to the muscles of the throat.

Treatment—At the time of injury, if the biting animal is known or suspected to be rabid, the bite should be scrubbed with soap and water and cauterized by pure phenol, followed immediately by 95 percent alcohol to remove the acid. Fuming nitric acid, neutralized promptly with copious quantities of sodium bicarbonate solution, may be used but is more painful.

If, after observation or examination, the biting animal is demonstrated to be rabid, Pasteur vaccine treatment should be initiated at once (see p. 322). In most instances when the biting animal is not available or the diagnosis of rabies is questionable, the physician would be well advised to institute the treatment.

Once symptoms occur, treatment is symptomatic and directed at control of excitement through the use of sedatives and anesthetics. Morphine may increase excitement and should therefore be avoided.

RUBELLA

Rubella (German measles) is an acute, infectious, epidemic, highly contagious, benign exanthematous disease presumably caused by a filtrable virus. The disease occurs most frequently in the first half of the year, with the peak in May and June. It is acquired by contact with infected discharges from the nasopharynx. The greatest incidence is in children between the ages of three and twelve. However, it occurs more frequently in adults than does measles. Infants under six months are attacked only rarely. One attack confers lasting immunity. There is no cross immunity between rubella and measles.

The incubation period varies from ten to twenty-two days but averages seventeen. In the prodromal period there may be a short, afebrile interlude of pharyngeal catarrh and malaise. The characteristic macular rash usually appears first on the face and neck, around the mouth or ears, or on the scalp. Sometimes it may be seen first on the trunk or extremities. At first morbilliform and in discrete spots, it tends to become scarlatiniform and general as it spreads downward. It does not cover the entire body at one time, as a rule. It usually is fully developed within twenty-four hours. A fine red enanthema may develop on the soft palate. Koplik's spots are not present. The temperature rises to 101°F. as the rash develops. The rash is present about three days and disappears in the order in which it appeared. Very moderate desquamation is sometimes seen.

Discrete enlargement of the occipital, postauricular, and posterior cervical lymph nodes is observed and subsides in two or three weeks. These may be tender. During the disease, the conjunctivae are pink and suffused.

Complications and sequelae generally are rare and inconsequential, although otitis, pneumonia, arthritis, nephritis, and encephalitis or meningoencephalitis have been observed. The occurrence of the disease during the first three months of pregnancy is believed to lead to severe congenital anomalies in the infant. Until this is confirmed or refuted, a pregnant woman exposed to rubella should be treated with immune globulin (p. 336) in an attempt to prevent or modify the infection.

The disease must be differentiated from measles (p. 24), exanthem subitum, scarlet fever (p. 9), pityriasis rosea (p. 235), infectious mononucleosis (p. 48), and secondary syphilis (p. 10).

Treatment—There is no specific therapy. Bed rest, adequate fluids, analgesics, and other symptomatic measures suffice for the uncomplicated case. The complications should be treated as if they were the primary disease.

Exposed individuals should be isolated from the tenth to the twenty-first day after exposure. Attempts to prevent or modify the disease with pooled convalescent serum or plasma or gamma globulin have given contradictory results. Ill individuals should be isolated and kept in bed until all symptoms disappear or for a minimum of seven days.

SMALLPOX

Smallpox (variola) is an acute, infectious, communicable disease characterized by a skin eruption progressing through stages of macule, papule, vesicle, pustule, and crust. It is caused by a specific virus and is transmitted by contact with the lesions or by air-borne droplets of a patient's nasopharyngeal secretions. Because of compulsory vaccination, epidemics rarely occur, although sporadic cases and small outbreaks are seen from time to time.

After an incubation period of eight to sixteen days, the first stage of the disease commences abruptly with chills, followed by high fever (sometimes reaching 106° F.), prostration, severe generalized aching, headache, and sometimes nausea and vomiting. Backache is a common complaint. In children, convulsions, delirium, and coma may occur. A fleeting scarlatiniform rash may develop.

On the third or fourth day the typical eruption begins, the temperature dropping as it develops. Red, raised macules appear, first on the face and wrists, and spread rapidly over the trunk and extremities. They are most numerous on the exposed surfaces of the body. The lesions may be either discrete or coalescent. The macules rapidly develop into firm, shotty papules two to four millimeters in diameter. Multilocular vesicles, usually umbilicated, begin to form on the fifth or sixth day of the disease.

By the eighth day, the vesicles have filled with cloudy fluid and become pustular. The lesions are surrounded by a red areola, have an infiltrated base, and are deep-seated. All of the lesions are approximately at the same stage of development at the same time. The mucous membranes of the mouth and respiratory tract frequently are involved. The temperature rises with pustulation and does not return to normal until crusts are well formed. The thick, brownish-yellow crusts are shed in the period of ten to forty days following the appearance of the lesions. Sometimes the pustules become hemorrhagic, in which case the outlook is grave. When the lesions heal and the crusts drop off, a pockmark, or pit extending into the corium of the skin, remains. This does not always occur with mild infections. The infectious period lasts from the prodromal stage until the last crust has disappeared.

Variola minor (alastrim) is a mild, not uncommon variety of smallpox which may cause difficulty in diagnosis. "Varioloid" is the term applied to smallpox occurring in an individual successfully immunized. The course of the disease is shortened considerably, the lesions are discrete, and they usually involute very early. They are easily confused with those of chickenpox.

A mild leukopenia or normal white count is usual during the pre-eruptive stage; but with the appearance of the rash and during the pustular stage, a polymorphonuclear leukocytosis develops.

The complications of smallpox usually are due to secondarily invading organisms, such as streptococci and staphylococci. Abscesses, septicemia, nephritis, erysipelas, pneumonia, corneal ulcers, and pustules of the eyelids may occur. In children, otitis media and diarrhea are infrequent but important. In adults, hemiplegia, polyneuritis, and encephalitis may be seen occasionally.

The disease must be differentiated from chickenpox (p. 19), scarlet fever (p. 9), pustular syphilid (p. 10), and sometimes septicemia. Diagnosis may be aided by complement-fixation tests or by the intradermal injection of heat-killed cowpox vaccine in patients who have not been vaccinated. In the latter test, the presence of smallpox is indicated by a local reaction which appears at the site of the injection within a few hours and becomes maximal in twenty-four hours. The virus can be cultured and identified by inoculating embryonated chicken eggs.

Treatment—There is no specific treatment. Vaccination of nonimmune individuals may prevent or modify the disease if carried out before the sixth day of exposure. The sulfonamides and antibiotics may be of assistance in combating the secondary infections. Complete bed rest, strict isolation, sterilization of all articles used by the patient, and disinfection of the sickroom after recovery are necessary.

One attack of smallpox confers immunity. Vaccination (p. 321) offers the only effective method of prevention and control.

PROTOZOAL DISEASES

AMEBIASIS

Amebiasis is infection with *Endamoeba histolytica*. This organism is the most frequently encountered pathogen of the various amebae found in the human intestinal tract. Geographical distribution is wide, including tropical, subtropical, and temperate regions. It is estimated that between 14 and 20 percent of the population of the United States are infected as carriers.

The disease is acquired by ingestion of food contaminated with feces containing motile amebae or cysts. It may take a number of forms, varying from acute dysentery to an asymptomatic carrier state. Amebae may enter the blood stream and be transported to the liver with consequent hepatitis or abscess.

From the intestinal tract the amebae penetrate the tissues of the host, principally the mucosa of the colon and rectum, producing necrosis without inflammatory reaction. As the disease progresses, extension to the submucosa may occur, with bottleneck ulceration and secondary bacterial infection.

In the acute form of amebiasis, which is relatively infrequent, the patient complains of headache, nausea, griping abdominal pain, and frequency of bowel movements, usually fifteen to twenty each twenty-four hours. There is low fever and, in the absence of secondary infection, slight or no elevation of the white blood count. Examination of the abdomen reveals an increase in peristalsis, with generalized tenderness. Stools are characteristically fluid, containing specks of bloody mucus.

When the disease is mild, symptoms may be atypical and not necessarily indicative of intestinal infection. The patient with chronic amebiasis may complain of undue fatigability and lassitude and may be considered neurotic. As the physician encounters these and other vague symptoms such as flatulence, sense of fullness in right lower quadrant, and loose stools followed by brief periods of constipation, he should keep in mind the possibility of amebiasis. On the other hand, there may be no symptoms, and a carrier stage may last indefinitely, with the individual in apparent good health until the complications of hepatitis or liver abscess suddenly appear.

Amebic hepatitis may appear early or after a chronic or subclinical infection, or it may develop during an acute stage or a remission of the disease. The patient complains of severe pain in the hepatic region, has fever, and is prostrated. Upon examination, the liver is found to be enlarged and tender. The temperature may be variable, with chills and profuse sweats suggesting malaria. The white blood count is elevated to 25,000 or 30,000 with a polymorphonuclear leukocytosis of 70 to 80 percent.

Amebic abscess of the liver may develop within a few months after the initial infection, although it is more commonly seen as a late complication. When it occurs with active dysentery, the abscess is usually acute and multiple. When the infection is of long standing, the abscess is usually single, large, and chronic. The clinical picture of acute amebic hepatitis is easy to confuse with that of acute amebic abscess. A therapeutic trial with emetine is usually diagnostic, however; for fever, pain, tenderness, enlargement of the liver, and disproportionate leukocytosis subside with hepatitis and persist with abscess.

Chronic abscess occurs more commonly in the right lobe of the liver. Symptoms vary, depending on the size of the lesion, its situation with relation to other structures, and the degree of infection. There may be asymmetric enlargement, the right lobe edge being easily palpable and tender. The diaphragm may be affected, as shown by pain on heavy percussion of the chest wall. With peripheral extension, intercostal tenderness may appear. Small abscesses may cause slight elevation of the white blood count with an increased percentage of polymorphonuclear leukocytes. Large abscesses may produce no leukocytosis. With chronic abscess there may be a variety of digestive complaints, gradual weight loss over a long period with or without low-grade fever, unproductive cough, pain on respiration, and pain referred to the right shoulder (due to involvement of the diaphragm and irritation of the basal pleura). Involvement of the pleura is often diagnosed erroneously as pneumonia, empyema, or tuberculosis. An untreated abscess may rupture and cause fatal peritonitis.

Amebiasis should be considered in all bloody diarrheas, in any case of acute bloodless dysentery not otherwise accounted for, and in any case of vague illness. Amebic abscess of the liver should be considered in any unexplained illness with symptoms referable to the lower chest, diaphragm, or upper abdomen. Positive diagnosis depends on recovery of motile forms or cysts of *E. histolytica* from rectal lesions, aspirated material, or feces. Obviously, the organism should be sought in any case of hepatitis.

Treatment—Carbarsone is the drug of choice for intestinal amebiasis. Its use is discussed on page 314. Emetine hydrochloride does not affect amebae in the epithelium or lumen of the intestine, but it has amebicidal action in tissues. It is therefore employed in early acute cases with dysentery. Dosage, dangers, and precautions appear on page 314. Various compounds containing iodine, oxyquinoline, and sulfonic acid groups (p. 315) are used as interim therapy between courses of carbarsone.

The antibiotics are valuable adjuncts to specific treatment in severe or resistant cases. It is believed that they have no direct amebicidal effect but act indirectly by destroying symbiotic organisms.

If amebic hepatitis or liver abscess is suspected, chloroquine diphosphate (p. 301) should be given by mouth. A priming dosage of 0.25 mg. four times daily for two days is followed by 0.25 mg. twice daily for two to three weeks. Hepatitis usually shows prompt improvement (two or three days). Absence of improvement suggests abscess. If the abscess appears to be in the right lobe of the liver, aspiration should be performed by means of an approved technic. The left lobe is never aspirated because of its proximity to the heart and stomach; it should be approached by means of laparotomy.

In acute abscess, the contents are usually semifluid and chocolate-brown in color. Old abscesses more often contain yellow or white material. Amebae are not present in the contents but are usually abundant in the wall. Removal of the contents of an abscess is usually followed by improvement in fever, leukocytosis, pain, and tenderness. With large abscesses, evacuation may have to be repeated.

The patient with intestinal amebiasis should be kept under treatment until at least three examinations (conducted not less than two days apart and the first one falling not less than ten days after the last course of treatment) have been negative. A convenient yet adequate routine is to administer a cathartic dose of magnesium sulfate in the office and to collect stool specimens. The first one, which will be semisolid, is examined by a flotation technic (p. 547) for cysts, and the second or third (watery) stool for motile amebae (p. 547). A follow-up set of examinations should be made at monthly intervals for not less than three months after presumed cure.

Amebiasis tends to recur despite vigorous treatment. However, when the symptom of diarrhea persists in the face of adequate therapy, some other cause should be sought.

Prevention of amebiasis involves the protection and sterilization of the water supply by boiling or through sand filtration; proper sewage disposal; the protection of food from insects and rodents; diagnosis and treatment of carriers; and avoidance of eating uncooked food in regions where the disease exists. Treatment of raw vegetables with various antiseptic solutions is of doubtful value.

MALARIA

Malaria is an acute and chronic infection caused by a parasite belonging to the Protozoa, genus *Plasmodium*, and transmitted from man to man by certain species of *Anopheles* mosquitoes. It is characterized by attacks of fever, anemia, splenomegaly, and, if untreated, cachexia and pigmentary degeneration, especially of the spleen, liver, and brain. It occurs epidemically or endemically wherever conditions favor the development of the parasite in the transmitting mosquitoes. Malaria has world-wide distribution but is most prevalent in tropical and subtropical countries between the latitudes 45° North and 40° South.

There are four species of organisms pathogenic for man: *Plasmodium vivax*, which causes tertian (benign tertian) malaria, is most widespread and is the prevailing species in temperate zones; *P. falciparum*, which causes estivo-autumnal (subtertian or malignant tertian) malaria, is largely confined to the tropics; both *P. malariae*, which produces the quartan form, and *P. ovale*, which causes a type clinically resembling that from *P. vivax*, are rare and of no importance in the United States.

All species of the genus *Plasmodium* go through an exogenous or sexual cycle in the mosquito (sporogony), the final form of which (the sporozoite) is introduced into man during the bite of an infected mosquito. In man, reproduction is by means of an endogenous or asexual cycle (schizogony). The sporozoites quickly disappear from the circulation, supposedly by gaining entrance into macrophages of the reticulo-endothelial system (exoerythrocytic or pre-erythrocytic stage). Here, development continues for a variable time which depends on the species of parasite. After this latent period, sporozoites reappear in the blood stream, penetrate red blood cells (erythrocytic stage), and pass through different phases of development, ending with small spore-like bodies (merozoites) which are liberated into the blood stream by destruction of the red blood cells. These penetrate fresh red cells, and the cycle is repeated.

Multiplication is in geometric progression. After about two weeks (incubation period), the number of parasites in the same phase of development is usually great enough so that the quantity of merozoites and toxic material released from the red cells with each generation is sufficient to cause a paroxysm of fever. When there are two generations of parasites, each completing its cycle at a different time, paroxysms may occur daily. In most broods of parasites, succeeding generations mature at the same time of day; but in some the time varies, with the result that paroxysms occur all around the clock. When irregularity is pronounced or when the parasite burden is low, clinical paroxysms may not occur.

In addition to the asexual cycle, there is in man an asymptomatic sexual cycle which produces male and female gametocytes. These are the only forms infective for the mosquito. The life cycle of vivax and falciparum parasites in the mosquito requires about a week to ten days for completion, after which time the mosquito can transmit the disease to man.

Infection can result also from the parenteral administration of blood containing the parasites, as during transfusion or with therapeutic malaria. However, when so introduced, the organisms may have an irregular reproductive cycle, and paroxysms may not occur or may be atypical.

The exact symptoms of malaria will vary, depending on the species of infecting organism, its virulence, and the degree of inherited or acquired immunity in the host. In benign tertian malaria (*P. vivax*), incubation requires ten to seventeen days, the organism segmenting in the blood every forty-eight hours. Patients may then have a remittent fever with general malaise, anorexia, and dull headache for the first three to five days, followed by occurrence of the typical paroxysm. Sensations

of chilliness spread from the spinal column to the extremities and give way finally to actual chill, with vigorous shaking of the body. The patient presents a pinched, cyanotic appearance and will request all possible coverings to counteract the cold. The pulse is rapid, urine is increased, and there may be nausea or vomiting. The cold sensation lasts for twenty to sixty minutes. Meanwhile, the body temperature is rising.

As the temperature reaches its peak, the hot stage of the attack sets in. During this phase the face becomes flushed, the pulse is more full, the eyes shine, and the patient may again suffer nausea or vomiting, headache, or slight delirium. Tension or pain may be felt in the region of the spleen, and there may be cough. The fever, which may reach 41°C. (106°F.) or higher, persists for one to four hours, whereupon the sweating stage begins. The pulse becomes slower, the temperature drops, and the patient, feeling relieved, falls asleep. The total paroxysm usually consumes eight to twelve hours. The patient awakens feeling well and able to resume his normal activities.

The anemia in *P. vivax* malaria is usually rapid in development but is not as severe as in falciparum infections, since the vivax parasites have a predilection for young red cells, particularly reticulocytes. The spleen enlarges during the attack and subsides between attacks. It may not be palpable during the first few attacks, but in subsequent attacks it becomes so. There may also be tenderness of the liver.

Other forms of malaria conform, with some deviations, to this pattern. In quartan malaria (*P. malariae*), the incubation period is about ten to eighteen days, and paroxysms usually occur at intervals of seventy-two hours, although overlapping or alternating broods may cause paroxysms to occur every day or to last as long as twenty-four hours. The average, however, is eight to ten hours. Splenic enlargement is not so great, headache is usually more intense, delirium more frequent, and the anemia slow in development (because of the slow growth and lesser density of the parasites). In general, the symptoms in quartan malaria are more severe than in tertian, and fatal infections are more frequent in children.

In falciparum malaria, incubation requires seven to fifteen days but may be protracted over many weeks or months. Symptoms are more varied. Most pernicious infections occur with this type of malaria. The term "intermittent malaria" is used to connote the typical irregularity of the temperature curve which this species produces. The paroxysms are often very sudden and prostrating; the severe chill is often absent, the patient complaining merely of chilly sensations or a general feeling of cold along the spine and in the extremities. The temperature rises rapidly during the first two hours to 104°F. or higher; then there is a period of oscillation in which the temperature drops slightly, a sign that is often mistaken for the crisis and is therefore called the "false crisis," since the temperature rises again to a point as high as before, if not higher. This peculiar irregularity of the temperature occurs in no other febrile condition and is so characteristic of *P. falciparum* as to constitute an important diagnostic sign. The anemia in falciparum malaria develops more rapidly than in other forms of the disease, because the parasites attack the erythrocytes of all ages. Since there is no depletion of iron stores, hemoglobin loss is rapidly restored during remissions unless the bone marrow is severely affected.

The prognosis in vivax malaria is good so far as danger to life is concerned, although in debilitated individuals death may occur. With *P. falciparum*, the parasitized red blood cells become sticky and adhere to the blood vessel walls, thus causing capillary embolism and infarction. Since this process may involve any organ, the symptoms of falciparum malaria are varied. There is constant danger that the infection may become pernicious, with extremely high fevers running up to 110°F. (about 43°C.) and resulting almost invariably in prompt coma and death. Frequently attacks start without the typical chill or rigor but go immediately into delirium or coma, or there may be sudden collapse with no other symptoms or with severe diarrhea, muscular cramps, and suppression of urine. The intense, rapid course may suggest cholera. One of the most common, although least dangerous, of the pernicious manifestations in malaria is bilious remittent fever, in which there may be extreme nausea followed by vomiting and bile-rich stools, with jaundice appearing on the second day.

In typical cases in endemic areas, the diagnosis of malaria may be obvious. In other regions and with atypical symptoms, it may be difficult. In any case, the diagnosis is established only by demonstration of the organisms in the blood. Standard technics are described on page 545. When examination by a technician experienced in malaria fails to show parasites in thick blood films taken morning or evening for three successive days, the patient will generally be found not to be suffering from clinical malaria. Presumptive evidence of malaria is justification for beginning treatment even while the search for organisms continues. Only occasionally will treatment have to be interrupted to allow a sufficient number of organisms to reappear in the blood to establish the diagnosis.

Malaria should be considered as a possibility whenever a patient presents a history or clinical evidence of one or more of the following:

1. Fever, high or low, intermittent or continuous (and which may or may not be preceded by prodromata of malaise), muscular pains, headache, and anorexia. Rigor may or may not have occurred, since often in the initial attack of benign tertian malaria a daily rise of temperature occurs for the first few days before the typical rigor and classical periodicity set in. When rigor has been suffered, there may be causes other than malaria for its occurrence.

2. Anemia, usually acute and progressive, and always hypochromic.

3. Enlargement of the spleen, which may be just palpable or may reach to the umbilicus.

4. Various cerebral manifestations which may include coma, delirium, or convulsions.

5. A history of one or more symptoms referable to the gastro-intestinal tract, such as persistent vomiting or loose stools.

6. Symptoms suggesting acute bronchitis or pneumonia.

7. Weak pulse and fainting.

8. Thrombosis, hemorrhages, edema.

9. Jaundice or nephritis.

10. Albuminuria, hematuria, hemoglobinuria.

11. Present or recent residence in an endemic area.

When prompt finding of the parasite is not possible and when in an endemic area all other signs point to malaria, any convincing combination of these symptoms should be basis enough for instituting therapy. Most important is the triad of fever, anemia, and splenomegaly.

Untreated primary attacks vary in duration, depending on the species of parasite and susceptibility of the patient. In the absence of remissions, an attack of vivax may last nine weeks. Interruption by the spontaneous remissions common with this species may increase the total duration to fourteen weeks. Falciparum infections last no longer than about six weeks.

The severity of the paroxysms in each species gradually lessens during these periods, and the temperature rises are diminished, the termination being similar to a lysis. In vivax infections that have been marked by early remissions therapeutically induced, there is a tendency toward resumption of clinical activity. In falciparum infections this may not last for more than a year, but in vivax it may persist for two or even three years. On this basis, it is important to observe that resumption of clinical activity within eight weeks of the end of the primary attack is a recrudescence while the parasites are still present in the peripheral blood. Any activity beyond this time, up to twenty-four weeks after the primary attack, is regarded as a relapse, and if longer still, as a recurrence. Relapses may occur in improperly treated cases, although newer drugs have diminished their incidence. Several theories are current to account for the relapsing nature of malaria. It seems most likely that relapses are due to emergence of the organisms from an asymptomatic exoerythrocytic stage of development in the reticulo-endothelial system.

In latent malaria, when the parasites may be present in the blood without paroxysms, the individual may show vague signs of illness, such as anorexia, malaise, headache, anemia, or alimentary tract disturbances. Children who survive their first or first few attacks tend to develop resistance to the disease as long as infection persists; they constitute the bulk of the carriers in endemic areas. Repeated infections may produce a partial immunity which is very specific and does not protect against reinfection with a different strain of the same species of *Plasmodium*.

Besides pigmentation, the principal damage which follows repeated attacks of malaria is related to the anoxia caused by destruction of red cells. Fibrotic enlargement of the spleen is common. Rupture on the slightest trauma is possible in severe conditions. The liver may also be enlarged. In cases of prolonged and severe chronicity, the skin is a dirty, earthy hue and may ulcerate readily from slight wounds. The patient may also suffer mental depression and deterioration of memory. In patients who survive a cerebral attack of pernicious malaria there may be delusional psychoses. Severely debilitated persons with cachectic malaria may also suffer from intercurrent infections, neuritis, and various gastro-intestinal disturbances. Such complications as meningitis, pneumonia, heart disease, acute or chronic gastritis or enteritis, nephritis, and cystitis are not uncommon with prolonged chronicity.

Treatment of malarial infection is aimed at cure of the clinical attack, management of the patient during the paroxysm, and prevention of relapses. The various drugs are discussed beginning on page 301. For treatment of the clinical attack, the selected drug should be given as soon as the diagnosis is made—or without waiting for the diagnosis in severe or comatose cases when the patient's life is in danger.

The patient with an acute attack of malaria should be put to bed and watched carefully for a possibility of serious developments. He should be kept on a diet of liquids only, frequent drinks of water or lemonade being recommended. For the nausea, sips of ice-cold alkaline mineral water or cracked ice may be given. A more ample normal diet may be allowed during intermissions of the benign forms. In the pernicious forms, hot-water bottles must be applied to the body, and special measures should be taken if convulsive seizures occur (see p. 147). Anemia should be treated (see p. 94).

Prophylactic measures which will benefit the community include the following:

Protection of the individual against the bite of the anopheline mosquito.
Destruction of anopheline mosquitoes.
Control of mosquito breeding areas.
Suppressive drug treatment when exposure to infection is likely.
Adequate treatment of clinical cases and gametocyte carriers.

METAZOAL DISEASES

ANCYLOSTOMIASIS

Ancylostomiasis (hookworm disease, uncinariasis) is found in tropical and subtropical countries and at times in temperate climates wherever there is warm, moist, fecal-polluted soil and barefootedness. In man, intestinal infection is due to two worms, *Necator americanus* and *Ancylostoma duodenale*; the cutaneous disease called "creeping eruption" is caused by the dog and cat hookworm, *Ancylostoma braziliense*, and others. Eggs deposited in feces on proper soil hatch within two days. The larvae feed for five or six days, during which time they molt twice to become nonfeeding, motile, infective filariform larvae. They may live at or near the soil surface for several weeks. When they come in contact with unprotected human skin, they rapidly penetrate it, enter the lymphatics and small blood vessels, and are deposited in the lungs. Here they break through into the alveoli, ascend the respiratory tract to the throat, and are swallowed. On reaching the small intestine, the larvae develop in four to seven weeks into mature worms firmly attached to the mucosa (females, 10 to 13 mm.; males, 8 to 11 mm. in length). More rarely, infection is acquired by the swallowing of infective larvae in contaminated water or food. In this case, the parasites penetrate the mucosa of the upper intestinal tract, proceed to the lungs, and continue development in the usual manner.

Clinical manifestations vary with the degree of infection and the physical condition of the patient. Dermatitis with intense itching ("ground itch"), erythema, edema, and a papular or vesicular eruption may develop on the feet or wherever the filariform larvae penetrate the skin. This frequently follows infection by *N. americanus* but is less common in the case of *A. duodenale*. The eruption heals in about two weeks. Pulmonary involvement causes symptoms similar to but less severe than those in ascariasis. Light intestinal infections are usually asymptomatic but may cause vague digestive upsets and asthenia. Larger worm burdens result in headache, vertigo, indigestion, eructations, anorexia, pica, epigastric pain and tenderness, chronic fatigue, mental torpor, and anemia. In the more severe infections there are, in addition, alternating diarrhea and constipation, cardiac palpitation, shortness of breath, protuberant abdomen, profound anemia, hemic murmurs, paresthesias, and subcutaneous edema. Growth and mental development in children are depressed.

Diagnosis is made by microscopic identification of hookworm ova in the stools. Recovery of adult worms from the feces is sometimes possible.

Treatment—The drug of choice is tetrachloroethylene (p. 312). Hexylresorcinol (p. 312) is also used. If both the ascaris and hookworm are present, hexylresorcinol should be administered one week before tetrachloroethylene is given, to avoid possible intestinal obstruction. General measures include dietary correction, administration of iron and vitamin supplements, prevention of fecal pollution by sanitary measures, and education in hygiene.

The larvae of creeping eruption may be killed by thoroughly freezing an area 4 to 5 cm. in diameter at the advancing end of the lesion with ethyl chloride spray applied for about thirty seconds. Repetition may be necessary. Freezing should not be employed on severely excoriated or secondarily infected areas. Carbon-dioxide snow can be used but produces more secondary reaction. If the larvae can be located by examination with a magnifying lens after cleansing of the skin with alcohol and application of cedar oil, one treatment with galvanic cautery under local anesthesia, sufficient to produce a small second-degree burn, is a painless and effective treatment. Systemic treatment with Fuadin, an antimony compound, has not given consistently good results.

ASCARIASIS

Ascariasis (*Ascaris lumbricoides* infection) is a very common helminth infection in man; children are particularly susceptible. It is highly endemic wherever soil pollution with human feces occurs. Infection is acquired directly by ingestion of ova

containing viable embryos. The larvae are liberated in the small intestine, penetrate the wall, and enter the blood stream either directly into the portal circulation or by way of the thoracic duct. They pass through the right heart and are deposited in the lungs, where many of them perforate into the alveoli. After a period of growth, the larvae migrate up the respiratory passages to the epiglottis and are swallowed. At this stage they are 1 to 3 mm. long. The adult worms develop in the small intestine; the females are 20 to 35 cm. long, the males somewhat shorter. Numerous eggs are produced, some being fertilized and others not. The embryos are not fully developed when the eggs are passed, but under favorable conditions they become infective in about two weeks. The entire life cycle requires approximately sixty to seventy-five days.

Clinical manifestations may be caused by migrating larvae, by adult worms, or by the excretions of either form. In light infections, symptoms are absent or insignificant. The larvae cause minute alveolar hemorrhages and inflammation in the lung, which, if extensive, result in pneumonitis and even consolidation, with fever, cough, and hemoptysis. In heavy infections, embolic phenomena sometimes occur from larvae which enter the arterial circulation. Urticarial rashes may be noted. Large numbers of adult worms in the intestine may cause abdominal discomfort, nausea, anorexia, colic, toxemia, and intestinal obstruction. Adult worms are rarely found outside the bowel lumen but may invade the appendix, biliary tract, or peritoneal cavity.

Diagnosis is made by microscopic identification of the characteristic eggs in the feces; occasionally an adult worm is recovered. In pulmonary ascariasis, larvae may be found in the bloody sputum.

Treatment—The drug of choice is crystalline hexylresorcinol (p. 312). Chenopodium Oil is effective but dangerously toxic. In the presence of mixed infection, the ascaris should be treated before other vermifuges are employed. In some instances, prophylactic measures and correction of malnutrition alone cause the worms to disappear in a year or so.

GIARDIASIS

Giardiasis (lambliasis, infection with *Giardia lamblia*) is common throughout the world, particularly in warm climates. The organism lives in the upper intestine. Man is the natural host and acquires infection by swallowing cysts. These pass through the stomach unharmed and excyst in the duodenum. The parasites differ from other intestinal protozoa in that they live in a liquid or semiliquid medium and, therefore, are not found in the colon except in the presence of diarrhea. They have been recovered from the gall bladder and appendix. The stools of infected individuals intermittently contain large numbers of cysts.

Clinically, there is evidence that this parasite may cause intestinal disturbances, although many infected individuals do not have symptoms. No significant lesions of the intestinal tract or gallbladder mucosa have been demonstrated. The manifestations consist of vague intestinal disturbances, with flatulence, abdominal distention, epigastric tenderness, mild diarrhea alternating with constipation, and, at times, evidence of low-grade chronic cholecystitis. The stools may contain mucus, but rarely blood.

Diagnosis is readily made by microscopic identification of the motile trophozoites either in liquid stools or in material obtained by duodenal aspiration. When stools are formed, concentration technics facilitate demonstration of the cysts.

Treatment—Quinacrine (p. 301) has superseded all other therapeutic agents because of its high efficacy. It is given in the same manner as for malaria: 0.1 Gm. of the hydrochloride three times daily after meals for five to seven days. One course of treatment is usually sufficient.

OXYURIASIS

Oxyuriasis (*Enterobius vermicularis*, pinworm, or seatworm infection) is cosmopolitan in distribution and probably is the most common helminth infection of man. It is prevalent in warm climates, in children of school age, and particularly in inmates of institutions. Usually all members of a family are infected once the parasite is introduced into the household.

Infection is acquired directly by ingestion of embryo-containing ova. The eggs hatch in the upper intestine and release larvae, which descend to the ileum where they mature. Following copulation, the females migrate to the cecum and attach themselves to the mucosa. When the eggs are fully developed, the worms detach, pass down the colon, and eventually emerge through the anus onto the perianal skin, where the eggs are actively discharged. The eggs become infective within a few hours. Heaviest infections are caused by finger-to-mouth transmission; finger-contaminated food pro-

duces variable severity; air-borne eggs may be inhaled or swallowed; and rarely, if at all, eggs may hatch on the perianal skin and the larvae migrate through the anus to the colon. The entire cycle requires four to seven weeks. Adult female worms measure 8 to 13 mm. in length; males, 2 to 5 mm.

Clinical manifestations may be absent; itching of the perianal region often is pronounced and may provoke scratching, which leads to eczema and pyoderma. Heavy infections may cause anorexia, insomnia, nervousness, abdominal pain, and weight loss.

Diagnosis is made by microscopic identification of the eggs obtained from the perianal skin by means of swabs made of cellophane or Scotch Cellulose Tape. Recovery of adult worms from the skin or feces is sometimes possible.

Treatment—Gentian violet (medicinal) is the drug of choice; for dosage and administration, see page 311. It is important to treat all infected members of a household simultaneously and to repeat the course of treatment at least once after a rest period of one week. General treatment includes antipruritics (p. 480) and local antiseptics (p. 304); mechanical measures to prevent contamination of the hands, such as wearing tight-fitting trunks at night, frequent cutting of the fingernails, and thorough scrubbing of the hands and nails; daily changes of bed and personal linen; and frequent washing of toilets with soap and water or a suitable disinfectant.

STRONGYLOIDIASIS

Strongyloidiasis (strongyloidosis, *Strongyloides stercoralis* infection) is widely distributed in tropical and subtropical regions and is fairly common in the southern United States. The usual mode of infection is penetration of the skin by larvae in the manner of hookworm. Rarely, parasites may be ingested. Larvae which reach the blood stream are carried to the lungs, where they break through into the alveoli and in a few days develop into adolescent males and females. The females are fertilized in the lungs, after which they usually migrate to the upper intestines by way of the trachea and esophagus. Under certain conditions of massive infection they may mature and deposit eggs in the lungs, from which larvae hatch and produce pulmonary strongyloidiasis. The gravid females, on reaching the duodenum and upper jejunum, bore into the mucosa and begin to deposit ova about two weeks after penetration of the skin.

These eggs, which resemble those of hookworm, hatch in the tissues. The motile larvae (200 to 250 microns long) escape into the intestines and are passed with the feces. If deposited on warm, moist soil, development proceeds in one of two ways. Under certain conditions, they transform within twenty-four hours into the skin-penetrating, filariform larvae. In other circumstances, a free-living generation of adults develops; these produce eggs that hatch in a few days into infective larvae, or the adult phase may be repeated. At times, hyperinfection may occur if filariform larvae develop in the intestinal tract. These penetrate the mucosa or the perianal skin and proceed to the lungs in the usual manner.

Clinical manifestations are not constant. A papulovesicular skin eruption with petechial hemorrhages and inflammation, swelling, and intense pruritus at the site of entry may be noted. In twenty-four to forty-eight hours there appear mild fever, malaise, anorexia, headache, cough, and signs of pulmonary inflammation. Chronic pneumonitis may persist for years. The pulmonary and, at times, the intestinal phase may be accompanied by a polymorphonuclear leukocytosis and pronounced eosinophilia. Light infections of the intestinal tract are often asymptomatic. With heavier infections, there may be abdominal pain and attacks of diarrhea often alternating with constipation. The stools may contain mucus but rarely gross blood. Hyperinfection causes ulceration and sloughing of the intestinal mucosa, which is manifested by profuse diarrhea, colicky pains, fever, emaciation, cachexia, vomiting, and sometimes death.

Diagnosis is made by identification under the microscope of the motile rhabditiform larvae in aspirated duodenal contents or diarrheal stools. Ova are rarely found. Stool concentration facilitates examination. *Strongyloides* larvae may at first be confused with hookworm larvae, but differentiation is actually not difficult. *Strongyloides* larvae are sometimes present in the sputum.

Treatment—Gentian violet (medicinal) is the drug of choice, even though it often fails to eradicate the parasites completely; for dosage and administration, see page 311.

TAPEWORMS (TAENIASIS)

Hymenolepis Nana (dwarf tapeworm) is widely distributed in warm countries and is the most common tapeworm of children in the southern United States. The adult worm averages 20 mm. in length. Infection commonly occurs directly from ingestion of food or water contaminated with human feces containing viable ova. No intermediary or reservoir hosts are required for transmission. Symptoms are usually lacking, although heavy infection may cause abdominal pain, diarrhea, asthenia, dizziness, headache, and nervous disturbances. Anemia and eosinophilia are sometimes noted. Diagnosis is made by demonstration of the characteristic ova in the stool. Occasionally it is possible to identify expelled segments of the worm.

Taenia Saginata (beef tapeworm) occurs wherever raw or inadequately cooked beef is a popular item of diet. It is one of the longest tapeworms (4 to 10 meters or more) and the second most common in man. Cattle act as intermediate hosts and become infected by ingesting human feces containing viable ova. The embryos hatch in the upper intestinal tract and penetrate into the tissues of the animal, where they develop into quiescent larvae, or cysticerci. When man consumes an intact cysticercus, it develops into an adult worm in eight or ten weeks. It is doubtful that the cysticercal form occurs in human beings. Human infection is usually, but not necessarily, limited to one worm. The parasite causes little or no damage except slight irritation of the mucous membrane at the point of attachment and, rarely, intestinal obstruction.

Leukocytosis with eosinophilia may be detected early in the infection. Symptoms more often are psychic in origin and date from identification of segments in the stool. Minor digestive disturbances, weight loss, and nervous manifestations are described. Eggs appear irregularly in the stools but cannot be differentiated from those of other species. A few gravid segments usually can be found after purgation, and, when pressed between glass slides and examined with a hand lens, the lateral arms of the uterus can be counted. Beef tapeworm has from fifteen to eighteen on each side; the pork tapeworm has seven to thirteen.

Prophylaxis involves treatment of infected individuals, prevention of cattle-grazing on contaminated land, beef inspection, refrigeration (freezing at −10°C. kills cysticerci within five days), and thorough cooking or pickling.

Taenia Solium (pork tapeworm) is somewhat less common than the beef tapeworm but is found wherever raw or inadequately cooked pork is eaten. The length of the adult worm varies from two to four meters. Hogs are the most common intermediate host. The cysticerci in these animals are ellipsoidal, translucent cysts, measuring about 10 by 5 mm. They may be found in any tissue but are most common in the striated muscles of the tongue, neck, and shoulder; they also occur in the intercostal, abdominal, psoas, femoral, and posterior vertebral muscles.

Man may be infected not only by ingestion of cysticerci in pork, but also by consumption of viable eggs in contaminated food or water and by regurgitation of ova into the stomach as a result of reverse peristalsis. In either case, cysticerci develop and may invade any tissue or organ of the body. Intestinal taeniasis does not cause any characteristic symptoms. The manifestations of cysticercal disease vary, depending upon the location of the lesions. Serious consequences result from involvement of the brain, spinal cord, eyes, or heart. With these exceptions, the life cycle and clinical features of *T. solium* are essentially the same as those of *T. saginata*.

Diphyllobothrium Latum (fish tapeworm) occurs in the lake region of the North Central States and Canada. Infection is acquired from eating raw or inadequately cooked fish containing viable larvae. Man and certain fish-eating animals serve as definitive hosts. When tapeworm eggs are passed in the feces and deposited in fresh water, free-swimming ciliated larvae are released. These are ingested by certain small copepods, or water fleas, in which the second larval stage develops. The cycle is continued when the copepods are eaten by certain fresh-water fish (burbot, pickerel, pike). The larvae penetrate the intestinal tract and enter the blood stream, eventually lodging in skeletal muscle and viscera, where they transform into wormlike encysted larvae, or spargana, 10 to 20 mm. in length. When an infected, inadequately cooked fish is eaten by a susceptible host, the sparganum passes unharmed through the stomach and adheres to the wall of the small intestine, where it develops into a mature worm in about three weeks. Adult worms may measure ten meters or more in length. The entire life cycle requires eight to fifteen weeks. Infection in man is essentially asymptomatic or, rarely, may be evidenced by vague complaints of weakness, abdominal pain, diarrhea, and weight loss. Diagnosis depends upon identification of the characteristic operculate eggs in the stool. Segments of the worm may be recovered and identified following a saline purge.

Treatment of Tapeworms—The drug of choice for all tapeworms is Aspidium Oleoresin (male fern, filix-mas) (p. 313). Refractory cases of dwarf tapeworm have been relieved by small doses of quinacrine (1 mg. of the hydrochloride per Kg. of body weight) three times daily for ten days; hexylresorcinol (p. 312) has also been used. There is no specific medical treatment for the cysticercus stage.

TRICHINOSIS

Trichinosis (trichiniasis, *Trichinella spiralis* infection) is found throughout the world wherever raw or insufficiently cooked pork containing viable larvae is consumed; it is particularly prevalent in the United States. Development of the parasite is the same in man and animals. When infected meat is eaten, encysted larvae pass to the small intestine and are released by digestion of the protective capsule. They invade or attach themselves to the mucosa for a few days until mature. Adult worms are small—the females 3 to 4 mm., the males 1.5 mm. in length. After copulation, the males die and the females burrow into the mucosa, where thousands of living larvae are produced by each worm during the following three to six weeks. These penetrate the lymphatics and venules, pass through the liver and lungs, and reach the general circulation, which disseminates them to all parts of the body. Beginning eight or nine days after infection, the larvae may be found in striated muscle; there they encyst and attain a length of 0.8 to 1 mm. As a rule, the diaphragm, intercostals, and muscles of the neck, larynx, tongue, and eyes are most heavily infected. Calcification of the cysts occurs eventually, as early as six months in man, but in swine and other animals the encysted larvae may remain alive for years.

Clinical manifestations are variable, being altered by age, physical status, and susceptibility to toxins of the host, the number of parasites present, and the parts of the body invaded. Many infections are asymptomatic. About twenty-four hours after infection a few cases may develop nausea, vomiting, abdominal pain, fever, and sometimes severe dysentery. About one week later, during migration of the larvae, malaise, weakness, remittent or intermittent fever, myalgia, profuse sweating, periorbital and facial edema, dermatitis (erythematous or urticarial), laryngitis, painful swallowing, striate hemorrhages beneath the fingernails, eosinophilia, and cardiac and respiratory difficulty may be present in varying severity. Death may occur. Meningitic and encephalitic manifestations are encountered but are uncommon. After one to three weeks the acute illness subsides gradually.

Recovery is complete, although vague muscle pains and susceptibility to fatigue may persist for months.

Diagnosis is often difficult. The intradermal skin test using trichinella extract is the greatest single aid in diagnosis. A positive reaction indicates sensitivity to trichinae, but since hypersensitivity is retained for years, it may be impossible to tell whether infection is recent or not. A negative test is of considerable diagnostic significance. Usually the test becomes positive in the second or third week after onset of illness. The blood precipitin test becomes positive in the fourth week and may be used to confirm the skin test (infectious mononucleosis may cause a false positive precipitin test). Larvae may be identified in muscle biopsies pressed between glass slides or digested in artificial gastric juice. Rarely they may be obtained from spinal fluid or blood. Fecal examination is of no value. An increasing eosinophilia is presumptive evidence of infection.

Treatment is symptomatic and supportive. When gastro-intestinal symptoms follow the eating of inadequately cooked pork, active purgation with magnesium sulfate should be tried in the hope that some of the parasites will be evacuated. It is of no use once the migration of larvae has started. General measures include bed rest and frequent administration of sedatives (p. 390), analgesics (p. 405), and fluids. Intravenous injection of calcium salts may relieve the muscle pain. Sandbags and the strapping of involved muscles may be tried. If the pain cannot be controlled otherwise, codeine and even morphine may be required; but they should be avoided as much as possible, because the illness is prolonged and addiction may result. The diet should be well balanced and supplemented with vitamins and iron. Blood or plasma transfusions are needed for severe cases.

TRICHURIASIS

Trichuriasis (trichocephaliasis, whipworm infection) is caused by *Trichuris trichiura*, a common intestinal nematode. Infection follows the swallowing of infective ova obtained directly or indirectly from fecal-polluted soil. The eggs hatch in the upper duodenum, and the motile larvae pass down to the cecum and attach themselves to the bowel wall. They mature in about three months. The adult worms (male, 30 to 45 mm.; female, 35 to 50 mm.) penetrate the mucosa with an anterior spearlike projection and become firmly anchored as though sewed in the mucosa. The female produces a thou-

sand or more eggs daily, which are readily identified in the feces by their barrel shape and the small pluglike blister at each pole. When deposited on shady, warm, moist soil, the enclosed larvae develop and become infective in about three weeks.

There are no outstanding clinical manifestations. In many instances the infection is silent. Heavy infections may cause indigestion, insomnia, emotional irritability, urticaria, and low-grade anemia.

Diagnosis is made by demonstrating the ova by microscopic examination either of direct fecal smears or, preferably, of specimens obtained by concentration methods.

Treatment is unsatisfactory. In Central and South America, *leche de higuerón*, or higuero latex (30 cc. in the morning on an empty stomach, preceded the night before by a sodium sulfate purge), has been effective. The active principle of higuero latex is an unstable enzyme. It is not available in the United States. Hexylresorcinol (p. 312) is second choice. In addition to oral administration, it may be given as retention enemas in 1:1,000 solution. Santonin is effective but toxic. A mixture of tetrachloroethylene (p. 312), 2.7 cc., and Chenopodium Oil, 0.3 cc., has been recommended.

FUNGUS DISEASES*

ACTINOMYCOSIS

Actinomycosis is a chronic and extremely destructive infection due to the fungus *Actinomyces bovis* (also called *hominis* and *israeli*), which in cattle causes "lumpy jaw." The organism is widely disseminated, and there are many strains with varying cultural and staining characteristics.

The tissues of the face and neck are most commonly involved, the organism gaining entry apparently about the teeth or through the tonsils. Hard inflammatory nodules appear and eventually suppurate, forming a series of communicating sinuses. The abdominal viscera and the lungs are the other common sites of localization, and the disease may be mistaken for sarcoma (of the face or jaw), chronic bronchitis, tuberculosis, chronic peritonitis, osteomyelitis, or syphilis.

Diagnosis is difficult and depends on demonstration of the organisms in discharges or biopsy from the infected tissues. The presence of characteristic "sulfur granules" is diagnostic. If sulfur granules are absent, the organisms can often be demonstrated on cultivation.

* For fungus diseases limited to the skin, see page 229.

The prognosis depends on the location of the lesions, the cervicofacial type being most responsive to therapy and the pulmonary type least so.

Treatment has in the past consisted principally in administration of iodide (p. 506) in graduated doses to the limit of tolerance, usually 5 to 10 Gm. daily. This may be given as saturated solution of sodium or potassium iodide by mouth, or partly or wholly as ethyl iodide (usually not in excess of 1 cc. three times daily) by inhalation.

At present, penicillin (p. 288) appears to be the most effective agent. It must be given in very large doses for a prolonged period.

When total excision of the lesion is possible, it should be employed, but curettage and partial excision may serve merely to spread the infection. In open lesions, wet dressings of one of the solutions of iodine (p. 306) or a 33 percent solution of thymol (p. 305) in olive or cottonseed oil may be beneficial. Judicious x-ray treatment may promote resolution and healing.

The chronic and indolent nature of actinomycosis may lead to long-delayed response to therapy, but intelligent persistence over many months may bring great rewards.

BLASTOMYCOSIS

North American blastomycosis (Gilchrist's disease) is a relatively uncommon, chronic granulomatous infection caused by the organism *Blastomyces dermatitidis*. It occurs mostly in those who work about cellars, stables, and other dark, moist places. The organism has not been positively identified in nature.

Blastomycosis may be either local or systemic. In blastomycosis limited to the skin, the organism enters through a scratch or abrasion. The local lesion starts with a papulopustule on some exposed area, usually the face, ankle, wrist, arm, or leg. It soon ruptures, discharging purulent or sanguino-purulent material, microscopic examination of which reveals single or budding, round or ovoid, yeastlike cells that are 8 to 15 microns in diameter and have thick refractile walls. The lesion spreads peripherally, showing a raised verrucous or papilliform border and a granulating center covered with pinkish-gray exudate. As the lesion spreads, there is central healing with a paper-thin scar. The primary cutaneous form may or may not become systemic.

Systemic blastomycosis usually results from inhalation of the organism, and the lungs are almost always involved. Initial symptoms are not localized and are similar to those of other chronic infections such as tuberculosis (p. 12). The patient may have dry hacking cough, pain in the chest, fever, and occasional dyspnea. X-ray of the lungs shows multiple small pulmonary shadows, suggesting miliary tuberculosis, or dense masses with irregular outlines, resembling neoplasm. Cavities, when present, may be small with hazy outlines. As the disease advances, however, multiple lesions develop which suggest a mycotic infection.

After the lungs, the skin, subcutaneous tissues, and bones are most commonly affected. The skin lesions originate deep in the corium but later come to resemble those of primary cutaneous origin. Of the bones, the vertebrae and ribs are most frequently involved. There may be lesions in the kidneys or, rarely, meningoencephalitis. Collapse of vertebrae may result in compression of the spinal cord and paralysis.

The diagnosis may be suspected from the nature and history of the lesions, but it is established only by demonstration of the organism in the sputum, spinal fluid, or the pus of local lesions. The course of the disease is progressive. The systemic form is more fatal than tuberculosis and more resistant to treatment. The cutaneous form usually responds to treatment and may be only slowly progressive without treatment.

Treatment—Infection limited to the skin usually responds to systemic administration of iodide. Before such treatment is started, however, the patient should be tested with *Blastomyces* vaccine, 1:1,000, the test being performed in the same way as the tuberculin test (p. 339). If the reaction is less than 1 cm. in diameter, the patient is not considered to be unduly sensitive, and treatment with iodide can be begun (p. 506).

If the reaction is larger than 1 cm., the patient should be hyposensitized with the vaccine. The latter is diluted 1:100 to 1:1,000, depending on the size of reaction. The initial dose is 0.1 cc. of diluted vaccine, and the dose is increased each time by 0.1 cc., the injections being given on alternate days. When the dose reaches 1 cc., a dilution of ten times greater strength is substituted, and dosage is begun again at 0.1 cc. Should the patient develop fever or any exacerbation of symptoms, treatment is suspended until the reaction subsides and is then begun again at the last dose which caused no reaction. The dose is increased more slowly than before. It is not carried higher than 1 cc. of original vaccine.

After two weeks of such therapy without reactions, iodide can be started, beginning with small doses (see p. 506). Iodism must be distinguished from reaction to the vaccine. The speed of response of the disease is variable, and treatment may have to be continued for months or years.

The skin lesions should receive the same care as any chronic open lesion. They should be kept clean. Sulfonamides or penicillin may be applied locally to control secondary infection. X-ray therapy has speeded healing in some instances.

Iodide therapy may be tried in systemic blastomycosis, but the prognosis is poor.

COCCIDIOIDOMYCOSIS

Coccidioidomycosis is a systemic infection, clinically resembling histoplasmosis and tuberculosis, caused by the fungus *Coccidioides immitis*. Its distribution appears to be limited chiefly to the southwestern portion of the United States. It has been particularly studied in the southern part of the San Joaquin Valley of California.

The causative fungus has a yeastlike and a mycelial phase. The former is seen in tissues and appears as a spherule 5 to 80 microns in diameter with a thick double-contoured refractile capsule. As the spherule matures, it enlarges and its granular protoplasm breaks up into a large number of endospores which are released when the spherule bursts. The endospores thus released enlarge independently to repeat the cycle. The mycelial phase forms characteristic chlamydospores. These are found widely disseminated in the endemic areas, and infection is believed to occur through the respiratory tract by inhalation of dust containing chlamydospores. As might be expected, the highest incidence of the disease is during the dusty dry season, and the initial infection is always respiratory.

Coccidioidomycosis occurs in several forms:

1. As a mild, even asymptomatic, infection, the only later evidence of which may be a positive skin test with coccidioidin.

2. In the more common form of an acute respiratory infection of the nature of pneumonitis, bronchitis, or pleuritis. It is self-limited and is seldom distinguishable clinically from the common respiratory infections except when, as frequently happens, it is accompanied by erythema nodosum or erythema multiforme. As a rule, there is complete recovery without sequelae; however, about 10 percent show asymptomatic residual lesions which may include nodules or cavitation in the lungs. The benignity of these residual lesions is in great contrast to the more serious nature of similar lesions occurring in tuberculosis.

3. As the progressive disseminated disease of rare occurrence which was recognized many years ago and was termed coccidioidal granuloma. In such cases the initial infection does not subside; rather, it spreads either through the lungs or by the blood or lymph stream to practically all organs, but more particularly to lymph nodes, meninges, bone, liver, and spleen. The course is usually protracted, and the mortality is about 50 percent. In contradistinction to tuberculosis, a primary and a secondary stage cannot be distinguished. If recovery takes place, reinfection is unknown.

The most positive diagnosis depends upon recovery of the organism, which is very difficult in acute primary disease. Complement-fixation tests are highly specific and can be expected to be positive early in the course of the disease. Skin tests with coccidioidin are entirely analogous to those with tuberculin (p. 339). Like the tuberculin test, the positive coccidioidin skin test indicates that the person has been infected at some time but does not necessarily indicate activity at the time of the test. One-tenth cc. of 1:1,000 coccidioidin is given intradermally, and the test is read in forty-eight hours exactly as a tuberculin test would be. The chest lesions as seen by x-ray fall mainly into four groups: adenitis, pneumonitis, the residual lesions following cavitation, or nodules. The differential diagnosis from common respiratory infections may be very difficult. The following factors may be helpful in establishing the diagnosis of coccidioidomycosis: recent residence in an endemic area, serial x-ray examinations of the chest, and, most importantly, a positive complement-fixation or coccidioidin skin test.

Treatment—There is no specific treatment for coccidioidomycosis. In the acute primary disease, the patient should be confined to bed until the chest is clear by x-ray and the blood sedimentation rate has returned to normal. On the average, this period is about one month. There is no satisfactory treatment for the granulomatous lesions.

HISTOPLASMOSIS

Histoplasmosis is an infectious disease caused by the fungus *Histoplasma capsulatum*. Although the pathogenicity of the organism has been known for many years, it is only now that the distribution, frequency, and varied forms of the disease are being recognized. Of greatest significance is the observation that it may produce hilar and peripheral pulmonary calcifications indistinguishable in x-ray films from those of tuberculosis.

The disease occurs most commonly in the Mississippi and Ohio river basins, the incidence diminishing as one travels upstream or downstream from the confluence of the two rivers. There are, however, great local variations. Among children and adolescents in the center of this region, histoplasmosis is much more common than tuberculosis as a cause of pulmonary calcification.

Histoplasmosis may occur in a wide spectrum of local and generalized disease. Most common is the benign form which closely resembles primary tuberculosis. The resulting pulmonary calcifications in the two diseases may be indistinguishable radiologically. More characteristic of histoplasmosis are multiple parenchymal calcifications or massive calcifications of the hilar lymph nodes, often two to three centimeters in diameter and commonly composed of clusters of smaller calcifications giving a mulberry appearance. It is believed that some of these calcified lesions may later be absorbed. The active process, of which these calcified lesions are the final result, is usually completely asymptomatic.

As compared with the benign form, acute or subacute disseminated infections are relatively uncommon. They may involve any organ or combination of organs. Pulmonary infection may resemble the adult type of tuberculosis. The infection may also involve the skin, mucous membranes, and gastro-intestinal tract, with ulcerative lesions. The most common signs and symptoms in the order of decreasing frequency are fever, hypochromic anemia, hepatomegaly, splenomegaly, and lymphadenopathy. Anorexia and loss of weight are common.

The most conclusive diagnosis is established by demonstrating the organisms in, or cultivating them from, superficial lesions, sputum, blood, sternal bone marrow, lymph nodes, or other biopsy materials. The organisms are rarely found extracellularly in any tissue. They are also rarely found in sputum.

H. capsulatum occurs as a yeastlike phase which grows at body temperature and as a mycelial phase which develops at room temperature. Since the fungus grows very slowly, cultures should not be discarded in less than five weeks. Blood should be added to the medium. Cultures should be handled with great care because the mycelial form is infectious. To avoid dissemination of spores, surface growths should be wetted down with a strong germicide before disposal.

The yeastlike phase as it occurs in human and animal tissues is a small oval organism, 1 to 5 microns in diameter, surrounded by a clear capsule. The organism is a parasite of the reticulo-endothelial system and is therefore found where the cells of this system are most numerous—namely, in the bone marrow, spleen, liver, lymph nodes, lungs, and adrenal glands—and in the macrophages of the blood. The response of the tissue is a granulomatous reaction very similar to that seen in tuberculosis or coccidioidomycosis.

In histoplasmosis, allergy develops analogous to that in tuberculosis (p. 12). Two serologic tests have value. In the benign form of the disease, the skin test with histoplasmin is highly specific; 0.1 cc. of 1:1,000 histoplasmin is injected intradermally, usually in the forearm, and the test is read after forty-eight to seventy-two hours. A positive test is indicated by induration or edema 0.5 cm. or more in diameter. Erythema is not considered, and earlier reactions are deemed nonspecific. The syringe and needles used for histoplasmin should not be used or have been used for any other purpose. Occasionally, severe reaction occurs with local tissue necrosis or regional lymphadenopathy. With high doses there is some cross reaction with other mycoses, but these can be ruled out by tests using serial dilutions of the various antigens. The histoplasmin skin test may be negative in acute active forms of histoplasmosis. The complement-fixation test is positive in active histoplasmosis and negative in the benign form. The two tests therefore complement each other.

Histoplasmosis should be suspected in febrile patients with anemia and leukopenia, particularly in the presence of lymphadenopathy, splenomegaly, or hepatomegaly. In the regions of known endemic occurrence, children with pulmonary calcifications should have the histoplasmin as well as the tuberculin test. With pulmonary lesions the differential diagnosis is the same as for tuberculosis. The picture may be confusing for the reason that the two diseases may coexist. Cutaneous and oral lesions must be differentiated from other mycoses and tuberculosis. When lymphadenopathy is present, leukemia (particularly in the aleukemic phase), lymphosarcoma, and Hodgkin's disease must be considered. Histoplasmosis and Hodgkin's disease may exist simultaneously.

Treatment—There is no specific treatment. Patients with symptoms or with advancing disease should be handled according to the same general principles (but excluding antibiotic therapy) that are employed in tuberculosis (p. 12). The disease may be rapidly fatal, but some instances of advanced pulmonary disease have gone on to recovery. The benign form requires no treatment.

DISEASES OF UNKNOWN ETIOLOGY

RHEUMATIC FEVER

Rheumatic fever is a systemic, nonsuppurative, inflammatory disease which is caused directly or indirectly by the Group A hemolytic streptococcus. The pathogenesis is unknown, but there is a strong possibility that rheumatic fever represents a type of allergy analogous to that in glomerulonephritis, periarteritis nodosa, and other conditions characterized by sensitization of mesenchymal tissues.

Rheumatic fever is the leading cause of death between the ages of five and eighteen years and is the most common cause of heart disease under the age of forty. The greatest incidence occurs between five and fifteen years of age, although probably one-third of all cases occur between fifteen and forty. Rheumatic fever is most prevalent in temperate zones where rain, cold, and dampness prevail. The seasonal incidence varies in different localities. A high familial incidence has been noted, but probably the factors are environment and exposure to infection rather than heredity. The disease is most common among the poorer economic classes. Epidemics are unusual, but they occur.

Acute attacks frequently are preceded by upper respiratory infections with Group A hemolytic streptococci, although trauma, cold, and fatigue may also initiate them. The attack of rheumatic fever may follow a latent period of one to three weeks, or it may develop within a few days.

The characteristic tissue reaction involves primarily the collagen, the fibers of which swell and fuse. Later they may fragment. There is cellular infiltration with large round cells and Aschoff cells (large cells with abundant basophilic and irregularly outlined cytoplasm and one or more prominent vesicular nuclei, each containing a barlike or round central nucleolus). A network of reticulin fibers appears between the cells. Healing (which requires four to six months) leaves a small focus of scar tissue. The lesion is known as an Aschoff body and is found in no other condition than rheumatic fever.

In the acute stages, an inflammatory, exudative process usually involves one or more joints or tendon sheaths. The joint or sheath cavities become distended with turbid, yellowish fluid, and the synovial membrane, capsule, and adjacent tendons are injected. Permanent damage almost never occurs. Characteristically, the joints and tendon

sheaths recover quickly while others become involved in rapid succession. All degrees of severity may be present, from slight soreness on movement to pronounced inflammation and swelling with excruciating tenderness. The larger joints of the extremities are most frequently involved.

Myocarditis and endocarditis are common and, when present, lead to damage of the mitral valve in nearly all cases; the aortic is involved about one-half as often; the tricuspid, about one-third; and the pulmonary valve, only rarely. Mitral stenosis and aortic insufficiency tend to develop, more commonly in young individuals and after repeated attacks. Permanent heart damage is found in about one-third of cases.

Involvement of the serous cavities may give rise to pericarditis, pleurisy, or peritonitis. Meningitis may occur. Pneumonitis is an uncommon but serious (sometimes fatal) complication. Arteritis, periarteritis, and obliterative endarteritis develop and give rise to various clinical manifestations which depend upon the severity and site. Proliferative lesions in the subcutaneous tissue may take the form of small nodules (usually 1 to 10 mm. in diameter). These are loosely attached to periarticular ligaments, tendon sheaths, superficial aponeuroses, or periosteum; they are found particularly on the back and about the elbows, knees, and ankles. Somewhat similar lesions occur in acute rheumatoid arthritis (p. 247).

In adults, the onset is usually abrupt, with fever, prostration, pallor, copious sweating, and pain and tenderness in the joints. In children, the onset may be insidious, with "growing pains." Joint involvement is less common and less severe than in adults. Epistaxis, frequently without trauma, may be troublesome. Fatigability and failure to gain weight persist as long as there is carditis. The attack may last several weeks and abate completely (monocyclic). There may be recurrence just as improvement begins (polycyclic). The symptoms may persist unabated for many months (continuous). Repeated attacks are the rule, particularly in children, of whom about 85 percent will suffer recurrence within a few years. Therefore, any illness in a patient who has had rheumatic fever or rheumatic heart disease should be considered a reactivation until proved otherwise.

In that minority of cases in which subcutaneous nodules occur, a biopsy with characteristic microscopic findings is proof of the disease. Otherwise, there are no absolute diagnostic criteria. For purposes of diagnosis, manifestations may be classed as major or minor. A useful rule is to accept at least two major manifestations or one major and two minor manifestations as diagnostic. Any manifestation receives added weight if it follows by two or three weeks a known streptococcus infection.

Major manifestations:

1. History of previous rheumatic fever—either an authenticated history or the detection before or during the present illness of typical rheumatic heart disease or heart lesions.
2. Characteristic active inflammation of joints, multiple and migratory, with restoration of function without residuals on recovery.
3. Carditis. Early in the disease the pulse rate is proportional to the fever; later it is proportional to the degree to which the heart is affected. A rapid pulse rate may herald a recurrence involving only the heart. Gallop rhythm is an unfavorable prognostic sign. Usually one or more of the following are required.
   a. Pericarditis—fibrinous or with effusion.
   b. Significant cardiac enlargement during acute illness.
   c. Cardiac failure during acute illness.
   d. Cardiac murmur appearing during acute illness or changing in quality from day to day.
   e. Significant changes in the electrocardiogram, especially prolongation and variation in length of the P-R interval. A changing pattern is of especial importance, not only for diagnosis but also as indicating an increase in cardiac damage. Premature contractions, auricular fibrillation, and, less frequently, heart block may occur. Terminal-segment changes alone are not acceptable proof of rheumatic fever.
4. Subcutaneous nodules (see text above).
5. Sydenham's chorea (p. 48).

Minor manifestations:

1. Fever. This has low specificity unless persistent and accompanied by other diagnostic features.
2. Erythema multiforme, especially erythema marginatum. None of the cutaneous manifestations is diagnostic.
3. Abdominal pain, especially if occurring early in the attack. Mild gastroenteritis may precede an attack. Occurring later during the course of the disease, gastroenteritis may be due to intoxication, cardiac failure, or drug irritation.
4. Precordial pain, especially in a young person.
5. Repeated nontraumatic epistaxis.
6. Purpura or petechial rash.
7. Pneumonitis, with or without pleurisy (in 5 to 10 per cent of cases).
8. Laboratory tests; these are not specific.
   a. Increased sedimentation rate is the most useful and may be considered a minor manifestation.

If the sedimentation rate is not increased, at least two of the following tests should be positive to be considered as a minor manifestation.
   b. Repeated antistreptolysin titers showing a persistent or rising titer (evidence of a persistent streptococcus infection).
   c. Persistent definite leukocytosis up to 15,000 to 20,000.
   d. Anemia, which may be mild in degree and hypochromic in type.

Treatment—It is possible that the treatment of rheumatic fever may be revolutionized within the next few years. In a few cases, attacks have been abruptly terminated by administration of cortisone (p. 462) or adrenocorticotrophic hormone (p. 473). However, until more experience is gained, the safety and ultimate value of such treatment will not be known.

At present, the foundations of treatment are rest, relief of pain, attention to nutrition, psychological support, and regulated convalescence, preferably in a suitably equipped sanatorium. Until the sedimentation rate approaches normal levels, complete rest in bed, large amounts of fluid, high-caloric and high-vitamin diet, and good nursing care are essential. For the second period of treatment, bed rest is continued for one month after the sedimentation rate approaches normal. If at the end of this period the sedimentation rate is normal and gradual withdrawal of drugs produces no recurrence of pain, the third period of treatment (about six weeks) commences and consists in gradual resumption of activity and initiative. The fourth period, indicated by successful completion of the previous three and a normal pulse rate and pulse response, is one of reconditioning.

Drug therapy is aimed at relief of pain and prevention of recurrences. For the former, the drug of choice is salicylic acid, either as the sodium salt or aspirin (see p. 405), in amounts sufficient to keep a constant blood concentration of 35 mg. per 100 cc. Children require 0.08 to 0.10 Gm. per Kg. of body weight per day in divided doses spaced equally in the twenty-four hours. Between 10 and 16 Gm. per day are needed for adults. Vitamin K should be given concurrently to combat hypoprothrombinemia. About 1 mg. of menadione or its equivalent (p. 499) is given for every gram of salicylate. Sodium bicarbonate tends to lower salicylate blood levels but at times must be employed to overcome gastric intolerance or acidosis. Aluminum hydroxide (p. 382) may be more satisfactory for combating gastritis.

Neither sulfonamides nor antibiotics are effective during the acute attack. There is evidence that sulfonamides may aggravate the disease when given during this stage. Antibiotics, particularly penicillin, are indicated in the treatment of any superimposed, susceptible bacterial infection. Congestive heart failure is treated in the usual way (see p. 63).

During the second period of treatment and continuing through the fourth, sulfadiazine (0.5 to 1 Gm. per day) has been effective in reducing recurrence of a streptococcus infection. Routine prophylactic treatment is not approved by all rheumatologists. Some believe that it should be used only when it is impossible to obtain adequate diets and wholesome living conditions. Penicillin administered orally (100,000 units morning and night on an empty stomach) or in the form of troches (5,000 units three times daily, one hour after meals) also has reduced recurrences of acute attacks. Routine tonsillectomy is of doubtful value in preventing recurrences. However, if the tonsils are diseased and apparently harbor Group A streptococci, they may be removed, but only when the disease is inactive.

It is essential that the physician supply good psychological support for the patient to prevent the development of a cardiac neurosis. Limitation of physical activity after successful recovery from the disease is not helpful in protecting against additional attacks and subsequent heart disease. Physical exercise should be encouraged within limits imposed by residual cardiac lesions.

CHOREA

Chorea (Sydenham's chorea, chorea minor, chorea anglorum, St. Vitus's dance) is an acute disease of the central nervous system characterized by emotional instability, muscular weakness, and coarse, asymmetrical, in-co-ordinated, purposeless muscular movements. The causative agent has not been identified but is probably related to that of rheumatic fever (p. 46). The disease is most prevalent between the ages of five and ten years and is uncommon in infancy and after adolescence. The duration varies from a few weeks to several months. Recovery is usually complete, but recurrences are frequent, and rheumatic complications are prone to occur.

The choreic movements are aggravated by excitement, by fatigue, and by attempts to perform co-ordinated acts. They usually disappear during sleep. Their severity varies from infrequent, casual motions to continuous, exhausting hyperactivity. Bodily injury may occur.

Fever or other evidence of infection is unusual except in the presence of rheumatic complications. Eosinophilia is frequent. Diagnosis may require differentiation from habit spasm, encephalitis, tuberculous meningitis, athetosis, congenital tremor, and possibly localized brain lesions, cerebral degeneration, petit mal epilepsy, poliomyelitis, and syphilis.

Treatment—There is no specific treatment. Measures which tend to prevent rheumatic fever are thought to be effective in prophylaxis. Routine tonsillectomy is of doubtful value.

Physical and mental rest is essential. Comfortable restraints, sideboards, and padding of the bed may be necessary to prevent injury when activity is extreme. There is need of a liberal diet, which, during the acute stage, should be fed by an attendant. Carefully supervised occupational therapy is desirable.

Sedatives are of considerable value, but they do not appreciably shorten the course of the disease. Barbiturates are generally preferred (p. 390). Dosage and frequency of administration will depend upon age, severity of the disease, and the clinical response. As a rule, satisfactory results will be obtained with oral or rectal doses of 3/4 to 1 1/2 grains repeated at three or four-hour intervals. Very severe cases with maniacal tendencies may require administration of scopolamine (hyoscine) hydrobromide (1/500 to 1/100 grain hypodermically). Bromides and chloral are less commonly used.

In the presence of rheumatic manifestations, salicylates (p. 405) are indicated in doses just short of those producing salicylism. Chemotherapy with sulfonamides, penicillin, or arsenicals has not proved effective.

Artificial-fever therapy (p. 336) may shorten the course of the disease. Its use should be limited to hospitalized cases.

Vitamin supplements are often indicated during the acute and convalescent phases. Anemia is a common complication, for which iron compounds should be given (p. 368).

INFECTIOUS MONONUCLEOSIS

Infectious mononucleosis (benign lymphadenosis) is an acute benign infection characterized by (1) an absolute lymphocytosis due to the presence in the peripheral blood stream of a large number of abnormal, though mature, lymphocytes; and (2) one or more of the following symptoms and signs: irregular fever, sore throat, skin eruptions, lymphadenopathy, and splenomegaly. During the weeks following onset, the blood serum usually develops antibodies against sheep erythrocytes. The disease is considered a specific infection, but the causative agent is unknown.

The importance of infectious mononucleosis lies in the large number of serious conditions which it may simulate. The lymphadenopathy may suggest syphilis, Hodgkin's disease, or lymphoblastoma. The sore throat, sometimes with ulceration, may lead to confusion with diphtheria, follicular tonsillitis, herpetic pharyngitis, or aphthous stomatitis. Cutaneous manifestations may resemble those of scarlet fever, rubella, or erythema nodosum. The fever and systemic symptoms may suggest typhoid fever, undulant fever, influenza, possibly bacterial endocarditis, or even acute rheumatic fever. Occasionally, signs and symptoms of meningeal irritation and abnormalities in the cerebrospinal fluid make it necessary to rule out pyogenic or benign lymphocytic meningitis, encephalitis, and poliomyelitis. There may be false positive serologic tests for syphilis, typhoid fever, or undulant fever. A lymphocytosis, relative or absolute, may be found also in leukemia, agranulocytosis, Vincent's angina, tuberculosis, tularemia, pertussis, dengue, mumps, chickenpox, rubella, typhoid fever, catarrhal jaundice, and serum disease.

Infectious mononucleosis may at first suggest early lymphatic or myelogenous leukemia (p. 103). The distinction is ultimately made by the benign course, positive Paul-Bunnell test, and absence of immature lymphocytes in the former, in contrast to the fatal course of the latter, with eventual appearance of immature leukocytes in the peripheral blood, anemia, thrombocytopenia, and hemorrhagic phenomena.

A helpful diagnostic procedure is that of Paul and Bunnell. It is based on the presence of agglutinins against sheep red cells in the serum of patients having infectious mononucleosis. Agglutination at a dilution of 1:64 or higher is considered positive, but this titer may not be reached for two or three weeks. The test is ultimately positive in as high as 92 percent of cases. A positive Paul-Bunnell test may be encountered in persons who have been treated with horse serum, and possibly after the intramuscular injection of liver extract. These are the only known exceptions to the specificity of the test.

Treatment—There is no specific therapy. Patients are given general and symptomatic treatment as in any febrile illness.

SYSTEMIC DISEASES

BODY WATER

Disturbances of Fluid and Electrolyte Balance

The body fluid constitutes the "internal environment" in which the body cells actually live. Protoplasm exists as a solution. It communicates across the cell membrane with the interstitial fluid, which in turn is in contact with the blood plasma through the endothelium of the capillaries.

The composition of the various partitions of the body fluid is shown in Figure 1 (p. 50). It will be noted that only a small fraction of the dissolved matter in extracellular fluid is in the form of nonelectrolytes, that is, substances which are not ionized and dissociated in solution.

The capillary endothelium is permeable to all normal constituents of the plasma except protein, so that, at equilibrium, plasma and interstitial fluid are very similar in composition except for the virtual absence of protein in the latter. Plasma and interstitial fluid together are known as extracellular fluid. Sodium is the principal basic ion and chloride the principal acidic ion.

In contrast to capillary endothelium, the cell membrane is freely permeable only to water, hydrogen ions, and perhaps dextrose, amino acids, urea, and ammonia. Thus, although osmotic equilibrium is maintained between intracellular and extracellular fluid, the composition of the two fluids is very different. In intracellular fluid the basic ions are principally potassium and magnesium, and the acidic ions are phosphate and sulfate; there is a high percentage of protein.

In the normal adult, body water is subdivided approximately as indicated in Table 2. The equilibrium between these various compartments of body fluid is highly dynamic; there is a rapid and continuous interchange through the dividing membranes, and over-all constancy is maintained only when the rate of passage in one direction exactly equals the rate in the opposite direction.

Fluid and electrolytes are lost by a number of routes. Some of the loss is obligatory (that is, it is necessary for continued health or it cannot be

TABLE 2 — *Partition of Body Fluids*

	Fraction of body weight	Volume in a 70-Kg. man
Intracellular fluid...	50%	35 liters
Extracellular fluid		
Interstitial fluid...	15%	11 liters
Blood plasma.....	5%	3 liters
Total........	70%	49 liters

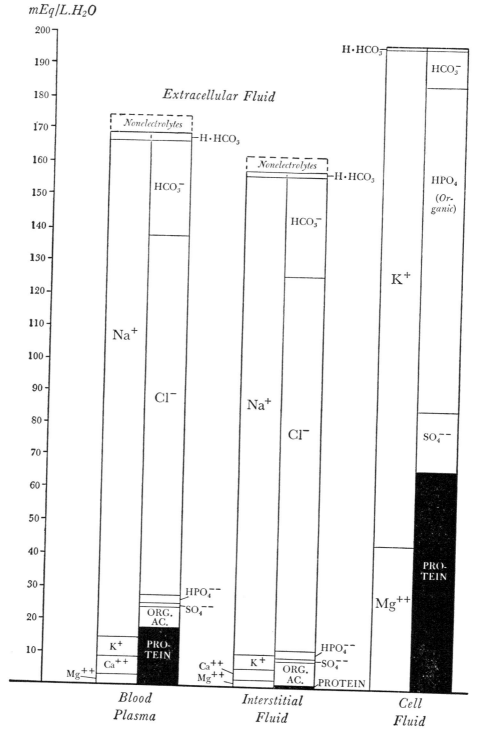

FIGURE 1—*Composition of Certain Body Fluids* (After Gamble, J. L.: *Chemical Anatomy, Physiology and Pathology of Extracellular Fluid*, Ed. 5. Cambridge, Mass.: Harvard University Press, 1949)

avoided at all); the rest is disposal of excess. The quantity of obligatory water loss is more closely related to total caloric expenditure than to body weight or surface area. Data on the normal routes of loss are given in Table 3. The values are only approximate and cannot be considered to apply rigidly to all individuals and under all circumstances. Output will be increased, beyond that indicated, by sweating, fever, relatively high intake of salt or protein (which increases urinary solids) or by diarrhea, vomiting, drainage from wounds or fistulas, or other abnormal source of loss.

TABLE 3 — *Minimum Fluid Loss in Health*

Route	Nature of loss	Principal substance lost	Rate of water loss, Gm. per 100 Cal. metabolized	Approx. total water loss per day in cc.			
				Adult, 2,500 Cal.,* urine sp. gr. 1.025	Adult, 2,500 Cal.,* urine sp. gr. 1.015	Adult, 2,500 Cal.,* urine sp. gr. 1.010	Baby, 300 Cal.,* urine sp. gr. 1.015
Insensible loss (skin and lungs)	Obligatory	Water	44	1,100	1,100	1,100	130
Stool	Obligatory	Water	3 to 5 (for adults)	100	100	100	30
Growth	Obligatory in children	Water, salts	4	0	0	0	10
Sweat	†	Water, salts	0 to 100	0	0	0	0
Urine	Largely elective	Water, salts	Obligatory loss varies with sp. gr. and urinary solids	425‡	675‡	875‡	80‡
Total, assuming no food intake other than dextrose or breast milk				1,625	1,875	2,075	250
Additional urine volume required if on ordinary diet or artificial infant feeding				425	675	875	30
Total, assuming ordinary diet or artificial feeding				2,050	2,550	2,950	280

*The figure refers to calories metabolized rather than to caloric intake.

†Not influenced by state of water metabolism; obligatory for heat loss.

‡For each Gm. of urinary solids per 100 calories metabolized. This factor depends on type of diet and salt intake. It is somewhat oversimplified here.

The amount of electrolyte accompanying the insensible water loss is very minute. In the absence of diarrhea, the salt loss in the feces is very small. Except for what is necessary to neutralize an excess of fixed acid or base, electrolyte loss in the urine is normally elective and can, in case of need, be reduced almost to zero by normal kidneys. However, in various disease states, either the selective or the total excretory capacity of the kidneys, or both, may be greatly impaired, with serious or sometimes disastrous effects on the control of fluid and electrolyte balance. In health, the greatest obligatory electrolyte loss is in sweat, which may contain from 0.06 to 0.3 percent (about 10 to 50 millimoles per liter) of sodium chloride and as much potassium as does interstitial fluid. Electrolyte loss is important also in abnormal fluid losses, such as in vomiting, diarrhea, exudates, and discharges. An adequate daily allowance of sodium chloride for maintenance in resting, non-sweating, well individuals is 1 Gm. for infants, 3 Gm. for children, and 6 Gm. for adolescents and adults.

TABLE 4 — *Minimum Water Intake in Health*

Source of water	Gm. per 100 Cal.	Approx. total water intake per day in cc.			
		Adult, 2,500 Cal.,* urine sp. gr. 1.025	Adult, 2,500 Cal.,* urine sp. gr. 1.015	Adult, 2,500 Cal.,* urine sp. gr. 1.010	Baby, 300 Cal.,* urine sp. gr. 1.015
Preformed water in food	Variable	900†	900†	900†	300†
Water of oxidation of food	12	300*	300*	300*	35*
Minimum requirement of fluid as such Assuming no food other than dextrose or breast milk	——	425	675	875	——
Additional requirement if on ordinary diet or artificial infant feeding	——	425	675	875	——
Total		1,625 or 2,050	1,875 or 2,550	2,075 or 2,950	335

*Based on food metabolized.
†Based on food intake.

Water and electrolyte losses are normally replenished by food and drink. Table 4 gives data on minimal water intake necessary to balance minimal output as indicated in the preceding table. It cannot be emphasized too strongly that the correspondence between urine volume and minimum intake of fluid as such is a coincidence not based on any actual relationship. It fails to hold if caloric intake is altered or if there are additional sources of fluid loss, such as sweating, diarrhea, vomiting, or loss through wounds or burns. *Urine volume cannot be taken as a quantitative guide to fluid intake.* Perhaps the best guide to fluctuations in fluid balance under many circumstances is the day-to-day variation in body weight. The simplest clinical sign of adequate fluid intake is a urinary specific gravity well below the maximum which the patient's kidneys are capable of achieving.

The volumes and electrolyte concentrations of the three compartments of body fluid are mutually interdependent and are affected by many factors. A basic control is exercised by the kidneys under the influence of renal blood flow, posterior pituitary hormone (which controls reabsorption of water in the distal convoluted tubules and is secreted under regulation of the hypothalamus), and steroid hormones from the adrenal cortices, ovaries, and testicles (which influence reabsorption of sodium in the proximal convoluted tubules).

The factors governing plasma volume also include the quantity of albumin maintained in the plasma by the liver and the average tissue demand for blood flow in accord with the factors listed under heading II in Table 8 (p. 64). Changes in blood volume (cells and plasma) may also be mediated through the nervous system, for polycythemia has been observed with cerebellar tumors. The volume of interstitial fluid seems to depend largely on the amount of sodium in the body, which is in turn normally regulated by the kidneys (see preceding paragraph).

Since the capillary walls are permeable to all normal constituents of plasma except protein, the partition of fluid between plasma and interstitial fluid depends on the balance between the inpulling colloid osmotic pressure of the plasma (due to the plasma proteins, especially the albumin fraction) and the net outpushing hydrostatic pressure in the capillaries (capillary pressure minus tissue pressure). Hydrostatic pressure diminishes progressively

TABLE 5 — *Disturbances of Fluid and Electrolyte Balance*

Deficiency
    Of fluid . . . . } { see Dehydration, p. 56, Shock, p. 90, Acute Blood Loss;
    Of electrolyte . . . . } { p. 94, and Heat Prostration, p. 273
       Total . . . . } } see Acidosis, p. 59, and Alkalosis, p. 61
      Acid-base balance . . . . . . }

Excess
    Of fluid (see Water Intoxication, p. 62)
    Of fluid and electrolyte (see Edema below)
    Of electrolyte (see Sodium Excess, p. 341)

Expansion of one compartment at expense of others
    Interstitial fluid (see Burns, p. 270, Shock, p. 90, and Acute Blood Loss, p. 94)

along the course of a capillary from about 30 mm. Hg at the arterial end to about 10 mm. at the venous end. As long as this pressure exceeds the sum of tissue pressure and effective colloid osmotic pressure (normally about 22 mm. Hg), fluid passes from the capillary into the interstitial space. Toward the venous end of the capillary, where the hydrostatic pressure is lower and the osmotic pressure is higher (from loss of fluid but not of protein), fluid passes from the interstitial space into the capillary. When transudation exceeds the sum of reabsorption and lymphatic drainage, the volume of interstitial fluid increases until the tissue pressure rises sufficiently to restore equilibrium.

Fluid and electrolyte balance may be disturbed in a number of ways, the more important of which are indicated in Table 5. The mechanisms, diagnosis, and treatment of these disturbances are discussed under the headings listed in the table.

EDEMA

When the volume of interstitial fluid exceeds normal by more than about 50 percent, the fluid is more or less readily displaced by pressure (as from the physician's thumb), and edema is said to be present. Usually, an adult must retain 10 to 20 lb. of extra fluid before generalized edema appears.

Edema is thought to be due to one or more of the factors listed in Table 6. It should be stated,

TABLE 6 — *Factors in Genesis of Edema*

1. Diminished effective colloid osmotic pressure of the plasma
    Diminished plasma protein level (particularly albumin)
    Increased protein level in interstitial fluid

2. Increased average hydrostatic pressure in the capillaries
    Increased venous pressure
      Systemic
        Increased blood volume
          Heart failure
          Other causes
      Local
        Venous obstruction
        In legs due to erect posture

3. Sodium retention
    Increased sodium intake beyond normal excretory capacity of kidneys
    Diminished renal excretory capacity in presence of normal intake
      Kidney disease
      Excess of sodium factor of adrenal cortex
      Excess of estrogen, progesterone, or androgen
    Reduced renal blood flow
      Heart failure
      Crush syndrome

4. Increased capillary permeability
    Bacterial toxins, histamine, and other agents
    Increased temperature
    Reduced oxygen supply

however, that there are cases in which none of the given factors seem to apply. It is likely that the next few years will bring considerable change in fundamental concepts.

In the absence of other contributing factors, edema may appear in adults when the total plasma protein level falls to or below 5 to 5.5 percent (albumin fraction, 2.5 percent); in children the critical level is 4 to 4.5 percent total protein or 1.5 percent albumin fraction.

When sodium accumulates in the body as the result of disparity between intake and excretion, water is also retained by the kidneys (1 L. of water for each 9 Gm. sodium chloride). This extra salt and water is distributed between plasma and interstitial fluid. It should be emphasized that in all cases water retention is secondary to and dependent on sodium retention. Regardless of the underlying cause of edema in a given case, sodium excess enhances edema and sodium restriction limits it.

Protein and other colloids cannot be removed from the interstitial fluid by the capillaries. This function is performed by the lymphatics. If these become obstructed, the protein concentration in the interstitial fluid becomes high even when capillary permeability remains normal. As a result, the colloid osmotic pressure of the fluid becomes high, favoring transudation from the capillaries and hindering reabsorption. This type of edema is called lymphedema.

Accumulations of fluid in the body cavities have the same significance as edema. It should be noted that inflammatory changes involving the pleura (tuberculosis or pneumonia) commonly cause hydrothorax (pleural effusion) while local portal venous obstruction (cirrhosis of the liver or metastatic cancer) may cause ascites.

Cardiac Edema is the end result of a chain of causes and effects. When cardiac output is insufficient to meet circulatory demand (see Heart Failure, p. 63), there is an early compensatory increase in venomotor and vasomotor tone. The first causes a rise in venous pressure, and the second causes, among other things, a reduction in blood flow to the kidneys. There is gradual retention of sodium and water, probably effected through a complex mechanism involving the hypothalamus, posterior pituitary gland, and adrenal cortex; and plasma volume increases. Hemoglobin level and red cell volume may increase as well.

If the relative cardiac insufficiency was due to hemorrhage, blood flow will again become adequate as blood volume increases to normal and the stimulus ceases to operate. If, however, the cardiac insufficiency is due to myocardial weakness (see p. 63), increase in blood volume does not restore blood flow to the level demanded by the tissues. The stimulus to sodium and water retention continues to operate, blood volume and venous pressure continue to increase, and edema develops. In the past, the immediate mechanism of such edema has been considered to be increased hydrostatic capillary pressure, but the relationship may actually be more complicated.

Treatment of cardiac edema should be primarily treatment of the heart failure that causes it (see p. 65). Sometimes, however, edema persists after what would seem to be an adequate period of bed rest, oxygen administration, low sodium intake, adequate medication with digitalis, and treatment of those factors responsible for increased circulatory demand. Except as edema, hydrothorax, and ascites directly embarrass respiration, they are probably not of themselves seriously harmful. Their significance appears to lie, rather, in the relatively high blood volume which accompanies them and which may be reducing cardiac output by overfilling the heart in diastole.

In this situation an active campaign of sodium depletion is in order. The sodium intake should be kept at the very low level of less than 0.5 Gm. daily until edema has disappeared. It may then be increased by degrees to 2 or 3 Gm. daily. If edema recurs, sodium intake is reduced. Water intake must be sufficient to prevent intracellular dehydration. The patient can be allowed what fluid he wants, up to a maximum of 2 or 3 liters, depending on extent of perspiration and other sources of fluid loss. Beyond a low-sodium diet, the simplest sodium-depleting measure is administration of one of the diuretic salts (p. 350) in doses of 6 to 12 Gm. (90 to 180 grains) daily.

The only contraindication to sodium depletion is extremely severe renal failure, in which the kidneys have lost their power of reabsorbing sodium. However, such patients are rarely edematous. It should be emphasized that extreme sodium restriction is limited to the period of edema. Once this has disappeared, sodium intake is to be increased to at least 1 Gm. daily, or more if the patient does not retain it (as indicated by weight gain). Continued extreme restriction in the absence of edema may lead to the syndrome of sodium deficiency (p. 342).

If diuresis and recession of edema do not follow administration of diuretic salts or if they do not persist long enough, the salts can be supplemented with either a xanthine or a mercurial-xanthine diuretic (pp. 358 and 351). The mercurial diuretics are the more powerful, but they carry slightly more hazard of side reactions. In many cases, the administration of diuretic salts and mercurials without digitalis will reduce blood volume to normal and thus eliminate the clinical manifestations of congestive heart failure. Such a demonstration serves to emphasize the importance of sodium retention as a cause of symptoms in heart failure. It has not yet been demonstrated that such treatment is an adequate substitute for that recommended on page 65; it is, however, very useful as a supplement. Many patients with only a small myocardial reserve can remain ambulatory and free of edema when given mercurial diuretics once or twice a week in addition to digitalis.

When edema and visceral congestion are very prominent in heart failure, active sodium depletion may be undertaken at the beginning of treatment without waiting to see the response to other measures.

Edema fluid may hold stores of drugs. Instances are known in which digitalis intoxication was due to rapid reabsorption of edema fluid containing digitalis. When any potent drug has been given long enough to have become distributed in edema fluid, caution must be exercised in inducing rapid reabsorption.

Nephritic Edema may have a number of causes, depending on the stage in which it occurs. In the onset phase of acute glomerulonephritis, edema is believed to be partly inflammatory and due to capillary damage. It is usually nonpitting. Reduction in glomerular filtration may lead to sodium retention which contributes to the edema. There is no satisfactory treatment for the edema of acute nephritis. Attempts to produce diuresis are likely to be more harmful than beneficial.

In chronic glomerulonephritis, edema is largely osmotic and may be due to one or both of two factors: (1) a low level of plasma albumin which permits excessive transudation from capillaries of normal permeability; and (2) sodium retention due to reduction in glomerular filtration. Such edema pits on pressure. In terminal nephritis, renal edema usually disappears because the level of plasma protein rises and tubular damage becomes too extreme to permit sodium retention. Sometimes, however, earlier in the course of chronic glomerulonephritis, tubular damage may be relatively greater than glomerular damage, and edema due to low plasma protein may be associated with sodium depletion rather than sodium retention.

If the edema of chronic nephritis is due primarily to a low level of plasma protein, temporary, and occasionally prolonged, improvement may follow intravenous infusion of blood plasma or its albumin fraction—measures which tend to increase the osmotic pressure of the plasma. To the extent that edema is due to sodium retention, it will be benefited by a regimen of sodium depletion (see under Cardiac Edema above). However, if sodium depletion does not diminish the edema and results instead in the development of weakness, apathy, vasomotor instability, shock, or other signs of either sodium deficiency or adrenocortical deficiency (p. 183), it is evident that the patient was not originally retaining sodium. Under these circumstances, the sodium stores should be replenished at once (see p. 57), and the intake should be maintained at an adequate level to maintain sodium balance until the reabsorbing power of the renal tubules may have improved.

Allergic Edema—The localized edemas of allergy, such as urticaria, angioneurotic edema, and the bronchial edema of asthma, are thought to be due to local increase in capillary permeability probably caused by the release of a histamine-like substance. The prompt effect of vasoconstrictors such as epinephrine and ephedrine is possibly explained on the basis of a lowering of hydrostatic capillary pressure.

Nutritional Edema seems to be of two types: one associated with a low plasma protein level, the other with deficiency of thiamin. The first type disappears promptly with restoration of normal plasma protein concentration by means of an adequate diet. The second type is diffuse and generally nondependent and resembles clinically the edema of chronic glomerulonephritis or toxemia of pregnancy. It may occur in the absence of heart failure. Its mechanism is unknown. It disappears rapidly in most cases following massive doses of thiamin (p. 484); in a few cases, other factors of the B complex must be given in addition.

Toxic or Inflammatory Edema, due to bacterial toxins or various poisons, may be local or general. The mechanism is apparently a combination of (1) increased capillary hydrostatic pressure from reflex dilatation of the arterioles and (2) increased capillary permeability from the toxins (for further discussion, see Burns, p. 270, and Shock, p. 90). Treatment is that of the underlying condition unless the accumulation is sufficiently rapid or great to disturb fluid and electrolyte balance.

DEHYDRATION

For convenience, the term "dehydration" is commonly applied to deficiency of either water or electrolytes or of both. Actually, pure water deficiency presents a very different picture from that of pure electrolyte deficiency. Because a certain amount of water loss is obligatory, water deficiency can be produced by water deprivation, as in fasting. In contrast, electrolyte deficiency is usually the result of abnormal losses.

In pure water deprivation, the obligatory losses first affect the blood plasma, which is reduced in volume, with concentration of its constituents. As the plasma begins to become hypertonic, water passes into it from the interstitial fluid, which in turn becomes slightly hypertonic and extracts water from the cells. At equilibrium, all three compartments of body fluid share the deficiency about equally. As carbohydrate, fat, and protein stores are metabolized, a certain amount of tissue-held water is released and water of oxidation is formed. This retards but is not sufficient to prevent deficiency. The urinary excretion of electrolyte falls to a low level, and the urine becomes small in volume, with as high a specific gravity as the concentrating power of the kidneys will permit. However, the need for excretion of metabolic waste products often maintains urine secretion after dehydration has become extreme, so that the degree of oliguria does not always parallel the severity of dehydration. Even so, the urine volume is usually insufficient to carry away metabolic waste products, and the nonprotein nitrogen concentration of the blood increases. Unless water losses are extreme, hemoconcentration is usually slight, and the efficiency of the circulation is only slightly impaired. The obligatory water loss and oxidation of food stores result in progressive weight loss. The outstanding symptom of pure water deficiency is thirst.

In pure electrolyte deficiency, such as may be produced by a combination of continuous jejunal drainage through a Miller-Abbott tube and intravenous infusions of dextrose solution, the loss of sodium and chloride makes it impossible for the body to retain water. As the sodium and chloride levels of the plasma fall, the kidneys reabsorb these ions almost completely from the glomerular filtrate, at the same time discontinuing all active reabsorption of water. Thus, even as plasma volume diminishes, relatively large volumes of very dilute urine may be formed. As opposed to the low levels of sodium and chloride in the plasma, there is an increase in hemoglobin concentration, red cell count, and hematocrit reading. Protein disappears from the plasma, so that the rise in concentration is absent or is disproportionately small. Electrolytes and water are drawn into the plasma from the interstitial fluid; as the deficiency continues, water, potassium, and small amounts of chloride pass from the cells into the interstitial fluid. The excess of potassium which leaves the cells is replaced by an equivalent amount of sodium from the extracellular fluids.

In electrolyte loss, however, in contrast to water loss, it is the plasma compartment of body fluid which is most severely depleted. This greatly reduced plasma volume alters the hydrodynamics of the circulation. Venous (and possibly capillary) pressure falls, cardiac filling and output diminish, and there is systemic vasoconstriction. As reduction in plasma volume progresses, cardiac output may fall to the point where even maximal systemic vasoconstriction is incapable of maintaining blood pressure and blood flow, and shock ensues. As in shock from other causes (p. 90), there will be oliguria or anuria.

Thus, pure electrolyte deficiency is characterized clinically by circulatory failure and, up to its last stages, adequate urine volume. The nonprotein nitrogen of the blood is normal or low instead of high. The outstanding symptoms are weakness, apathy, anorexia, and faintness or actual fainting on sitting up or standing. Thirst is conspicuously absent.

In practice, pure water or pure electrolyte deficiency is rarely seen. Almost always a mixed type is encountered, although one or the other phase may predominate. The most important ions involved in dehydration are the basic ones, sodium and potassium, and the acidic ion, chloride. The principal causes of dehydration are listed in Table 7, with substance predominantly lost and effect on acid-base balance given in parentheses following.

When kidney function is not too much impaired by dehydration or renal disease, ions are selectively excreted or retained in such a way as to bring about certain general patterns in the body fluids. Sodium deficiency leads to acidosis, and vice versa. In the presence of sodium deficiency and acidosis, intracellular sodium tends to be low and intracellular potassium normal or high. In chloride deficiency and its corollary, alkalosis, intracellular sodium is high and intracellular potassium low. The relationship holds in any direction, so that extracellular chloride deficiency, alkalosis, and intracellular potassium deficiency occur together, regardless of which is primary, assuming always a moderate

TABLE 7 — *Principal Causes of Dehydration, with Substance Predominantly Lost and Effect on Acid-Base Balance*

Water deprivation (water; mild acidosis from accumulation of acid metabolites)

Persistent vomiting or its equivalent, drainage of gastric or duodenal contents through an indwelling tube (water and chloride; alkalosis)

Prolonged diarrhea (water and sodium; acidosis)

The combination of preliminary fasting, excessive sweating in the operating room, and loss of blood at operation (water and sodium; acidosis)

Excessive sweating (water, sodium, and chloride; none)

High intake or formation of fixed acid, as in severe uncontrolled diabetes mellitus (sodium; acidosis)

High intake of fixed base, such as alkalies in peptic ulcer (chloride; alkalosis)

Urinary excretion of nonelectrolytes, such as dextrose in uncontrolled diabetes mellitus and other sugars after intravenous injection in hypertonic solution (water; none)

Extensive burns; drainage from sinuses, fistulas, wounds, or denuded areas (water and sodium; acidosis)

Addison's disease (sodium; acidosis)

Terminal glomerulonephritis, when the kidneys lose their power of reabsorbing electrolyte from glomerular filtrate (sodium; acidosis)

degree of renal function and sufficient time for the readjustment to be accomplished.

When the ionic deficit is multiple and severe and when anuria or extreme oliguria renders adjustment by the kidneys impossible, the relationships do not hold. In such conditions, patients are usually extremely unstable clinically. This situation is seen most commonly in diabetic acidosis and in severe diarrhea in infants.

The clinical manifestations of dehydration are the natural consequences of the physiological changes. Deficiency of water leads to thirst, oliguria, and nitrogen retention. The relatively greater reduction of plasma and interstitial fluid volume which accompanies electrolyte loss gives rise to circulatory failure, which in its mildest form may be represented by weakness, apathy, and vasomotor instability, and in its most severe form by shock. The slowing of the circulation may impair heat dissipation, and fever may develop, especially in infants. The loss of interstitial fluid causes dryness, looseness, and wrinkling of the skin, which give a pinched appearance to the features. The tongue is dry and usually coated. Intraocular tension is reduced, the eyeball may recede, and in infants the anterior fontanel may be depressed.

The history of the nature, duration, and severity of the preceding illness and fluid losses, and the degree of weight loss, make possible an estimate of the type and severity of dehydration and the probability of acidosis (p. 59) or alkalosis (p. 61). The signs of acidosis, alkalosis, and potassium deficiency (p. 343) should be sought for.

The volume and specific gravity of the urine should be noted. The urinary pH is not necessarily an index to acidosis or alkalosis; urinary tract infection may cause the urine to be alkaline in acidosis, and when the plasma sodium level is below normal, the urine may be acid in alkalosis.

Except in very mild dehydration, the following laboratory tests should be made before treatment is started and at intervals thereafter: plasma protein, plasma chloride, hemoglobin, and carbon-dioxide combining power (plasma bicarbonate is better if it is available). Other determinations which are sometimes helpful include plasma sodium and potassium, hematocrit reading, and red cell count. These tests are useful as guides to treatment. Compensatory changes may make them unreliable or even misleading in the *diagnosis* of dehydration.

Treatment—In principle, the treatment of dehydration consists in replacing the water and ions that are deficient and, if ketosis is present, providing enough carbohydrate to allow oxidation of the ketone bodies. Consideration must be given to previously incurred deficits, current abnormal losses, and current normal needs. Deficits and losses of electrolyte must be restored with electrolyte solutions. Since normal kidneys can, if necessary, excrete urine containing almost no electrolyte, the size of "normal" needs of electrolyte depends on the state of renal function. Deficits and current losses and needs of water cannot always be met by electrolyte solutions. In particular, the obligatory water of the urine (see p. 51) and the insensible perspiration (and, to a certain extent, sweat) should be provided as water free of electrolyte. *Therefore, two types of fluid therapy are always necessary, electrolyte solutions and water free of electrolyte* (usually given as dextrose solution).

Since there is no current means of predicting accurately the quantities required, therapy must, in the words of Butler and Talbot, "reflect common sense, careful clinical observation, and a tolerance indicative of an enlightened awareness of ignorance." The history of type, duration, and degree of fluid loss permits a rough estimation of the nature and extent of the deficit. Other factors to be considered include the clinical disturbance present, the state of renal function, and the reaction as treatment progresses.

Close observation of the patient is particularly important because the initial apparent condition may change rapidly during therapy. The physician should examine the patient frequently, the nurse should note carefully fluid intake and output and changes in signs and symptoms, and each urine specimen should undergo determination of volume and specific gravity.

As long as the patient is vomiting or has diarrhea, nothing should be given by mouth except medication for diarrhea. When the oral route can be used, it is preferred because of its simplicity and because oral administration of potassium salts practically never leads to potassium intoxication except in the presence of renal failure. Intravenous drip is, in general, more satisfactory than hypodermoclysis in the treatment of dehydration.

In spite of the fact that estimates based on rules cannot be relied on, they may be useful as general guides. Darrow suggests that the basic daily fluid intake for current needs should be 100 to 150 cc. per 100 calories *metabolized* (for a patient at bed rest, increase by 25 percent the basal metabolism as calculated from the nomogram on p. 569). The larger quantity is given if the abnormal fluid loss is high and the concentrating power of the kidneys is poor.

For restoration of fluid and electrolyte deficit, electrolyte solution may be administered in quantities of 40 to 80 cc. per *Kg. of normal body weight* (18 to 35 cc. per lb.). Unless deficiency is mild, this quantity of fluid is added to the basic intake instead of being included in it. Whatever volume of fluid is given beyond the electrolyte needs should be made up of blood, plasma, or solutions of amino acids (p. 260) or 5 to 10 percent dextrose (p. 349).

If the patient is in shock, he should first receive whole blood, if that is available, in quantities of 10 to 30 cc. per Kg. (5 to 15 cc. per lb.) of body weight. If blood is not available, plasma should be given, although it is less effective. Even if blood or plasma has not been given initially, daily determinations of hemoglobin and plasma protein are useful to indicate need for them.

If fluids still cannot be taken by mouth after twelve to twenty-four hours of treatment, the basic fluid intake should be continued parenterally plus sufficient additional fluid to replace evident losses, the patient's response to previous therapy always being taken into account. Continued loss or persistent deficit of electrolyte is an indication to give 25 to 35 percent of the total fluid intake as electrolyte solution. Plasma is, of course, an electrolyte solution, and preparations of amino acids may contain electrolyte which should be calculated in the day's ration. *At least 65 percent of the fluid intake should be without sodium salts.*

If electrolyte solutions are given by hypodermoclysis, the blood, plasma, amino acid, or dextrose solutions are given slowly by vein. If all are given intravenously, the electrolyte, amino acid, and dextrose solutions should be mixed.

The choice of electrolyte solution depends on personal preference, on the acid-base balance, and on the state of renal function. A discussion of such solutions begins on page 348. Potassium deficiency and its treatment are dealt with beginning on page 343.

Especial care should be taken to avoid *over*dosage of electrolyte, and particularly sodium, in patients who have been injured or operated upon. It has been shown that for two to four days after injury or operation, injected salt solutions tend to cause localized edema in the traumatized regions, delaying healing and in some instances interfering with function. In fact, in the first few postoperative days a *slight* sodium deficit seems preferable to any excess. Thus, during this period, dextrose solutions seem to be the best parenteral sources of fluid. However, such a policy carries the obligation of especial vigilance for signs of sodium deficit. If these appear, because of external sodium loss or internal shift, vigorous saline therapy must be instituted without regard for the consequences of local edema. Some investigators recommend replacement of any large loss of digestive fluids without waiting for evidence of sodium deficit.

When renal function is adequate, the kidneys can be depended on to reject any excess of basic or acidic ions. However, electrolyte deficiency and trauma (see Crush Syndrome, p. 222) of themselves induce renal failure. When anuria or oliguria is due to water or electrolyte deficiency, ample quantities of these substances should be supplied. However, when urine output diminishes because of a defect within the kidneys (crush syndrome, nephritis, etc.), the forcing of fluids may be dangerous. Under these circumstances, the effort should be to keep the body water and electrolyte concentration at normal levels. The data on water losses (p. 51), and daily determinations of body weight, give an idea of the amount of water to administer, and the levels of serum electrolytes indicate needs for those substances.

ACIDOSIS

Acidosis is that condition in which the body fluids contain a relative excess of acidic ions and a relative deficiency of basic ions. It may arise from excessive intake or production of actual or potential acid or from undue loss of basic ions. The effect is to decrease the bicarbonate content and eventually the pH of the body fluids. Since undue loss of basic ions is usually accompanied by some loss of acidic ions and water, acidosis is ordinarily associated with dehydration and electrolyte deficiency (see preceding section).

Additions of acid may be due to:

1. Ingestion or injection of acids, or of acid salts such as ammonium chloride.
2. Excessive muscular exertion, with accumulation of lactic acid.
3. Ketosis, as in diabetes mellitus, starvation, following ether or chloroform anesthesia, and as a result of excessive catabolism of protein and fat in severe fevers (for further discussion, see Diabetic Acidosis below).
4. Nephritis, with retention of acidic ions, particularly sulfate and phosphate.
5. Infectious diseases, severe burns, general anesthesia, and pregnancy, with formation of unidentified acid metabolites.

Withdrawal of base is most likely to accompany diarrheal diseases. It also occurs as the result of inadequate reabsorption of base in the renal tubules in advanced nephritis. Often acidosis will result from a combination of several factors.

Severe acidosis is characterized by a peculiar rapid and deep breathing (Kussmaul). Symptoms of less diagnostic value include malaise, weakness, drowsiness, and headache. Early or mild cases can be recognized only by examination of the blood. Most commonly the carbon-dioxide combining power of the plasma is measured (p. 535). Values below 55 volumes per 100 cc. are indicative of acidosis.

Diabetic Acidosis—The acidosis that occurs in diabetes mellitus, starvation, and the other conditions listed in the third category above has certain features of its own. Its fundamental characteristic is ketosis—the accumulation in the blood of significant quantities of the ketone bodies, beta-hydroxybutyric acid, acetoacetic (diacetic) acid, and acetone.

In the absence of sugar utilization, the metabolism of fats and proteins is increased to meet the energy requirements of the body, and there is greater production of ketones by the liver for distribution to the tissues for complete combustion. The actual production of ketones may be subject to regulation by the glycogen level in the liver itself. When the rate of ketogenesis in the liver exceeds the rate of oxidation of ketones in the tissues, ketonemia and ketonuria ensue, and the excess is excreted in the urine as acetone and diacetic acid. Thus, ketogenesis indicates either a relative or absolute shortage of carbohydrate for fuel.

Some of the ketones are excreted as free acid; other portions are neutralized by increased ammonia production and by the buffer action of the blood in which the ketones displace carbon dioxide from the bicarbonate of the plasma. Fixed base, chiefly sodium, is lost when the ketosis is severe, and dehydration and hemoconcentration occur. Compensatory mechanisms are overwhelmed, and several outstanding alterations from normal gradually appear: (1) The carbon-dioxide combining power of the blood is reduced in proportion to the severity of the acidosis; (2) continued loss of fixed base entails a reduction in sodium chloride and electrolyte concentration, lowered alkali reserve, diuresis, and dehydration, accentuated by vomiting; (3) acetone and diacetic acid appear in the urine in large quantities; (4) hemoconcentration develops; (5) the pH of the blood shifts toward the acid side; (6) Kussmaul breathing ("air hunger") and fall in blood pressure occur and may be followed by circulatory collapse, depression of renal activity, retention of nonprotein nitrogen in the blood, subnormal temperature, and finally death.

The term "diabetic coma" is unfortunate because occasionally consciousness is retained to the last, whereas more often it is lost when the degree of acidosis is less extreme. Usually an arbitrary value of 20 to 25 volumes percent for the CO_2 combining power of the plasma serves as a criterion for classification of cases. Above this value, the term "acidosis" is used; the term "coma" may be applied when lower values are found. The usual causes of diabetic acidosis and coma are dietary imbalance, too little (or sudden withdrawal of) Insulin, and infection.

Acidosis should be suspected whenever any unusual symptom or sign makes its appearance in a known diabetic patient. Frequent early symptoms are weakness, headache, thirst, loss of appetite, vomiting, and pains in the legs, back, or abdomen. Later, deep breathing (Kussmaul), somnolence, and coma may follow. The appearance of the patient is usually characteristic. The face is flushed, the skin and mouth are dry, and the eyeballs become soft. The characteristic odor of acetone may pervade the entire room. Diagnosis should be verified by examination of the urine, which almost invariably contains large quantities of sugar (p. 517) and gives a strongly positive test for diacetic acid with ferric chloride (p. 519). Both protein and casts appear with regularity in diabetic acidosis. The blood-sugar level is usually greatly elevated, and the carbon-dioxide combining power of the plasma (p. 535) is reduced. Symptoms are usually intense if it falls below 20 volumes percent. Leukocytosis is the rule, and the presence of abdominal pain may lead to the suspicion of appendicitis. A few hours' intensive treatment of the acidosis will usually settle this question.

Treatment of Acidosis must be directed toward the underlying cause (see listing above). In all forms, fluids and electrolytes are given in large quantities (see Treatment of Dehydration, p. 56). In very mild acidosis, or when much of the chloride of the plasma has been replaced by other fixed acids, Isotonic Sodium Chloride Solution, U.S.P., or Ringer's Solution, U.S.P., may suffice. They are given by slow intravenous injection or by hypodermoclysis in sufficient quantity to restore the plasma carbon-dioxide combining power to normal and also to replace absolute deficiencies.

Usually a solution containing sodium lactate is preferred because this compound provides the needed basic ions unencumbered with fixed acidic ions which must be excreted. Lactated Ringer's Solution, U.S.P., one-sixth-molar sodium lactate solution, or mixtures of the latter with Isotonic Sodium Chloride Solution or Ringer's Solution may be employed. For moderate acidosis, the average dose of Lactated Ringer's Solution (*the diluted form, not the concentrated solution as ordinarily supplied*) is 20 to 30 cc. per Kg. (10 to 15 cc. per lb.) of body weight. Injections are repeated until fluid and electrolyte balance are restored to normal. Some clinicians prefer a mixture of 1 part one-sixth-molar sodium lactate solution and 3 parts isotonic salt or Ringer's Solution. Such a mixture provides about half again as much unencumbered base as does Lactated Ringer's Solution.

For severe acidosis, the one-sixth-molar solution

of sodium lactate is preferred (*the one-molar solution as supplied must be diluted before use*). Since there is usually a total electrolyte deficiency in severe acidosis, it may be well to give the sodium lactate solution mixed with an equal volume of Isotonic Sodium Chloride Solution or Ringer's Solution.

When the plasma carbon-dioxide content, as distinguished from the CO_2 combining power, is known, the dose of sodium lactate necessary to restore the carbon dioxide of the body fluids approximately to the normal value of 60 volumes percent within a period of from two to four hours may be calculated as follows: Dose in cubic centimeters of *concentrated* sodium lactate equals (60 minus plasma CO_2 content) times (0.3 body weight in kilograms).

In acidosis due to chronic nephritis, the amount of sodium lactate needed is very close to the above calculation. In diarrheal acidosis, somewhat less than the expected rise in carbon-dioxide content usually results. In diabetic acidosis, a somewhat larger increase may be expected because of synergistic Insulin action.

When the plasma carbon-dioxide content is not known but the patient otherwise presents the findings of severe acidosis, a safe but effective dose is 10 cc. of the *concentrated* solution (60 cc. of the diluted solution) per kilogram of body weight. Such a dose would be expected to increase the plasma carbon-dioxide content by 25 to 35 volumes percent.

In very dehydrated patients, it is most effective to give from one-third to one-half the total dose of lactate solution intravenously (i.e., 20 to 30 cc. of the diluted solution per kilogram of body weight) and the rest subcutaneously or intraperitoneally.

Sodium bicarbonate is also used in treatment of acidosis. It is positively indicated in the presence of severe impairment of liver function, when oxidation of lactate may not occur. With this exception, the lactate is generally preferred because overdoses are much less likely to be injurious.

Severe acidosis (particularly diabetic acidosis) usually involves intracellular potassium deficiency. When such deficiency is suspected, potassium salts should be administered as outlined on page 344.

Treatment of Diabetic Acidosis—In ketosis (acidosis due to inadequate carbohydrate *utilization*, actual or relative), the administration of fluid and electrolyte is likewise essential, but it *must* be accompanied by restoration of carbohydrate utilization by means of Insulin. In nondiabetic ketosis, the administration of 5 to 10 percent dextrose solution may be sufficient. Such a solution may be mixed with any volume of Lactated Ringer's Solution,

Ringer's Solution, or Isotonic Sodium Chloride Solution if desired. Sufficient fluid should be given to maintain the urinary output at approximately 1,500 cc. every twenty-four hours and the specific gravity of the urine well below the maximum of which the kidneys are capable. If signs of dehydration are apparent, from 3,000 to 6,000 cc. of fluid may be needed in the first twenty-four hours (see p. 57).

Diabetic coma is a first-rank medical emergency. Success depends upon the promptness with which treatment can be instituted; in a critical case, the first three hours will spell the difference between success and failure. Each case is an individual problem, and the response to initial treatment must serve as a guide to the intensity with which ensuing measures will need to be pursued.

INSULIN—The more profound the coma, the greater the dose required. In a mild case, 30 to 90 units may be ample. Recovery of a severe case may not infrequently necessitate administration of several hundred units and, in exceptional circumstances, even in excess of a thousand. Insulin must be given for its effect as disclosed by lowering of blood sugar and diminution of glycosuria. Since rapid action is desirable, the preparation should be unmodified (either amorphous or crystalline) Insulin. The first dose may vary from 20 to 100 units intravenously and a like amount subcutaneously, and may be accompanied by a single dose of Protamine Zinc Insulin of 50 units or more to act as a bridge over the gaps in effect between doses of unmodified Insulin. Some prefer to give doses based on the patient's weight, e.g., an initial dose of 1 unit per Kg. of body weight. Doses should be repeated subcutaneously at intervals of thirty to sixty minutes until there is clinical and laboratory evidence of improvement.

SALT—An initial intravenous infusion of 1,000 cc. of electrolyte solution (p. 348) may be given fairly rapidly and should be followed by additional fluids by mouth, by hypodermoclysis, and by proctoclysis. Large volumes are sometimes required. Hypertonic solutions (50 cc. of 10 percent sodium chloride, repeated if necessary) are sometimes used to overcome anuria.

DEXTROSE—The intravenous administration of dextrose at the onset of treatment must still be regarded as controversial. Experience at the Baker Clinic indicates that it may be detrimental. It should probably be given only later, after the initial hyperglycemic level has been reduced below 200 mg. per 100 cc., or the urine shows 1 plus to negative when tested by Benedict's solution, which

may occur while acidosis is still severe. By this time it is often possible to begin oral feedings of orange juice or ginger ale. Approximately 300 Gm. or more of carbohydrate will be required during the first twenty-four hours if the glycogen stores of the body are to be returned to near normal.

ALKALI—Although clinical opinions differ concerning the value of alkali, it is obvious that most cases do not need it. Alkali therapy may well be reserved for cases of severe ketosis with extreme hyperpnea and CO_2 combining power below 15 volumes percent. In such instances, sodium lactate may be given intravenously as outlined on page 349.

Record the blood pressure and all laboratory and clinical findings hourly. If systolic blood pressure falls below 80 mm., circulatory collapse and anuria are impending and can best be averted by restoration of blood volume by electrolyte solution or blood transfusion. The first few hours and days following recovery from diabetic coma are critical ones. Remember that coma is usually precipitated by some complication, especially infection, and continue to look for it.

ALKALOSIS

Alkalosis is that condition in which the body fluids contain a relative excess of basic ions and a relative deficiency of acidic ions. It may arise from excessive intake or production of actual or potential alkali or from undue loss of acidic ions. Since undue loss of acidic ions is usually accompanied by some loss of basic ions and water, alkalosis is ordinarily associated with dehydration and electrolyte deficiency (see Dehydration, p. 56). Alkalosis of more than brief duration leads to intracellular potassium deficiency, which must be treated on its own merits (see p. 343).

Alkalosis is most frequently due to either persistent loss of gastric juice (from vomiting or by tube drainage) or repeated ingestion of alkali, as during treatment of peptic ulcer. Acute alkalosis may result from overbreathing, which washes carbon dioxide from the lungs and alters temporarily the bicarbonate-carbonic acid balance of the blood.

In acute alkalosis from overbreathing, anxiety and general tingling sensations occur, with tetany and often carpopedal spasm. In the more chronic forms of more gradual onset, there is first distaste for food, then gastric discomfort progressing to nausea, vomiting, and abdominal pain. There may also be nervousness, irritability, hyperesthesia, tinglings, dizziness, and headache; muscle and joint pains, hyperactive reflexes, fibrillary twitchings, and muscle spasms; low fever, tachycardia, slow respiration, prostration, and coma. Severe alkalosis may be fatal if untreated.

Laboratory findings in severe cases include alkaline urine of large volume and low, fixed specific gravity, with granular casts and a trace of protein; diminished or absent urinary excretion of chloride and ammonia; impaired renal function; low blood chloride (p. 347); high blood urea or nonprotein nitrogen; carbon-dioxide combining power of the blood (p. 535) elevated beyond 65 volumes percent, often to 75 or more.

Treatment is simple and promptly effective. For acute overbreathing the patient may breathe a mixture of carbon dioxide and oxygen. The same end is accomplished by having him rebreathe from a large paper bag closely pressed about the mouth with the nares closed.

In the chronic forms with vomiting and tetany, all foods and alkalies are withheld, and isotonic or slightly hypertonic salt solution is given intravenously or rectally to a total of 20 Gm. of sodium chloride daily. The salt is taken by mouth when possible. Associated fluid and electrolyte deficiency is treated according to the principles set forth beginning on page 56.

Total urinary output of chloride is determined daily and blood chloride occasionally. When excretion and blood level have returned to normal, treatment is discontinued. When alkalosis is severe, ammonium chloride, 10 Gm. daily, may be given in place of sodium chloride. In emergency when the usual laboratory data are not available, a 0.9 percent solution of ammonium chloride may be injected by vein very slowly until carpopedal spasm and hyperpnea are relieved.

As the condition improves, a high-carbohydrate, high-salt, low-protein diet is given.

WATER INTOXICATION

Water intoxication is a rare condition due to an absolute excess of water in the body. Since the ability of normal kidneys to excrete water is very great, water intoxication is seen clinically only when renal function is seriously impaired, as following hemorrhage, deep anesthesia, or traumatic or postoperative shock (see Crush Syndrome, p. 222) or during treatment of diabetes insipidus with posterior pituitary extract (p. 194). Such impairment of renal function must be accompanied by excessive ingestion or administration of water or dextrose solution.

In water intoxication all the body fluids become hypotonic, and the cells imbibe extra water. In severe experimental water intoxication, hemolysis and hemoglobinuria may occur. Symptoms apparently have two origins. Increased intracranial pressure (presumably from edema of the brain) produces increased spinal-fluid pressure, papilledema (after a latent period of thirty-six hours), headache, dizziness, restlessness, elevation of blood pressure, nausea and vomiting, muscular twitchings, and, in experimental animals, ataxia, convulsions, coma, and death. Increased extrarenal excretion of water is involved in the vomiting and also in diarrhea, salivation, lacrimation, and sweating. There is a peculiar intracutaneous edema (demonstrated by pressure over bones) but no definite subcutaneous edema.

Treatment consists in intravenous administration of hypertonic (10 percent) sodium chloride solution. Dosage is not definitely established, but probably 100 cc. can be given slowly at hourly intervals until symptoms disappear. If no improvement follows the second injection, other possible diagnoses should be strongly considered.

CARDIOVASCULAR SYSTEM
Heart Disease
ORGANIC HEART DISEASE

Intrinsic organic disease of the heart may involve the pericardium, myocardium, endocardium (including the heart valves), coronary arteries, or a combination of them. Approximately 90 percent of organic heart disease is due to arteriosclerosis, hypertension, rheumatic fever, or syphilis.

Arteriosclerosis (p. 74) and hypertension (p. 80), often working in combination, are the prevailing causes of cardiac disability in middle and later life. Sclerosis of the coronary arteries impairs coronary circulation, and hypertension increases the work of the heart. Angina pectoris or coronary occlusion may result from coronary sclerosis; cardiac hypertrophy and later failure may result from coronary sclerosis or hypertension or both. A contributory factor in this period is a seeming diminution in recuperative power between beats. This is apparently the condition which older clinicians termed "chronic myocarditis"; it has more recently been called "myocardial senescence."

Rheumatic fever (p. 46) causes pericarditis, myocarditis, and endocarditis, the last involving the heart valves. The lesions may heal with scarring or may become chronic. The valve most commonly involved is the mitral, with stenosis or insufficiency or both. Fairly common is aortic insufficiency of mild degree. Rather uncommon are aortic stenosis and tricuspid stenosis. The pulmonic valves are very rarely involved in the rheumatic process.

Syphilis (p. 10) may cause myocarditis, but the frequency of syphilitic myocarditis is a matter of debate. Typically, syphilis involves the heart secondarily to the aorta. Aortitis may spread to the aortic valves, producing aortic insufficiency, or to the orifices of the coronary arteries, leading to impairment of coronary circulation and anginal symptoms.

Congenital defects of the valves and septa of the heart, and persistence of the ductus arteriosus, may seriously impair cardiac function and predispose to bacterial endocarditis.

Hyperthyroidism (p. 180) greatly increases the work of the heart as well as its metabolic rate, and chronic hyperthyroidism often leads to auricular fibrillation (p. 71) and heart failure (see below). Beriberi (p. 486) may be accompanied by cardiac dilatation and failure, and severe anemia (p. 94) or pulmonary emphysema (p. 121) may also lead to decompensation.

If the presence of heart disease can be recognized in its early stages, a great deal can often be done to prolong the period of useful life. When possible, therapeutic measures are taken to combat the underlying cause. The patient must be educated to live with his condition, a process often requiring great tact and patience on the part of the physician. Moderation is, of course, the keynote, but it need not be a fetish; perhaps the best general rule is that the patient may do anything which does not bring on shortness of breath or fatigue.

Before compensation is broken, the assessment of the extent of cardiac damage is often difficult. The character of the heart sounds and murmurs, if any, the rate and rhythm, the blood pressure, the vital capacity, and the size and configuration of the heart all give useful information. On the last point, the x-ray often tells much more than can be gleaned from physical examination.

HEART FAILURE

Heart failure (myocardial insufficiency, cardiac decompensation) has been defined by Dock as "a loss of organic function sufficient to produce symptoms apparent to the patient, or signs apparent to

---

Concepts of the mechanism, interpretation, and treatment of heart failure are currently undergoing great change. The discussion below reflects those new developments which seemed to be reasonably well established at the time this book went to press. If those schooled in the older concepts find themselves on unfamiliar ground, it is recommended that they study several times and correlate the following discussions:

Heart Failure, including the table on page 64
Disturbances of Fluid and Electrolyte Balance:
Introduction (p. 49)
Edema (p. 53)
Dehydration (p. 56)
Urinary Tract: Introduction (p. 218)

---

the unaided eyes of a trained observer." When these symptoms or signs appear with work loads which are less than the minimum observed in normal subjects, the loss of functional capacity is probably greater than 90 percent. If symptoms occur when the load is two to five times the normal basal level, loss of function is probably more than 50 percent.

Heart failure is, fundamentally, the result of a discrepancy between the cardiac output and the flow of blood necessary to satisfy the circulatory needs of the body. Factors influencing the relationship are outlined in Table 8 (p. 64). One factor alone may lead to heart failure, or, more commonly, several may contribute.

It will be noted that some conditions may act simultaneously in several different ways (e.g., pulmonary emphysema tends to induce heart failure by increasing resistance in the pulmonary circuit, reducing oxygen supply to the myocardium through production of arterial anoxia, and increasing blood flow to compensate for the arterial anoxia). Sometimes, in spite of an adequate myocardium, blood flow to the tissues is insufficient because of restricted ventricular filling during diastole. The term "circulatory failure" has been applied to this condition to distinguish it from "heart failure," in which myocardial inadequacy is a significant factor.

If average intrathoracic pressure remains constant, increased venous pressure results in increased filling of the ventricles during diastole. Up to the maximum working capacity of the heart, such increased ventricular filling causes increased cardiac output. When the ventricles are filled beyond their expulsive capacity, however, they of necessity dilate, and their efficiency is reduced. When such dilatation and inefficiency are present, cardiac performance is improved by a *reduction* in venous pressure.

TABLE 8 — *Factors in Heart Failure*

I. Factors which tend to diminish effective cardiac
   output
   A. Myocardial weakness
      1. Myocardial lesions
         a. Myocardial senescence
         b. Cardiac infarction
         c. Rheumatic or other myocarditis
         d. Beriberi
      2. Inadequate oxygen supply
         a. Coronary arteriosclerosis
         b. Arterial anoxia
            (1) Severe anemia
            (2) Pulmonary disease
               (a) Extensive pneumonia
               (b) Emphysema
   B. Valve lesions
   C. High resistance in the pulmonary circuit
      1. Mitral stenosis
      2. Pulmonary emphysema
      3. Massive pulmonary embolism
   D. High resistance in the systemic circuit
   E. Ventricular *over*filling during diastole
      1. Elevated venous pressure
         a. Increased blood volume (see below)
   F. Restriction of ventricular filling during diastole
      1. Constrictive (chronic adhesive) pericarditis
      2. Cardiac tamponade
         a. Pericardial effusion or hemorrhage
      3. Overly brief diastole
         a. Ventricular rate in excess of 180 to 200 beats
            per minute
         b. Disturbances in intraventricular conduction
            which lengthen systole and shorten diastole
      4. Greatly reduced blood volume
         a. Severe dehydration (p. 56)
         b. Shock
         c. Hemorrhage
II. Factors which tend to increase blood flow greatly
   A. Increased tissue demand for oxygen and food-
      stuffs
      1. Physical exertion
      2. Fever
      3. Hyperthyroidism
   B. Arterial anoxia
      1. Severe anemia
      2. Pulmonary disease
         a. Extensive pneumonia
         b. Emphysema
   C. Beriberi
   D. Arteriovenous shunt
      1. Arteriovenous fistula
         a. Uterus in late pregnancy
      2. Bones in Paget's disease and hyperparathy-
         roidism
      3. Patent ductus arteriosus

Increased venous pressure may be due to increased
blood volume, which, with its corollary, edema, is
seen in such diverse conditions as hyperadrenalism
(or overdosage of adrenocortical hormone) and
beriberi. There is a question as to whether this in-

creased blood volume can be the sole cause of the
heart failure that may accompany these conditions.

In very acute heart failure (such as may be associated with extreme ventricular tachycardia, a
large myocardial infarction, or massive pulmonary
embolism) shock and pulmonary edema are usually
the predominant manifestations. When failure
comes on in the course of a day or two, as in a
prolonged bout of paroxysmal auricular tachycardia, shock may be less prominent, and pulmonary
and hepatic congestion and edema of the legs may
precede the full-blown picture of heart failure.

When the discrepancy between cardiac output
and circulatory need is small but persistent, there
is a gradual rise in blood volume, hemoglobin level,
and red cell count, (see p. 92) apparently brought
about by the same compensatory mechanism which
increases these entities after hemorrhage or ascent
to a high altitude. When the increase becomes too
great, the first result is engorgement of the veins
and viscera. Up to the work capacity of the heart,
the resulting increased cardiac filling increases cardiac output and tends to reduce the stimulus for
further increase in blood volume. Myocardial hypertrophy may take place. When the work capacity
of the heart is exceeded, the ventricles are able to
expel a progressively smaller proportion of the blood
they contain at the end of diastole. The result is
cardiac dilatation, loss of myocardial efficiency,
and continuation of the stimulus for increase in
blood volume. As venous and visceral engorgement
increases, the increased pressure progresses back
through the circulatory system, causing edema
(from increased capillary pressure) and possibly
arterial hypertension.

In heart failure that comes on slowly, the earliest
symptoms are likely to be fatigability and (in relatively active persons) dyspnea on exertion or (in
sedentary persons) nocturnal dyspnea, sometimes
termed "cardiac asthma."

The full-blown picture with very high blood
volume includes some or all of the following:

Dyspnea—on exertion or aggravated by exertion
Orthopnea
Increased venous pressure (distended neck veins
   when patient is erect), especially on exertion
Cardiac dilatation (lesser degrees are best re-
   vealed by x-ray)
Enlarged liver—usually tender when failure has
   developed over a relatively short period of time
Dependent edema (see p. 53)
Hydrothorax
Ascites
Cyanosis

From the point of view of prognosis in heart failure, it is desirable to estimate the degree of failure and the relative importance of those contributing factors which can be reduced or eliminated. The degree of failure is judged by the load which brings on symptoms and signs. All the factors listed in Table 8 should be sought for and evaluated by means of careful history and physical examination. In addition, the following are helpful in appraising various aspects of the situation.

Heart volume as shown by x-ray is a direct index of the degree of overloading of the heart.

The improvement in signs and symptoms on bed rest, together with the history of activity, suggests the influence of physical exertion.

The level of venous pressure,* degree of visceral engorgement, and amount of edema, ascites, and hydrothorax are indices of the rate of increase in blood volume and, to a lesser extent, of the amount of increase. Their response to treatment suggests the patient's recuperative ability.

The level of systemic arterial pressure can be measured directly; the intensity of the pulmonic second sound suggests the level of pulmonary arterial pressure and the resistance in the pulmonary circuit.

Especially important is recognition of relatively high or relatively low cardiac output. A high output accompanies dilatation of the peripheral vascular bed and is evidenced by normal or high skin temperature (for clinical purposes the physician's hand is an adequate thermometer), large pulse pressure relative to systolic pressure (in the absence of murmurs signifying aortic valve disease), and vigorous heartbeat. "High-output failure" is seen in aortic insufficiency and in those conditions marked by increased blood flow (see under II in table). Low cardiac output is accompanied by a normal or increased degree of peripheral vasoconstriction, and this is manifested by normal or low skin temperature, small pulse pressure, and faint heartbeat. "Low-output failure" is seen typically in myocardial senescence, myocarditis, and coronary arteriosclerosis. Obviously, there is a greater demand on the heart in high-output failure than in low-output failure, and, in the former, compensation will accordingly break at a higher level of myocardial performance. The distinction is important for therapy as well as for prognosis.

Treatment of heart failure is directed to two general ends: reduction to a minimum of the demands on the heart, and improvement in the effectiveness of cardiac function. The causative factors in heart failure listed in the table should be sought for and evaluated, and, whenever possible, they should be ameliorated or removed altogether.

Physical exertion can be minimized very quickly. The patient is put to rest with head and shoulders elevated in the position which is most comfortable for him. He should not do anything for himself that can be done for him by others. A commode at the bedside will usually cause less total exertion than a bedpan. If respiration is embarrassed by ascites, the fluid should be withdrawn by paracentesis. The same may be said of hydrothorax, except that thoracentesis carries some risk to the patient.

Rest and sleep should be insured, and it is usual in the first few days to administer morphine sulfate, 15 mg. (1/4 grain) hypodermically in the evening—a dose which may be repeated if the patient does not sleep. It may be given every four hours day and night for a few days if needed. Later on, the barbiturates (p. 390) may be useful to provide mild sedation during the day and sleep at night. In some patients, however, insomnia and even mild delirium may be due to cerebral hypoxia; in such cases the patient will be made more restless and wakeful by sedatives but, paradoxically, may fall asleep on administration of oxygen or xanthine preparations (p. 358).

If the case seems to be one of low-output failure in which exertion is the only factor present that may increase the demand for blood flow, then measures to increase cardiac efficiency can be expected to be most effective. When the degree of venous congestion, edema, and visceral engorgement and the size of the heart shadow are such as to indicate that cardiac efficiency is being reduced by overfilling, then usually the greatest immediate benefit is obtained by reducing venous pressure. The time-honored method of accomplishing this is by removal of 600 to 800 cc. of blood by venesection (femoral if the arm veins are collapsed and the limbs cold). The same effect can be obtained by applying blood pressure cuffs to the extremities and keeping them inflated to a pressure just below the arterial diastolic. Since reduction of blood volume or of venous return may be harmful in the presence of cyanosis due to chronic pulmonary emphysema, pallor from anemia, or any acute cardiac damage such as coronary occlusion, no attempt is made to reduce venous return when their presence is ob-

---

* Inspection of the neck veins and palpation of the liver give a rough idea of venous pressure; if measurements of venous pressure are to be of prognostic value, there must be serial determinations with a needle in a vein attached to a manometer.

vious. If there is some question, a test with blood pressure cuffs may precede venesection.

The next emergency measure in importance is administration of oxygen, which should be continued without pause for at least several days and until considerable recovery has occurred. Intermittent administration and premature discontinuance are unwise. In the presence of pulmonary edema, oxygen should be given from a pressure mask.

Next in importance in low-output failure is administration of digitalis, which increases myocardial efficiency and also diminishes venous return. It is given intravenously if the case is urgent, by mouth if not. The contraindications to venesection apply also to digitalis. A discussion of choice of preparation, dosage, and administration begins on page 356.

In high-output failure, it is of the utmost importance to seek out and remove the causes of the excessive demand (see list on p. 64). Because failure is due much more to such excessive demand than to subnormal performance, less can be expected from measures that increase cardiac efficiency, and neither venesection nor digitalis administration is likely to be beneficial. Beyond reducing demand, best results are usually obtained with oxygen, rest, and sedation.

In both types of heart failure, it is of fundamental importance to reduce blood volume to the point where it does not lead to cardiac overfilling. This is accomplished by sodium depletion (see Edema, p. 53).

The most important feature of the diet is that it should be very low in sodium (see pp. 341 and 585). Within this restriction it should be simple. In chronic failure, an intake of 50 Gm. protein, 50 Gm. fat, and 150 Gm. carbohydrate is an adequate goal unless the patient is obese, in which case the fat may be cut to 30 Gm. and the carbohydrate to 80 Gm. The patient should be allowed as much water as he desires, but it must be practically sodium-free. In regions where the water has a higher sodium content than 10 mg. per 100 cc. (10 parts per 100,000), distilled water should be taken. Hard water which has been softened chemically is contraindicated because of its sodium content.

Acute emergencies in the form of pulmonary edema, paroxysmal dyspnea, or cardiac asthma require prompt and energetic action. For the first, immediate venesection, or high caudal or spinal anesthesia, is the best remedy. A hypodermic injection of morphine sulfate, 15 mg. (1/4 grain), and atropine sulfate, 0.6 mg. (1/100 grain), should also be given. This medication is helpful in the other two conditions as well, but they are usually quickly controlled by slow intravenous administration of 'Monotheamin' or aminophylline, 0.5 Gm. in 20 cc. of water.

As symptoms recede and compensation returns, an additional period of bed rest is advisable to enable the myocardium to build up some reserve capacity. Restrictions are relaxed only gradually, with careful observation to make sure the patient is not overtaxing himself. Undue haste invites relapse. Convalescence is usually a difficult period for the patient because of its slowness. By careful supervision and explanation, the physician can aid greatly in rehabilitation. Many patients can again become useful and happy for years after a bout of cardiac decompensation if they can be educated to avoid whatever causes shortness of breath and fatigue. Proper handling will also reduce to a minimum unnecessary fears and invalidism. Of course the extent to which a given patient can resume full activity must be assessed as convalescence progresses. In any case, the patient should never encroach to any extent upon his reserve energy.

If the attack of heart failure was caused by factors which are likely to recur and if digitalis exerted a favorable effect, it is considered advisable to continue maintenance doses of this drug indefinitely as a precautionary measure. Sodium depletion should also be continued, but only to the extent necessary to control the volume of blood and interstitial fluid (edema). Excessive sodium depletion is dangerous (see p. 342). In patients having coronary disease, the xanthines (p. 358) may have value. The diet should continue moderately low in protein (about 50 Gm. daily), and the caloric value should be sufficiently low to maintain body weight at "ideal" or less (p. 568).

ANGINA PECTORIS

Angina pectoris is a syndrome characterized by paroxysmal pain or discomfort associated with increased demands on the heart. It is a concomitant of coronary artery disease, usually of arteriosclerotic origin after the age of forty, sometimes of syphilitic origin before. The sensation may be of pain, burning, heaviness, fullness, numbness, or constriction, or the patient may not be able to define it better than an uneasiness or discomfort. The distribution is also variable, involving, in order of frequency, the substernal region, precordium, medial aspect of the arm (usually the left), various parts of the head and neck, and epigastrium. It is in most cases brought on by factors which increase the demands on the heart, such as exercise, emotion, distention of abdominal viscera with food or gas, or a combination of these factors.

The immediate cause of angina pectoris seems to be myocardial anoxia or spasm of the coronary arteries or both. Pain of the same distribution may be due to dilatation or a dissecting aneurysm of the aorta, both of which are most often due to syphilis.

With atypical distribution and occurrence of the pain, angina pectoris may be misdiagnosed as gastro-intestinal disorder such as peptic ulcer or "indigestion," gall-bladder disease, intercostal neuralgia, or root pain from mediastinal tumor, vertebral tuberculosis, or osteoarthritis. Sometimes the differential diagnosis from coronary occlusion is very difficult. In fact, the mechanism of the two is apparently similar, and they differ only in the extent to which myocardial function is disturbed.

The course of angina pectoris is extremely variable. Sudden death from coronary occlusion may occur at any time. On the other hand, improvement is common, with development of collateral circulation in the heart, and the patient may live many years. The condition of the cardiovascular system, the temperament of the patient, and the care with which he follows directions are all important factors in determining the outcome.

Treatment follows the same general principles as in heart failure. Adequate rest and the avoidance of exertion and excitement are of fundamental importance in controlling pain and restoring cardiac function. The factors which contribute to the production of pain must be carefully analyzed and the patient shown how to avoid or minimize them. A simple diet should be taken, and overeating and foods which disagree are to be avoided. The weight should be reduced gradually to the minimum which is compatible with a feeling of well-being. Complicating factors such as diabetes mellitus, infections, prostatic hypertrophy, and anemia should be sought and treated (but judiciously). In the treatment of diabetes in patients subject to angina, hypoglycemia or rapid reduction in blood-sugar level is to be avoided, since either one may induce coronary occlusion.

The most valuable drugs for the immediate relief of angina pectoris are the nitrites (p. 364). Hypodermic Tablets Nitroglycerin, 0.4 or 0.6 mg. (1/150 or 1/100 grain) or more, allowed to dissolve under the tongue, are usually promptly effective. Less so is amyl nitrite, 3 to 5 minims, inhaled from a handkerchief. Ineffective for immediate relief but valuable for the prevention of attacks is erythrityl tetranitrate or mannitol hexanitrate, 0.03 to 0.06 Gm. (1/2 to 1 grain) every four to six hours.

There is increasing evidence also that the xanthines (p. 358) and papaverine (p. 363) are useful in angina pectoris, as they are in coronary disease without angina.

CORONARY OCCLUSION

Coronary occlusion (coronary thrombosis, myocardial infarction), except for those rare instances in which it results from embolism, occurs as a complication of coronary artery disease. The occlusion is believed to be due to coronary sclerosis, thrombosis, or spasm or a combination of them. It is apparently an extension of the mechanism of angina pectoris to the point where anoxic necrosis of a portion of the myocardium results. At one extreme, death may be instantaneous; at the other, the patient may recover and live comfortably for many years.

Typically, the patient experiences pain or other unpleasant sensation of the same general character as in angina pectoris, except that it is much more severe and prolonged and has a greater radiation. Rest and nitrites do not relieve it. Shock and fall in blood pressure may develop rapidly. Sometimes, however, symptoms are mild or absent. Within a few days, fever and leukocytosis usually develop; and if the infarcted area reaches to the outer wall of the heart, a transient pericardial friction rub may be present.

A number of cardiac and vascular disturbances may follow coronary occlusion. The most frequent are thromboembolic phenomena, such as pulmonary or peripheral emboli, extension of the myocardial infarction, or phlebothrombosis; heart failure; disorders of the heartbeat such as bundle branch block, heart block, auricular or ventricular fibrillation, or ventricular tachycardia; and rupture of the myocardium.

In the typical case, the characteristic pain and shock make the diagnosis obvious. When the symptoms are mild or atypical, the course of the disease is significant. Fever, leukocytosis, rapid red-cell sedimentation rate, persistence of a lower blood pressure than before the attack, the hearing of a pericardial friction rub, alterations in character and rhythm of the heart sounds, and, particularly, characteristic findings or rapid changes in the electrocardiogram establish the diagnosis and differentiate it from angina pectoris.

Coronary occlusion should be considered in any individual over forty who has a severe attack of what may appear to be indigestion, biliary colic, acute pancreatitis, or perforating peptic ulcer.

Differential diagnosis should also include acute pneumothorax, pulmonary embolism, dissecting aneurysm, rupture of the aorta into the pericardial sac, and acute pericarditis from other causes. The prognosis is always uncertain because of the ever-present possibility of sudden death.

Treatment may be extremely important in affecting not only immediate survival but also the subsequent course of the attack. The patient is first put at absolute rest with head and shoulders elevated, and then the pain is relieved as quickly as possible. Although morphine is the traditional drug for emergency use in coronary occlusion, recent evidence has indicated that papaverine is an excellent initial medication because of its coronary vasodilator action and favorable effect on abnormalities of conduction; 0.1 to 0.2 Gm. of the hydrochloride is given, intramuscularly if symptoms are mild, intravenously (dissolved in 50 cc. of 5 percent dextrose solution) if they are severe. Five to ten *minutes* should be taken for the intravenous injection. Intramuscular injections of papaverine should be repeated at intervals of three to four hours for the first few days of the acute phase. After that the drug may be given by mouth if desired.

If the patient is not substantially relieved by papaverine, morphine sulfate should be given in whatever quantity is required. For mild residual symptoms the usual dose is 16 mg. (1/4 grain) hypodermically. For more severe symptoms, the drug is given very slowly by vein until relief is obtained, the necessary dose usually lying between 10 and 16 mg. (1/6 and 1/4 grain). Both morphine and papaverine may be used freely during the acute phase.

In the presence of dyspnea or cyanosis, oxygen should be administered continuously in full strength with a face mask. Later, the tent or nasal catheter can be substituted when lower concentrations suffice. If the patient is too ill to be removed to a hospital, the oxygen should be given him at home. Sometimes oxygen will afford relief of pain not controlled by morphine and papaverine.

Bed rest should be continued for several weeks, for myocardial infarcts require that long to become fibrosed. At first, bed rest should be as nearly complete as the patient will tolerate without too much persuasion. The use of a commode at the bedside (with help in getting on and off) may entail less total exertion than use of a bedpan. The patient is fed by an attendant unless he insists on feeding himself. The bowels are left to nature. The routine of daily bath and change of linen can be omitted for a few days unless the patient requests them.

After the first week, if he is doing well, he may be permitted somewhat more activity in bed. If the bowels do not move every two to four days, they are aided by enemas or gentle laxation. Upward massage of the legs is given two or three times daily to protect against phlebothrombosis. During the third and fourth weeks, passive leg raising is done (ten or twenty elevations two or three times daily) to improve the condition of the leg muscles and to give the patient a sense of progress; some physicians permit him to sit up in a chair at intervals. At about the end of the fourth uneventful week, he may progress gradually to walking. The rate of increase in activity depends upon the patient's physical and psychological condition. The optimal level of activity is usually reached in about three months.

As soon as the patient wishes food, he may be given a light and easily digested diet. He may have fluids in ordinary quantities as desired. After about ten days the allowance of food may be increased, but the latter should remain easily digestible.

The demonstration of the role of reflex collateral vasospasm in increasing the area of gangrene in peripheral arterial occlusion in man and in experimental coronary occlusion in animals has led to the use of vasodilators in the treatment of coronary occlusion. Papaverine (p. 363) has a powerful vasodilator effect which is particularly useful for relief of the initial pain as well as for any possible action in minimizing the size of the infarcted area. The xanthines (p. 358) are less powerful as vasodilators, but they are commonly given for the following additional effects: as myocardial stimulants to minimize the possibility of congestive failure, as diuretics to forestall the occurrence of edema, and as protectives against cardiac arrhythmias. 'Monotheamin' or aminophylline, 0.5 Gm. intravenously in 50 cc. of 5 percent dextrose solution, may be effective against the initial pain. Many cardiologists give one of these drugs routinely, 0.1 or 0.2 Gm. three or four times daily by mouth or rectum during the first two or three weeks. Often it is desirable to continue administration indefinitely.

Shock is often a very early complication of coronary occlusion. It can be minimized by prompt relief of pain and administration of oxygen. Beyond that, it is treated by supporting the circulation with intravenous blood plasma and, if dehydration is present, slow administration of isotonic salt or dextrose solution or both (p. 56). Sympathomimetic drugs, such as epinephrine, are not of value.

Thromboembolic complications may be expected to appear in about 25 percent of cases. The thrombosis may extend in the coronary arteries, causing additional myocardial necrosis. Pulmonary or systemic embolism may occur from the breaking loose of a clot formed on a necrotic area of endocardium. More commonly, pulmonary embolism arises from thrombi formed in the veins of the legs and abdomen as a result of circulatory stasis.

Early, prolonged, and adequate therapy with anticoagulants has reduced the number of patients developing these thromboembolic phenomena by 55 percent, the actual occurrence of such phenomena by 65 percent, and the death rate in the first six weeks by 30 percent. Either heparin (p. 374) or Dicumarol (p. 375) may be used.

For best results, administration is begun as soon as practicable and is continued for a minimum of thirty days, or for thirty days after any thromboembolic complication. If Dicumarol is given, the prothrombin time should be maintained in a range of 30 to 50 seconds as measured by the Link-Shapiro modification of the Quick one-stage technic (p. 529). If heparin is used, the clotting time of whole blood should be prolonged to three times the normal value by the Lee-White technic (p. 529). About 6 percent of cases of coronary occlusion show hemorrhagic phenomena in the absence of anticoagulant therapy. In the presence of such therapy the incidence is about doubled; however, if the drugs are withheld from those in whom they are contraindicated (see p. 375), if the prolongation of clotting is not allowed to become excessive, and if the drug is stopped promptly and suitable countermeasures are taken (see p. 376) on the occurrence of hemorrhage, no serious consequences are likely to result.

Congestive heart failure may develop following coronary occlusion. It is treated in the usual manner (p. 65). There has been considerable difference of opinion as to whether digitalis should be administered in the presence of coronary occlusion. It is the general opinion that this drug should not be given in the absence of failure or to prevent failure, but the weight of evidence seems to favor its administration once decompensation has set in. Although digitalis tends to increase the irritability of the myocardium, the possibility of inducing cardiac arrhythmia seems small as compared with the benefits of the drug in the treatment of failure, provided that intoxication is not produced. Especial caution should be exercised in the matter of dosage, and, as a general rule, only about three-fourths the usual quantity should be given.

A number of cardiac arrhythmias may occur. Auricular fibrillation is not uncommon in the early stages. It is usually transient, needing no specific treatment unless a high ventricular rate threatens or actually produces failure. It is then treated with digitalis and quinidine (p. 71). Later, ventricular tachycardia or fibrillation may occur. The latter is usually fatal within a matter of minutes. Ventricular tachycardia is treated with quinidine, orally or intravenously (p. 360) as the urgency of the situation demands. Ventricular extrasystoles are not uncommon and indicate an excessive myocardial irritability that predisposes to the more serious arrhythmias. When ventricular extrasystoles are present, some cardiologists recommend oral administration of quinidine sulfate, 0.2 to 0.4 Gm. daily in divided doses, as a prophylactic.

Rupture of the heart is not an uncommon fatal complication. Its incidence is highest toward the end of the second week, when the necrotic infarcted zone of the myocardium has softened considerably and the new fibrous tissue is not yet fully formed. It is best prevented by complete bed rest and the avoidance of sudden strains, such as coughing, lifting, straining at stool, or even loud talking or calling.

In addition to the patient's symptoms and physical findings, certain laboratory aids are helpful in diagnosis and prognosis and in assessing progress. Serial white blood counts help in judging the extent of myocardial necrosis and the rate of repair. An even more delicate index is the red cell sedimentation rate (p. 525). In the presence of a mural thrombus, however, the sedimentation rate may remain accelerated long after healing is complete in the myocardium. Serial electrocardiograms aid in determining the presence and location of an infarct.

DISORDERS OF THE HEARTBEAT

Sinus Arrhythmia is a simple repeated increase and decrease in heart rate. It is correlated with respiration, and the relationship, when not clear, becomes so if respiration is deepened. It occurs during high vagal tone, when the pulse is relatively slow, and is in fact due to small variations in that tone. It usually disappears as the pulse rate approaches and exceeds 100. It is very common and should not be regarded as abnormal. Its only importance lies in its possible confusion with serious arrhythmias.

Extrasystoles are premature beats which may arise in auricles or ventricles. They may occur intermittently or regularly. In the latter case they may be spoken of as coupled beats. When extrasystoles are of ventricular origin, the ventricle is usually in its refractory period at the time the next auricular impulse reaches it, and there is thus a compensatory pause. In auricular extrasystoles, the next normal beat usually follows the extrasystole after a normal interval. Extrasystoles are distinguished from other irregularities by the electrocardiogram and, at the bedside, by the prematurity of the beat and, when the latter is weak enough, by the absence of a second heart sound. As the heart rate increases, extrasystoles tend to disappear. In case of difficulty in bedside diagnosis, the patient may be exercised sufficiently to cause them to disappear, and their return is listened for over the apex impulse. If the first irregularity is a premature beat, the diagnosis is extrasystoles; and if it is an unusually long pause, the diagnosis is heart block.

Extrasystoles may produce palpitation—from rapidly coupled beats or from the unusually vigorous systole which follows the compensatory pause. Extrasystoles are very common, usually occurring after exercise, following heavy meals, or a short time after going to bed. They may be brought on by nervous tension, by smoking, or by digitalis. In the absence of organic heart disease, they are of no significance. They may at times serve to call attention to the heart when it is diseased, but they are not of diagnostic or prognostic importance except possibly following coronary occlusion (p. 67), when they may be considered as an indication of excessive myocardial irritability.

Treatment is indicated only when the patient is very much disturbed by the beats. Quinidine sulfate (p. 360), 0.1 to 0.3 Gm. two or three times daily, will often stop them. Mild sedation (p. 390) may be equally effective in the absence of serious organic heart disease. Digitalis should not be given, since it may bring them on or make them worse.

Paroxysmal Auricular Tachycardia arises from an abnormal focus in the auricles. The heart rate is usually between 160 and 200 beats per minute, but it may be as low as 110 or as high as 250. The characteristic features of the condition are (1) abrupt onset and termination, and (2) absolute invariability in the rate.

Paroxysmal auricular tachycardia may occur at any age but is most common in young adults. It usually occurs in otherwise healthy individuals and is rarely associated with organic heart disease. Sometimes attacks are initiated by certain sudden movements, or even thoughts, but often there is no such correlation. Attacks may be of any frequency or duration. Sometimes they may be accompanied by gastro-intestinal symptoms. Usually they cause no great disturbance in the peripheral circulation, but when the heart rate is over 200 for a prolonged period, congestive failure may develop.

Treatment—Patients themselves sometimes discover postures or maneuvers that stop the attack. Drinking ice water, holding a deep breath as long as possible, or pressure on the eyeballs is often successful. A more complicated but frequently effective maneuver is stimulation of the carotid sinus. The patient lies recumbent, with a small pillow under the neck and shoulders so that the head is somewhat hyperextended on the neck. The physician palpates the carotid artery (usually the right one first) lateral to and deeper than the trachea. The carotid sinus is usually at the level of the upper margin of the thyroid cartilage, beneath the angle of the jaw. Using the thumb, one compresses the sinus backward and inward and massages it against the vertebral column, meanwhile observing carefully the pulse rate and facial color of the patient. Stimulation is discontinued immediately when a response is obtained; this usually occurs in a few seconds and consists in termination of the attack or a considerable change in the patient's color or appearance. Occasionally there is response only to stimulation on the left side. Carotid sinus stimulation must be applied cautiously, however, for in some individuals there may be an exaggerated reaction, with cardiac standstill and anoxic convulsions or hemiplegia. Particular care is also necessary in middle-aged or elderly persons with evidence of arteriosclerosis, and in those under the influence of digitalis.

When the attack resists all the above measures, a trial of drugs may be made if the patient's condition warrants it. Most effective is methacholine (p. 417), which acts as a powerful vagus stimulant. It is given subcutaneously, the dose being 15 to 50 mg., depending on the age and weight of the patient.

Quinidine (p. 360) is sometimes effective, but because of its danger it is reserved for desperate cases in which other means have failed. Under these circumstances it is given intravenously, 0.3 Gm. of a salt being prepared and injected very slowly while someone listens over the patient's precordium with a stethoscope. As soon as the attack ceases, the injection is stopped.

Digitalis in full doses (p. 353) may occasionally be effective when other measures fail.

If it is extremely important to prevent attacks, the patient may be placed on quinidine sulfate, 3 to 5 grains by mouth three times daily, or on full doses of digitalis. Any factor which the patient considers contributory should receive attention.

Auricular Flutter is a condition in which an impulse to contraction moves regularly around the auricles without dying out. The rate of propagation is usually 250 to 350 cycles per second. Since the ventricles cannot respond so frequently, there is always at least a 2:1 block. The ventricular rhythm of untreated cases is usually regular; but sometimes in untreated cases and more often after treatment, the ventricular rhythm may be irregular because of change in the degree of block between auricles and ventricles.

Auricular flutter occurs usually, but not necessarily, in the presence of organic heart disease. Attacks tend to persist for long periods or permanently unless treated. In diagnosis, the electrocardiogram is conclusive. However, the condition can usually be diagnosed at the bedside. The ventricular rate is very constant under varying conditions, as in auricular tachycardia. However, in flutter the rate may change; when it does, the change is instantaneous, and the new rate bears a fractional relationship to the previous one (for instance, a ventricular rate of 160, representing a 2:1 block, may change to 107, representing a 3:1 block, or to 80, representing a 4:1 block). When the degree of block shifts rapidly, distinction from auricular fibrillation may be difficult. Changes in degree of block may be spontaneous, or they may be induced by exercise or carotid sinus stimulation (p. 70).

TREATMENT is directed first toward restoring normal rhythm. Digitalis (p. 353) is administered in full doses. The first result is an increase in the degree of block, with diminution in ventricular rate. At a 4:1 or 6:1 block, auricular fibrillation develops in some cases. Digitalis is then discontinued, and the rhythm frequently reverts to normal within a few days.

If the rhythm is not restored to normal following digitalis therapy, quinidine sulfate (p. 360) may be given. If it does not restore normal rhythm, the patient, whether in flutter or in fibrillation, is kept on sufficient dosage of digitalis to maintain a normal ventricular rate.

Auricular Fibrillation is characterized by the presence of irregularly wandering contractile impulses in the auricles. Since these reach the auriculoventricular node in no regular pattern, the ventricular rate is totally arrhythmic. When the rate is 140 or more, the irregularity may be difficult to detect.

Auricular fibrillation may be paroxysmal or permanent. It occurs rarely in the absence of disease and sometimes in the presence of apparently unrelated extracardiac disease, but it is usually seen in rheumatic heart disease, arteriosclerotic or hypertensive heart disease, and hyperthyroidism. It may occur as a complication of coronary occlusion.

Diagnosis is seldom difficult, the absolute arrhythmia being characteristic. The electrocardiogram is also diagnostic.

Treatment has two aspects: maintenance of a reasonably slow ventricular rate and resumption of normal rhythm. When the rate is so rapid that palpitation is severe or the circulation becomes embarrassed, digitalis should be administered in sufficient dosage to maintain a rate of 80 or somewhat below (in the febrile patient, more rapid rates are allowed). Digitalis administration and dosage are discussed beginning on page 353.

When there is a history of previous transient attacks and the circulation is adequate, it may be necessary to do no more than put the patient at rest, administer morphine or a sedative, and await the resumption of normal rhythm.

When auricular fibrillation is associated with hyperthyroidism, there is a good chance that a normal rhythm will be resumed spontaneously after the hyperthyroidism has been controlled (p. 180). If the heart is not badly damaged and the rhythm has not reverted after a week or two of normal metabolism, one may attempt restoration by the administration of quinidine. If the ventricular rate is rapid, it is of course first controlled by digitalis. If the rate is slow, some cardiologists give digitalis anyway as a preparatory drug, whereas some do not. The administration and dosage of quinidine are discussed beginning on page 360. Quinidine may also be indicated as a prophylactic in cases of recurrent paroxysmal auricular fibrillation.

If the patient has moderately advanced or severe organic heart disease, it is generally considered inadvisable to attempt to restore normal rhythm. The ventricular rate is simply controlled by digitalis.

Ventricular Tachycardia is a serious disorder in which the beats arise from an abnormal focus in the ventricle itself. It is almost always associated with severe organic heart disease, usually coronary thrombosis.

As in other types of abnormal heart action, the onset and offset of an attack are abrupt. The ventricular rate is usually 150 to 200. In ventricular tachycardia the rhythm may be absolutely regular for many seconds or minutes, but careful auscultation will disclose occasional slight irregularities. These help distinguish the condition at the bedside from auricular tachycardia, in which the rhythm never varies, and from auricular flutter, in which the rhythm, when it changes, does so to a very different rate which has a fractional relationship to the previous rate. A second point of distinction is that in ventricular tachycardia the first heart sound will occasionally vary in quality or intensity. Further, the auricular rate, as manifested by pulsations in the jugular vein, will be less than the ventricular rate. Finally, carotid sinus stimulation (p. 70) or other measures which activate the vagus nerve have no effect on ventricular tachycardia. The electrocardiogram is characteristic.

Treatment consists in the administration of quinidine (p. 360) — intravenously if the situation is urgent, orally if it is not. The necessary oral dose varies widely in different patients and must be determined by trial. Digitalis aggravates ventricular tachycardia and is absolutely contraindicated.

Ventricular Fibrillation is characterized by the continuous passage of abnormal impulses over the ventricles in such a way that no co-ordinated contractions are produced and the cardiac output is reduced to zero. Unconsciousness is immediate. Ventricular fibrillation is undoubtedly a common cause of sudden death in coronary arteriosclerosis and after coronary occlusion, and it may be the cause of death in some cases of electrocution. Rarely, recovery takes place, and thus ventricular fibrillation may be a cause of the Adams-Stokes syndrome (p. 73). Quinidine (p. 360) appears to have some value in prophylaxis if the possibility of ventricular fibrillation can be anticipated.

Heart Block is a term applied to abnormalities of conduction of the impulse which initiates myocardial contraction. There are a number of grades and varieties of heart block.

Sinoauricular block may occur, in which one or more impulses originating in a normal sinus node may be blocked before reaching the auricular musculature. One or more complete heart cycles are thus lost. It occurs under the same conditions as auriculoventricular block, and treatment, when needed, is the same.

Auriculoventricular block is the most common form. It occurs in the junctional tissue, auriculoventricular (A-V) node, or the bundle of His. In the so-called "first-degree heart block" (delayed conduction time), impulses reach the ventricles, but only after an abnormally long interval. A gallop rhythm is sometimes present; but since there are other causes of gallop rhythm, first-degree block cannot be diagnosed, and may not even be suspected, without the electrocardiogram.

Second-degree heart block (partial heart block) involves a greater defect, in which each successive impulse is progressively more delayed until one or more are blocked altogether. The degree of partial heart block is usually described in terms of the relative numbers of P waves and ventricular complexes, such as 7:6, 5:3, 2:1. Partial heart block can usually be recognized at the bedside by careful auscultation of the heart and observation of auricular waves in the jugular veins, both with the patient at rest and after attempts to disturb the rate by exercise, deep breathing, carotid sinus pressure (p. 70), or drugs such as nitrites (p. 364) or atropine. The electrocardiogram is the final diagnostic appeal. Differential diagnosis includes extrasystoles, normal bradycardia, and complete block.

In third-degree heart block (complete heart block), no auricular impulses get through to the ventricles, and the rhythm of the two parts is independent, the ventricles responding to a pacemaker just below the defect in the A-V node or the bundle of His. Since the inherent rhythm of the ventricles is slow, the ventricular rate is regular and slow—30 to 50—depending on the location of the pacemaker.

The same methods are used in recognizing complete as in diagnosing partial heart block. The same differential diagnosis is involved. There is no other condition that is likely to give a regular rhythm slower than 35; and regardless of rate, complete heart block is accompanied by a pathognomonic series of changes in quality and intensity of the first heart sound which are due to the changing intervals between auricular and ventricular systole.

Heart block of any degree is usually due to one of three causes. Digitalis is the commonest cause, particularly of delayed conduction. Diphtheria and rheumatic fever (rarely other infections) may cause heart block. Delayed conduction time is especially common in rheumatic fever (p. 46) and may be the only positive evidence of the disease. The third cause is chronic organic heart disease, particularly coronary arteriosclerosis and, less commonly, rheumatic valvular disease, hyperthyroidism, or syphilis.

Delayed conduction time and partial heart block need no specific treatment. Obviously, the underlying cause should be dealt with. Patients with chronic heart failure and partial heart block should be given digitalis very cautiously.

In contrast, complete heart block, although not necessarily incompatible with a long life and the performance of hard physical work, nevertheless is usually a serious condition because of the tendency to syncopal attacks (Adams-Stokes syndrome). At the onset of complete block, there may be a period of ventricular standstill before the idioventricular rhythm begins. Similar periods of ventricular asystole may follow changes in location of the ventricular pacemaker (with alteration of the subsequent rate), or they may occur without obvious cause. The pauses come without warning. The ensuing symptoms depend on their duration and may vary from a transient feeling of faintness through syncope and convulsions to death.

Treatment of complete heart block is directed toward prevention of ventricular standstill. The slow rate in complete block is not harmful, but the patient must be warned against exertion; for syncope may result from anoxia because the slow fixed heart rate limits the increase in cardiac output which is the normal response to exertion. When attacks of standstill occur several times a day (as may be the case in acute coronary occlusion), epinephrine hydrochloride, 0.3 to 0.5 cc. of 1:1,000 solution every two hours, may be lifesaving. In ambulatory patients, ephedrine sulfate, 25 mg. (3/8 grain) two or three times daily by mouth, is often effective. Sometimes barium chloride, 30 to 60 mg. three or four times daily by mouth, will prevent attacks when ephedrine will not. Quinidine is contraindicated. When attacks occur very infrequently, the problem of prevention is more difficult because of the need for continuous medication and the question of whether cessation of attacks is actually due to the drug.

FUNCTIONAL HEART DISEASE

The term "functional heart disease" has been applied to those cases in which symptoms referable to the heart are not accompanied by actual disease of that organ. In some such patients the symptoms may be referable to disturbances of rate or rhythm (see preceding pages) without evidence of structural change in the heart or, in fact, any bodily disease whatsoever. Obviously, the search for organic disease should be thorough.

In other patients, disturbances of rate or rhythm are either lacking altogether, or the symptoms are disproportionately severe in relation to the abnormalities found. In such cases the complaints are likely to be palpitation, weakness, faintness or giddiness, pain referred by the patient to the heart, shortness of breath, or some combination of these. Investigation usually discloses that the palpitation is not accompanied by changes in cardiac rhythm or more than slight acceleration in rate, the pain is not related to exertion, and the dyspnea is reported to occur at rest and during emotional stress rather than on exertion (the "dyspnea" commonly consists of a feeling of need for deeper respiration than the patient can accomplish; it is quite different from the dyspnea of cardiac failure or asthma).

In such patients the differential diagnosis usually lies between hyperthyroidism (p. 180), incipient tuberculosis (p. 12), and neurosis (p. 150). A special pattern of neurosis with cardiovascular manifestations is perhaps more common in armies than in civilian life and has been variously designated as neurocirculatory asthenia, soldier's heart, irritable heart, and D.A.H. (disordered action of the heart).

BACTERIAL ENDOCARDITIS

Acute bacterial endocarditis is usually secondary to some other disease, such as pneumonia, carbunculosis, puerperal sepsis, or gonorrhea, and is most commonly due to hemolytic streptococci, pneumococci, *Staphylococcus aureus*, or gonococci. The onset of endocarditis may be insidious or well defined. Initial manifestations may include chills and increase in fever, prostration, new heart murmurs, splenomegaly, leukocytosis, proteinuria, and sometimes microscopic or gross hematuria. Later, petechiae may appear, and there may be arterial occlusions in various organs. Treatment is that of the primary disease. The prognosis is generally unfavorable.

Subacute bacterial endocarditis is more common than the acute form and is generally due to *Streptococcus viridans*. Most cases occur in the presence of congenital anomaly of the heart or chronic valvular disease such as may follow rheumatic fever. Older children and young adults are the most common victims.

The onset is usually insidious, with fatigability and perhaps aches and pains. Sooner or later there is afternoon fever and possibly chills or sweats. Embolic phenomena may occur, anemia is usual, and often there is an associated glomerulonephritis (p. 218). Early in the disease it may be confused with tuberculosis, typhoid fever, undulant fever, or malaria, and it must be considered in the differential diagnosis of any case of obscure fever or obscure debilitating illness. The presence of congenital or valvular heart disease and the occurrence of petechiae and of transient tender areas in the pulp of the fingers and toes point toward endocarditis; positive blood cultures are conclusive.

Treatment—Although the eventual mortality rate is still high, it has been reduced from the previous figure of almost 100 percent by vigorous treatment with penicillin (p. 288). For best results, the sensitivity of the organism should be ascertained before antibiotic therapy is begun. The aim is then to maintain the blood level of penicillin above the lethal concentration as determined in vitro. The daily dosage may vary from 500,000 to several million units.

Eight weeks is a minimum period of administration. Because of variation in healing rate, some patients must be treated longer. The exact method of administration—intramuscular or intravenous, intermittently or by continuous drip—is immaterial. When relapses occur, they are usually within the first month and result from inadequate dosage or insufficient duration of treatment. The occurrence of heart failure or of cerebral hemorrhage or embolism is a poor prognostic indication. If patients survive one year, they usually remain well.

DISEASE OF THE PERICARDIUM

Pericarditis is usually due to rheumatic fever, pneumonia, tuberculosis, chronic glomerulonephritis, or coronary occlusion. It may also occur in the course of any severe systemic infection or as a terminal event in any chronic disease.

Acute Fibrinous Pericarditis is the commonest and mildest form, and the fibrinous exudate is the most prominent feature. Symptoms may be absent or confused with those of the primary disease. When they occur, the most frequent is precordial pain which may radiate to the neck or shoulder. If the diaphragm is involved, the pain may be abdominal. It may be sharp or stabbing and may be aggravated by change of position, deep breathing, or cough. Dyspnea or cough or both are occasional symptoms. The most distinctive physical finding is a friction rub, which may be felt or heard anywhere over the precordium or in the midback to the left of the vertebral column. It may vary greatly in character and intensity from hour to hour. Pericardial effusion may alter or abolish it. Treatment is directed toward the primary condition. An ice bag over the precordium sometimes relieves pain, but analgesics may be necessary.

Pericarditis with Effusion may be a sequel to fibrinous pericarditis. The volume of fluid may reach two liters, and it may be serofibrinous, purulent, or hemorrhagic. A hemorrhagic fluid suggests tuberculosis or malignancy. When the volume of fluid is sufficiently large, it impedes filling of the heart during diastole. Cardiac output is thus reduced, and dyspnea may result. Dyspnea and pain are the chief symptoms.

In pericarditis with effusion, the area of cardiac dullness is enlarged, and the area shifts with change of posture. A friction rub may or may not be present. X-ray findings are characteristic. In the presence of dyspnea, there are likely to be distention of the neck veins and evidence of compression of the lower lobe of the left lung. The pulse pressure is usually low and may fall almost to nothing on inspiratory effort (paradoxical pulse). Again, treatment is directed chiefly toward the primary condition; but if cardiac function is embarrassed, paracentesis should be performed as often as necessary. However, suspicion of *purulent* exudate should lead to immediate exploratory tap; and if pus is found, the pericardial sac should be drained surgically.

Chronic Adhesive Pericarditis usually develops as a sequel to acute pericarditis of rheumatic, pneumococcal, or tuberculous origin. Myocardial infarction may lead to localized adhesions. The heart is fixed in position, and filling may be greatly impeded. Heart failure is common. X-ray is of great diagnostic assistance.

Treatment is primarily directed toward conserving cardiac function (pp. 63 and 65) and relieving ascites. Some patients without ascites and with fair cardiac function are greatly helped by the Brauer operation.

Arterial Disease

ARTERIOSCLEROSIS

Arteriosclerosis is a chronic degenerative process of the arteries. The lesions have three components:

1. Atheroma, consisting of plaques of subintimal lipoid deposits which may later ulcerate and calcify. Atrophy of the media may follow.
2. Degeneration, loss of elastic tissue, and calcification of the media.
3. Thrombosis, arising principally from atheroma.

All three components may be present in the same artery, or one may predominate. The term "atherosclerosis" has been applied to the atheromatosis commonly found in the aorta and smaller arteries. "Diffuse arteriolar sclerosis" refers to a degeneration of the elastic and muscular coats of arterioles by which the vessel wall is weakened and may be subject to rupture and hemorrhage. It is a frequent accompaniment of hypertension. Mönckeberg described a type of sclerosis involving medium-sized arteries which was characterized by medial degeneration and calcification without atheroma. It is of little clinical importance.

The cause of arteriosclerosis is unknown. A certain amount of it appears to be a natural concomitant of the aging process, but there is evidence that some disturbance of lipid metabolism also plays a part.

The symptoms and signs caused by arteriosclerotic lesions represent a deficiency of blood flow to the organs or regions supplied by the arteries involved. They may develop suddenly or gradually. When extremities are affected, the patient complains of fatigue, numbness, paresthesias, cramps, pain, weakness, or coldness; finally, trophic ulcers and gangrene may develop. Arterial pulsation is diminished or absent. The skin is cool and its color is altered toward pallor or lividity, and sometimes there is atrophy. The sclerotic vessels may be visible on x-ray examination.

Arteriosclerosis of the brain is manifested by dizziness, syncope, impaired memory, slowed cerebration, and personality changes (see p. 157). Later there may be cerebral hemorrhage or thrombosis, or psychosis. When arteriosclerosis involves the heart, angina pectoris, acute coronary insufficiency, coronary occlusion, or valvular changes may occur. Loss of elasticity of the aorta and peripheral arteries may result in a mild elevation of systolic pressure with little change in diastolic (senile hypertension). The aorta may be the site of a dissecting aneurysm. Diffuse vascular disease of the kidneys is manifested by albuminuria, cylindruria, and impaired function.

Perhaps the best method of detecting early arteriosclerotic change is by the ophthalmoscope, for the retinal vessels are easily seen. Here the earliest sign, arterial narrowing, is found. Later the veins appear to be constricted where the arteries cross them (a-v nicking), and the arteries become tortuous.

Since arteriosclerosis is of such universal occurrence, the clinician must assess carefully the importance of its presence in each case. In the absence of signs and symptoms such as those mentioned above, the finding of arteriosclerotic vessels may be only incidental and of no clinical significance.

When arteriosclerosis results in atheromatosis which is severe enough to lead to progressive or episodic occlusion of arterial lumina, the term "arteriosclerosis obliterans" (or "occlusive arteriosclerosis") may be applied. Arteriosclerosis obliterans is responsible for most peripheral occlusive arterial disease (see p. 77). It tends to occur in men, but not exclusively (ratio of men to women, 5:1); it almost always has its onset after the age of forty; the upper extremities are rarely involved; thrombophlebitis is never a concomitant or antecedent event; calcification of the arteries, as shown by x-ray, is common, as are hypertension and diabetes mellitus; and blood cholesterol and total blood lipids are frequently elevated, particularly in younger patients.

The differential diagnosis is usually from thromboangiitis obliterans (see below). In the latter disease, in contrast to arteriosclerosis obliterans, men are almost exclusively attacked (ratio of men to women, 100:1); the onset is almost always before the age of fifty; the upper extremities are commonly involved; thrombophlebitis is frequent; the arteries are not calcified; hypertension and diabetes are rare in the early years of the disease; and blood lipids are usually normal.

Treatment—There is no present positive means of preventing, reversing, or even arresting the progress of arteriosclerosis. Iodides (p. 506) have long been prescribed in the hope that they would "soften the arteries." However, there is no good evidence that they do this. In those instances in which arteriosclerosis is causing symptoms, the physician can do no more than aid the patient to make the best of a damaged arterial circulation, as by relief of vasospasm and improvement of collateral circulatory channels.

Probably the greatest progress has been made in the symptomatic relief of arteriosclerosis obliterans. The same protective measures should be taken as in thromboangiitis obliterans (see below). A warm environment and plenty of rest are the key factors. The feet must be given scrupulous care (see under Diabetes Mellitus, p. 176). Obesity should be avoided or eliminated (p. 260). Diabetes mellitus should be brought under control (p. 174). Tobacco should be interdicted, even though it is not as important in arteriosclerosis as in thromboangiitis. Postural exercises, as in thromboangiitis obliterans, may possibly have value; other forms of passive vascular exercise are rarely helpful.

The treatment of peripheral arterial occlusion is discussed on page 78. Arteriosclerosis involving the heart is discussed under Angina Pectoris (p. 66) and Coronary Occlusion (p. 67).

THROMBOANGIITIS OBLITERANS

Thromboangiitis obliterans (Buerger's disease) is a progressive disease of the blood vessels which is characterized by the presence of numerous small inflammatory areas in the walls of arteries and veins, intimal proliferation, thrombosis, and subsequent partial recanalization. Though the extremities are most commonly affected, the disease may involve any part of the vascular system. In the early stages, reflex vasoconstriction may aggravate the circulatory impairment which is caused by structural changes. Thrombophlebitis occurs in about one-fourth the cases. In the terminal stages, infection of the extremities develops, along with chronic ulceration and gangrene. The lower limbs are most commonly affected. The disease is seen principally in young adult males.

The cause is unknown. Although smoking definitely aggravates the disease, thromboangiitis obliterans is seen in nonsmokers. The symptoms result from diminution of blood supply to the affected parts or from reflex disturbances of the collateral circulation. The prognosis depends upon the efficiency with which collateral circulation can be established. Early symptoms are vague, consisting usually of fatigue, coldness, numbness, or the appearance of painful areas of skin and subcutaneous tissue resembling superficial thrombophlebitis. Patients complain of indefinite pains in one foot or of the sudden onset of cramplike pains in the calf after exercise (intermittent claudication). As circulatory impairment progresses, the peripheral arterial pulses diminish and disappear. If the condition is not controlled, the patient will develop trophic disturbances of the extremities, ulceration, pain, color changes, and gangrene.

The diagnosis of early thromboangiitis obliterans is difficult because of the indefiniteness of the symptoms. In advanced cases the picture is usually characteristic. Differential diagnosis includes arteriosclerosis obliterans, diabetic arteritis, and Raynaud's syndrome. Distinction from arteriosclerosis obliterans is discussed under Arteriosclerosis, above. Diabetic arteritis is detected by appropriate laboratory studies for diabetes mellitus (p. 173). Raynaud's disease (p. 86) occurs more frequently in women, color changes are more definite, and the upper limbs are more commonly involved. Pain is usually less intense.

Treatment of thromboangiitis obliterans is not curative, but in some instances the rate of progress of the disease may be slowed. Unless the patient stops smoking completely, no form of therapy is of benefit. It is recommended, however, that the patient continue to smoke until (1) the diagnosis of thromboangiitis obliterans is irrefutably established, and (2) the patient has had time to realize, with the aid of the physician, that he has no choice if he is to be helped. The first time he stops smoking is the one most likely to succeed, and the physician should set the stage for success in every way possible.

Care of the feet is of utmost importance, and the same regimen should be employed as in diabetes mellitus (p. 176). During cold weather the patient should take particular care to keep his feet and lower legs warm. Tight garters are forbidden. Shoes must be fitted properly. Moderate exercise is permitted if the patient tolerates it.

Various forms of physical therapy may be of value. Postural exercises are recommended: The patient elevates his limb at a 45-degree angle for one or two minutes, then drops it over the side of the bed for a similar period; this sequence is continued for fifteen to twenty minutes at a time. Ultraviolet therapy, used empirically, is often of considerable benefit. Massage, in general, should be discouraged.

Passive vascular exercise with the pavex machine has been of some benefit in relieving pain and encouraging the development of collateral circulation. It is most useful in early cases. Periodic venous compression and oscillating beds may also be helpful.

In the early stages, measures to combat vasospasm may result in great improvement in the circulation and relief of symptoms. The most effective of these measures is sympathetic ganglionectomy. This formidable surgical procedure is undertaken only after preliminary sympathetic block (by the paravertebral, high spinal, or high caudal technic) has demonstrated a satisfactory degree of temporary improvement. The operation probably does not modify the eventual course of the disease; therefore, its possible symptomatic value must be balanced against its hazards.

Of the various drugs which produce vasodilation, papaverine hydrochloride (p. 363) is probably the most effective in thromboangiitis obliterans. In acute cases it may be given intravenously in doses of 0.065 Gm. or more every four hours until ten doses have been given. It may be administered by mouth in larger doses (see p. 364), either alone or together with a xanthine preparation (p. 358) and possibly a barbiturate (p. 390). Methacholine chloride (p. 417) is beneficial in some cases when administered by iontophoresis.

Typhoid vaccine (p. 336), given intravenously once or twice a week in amounts just inadequate to produce a chill, may be combined with other measures. The exact mechanism of improvement is unknown but may include vasodilation. Other nonspecific therapy which has been followed by symptomatic improvement includes intravenous administration of ether (10 to 20 cc. in 200 cc. of Isotonic Sodium Chloride Solution), sodium citrate (20 cc. of 12.5 percent solution), or hypertonic sodium chloride solution (250 to 300 cc. of 3 to 5 percent). One of these is given every other day in the acute stages, then twice weekly, and later once a week for an indefinite period.

PERIARTERITIS NODOSA

Periarteritis nodosa is a rare disease of uncertain etiology, characterized by widely disseminated necrotizing lesions of middle and small-caliber arteries and veins. Since similar lesions have been found in serum sickness and following the administration of sulfonamide drugs, it is thought that some form of hypersensitivity may be responsible.

Patients may succumb quickly to an acute fulminating form of the disease, or they may develop a more chronic type of illness and survive for years. Renal and cardiac insufficiency are common late eventualities.

Because the lesions may involve any organ of the body, the manifestations may take almost any form. The complex symptomatology, corresponding to no system disease, may itself suggest a correct diagnosis. If the characteristic blood-vessel lesions are found by muscle biopsy, the diagnosis may be established. The possibility of periarteritis nodosa must be considered in the case of any patient who presents the picture of an obscure febrile illness, nephritis, or cardiac disorder accompanied by unexplained findings such as anemia, anorexia, asthenia, myalgia, weight loss, precordial distress, hypertension, peripheral neuritis, or paresthesias.

Treatment—There is no specific treatment for periarteritis nodosa. Cortisone (p. 462) and adrenocorticotrophin (p. 473) have produced dramatic regression in some cases, but the eventual results are not known. Since the disease is thought to be of allergic origin, administration of antihistaminic drugs and careful search for an allergen may be carried out. It is likely, however, that by the time the diagnosis is established, the disease process will have become irreversible or, at least, unresponsive to conventional desensitization technics. Papaverine

hydrochloride, 0.03 to 0.06 Gm. orally every four to six hours, may be useful as a vasodilator for the relief of peripheral arterial spasm.

ARTERIAL OCCLUSION

Arterial occlusion may result from either embolism or thrombosis. The consequences depend on the location and distribution of the artery, the state of the collateral circulation, and the treatment. Coronary and pulmonary occlusion are discussed elsewhere (see pp. 67 and 119).

Emboli lodging in a peripheral artery originate in the left side of the heart or, rarely, in the arterial tree proximal to the site of occlusion. The most common cardiac origin is the left auricle during chronic auricular fibrillation. Sometimes dislodgment does not occur until normal rhythm is restored, as by quinidine therapy. Emboli may also arise from mural thrombi in the left ventricle, usually during the second or third week following a myocardial infarction which has reached the endocardium. Thrombi may separate from diseased mitral or aortic valves during the course of endocarditis. Emboli consisting of groups of malignant cells may stimulate local thrombosis.

Because of the effective collateral circulation in most parts of the body, peripheral arterial embolism may in some instances remain silent. Commonly, however, the embolus proves irritating to the arterial wall, and there is spasm of the involved artery and reflexly of the collateral circulation as well. It is this collateral vasospasm that is largely responsible for the symptoms.

Arterial thrombosis *in situ* is the result of injury or disease affecting the local endothelium or the coagulability of the blood or both. Common causes are thromboangiitis obliterans (p. 76), arteriosclerosis obliterans (p. 75), periarteritis nodosa (see above), localized arteritis secondary to systemic bacterial infection, trauma of various kinds (including pressure on the vessel), and conditions leading to increased coagulability of the blood. Sometimes no cause can be discovered. In thrombosis, as in embolism, it is commonly the collateral vasospasm that leads to symptoms except when the thrombosis is extensive enough of itself to block a considerable fraction of the collateral circulation.

The symptoms of arterial occlusion are extremely variable, and unless the physician is aware of the possibility, the diagnosis may be overlooked. Even when the occlusion itself is sudden, the onset of symptoms may be insidious. Pain is the initial symptom in only about half the cases. In others the first thing noted may be numbness (with or without tingling), coldness, cramps, pallor, burning, or even itching. Sudden severe pain, pallor, and coldness distal to the occlusion are the classic manifestations. However, any of the symptoms listed may appear in any order and to any degree.

The most important diagnostic sign is absence of pulsation in some of the arteries of an extremity in which pulsations were previously present. The arterial pulses should be routinely checked in any patient who complains of distress referable to an extremity. It is also wise to examine and record for reference purposes the state of the arterial pulsations in the extremities of any individual whose condition predisposes him to arterial occlusion. If an absence of previously present pulsations is accompanied by unusual local pallor and reduction of surface temperature, the diagnosis of arterial occlusion is certain. Other manifestations may include hyperesthesia, anesthesia, and muscular weakness.

The outcome of arterial occlusion depends on the suddenness of occlusion, the location and distribution of the artery, the presence or absence of previous vascular disease, and the amount and duration of collateral vasospasm. If local anoxia is too great in degree or duration, the vascular endothelium is damaged, and widespread thrombosis may follow later restoration of the circulation. In the absence of treatment, the main symptoms persist one to three days. The patient may then recover, or, if endothelial or tissue damage has been too great, gangrene sets in. In case of recovery, vasomotor symptoms may persist, as following injury due to cold (see p. 273).

Treatment is of the utmost importance in determining the outcome. For this reason, early suspicion and diagnosis are essential. If the signs point to a large embolus at an accessible location, immediate embolectomy may be undertaken. If this is not the case, pain is relieved by the administration of morphine or an analogue (p. 399). At the same time, measures are taken to relieve arterial spasm. The patient is placed in a warm room (85° to 90°F.), and warm packs are applied to all the extremities *except* those involved. Papaverine hydrochloride (p. 363) is given slowly by vein; if 0.13 Gm. (2 grains) is not effective, there is no point in giving more. Alcohol by mouth promotes vasodilation, and the quantity should be liberal.

The involved extremity is wrapped loosely in cotton to conserve the natural warmth, and it may be placed in a cradle with one or two lights. *The temperature of the air about the limb should never exceed 92°F., and the limb should never be elevated.* In fact, the head of the bed should be elevated if a leg is involved, and the patient should assume a semisitting posture in the case of an arm. The Sanders oscillating bed may be used if it is available; it is set for maximal low foot and minimal low head positions.

To prevent extension of thrombus formation, anticoagulant therapy with heparin or Dicumarol should be instituted promptly (p. 374).

To achieve maximum vasodilation, sympathetic block has been employed. This is most easily accomplished by high spinal or epidural anesthesia for the legs and abdominal viscera, by brachial plexus block for the arms, and by stellate ganglion block for the head. Its precise role has not yet been established. The anesthesia obtained may obviate the need for opiates. The availability of continuous technics makes possible continuation of the block for several days.

If immediate embolectomy was either not indicated or not feasible, if subsequent medical treatment is not effective in greatly improving the circulation in six to twelve hours, and if there is still a reasonable chance to save a limb, the possibility of embolectomy should again be considered.

Disturbances of Arterial Pressure

The arterial tree is essentially a branched tubular elastic conduit with a pump (the heart) at one end and a series of small faucets (the arterioles) at the other. Through the conduit flows a somewhat viscous suspension (the blood). When the blood is moving, its pressure and velocity are determined by the laws of hydrodynamics, which are extremely complicated as they apply to branched elastic pipes. When it is stopped, as proximal to an inflated blood-pressure cuff, the laws of hydrostatics apply. Other factors remaining constant, the pressure of the blood in the arterial tree is determined by the balance between force of contraction of the left cardiac ventricle and peripheral resistance, which for the most part resides in the arterioles. Additional factors of less importance in determining blood pressure are the viscosity of the blood, the elasticity of the arterial walls, and, under certain circumstances, the total blood volume.

The cardiac output of blood (aortic input) is intermittent, whereas the peripheral outflow is continuous. The volume of blood in the arterial tree (and consequently the intra-arterial pressure) at a given point therefore reaches a maximum immediately after cardiac systole and a minimum at the end of cardiac diastole; hence the terms "systolic" and "diastolic" for the maximum and minimum points of the cycle of arterial pressure. (Obviously, the phases of the cycle require time to pass peripherally from the ascending aorta.) The difference between the maximum and minimum pressures is termed the "pulse pressure" because without such a difference the arteries would not pulsate.

Pulse pressure is influenced by the elasticity of the arterial walls; but in a given individual over a period of days or weeks, variations in pulse pressure are determined principally by cardiac stroke volume (the quantity of blood expelled from the left ventricle during each contraction). Total cardiac output (minute volume) is the product of stroke volume and heart rate; and, correspondingly, the product of pulse pressure and pulse rate can be used as an index to, but not an exact measure of, cardiac output.

Normally, cardiac output is adjusted to tissue needs by a series of complex mechanisms. If cardiac output increases, either pulse rate or stroke volume (pulse pressure) or both must increase, or one must increase sufficiently to compensate for any decrease in the other. When the pulse rate remains constant during changes in cardiac output, the necessary alteration in pulse pressure is accomplished by a change in systolic pressure; diastolic is little affected. If cardiac output is to remain constant, any change in heart rate must be balanced by an opposite change in pulse pressure. Such a change in pulse pressure is accomplished by alteration of the diastolic pressure; the systolic remains almost constant. Changes in peripheral resistance are reflected mainly in the diastolic pressure, but the systolic changes also in the same direction as the diastolic.

Human arterial blood pressure is ordinarily measured in the left brachial artery with the subject comfortably seated. There is often a variable and unpredictable difference between the readings in the two arms. The use of standard equipment, technic, and precautions will minimize variations of extraneous origin. The joint recommendations of the American Heart Association and the Cardiac Society of Great Britain and Ireland were published in the *American Heart Journal, 18:*95, 1939.

Opinions differ as to the limits of the normal range of human blood pressure. In resting adults, anything between 90 and 120 mm. Hg systolic and 60 and 80 diastolic must be considered normal. Pressures between 120/80 and 140/90 are possibly abnormal; pressures of 140/90 to 150/100 are prob-

ably abnormal; and any figure over 150/100 is certainly abnormal. Pressures below 90/60 are not necessarily abnormal if the circulation is adequate. Within the normal range, the diastolic pressure is usually about two-thirds the systolic. Outside the normal range, the ratio does not hold. Average readings in children increase from 80 systolic at the age of one month to 105 at twelve years.

The blood pressure as determined in the femoral artery is normally much higher than that in the brachial artery. This difference is probably due to hydrodynamic factors, the chief of which may be the relatively large mass of blood in the aorta and iliac artery proximal to the site of blood pressure determination. In a series of comparative readings, Wendkos and Rossman found that in healthy young men the blood pressure in the thigh, as determined by the standard cuff technic but with the subject lying down, averaged 155/92 as against 118/71 in in the arm. The readings in both thigh and arm appeared to be elevated by increase in thickness of the limb.

Statistically, the blood pressure rises slightly but progressively with age. It seems probable that such a rise is not a normal phenomenon but results from the inclusion in the data of cases of unrecognized mild hypertension. On the average, women have a somewhat lower (average, 5 mm. Hg) blood pressure than men prior to the menopause; after the menopause, the blood pressure of women averages slightly greater than that of men. Obesity is associated with a small elevation (7 to 8 mm. Hg), as is a broad build in contrast to a slender build.

Both systolic and diastolic pressures vary with the phases of respiration, falling during inspiration and rising during expiration. These cyclic changes are due to similar variations in diastolic filling of the left ventricle secondary to changes in pulmonary venous pressure which are in turn caused by alterations in capacity of the pulmonary vessels incident to expansion and contraction of the lungs during respiration.

Posture has a small but definite effect on brachial blood pressure. The diastolic pressure is lowest during recumbency, higher in the sitting posture, and highest when the subject stands. The systolic pressure usually changes in the same direction but to a less extent, with the result that pulse pressure is less in the erect than in the recumbent posture. Individuals whose blood pressure is habitually low may have a fall rather than a rise in systolic pressure when standing.

Strong emotional influences lead to rises in systolic pressure which may be very great. Release of epinephrine from the adrenal medulla is often a factor. Restful sleep causes a fall of 15 to 30 mm. in systolic pressure during the first hour, after which there is a gradual rise to waking levels. On the other hand, disturbed sleep with dreams of motor activity may be accompanied by extreme rises in pressure.

Exercise or even the immediate contemplation of exercise initiates a rise in blood pressure corresponding to the extent of exertion. Mild exercise may cause an elevation of a few millimeters limited to the systolic pressure. Strenuous effort may be associated with pressures of 180 to 200 systolic and 100 to 110 diastolic. Immediately after cessation of exercise the pressure falls to normal or below (probably because of a shift in venous reservoirs) and then rises rapidly to the previous level, from which it declines to normal over a period of less than five minutes in healthy individuals at ordinary altitudes. At high altitudes the decline is slower.

In contrast to the peripheral blood pressure as measured in the conventional manner, the normal mean arterial pressure (average of systolic and diastolic pressures) in the pulmonary artery is apparently 18 to 20 mm. Hg. This pressure falls during ordinary inspiration and rises during expiration. The resistance of the pulmonary vascular bed is relatively low. When it is increased—as in pulmonary emphysema or mitral stenosis or during an attack of asthma—pulmonary arterial pressure rises. When such an increased pressure is due to bronchoconstriction (asthma), it is greatly reduced by the xanthine drugs (p. 358).

HYPERTENSION

Hypertension may be defined as a persistent elevation of the arterial blood pressure above the accepted range of normal. Abnormal elevation of the systemic blood pressure is associated with many different diseases (see Table 9) and undoubtedly may be produced through a number of different mechanisms. Thus, high blood pressure is not a disease entity but rather a physical sign of disorder affecting the vascular system.

Hypertension may be established and maintained by one or more of three types of mechanism: mechanical, neural, and humoral. The mechanical is exemplified by coarctation of the aorta (Table 9, II E), in which a high arterial pressure is required to push an adequate blood supply through the tortuous compensatory channels to the tissues below the level of the coarctation. The neural mechanism operates through stimulation of the vaso-

TABLE 9 — *Common Types of Hypertension*

I. Essential hypertension
II. Hypertension secondary to
  A. Renal disease
    1. Glomerulonephritis (p. 218)
    2. Pyelonephritis (p. 221)
    3. Polycystic disease
  B. Toxemia of pregnancy (p. 212)
  C. Oversupply of adrenocortical steroids (p. 462)
    1. Hyperadrenalism
    2. Cushing's syndrome
    3. Adrenal cortical tumors
    4. Therapeutic overdosage
  D. Oversupply of epinephrine from adrenal medulla
    1. Pheochromocytoma
  E. Coarctation of the aorta
  F. Periarteritis nodosa (p. 77)
  G. Increased intracranial pressure

motor center; the humoral, through vasoconstrictor substances which circulate in the blood and act directly on the arteriolar musculature.

A number of different vasoconstrictor substances have been found in the blood in certain types of human hypertension and in experimental hypertension in animals. Their relationship to clinical disease is still controversial. One of these humoral mechanisms which has been well studied operates in the hypertension that occurs in the dog following constriction of a kidney or partial occlusion of a renal artery. It has also been found in the blood of patients with hypertension due to chronic glomerulonephritis and pyelonephritis. It involves three substances: (1) renin substrate (hypertensinogen), an alpha$_2$ globulin which is produced in the liver and which is constantly circulating in the blood under normal conditions; (2) renin, a proteolytic enzyme of great specificity which is formed in the cells of the renal tubules and which is released from them when renal circulation is impaired; and (3) angiotonin (hypertensin), a polypeptide which is released from renin substrate in the blood by the action of the enzyme renin. Angiotonin causes generalized arteriolar constriction and, at the same time, a more forceful beating of the heart. These two factors act together to increase arterial pressure without significantly altering peripheral blood flow. Renal blood flow may, however, be reduced.

A renal pressor system such as the foregoing is very possibly the mechanism (humoral) of hypertension in chronic primary renal disease (Table 9, II A). In pheochromocytoma (Table 9, II D 1), the epinephrine is a humoral agent which constricts the arterioles by direct action.

Increased intracranial pressure (Table 9, II G) increases intracranial resistance to blood flow and may result in cerebral hypoxia involving the vasomotor center. The hypoxia stimulates the center to produce generalized vasoconstriction and hypertension (a compensatory neural mechanism).

The mechanism of hypertension in toxemia of pregnancy (Table 9, II B) has not been established; however, the final step is apparently neural, for the hypertension is promptly abolished by extensive sympathetic nerve block (see p. 440).

The means by which the adrenocortical steroids produce hypertension is unknown, as is the mechanism in periarteritis nodosa.

Essential Hypertension (primary hypertension, hyperpiesia) constitutes 80 to 85 percent of all cases exhibiting hypertension. It is the most common lethal disease of adult life. Essential hypertension probably does not arise in any case from a single cause but rather from the interaction of a number of factors, the importance of each of which may vary from one patient to another. Hereditary, endocrine, emotional, and possibly other types of factors are concerned. It has been shown that many patients with essential hypertension are chronically inhibited in their expression of aggressiveness and self-assertion, and it is believed that in such patients the frustration may be the trigger factor in the genesis of hypertension.

In early hypertension, the body changes are entirely functional and apparently reversible. At first there may be no more than an exaggerated response of the systemic blood pressure to ordinary stimuli. This hyperreactivity may be present from early life and for many years before clinical hypertension can be demonstrated. It is possibly inherited and may be considered a constitutional predisposition which may or may not be followed by clinical hypertension.

As time goes on, the blood pressure may persist at an elevated level for hours or days after removal of the stimulus, and the individual will have intermittent periods of hypertension. Eventually the elevation of blood pressure may become permanent, especially in those who are overweight and exhibit tachycardia. At this stage, there are still no organic changes.

Peripheral blood flow is normal in early essential hypertension. This can be true only if there is an increase in both peripheral resistance (believed in essential hypertension to be due to arteriolar spasm) and the force of myocardial contraction. There is some question as to which of these two factors is primary and which compensatory in elevating the blood pressure.

The dynamic factors which normally control arterial pressure continue to act in hypertension, and they may lead to considerable variation in the level of blood pressure—a variation which is not directly related to changes in the underlying disease process. The exact level of blood pressure is not a reliable index to the severity of the disease.

Symptoms are usually absent in early hypertension. When they occur, they are generally indicative of vasomotor instability; typical are dizziness, flushing, and cold extremities. Headache of a bursting or constricting nature may be present. Nosebleeds may occur. Neurotic manifestations of underlying emotional conflict may be prominent (see p. 150). Generally there is no relationship between the severity of the symptoms and the degree of hypertension.

As the disease progresses, organic changes are superimposed on the spasm in the arterioles. First, there is hypertrophy of the arteriolar muscle. Later, this muscle degenerates and is eventually replaced by tough fibrous tissue. It is the ischemia produced in various organs by this arteriolar sclerosis that is responsible for the symptoms and signs of advanced hypertensive disease. The organs most seriously affected are usually the heart, brain, and kidneys.

The systolic pressure in established hypertension ranges from 150 to 300 mm. Hg or more; the diastolic, from 90 to 180. Readings vary greatly among different individuals and at different times in the same individual. Repeated measurements must often be made before the customary levels for a given patient are discovered, uninfluenced by excitement, exertion, or fatigue. The systolic level is far less important than the diastolic in connection with damage to heart, arteries, and kidneys. A change of a few millimeters in the level of diastolic pressure is of more significance than several times that much change in systolic level. It is to be emphasized that this statement applies to levels and not to isolated readings.

Hypertension affects the heart directly in two ways: by imposing an increased work load on the left ventricle, and, later, by impairing the blood supply through coronary arteriolar sclerosis. Hypertrophy of the left ventricle (demonstrable by x-ray before it is evident on physical examination) is the first clinically recognizable effect of hypertension on the heart. Such hypertrophy may be present for years, however, without giving rise to symptoms. As the heart size increases and the left ventricle and aorta dilate because of the excessive pressure, apical and aortic systolic murmurs may appear. In still more advanced cases, an aortic diastolic murmur indicative of aortic insufficiency may be heard. Gallop rhythm is a frequent and serious indication of cardiac dilatation and failure.

The electrocardiogram in hypertensive heart disease frequently shows left axis deviation. Other abnormalities include left bundle-branch block, a low or inverted T_1 or T_2 wave, and alterations in the ST segments.

In the presence of hypertensive heart disease, the blood pressure generally remains high. Sometimes, however, it may fall to normal or nearly normal levels because of spontaneous remission, heart failure, coronary occlusion, or general vasomotor collapse. In such cases the diastolic pressure may be maintained at a somewhat high level even though the systolic has fallen to 150 or less.

When cardiac symptoms arise in the course of hypertensive heart disease, they are usually those of heart failure which is due to inability of the left ventricle to maintain against the increased arterial pressure an output of blood adequate for tissue needs. Heart failure may be precipitated by the complications of auricular fibrillation or flutter, coronary occlusion, or relative myocardial ischemia. When heart failure results from relative myocardial ischemia, the onset may be very gradual. The most common early symptoms are fatigability and dyspnea. The latter may take the form of breathlessness on exertion or of paroxysms occurring during rest (paroxysmal nocturnal dyspnea, cardiac asthma). Precordial aching or oppression, palpitation, and arrhythmias are found in more advanced failure. For a general discussion of heart failure and its treatment, see Organic Heart Disease and Heart Failure, pages 62 and 63.

About one-third of cases of hypertension develop cerebral complications, which most often terminate as hemorrhage into the internal capsule (see Apoplexy, p. 169). Preceding the final disaster, minor strokes (due possibly to minute hemorrhages or thrombosis of small vessels) are common. These may be manifested only by such indefinite symptoms as increased irritability, forgetfulness, tinnitus, dizziness, fatigue, paresthesias, or anxiety states. There may be brief episodes of minor aphasias, pareses, or speech disorders. In some instances there may be convulsive seizures which are followed by hours or days of clouded consciousness.

Perhaps the most common manifestation of vascular encephalopathy in hypertension is headache. Typically, it occurs during the night or early morning while the patient is in bed, often increasing in severity over a period of hours. It may become intolerable. The headache is usually occipital, but it may have a hemicranial distribution, resembling migraine.

Examination of the eye grounds is especially important in hypertension for two reasons. The reactions and state of the retinal vessels are believed to parallel closely those of the cerebral vessels; and the retinal arterioles are the only ones which can be observed directly in the living, intact patient. The retinal vessels are therefore believed to afford a clue to the state of the cerebral vessels and, to a much less extent, of the arterioles in general. The earliest characteristic sign of hypertensive vascular disease is reduction in caliber of the retinal arterioles and irregularities in their light streak (the shiny reflection which extends along the center of the arteriole). Later, the arterioles become copper-colored and tortuous, the light streak disappears, and the veins are indented at the points of crossing. There may be hemorrhages and lipoid degeneration of the retina and, finally, edema of the optic disk. However, retinal vascular changes alone are not a sure indication of either the tempo or severity of hypertensive disease.

Disturbances of vision are common in the course of hypertensive disease. There may be blurring or sudden loss of vision in one or both eyes. The blindness may be permanent, but more often it is only transitory.

Structural changes are usually present in the small arteries and arterioles of the kidneys in patients who die in the course of hypertensive disease. These vascular changes may not be accompanied by any clinical manifestations, but usually the urine concentration test (p. 520) will reveal impairment of tubular reabsorptive power. Functional insufficiency is likely to occur much earlier in the heart or brain than in the kidneys, and death from renal insufficiency is rare except in the rapidly progressive, acute phase of the condition known as malignant hypertension. Further discussion will be found under Nephrosclerosis (p. 221).

Nocturia is a common symptom throughout the course of hypertension. Very early, the total nocturnal urine volume is not increased, and the nocturnal frequency is believed to be no more than an indication of emotional tension. Later, nocturia with increased volume may be due to loss of reabsorptive power in the renal tubules.

Hypertension, even of extreme degree, may be present for years without producing symptoms or disability. The prognosis is necessarily poor only when there is a well-established associated cardiac or renal disease. In general, the younger the patient when hypertension develops, the more likely he is to succumb early to the disease. Conversely, hypertension which begins in old age is usually not serious unless coronary disease or cerebral arteriosclerosis complicates the condition. A persistently high diastolic pressure, cardiac arrhythmia, paroxysmal nocturnal dyspnea, and cardiac failure are unfavorable signs. Most hypertensive patients die of heart failure; cerebral hemorrhage, coronary insufficiency or occlusion, and renal insufficiency are, in that order, the next most common causes of death. It should be emphasized that the natural course of essential hypertension is extremely variable and unpredictable. Therefore, hope and effort should never be abandoned, although, on the other hand, an unqualifiedly optimistic prognosis should be avoided.

Malignant Hypertension (malignant nephrosclerosis) is not a separate entity but a severe degree of essential hypertension with a rapidly fatal course. Its chief characteristics are a diastolic pressure of 140 or higher, headaches, visual impairments, abnormal eye grounds, proteinuria, hematuria, and terminal uremia or cardiac failure.

Diagnosis—A single elevated blood-pressure reading does not justify a diagnosis of hypertension. Repeated determinations must be made with the patient in a relaxed, resting state to rule out the effects of exercise and emotion. If high readings are obtained intermittently, the possibility of pheochromocytoma or the early stages of essential hypertension should be considered. In the presence of a blood pressure more or less fixed at a high level, the causes of secondary hypertension (Table 9, p. 80) should be investigated before it is concluded that the hypertension is primary, or essential. In addition, the patient as a whole may have to be studied for a considerable period before the diagnosis of essential hypertension can be made with a reasonable degree of certainty.

Some patients with organic heart disease whose blood pressures have previously remained within normal limits may develop slight elevations (such as 160/100) when congestive failure sets in. On restoration of compensation, the blood pressure returns to normal. Such elevations are believed to be related to increase in blood volume (see Heart Failure, p. 63) and are not indicative of true hypertension. Likewise, the increased blood flow which occurs in hyperthyroidism and in the presence of a large arteriovenous fistula leads to an elevation of systolic pressure and frequently a lowering of diastolic pressure. These changes are compensatory (see p. 79) and do not constitute hypertension.

It should be emphasized that the diastolic pressure is much more important than the systolic in evaluating the presence and significance of hypertension. Many patients with sclerosis of the larger arteries have a high systolic pressure but only a slight elevation of diastolic pressure. The systolic elevation in such patients is due to loss of elasticity of the arterial tree and is not of great significance.

Treatment—In secondary hypertension, the treatment is that of the underlying disease. In essential hypertension, therapy is difficult and frequently unsatisfactory, if only because the fundamental etiology is unknown. However, it seems certain that conscientious management and unflagging effort along the lines discussed below will in many cases slow the progress of the disease, lead to significant and prolonged improvement, or even, if the disease is recognized early enough, cause its disappearance. It is obviously of the utmost importance to begin treatment before the hypertension is fixed or irreversible organic changes have taken place.

Even though the underlying cause of essential hypertension cannot yet be reached, two important contributing factors may be susceptible of control: emotional tension and obesity. Emotional tension should be managed according to the principles outlined beginning on page 151. External contributing emotional factors, such as domestic or financial difficulties, are easier to discover and deal with than are internal factors. The physician should be constantly alert for indications of the extent and depth of internal emotional conflicts, particularly as to inhibition of self-assertive impulses. (Emotional conflicts are discussed further under Anxiety, p. 149, and The Neuroses, p. 150.) Younger patients with evidence of deep emotional conflicts who are in the early, potentially reversible stages of hypertension may be greatly helped or, occasionally, cured by psychoanalysis or a comparable form of psychotherapy. In most patients, tension can be substantially reduced by explanation, reassurance, redirection of interests and activities, and other psychotherapeutic measures which are available to any physician who is sufficiently interested and will give the necessary time.

Excessive weight of itself appears to cause a certain elevation of blood pressure. In addition, it increases the work of the heart. In overweight persons, resting cardiac work may be greatly reduced by weight loss. The treatment of obesity is discussed on page 260. Particularly in the presence of hypertension, drug and endocrine therapy of obesity are undesirable and may be dangerous because the drugs employed tend to increase nervous tension, the work of the heart, or even the blood pressure itself.

Apart from control of obesity and specific emotional factors, the patient may be greatly benefited by the maintenance under close supervision of the many aspects of personal hygiene that contribute to well-being. Both the hours and the intensity of work should be reduced. The patient should spend nine or ten hours in bed each night and take an hour's rest in the horizontal position before or after lunch. A program of leisure should be established, with frequent vacations of a week end or longer. Ordinary noncompetitive exercise is usually well tolerated in uncomplicated hypertension. Tobacco should be entirely abandoned because it tends to produce arteriolar constriction. Coffee, tea, and alcohol in moderation are not harmful.

The role of diet in hypertension (other than for weight reduction) is highly controversial. The low-protein diet which was advocated at one time now appears to have no sound basis. The protein content of the diet should probably be normal (see p. 259). Certain hypertensive patients with evidence of sodium retention may improve both symptomatically and in blood pressure levels on a very low sodium diet (0.5 Gm. per day or less; see p. 585). The beneficial effects can often be augmented by concomitant use of mercurial diuretics. The regimen must be employed judiciously to avoid sodium depletion (p. 342). However, even the low-sodium diet alone should not be continued more than three to four months in the absence of improvement; for it is unpalatable and difficult to prepare, and when it is rigid enough to be beneficial, it carries the danger of sodium depletion if the patient is not watched closely.

Much interest has been aroused by the rice diet originated by Kempner. There is a growing body of opinion that the important feature of the rice diet is its low sodium content and that, as a diet, it has the same value and disadvantages as other types of low-sodium diets.

Mild sedation is often valuable in helping to allay tension and anxiety. Many drugs are suitable (see p. 390). Barbiturates such as 'Amytal' or phenobarbital may be employed in doses of 15 to 30 mg. (1/4 to 1/2 grain) with meals and at bedtime. A short-acting barbiturate such as 'Seconal

Sodium' may be added at bedtime if insomnia is a problem.

Potassium thiocyanate is of great value in many cases because of the symptomatic relief it affords, particularly of hypertensive headache. The drug must be used carefully, however, and it frequently has no significant effect on the level of blood pressure. Further discussion and details of administration will be found on page 512.

When essential hypertension does not respond to the measures outlined above, the operation of sympathectomy should be considered. Sympathectomy is not a cure for hypertension; it does not remove the cause or arrest the progress of the disease. However, in many cases it gives a great measure of symptomatic relief. Patients must be carefully selected for operation. No test has yet been found which will differentiate satisfactorily between those patients who do and those who do not benefit by the operation. It has been observed, however, that favorable response is most common in patients with labile blood pressure as determined by frequent readings at rest and after barbiturates or high sympathetic block (high spinal anesthesia). Patients under the age of fifty usually respond better than do those who are older.

In favorable cases, sympathectomy is followed by relief of headache and cardiac symptoms out of all proportion to the hypotensive effect. However, the operation is always a major one, and convalescence is long. Postoperative complications may include postural hypotension (p. 85), vasomotor imbalance, and impotence in men.

Prompt sympathectomy should be urged for patients with early malignant hypertension. Even though the effect is only palliative, symptomatic improvement may be very great while it lasts, and other forms of treatment are usually ineffective.

Vasodilators have been employed for many years in the treatment of hypertension. Their use appears to have no sound basis, and they are seldom effective. The entity hypertension is called by that name only because elevation of the arterial blood pressure is the most easily demonstrable feature. Actually, the elevated blood pressure appears to be a derivative and resultant manifestation rather than an underlying factor, and in many patients a forcible direct reduction of blood pressure level initiates symptoms or aggravates those already present. Of the vasodilators, the nitrites (p. 364) have the greatest effect on the blood pressure in hypertension. Their use is generally unsatisfactory, and they have the disadvantage of relatively short duration and induction of headache and more serious side-effects. Equally unsatisfactory in hypertension are the xanthines (theophylline, aminophylline, theobromine, and related compounds marketed under many names), tetraethylammonium compounds (p. 433), methacholine (p. 417), aconite, histamine, Priscoline, veratrum viride, extracts and concentrates of garlic and parsley, and pyrogenic substances.

HYPOTENSION

Hypotension, like hypertension, is a clinical sign rather than a disease entity. Actually, when the blood pressure is low, the level of pressure is far less important than the rate of blood flow. Symptoms occur in association with low blood pressure only when blood flow is inadequate.

Hypotension may be secondary to many other conditions. Acute hypotension occurs during primary or secondary shock and following extensive blood loss. Hypotension is common in the course of and during convalescence from any debilitating disease such as rheumatoid arthritis, tuberculosis, chronic anemia, and severe infections. It may also accompany chronic malnutrition from any cause. Hypotension is an important diagnostic criterion of adrenocortical insufficiency (Addison's disease, p. 183). Persistent systolic pressures below 80 mm. Hg should lead to investigation of such a possibility. Hypotension may also be observed as a result of extensive myocardial degeneration following coronary occlusion. It is sometimes observed in myxedema or severe hypothyroidism.

Postural (Orthostatic) Hypotension is an entity in which assumption of the erect posture is regularly followed by a sharp drop in both systolic and diastolic blood pressures with a reduction in cerebral blood flow sufficient to induce weakness or fainting. Postural hypotension may be a feature of organic disease of the central nervous system affecting the spinal cord (such as tabes dorsalis), or it may occur without known cause.

In those cases not secondary to organic disease, other abnormalities are also generally found: (1) failure of the pulse rate to undergo the acceleration which normally accompanies assumption of the erect posture (in some cases, however, there may be an exaggerated acceleration [orthostatic tachycardia]); (2) deficient localized or generalized sweating; (3) greater urine secretion during recumbency than while erect; and (4) accentuation of symptoms in hot weather. Other manifestations sometimes encountered include (1) a more

youthful appearance than average for the chronological age; (2) pallor; (3) impotence and loss of libido; and (4) a blood nonprotein nitrogen level at the upper limit of normal.

The fundamental defect in primary postural hypotension seems to be a lack of responsiveness of the autonomic nervous system involving both sympathetic and parasympathetic branches. The diminution in blood flow and fall in blood pressure are due to failure of vasomotor response of the splanchnic blood vessels to the shift in the venous blood pool which occurs on change of posture. It is the veins and venules rather than the arterioles which are involved. When the patient rises, there is a pooling of blood in the splanchnic veins in the absence of splanchnic venoconstriction, and cardiac filling is drastically reduced. Postural hypotension is not a progressive condition, and it has no consequences other than those described above.

Treatment—Hypotension that is secondary to an underlying condition needs no treatment; it is the cause which should be attacked. Asymptomatic hypotension with adequate circulation cannot be considered a disease and should not be treated.

In postural hypotension, those symptoms due to lack of vasomotor control can usually be prevented by administration of a vasoconstrictor drug which acts on venules and veins as well as arterioles. Ephedrine sulfate or hydrochloride is usually satisfactory in oral doses of 25 to 50 mg. every two to four hours, beginning an hour before rising and continuing for the period of physical activity. Other systemic vasoconstrictor drugs may also be effective (p. 362). Wakefulness and other side-effects may be combated by barbiturates (p. 390) and by giving the last daily dose of vasoconstrictor not later than 4 or 5 p.m. The other manifestations cannot be successfully treated.

Vasomotor Disturbances

The over-all resistance to blood flow and the relative flow to different areas are controlled by the degree of constriction of the smooth muscle in the walls of the arterioles in the vascular bed as a whole and in the various regions of the body. This vasomotor control is exercised through the sympathetic nervous system by means of impulses originating in (1) the vasomotor center in the floor of the fourth ventricle of the brain, and (2) local and regional reflexes. Such regional reflexes are responsible for the local vasospasm and resulting circulatory disturbances in arterial occlusion (pp. 77

and 67), thrombophlebitis (p. 87), injury due to cold (p. 273) or following trauma, and peripheral arterial disease (p. 74). Vasomotor disturbance is, then, a factor in disability from the above conditions. Vasomotor disturbance is the principal manifestation in Raynaud's disease, the only syndrome discussed in this subsection.

RAYNAUD'S DISEASE

Raynaud's disease is a condition in which the fingers, occasionally the toes, and rarely the ears and nose undergo specific attacks of vascular spasm in response to cold or apprehension. During an attack, the fingers are pale or livid, cold, and numb. After a period which may vary from a few minutes to an hour, the spasm relaxes and compensatory hyperemia sets in, with local flushing and sensations of heat and burning. The underlying factor is believed to be a psychosomatic disturbance involving (1) chronic partial local vasospasm and (2) extreme sensitivity to cold and anxiety as stimuli to extreme angiospasm.

The anoxia of repeated attacks injures the vascular endothelium, setting up a nonspecific endarteritis which slows blood flow still further and may lead to small areas of thrombosis and tissue necrosis in the fingers. Skin changes secondary to inadequate blood flow may be severe and irreversible, with atrophy, scarring, and deformities.

In differential diagnosis, Raynaud's syndrome may be suspected whenever *all* of the following conditions are found: (1) the typical coloring of the skin is noted (2) following exposure to cold or apprehension (3) in recurring episodes appearing over a period of at least two years (4) without evidence of gross arterial occlusion, primary cold injury (p. 273), or other organic cause. The disease occurs almost exclusively in women. A useful criterion in diagnosis is that the involvement is always eventually bilateral. Unilateral cases are suspected of being in an early stage.

Treatment has two phases: immediate protection against attacks, and correction of the underlying predisposition. In cool or cold weather the patient should wear two pairs of ordinary gloves or one pair of heavy woolen ones. All should fit loosely to avoid mechanical constriction. Spasm may be relieved by intravenous administration of 60 to 120 mg. of papaverine hydrochloride three or more times weekly (for precautions, see p. 363). General good hygiene should be instituted, and tobacco should probably be discontinued entirely.

The approach to underlying factors should be similar to that in the neuroses (p. 150), of which Raynaud's disease may possibly be a form. A sympathetic general physician can often be helpful in adjustment of social and personality problems; but in many, if not most, instances, psychiatric treatment may be necessary for maximum improvement. In extremely stubborn cases, sympathectomy has been employed, but the degree of improvement is not always commensurate with the seriousness of the operation.

Diseases of Veins

VARICOSE VEINS

The development of varicosity in veins appears to depend on the combination of incompetent valves, lack of support from the surrounding tissues, and high hydrostatic internal pressure. Man's erect posture makes the veins of the legs subject to the greatest internal pressure. Because of their course through the subcutaneous tissue without external support, the saphenous veins of the legs are, as might be expected, the most common sites for varicosity.

A weakness or defect of the valves appears to be inherited. Varicosity may, however, be precipitated or aggravated by factors which increase venous pressure in the legs or reduce the pumping effect of movement of the legs, such as habitual prolonged standing, heavy labor, pregnancy, and phlebitis.

Varicose veins appear as dilated, tortuous vessels along the medial and posterior surfaces of the legs and thighs. They become more distended on assumption of the erect posture. Varicose veins may cause no symptoms, or they may give rise to tired and heavy sensations and aching in the legs, swelling of the ankles and feet, and cramps in the legs, especially at night or when immersed in cold water.

Untreated varicosity tends to become progressively more severe and to disturb the local circulation. Brown pigmentation and atrophy of the skin of the lower leg are common. There is usually itching. Eczematoid dermatitis may develop. Subcutaneous fibrosis may give the persistent edema a brawny character. The combination of trauma and chronically impaired circulation may result in varicose ulcers on the medial aspects of the lower legs. Varicose ulcers must be differentiated from those due to peripheral arterial vascular disease (see Arterial Disease, p. 74), syphilis, and tuberculosis.

Varicose veins must be distinguished from multiple arteriovenous fistulas and from compensatory venous dilatations subsequent to deep venous thrombosis. The last do not follow the course of the saphenous veins and are not of the same pattern as varicose veins. Flat feet and sacroiliac or spinal arthritis may give rise to pain or discomfort resembling that from varicose veins.

A number of tests are useful in establishing the diagnosis of varicose veins and deciding upon treatment. In the simplest of the Trendelenburg tests, the patient lies supine while the foot is raised until the suspected varix empties and collapses. He then rises and the vein is observed. A varicose vein fills from above; a normal vein, from below. A second test is started in a similar manner. After the suspected varix has emptied, a tourniquet is applied about the mid-thigh before the patient stands. If the greater saphenous vein fills within one-half minute after the patient stands, the communicating veins are incompetent; if it requires longer than one-half minute to fill, the communicating veins are competent. Another simple test is to have the patient walk about for a few minutes barelegged and barefooted. If the foot becomes swollen and cyanotic, the deep veins are incompetent.

Treatment depends on a number of factors. If the greater saphenous vein has filled from above in the first Trendelenburg test, the most satisfactory procedure is ligation of that vein at its junction with the femoral and resection of several centimeters to prevent re-establishment of the channel. When the communicating veins are also incompetent, they are ligated three to six weeks later. Incompetence of the lesser saphenous vein is likewise best treated by ligation in the popliteal space. Ligation is generally contraindicated by extreme age, infirmity, prejudice of the patient, or the presence of arthritic pain in knee or ankle.

Injection of varicose veins with a sclerosing solution is indicated under the following circumstances:

1. Recurrence after ligation of the greater saphenous vein.

2. Persistence of enlargements in the lower leg after ligation of either the greater or the lesser saphenous vein.

3. Arthritic pain in knee or ankle which contraindicates ligation.

4. Thin-walled varicosities in young women who have no abnormality in the greater saphenous vein in the thigh.

5. Lesions limited to small bursts of painful or disfiguring superficial varicosities in the thigh or calf.

Injection treatment is contraindicated for about six months after thrombosis or phlebitis and after the sixth month of pregnancy.

When properly carried out, the injection treatment of varicose veins is a relatively safe procedure. Sloughs or ulcerations are a possible complication. Sclerosing solutions are discussed on page 367.

Palliative treatment may be employed when more active therapy is contraindicated. It involves the use of an elastic support, which may be provided by means of an elastic bandage, a stocking made of elastic yarn, or Unna's paste boot. A bandage or stocking should extend to the groin or at least well above the level of valvular incompetence. Paste boots are not extended above the knee and consequently are effective only for lesions below the knee.

In the presence of varicose ulcers, the leg should be kept elevated and secondary infection should be combated by local application of anti-infective agents or antiseptics. After the lesion is clean, healing may be promoted by application of ultraviolet radiation. Ordinarily, varicose ulcers recur unless the varicose veins are controlled.

THROMBOPHLEBITIS AND PHLEBOTHROMBOSIS

Thrombophlebitis and phlebothrombosis both involve intravenous clotting, and both occur principally in the legs and pelvis. In their later stages they may become indistinguishable, but in the early phases they appear to be different in etiology, pathology (including type of clot), and symptomatology, and distinction between them is held by many to be of importance because of a difference in prognosis and treatment (see Table 10, p. 88).

Thrombophlebitis is primarily an inflammation of the vein wall, and the clot which forms on the damaged endothelium is buff-colored or layered, thin, tough, and adherent. Phlebothrombosis is primarily an intravascular clotting due to local circulatory stasis or an increased tendency of the blood to clot, or both. The thrombus is red, soft, and nonadherent, and it is easily dislodged to produce a pulmonary embolus (p. 119). In fact, palpation of the vein may on occasion be enough to free the clot.

The onset of phlebothrombosis is usually insidious, and a massive pulmonary embolism may be the first gross indication of its presence. Prophylaxis is therefore of greatest importance. Predisposing factors include bed rest; debilitation; immobility due to pain, tenderness, or weakness; local or general circulatory stasis; abdominal distention; dehy-

TABLE 10 — *Comparison of Thrombophlebitis and Phlebothrombosis*

Thrombophlebitis	Phlebothrombosis
Etiology	
Injury to vascular endothelium by bacteria or by mechanical or chemical means	1. Local or general circulatory stasis 2. Increase in clotting tendency of blood
Pathology	
Inflammation of vessel wall; clot firmly attached	Little or no inflammation; clot loosely attached
Symptomatology	
1. Local inflammation (pain and tenderness and, if superficial, swelling, heat, redness) 2. Early impairment of regional circulation due to collateral vasospasm 3. If severe or extensive, fever and toxemia 4. Embolism extremely rare	1. Clot palpable if vein is superficial; little or no inflammation 2. Gradual development of venous obstruction and, distal to it, circulatory stasis 3. No systemic manifestations 4. Embolism very common
Prophylaxis	
None	1. Early ambulation and avoidance of complete bed rest 2. Maintenance of local circulation by frequent change of posture and by massage 3. Prevention of abdominal distention 4. Possible use of anticoagulants (see text)
Treatment	
If superficial, elastic bandage plus ambulation If deep, relief of collateral vasospasm by sympathetic block	1. Anticoagulants 2. Ligation or removal of thrombosed vein (see text)

dration; and increased tendency of blood to clot.

Early signs of phlebothrombosis include pain and soreness on stretching the calf muscles; small areas of tenderness, with or without induration, in the calf, about the heel, or deep in the sole of the foot; deep tenderness along the course of a principal vein; and slight increase in minimum circumference at the ankle or maximum circumference at the turn of the calf. Patients subject to any of the predisposing factors, and particularly those who have undergone operations in the presence of malignant disease, should have their legs examined daily for early signs of phlebothrombosis. Most fatal pulmonary emboli come from the deep veins of the legs, and they can be prevented by early treatment of the phlebothrombosis.

The earliest manifestations of thrombophlebitis may be local (see Table 10) or systemic (chill, fever, malaise). If only the superficial veins are involved, the local symptoms usually predominate. In the more common deep thrombophlebitis (phlegmasia alba dolens), the systemic manifestations are likely to be more prominent. In fact, the onset may be marked by chill and fever. Swelling, pallor, coldness, and pain, involving the limb as a whole, are due not to the inflammation but to an associated

venous and arterial vasospasm of the collatera circulation, as in arterial occlusion (p. 77). Deep thrombophlebitis that runs its course may be followed by persistent edema and recurrent ulcerations and erysipeloid infections.

Treatment

PHLEBOTHROMBOSIS—The incidence of phlebothrombosis can be reduced by attention to the factors listed under Prophylaxis in Table 10. If prothrombin time (p. 529) is reduced (i.e., prothrombin activity is increased) during the existence of predisposing factors as listed above, the prophylactic administration of anticoagulants should be considered (see p. 374). In patients over fifty, prophylactic bilateral ligation of the femoral veins distal to the deep branch may be worth while in preparation for serious abdominal or pelvic operations (particularly for cancer) or, in the affected leg, when a fracture is going to require prolonged immobilization.

The treatment of established phlebothrombosis is undergoing change. Ligation or removal of the thrombosed vein has an established place, but its success depends on early diagnosis and exact localization of the thrombus. Therapeutic administration of anticoagulants has an increasing number of advocates. However, recurrent thrombosis and embolism may follow withdrawal of therapy.

THROMBOPHLEBITIS—Measures for the prevention of thrombophlebitis are not known. In superficial thrombophlebitis without evidence of disturbance in the collateral circulation, treatment consists in (1) application of an elastic compression bandage to the entire limb and (2) maintenance of ambulation. If the process extends into the long saphenous vein above the knee, this vein should be ligated at its junction with the femoral vein.

In deep thrombophlebitis, the most important treatment is vasomotor block which is either continued or repeated until fever is gone. Such a vasomotor block ordinarily shortens the course to a matter of hours or days instead of weeks or months. It may be established by high spinal or epidural block or by direct paravertebral block of the sympathetic chain in the case of the legs or pelvis, or by brachial plexus block for an upper extremity. A compression bandage is applied to the entire limb (if it is a limb which is involved), and the patient is made to contract his muscles against resistance. In deep thrombophlebitis, he remains horizontal in bed until well.

When thrombophlebitis is secondary to bacterial infection, there is always the possibility that organisms may cause liquefaction of the clot and lead to septic embolism. Under these circumstances, proximal ligation of the affected veins should be undertaken. Successful chemotherapy of the primary infection prevents this complication.

Diseases of the Lymphatic System

The lymphatic system is a closed network of vessels which exist wherever blood vessels are found but which have no direct communication with either blood vessels or tissue cells. The lymphatic system drains from the interstitial spaces the excess fluid which is filtered from the capillaries and not reabsorbed by them. When the interstitial fluid is locally rich in protein, as during inflammation, the lymph is correspondingly rich in protein. Dead or foreign particulate matter, such as bacteria, cell debris, cancer cells, fat droplets from the intestinal mucosa (following absorption of fat), and carbon particles deposited on the bronchial mucosa from inspired air, also finds its way into the lymphatic system by means that are incompletely understood.

The lymphatic capillaries form a network which drains into vessels that are much like veins in structure. At intervals along these lymphatic vessels occur chains and groups of beanlike bodies, the lymph nodes, which filter the lymph through a series of sinuses packed with lymph cells, or lymphocytes. Material which cannot be phagocytized remains as a permanent deposit in the nodes.

The lymph vessels are richly supplied with valves which allow only centripetal movement of the lymph. Eventually, the vessels join and empty into the great veins at the base of the neck. The largest and most constant of these terminal lymph vessels is the thoracic duct, which extends from the second lumbar vertebra along the spinal column and aorta to the junction of the left (usually) subclavian and internal jugular veins. It drains the lymph from below the diaphragm, from the left half of the body above the diaphragm, and from all of the dorsal portion of the chest wall.

It is clear from the above description that the lymphatic system is likely to be involved in all types of wounds, injuries, and infections.

LYMPHANGITIS

Acute lymphangitis occurs secondarily to local infection, usually of the skin and subcutaneous tissue. The commonest organisms in acute lymphangitis are streptococci or staphylococci. The spreading pink or red blush that surrounds an infected wound is actually a *reticular lymphangitis* involving the reticular network of lymphatics in the skin. Erysipelas (p. 5) represents a severe form of reticular lymphangitis. When the tubular lymphatic vessels (as opposed to the reticular network) are involved, the condition is termed *tubular lymphangitis*. Tubular lymphangitis of the skin is seen as one or more tender red streaks extending up (usually an extremity) to or beyond the first set of lymph nodes. The regional lymph nodes are enlarged and tender. Chronic lymphangitis is manifested by recurrences of the acute form; it is usually secondary to inadequate treatment of the original acute attack. Lymph stasis may be a contributory factor.

Acute lymphangitis is a sign that the infection has penetrated the body's first line of defense. It may be a forerunner of septicemia. As such, it should be vigorously treated. The involved part should be elevated and kept at rest. A plaster cast is often the best means of maintaining a fixed position. The original infection is treated locally or systemically or both with anti-infective drugs (p. 286). Heat often relieves pain, but it is contraindicated because it increases lymph production. Chronic lymphangitis may require excision of the infected part or even of the involved area of lymphatics.

LYMPHADENITIS

Lymphadenitis is inflammation of lymph nodes. Acute lymphadenitis occurs in the course of many different types of infection. In the mildest forms, the inflammation is due to toxic products of the infection rather than to the presence of organisms in the nodes. Sometimes organisms are carried through lymph channels to nodes, where they set up active infection without involvement of the vessels which were traversed. Such acute infections are usually due to streptococci or staphylococci. Chronic lymphadenitis may be due to tuberculosis, syphilis, cancer, or organisms of low virulence. Acute lymphadenitis occurs usually in the groin, axilla, or neck.

Treatment is directed first toward the primary infection. If acute suppuration occurs, the node should be incised and drained according to the same principles as any abscess (see p. 1). The treatment of chronic lymphadenitis depends on the cause.

LYMPHEDEMA

Lymphedema is the condition which results from chronic interference with the flow of lymph. It may be caused by fibrotic obstruction secondary to a chronic skin infection, thrombophlebitis, or cancerous infiltration, or it may be due to the presence of filariae or to interruption of the lymph channels as in block dissection of the axillary lymph nodes. The edema is due to accumulation of lymph distal to the obstruction. The distended lymph vessels dilate (lymphangiectasis), and eventually there is fibrosis. When such fibrosis is well advanced, the condition is termed "elephantiasis."

Phlegmasia alba dolens (milk leg) is a form of lymphedema which is associated with and secondary to deep pelvic thrombophlebitis following childbirth. The name was applied because it usually appears about ten days postpartum. The lymphedema makes the leg swollen, tense, pale, and shiny and obscures evidences of thrombophlebitis.

Lymphedema must be differentiated from hereditary edema (Milroy's disease), in which there is a family history and absence of evidence of lymphatic obstruction.

Early, mild cases of lymphedema secondary to thrombophlebitis respond to rest, elevation, massage, and support by bandaging. For treatment of thrombophlebitis, see page 87. In more advanced and resistant cases, a regimen of sodium depletion and mercurial diuretics may be tried (see Edema,

p. 53). In extreme cases the Kondoléon operation may be of value.

Shock

Shock is a condition of collapse or prostration which is (1) induced by any of a number of factors, (2) accompanied by signs and symptoms of peripheral circulatory impairment or failure, and (3) characterized by a progressive reduction in the circulating blood volume.

Customarily, shock is divided into primary and secondary types. Primary shock is a temporary depression of the sensorium resulting from sudden extreme emotion, as in profound fear, excruciating pain, intensely disagreeable sights, or tragic news. It may result in fainting. The circulatory disturbances are temporary, and recovery is usually very prompt.

Secondary shock (surgical shock, traumatic shock) is a severe disturbance of body function which, unless treated promptly and vigorously, frequently results in death. The immediate cause of secondary shock is reduction in the volume of circulating blood. Factors in such a reduction are:

1. Most importantly, escape of blood plasma because of increased capillary permeability.

2. Loss of plasma or other body fluid and electrolyte.

3. Loss of vasomotor or venomotor tone, with consequent pooling of blood in the veins of the abdominal viscera.

The reduction in circulating blood volume first reduces venous pressure and diastolic filling of the heart. The result is a reduction in cardiac output. Immediate fall of blood pressure is prevented by reflex generalized arteriolar constriction (for discussion of blood pressure regulation, see p. 78). There is a diminution in blood flow which early affects the kidneys, causing reduction or cessation of urine formation. As blood flow progressively diminishes, two things happen: Even maximal arteriolar constriction no longer suffices to maintain blood pressure, which then begins to fall; and tissue hypoxia develops. This hypoxia is the damaging feature of shock, and its most important effects are on the cardiovascular and central nervous systems. As hypoxia progresses, it causes further increase in capillary permeability which further exacerbates the shock. A vicious cycle is set up. The hypoxia also progressively impairs the functional capacity of the myocardium and brain. If it is too severe or lasts too long, the tissue changes are irreversible and death becomes inevitable.

The most important factors in the production of shock are:

1. Severe trauma, particularly crushing injuries, with loss of plasma and blood into the tissues and perhaps with absorption of toxic products. Surgical procedures are included.
2. Loss of plasma, which occurs particularly in severe burns but may occur as the result of any injury to the capillaries, such as that caused by chemical and bacterial irritants, direct mechanical trauma, and tissue anoxia.
3. Loss of water and electrolytes, as in loss of body fluids or inadequate intake of water and salt.
4. Reflex falls of blood pressure such as may occur when the contents of the upper abdomen are manipulated during a surgical operation.

Aggravating factors include the following.

1. Anesthesia, including spinal anesthesia.
2. Loss of muscle tone, which removes an important force in venous return.
3. Reflex vasoconstriction.
4. Cold.
5. Pain.
6. Psychic influences, including fear.
7. Hypoxia.
8. General factors such as advanced age, presence of disease, anemia, and generally lowered vitality.
9. Duration, since an irreversible point may be reached.

The patient in shock is prostrated and appears to be seriously ill. The face is ashen or livid in color, anxious in expression, and moist with cold sweat. Usually there is circumoral pallor (a sign of peripheral compensatory vasoconstriction). The eyes appear to be sunken. The pulse is rapid, feeble, and of small volume. Frequently, the pulse is difficult if not impossible to obtain. Respirations are usually shallow, but there may be frequent sighs and signs of air hunger. The extremities are cold and clammy. The patient may be depressed and restless. Vomiting may occur. Diarrhea is sometimes seen. Not infrequently the patient complains of thirst. The urine is scanty or absent. The blood pressure declines progressively, the systolic usually falling more rapidly than the diastolic. As the systolic pressure drops below 80 mm. Hg, the possibility of reversal of the shock becomes progressively less good. Consciousness usually is retained until late, but there is gradual loss of reflexes, suppression of body functions, and eventually unconsciousness and death. Shock may run a course of hours to days. If the condition is not treated vigorously or with sufficient promptness, changes become irreversible and death is inevitable.

Laboratory findings are of less importance than careful observation of the patient in diagnosis and treatment of shock. Repeated estimations of the degree of hemoconcentration (by hematocrit, plasma protein, or blood specific-gravity determinations) are helpful in following the response to therapy, but they are not of diagnostic value. In shock, the nonprotein nitrogen level of the blood is usually elevated, whereas chloride is low. The urine, if present, is concentrated and contains protein, bile, red cells, and debris.

Treatment—Shock is more easily prevented than treated and, once developed, is more easily treated early than late. When an individual has been exposed to conditions likely to induce shock, all contributory or aggravating factors should be removed insofar as possible (see listing above). Fluid losses should be replaced, and fluid balance and urine volume should be maintained. Severely traumatized or burned patients should receive blood or plasma prophylactically.

The first aim of treatment is maintenance or quick restoration of the circulating blood volume. The most important therapeutic substances are blood and blood derivatives. The amount to be given depends on the stage of shock and, later, on the response to early therapy.

As prophylaxis and in early shock (cold moist skin, grayish-blue color, rapid pulse, unchanged or only slightly lowered blood pressure), 250 to 750 cc. of plasma or 500 to 1,500 cc. of whole blood should be given intravenously as early as possible. If the history or findings suggest dehydration (p. 56), 500 cc. of electrolyte solution (see p. 348) should be given with the first dose of plasma or blood. The efficacy of the initial treatment is judged by the patient's general demeanor and by the extent of restoration of normal skin color, pulse, respiration, and blood pressure. If the patient's response is not satisfactory, additional doses of 250 cc. of plasma are given as may be required.

If shock is more severe (as when it has gone untreated for some time, or as evidenced by considerable drop in blood pressure [particularly in pulse pressure], rapid thready pulse, cold clammy skin, collapsed veins, thirst, and hemoconcentration), 1,000 to 1,500 cc. of whole blood should be given rapidly by vein, followed at once by 1,000 to 2,000 cc. of plasma. Whole blood is much more effective than plasma; if it is unavailable, the dose of plasma should be doubled. Electrolyte solutions should not be given early to patients with severe or long-standing shock. If the veins are so collapsed as to render insertion of a large needle impossible, they should be cut down on without hesitation. Once the needle or catheter is in place, it should be kept open by administration (between doses of blood or plasma) of 5 percent dextrose in electrolyte solution dripping in at the rate of 20 to 40 drops per minute.

Additional blood or plasma or both should be given freely until shock is controlled.

Once administration of blood or plasma has begun, other measures should be undertaken. Pain may be controlled by administration of not more than 32 mg. (1/2 grain) of morphine sulfate. Fractures or severe injuries of the extremities should be immobilized until such time as the patient's condition warrants specific treatment. Moderate heat should be applied to the body by means of blankets, hot-water bottles, or electric cradles. The patient may be placed in the shock position (elevation of the foot of the bed). In severe shock, administration of oxygen by means of a face mask is advisable.

If operation is required, it is delayed until shock has been controlled. Infiltration or nerve block anesthesia (pp. 440 and 441) is employed whenever possible. If general anesthesia is necessary, cyclopropane (p. 413) is a good agent because it is effective with high concentrations of oxygen. Nitrous oxide is disadvantageous because it requires a lower oxygen concentration for efficacy. Spinal anesthesia should not be employed in patients who have suffered severe shock.

Once the patient is well along the road to recovery from shock, sufficient water and electrolyte are given to maintain an adequate urine output (see p. 52). If the red blood cell count drops to low levels as blood volume is restored to normal, whole blood should be given intravenously to restore the red count to 3.5 to 4 million.

Cardiac and circulatory stimulants and vasoconstrictor drugs are not useful in the treatment of shock, either early or late, and they may be harmful. The value of adrenocortical steroids or extracts is at present questionable.

BLOOD AND BONE MARROW

The blood* is the internal transportation system of the body. It is a complex fluid carrying formed elements, the blood cells, in suspension. Blood constitutes about 1/11 of the body weight and plasma (the liquid portion) about 1/20. Normally, about 55 percent of the blood (v/v) is plasma. Plasma, in turn, consists of water and 8 to 9 percent (w/v) of dissolved substances which include protein (albumin and several types of globulin), inorganic salts (for details, see p. 50), dextrose, neutral fats, other lipid materials, amino acids, urea and other nonprotein nitrogenous substances, and many other types of constituents.

_____
* Plates 29 to 42 (Section 3) depict the blood in health and disease.

The blood transports oxygen and food materials to the body cells and removes waste products. It also carries many other things less constantly needed, such as antibodies and chemical messengers (hormones). It maintains a constant dynamic osmotic and fluid balance with the tissue (interstitial) fluid through the walls of the capillaries. In addition, the blood serves to equalize temperature in the various parts of the body and to deliver excess heat to the skin for radiation.

The formed elements of the blood consist of red cells (erythrocytes), white cells (leukocytes), and platelets (thrombocytes). The lymphocytes (nongranular leukocytes) originate in lymph nodes, and the monocytes (also nongranular leukocytes) in the reticulo-endothelial system. The red cells, granular leukocytes, and platelets are formed in the red bone marrow.

Red bone marrow occurs in the ends of the long bones and also in the ribs, skull, vertebrae, sternum, and pelvic and other bones. _In toto_, the red bone marrow is a relatively large organ which weighs 1,400 to 3,700 Gm. The red cells contain hemoglobin, which carries oxygen from the lungs to the capillaries; from the capillaries, oxygen passes to the body cells by diffusion. Low oxygen tension in the arterial blood stimulates increased formation and release of red cells. In iron-deficiency anemia and pernicious anemia, the volume of active bone marrow increases greatly.

The average life of a red cell is normally about 110 to 130 days; this means that in an average normal adult the red cells in about 40 to 50 cc. of blood are destroyed and replaced daily. Destruction takes place largely in the blood stream and is apparently mechanical—from the physical stresses of circulation. The debris is removed for the most part by the spleen.

Red cell production is normally controlled so as to maintain a very constant concentration of red cells and hemoglobin in the blood. Normal values for red cells, hemoglobin, and hematocrit (relative volume of packed red cells in blood) are shown in Table 11. The factors determining the level are poorly understood. Higher levels are maintained in persons living under subnormal oxygen tensions (at high altitudes) and in patients with chronic heart failure or advanced pulmonary emphysema. In certain species of animals, high levels of circulating estrogen lower the levels of red cells and hemoglobin; but such effects have not been established in the human species, even though they would explain the "anemia" of pregnancy and the lower normal levels in women as compared with men. Administration of androgen raises the red count and hemoglobin.

The granular white cells (polymorphonuclear leukocytes) occur in three forms which are distinguished according to whether their staining reactions are neutrophilic, eosinophilic, or basophilic. The neutrophilic granulocytes have as their function the destruction and removal of foreign matter, including bacteria. They are the body's principal defense against infection. They are able to insinuate themselves through the capillary walls, and they gather at the site of infection or injury to form a protective coating. Pus consists mostly of dead neutrophilic polymorphonuclear leukocytes. Young forms have a single nucleus, and the number of nuclei increases as the cells become older.

TABLE 11 — *Normal Values for Red Blood Cells and Hemoglobin*

	Red Blood Cells, in Millions per cu. mm.	Hemoglobin, in Gm. per 100 cc. of Blood	Hematocrit Reading, in Percent
Men	5.4 ± 0.8	16 ± 2	47 ± 7
Women	4.8 ± 0.6	14 ± 2	42 ± 5

Eosinophilic granulocytes are only slightly motile and phagocytic. Their function is unknown. Their concentration in the blood is greatly increased in allergic states and in certain infections and infestations (notably asthma, anaphylactic shock, certain skin diseases, trichinosis, hookworm disease, and other types of intestinal parasitism). They are present in large quantities in secretions of allergic origin. Their number in the blood is greatly reduced by the gluco-corticoid hormones (see p. 462). The function of the basophils is likewise unknown.

The platelets have as their best-known function the liberation of thrombokinase in connection with the clotting of blood. They probably serve other purposes as well, such as sealing leaks in capillaries and covering rough places or foreign bodies, including bacteria.

Little is known of the function of the lymphocytes, although it has been surmised that they have to do with processes of repair and of resistance to chronic infection and possibly to cancer. They constantly appear on mucous membranes in very large numbers. The monocytes are scavenger and repair cells.

The number of white cells in the blood at any one time represents a balance between accession and disappearance. The number of polymorphonuclear neutrophils normally varies in cycles of ap-

proximately an hour (e.g., if a count is taken at a maximum of the cycle, a count a half hour later will be several thousand lower, and a count after an additional half hour will be fairly close to the maximum). The neutrophil count reaches a maximum in the afternoon, regardless of whether food has been taken. The lymphocytes have a similar rhythm, but the cycle requires only about half an hour, and there is no general afternoon rise.

The total white count is thus seen to represent for the most part the sum of two independent variables. As a matter of observation, the maximum total white count (in the afternoon) is usually about twice the minimum for that individual. Maxima as high as 14,000 are undoubtedly normal for some persons; their minima would be around 7,000. Others, who might have maxima of about 8,000, may have normal minima of around 4,000. It is clear, then, that single white blood counts must be interpreted cautiously.

The differential count is likewise variable. As determined in fixed smears, the percentage may normally vary about as follows: polymorphonuclear neutrophils, 40 to 65; eosinophils, 0 to 5; basophils, 0 to 1.6; lymphocytes, 14 to 36; and monocytes, 2 to 10.

Tissue damage or infection of certain types (notably with streptococci or staphylococci) calls forth an immediate increase in the number of circulating polymorphonuclear neutrophils, and particularly of young forms. There is thus an increase in total white count and in percentage of polymorphonuclear cells and a shift in distribution according to number of nuclei. An increase in the percentage of younger cells (with fewer nuclei) has been termed "a shift to the left" in accordance with a classification proposed by Arneth and modified by Schilling. An increase in number of polymorphonuclear neutrophils may also occur during pregnancy, parturition, and menstruation, in the presence of cancer, during muscular exercise, and after administration or release of epinephrine (as in fear, pain, or anger).

The number of lymphocytes may be increased during chronic infections (such as tuberculosis or syphilis); the rise is especially noteworthy in whooping cough. Small children normally have higher lymphocyte counts than adults.

Reduction in white count (leukopenia), involving mainly the polymorphonuclear neutrophils in most instances, is seen in some infections (notably typhoid fever and certain virus infections), in anemia, and as a toxic or allergic reaction to certain drugs (see Agranulocytosis, p. 102).

Anemia

When red blood cells are lost or destroyed more rapidly than they are formed, anemia develops. The normal levels, below which anemia is said to be present, appear in Table 11. The factors which may cause anemia are outlined in Table 12.

The anemias may be subdivided into types by the use of two indices:

1. Mean Corpuscular Volume (M.C.V.), which is hematocrit reading (volume of packed red cells in cc. per 100 cc. blood) divided by red cell count in millions per cu. mm. and multiplied by 10. The resultant figure represents the volume in cubic microns of the average red cell; the normal value is 87 ± 5.

2. Mean Corpuscular Hemoglobin Concentration (M.C.H.C.), which is hemoglobin concentration in Gm. per 100 cc. divided by hematocrit reading (volume of packed red cells in cc. per 100 cc. blood) and multiplied by 100. The resultant figure represents Gm. of hemoglobin in 100 cc. of red cells; the normal value is 34 ± 2.

TABLE 12 — *Causes of Anemia*

I. Blood loss or destruction
  A. Hemorrhage
    1. Acute
    2. Chronic
  B. Abnormal destruction
    1. Infection (e.g., *Streptococcus pyogenes, Str. mitis* [viridans], *Clostridium perfringens*)
    2. Parasites (malaria)
    3. Intoxication (e.g., severe burns, snake bite, lead, benzene, toluene, amino and nitro derivatives of phenol and toluene [phenylhydrazine, trinitrotoluol], hydrogen sulfide)
    4. Unknown causes, as in congenital or acquired hemolytic jaundice, sickle-cell anemia, Mediterranean anemia, or paroxysmal nocturnal hemoglobinuria
II. Inadequate blood formation
  A. Lack of necessary materials
    1. Protein or vitamins or both (nutritional anemia)
    2. Iron (iron-deficiency anemia)
    3. Maturation factor found in liver (pernicious anemia)
    4. Folic acid
  B. Toxic states
    1. Chronic infection
    2. Malignancy
    3. Chronic nephritis
  C. Occupation of bone marrow by other than hematopoietic tissue
    1. Carcinoma metastatic to bone marrow
    2. Multiple myeloma
    3. Myelosclerosis
    4. Osteopetrosis (osteosclerosis, "marble bones")
    5. Hodgkin's disease
    6. Gaucher's disease
    7. Leukemia
  D. Unknown causes
    1. Idiopathic aplastic anemia

The types of anemia are as follows:

1. *Macrocytic anemia* (cells larger than normal), in which the M.C.V. is greater than 94 and the M.C.H.C. is greater than 30.

2. *Normocytic anemia* (cells of average size), in which the M.C.V. is between 80 and 94 and the M.C.H.C. is greater than 30.

3. *Microcytic hypochromic anemia* (cells smaller than normal and containing less hemoglobin), in which the M.C.V. is less than 80 and the M.C.H.C. is less than 30.

The majority of macrocytic anemias respond to the antianemia principle of liver or to folic acid, whereas most microcytic hypochromic anemias respond to iron. The normocytic anemias are a heterogeneous group for which there is no single type of therapy.

Because the chief function of the red blood cells is to carry oxygen, the symptoms of anemia per se are those of hypoxia. They are common to all anemias, regardless of cause or type, and include weakness, fatigability, dyspnea and palpitation (and sometimes angina) on exertion, vertigo, and fainting attacks. The patient may exhibit pallor, tachycardia, and edema. Signs and symptoms are usually proportional to the severity of the anemia; but if the latter develops very slowly, there may be few or no symptoms in spite of a very low level of hemoglobin.

ACUTE BLOOD LOSS

Acute blood loss is ordinarily due to hemorrhage from the circulatory system following rupture or gross injury of a blood vessel. The hemorrhage may be external, or it may be internal (into the tissues or the lumen of a viscus). A significant acute loss of blood from the circulation causes clinical signs like those of secondary shock (p. 90). When there is obvious hemorrhage, the situation will be clear. In the absence of an external loss of blood, hemorrhage can be differentiated from shock due to other factors by the rapid hemodilution which follows hemorrhage and is proportional to the amount of blood lost. Death is likely to follow sudden loss of half or more of the total blood volume, although the exact tolerance depends on the age and state of health.

Following hemorrhage, active blood regeneration begins at once under normal circumstances. If iron stores are normal, there is complete restoration within two to four weeks, depending on the amount of blood which has been lost.

Treatment—The most important aspect of treatment is that it be initiated with all possible speed. Whole blood given intravenously is the therapeutic agent of choice, but plasma should be employed if whole blood is not immediately available. If the hemorrhage has not stopped at the time treatment is begun, whole blood should be obtained as soon as possible; plasma is given during the interval.

The quantity of either whole blood or plasma to be administered is that which re-establishes and maintains a normal circulating volume. The initial injection is usually 500 cc. Additional quantities of 250 to 500 cc. are given as required. In severe hemorrhage, 2,000 to 3,000 cc. may be needed. Hematocrit determinations should be made to be certain that the red count is maintained at a level sufficient to assure an adequate oxygen supply to the tissues. The blood pressure also should be followed closely; restoration to a normal level is a favorable sign.

Once measures to restore blood volume have shown evidence of success, location and repair of injured vessels may be undertaken. The remainder of the treatment is the same as that for shock.

CHRONIC BLOOD LOSS

Severe anemia may result from repeated small hemorrhages, such as may occur in excessive uterine bleeding, hemorrhoids, peptic ulcer, hookworm, or cancer of the gastro-intestinal tract. The anemia is dependent on depletion of iron stores. Anemia of similar character may result from (1) inadequate dietary intake of iron, (2) high demand for iron, as during growth, pregnancy, or lactation, (3) impaired absorption of iron, as in hypochlorhydria, achlorhydria, or chronic diarrhea, or (4) chronic infection.

The constant and characteristic feature of this type of anemia is diminution in hemoglobin concentration. It is thus a microcytic hypochromic anemia, in which the red cells are small and contain subnormal quantities of hemoglobin, even though the total red cell count may be normal or nearly normal (see Plate 30). The bone marrow shows a normoblastic hyperplasia.

Treatment consists in stopping the blood loss or other abnormal conditions and administering iron. Of course, if there are indications of oxygen want, transfusions are given as for acute blood loss (see above). Transfusion may be indicated also as preparation for surgical control of the blood loss, as in hemorrhoids or peptic ulcer. Continued action of the causative factor, such as persistent hemorrhage, may slow or prevent response to therapy. Once the causes have been eradicated, the patient usually responds rapidly to administration of iron. Sometimes it is necessary to correct the anemia before direct treatment of the cause is advisable.

Many preparations of iron are available (see p. 368). Ferrous sulfate, 0.3 to 0.6 Gm. three times daily by mouth after meals, is usually satisfactory from the point of view of both response and tolerance.

IDIOPATHIC HYPOCHROMIC ANEMIA

Idiopathic hypochromic anemia (simple anemia, simple achlorhydric anemia, chronic microcytic anemia) is a chronic microcytic hypochromic anemia which occurs almost exclusively in women between the ages of twenty and fifty years who have little or no hydrochloric acid in the gastric secretion. There is usually a history of anemia, including pernicious anemia, in the family. The patient herself may later develop pernicious anemia.

Women with idiopathic hypochromic anemia invariably have excessive menstrual bleeding which is often unnoticed by them. The few men having the condition usually have bleeding hemorrhoids. Frequently, other factors than chronic blood loss are present, such as deficient iron intake, decreased absorption of iron (due to the low gastric acidity), or frequent pregnancies. The points of distinction in this anemia that justify the term "idiopathic" are (1) the background and associated disturbances in these patients, and (2) the fact that other individuals with as much blood loss or as deficient an iron intake do not develop anemia.

Patients with idiopathic hypochromic anemia usually complain of a long period of vague gastrointestinal symptoms, asthenia, nervousness, and mild paresthesias of the extremities. When dysphagia is present, the condition is known as the Plummer-Vinson syndrome (p. 126). There is usually pallor, either glossitis or atrophy of the mucous membrane of the tongue, and trophic disturbances of the nails (brittleness, dullness, longitudinal ridges, and occasionally spoon-shaped nails). The hemoglobin is often greatly reduced; the red count may be at or near normal levels. The appearance of a typical stained blood smear is shown in Plate 30.

Treatment is essentially the same as in chronic blood loss (see above). In addition to iron, however, the patient should take a high-calorie, high-protein, high-vitamin diet. If gastro-intestinal symptoms persist or if the hemoglobin fails to rise, hydrochloric acid should be administered (as Diluted Hydrochloric Acid, U.S.P., 4 cc., or 'Acidulin,' 4 pulvules, three times daily with meals). Iron medication should, of course, be continued until excessive demands are no longer present. Some patients require iron therapy throughout life if their hemoglobin is to be maintained at a normal level.

PERNICIOUS ANEMIA

Pernicious anemia (Addisonian anemia, primary anemia, Addison-Biermer anemia) is a chronic, recurrent, macrocytic anemia usually occurring in middle or later life. Actually, the anemia is only a part of the clinical picture and is the final result of a chain of conditions.

The primary lesion in pernicious anemia is inflammation and later atrophy of the mucosa of the alimentary tract. Sore tongue is a frequent early symptom, and papillary atrophy of this member is a constant later finding. The presence of inflammation of the stomach and intestines early in the disease is difficult to establish, but atrophy of the gastric mucosa is the rule, and deficient or absent gastric secretion occurs so regularly as to raise a question as to whether true pernicious anemia can be present in a patient whose gastric secretion contains free acid.

Red blood cell production in pernicious anemia is deficient because of lack of a maturation factor which is necessary for continued development of red cells beyond the stage of megaloblasts. This maturation factor is present in liver, and there is a possibility that it may be vitamin B_{12}. The factor or its precursor (the so-called extrinsic factor) is normally present in food, and it is acted on by an intrinsic factor (a thermolabile, enzyme-like substance normally secreted in gastric juice) which either makes possible absorption of the extrinsic factor or alters it to the maturation factor. It is failure of absorption of the maturation factor, in turn due to lack of intrinsic factor in the gastric secretion, that brings on the anemia of pernicious anemia.

The red cell maturation factor is apparently also necessary for the integrity of the nervous system, for in a high percentage of cases of pernicious anemia there are degenerative changes in peripheral nerves and in the posterior and lateral columns of the spinal cord (subacute combined degeneration of the spinal cord; see p. 173).

Pernicious anemia is a relatively common disease in the United States, having an incidence of approximately seven per one hundred thousand population. It is seen most frequently in blond, blue-eyed individuals, but it does occur in others and has even been reported in Negroes. There is a high familial incidence of the disease. Not only are there frequently several members of a family with the disease, but others in the family may have idiopathic hypochromic anemia. In addition, there is likely to be a high incidence of achylia gastrica in the remainder of the family.

The onset of symptoms in pernicious anemia is usually insidious. In about one-third of cases, the earliest symptoms are those of anemia (see p. 94). In another third they are concerned with the gastro-intestinal tract: recurring glossitis, mild indigestion, capricious appetite, nausea and vomiting, constipation or diarrhea, and periods of alternating diarrhea and constipation. Symptoms referable to the nervous system occur first in about one-fourth the cases; they include paresthesias (such as numbness and tingling of the extremities), weakness, difficulty in walking (in-co-ordination), stiffness of the limbs, lack of concentrating power, irritability, depression, and even spastic paraplegia with loss of bladder and rectal sphincter control. In about one patient in ten, cardiac symptoms (secondary to anemia) are the earliest.

Physical examination reveals pallor, a characteristic lemon-yellow color of the skin, and slight icterus of the sclera. The tongue often has a smooth appearance due to atrophy of the papillae, but it is fiery red if glossitis is present. The liver and spleen may be palpable. If the peripheral nerves and posterior columns only are involved, the patellar and ankle jerks are diminished or absent and there is a loss of vibratory sense and the sense of position in the lower extremities. Spastic paraplegia, exaggerated deep reflexes, and bilateral Babinski reflexes result from involvement of the lateral columns.

During a relapse, the red blood count usually is below 2 million per cu. mm. The hemoglobin is not decreased in proportion to the red count, and the color index (p. 525) is over 1. Examination of the stained smear reveals the characteristic large, round or oval, well-stained red blood cells (see Plate 33). Mean corpuscular volume is increased to between 100 and 130 cubic microns (see p. 94). Reticulocytes are usually present but seldom in greater ratio than 1 percent. Nucleated red blood cells may be seen but are rare except during the reticulocyte response following an induced or spontaneous remission. The blood platelets are nearly always reduced in numbers, and they may be so few that purpura occurs. The white blood cell count is usually low. Absence of free hydrochloric acid in the gastric contents is a constant feature of the disease. It has been shown that the achlorhydria not only precedes the anemia by many years and persists after adequate treatment of the anemia but probably exists from birth. The serum bilirubin (as measured by the icterus index or van den Bergh reaction) is always increased in pernicious anemia when the red count is low.

If untreated, pernicious anemia runs an unpredictable but downhill course, with remissions and exacerbations. Eventually the disease proves fatal. The most common complications are chronic cholecystitis and infection of the urinary tract. Cancer of the stomach is not infrequent and should be watched for during the prolonged treatment of the disease.

Macrocytic anemias resembling pernicious anemia insofar as the blood and bone marrow are concerned occur when the supply of maturation factor is inadequate for other reasons than lack of the intrinsic factor of gastric juice. The diet may be inadequate in extrinsic factor (vitamin B_{12}?), as in certain cases of sprue (p. 133) and macrocytic nutritional anemias; the maturation factor may not be absorbed adequately, as in intestinal anastomoses or stenoses or severe chronic diarrheas; or the liver may be unable to store the maturation factor, as in advanced cirrhosis. It has been suggested that in some individuals the bone marrow may be unable to utilize the factor (achrestic anemia). It would appear, however, that not all nutritional macrocytic anemias are due to deficiency of extrinsic factor; some do not respond to liver extracts concentrated for the maturation factor but do respond to relatively crude preparations administered either by mouth or by injection.

Treatment—Adequate amounts of liver or of liver extract provide complete therapy in pernicious anemia. Preliminary studies suggest that vitamin B_{12} is similarly effective. If adequate treatment is begun before lesions of the central nervous system are too far advanced, patients can be expected to live out their normal life span.

Treatment is adequate only if it accomplishes the following:

1. Return of the red blood cell count, red blood cell size, and hemoglobin concentration to normal levels and maintenance at such levels.
2. Disappearance of symptoms referable to the alimentary tract.
3. Cessation of progress in the lesions of the nervous system.

The amount of therapeutic agent required for these accomplishments varies from one patient to another and in the same patient from time to time. In general, older patients with moderate to advanced arteriosclerosis, lesions of the nervous system, or infection require larger doses than younger individuals who are free from infection and nervous-system involvement.

Because of the large quantity which must be consumed daily, liver itself is an impractical therapeutic agent. Effective agents include liver extracts given by injection or by mouth; desiccated, defatted hog stomach and liver-stomach concentrates administered orally; and vitamin B_{12} given by injection. These substances are discussed beginning on page 369. Folic acid (p. 371), a member of the vitamin B complex, produces a remission (sometimes temporary) in the blood. However, it is not the extrinsic factor or the maturation factor. Furthermore, it does not have any favorable action on the lesions of the nervous system, and in some instances it has appeared to exacerbate them. Folic acid alone is now considered an unsuitable agent for the treatment of pernicious anemia.

In pernicious anemia, therapy must be continued for life. If treatment is stopped, a relapse of the blood is certain to occur sooner or later. During such a relapse, lesions are likely to develop in the nervous system which may cause permanent and irrevocable damage.

If the blood count is below 1 million when the patient is first seen, it is advisable to transfuse him at once with 500 cc. of whole blood to tide him over until specific therapy takes effect.

Iron therapy is not indicated in pernicious anemia unless the hemoglobin percentage lags behind the red cell count. If this occurs, the patient should receive an iron preparation (such as ferrous sulfate, 5 grains by mouth three times daily after meals).

The diet in pernicious anemia should be ample, with a high protein content made up mostly of meat, eggs, and milk. Dilute hydrochloric acid with meals (see p. 384) may help to relieve gastrointestinal symptoms.

APLASTIC ANEMIA

Aplastic anemia (hypoplastic anemia, refractory anemia) results from decreased blood formation due to the toxic effects of certain medicinal or industrial agents or to unknown causes. It is characterized by severe anemia of normocytic normochromic character associated with granulocytopenia, thrombocytopenia, and purpura.

The condition may be caused by benzene and related hydrocarbons, arsenicals, mustard and other war gases, gold, sulfonamides, some insecticides and hair dyes, and exposure to radioactive substances. In aplastic anemia, most of the red-blood-cell-forming portions of the bone marrow disappear and are replaced by fat and fibrous tissue containing a few lymphocytes. Clinically and pathologically, there is no difference between the idiopathic and the secondary types except that the secondary aplastic anemias usually recover following removal of the causative factor. If the cause cannot be ascertained, the ultimate prognosis is very poor.

In addition to the symptoms of anemia (see p. 94), there may be purpura (with bleeding from the mucous membranes and into the skin and internal organs) and, as a grave consequence of the granulocytopenia, infections of mucous membranes, especially of the mouth and throat. Points of diagnostic importance include history of exposure to toxic substances; absence of anorexia or weight loss, lymphadenitis, or splenomegaly; granulocytopenia; thrombocytopenia with purpura; normocytic type of anemia; lack of abnormal white blood cells in either the blood stream or bone marrow; a decrease in reticulocytes; normal red cell fragility; a high level of plasma iron; and hypoplasia of all elements of the bone marrow.

Patients with clinical and hematological findings characteristic of aplastic anemia but having normal or hyperplastic bone marrow have often been included in this group of anemias. However, they probably should be excluded inasmuch as they often run a more prolonged course and experience longer periods of remission. The inability to produce erythrocytes in these cases has been attributed to a "maturation arrest." They have also been designated as pseudoaplastic anemias.

Treatment—There is no curative treatment known at present. The condition may be rapidly fatal or may be prolonged for many months. Thorough study should be made to determine and eliminate or control, if possible, the cause of the condition. Repeated transfusions of fresh whole blood may give temporary relief and diminish for a time the hemorrhagic tendency. Large intramuscular injections of liver extract and the various vitamin preparations may be given, but without much hope of improving the condition. In the more chronic cases, and especially in the so-called pseudoaplastic anemias, all types of therapy should be used in the hope that something will be of benefit and that the patient can be kept alive until the bone marrow returns to normal function.

CONGENITAL HEMOLYTIC ANEMIA

Congenital hemolytic anemia (congenital hemolytic jaundice, spherocytic anemia, spherocytosis, chronic acholuric jaundice, chronic familial jaundice) is a chronic, usually hereditary disease characterized by periods of excessive hemolysis, spherocytosis (a tendency of the red blood cells to be more spherical), increased fragility of red blood cells, splenomegaly, and varying degrees of icterus.

Most investigators believe the disease is the result of a hereditary defect of the red blood cells. The more spheroidal shape of the cell is generally accepted as being responsible for the main features of the clinical disease, such as increased blood destruction, increased fragility to hypotonic salt solution, icterus, anemia, reticulocytosis, and splenomegaly. The condition is transmitted as a dominant Mendelian characteristic. The fact that normal red blood cells transfused into a patient with congenital hemolytic anemia have a normal life span, whereas the cells of a hemolytic-anemia patient are short-lived when transfused into normal individuals, suggests that the red blood cells are primarily at fault.

All patients with the disease are subject to recurring hemolytic crises, during which they develop fever, abdominal pain, nausea and vomiting, increasing icterus, and a rapid fall of the red blood count. The jaundice and anemia are usually slight between crises. The cause of the crises is unknown, and the period between crises varies considerably. The onset of the disease is usually during childhood or early adult life. The younger the patient at the time of the first crisis, the more severe the disturbance tends to become. Adults with the disease are more jaundiced than sick and may show few symptoms or signs other than mild anemia, splenomegaly, and varying degrees of icterus for a great number of years. The anemia is always one of the most striking features of the disease in young infants and may be severe. Gallstones are a frequent complication of the disease.

A history of recurrent anemia or jaundice over a period of years and a positive family history are usually present and help to confirm the diagnosis, but their absence does not exclude it. Diagnosis is based on finding (1) an anemia (2 to 3.5 million red blood cells and 6 to 11 Gm. of hemoglobin) of the hemolytic type (increased blood bilirubin with increased excretion of urobilin and evidence of increased blood regeneration as manifested by an increase of reticulocytes in the peripheral blood),

(2) spherocytosis (decreased cell diameter and increased cell thickness; see Plate 36), (3) an increased susceptibility of red blood cells to hemolysis by hypotonic salt solution, (4) an increased rate of hemolysis of blood in vitro on incubation at 37°C., and (5) splenomegaly in which engorgement with blood is the outstanding feature.

Treatment—The only satisfactory treatment is splenectomy. Following this operation, the reticulocyte count returns to normal, the icterus disappears, and the anemia subsides. The spherocytosis (and often the increased cell fragility) persists. Since one hemolytic episode is usually followed by others, splenectomy is recommended for all individuals who have had one such episode. Emergency splenectomy may be necessary as a lifesaving measure during a severe crisis. Transfusions of whole blood may be required before operation; but they are best avoided, if possible, because of the occurrence of severe reactions despite careful matching of blood.

Splenectomy is not recommended for those individuals having a subclinical disturbance with few or no symptoms, for they may live out their normal expectancy with little or no discomfort.

SICKLE-CELL ANEMIA

Sickle-cell anemia is a chronic, hereditary, familial, hemolytic anemia, confined almost exclusively to Negroes, in which a high percentage of the red blood cells have an elongated crescent, or sickle, shape. The blood of approximately 10 percent of all Negroes has the sickle-cell trait, but only a small percentage of these Negroes develop an anemia.

The condition is usually noted early in life and is associated with recurring acute hemolytic episodes. Between the crises, there is usually a moderate anemia, with symptoms. During the acute crises, the condition is often confused with acute rheumatic fever because of the fever, severe bone and abdominal pains, the presence of hemic murmurs, and an enlarged heart (the result of the chronic severe anemia). Chronic ulcers above the ankles are very common and usually have a punched-out appearance. The spleen and liver usually become enlarged. Roentgenographic changes in the skull and other bones may occur.

The sickling of the red blood cells may be noted on a stained smear, but it is more readily observed by the use of special technics. In sealed wet films, sickling reaches a maximum in six to twenty-four hours. If a drop of blood is mixed with a drop of fresh 2 percent sodium bisulfite solution on a glass slide, covered with a cover slip, and examined under the microscope (high dry objective), any tendency toward sickling will become obvious within fifteen minutes. Examination of wet films should be undertaken in all Negro patients having anemia.

Treatment is unsatisfactory; there is no known method of correcting the sickling defect. During hemolytic crises, transfusion of whole blood may be lifesaving, even though severe reactions may occur.

ERYTHROBLASTOSIS FETALIS

The term "erythroblastosis fetalis" includes the syndromes formerly known as hydrops fetalis, icterus gravis, and congenital hemolytic anemia of the newborn. These syndromes are actually no more than different degrees of the same process. Infants with the disease may be stillborn with extreme anasarca, or they may develop a progressive icterus and anemia shortly after birth. The condition may be fatal unless proper treatment is instituted.

The chain of events in erythroblastosis fetalis is complicated. It starts with the mating of a man whose red blood cells contain an agglutinogen distinct from those responsible for the normal blood groups and a woman whose red cells lack that particular agglutinogen. If the child inherits the mother's lack of agglutinogen, nothing happens. If, however, the child inherits the father's agglutinogen, there is a chance that a sufficient number of fetal red cells (containing the agglutinogen) will escape through the placenta into the mother's circulation to stimulate the production of antibodies (agglutinins). These antibodies may then, in turn, pass through the placenta from the mother to the fetus, in whose circulation they will agglutinate and destroy red cells and produce a hemolytic anemia (see Plate 32).

Slightly more than 90 percent of cases of erythroblastosis fetalis are due to a group of agglutinogens collectively called the Rh factor because the first one was found in rhesus monkeys. The remainder are due to other agglutinogens. In every case, however, in order for erythroblastosis to develop, the agglutinogen must be present in the blood of the fetus but not of the mother, and the mother must become sensitized to the agglutinogen.

About 85 percent of people are Rh positive (i.e., have the Rh agglutinogen in their blood). Unless an Rh-negative woman has been sensitized by transfusion or intramuscular injection of Rh-positive blood, at least one pregnancy is required to initiate sensitization. The severest form of the disease is seen when an Rh-negative woman previously sensitized by transfusion becomes pregnant with an Rh-positive baby. A single transfusion of Rh-positive blood given in childhood may sensitize an Rh-negative woman for life. On the other hand, erythroblastosis actually occurs in only a fraction of those pregnancies in which it is possible. The combination of an Rh-positive infant and an Rh-negative mother is found in about 8 percent of pregnancies, whereas laboratory evidence of erythroblastosis is present in only about 0.6 percent of pregnancies and clinical erythroblastosis in about 0.25 percent. Apparently the placental barrier holds in most instances. In others, the mother may not develop antibodies. Once immunized, however, a woman remains so for life, and her chance of subsequently having a normal Rh-positive baby is very slight.

The effect of the hemolytic anemia on the baby depends on its duration and intensity and on the response of the baby's bone marrow. In the mildest form, the baby is anemic at birth or develops anemia within the first day or two. The blood count is usually minimal about the eighth day, after which it begins to improve. The child has the usual symptoms of anemia (p. 94). If it is severe, the child may die of anoxia (usually within the first two days) or it may develop severe purpura or hemorrhage because of thrombocytopenia or prothrombin deficiency or both.

If blood destruction has begun before term, jaundice may be present at birth or develop within a day or so. In severely anemic or jaundiced patients, there may be permanent damage (probably anoxic) to various parts of the brain, with death or with residual mental retardation, extrapyramidal spasticity, or choreoathetosis. Sometimes there is cirrhosis of the liver or enlargement of the liver and spleen.

The most severe form of erythroblastosis occurs when fetal blood destruction begins early in pregnancy. Abortion or stillbirth usually results, and the fetus is malformed, often with severe generalized edema.

Treatment—Ideal therapy for erythroblastosis fetalis would be prevention of antibody formation by the mother. No satisfactory method of achieving this has yet been found.

The next best approach is to be prepared to treat the infant immediately after birth in those instances in which the disease is possible or probable. A history of several pregnancies ending prematurely or at term in jaundiced or anemic infants suggests strongly that subsequent pregnancies may have a similar or worse outcome. In the absence of such a history, the mother's blood may be tested for Rh factor. If she is Rh positive, erythroblastosis is not possible from this factor, but it may occur from other agglutinogens.

Regardless of the outcome of other tests, the mother's and father's blood should be matched for incompatibility, evidence of which suggests the presence of antibodies which might cause erythroblastosis in the fetus.

If the mother is Rh negative, then the father's blood should be tested for this factor. If his blood is Rh positive when the mother's is Rh negative, the possibility of erythroblastosis exists, and the mother's blood should be tested at once for anti-Rh agglutinins. If the test is performed early in pregnancy, any antibodies present will be the result of previous pregnancies or transfusions. The test is repeated at seven months and just before delivery. Continued absence of antibody usually precludes the possibility of hemolytic disease.

If the original test is positive and subsequent tests show a decrease in titer, it is clear that the fetus is not immunizing the mother and is not being affected by the antibody present in the mother's blood. If the titer increases or antibody develops during pregnancy, one must assume that the mother is being immunized and that some degree of hemolytic disease may be expected in the infant. The earlier in pregnancy immunization begins, the more likely is the fetus to be involved.

The administration of 5 Gm. methionine daily to immunized mothers is said to aid the fetal and maternal livers to secrete the products of fetal hemolysis and thus make it possible for mothers showing mounting antibody titers to give birth to babies either free from the disease or showing only anemia without liver embarrassment.

Specific treatment for the newborn infant is early substitution transfusion. By this method of therapy, about 90 percent of the infant's antigen-containing red cells and a larger amount of the maternal antibody are removed. Some investigators recommend that blood substitution be performed at birth, regardless of clinical findings. However, most clinics do not consider this necessary. The infant is closely watched for two days and is treated only if anemia or jaundice develops.

In all cases, blood from the umbilical cord should be tested for maternal antibody and by the Coombs technic for sensitization of the red cells (serum for the Coombs test is available on the market). A negative Coombs test (demonstrating that the red cells have not been affected by maternal antibody) is rarely followed by severe hemolytic disease. If the Coombs test is positive, a red cell count should be performed and the icterus index determined every two hours for the first day or two. If jaundice appears and progresses during the first twenty-four hours, substitution transfusions should be performed. If the red count falls below 2.5 million, a transfusion of 75 to 100 cc. of compatible Rh-negative blood is given. Dehydration is treated by administration of lactose water by mouth or dextrose and electrolyte solution parenterally (see p. 57). One gram of methionine (p. 257) or choline (p. 504) may be added to the lactose water for possible protection to the liver.

In substitute transfusions, about 500 cc. of the baby's blood are withdrawn from one site while about 600 cc. of compatible Rh-negative blood are introduced at another. It has been suggested that blood from a woman is preferable to that from a man. The physician should familiarize himself with details of the chosen technic before attempting substitute transfusions.

Even after blood replacement, slight anemia may develop after four to six weeks. It should be treated by transfusion.

Erythremia

Erythremia (polycythemia [rubra] vera, splenomegalic polycythemia, Vaquez's disease, Osler's disease) is a rare, chronic, progressive disease due to overproduction of all the blood cells formed in the red bone marrow—red cells, granular leukocytes, and platelets. The cause is unknown; perhaps the most plausible theory is that the disease represents a benign neoplasm of the bone marrow. The onset is usually in middle age.

The average life span of the red cells is normal in erythremia, and consequently the excessive formation leads to an increase in red cell count; 7 to 10 million per cu. mm. is common, and 15 million has been recorded. Hemoglobin is less greatly increased (16 to 25 Gm. per 100 cc. are usual), largely because the red cells are small (low mean corpuscular volume). Plasma volume remains normal or is only slightly increased, but the increased numbers of red cells very greatly raise the total blood volume. The true measure of the increase in red cells is the red cell mass per unit of body weight, which is derived by multiplying the red cell count by the total blood volume and dividing by body weight. In erythremia, the hematocrit reading may

reach 65 to 85 percent, the total blood volume may be two to three times normal, and the red cell mass per unit of body weight may be four or five times normal.

Most of the signs and symptoms of erythremia are due to the increased mass of red blood cells, which distends blood vessels and organs, increases the viscosity of the blood, and slows the rate of circulation. The patients look plethoric. There is splenomegaly and usually a moderate hypertension and an arterial degeneration that resembles thromboangiitis obliterans but may occur in any part of the body, including the brain. There may be headache, vertigo, tinnitus, surging and congestive sensations, dyspnea, weakness, priapism, and gastrointestinal symptoms. Thromboses are common. Pains in the bones may be excruciating and are apparently due to pressure of the hyperplastic bone marrow. There may be hypermetabolism simulating hyperthyroidism.

Erythremia must be distinguished from polycythemia secondary to hypoxia (as in pulmonary emphysema or chronic heart failure). In erythremia, the increase in red cell mass is greater and there is an increase in white blood count (to as many as 50,000 per cu. mm., due to granular leukocytes) and in platelet count (to 1 to 6 million per cu. mm.); arterial oxygen saturation is normal. In secondary polycythemia, the increase in red cell mass is not so great and there is no increase in white cells or platelets; arterial oxygen saturation is diminished. Erythremia must also be differentiated from primary cardiovascular disease and from hyperthyroidism.

After a variable number of years, patients with erythremia may succumb to cardiovascular complications. If these are survived, the bone marrow may gradually diminish in activity and become fibrosed. Red cell production takes place in the spleen (which may become very large) and in other organs; in spite of this, however, anemia, leukopenia, and thrombocytopenia develop and eventually prove fatal.

Treatment is a long-term project which is capable of greatly prolonging the period of usefulness, comfort, and even life itself, despite the impossibility of cure. Two approaches are possible: reduction in bone-marrow activity, and removal of the excess blood from the circulation. The latter approach is the more conservative. Venesections of 500 cc. are performed twice weekly until the hematocrit reading (red cell volume) is reduced to normal (see p. 525). Six to eight bleedings are usually required.

Hemoglobin levels usually parallel hematocrit readings in a rough way and may be employed as a guide to bleeding if hematocrit readings are not obtainable.

Because of the viscosity of the blood, a large needle is recommended for the venesection. Although there have been some objections, many investigators are convinced of the value of erythremic blood for transfusion, both for its high red cell concentration and for its high platelet count (of particular value in purpura). Maintenance bleedings are undertaken as indicated by a rising hematocrit and recurrence of symptoms, usually at intervals of six to eighteen months. The patient should be placed on a low-iron diet (curtailment of intake of red meat, liver, eggs, shellfish, green vegetables high in iron, and whole-grain cereals). Such a diet reduces the need for venesection, but it or an associated deficiency of extrinsic factor may give rise to glossitis.

For those patients in whom depletion is not satisfactory for one reason or another, reduction in bone-marrow activity may be undertaken. Perhaps the best method at present is administration of radioactive phosphorus (P^{32}). It is not accompanied by the increase in platelets and thrombotic tendency that may follow bleeding. It does not deplete the blood protein. On the other hand, it is not generally available, and there is a suggestion that it may tend to induce leukemia later in the course of the disease. As an alternative to radioactive phosphorus, generalized x-ray treatment ("spray therapy") may be employed. Its effect is similar to that of radioactive phosphorus, but it may produce severe radiation sickness.

Phenylhydrazine, $C_6H_5 \cdot NH \cdot NH_2$, was at one time used in treating erythremia. The drug acts by destroying hemoglobin and thus inducing destruction of the affected red cells. It is toxic and uncertain in action and can no longer be recommended.

Agranulocytosis

Agranulocytosis (granulocytopenia, malignant neutropenia, agranulocytic angina) is a condition characterized by complete or almost complete disappearance of granular leukocytes from the bone marrow and peripheral blood. Less mature forms persist in the bone marrow and may undergo hyperplasia. In a few instances, there may be anemia and thrombocytopenia in addition to granulocytopenia.

Agranulocytosis appears to be an allergic phenomenon. In many instances no cause can be found, but in many others the condition is clearly due to a drug which also produces side-effects of unquestionably allergic nature. Drugs known to cause agranulocytosis include aminopyrine, antipyrine, thiouracil and its derivatives, sulfonamides, barbiturates, benzene, organic arsenicals, and gold salts. Radioactive phosphorus may also produce it, but probably through a different mechanism.

A chronic recurrent type has been described which is apparently unrelated to drugs and is cured permanently by splenectomy.

Only a small percentage of individuals taking the certain drug develop agranulocytosis. In some cases the condition may follow the first dose, whereas in others it may occur only after many years of therapy. The dosage which initiates it may be very small.

Agranulocytosis may have a sudden onset, or it may be the result of a slowly progressive leukopenia. In some instances the onset is silent; in others it is accompanied by chill, fever, and prostration. Usually there have been prodromal symptoms of fatigue and weakness. In some cases there is ulcerative stomatitis, pharyngitis, vaginitis, or proctitis which may or may not be due to secondary infection. Infection occurs sooner or later in untreated agranulocytosis and is the cause of the very high mortality rate.

In true agranulocytosis, the white count is usually below 2,000 per cu. mm. The reduction is mainly at the expense of the granulocytes, but the lymphocytes may be reduced also. In very severe cases, the count may fall below 1,000 and the granulocytes may disappear completely.

Treatment—Some aspects of the treatment of agranulocytosis are still controversial, but several points are clear. It is of utmost importance to discover and discontinue the offending drug at once. There is some evidence that the longer such a drug acts after the onset of agranulocytosis, the poorer is the prognosis. The next thing is to administer chemotherapy, even if there is no evidence of infection. Penicillin should be given in total daily doses of 500,000 to 1,000,000 units, supplemented by the sulfonamides and other antibiotics if infection fails to respond to penicillin. Chemotherapy is continued until a normal blood picture returns and infection has subsided. If the offending drug is stopped promptly and adequate chemotherapy is administered, the mortality rate is very low. In untreated or late cases, it is 80 to 90 percent.

Attempts have been made to speed return of the leukocytes by stimulating the bone marrow. Results that are apparently good have been reported from the use of Pentnucleotide, liver extracts, pyridoxine, extracts of yellow bone marrow, and repeated blood transfusions. However, some investigators have not been impressed. Dosage and administration are discussed on page 372.

Early discovery of agranulocytosis is sufficiently important to make it incumbent on the physician to warn the patient for whom he prescribes drugs which may induce the condition. Prescriptions should be marked "nonrefillable," and the patient should be told to report at once any unusual fatigue, weakness, or sore throat or any evidence of illness or infection. Should any of these symptoms appear or should the patient suffer an intercurrent illness, total white and differential counts should be made frequently until the patient is well.

Leukemia

Leukemia (leukanemia, leukocythemia) is a uniformly fatal disease due to abnormal proliferation of white blood cells and infiltration of masses of these cells into the tissues of the body. Abnormal white blood cells are always present in either the bone marrow or the lymph glands and can usually be found in the peripheral blood.

The cause of leukemia is unknown, but it is generally considered to be of neoplastic origin. However, there are features of the disease which suggest that it is of infectious origin. Leukemia has been divided into types according to the characteristics of the predominating cell type. The three main groups are myelogenous, lymphatic, and monocytic, in which the parent cells are respectively myeloblasts, lymphoblasts, and histioblasts. These types are further divided into acute and chronic varieties. A subleukemic stage of these varieties (that is, with normal total white blood count) may occur during the course of the disease, or the disease may run a subleukemic course throughout. In a subleukemic phase, close inspection of a stained smear will usually reveal the abnormal cells, even though the total white cell count is within normal limits.

The various types of leukemia may occur at any age. However, chronic myelogenous leukemia tends to occur before sixty, whereas chronic lymphatic leukemia is more likely to begin after that age. The acute leukemias occur predominantly before twenty-five years. Acute myelogenous is seen most often during the first ten years of life; the acute lymphatic occurs more frequently between the ages of ten and twenty-five.

ACUTE LEUKEMIA

Regardless of type, the clinical picture of acute leukemia is generally the same. There is usually an acute onset, with fever, toxemia, and prostration. Anemia develops rapidly. Thrombocytopenia leads to purpura and hemorrhages from the mucous membranes, especially of the nose. The clinical picture may resemble an acute, overwhelming infection. In some cases the rapidly developing anemia is the outstanding clinical feature. The lymph glands may be enlarged slightly, as may the spleen. Gangrenous stomatitis or ulcerative lesions of mucosa of the mouth may dominate the picture. Extreme proliferation of the gums may be present. It has been said that enlarged glands are more common in acute lymphatic, enlarged spleen in acute myelogenous, and ulcerative lesions of mouth and pustular skin lesions in acute monocytic leukemia; however, this is not a fast rule.

Examination of blood usually confirms the diagnosis, but, in occasional cases, bone-marrow studies are required. The normocytic anemia is usually outstanding and progressive and may be very severe. The white blood cell count, which is usually elevated but rarely more than 60,000, may be normal or below normal. Abnormal cells can generally be found on stained smear, and the predominating cells are often myeloblasts, lymphoblasts, or histioblasts (see Plates 37, 41, and 42). The predominance of blast cells differentiates the acute varieties from the chronic, in which only a few such cells are present except during acute exacerbations. It may be difficult or impossible to differentiate on stained smears the type of blast cell that is present. The finding of a fair percentage of myelocytes, metamyelocytes, and polymorphonuclear leukocytes along with the blast cells indicates that the condition is acute myelogenous leukemia. The association of adult lymphocytes with blast cells suggests an acute lymphatic leukemia. Mature monocytes will be seen with the blast cells in acute monocytic leukemia. In the occasional case, a diagnosis of stem-cell or blast-cell leukemia will have to be made unless the blood is studied by supravital staining technic.

Treatment—Acute leukemia is usually fatal within a few weeks. Treatment is at present only palliative. Radiation therapy is contraindicated inasmuch as it may hasten the fatal outcome, especially if hemorrhagic manifestations are present. Frequent transfusions of whole fresh blood (500 to 800 cc. daily) may produce temporary improvement.

Aminopterin and A-Methopterin, folic acid antagonists, have been used experimentally in the treatment of the acute leukemias. A temporary remission is reported in a moderate percentage of patients. However, aminopterin is quite toxic and is often followed by the development of stomatitis, hemorrhagic manifestations, and bloody diarrhea. The recommended dose is from 0.5 to 1 mg. daily by subcutaneous injection. It is discontinued on development of toxic symptoms. Maintenance dosage is 0.5 mg. daily or at less frequent intervals as indicated by the clinical condition of the patient. A-Methopterin is less toxic. The dose is 5 mg. daily by mouth. The response to repeated courses of either drug is often less satisfactory than to a first course.

CHRONIC MYELOGENOUS LEUKEMIA

Chronic myelogenous leukemia (chronic myeloid leukemia, chronic splenomyelogenous leukemia) is often insidious in onset. The greatly increased white blood count or enlarged spleen may be found during a routine examination before the onset of any symptoms. The first overt manifestation may be a sensation of weight in the left upper quadrant of the abdomen or the finding of a mass in this region by the patient. Eventually, symptoms develop as a result of the increased metabolism and anemia. These include weakness, loss of weight, pallor, dyspnea, vertigo, palpitation, and fatigability.

Great enlargement of the spleen is a conspicuous finding in chronic myelogenous leukemia. The size alone may produce symptoms, and there may be local pain and tenderness because of splenic infarction and perisplenitis. There is also pallor of the skin and mucous membranes, retinal hemorrhages, enlarged liver, and evidence of weight loss. The lymph glands are slightly if at all enlarged, and hemorrhagic manifestations usually do not occur until late.

Early in the disease, there is usually a normocytic anemia (2 to 3 million). The outstanding finding is the greatly increased white blood count, which is usually between 100,000 and 200,000 per cu. mm. Counts of more than a million have been recorded. On stained smears a great preponderance of granular cells is found, and usually 30 to 40 percent of them are neutrophilic myelocytes (see Plates 38, 41, and 42). The polymorphonuclears, metamyelocytes, eosinophils, and basophils are also increased in absolute number. One to 3 percent are usually myeloblasts. The basal metabolism is likely to be considerably increased, especially in the more

rapidly progressing conditions. Diagnosis rests on the finding of an enlarged spleen, anemia, and the characteristic blood picture.

Treatment is only palliative, and death usually occurs within two or three years after the onset of symptoms. However, x-ray therapy often produces a temporary remission of the disease, with improvement of anemia, decrease in the white blood cell count, and decrease in the size of the spleen. Individual responses vary greatly. X-ray should be interrupted when the white blood count falls to 30,000, for severe leukopenia may then follow additional treatment. Since the condition eventually becomes resistant to x-ray, it is often advisable to withhold irradiation until it is made necessary by the anemia or by the symptoms which result from the greatly enlarged spleen.

Recently, urethane has appeared to be a helpful adjunct to irradiation. Its use is discussed on page 372. Radioactive phosphorus has also been employed, but without success. Transfusion of whole blood is the only known treatment for the anemia and the hemorrhagic manifestations.

CHRONIC LYMPHATIC LEUKEMIA

Chronic lymphatic (lymphocytic) leukemia usually begins insidiously, and the earliest finding is commonly the painless, often generalized lymphgland enlargement. As the disease progresses, symptoms result from the accompanying anemia and increased metabolism. The lymph glands vary in size up to several centimeters in diameter. They are not tender and do not adhere to each other or to the skin. They may produce pressure symptoms, depending on their location. The spleen is usually enlarged, but not greatly so. The white blood cell count is rarely elevated over 200,000 and is usually between 60,000 and 100,000 per cu. mm. Up to 90 percent of the white blood cells may resemble normal lymphocytes, but there are usually a small number of lymphoblasts present (see Plates 39, 41, and 42). The normocytic anemia is slowly progressive. Length of life after the onset of the condition averages four to five years.

Lymphosarcoma-cell leukemia is often considered a form of lymphatic leukemia; actually, it seems to be a different entity. It arises during the course of lymphosarcoma (p. 107), after the lymphgland involvement has remained localized for some time. The breaking over of the neoplastic cells into the blood stream is usually a terminal process. With the onset of the leukemic phase, signs and symptoms of anemia and generalized lymph-gland enlargement become superimposed on the symptoms referable to the localized tumor mass. The sarcoma cells in the peripheral blood usually differ greatly in appearance from the normal lymphocytes present. They are large cells with a small amount of deep-blue-staining cytoplasm. There is usually one eccentrically placed light-blue-staining large nucleolus in the nucleus.

Treatment is the same as for chronic myelogenous leukemia (see above).

MONOCYTIC LEUKEMIA

Monocytic leukemia, formerly thought to be quite rare, is now being diagnosed much more frequently. It has been divided into two types on hematological grounds. In the Naegeli type, which is thought to be of myelogenous origin, there are myeloblasts and early myelocytes in addition to the monocytes. The Schilling type has only increased numbers of monocytes and histioblasts (monoblasts) (see Plates 40, 41, and 42). The monocytes in monocytic leukemia apparently develop from the reticulo-endothelial system.

Acute and chronic varieties have been described, but often the condition runs a chronic course until there is an acute exacerbation preceding the termination of the disease. Signs and symptoms include those referable to the anemia, moderate splenomegaly, fever, loss of weight, ulcerative lesions of the mouth, hypertrophy of the gums, and purpura. Skin lesions may develop. Lymph-gland enlargement is usually confined to the cervical region. The average length of life is about two years.

Treatment, as in other types of leukemia, is palliative. Chief reliance is on blood transfusions, however, for the condition does not respond to radiation as well as do the other types of leukemia.

MULTIPLE MYELOMA

Multiple myeloma is a neoplastic-like disease involving destructive lesions of the bones. It is accompanied by an anemia and the presence of Bence-Jones proteins in the blood and urine. It is generally considered that the neoplastic process involves the myeloid cells derived from the bone marrow which are closely related to, if not identical with, plasma cells. Clinically, the outstanding findings are anemia, severe bone pain, pathological fractures, x-ray evidence of punched-out areas of bones, the finding of Bence-Jones proteins in the urine, and high plasma protein. The increase in plasma protein is due to globulin. Autohemagglutination and greatly increased sedimentation rate often result from this hyperglobulinemia. The moderately severe anemia is usually macrocytic in character. There may be a few plasma cells in the blood stream; but in those rare cases in which there is infiltration of the tissues of the body with plasma cells, a true plasma-cell leukemia is present. In such cases the blood count may reach 50,000, with 20 to 50 percent of the cells being plasma cells.

Diagnosis rests in x-ray findings, the presence of Bence-Jones proteins in the urine, and high plasma protein. The bone-marrow findings are often characteristic. Great numbers of plasma cells are usually present; they may constitute as much as 90 percent of the nucleated cells. One or more nucleoli are present in many of the plasma cells. However, plasma cells may be found in increased numbers in the bone marrow in other conditions (cirrhosis, Hodgkin's disease, and chronic infections). Multiple myeloma is always fatal but usually lasts for two to three years.

Treatment—X-ray therapy may be followed by relief of pain. Frequent transfusions are necessary to combat the anemia. Urethane may be beneficial (see p. 372).

Purpura

Purpura is characterized by bleeding into and under the skin, into and from the mucous membranes, into the tissues of internal organs, and sometimes into the joints. The causes and mechanism of purpura are poorly understood. Reduction in the number of circulating platelets (thrombocytopenia) is sometimes a factor, but purpura from a given etiological agent may at one time be associated with thrombocytopenia and at another time with a normal platelet count. On the other hand, thrombocytopenia may occur without hemorrhage.

In spite of these apparent inconsistencies, the purpuras are usually classified according to the platelet count, as indicated in Table 13. It is generally thought, however, that some sort of injury to capillary walls is at least as important as the behavior of the platelets in the genesis of purpura.

Thrombocytopenic Purpura is marked not only by a low platelet count (the normal varies with the method; for one method, see p. 527), but also by

TABLE 13—*Types of Purpura*

I. Thrombocytopenic
   A. Idiopathic (purpura haemorrhagica), without known cause; characterized by an increased number of megakaryocytes (the apparent precursors of platelets) in the bone marrow
   B. Toxic; characterized by greatly reduced numbers of megakaryocytes in the bone marrow
      1. Certain infections, such as typhoid fever, typhus, scarlet fever, measles, smallpox, subacute bacterial endocarditis, and other septicemias
      2. Drugs (allergic?), including organic arsenicals, gold salts, benzene, snake venoms, and certain sedatives
      3. Irradiation, as with x-ray or administration of radioactive phosphorus
   C. Allergic; drugs (see above), foods, or cosmetics
   D. Associated with blood disorders
      1. Aplasia of bone marrow, as in anemias
      2. Replacement of bone marrow, as in leukemia, multiple myeloma, Hodgkin's disease, and metastatic cancer
      3. Splenic disorders, such as Gaucher's disease, Felty's syndrome, and hemolytic jaundice
   E. Miscellaneous

II. Nonthrombocytopenic
   A. Toxic
      1. Certain infections, including those listed above
      2. Chronic wasting diseases, such as chronic renal, cardiac, or hepatic disease
      3. Drugs, including iodides, belladonna, quinine, bismuth, mercurials, salicylates, chloral hydrate, and snake venoms
   B. Avitaminosis C (scurvy)
   C. Allergic; purpuras of Henoch and Schönlein
   D. Miscellaneous

prolonged bleeding time (but normal coagulation time), delayed clot retraction, and increased capillary fragility. The onset of an attack may be sudden. Purpuric lesions of the skin are the most common symptoms, but any type of hemorrhagic manifestation may occur. The spleen may be slightly enlarged, but there is no constant physical finding. Changes in the red and white blood cell counts are incidental to hemorrhage or to the primary disease. The bone marrow shows an increased or decreased number of megakaryocytes (see Table 13). Tests have been proposed for determining capillary fragility (e.g., the Rumpel-Leede test), but none is of particular value.

The possible cause of thrombocytopenic purpura should always be sought (see Table 13). Idiopathic disease (purpura haemorrhagica) is a chronic dis-

order of spontaneous relapses and remissions. It tends to occur in families and usually has its onset in childhood or early adult years. Ready bruising is a common observation. The disease may be fulminating, with fatal outcome. Idiopathic thrombocytopenic purpura is distinguished from secondary types by (1) increase in megakaryocytes in the bone marrow, (2) slight or no lymphadenopathy or splenomegaly, (3) absence of abnormal cells from the blood and bone marrow, (4) absence of anemia which cannot be explained by blood loss, (5) normal or only slightly increased white blood count, and (6) no history of recent ingestion of drugs or occurrence of infections known to produce purpura.

TREATMENT—The patient should be put to bed for the duration of an attack. The diet should be rich in hemoglobin-building and vitamin-containing foods such as liver, kidneys, chicken gizzard, eggs, apricots, peaches, and other fruits and vegetables. If there is hemorrhage, the patient should receive transfusions of 500 to 1,000 cc. (for an adult) of fresh whole blood. The effect of such a transfusion usually lasts two or three days.

The distinction between idiopathic and secondary purpura is important in treatment as well as for prognosis. The cause of secondary purpura should be sought and removed or treated. Aside from transfusions, there is no satisfactory direct treatment of secondary purpura as such.

The natural tendency toward improvement during attacks of idiopathic thrombocytopenic purpura makes evaluation of therapy difficult. If recurrences continue or if they are not controlled by transfusions, splenectomy may be performed. However, it is not a cure-all and should not be undertaken lightly. It is a dangerous procedure in acute purpura, and it is not indicated in secondary purpura as a treatment of purpura itself.

Many drugs have been tried in thrombocytopenic purpura with controversial results. Vitamin C has been recommended (200 to 300 mg. daily), as have preparations with vitamin P activity (p. 501).

Nonthrombocytopenic Purpura may be of toxic origin, in which case the primary cause is usually clear (see Table 13); it may be part of the picture of scurvy (p. 491); or it may be allergic. Allergic nonthrombocytopenic purpuras are often associated with other allergic manifestations such as erythema, urticaria, effusions, and edemas. Purpura may occur as part of angioneurotic edema, erythema nodosum, erythema multiforme, and the like.

"Henoch's purpura" is the name given to a type in which there is urticaria of the intestinal wall, with effusion of tissue fluid and blood. Transient or severe colic is the most common symptom. The abdomen is tender but not rigid. There may be vomiting. Constipation is the rule, and it may be associated with obstruction. Although uncommon, diarrhea may be observed; it may be bloody. Moderate, irregular fever is common. Rheumatoid pains often precede the attack. When the abdominal symptoms precede the skin eruption, Henoch's purpura may be difficult to distinguish from a surgical abdomen.

In "Schönlein's purpura," there are periarticular effusions as well as purpura of the skin. The lower extremities are most commonly affected. Slight fever may be present. When the skin lesions are late in appearing, the condition may be confused with rheumatic fever. However, it is not affected by salicylates.

In the nonthrombocytopenic purpuras, hemorrhage is rarely sufficient to cause anemia. There may be neutrophilic leukocytosis and sometimes eosinophilia. The platelet count is normal, as are bleeding and coagulation times and clot retraction.

TREATMENT of the attack itself is symptomatic. Vasoconstrictor drugs such as epinephrine and ephedrine (p. 422 *et seq.*) may be of value. Antihistaminic drugs (p. 509) may be tried. Preparations having vitamin P activity (p. 501) have been recommended. Basic treatment is discovery and eradication of the underlying cause. This may be difficult in allergic purpura.

Hodgkin's Disease

Hodgkin's disease (lymphoblastoma, malignant lymphoma, malignant lymphogranuloma, or pseudoleukemia) is a uniformly fatal condition, often running a chronic, prolonged course marked by painless and progressive enlargement of lymph glands. These show characteristic histological changes and are temporarily radiosensitive.

Three clinically and histologically distinct types have been described. The most benign form, Hodgkin's paragranuloma, is compatible with a practically normal life for many years and seems to be an infectious process. It may or may not be transformed into the more malignant type, Hodgkin's granuloma. This is the classic type of the disease and has been considered to be neoplastic, although there is increasing evidence that it may be infectious. The third and most malignant, Hodgkin's sarcoma (lymphosarcoma), has all the features of a highly invasive neoplasm and tends to occur in an older age group.

Widespread involvement of lymph glands usually occurs eventually, although in a majority of cases the glands of one side of the neck are involved first. The glands are firm and freely movable and neither tender nor adherent to the skin or adjacent glands. The lymph-gland enlargement may be the only early symptom, but sooner or later constitutional symptoms develop. These include loss of weight, weakness, pruritus, symptoms of anemia (which develops during the course of the disease), and fever, often of characteristic recurring character (Pel-Ebstein type). Symptoms may also result from pressure of enlarged glands on nerves, blood and lymph vessels, and organs of the body. Abdominal symptoms are common, and in some cases all manifestations are restricted to the abdomen. Splenomegaly is usually a late phenomenon.

The development of painless, enlarged lymph glands is most suggestive of Hodgkin's disease, but the diagnosis rests primarily on finding the characteristic microscopic picture in a biopsy of the involved glands. Changes in the blood occur but are not of diagnostic value.

Treatment—At present, symptomatic local x-ray treatment is the best available therapy. It prolongs life in a majority of individuals but does not cure the condition. X-ray should be given only when the patient's symptoms demand it, for the disease process becomes resistant to x-ray after one or two treatments.

One of the nitrogen mustards, Mechlorethamine (bis-beta-chloroethylmethylamine), which has the formula $(ClCH_2 \cdot CH_2)_2 : N \cdot CH_3$, appears to be useful as an adjunct to irradiation. It is of value after the patient has become refractory to the latter, and in some instances it has appeared to restore susceptibility. It is given as the hydrochloride, in courses of one to seven daily intravenous injections of 0.1 mg. per Kg. of body weight. Serious delayed toxic effects may occur, including lymphocytopenia, granulocytopenia, and thrombocytopenia.

Anemia is best treated by transfusion of whole blood. Iron and liver may be tried, but they are seldom effective.

Hemorrhagic Diseases

HYPOPROTHROMBINEMIA

There are five main situations in which a low blood level of prothrombin is found: (1) deficiency of vitamin K (see p. 499), (2) inadequate absorption of vitamin K from the gastro-intestinal tract, (3) poor utilization of vitamin K by the liver, (4) action of drugs, and (5) idiopathic.

Deficiency of Vitamin K—True dietary deficiency of vitamin K is highly improbable because of its wide distribution in food and its synthesis by the normal intestinal flora. However, in newborn infants there is a high incidence of vitamin K deficiency.

Hemorrhagic disease of the newborn occurs in about 1 percent of infants. It is due directly to lack of vitamin K and is the only clinically recognized form of primary deficiency. The newborn infant has received prothrombin from its mother antenatally. During the first seven to ten days of life there is no natural source of the vitamin, since the bacterial flora of the intestinal tract are not well established and no vitamin K is obtained from colostrum or breast milk. Consequently, all infants will show a fall in blood prothrombin; in an occasional one, this becomes severe enough to depress the clotting mechanism to hemorrhagic levels. Usually such hemorrhage develops between the second and sixth days. There is no critical prothrombin level below which bleeding is inevitable. There is a potential risk when activity is below 70 percent of normal; if it is below 40 percent of normal, hemorrhage is usually severe when it does occur. The prothrombin tests are described on page 529.

Aside from the actual amount of prothrombin with which the infant is born, there are other factors which, though controversial, have appeared to affect prothrombin level. Asphyxia neonatorum is frequently associated with abnormally low levels and coincident intracranial hemorrhage. Obstetrical trauma is, of course, a direct cause of cerebral vascular accidents; but in some cases it may play a secondary role, and the defect in the clotting mechanism may be directly responsible. Many believe this explains the slow, oozing type of hemorrhage which does not become clinically evident until the fifth or sixth day of life. Barbiturates given to produce analgesia during labor, even when given in small doses, are said to depress maternal prothrombin unless vitamin K is given. Inhalation anesthesia, particularly when prolonged or repeated, may be a factor.

The clinical manifestations of hemorrhagic disease of the newborn depend upon the site and extent of the bleeding. This commonly occurs in the gastro-intestinal tract (giving rise to melena or hematemesis); from the umbilical cord, nose, mouth, or genito-urinary tract; or into cephalohematomas. Exsanguination and death may occur in severe cases by the fourth or fifth day.

Prophylactic administration of vitamin K to the mother before delivery is the treatment of choice. This may be accomplished with daily oral doses of menadione, 1 to 2 mg., during the last two to five weeks of pregnancy. Single large doses of 5 to 10 mg. given at the onset of labor may be employed. There is evidence that some response is obtained when the drug is given as late as an hour or two before delivery. If water-soluble preparations are used, doses should be adjusted according to potency (p. 499). Parenteral administration is generally preferred for prophylaxis when labor is already in progress; and if labor should be prolonged, a second dose in eighteen to twenty-four hours is recommended.

Vitamin K may be given prophylactically to the infant immediately after delivery. There may be some delay in response because of slow absorption or temporary depression of liver function. Oral or parenteral doses of 1 to 2 mg. menadione or its equivalent are sufficient. Routine administration to both mother and infant is sometimes preferred. The vitamin should be administered prophylactically to all infants requiring surgical procedures during the first seven to ten days of life. In the presence of hypoprothrombinemia and hemorrhage, active treatment should be started immediately, the above doses being given once or twice daily. They are continued until prothrombin returns to normal. Severe anemia may require transfusion of 50 to 100 cc. of whole blood.

Therapeutic doses are nontoxic, and amounts several times those recommended do not cause untoward side-effects. Vitamin K is of no value in erythroblastosis fetalis, hemophilia, or hemorrhage from causes other than deficiency of prothrombin.

Inadequate Absorption of Vitamin K—Vitamin K is absorbed from the intestine only in the presence of bile salts. In obstructive jaundice and in bile fistulas, when no bile reaches the intestines, a great decrease in the blood level of prothrombin results and is followed by the well-known hemorrhagic tendency in these conditions. Oral administration of vitamin K and bile salts or the parenteral injection of synthetic preparations of vitamin K cures this hypoprothrombinemia. In sprue, ulcerative colitis, other conditions associated with chronic diarrhea, intestinal anastomoses, intestinal obstruction, intestinal fistula, and the like, there may be a decreased absorption of vitamin K and resultant abnormally low blood level of prothrombin. In these conditions, parenteral administration of vitamin K may be necessary (see p. 499).

Poor Utilization of Vitamin K by the Liver — Prothrombin is synthesized in the liver, and consequently a deficiency of prothrombin may accompany any severe disease of this organ, such as advanced cirrhosis, severe hepatitis, or cancer of the liver. Because the liver is *unable* to synthesize prothrombin in these conditions, the administration of vitamin K does not increase the prothrombin content of the blood and does not relieve the hemorrhagic tendency.

Action of Drugs — A few drugs are able to reduce the prothrombin level of the blood. Perhaps the most powerful is Dicumarol, which is employed clinically in prevention and treatment of thrombosis and embolism. The drug and its uses are discussed on page 375.

Salicylates (which are related chemically to Dicumarol) produce in rats hypoprothrombinemia which is overcome by vitamin K. They are considered by some investigators to have the same action in man, and it has been suggested that 1 mg. of menadione (see p. 499) be administered prophylactically for each gram of salicylic acid.

Idiopathic Hypoprothrombinemia is a rare disease, formerly classified as atypical hemophilia, in which there is a severe hypoprothrombinemia for which no cause can be found. The condition usually becomes manifest in infancy and is characterized by frequent recurrent hemorrhages following trivial injury. The only abnormality of blood coagulation is the increased prothrombin time. Administration of vitamin K does not correct the hypoprothrombinemia. The only treatment is repeated transfusions.

HEMOPHILIA

Hemophilia is a hereditary disease, occurring only in the male but transmitted only by the female, in which the coagulation of the blood is much prolonged. This disease usually becomes manifest in infancy. The outstanding symptom is hemorrhage following trauma which would not normally cause bleeding. The bleeding usually continues for hours or days and tends to be of a persistent, oozing character which results in severe anemia and even death if not stopped. The bleeding time is normal, for bleeding from a pinprick stops in normal time. One of the common complications is deformity of joints following hemorrhage into them. Few individuals with hemophilia reach adult life; more than half die during the first five years.

It has been suggested that the essential defect in hemophilia is a deficiency in some activity associated with the globulin fraction of the plasma protein. The chemical identity of this factor is not known, but it may be a precursor of thromboplastin. It has been designated "antihemophilic globulin." It is present in normal individuals and is essential for coagulation. The addition of this antihemophilic globulin from normal individuals to hemophilic blood in vitro causes the hemophilic blood to clot. It is also capable of bringing the coagulation time of hemophiliacs to normal in vivo.

The diagnosis of hemophilia is based on (1) family history, (2) occurrence of repeated protracted hemorrhages, (3) joint manifestations, and (4) prolonged coagulation time of the blood.

Because of the lack of thromboplastin in the plasma, very little of the prothrombin is converted into thrombin during the process of clotting. This decreased utilization or conversion of prothrombin can be determined in the laboratory. Quick considers this test to be more reliable than the determination of coagulation time in the diagnosis of hemophilia.

Treatment — The aim of treatment is to supply the deficient factor that is necessary for normal clotting of the blood. Transfusion of whole blood or plasma will temporarily bring the coagulation time to normal. In the past, this procedure has been reserved for emergencies. The transfusion of 100 cc. of whole blood will reduce the coagulation time to normal for several hours. In case of emergency, transfusions of 500 to 1,000 cc. are in order. The degree of anemia influences the amount of blood required. Within three to four days the coagulation time returns to its original level, but meanwhile hemorrhage has been stopped and the tissues have healed sufficiently to prevent further bleeding. Major surgical operations can be done if the patients are transfused (1,000 cc.) before surgery and while healing is occurring.

It has recently been found possible to maintain the coagulation at near normal by repeated prophylactic transfusions. Apparently, some patients become refractory to this type of therapy, but others can be maintained for long periods of time, during which they can lead normal lives. The amount of blood or plasma and frequency of their injection must be determined for each individual patient. After fractionation of plasma, it has been shown that 200 to 600 mg. of Fraction I (Cohn and associates) of the plasma proteins, given intravenously in 10 to 20 cc. of isotonic salt solution, are as effective as 80 to 100 cc. of plasma or 100 cc.

of whole blood in reducing the coagulation time. Patients receiving these purified fractions, however, have been reported to become resistant to further therapy, and antibodies against the purified globulin fractions have been demonstrated in their blood.

It has been shown that the antihemophilic globulin substance acts as a local hemostatic when applied in dry form with adequate dressings to the bleeding point. Local hemorrhage may be arrested by such preparations in a few minutes. Instantaneous arrest of hemorrhage can, however, be obtained by local application of another globulin preparation obtained from human, bovine, rabbit, or porcine plasma by a salting-out procedure. This "hemostatic globulin," which is thrombic in nature, has been used in local control of hemorrhage following amputations, débridements, and dental extractions in hemophiliacs.

In emergency, gauze dressings soaked in normal blood can be used to control local hemorrhage.

PSEUDOHEMOPHILIA

Pseudohemophilia is a hereditary disease occurring in both males and females. The cause appears to be a disturbance in contractility of the capillaries following trauma. Such a defect can be demonstrated by direct visualization of the capillaries in the nail beds of patients having the disease. The result is a prolonged bleeding time. Coagulation time, platelet count, and clot retraction are normal.

The patient with pseudohemophilia usually complains of excessive bleeding over a long period—often since childhood. Although bleeding may be completely spontaneous, it usually occurs following a slight cut or other trauma. Severe postoperative bleeding is common but inconstant, occurring in connection with one operation but not with another. Bleeding may occur from the nose, gums, gastro-intestinal tract, or uterus or into the skin, urinary tract, or joints. Hemorrhage following dental extraction is common and may be the first indication of the disease. Increased capillary fragility can be demonstrated in about half the cases; nevertheless, ecchymoses occur more frequently than petechiae. Death from hemorrhage is rare.

The diagnosis depends on the history of hemorrhage, a positive family history, and prolonged bleeding time in the presence of normal coagulation time, platelet count, and clot retraction.

Treatment is unsatisfactory. During active bleeding, the only reliable measures are pressure and local application of fibrin foam. Operations should be avoided insofar as possible. Transfusions may be necessary to replace blood loss.

RESPIRATORY SYSTEM
Nose and Throat
EPISTAXIS

Epistaxis, or nasal hemorrhage, occurs most frequently from these areas: Kiesselbach's area, which lies on the anterior part of the nasal septum above the intermaxillary bone and is richly supplied with capillaries; the upper portion of the nose near the root of the middle turbinate; the convex area of the inferior turbinate from the floor of the nasal passage posteriorly; the middle of the septum; and nevi, which may occur anywhere.

Epistaxis may be due to local causes, such as trauma, irritation, inflammation, abnormality of a small blood vessel, or tumor. It may be secondary to systemic disturbances, such as generalized infection, blood dyscrasia, scurvy, cardiac or vascular disease, or to violent exertion, especially at high altitude.

Diagnosis is rarely difficult, except perhaps in an occasional patient whose nasal hemorrhage is far enough posterior so that the blood is unconsciously swallowed. The anterior nasal area should be examined thoroughly in any patient who shows blood in the pharynx.

Treatment—The patient should be propped in a sitting posture. Mild epistaxis of local origin may be checked by one of the following measures:

1. An ice pack to the nose.

2. Application to the bleeding area of a cotton pledget soaked with a solution of epinephrine hydrochloride, 1:1,000 (p. 422).

3. Local cauterization by heat, surgical diathermy, or chemical agents. For the last, a topical anesthetic (p. 441) is first applied, then a drop of chromic acid, trichloroacetic acid, or silver nitrate solution or stick. The use of acid is followed at once by thorough application of saturated solution of sodium bicarbonate, and the use of silver nitrate is followed by thorough application of sodium chloride.

4. Packing of the nose with gauze, or the insertion of a lubricated condom which is then inflated with air.

Nasal hemorrhage in patients having hemophilia, purpura, septicemia, leukemia, scurvy, or polycythemia vera is a serious complication, and active measures must be used promptly. Local treatment should be given as suggested above, in addition to the institution of every measure possible to correct the underlying cause.

Among the drugs having a general systemic effect and used as adjunct therapy in the treatment of epistaxis are morphine (p. 399) to quiet the patient and calcium salts intravenously (p. 344) for possible effects on blood coagulation.

As yet, there is no known good coagulant which can be administered systemically. However, in chronic epistaxis, moccasin snake venom has been reported upon favorably. The best results were obtained in patients who had telangiectasia, ulceration, or hemangioma of the nasal septum, not associated with blood dyscrasia. The venom is diluted 1:3,000 with isotonic salt solution and preserved with a 1:10,000 dilution of 'Merthiolate.' Beginning with an initial dose of 0.5 cc. of the 1:3,000 dilution, injections are given twice weekly as the dosage is rapidly increased to 1 cc. as a maximum. In children the recommended initial dose is 0.3 cc.; and the maximum, 0.8 cc. The duration of therapy depends upon the results.

In severe cases, blood transfusion may be indicated, and thorough and continuous suction may be necessary to determine and cauterize the bleeding point.

CHRONIC RHINITIS

Chronic rhinitis (chronic rhinopharyngitis, hypertrophic rhinitis) is an inflammatory condition of the nose due to prolonged irritation of the nasal mucosa from chronic obstruction, latent sinus disease, recurrent acute nasal infections, nasal allergy, or constant or recurrent exposure to dust or irritating chemicals. Exposure to cold and drafts, rapid climatic changes, and other unhygienic conditions may be important contributory factors.

Clinical manifestations include repeated attacks of coryza, diminution or absence of sense of smell, chronic nasal obstruction (often on alternate sides), altered nasal secretion, crusting, hyperplasia of mucosa and submucosa, hypertrophied turbinates, and postnasal discharge.

Treatment should aim at correcting the underlying cause. Deformities causing significant nasal obstruction should be corrected surgically. Symptomatic relief may be afforded by inhalants and solutions containing vasoconstrictors (p. 376). When long-continued use is anticipated, administration by atomizer or vapor inhalation is preferred.

ATROPHIC RHINITIS

Atrophic rhinitis (ozena) is a chronic disorder characterized by atrophy of the nasal mucous membrane and the presence of thick discharge and crusts which usually have a foul odor. The atrophy may involve the olfactory area and cause loss of the sense of smell. The disease usually has its onset before or during adolescence. The cause is unknown.

Treatment—Cleanliness is essential and may be attained by using a nasal douche containing 1 teaspoonful of salt and 2 teaspoonfuls of sodium bicarbonate to a pint of warm water. The level of fluid in the douche bag should be no more than three inches above the nose. The treatment may be repeated once or twice daily. Odor and crusting are often reduced by application of a hygroscopic solution such as corn syrup or 25 percent dextrose in glycerin.

Temporary improvement follows local hyperemia, which can be induced by increasing the acetylcholine content of the nasal tissues. This can be accomplished by:

1. Inhibition of cholinesterase with neostigmine methylsulfate (p. 419). The usual procedure is to spray into each nostril, four times daily, 0.25 cc. of a 1:2,000 solution.

2. Increase in the liberation of acetylcholine with estrogens (p. 463). An oil solution of estrogen, 1,000 or 2,000 International Units per cc., is sprayed into each nostril two or three times daily in 0.25-cc. amounts. Ampoules estrone (p. 466) may be used to prepare the oil solution.

These treatments must be continued indefinitely.

In cases from which organisms of the *Klebsiella* genus can be cultured, considerable improvement may follow the administration of streptomycin, 1 to 2 Gm. daily, for periods up to fourteen days.

SINUSITIS

Sinusitis is an inflammation of the maxillary, frontal, ethmoid, or sphenoid air cavities communicating with the nose. Sinusitis occurs most commonly as the extension of an infectious process in the nose. Infection may also be blood-borne or may be secondary to trauma or to root abscesses of the teeth. Atopic or bacterial allergy, mechanical or chemical irritation, and hypothyroidism may be important contributing factors. Many clinicians are convinced that a close relationship exists between chronic nervous tension and chronic sinusitis.

Symptoms vary with the location and number of sinuses affected, virulence of the infection, severity of the inflammation, freedom of drainage, and duration of the disease. Nasal and ostial obstruction is usually present.

Acute sinusitis causes pain, tenderness, and unilateral or bilateral nasal discharge. This may be mucoid, mucopurulent, purulent, or hemorrhagic, and sometimes fetid. The symptoms of chronic sinusitis are similar but less intense.

Origin of the discharge may be determined by wiping out the nose and applying gentle suction or by lowering the head, thus increasing pressure within the sinuses. Examination will then reveal from which ostium the discharge is coming. The posterior ethmoid and sphenoid sinuses drain posteriorly into the superior meatus; the frontal, anterior ethmoid, and maxillary sinuses drain anteriorly into the middle meatus. If drainage is not maintained, rupture of the sinus wall with extension to adjacent tissue may occur. Diagnosis may require x-ray examination, transillumination, and, in chronic sinusitis, diagnostic puncture.

Treatment—The local and general measures employed are essentially the same as for the common cold (p. 18). In addition, steam inhalations and local application of heat or cold are helpful. Drainage may be increased by wiping out the nose, shrinking the mucosa with vasoconstrictors (p. 376), and applying gentle suction with the pharyngeal isthmus and opposite naris closed.

If there is no acute rhinitis present, Proetz displacement treatment is valuable. This procedure is described on page 377. Severe acute infections may require systemic anti-infective therapy.

AEROSINUSITIS

Aerosinusitis is an acute or chronic inflammation of one or more of the nasal accessory sinuses resulting from a difference in pressure between the gas in the sinuses and the air of the surrounding atmosphere.

This disease occurs in the same groups as those likely to contract aero-otitis media (p. 244) and from a similar cause, that is, interference with ventilation of the sinus. This may result from polyps or other tumors, accumulation of mucus or pus, or anatomic deformity which causes a block of the ostium. Frontal sinuses are most frequently affected.

The condition rarely occurs on ascent (pressure in the sinus higher than ambient pressure); when it does, return to ground level affords immediate relief. Most frequently the condition occurs on descent from altitude (relative negative pressure in sinus). Pain over the sinus, varying in intensity, is usually the most prominent symptom and persists for one to seven days. Fever and leukocytosis may occur. X-ray examination reveals a thickened lining, clouded by fluid or blood, and sometimes submucosal hemorrhage or stripping of the mucosa. Resolution usually requires seven to twenty-one days and may not be complete.

Treatment is aimed at equalization of pressure plus drainage of fluid. In milder forms of the condition, shrinkage of the nasal mucosa by vasoconstrictor drugs will usually allow normal evacuation of the sinus. The process is aided by external heat.

In severe cases, underlying pathological changes should be determined. Mechanical movement of the tissues forming the block may be required. Heat assists in fluid formation (which, by filling space, aids in equalizing the pressure) and in decreasing pain. Equalization of pressure usually results in normal drainage. Proetz displacement (p. 377) may assist in this equalization. Any predisposing condition should be corrected after the sinusitis has subsided.

ACUTE PHARYNGITIS

Acute pharyngitis is an inflammation of the pharyngeal mucosa and is often secondary to rhinitis, sinusitis, adenoiditis, or tonsillitis. It frequently accompanies the onset of such infectious diseases as scarlet fever, measles, diphtheria, septic sore throat, smallpox, typhoid fever, and typhus fever. Occasionally it is the result of chemical, mechanical, or thermal irritation. Sore throat, fever, malaise, anorexia, increased salivation, pharyngeal inflammation, and regional lymphadenopathy are common manifestations. These ordinarily persist for a few days but may last as long as two weeks.

Treatment is essentially the same as for acute tonsillitis (p. 9). Local applications are of doubtful value, except when they provide symptomatic relief. Appropriate treatment of existing primary disease is essential.

Larynx, Trachea, and Bronchi
ACUTE INFECTIONS

In Adults, acute infections of the larynx, trachea, and bronchi are usually, but not always, secondary to the common cold, sinusitis, or other infection of the nose or throat. They may be due to any of the respiratory micro-organisms or to a virus. One or more of the parts of the tract may be involved. Predisposing factors to involvement of the laryngo-tracheobronchial tree include chilling of the body; breathing of cold, damp air; and inhalation of solid, liquid, or gaseous irritant agents.

Laryngitis produces hoarseness or loss of the voice, with a sense of local discomfort or even pain, and a dry cough. The mucous membrane is red and swollen. Constitutional symptoms are slight or absent. Tracheitis gives rise to a harsh, unproductive type of cough associated with substernal pain. Constitutional symptoms are ordinarily mild.

Acute bronchitis may be limited to the larger passages, or it may extend to the smallest ramifications or even into the alveoli, when it becomes pneumonia (e.g., hemolytic streptococcus pneumonia is primarily a bronchiolitis). The symptoms of bronchitis include cough, which is often not as prominent as in tracheitis but which is later productive of mucopurulent sputum; substernal soreness and tightness; malaise; and slight to moderate fever. Physical signs are found only if the smaller bronchi are involved, when there are bilateral roughness of breath sounds and râles (at first dry, later moist).

The differential diagnosis of acute bronchitis includes pulmonary tuberculosis, pneumonia (p.115), asthma (p.265), bronchiectasis (p.115), whooping cough (p.15), foreign body in a bronchus, mediastinal lymphadenitis, measles (p.24), and typhoid fever (p.14).

TREATMENT—For acute laryngitis, tracheitis, bronchitis, or any combination of them, the basic treatment is the same. The patient should remain in bed in a warm atmosphere of even temperature kept moist by a steam kettle to which may be added Compound Benzoin Tincture, menthol, eucalyptol, or other pleasant volatile substances. Useless cough should be controlled with codeine (p.403). Tobacco and alcohol are prohibited; and if there is laryngitis, the patient should try not to speak above a whisper. In laryngitis and tracheitis, cold or warm applications to the neck often afford relief.

Severe cases may require systemic anti-infective therapy (p.286). Febrile cases should be isolated. If there is little improvement in bronchitis after several days, one of the conditions listed under differential diagnosis should be suspected.

In Children, acute infections involving the larynx, trachea, and bronchi present different clinical pic-

tures and courses from those in the adult because of differences in anatomy and immunological status. This group of infections in children has been given the general name of "infectious croup." Rabe found that, in Connecticut, infectious croup had one of three causes: diphtheria (see p. 3), *Hemophilus influenzae*, type B (a bacterium not to be confused with influenza virus, type B), and an unidentified virus.

VIRUS CROUP was ten times as frequent as that due to *H. influenzae*, type B. It occurred most frequently in children under three years of age and seldom in those over seven. Seventy percent of the cases were in boys.

Virus croup follows an upper respiratory infection and is characterized by stridor with or without hoarseness. Except in the presence of severe respiratory obstruction over a period of days, signs of severe toxicity are lacking. There is much secretion in the larynx and trachea; as the infection persists, this becomes increasingly thick and tenacious, producing obstruction. The mortality rate increases with downward extension of the process, rising from 1 percent when only the larynx and trachea are involved to about 15 percent in those having pneumonitis.

Complications include pneumonia, respiratory obstruction from crusting of secretions, mediastinal emphysema, pneumothorax, septicemia, and otitis media.

Treatment is symptomatic. The child is kept in bed in a warm, moist atmosphere of even temperature. He is disturbed as little as is consistent with determining his condition. The principal question concerns tracheotomy. If the patient does not improve and if he is restless, shows severe retraction of the intercostal spaces on inspiration, and exhibits poor respiratory exchange on repeated auscultation, tracheotomy should be performed. The cannula is kept clear by frequent instillation of isotonic salt solution followed by suction with a small catheter. Those patients having severe respiratory obstruction in spite of tracheotomy are placed in an oxygen tent.

Maintenance of fluid balance (p. 49) is extremely important. Rabe suggests administration of sulfadiazine to severe cases. It has no effect on the croup but may prevent secondary bacteremia or pneumonia. An atmosphere of moist oxygen or a mixture of oxygen and helium is recommended to hasten resolution of emphysema.

CROUP DUE TO H. INFLUENZAE, TYPE B—In contrast to virus croup, that due to *H. influenzae*, type B, was found by Rabe to be most common in the age group of three to seven years. It was twice as common as virus croup in children over seven; but, as in virus croup, most of the patients were boys.

The clinical picture is typically a sudden severe sore throat, with laryngitis, fever, leukocytosis, and severe prostration out of proportion to the duration of obvious illness. A rapidly progressive course is characteristic. Rabe considers edema of the epiglottis and supraglottic region pathognomonic of the disease. He frequently found tender anterior cervical adenopathy. Ninety percent of cases had bacteremia, and the over-all mortality rate was 18 percent. The most common complication was emphysema.

Treatment has two purposes: to combat the toxemia and bacteremia, and to relieve respiratory obstruction. As Rabe states: "The paramount consideration is speed." The toxemia is treated by whole-blood transfusions and administration of type-specific rabbit antiserum. The infection itself is susceptible to sulfadiazine and streptomycin. Sulfadiazine is given, subdivided, in a total dosage of 0.2 Gm. per Kg. of body weight (0.09 Gm. per lb.) per day, the initial dose being half this amount. Severely ill patients may receive it by intravenous drip during the first day or two. For dosage of streptomycin, see page 290.

Severe respiratory distress is treated by tracheotomy. Intubation is definitely contraindicated because of the supraglottic edema. As in virus croup, patients are kept in a warm, moist atmosphere and are given moist oxygen for emphysema or pneumothorax. Maintenance of fluid balance (p. 49) is vital.

SPASMODIC CROUP

Spasmodic croup (false croup, spasmodic laryngitis) is an afebrile condition peculiar to children from two to six years of age. It is caused by adductor spasm of the laryngeal muscles. It is characterized by sudden nocturnal attacks of harsh, brassy cough, pronounced stridor and inspiratory dyspnea, hoarseness, and cyanosis. Vomiting, either spontaneous or induced, affords prompt relief; otherwise the acute phase lasts from a few minutes to three or four hours and is followed by sleep of exhaustion. By the next day, recovery appears complete, except possibly for slight residual hoarseness. If symptoms persist during the next day, the possibility of diphtheria (p. 3) should be eliminated. Second and third attacks on successive nights are common, but recurrence the same night is rare.

The disease occurs most frequently in the fall and spring during periods of sudden climatic change

accompanied by dampness and falling temperature. Although diagnosis is seldom difficult, there may be confusion with laryngeal diphtheria, acute catarrhal laryngitis, retropharyngeal abscess, laryngismus stridulus, acute laryngotracheobronchitis, and foreign body in the larynx.

Treatment—In the presence of slight cough or upper respiratory infection, susceptible children should be protected from exposure to cold night air and dampness. Active treatment includes transfer of the patient to a warm room, the atmosphere of which is kept saturated with moisture by means of one or more steam kettles. Other treatment is symptomatic.

CHRONIC LARYNGITIS

Chronic laryngitis may develop from repeated attacks of the acute form (p. 112). It is usually associated with inflammation elsewhere in the upper respiratory tract. Dry atmosphere, particularly when it is dusty, smoky, or overheated, predisposes to the chronic type, as does overindulgence in smoking and strong alcoholic beverages. Excessive use of the voice is a common primary cause. The low-grade catarrhal process gives rise to exacerbations of hoarseness, frequent clearing of the throat, irritative coughing, expectoration of scanty, tenacious mucus, sensation of rawness in the larynx, and susceptibility to voice fatigue. Since similar manifestations can result from tuberculosis, syphilis, and carcinoma of the larynx, prompt differentiation is important.

Treatment is often difficult. It involves avoidance or removal of predisposing factors, including sinus infection. Recovery from an acute exacerbation is assisted by the measures suggested for acute laryngitis (p. 113).

CHRONIC BRONCHITIS

Chronic bronchitis is a low-grade, long-standing inflammation of the bronchi, usually secondary to chronic pulmonary disease or chronic paranasal sinusitis. Chronic bronchitis almost never develops from a single attack of acute bronchitis; in the rare instances in which it is primary, it is usually the result of long-continued inhalation of irritant industrial gases or dusts. The infection occurs most frequently in older people and is more severe in winter. In children it may be secondary to chronic disease of the adenoids and tonsils.

Cough and expectoration are the outstanding symptoms. Systemic manifestations are rare.

Treatment is primarily that of the underlying disease. When cough is excessive, codeine may be employed. In older individuals with paroxysmal cough, large doses of potassium iodide (p. 506) may be helpful.

BRONCHIECTASIS

Bronchiectasis is a disease involving the branching portions of the bronchial tree; it is characterized by distortion and dilatation of the bronchi and chronic infection of them and the peribronchial tissues. The lower lobes of one or both lungs are usually involved; apical occurrence is unusual and suggests tuberculosis. Limitation of the condition to the left lower lobe suggests a congenital origin. Bronchiectasis usually causes chronic illness, with foul, purulent, and frequently hemorrhagic sputum. Hemoptysis is even more frequent in bronchiectasis than in tuberculosis.

Bronchiectasis is seen most frequently in the first decade. This predominance is largely accounted for by accidental introduction of foreign bodies into the bronchi and by the complication of acute bronchitis which occurs so often in childhood diseases such as whooping cough, measles, and influenza. These conditions favor bronchiectatic changes by obstructing and infecting segments of the bronchial tree. If the obstruction persists, the beginnings of chronic bronchiectasis are produced. Regardless of the causative factor, bronchiectasis is primarily a disease of childhood, even though the symptoms may not attract attention until later in life.

When a chronic cough exists, it should suggest bronchiectasis, particularly in those patients "subject to heavy chest colds." The course is irregular, and often exacerbations are accompanied by chills, fever, and patchy pneumonitis. Occasionally, large residual abscesses or acute empyema will follow such a flare-up. Copious, alarming hemorrhages may be the chief concern.

Wide variability in the outlook complicates the management of the individual case. Amyloid disease or a distant suppurating focus such as a brain abscess may be coexistent, particularly in the long-standing, severely septic cases. The presence of paranasal sinusitis, once considered to have a causal relationship with bronchiectasis, now suggests no more than another possible source of reinfection. Associated conditions arising within the chest also require consideration. These include bronchial neoplasm, mediastinal tumor, mediastinitis, and the presence of a foreign body. In general, bronchiectasis is a severe, progressive, and debilitating disease, ending fatally. Nevertheless, spontaneous recoveries or fairly good general health for many years in spite of the disease have been reported.

Treatment—During the past decade the results from lobectomy have been exceptionally gratifying, particularly in children. Hope must be offered with caution; and each case requires careful study of the cause, nature, and extent of the disease and presence or absence of complicating conditions before a plan of management is decided upon. If removal of the affected portions of the lung is thought to be inadvisable, conservative measures may alleviate the symptoms and prolong life. Such measures include (1) rest, (2) high-caloric and high-protein diet (pp. 584 and 259), (3) postural drainage, (4) medication, and (5) control of the infection in the upper respiratory tract. Postural drainage may be supplemented by occasional bronchoscopic aspiration and the instillation of iodized oil. Penicillin and the sulfonamides may be used to advantage, even though no specific organism has been isolated. If the sputum contains many fusiform bacilli and spirochetes, intravenous injection of neoarsphenamine (p. 297) may be helpful. Infections of the upper respiratory tract should be prevented or controlled if at all possible. It may be advisable to eradicate sinus disease and even to seek a change of climate.

When empyema or lung abscess develops as a complication of bronchiectasis and lobectomy is contraindicated, adequate drainage by thoracotomy may prove to be a lifesaving measure.

Lungs

PNEUMONIA

Pneumonia is an infectious disease characterized by the presence of exudate in one or more lobes of the lungs which produces a varying degree of consolidation. Pneumonia is principally an urban disease of winter in the temperate zone. The various causative organisms give rise to distinct types of pathological process and clinical picture.

Pneumococcus Pneumonia is often called by the descriptive name "lobar pneumonia" because of the characteristic lobar distribution of consolidation. It is usually secondary to upper respiratory infection. Predisposing factors include chilling of the body, breathing of cold, damp air, fatigue, hunger, debilitation, and alcoholism.

Thirty-three immunologic types of pneumococci have been recognized. Types I to VIII account for 80 percent of the cases. Although pneumococcus pneumonia has some tendency to recur, the same type organism is seldom found a second time. The right lower lobe is most commonly involved; the upper lobes alone, almost never. Pneumococcus pneumonia is endemic. It is not highly contagious except where living quarters are extremely crowded.

Onset is characteristically sudden, with definite chill, fever, pain in the side, cough, expectoration of rusty sputum, and rapid respiration. The temperature rises to 103° or 104°F., and when still higher may be accompanied by delirium. The pain, described as a "stitch in the side," is located frequently in the region of the nipple or at the base of the affected lung. Occasionally the pain may be referred to the abdomen and may be accompanied by tenderness which suggests appendicitis, colitis, or peritonitis. The cough, at first dry and hacking, gradually produces sputum which is rust-colored and tenacious; this becomes viscid by the third or fourth day and is later yellow in color and mucopurulent. Respirations are rapid, shallow, and labored, and these qualities are aggravated by pain and anoxia. The rate rises out of proportion to the fever. Cyanosis of varying degree appears early and increases in severity. Herpes (p. 21) may be seen on the lips. The beginning or course of the disease may be marked by nausea and vomiting. The most frequent and troublesome gastro-intestinal symptom is tympanites, which adds to the respiratory embarrassment. Deep jaundice indicates an associated toxic hepatitis.

If untreated, the disease runs a course of five to ten days, terminating by lysis or abruptly by crisis. Respirations become easier, toxic symptoms decrease and disappear, the pulse rate returns to normal, large quantities of mucopurulent sputum are expectorated, and the patient is more comfortable.

The physical findings may be insignificant for twenty-four to forty-eight hours, but careful examination will probably reveal premonitory physical signs. There is some limitation of movement of the affected side. Palpation and percussion may reveal slight dullness over the involved area. The breath sounds are characteristically quiet or suppressed, and at the end of inspiration or after a cough, showers of fine crepitant râles may be heard. Frank consolidation is usually well developed by

the second or third day. As the disease process resolves, vocal fremitus diminishes, the voice and breath sounds gradually return to normal, and many subcrepitant moist râles may be heard.

A gradual decline in blood pressure and less distinct heart sounds are indicative of progressive severity and poor prognosis. In fatal cases, the temperature remains high, the cyanosis and toxemia become more pronounced, and the immediate cause of death is circulatory failure.

The most common complications encountered are acute fibrinous pleurisy and pleurisy with effusion. The presence of the latter may be suspected by a rise in temperature, and aspiration may be required if the effusion is considerable in amount. The most frequent severe complication is empyema (p. 122), which should be suspected when the temperature rises abruptly after the patient has been afebrile for one or two days and leukocytosis, chill, dyspnea, and physical signs of fluid occur. More infrequent complications are pericarditis, endocarditis, meningitis, arthritis, and pneumococcal invasions of other organs. In children, otitis media is a not infrequent incident. In older individuals, the disease may continue in a more severe form, "unresolved pneumonia," for several weeks to months. Relapse may occur from invasion by another type of pneumococcus.

The sputum characteristically contains many of the causative organisms, but a careful microscopic examination also should be made to rule out tuberculosis. The sputum should be examined as soon as possible after collection but may be stored in the refrigerator for twenty-four hours if necessary. Typing of pneumococci is best accomplished by the Neufeld method. Two loopfuls of undiluted type-specific rabbit serum are added to a loopful of sputum smeared on a slide. One or two loopfuls of Loeffler's alkaline methylene blue stain (p. 547) are mixed thoroughly with the material. Mixtures of type-specific serums are used ordinarily, and single serums are then employed for isolation. The slides are examined under oil immersion. If the serums do not include the appropriate type, no capsule can be seen; but if an appropriate serum is used, the capsule appears and is swollen, greenish-gray in color, and sharply outlined.

If the sputum is scanty in amount, the pharynx may be swabbed and the swab with accumulated mucus incubated in a test tube containing 2 to 3 cc. of glucose blood broth. The culture may be used for typing. If insufficient pneumococci appear in the sputum, 0.5 cc. of saline-washed sputum may be injected into the peritoneal cavity of a mouse and the peritoneal exudate examined four to six hours later.

Blood cultures should be performed, because they give some indication of the severity and prognosis of the disease, persistent positive cultures indicating extensive lung involvement or particularly virulent infections.

The leukocyte count during the early course of the disease is usually 15,000 to 25,000 per cu. mm., with an increase in the proportion of young polymorphonuclears. The clotting time of the blood may be increased, and frequently the sedimentation rate is elevated. Early in the disease, x-ray examination may reveal only a small shadow around the hilus. This gradually extends, becoming dense and homogeneous, with a reversal of this process upon resolution. Frequently the diaphragm is elevated on the affected side. Mottling of the lung shadow may remain for some time after signs of consolidation disappear.

The differential diagnosis of pneumococcus pneumonia includes pneumonia from other organisms, acute bronchitis (p. 112), pleurisy (p. 121), influenza (p. 22), tuberculous pneumonia, and pulmonary infarction (p. 119). Occasionally the pneumococcus can produce "bronchopneumonia" (see following paragraph).

Hemolytic Streptococcus Pneumonia also takes a characteristic form. As with pneumococcus pneumonia, it is usually secondary to infection, such as measles or influenza, which affects the respiratory tract. The entire lower-respiratory tract is involved. The pharynx is usually red and swollen (a useful point in early distinction from pneumococcus pneumonia), and there is inflammation of the trachea and bronchi. The principal lesions, however, are in the bronchioles, the walls of which contain many organisms and are densely infiltrated with red blood cells and monocytes. The lumina are filled with exudate, and the inflammation and exudation may extend into the alveoli, giving rise to a patchy consolidation which has led to the descriptive term "bronchopneumonia." The lung bases are the most common sites for consolidation, which may, by confluence, involve an entire lobe. When infection reaches the surface of the pleura, empyema (p. 122) results.

Onset is marked by prostration, cough, and, very often, pain in the chest. Constant cough and dyspnea are usually more pronounced than in pneumococcus pneumonia. The sputum is characteristic, being at first pink and later yellow but not rusty.

On physical examination, dullness is seldom pronounced, and true bronchial breathing is rare. Moist râles are the predominant finding, and they may be heard even after the end of expiration.

The diagnosis may be suspected from the clinical picture. It is confirmed by the finding of *Streptococcus hemolyticus* in almost pure culture in the sputum. The differential diagnosis is the same as for pneumococcus pneumonia (see above).

Complications include empyema (p. 122), pericarditis (p. 74), atelectasis (p. 120), pneumothorax and metastatic focal infections, particularly about the joints or as solitary abscesses in muscle.

Virus Pneumonia has been recognized only recently. Its status is suggested by the title "primary atypical pneumonia, etiology unknown." The pathological process appears to be an inflammation of interstitial pulmonary tissues rather than a bronchitis or alveolitis.

Onset may be sudden or gradual, and the course mild and brief or severe and prolonged. Common early complaints are a dry, scratchy, or slightly sore throat and conjunctival irritation. Later there is gradual onset of fever, aching, hoarseness, and dry cough. There is little or no sputum. Physical examination of the chest shows, at most, suppressed breath sounds and a few râles. In contrast, the x-ray may show a large area of infiltration. The lesion may spread from one lobe to others. In some cases the severity of symptoms is far out of proportion to the area of lung involved. Complications and sequelae are rare; hemolytic anemia has been observed.

The diagnosis is made partly on the clinical picture and partly on elimination of other causative agents, the following results of laboratory tests being particularly important: normal white blood count, normal or only slightly increased blood sedimentation rate, absence of pathological organisms from the sputum, negative blood culture.

Differential diagnosis includes other forms of pneumonia, tracheobronchitis, influenza, psittacosis, typhoid fever, and tuberculous pneumonia.

Pneumonia Due to Other Organisms—Not uncommonly, pneumonia is produced by nonhemolytic streptococci, staphylococci, Friedländer's bacillus, or *H. influenzae*, and occasionally by other organisms. The disease in such cases is almost always secondary to infections of the upper respiratory tract (sometimes with the same organisms), specific infectious diseases, any chronic or debilitating disease, or mechanical or chemical irritation of the bronchial mucosa or alveolar epithelium. It may follow anesthesia, especially in those who have a mild upper-respiratory infection at the time.

As in streptococcus pneumonia (see above), the principal lesion is a bronchiolitis, the lower lobes are most commonly involved, and the consolidation is patchy. These forms of pneumonia are, therefore, bronchopneumonias. Symptoms are not specific or typical, those of the primary disease having engrafted on them more or less gradually those of pneumonia. Bronchopneumonia should be suspected when (1) fever is present for more than three or four days in the course of bronchitis; (2) an increase in fever and prostration with onset of cough occurs in the course of some other disease, particularly in older or debilitated patients; or (3) after exposure to respiratory irritant influences such as inhalation anesthesia. Physical signs are similar to those of bronchitis but are usually most prominent at the lung bases. Persistent râles over the lower lobes are strongly suggestive. X-ray may be helpful in diagnosis.

In children, the organisms under discussion may produce a primary pneumonia with the same clinical picture as that due to the pneumococcus.

The occurrence of bronchopneumonia stresses the importance of enforcing a proper period of convalescence from specific infections in children and the desirability of prompt treatment of upper respiratory infections. Secondary bronchopneumonia is always serious and is especially dangerous in infants and in the aged.

Treatment—The advent of systemic anti-infective agents has revolutionized the treatment and prognosis of the more common forms of pneumonia. If full advantage of the new agents is to be gained, the diagnosis must be made early and treatment started immediately. Bed rest is still of the utmost importance, and patients with pneumococcus pneumonia seem to fare better in a cool rather than a warm room. In any case, the temperature should be even. Patients with streptococcus pneumonia should be isolated.

There is a certain degree of incompatibility between accurate diagnosis of the causative agent and early institution of specific therapy. A satisfactory compromise might involve the following steps:

1. Taking of sputum for culture. In severe infections, blood culture also should be made.

2. Survey of pre-existing infection, nature of onset of the pneumonia, and physical findings for hints of the probable causative agent.

3. If it seems probable that the pneumonia is due to pneumococcus, hemolytic streptococcus, or staphylococcus, penicillin therapy should be started at once. If the cultures or the clinical picture subsequently indicates some other cause, treatment can be changed accordingly.

In pneumococcus and streptococcus pneumonia, penicillin is the most effective primary therapeutic agent. Adequate dosage for the average case is afforded by any of the following: procaine penicillin, 300,000 to 600,000 units once daily; crystalline penicillin—G, 300,000 units every twelve or twenty-four hours, or 100,000 units every eight to twelve hours, or 25,000 to 50,000 units every three to four hours.

Concomitant administration of sulfonamides is also advocated because of the belief that the greater penetration of these drugs into the cerebrospinal fluid may prevent the complication of meningitis. The sulfonamides may be given alone in those cases in which penicillin is contraindicated, or when the response to penicillin is unsatisfactory. The usual daily amount for an adult is 6 Gm. in divided doses, preferably of a sulfonamide mixture (p. 295). In severe cases, the first one or more administrations may consist of sodium sulfadiazine in the same dosage by the intravenous route (p. 296).

In pneumococcus pneumonia, adequate penicillin therapy typically produces an abrupt initial fall in temperature within eighteen hours; this is sometimes followed by a secondary rise to more than 100°F., with a return to normal in twenty-four to thirty-six hours. The sulfonamides produce a gradual fall in temperature over one or two days. Usually the white blood count returns to normal within four days, and resolution is complete both to physical examination and x-ray in two to four weeks.

With either penicillin or the sulfonamides, administration should be continued for one or two days after the temperature has returned to normal. In debilitated patients or those in whom complications might be especially dangerous, more prolonged administration may be indicated.

The effectiveness of antibiotics and the sulfonamides is such that antipneumococcus serum is rarely necessary. It is indicated only when systemic anti-infective therapy either fails or is for some reason contraindicated. The serum must be specific for the type of pneumococcus, and serum sensitivity tests (p. 334) should be made before injection. The initial dose is 50,000 to 200,000 units.

Aureomycin (p. 291) appears to be of value against virus pneumonia. Other anti-infective agents are indicated if complications arise from secondary bacterial invasion. The choice and dosage depend on the organism concerned (see p. 290).

In staphylococcus pneumonia, penicillin is the

agent of choice. Since the disease is often fulminating in character and the organism relatively resistant, initial dosage should be higher than in pneumococcus or streptococcus pneumonia; if procaine penicillin is used, it may be well to start treatment with two separate injections of 300,000 units at different sites. After this, the dosage outlined for the other two forms of pneumonia may be followed. Concomitant administration of sulfonamides is advocated by some.

In pneumonia due to *Hemophilus influenzae* or to Friedländer's bacillus, streptomycin and aureomycin may have value. Early treatment is extremely important. In those cases in which gram-negative organisms appear in the sputum only after administration of penicillin, the usefulness of streptomycin is uncertain. The usual dosage of streptomycin is 1 Gm. intramuscularly every four to six hours. In very severe infections, the initial dose may be administered intravenously dissolved in 20 cc. of isotonic salt solution. It is injected at a rate not to exceed 1 cc. per minute. After reasonable clinical improvement has taken place, the intervals between administrations can be lengthened. Dosage of aureomycin may be found on page 292.

PULMONARY EMBOLISM AND INFARCTION

Pulmonary emboli may be gaseous, liquid, or solid. To produce pulmonary embolism, air must enter the venous system quickly and in rather large volume. This sometimes happens in operations or wounds about the neck, shoulder, or thorax; in connection with placenta previa, induced abortion, or injections into the uterus; or under unusual circumstances during venoclysis. The air bubbles greatly increase resistance in the pulmonary circulation and tend to cause acute circulatory failure.

Fat embolism is due to fat globules liberated into the blood from traumatized fat or yellow bone marrow and may follow operation in obese persons, severe jarring of the skeleton, or fractures or operations on bone. The fat globules increase the resistance in the pulmonary circulation, which may in turn lead to diminished cardiac output, lowered arterial blood pressure, increased systemic venous pressure, pulmonary edema, and circulatory failure. A somewhat similar picture is produced by embolism from amniotic fluid which may enter the uterine veins during labor and delivery. Solid particles of meconium and of fetal sebum and epithelial debris act as multiple minute emboli and may produce "obstetric shock."

Solid pulmonary emboli are usually thrombi which have become detached from areas of phlebothrombosis in the systemic veins (see p. 87). Detachable thrombi may also form in the right auricle during chronic auricular fibrillation, on the wall of the right ventricle after myocardial infarction, or, rarely, on the tricuspid and pulmonic valves during endocarditis.

The effect of pulmonary emboli depends on their size and number and on the extent of reflex spasm of the collateral arterial bed. In pulmonary embolism, as in peripheral arterial embolism (see p. 77), spasm of the collateral pulmonary circulation may increase the degree of circulatory impairment far beyond that due to the embolus itself.

When a very large solid embolus blocks the pulmonary artery or one of its main branches, or when a number of smaller emboli block many smaller branches, the patient may die at once or in a matter of hours from acute circulatory failure (see Shock, p. 90). Fatal emboli usually originate in the deep veins of the leg and are particularly common in patients with malignant tumors, especially following abdominal surgery or during prolonged bed rest in elderly patients.

At the other extreme, very small emboli may cause obstruction and later fibrosis of the occluded vessel without seriously disturbing pulmonary blood flow or giving rise to clinical manifestations. Showers of such small emboli are probably more common in postoperative, postpartum, and cardiac cases than is generally realized.

Moderate-sized emboli disturb pulmonary blood flow and lead to localized hyperemia and edema. They may give the clinical picture of a small area of pneumonia and, if postoperative, may be falsely attributed to postanesthetic atelectasis. When there is pre-existing interference with the pulmonary circulation, moderate-sized pulmonary emboli cause infarction. If the interference tends to produce pulmonary congestion (heart disease or toxic or postoperative states), the infarct is hemorrhagic. If the interference has no such tendency (pulmonary emphysema or fibrosis), the infarct is more likely to be of the anemic type. Pulmonary infarction can be caused by thrombosis *in situ* as well as by embolism.

The classical picture of infarction of the lung is a sudden onset with severe pain in the chest, dyspnea, cough with bloody sputum, and, later, fever. There may be shock. However, parts of the picture may be lacking; and if pulmonary engorgement is already considerable, there may simply be an aggravation of previous symptoms.

The possibility of pulmonary embolism or infarction must therefore always be considered when predisposing conditions are present, and any occurrence of or increase in pulmonary symptoms should be immediately investigated. The development of a pleural friction rub and subcrepitant râles in the same part of the chest, with or without evidence of consolidation, supports the diagnosis. After the first day, x-ray is often confirmatory in showing a distinct, if not always the characteristic wedge-shaped, shadow at the site. Sometimes there is difficulty in distinguishing pulmonary embolism from coronary occlusion (p. 67).

The course is extremely variable. If the patient survives immediate shock, the symptoms usually subside in a matter of days or weeks, and the infarcted area scars. Complications include pleural effusion or, if the embolus or the bronchial tree is infected, lung abscess or empyema.

Treatment—Prevention is obviously of the utmost importance; it consists in the prevention and control of phlebothrombosis (see p. 87). The occurrence of severe pulmonary embolism or infarction is an emergency of the first order, for immediate and appropriate treatment can save life. In massive embolism, the ideal therapy would be immediate embolectomy. Unfortunately, it is seldom practicable. In the presence of any suggestive symptoms, the patient should be given by vein and at once 1 mg. (1/60 grain) of atropine sulfate and from 0.03 to 0.13 Gm. (1/2 to 2 grains) of papaverine hydrochloride. Either or both of these drugs may be repeated every four to six hours as needed. Oxygen therapy is important if there is shock or any evidence of anoxia. Other measures for shock are discussed on page 90. Anticoagulant therapy should be started or continued to prevent extension of the infarction or repetition of embolism; however, anticoagulants should not be given until forty-eight to seventy-two hours after an operation because of the danger of hemorrhage. The source of an embolus should be sought and ligated (see above). Block of the stellate ganglion *on the side of the lesion* has apparently been of benefit in minimizing collateral vasospasm.

Once response has been obtained to these emergency measures, they are continued or repeated as necessary. The occurrence of a second embolism is usually very serious.

ATELECTASIS

Atelectasis implies complete loss of air from a lung or portion thereof. If an entire lung is involved, the condition is known as massive collapse. The primary cause is obstruction of a bronchus which prevents air from entering the tributary alveoli. Since air already present is rapidly absorbed by the blood, the walls of the smaller bronchi and alveoli become approximated. Accumulation of thick, tenacious secretions after operative procedures (particularly in the upper abdomen) is considered the most common cause of obstruction. A foreign body or tumor in a bronchus may be a predisposing factor in atelectasis occurring as a complication of asthma or pneumonia. Contributing factors are ineffectual coughing and decreased respiratory movement.

Physical signs are râles, wheezes, diminished breath sounds, moderate dullness over the affected area, and increasing cyanosis. As a rule, a rapid rise in pulse, temperature, and respiratory rate occurs. The patient may cough in a guarded, ineffectual manner. X-rays usually show a shadow corresponding to the involved area with a shift of the mediastinum to the affected side.

Atelectasis must be distinguished from pulmonary embolism (p. 119).

Treatment—The contributing factors of oversedation, fixed position postoperatively, and tight binders should be avoided; deep breathing and coughing are encouraged. In some clinics, atelectasis following general anesthesia has been practically eliminated by bronchoscopic aspiration of secretions before termination of anesthesia.

Atelectasis should be suspected when a patient's postoperative condition suddenly becomes worse, with appearance of cyanosis, cough, or other respiratory symptoms. X-ray is usually diagnostic. Dramatic improvement ordinarily follows removal of the obstruction.

Bronchial catheterization according to the method of Haight may produce satisfactory results. In this procedure, with the patient recumbent and without anesthesia, a No. 16 French urethral catheter is introduced through the nose along the posterior wall of the nasopharynx until the arytenoids are felt. The catheter is then withdrawn slightly, and with the expiratory effort of a cough or the deep inspiration following it, the catheter is inserted quickly into the trachea. The foot of the bed is then elevated. Application of suction (preferably by a suction machine) through a connecting tube will remove collected secretions from the trachea. On farther introduction the catheter usually enters the right stem bronchus. If the patient is turned on the left side, the left stem bronchus is entered. In this way, both bronchi may be freed of obstructing secretion. With the catheter in this position, the outer end is three to four inches from the nose. The position of the catheter may be checked by fluoroscopy. If this procedure is not successful, bronchoscopic aspiration should follow as quickly as possible. Delay in removing the obstruction may result in serious pulmonary infection and possible fatal outcome.

PULMONARY EMPHYSEMA

Pulmonary emphysema is a condition in which the pulmonary alveoli become distended, coalesce, or rupture as a result of loss of elasticity of the lung structure. It may arise as a result of any of several factors:

1. Obstruction of the air passage, especially if there is greater interference with expiration than with inspiration, as in asthma, chronic bronchitis, whooping cough, mediastinal tumors, or partial obstruction of the larynx.

2. Enlargement of the thorax, allowing the lungs to expand and fill the increased thoracic space, as in Paget's disease or acromegaly.

3. Changes in pulmonary vessels affecting the elasticity of the lungs in Ayerza's disease.

4. Overexpansion of normal portions of the lungs when the affected areas are consolidated (pneumonia). This condition is always secondary and usually resolves, but it may become permanent if fibrosis occurs.

In spite of the increased rate and volume of respiration, an appreciable anoxia exists because of the actual loss of alveolar surface, the increase in residual air, and the consequent decreased alveolar ventilation.

The disease is insidious in onset and may be well advanced before symptoms occur. Shortness of breath on exertion, often with cyanosis, is frequently the first symptom. The cyanosis is usually out of proportion to the degree of dyspnea, and individuals with severe cyanosis are frequently ambulatory. If the emphysema is imposed on bronchitis, the condition may resemble asthma. As the disease progresses, embarrassment of the right heart leads to symptoms similar to cardiac decompensation. Death frequently results from intercurrent pneumonia. In obstructive emphysema, breathing is rapid and shallow, there is a mild cyanosis which increases with even slight exertion, and the chest is barrel-shaped and appears to be in an inspiratory position. The cardiac apex impulse often cannot

be seen, but there may be pronounced epigastric pulsation. The chest, being already in an inspiratory position, does not expand appreciably on inspiration and moves as if in one piece. On palpation, the cardiac apical impulse cannot be felt and tactile fremitus is feeble. Percussion reveals increased resonance not only in tone but in extent of area. On auscultation, breath sounds are feeble, expiration is prolonged, and the heart sounds are distorted, with frequently an accentuated pulmonic second sound. Harsh rhonchi may be heard, and breath sounds may be principally those of bronchitis. In emphysema dependent upon an increase in the thoracic capacity, the symptoms are not as severe as in the obstructive type, because the distention of the lungs is not so great. The senile type is marked by flattening of the thoracic spine, elevation of the ribs and thorax, abdominal breathing, and, in advanced cases, dorsal kyphosis.

Treatment consists in correction of the underlying predisposing factor or disease when that is possible. The condition tends to be progressive, and the amount of damage depends upon the stress to which the distended pulmonary tissue is subjected. In general, respiratory infections and their predisposing factors should be avoided or guarded against, and the patient should avoid heavy lifting and dusty occupations. Increase of abdominal pressure and elevation of the diaphragm by an elastic abdominal belt may give some relief. The cardiac symptoms are seldom relieved by digitalis.

Pleura

PLEURISY

Pleurisy is an inflammation of the pleura which varies in its clinical picture, implications, and treatment, depending on whether or not it is accompanied by effusion.

Dry Pleurisy (fibrinous pleurisy) is an acute inflammation of the pleura in which an exudate of fibrin covers both the visceral and parietal layers. It may be large or small in extent and is more common in the lower and lateral areas of the chest. Dry pleurisy is usually secondary to infection in the underlying lung. Tuberculosis is the most common cause; pneumonia, abscess, and cancer with secondary infection are less frequent causes. However, dry pleurisy may also occur in association with infections in more distant organs and particularly with upper-respiratory-tract infection.

The characteristic symptom is sharp, sticking pain in the side with dry, unproductive cough and often moderate fever. On physical examination there is usually a to-and-fro friction rub over the lower or lateral portions of the chest.

The immediate treatment of dry pleurisy is directed toward the control of pain. This is accomplished most effectively through immobilization by strapping completely around the entire lower part of the chest from the twelfth rib to the level at which the fifth rib crosses the midaxillary line. A protecting stockinet should be used under the encircling adhesive tape. Each strip of tape is wound snugly around the chest while the breath is held in deep expiration. This breathing maneuver is repeated for each strip of tape. Complete bed rest and the use of codeine (p. 403) and analgesics (p.405) may be combined with the strapping, particularly in the beginning of the disease.

It is extremely important to determine and treat the primary disease to which the pleurisy is secondary.

Pleurisy with Effusion may follow an attack of dry pleurisy or pneumonia, or it may appear insidiously with slight cough, fever, and dyspnea on exertion. When it develops without ascertainable cause, it is usually due to tuberculosis and should be so considered until proved otherwise. Frequently it constitutes the only manifestation of the disease at the time.

Sometimes a large effusion causes little discomfort. An effusion often leads to disappearance of the pain of dry pleurisy through separation of pleural surfaces.

Pleural effusion should usually be tapped for diagnostic purposes. Aspiration not only confirms the diagnosis of effusion, but the characteristics of the fluid often help in determining the underlying cause. The exudate of pleural effusion is rich in cells and protein, and it tends to coagulate on standing. The specific gravity is above 1.018. In contrast, the fluid in hydrothorax (transudate) contains very few cells and less than 2.5 percent of protein; it does not coagulate spontaneously, and the specific gravity is below 1.018. A bloody fluid is suggestive of tuberculosis or cancer.

When the fluid is an exudate rather than a transudate, it should be subjected to complete bacteriological study, including guinea-pig inoculation for tuberculosis. Smears should be stained for study of the cells. Bloody fluid should be centrifuged and the sediment fixed and examined for tumor cells.

Patients with pleural effusion should remain at bed rest. Small effusions may be absorbed during bed rest alone. Larger effusions, particularly those producing dyspnea, should be aspirated as necessary. The procedure should be carried out cautiously because of the possibility of accidents and difficulties, including even sudden death. No more than 1,500 cc. should be removed at a time; and the aspiration should be discontinued if the pulse becomes rapid or irregular, if fluid not previously hemorrhagic becomes so, or if the patient has severe pain, cough, or considerable distress or collapses. Following aspiration, it is often helpful to insert 10 to 20 cc. of air, since the resultant fluid level helps outline the exact extent of the effusion by x-ray.

As in dry pleurisy, it is extremely important to determine and treat the primary cause. Dry pleurisy usually subsides completely in two to three weeks. Pleurisy with effusion usually lasts much longer.

ACUTE EMPYEMA

Acute empyema is a serious disease of the chest in which pus is formed in the pleural cavity. It may be caused by any of the pyogenic bacteria, and it occurs most often as a complication of pneumonia. Since the advent of anti-infective agents, it has become relatively uncommon. Streptococcus empyema was a particularly dangerous complication of bronchopneumonia, appearing during the height of the disease and often resulting in large collections of turbid fluid which was slow to become frankly purulent. Sometimes lung abscesses or bronchiectatic suppurations would perforate into the pleural cavity and result in a mixed type of infection with peculiar necrosing properties. Empyema with mixed infection may also occur following trauma to the thoracic viscera or chest wall.

Empyema should be suspected whenever in the course of pneumonia or following trauma to the chest, signs of pleural fluid are found or the patient's course is unfavorable. Common examples are recurrence of fever after a few days of normal temperature in pneumococcus pneumonia or a sudden increase in fever and prostration during streptococcus pneumonia.

Physical examination may not reveal small collections of pus or those which are between lobes. When empyema is suspected, careful x-ray studies should be made to delimit the collection as accurately as possible, and a sample of pus should be removed if it is accessible. The finding of pus confirms the diagnosis, and culture ordinarily reveals the causative organism or organisms.

Empyema may be complicated by perforation of the chest wall, rupture into a bronchus with resulting bronchopleural fistula, suppurative pericarditis or mediastinitis, or distant metastatic abscesses.

Treatment—The occurrence of empyema implies either inadequate systemic anti-infective therapy of the primary infection or the presence of a resistant organism. The susceptibility of the organism, if not already known, should be determined by in-vitro tests.

Once empyema is present, treatment has two primary objectives: the saving of life and the prevention of chronicity. Since empyema is essentially an abscess, it is treated according to the same principles, the most important of which is adequate drainage after localization has taken place. Anti-infective therapy (p. 286) is pursued vigorously provided the causative organism is susceptible. During the maturing stage of the infection, pus is removed by frequent aspirations or drainage through a closed catheter. When the pus has become thick, and when it is apparent from x-ray and fluoroscopic observation that the infection is surrounded by a fairly stiff wall, rib resection and open drainage may be advisable. If open drainage is undertaken too early, the negative pressure in the pleural space is destroyed, a pneumothorax is established, and respiration may be seriously embarrassed. During the maturing period, it is important to maintain all phases of nutrition.

CHRONIC EMPYEMA

Chronic empyema is usually the result of inadequate drainage of acute empyema. Bronchial fistulas, foreign bodies, tuberculosis, and necrotic ribs may be other contributing causes. A radical unroofing of the cavity may result in a cure, but sometimes a thoracoplasty, muscle graft, or decortication of the thickened visceral pleura may be required to obliterate a long-standing cavity.

ALIMENTARY TRACT

Mouth and Throat

DENTAL CARIES

Dental caries is a degenerative disease of the teeth resulting in cavity-like lesions of the enamel and exposed cementum which often extend to involve the underlying dentine. If progression into the pulp cavity occurs, pain, alveolar abscess formation, and eventually devitalization of the affected teeth may result. Although the disease is almost universal, the cause has not been definitely established. It is generally accepted that the primary lesion is brought about by acid formation in the mouth. Among the factors promoting tooth decay are excessive intake of refined carbohydrate in the form of sugar and candy, congenital defects of development, nutritional deficiency of certain minerals and vitamins, poor dental hygiene, and lack of professional dental care.

Treatment—Since the tooth germs appear during the second month of fetal life, prophylaxis should begin early in pregnancy with ingestion of a well-balanced diet and increased amounts of calcium, phosphorus, and vitamins A, C, and D. Dietary supervision, including vitamin supplements, should be continued during infancy and childhood. Correct habits of oral hygiene should be established when the teeth erupt. Frequent brushing with vertical, rotary, and horizontal movements will remove retained food and debris from exposed surfaces. Use of a pleasant-tasting, noninjurious dentifrice aids in establishing this practice. Regular dental consultation is to be encouraged.

In children, topical application of sodium fluoride to the teeth after dental cleaning will reduce decay approximately 40 percent, although results vary considerably among individuals. Fluoride treatment will not stop decay once it has started. The value of similar treatment for adults may eventually be established. The procedure should be carried out by a qualified dentist. After cleaning, the teeth are thoroughly dried and a 2 percent solution of sodium fluoride is applied. Four treatments are given each year at the ages of three, seven, ten, and thirteen years, in order that all newly erupted permanent teeth may be treated. Fluorination of public water supplies is believed to prevent dental caries, but the method cannot be recommended until current studies are complete.

GINGIVITIS AND STOMATITIS

Inflammation of the gums and mucous membranes of the mouth may be the result of local irritation due to poor dental hygiene or Vincent's infection (p. 124), but usually it is related to systemic disease.

In the absence of proper nursing care during febrile and debilitating diseases, the "mouth of neglect" develops, leading to inability to eat, with accompanying malnutrition, and promoting serious local infections, gangrene, or parotitis. These secondary results of mouth neglect may eventually be determining factors in the fatal outcome of the primary disease.

Ulcerative stomatitis may be seen in debilitated children, but all patients with this condition should be studied for evidence of agranulocytosis (p. 102) and leukemia (p. 103). Pellagra (p. 488), ariboflavinosis (p. 487), pernicious anemia (p. 96), and idiopathic hypochromic anemia (p. 95) are frequently manifested by stomatitis. In general, wherever sore tongue and mouth are encountered, a deficiency disease should be considered unless the cause is self-evident.

Hypertrophy of the gums is seen in scurvy, leukemia (especially monocytic), and occasionally following the use of certain hydantoin derivatives.

Gingivitis and stomatitis are also seen in poisoning from lead, mercury, bismuth, silver, gold, copper, and arsenic.

Treatment—In the treatment of prolonged fevers and chronic diseases of all sorts, the importance of keeping the mouth clean cannot be emphasized too strongly. The mouth should be cleaned after each feeding and, if possible, rinsed frequently with a mild alkaline solution such as sodium bicarbonate and sodium chloride, 1 teaspoonful of each in 1 pint of warm water, or Alkaline Aromatic Solution, N.F., 1 part to 2 parts of water. Fissuring of lips and tongue may be prevented by the free application of a mixture of 3 parts White Petrolatum and 1 part glycerin. The stomatitides of pellagra, ariboflavinosis, pernicious anemia, idiopathic hypochromic anemia, and scurvy are cured by the specific therapy for the primary conditions. Small painful ulcerative lesions may be touched with silver nitrate.

The local treatment of gingivitis and stomatitis from inorganic poisons consists in the liberal use of mild alkaline lotions, such as Alkaline Aromatic Solution, N.F. (p. 382). For systemic treatment, see the section on Poisons and Antidotes (p. 551). Herpes labialis (fever blisters) (p. 21) occurring during various infections may be rendered less painful and prevented from spreading by early liberal application of a mixture of equal parts of Camphor Spirit and Myrrh Tincture.

VINCENT'S INFECTION

Vincent's infection is an acute, moderately contagious disease which may take several forms. One form, which is also known as Vincent's angina (pseudomembranous tonsillopharyngitis, fusospirochetal pharyngitis), is characterized by insidious onset, mild fever, sore throat, and fetid breath and usually by superficial ulceration of one or both tonsils with pseudomembrane formation and regional lymphadenitis. Oral sepsis, local trauma, and malnutrition are among the predisposing factors. The membrane is gray to grayish-yellow, friable, loosely attached, and covers a shallow ulcer with well-defined but ragged edges. The adjacent tissue is swollen and varies in color from dusky red to purple. The disease is usually mild and tends to resolve spontaneously in one or two weeks.

Two forms affect the gums and buccal surfaces of infants, young children, and occasionally adults. They appear sporadically, most often during the fall and winter months, but in closely confined groups may become epidemic. Actually, these two forms may be different diseases. The *nonulcerative type* occurs about twice as frequently in girls as in boys. Clinically, it is characterized by fever, severe gingivitis, oral fetor, and regional lymphadenitis. Fever of 101° to 102°F. (38.5° to 39°C.) usually precedes the gingivitis and is accompanied by myalgia, restlessness, and inability to eat. The gums are very tender and swollen, tend to bleed easily, and progress in color from red to purple.

The *ulcerative type* is about equally distributed between boys and girls. The lesions consist of marginal ulcerations of the gums and small, shallow, round or oval ulcers of the cheeks, tongue, lips, and occasionally the tonsils. The lesions are covered with a grayish-white membrane that is removed with difficulty. A tenacious mucoid material collects about the teeth and gives rise to the characteristic odor. As the mouth lesions reach their peak, fever and constitutional symptoms subside. Healing is complete in untreated cases about the tenth or twelfth day. In mild cases with little or no ulceration, it occurs earlier.

Diagnosis of any of the forms is made on the basis of clinical findings and identification of fusiform and spirilliform organisms in stained smears taken from the lesions. Although these organisms are thought to be secondary invaders, many clinicians consider the diagnosis doubtful in their absence. Possible sources of confusion in diagnosis of the gingival type are scurvy (p. 491), heavy-metal poisoning, aphthous stomatitis, syphilis, leukemia, and other blood dyscrasias. The pharyngeal type must be distinguished from diphtheria (p. 3), syphilis, infectious mononucleosis (p. 48), heavy-metal poisoning, and blood dyscrasias.

Treatment—Penicillin administered systemically for three to five days is the preferred treatment (for dosage and administration, see p. 289). Local therapy with penicillin troches, 20,000 units every two hours for twelve or more doses, may also be curative.

Sulfonamides (p. 293) are less effective than penicillin, but they may be a useful supplement in severe cases. They are applied to the lesions in powdered form every two hours or are administered as lozenges, 0.5 Gm. every two hours during the day and 1 Gm. every four hours at night.

In the pharyngeal type, symptomatic relief is usually obtained promptly with penicillin but may be enhanced by hot saline irrigations or gargles and by use of an ice collar.

In Vincent's gingivostomatitis, symptomatic relief may be obtained with mild, oxidizing mouthwashes and gargles (p. 382). However, if these are used oftener than two or three times daily, they may interfere with local chemotherapy. Iodine, chromic acid, and gentian violet have been employed locally, and arsenicals, bismuth, and antimony have sometimes been given systemically.

Nutritional deficiencies (especially scurvy and pellagra) predispose to the disease and, when suspected, should receive specific treatment. Therapeutic doses of ascorbic acid and nicotinamide and moderate doses of B complex vitamins will aid in recovery of certain cases.

Esophagus

Disorders of the esophagus which affect function have as their most common symptoms difficulty and pain on swallowing. Less often there is regurgitation or a sensation of actual impediment to the passage of food.

The most frequent disturbances affecting the esophagus are local: cancer, spasm, and stricture. Diverticula occur, but infrequently. Difficulty in swallowing is part of the clinical picture of bulbar and pseudobulbar palsy and may be a very early manifestation of tetanus. The diagnosis of disease of the esophagus depends in the main upon the history, x-ray studies with the heavy barium meal, and esophagoscopy.

STRICTURE OF ESOPHAGUS

Strictures usually follow the acute esophagitis resulting from ingestion of phenol, strong acids, or lye. The symptoms of obstruction develop gradually following the acute episode. The usual treatment of such strictures is mechanical dilatation, which is often prolonged and unsatisfactory. If obstruction threatens nutrition despite attempts at dilatation, gastrostomy may have to be performed.

DIVERTICULUM OF ESOPHAGUS

Diverticula of the esophagus are of three types. One, the pulsion, or pressure, diverticulum is caused by pressure within the esophagus. Another, the traction diverticulum, is due to contraction of scar tissue in surrounding structures which is adherent to the wall of the esophagus. The third, the traction-pulsion diverticulum, results from a combination of these factors.

The symptoms vary with the size of the diverticulum, its location, and its pressure on adjacent organs, including the esophagus itself. They are most frequently due to a hypopharyngeal pouch (pulsion) diverticulum. Regurgitation of food, and particularly of food eaten several days previously, is an important manifestation. The regurgitation often occurs on bending over. There may be pain and difficulty in swallowing due to pressure of the mass on the esophagus itself. A tumor may be seen and felt in the neck if the diverticulum is high. The disappearance of such a mass in the neck on regurgitation of food should always suggest an esophageal diverticulum. Diagnosis is made on history, x-ray, and esophagoscopy.

Operative intervention may be successful if the diverticulum is high. There is no other treatment.

SPASM OF ESOPHAGUS

Mild spasm of the esophagus occurs occasionally in many nervous individuals during periods of stress, but in some persons recurrent spasm of the lower end of the esophagus may become troublesome. The cause of this spasm is unknown. Although other nervous disturbances are usually present, the disease does not occur invariably in obviously psychoneurotic individuals. Histological examination reveals hypertrophy of the esophageal muscles just above the stomach, and in prolonged severe conditions there is considerable dilatation above this hypertrophy.

The condition occurs more often in women than in men and usually first produces symptoms in young adult or early middle life. It is manifested as a chronic recurring difficulty in swallowing. There is more difficulty with solids than liquids; and, during the periods of exacerbation of spasm, swallowing is accompanied by pain, usually referred to the epigastric notch. The intensity of the symptoms varies widely. In severe cases there may be periods of obstruction leading to stasis and regurgitation of food and to progressive dilatation above the spasm. Although malnutrition may develop in some individuals, patients may go on for years without serious impairment of health. Diagnosis is made on history, x-ray, and esophagoscopy.

Treatment—Medical management should be tried, but it is often unsatisfactory, especially in the more severe conditions. Patients should receive frequent small bland feedings plus sedative and antispasmodic medication, such as phenobarbital, 1/4 to 1/2 grain three or four times daily, and Belladonna Tincture, 1/2 to 1 cc. three times daily a half hour before certain feedings.

The most satisfactory results follow dilatation. Before the dilating procedure is undertaken, a careful x-ray study of the lower esophagus should be made, and open-tube esophagoscopy should be done. Ulceration in the hiatal portion of the esophagus is a contraindication to dilating the lower esophagus. The dilatation itself is usually accomplished by means of a bougie equipped with a rubber bag which is distended carefully with water after proper placing. The procedure requires skill and experience and is not without danger.

CANCER OF ESOPHAGUS

Cancer of the esophagus occurs fairly commonly and may develop in any part of the organ. Except when adenocarcinoma extends up the esophagus from the cardia, the tumors are squamous-cell epithelioma. Early in the condition the symptoms may be identical with those occurring in spasm of the esophagus, but eventually evidence of cachexia, fever, and anemia is added. The local lesion may be silent, so that the first symptoms may be referable to metastases or extension from the tumor. The disease is usually fatal within a year or two of the onset of symptoms, in contrast to the prolonged course of patients with spasm. Diagnosis is confirmed by x-ray and esophagoscopic studies with biopsy.

Treatment is very unsatisfactory. Great technical skill and considerable experience are required for surgical extirpation.

PLUMMER-VINSON SYNDROME

In idiopathic hypochromic anemia, glossitis and localized thickening of the mucous lining of the esophagus may be present, resulting in dysphagia. Iron apparently is essential for proper nutrition of epithelial surfaces, and its deficiency in this condition results in the above findings. Iron salts (p. 368) will cure the condition.

Stomach and Intestines

Concepts regarding disease of the gastro-intestinal tract have changed greatly in the past few years. It has been realized that practically all *symptoms* referable to the stomach and intestines are due to disturbances of motility in these organs. It has become apparent that anatomic and secretory disturbances produce symptoms only as they directly or indirectly alter motility. In addition, functional disturbances of the central nervous system, and diseases of other parts acting through the nervous system, commonly affect gastro-intestinal motility, sometimes giving rise to distinctive syndromes and at other times mimicking the symptomatology commonly associated with organic disease.

A number of conditions formerly considered pathologic are no longer so viewed. One of the casualties has been the diagnosis of gastroptosis, since it has been shown that in a large proportion of normal asymptomatic individuals the lower limit of the stomach may be well down in the pelvis. The pathologic status of hyperacidity and hypoacidity has been strongly questioned. These conditions are commonly found in certain diseases of the stomach, but they may also be present in normal persons without symptoms. In addition, identical disturbances of motility, and hence identical symptoms, may be associated with either, so that their distinction, or even existence, can be established with certainty only by gastric analysis.

It is thus readily apparent, both from the above discussion and from practical experience, that different diseases of the stomach and intestines may have identical symptoms and that similar symptoms may occur in connection with disease of other parts of the body or in the absence of organic disease. It is also clear that serious organic disease may be present in the stomach or intestine without causing symptoms, provided there is no alteration of motility.

Despite the above comments, careful questioning by an experienced physician will often reveal important evidence of a disease process actually present in the stomach, even though the history alone cannot be relied upon to reveal the correct diagnosis. Since the stomach is seldom accessible to physical examination, other means are therefore usually required to establish a diagnosis. They include gastric analysis, x-ray, and gastroscopy. These studies likewise are not infallible, and it may be impossible to make an accurate diagnosis until after a prolonged evaluation of the patient and all the clinical findings.

Fractional gastric analysis after histamine stimulation yields the most information that can be obtained by gastric analysis (p. 543). Histamine produces the greatest possible stimulus for secretion of acid, and the secretions obtained are free from the extraneous materials introduced into the stomach in the various test meals. The terms "achlorhydria" and "anacidity" as used in the literature are only relative, depending upon the indicator used for the free acid titration and the end point to which the titration is carried. Perhaps the most useful information can be gained if the secretions are titrated to pH 7 with phenol red rather than to the end point of pH 3.5 which is obtained with the commonly used Töpfer's reagent. When the gastric secretions are alkaline (pH greater than 7), pepsin and rennin are absent; when the secretions are acid, enzymes are present. Titration of gastric contents to pH 7 is of value in differential diagnosis and in prognosis as to possible improvement of the gastric secretions. For instance, patients having pernicious anemia always have a pH of gastric contents above 7, whereas patients with cancer of the stomach may have a pH over 3.5 but less than 7. Thus, if Töpfer's reagent is used, both patients with pernicious anemia and those with cancer of the stomach will be considered to have identical findings; but if the gastric contents are titrated to pH 7, a definite difference may be evident. Return of gastric secretions has not been demonstrated in patients whose gastric contents after histamine stimulation had pH values above 7. However, patients whose gastric secretions had values between 3.5 and 7 (no free HCl to Töpfer's) when first examined have, after treatment, shown considerable increase in secretions. It would, therefore, seem that if a true anacidity is present (pH above 7), the condition is permanent, but that improvement is possible if a small amount of titratable acid is present in gastric juices.

X-ray examination after ingestion of barium is often very helpful, but it must be remembered that organic disease of the stomach may in rare cases escape detection even after repeated examinations. In addition, it is too much to expect that the roentgenologist can always differentiate between benign and malignant ulcerations.

Gastroscopic examination has now become an important aid in both diagnosis and treatment of diseases of the stomach. As diagnostic measures, x-ray and gastroscopic examinations supplement each other, inasmuch as the one procedure may reveal lesions missed by the other.

INDIGESTION

Indigestion is one of the commonest complaints for which patients consult physicians. It consists of varying degrees of epigastric distress, sense of fullness and distention in the epigastrium (usually after eating), nausea, heartburn, fickleness of appetite, gaseous eructations, cramps, and intestinal distention with passage of flatus. It is usually associated with voluntary or involuntary aerophagia, which is responsible for the gaseous eructations and for much of the intestinal distention and flatus. Constipation or bowel irregularity may also be present, and the stools frequently contain an excess of mucus.

This symptom complex can occur as the result of a great variety of conditions, and the exact symptoms give no clue as to the underlying cause. Perhaps a majority of individuals experience symptoms of indigestion at times of stress, and many will be found on close questioning to have them very frequently without considering themselves abnormal.

The symptoms are due to a disturbance of gastrointestinal motility involving, in varying degrees, spasm of portions of the tract and flattening or partial reversal of the normal gradient from pharynx to anus.

The more common underlying causes of indigestion include (1) organic disease of the stomach, including chronic gastritis, peptic ulcer, and cancer of the stomach; (2) disease processes in other abdominal viscera, such as chronic cholecystitis or chronic appendicitis; (3) diseases of the heart, as coronary sclerosis and congestive failure; (4) reflexes not associated with disease of the stomach or any other organ. The last group is by far the largest. The vast majority of people with indigestion have no gross organic disease; the abnormal motility which produces their indigestion results from stimuli of nervous origin. The indigestion in such people is almost always related directly to nervous or emotional tension, with poor eating habits, especially rapid eating, a frequent auxiliary factor.

As is evident from the preceding discussion, considerable study may be necessary before the cause of indigestion becomes evident. It may be pointed out that there is no characteristic finding in the gastric secretion.

Treatment—Obviously, treatment of indigestion is most successful when it includes elimination of the underlying cause. In management of the symptoms themselves, the diet should not be drastically restricted. It is much more important that meals should be taken in an atmosphere of leisure and relaxation and that food should be eaten slowly and masticated thoroughly. Food should be well cooked and moderate in quantity. Only those few foods which actually upset the patient should be eliminated. The only real restriction should be the avoidance of *large quantities* of coarse, highly seasoned, or very hot or very cold foods.

Mild sedative and antispasmodic medication is often beneficial, such as the time-tried combination of Belladonna Tincture, 20 to 50 cc. (average 40 cc.), with Phenobarbital Elixir to make 240 cc., 1 teaspoonful, more or less, to be taken three times daily a quarter hour before meals.

Aerophagia, if present, can be controlled only after the patient is convinced that the air is swallowed and not generated in the stomach. In breaking the habit of swallowing air between meals, it may be helpful to have the patient insert between his teeth after the first belch an ordinary small wooden spool of the type used to carry thread. He is to keep his tongue away from the hole in the spool. Since air can be swallowed only if the mouth is entirely closed, the hole effectively prevents the swallowing of air and stops the vicious cycle of air swallowing and belching.

PEPTIC ULCER

Peptic ulcer is a common, chronic, recurring condition in which there is ulceration of the mucosa of the stomach or duodenum or, rarely, of the lower end of the esophagus or Meckel's diverticulum. It occurs usually in early or middle adult life, is often accompanied by indigestion and hemorrhage, and may result in pyloric stenosis or perforation. Gastric acidity is high in the vast majority of cases; in fact, the finding of low gastric acidity casts considerable doubt upon the diagnosis of peptic ulcer.

Duodenal ulcer is three to four times more common in men than in women, whereas gastric ulcer occurs slightly more often in women. The first portion of the duodenum and the lesser curvature of the stomach near the pylorus are the most common sites. The cause of peptic ulcer is not entirely agreed upon, but there is considerable evidence that, in most cases at least, the principal immediate factor is emotional, the ulcer tending to occur and recur at times of nervous and emotional strain.

A high percentage of ulcer patients complain of indigestion, but a few do not. The classical picture of peptic ulcer indigestion is the periodic occurrence of postprandial (one to three hours) epigastric discomfort that is relieved by food or soda. Epigastric distress which awakens the patient at one or two o'clock has also been considered characteristic. It is, however, important to remember that not all peptic ulcer patients have this classical picture, and that patients with other abdominal conditions or with no demonstrable disease may have identical symptoms. During severe exacerbations, vomiting and intense pain may result from pyloric spasm.

Most peptic ulcer patients bleed at some time or other, and about one in four has obvious clinical evidence of hemorrhage. The bleeding may be sudden and profuse with resulting shock, or repeated small hemorrhages may cause iron-deficiency anemia. The blood may be vomited, but tarry stools may be the first evidence of hemorrhage. In a few patients, severe hemorrhage is the first symptom of the disease. An increase in blood nonprotein nitrogen follows hemorrhage into the gastrointestinal tract.

In about 10 percent of ulcer patients, stenosis of the pylorus or first portion of the duodenum develops as the result of scarring or inflammatory reaction. Accumulation of food and gastric secretions may result, with eventual vomiting of large amounts of food residues. Food eaten several days before may be recognized by the patient. The efforts of the distended stomach to force the accumulated food through the obstruction may result in peristaltic waves which may be seen moving slowly across the epigastrium from left to right. This sign is characteristic of pyloric obstruction but is present only relatively early in the process, before the stomach loses its tone. X-ray examination after ingestion of barium confirms the diagnosis of obstruction and reveals its degree and the amount of dilatation of the stomach. Evidence of complete obstruction may at times be misleading, for the edema of an acute inflammatory process may cause a narrowed orifice to close completely for a time. If vomiting is long continued, dehydration and, later, alkalosis and nitrogen retention occur (see pp. 56 and 61).

Perforation of a peptic ulcer is a very serious complication. When there is perforation into the peritoneal cavity, intense generalized abdominal pain with extreme tenderness, rigidity of the abdominal wall, and signs of shock develop rapidly. As an aid in differential diagnosis, the x-ray may show free gas in the peritoneal cavity. If the perforation is sealed off by inflammatory tissue, only localized pain and tenderness may be evident. Perforation may occur at any time during the course of peptic ulcer, and it may be the first symptom of the disease.

Except in perforation, x-ray or gastroscopic examination is necessary before the diagnosis of peptic ulcer can be considered as established.

Treatment—Although psychiatric therapy has not in the past played a part in the management of peptic ulcer, it may do so in the future if there is confirmation and acceptance of the present evidence for the role of emotional maladjustment in the pathogenesis of the disease. Such treatment would have the virtue of attacking a fundamental underlying cause. Under the concepts of the past, treatment has been essentially palliative.

Even if the internal emotional strains are neglected, all agree that the external stresses should be eliminated insofar as this is possible. Tension and hurry must be avoided, especially at mealtime. The patient should eat slowly and chew all foods thoroughly. Liquids should be sipped. Excessive smoking and ingestion of alcohol should be eliminated. If symptoms are severe, a few days' rest in hospital may be necessary at the start of therapy.

Diet was for many years the prime therapeutic agent in the treatment of peptic ulcer, but most authorities now agree that, except for a few limitations, the details of the diet are not important. Coarse, highly seasoned, or spicy foods and perhaps a few which disagree with that particular patient should be eliminated, but otherwise the diet should be nutritious, well cooked, appetizing, and well balanced. The meals must not be large, and most patients feel better if small in-between-meal feedings are taken.

Belladonna, 0.3 to 1 cc. of tincture or 1/4 to 1/2 grain of extract, with phenobarbital, 1/4 grain, before meals to relax spasm is often of benefit. Antacids are unquestionably valuable in controlling severe acute symptoms, but many believe that continuous large doses of alkalies are not only futile but unwarranted and perhaps harmful. A great variety of antacids has been used. A comparison of them will be found on page 383. The following are effective and have the advantage of carrying little danger of alkalosis: aluminum hydroxide, 10 to 20 cc. of gel or 0.6 to 2 Gm. of powder; aluminum phosphate, 15 to 30 cc. of gel; magnesium trisilicate, 2 to 4 Gm.; calcium carbonate, 0.6 to 2 Gm. Aluminum hydroxide and magnesium trisilicate are often given in combination. The following are also effective but have the distinct disadvantage of tending to cause alkalosis (p. 61): sodium bicarbonate, 0.6 to 1 Gm.; magnesium oxide, 0.6 to 2 Gm.; magnesium hydroxide, 0.6 to 2 Gm. Sometimes these and calcium carbonate are combined in the form of Sippy powders, Nos. 1 and 2.

A certain degree of protection of the ulcerated surface may be achieved by administration of gastric mucin (prepared from hog stomach) in doses of 2.5 Gm. in water every two hours.

Severe hemorrhage from ulcer must be treated with bed rest as long as signs of bleeding persist. Morphine sulfate, 8 to 16 mg., is given by many clinicians when necessary to allay restlessness and apprehension; others oppose its use in gastrointestinal bleeding because they believe that its tendency to cause nausea and to increase gastrointestinal tone is undesirable. Shock should be treated with transfusions of whole blood (250 to 1,000 cc.), even though it is a rare occurrence for hemorrhage from ulcer to be fatal. There is a difference in opinion as to whether bleeding ulcer patients should be fed or not. Some authorities give nothing by mouth but sips of water for one to three days; others give a bland high-vitamin diet with added iron (p. 368) and vitamins (p. 483) from the start. Judicious feeding probably is preferred to starvation.

In patients with pyloric obstruction, body fluids should be restored to normal by large infusions (3 to 4 liters per day) of isotonic salt solution and of 5 percent dextrose solution. Rest, starvation, and daily lavage of the stomach may be followed by reduction of inflammatory swelling; but if obstruction persists more than a few days, it must be relieved by operation. Preoperative restoration of fluid balance (p. 56) and correction of alkalosis (p. 61) are absolutely essential.

Rupture of peptic ulcer is a surgical emergency and should be operated on as soon as possible.

Surgical treatment of peptic ulcer should be limited to the following indications: (1) perforation, (2) pyloric stenosis, or (3) failure of relief after an adequate trial of conservative treatment. Recently, a high degree of symptomatic relief has been reported to follow resection of the vagus nerve. Full evaluation of this procedure is not yet possible; but it has been shown that, if gastric retention is present, gastroenterostomy must be performed at the time of nerve resection if serious malfunction is to be avoided. Some recommend that all chronic *gastric* ulcers be excised because of the high incidence of malignancy in this condition.

GASTRITIS

Acute gastritis results from chemical irritation or necrosis, as following ingestion of phenol, bichloride of mercury, acids, strong alkali, excessive quantities or concentrations of alcohol, and perhaps highly seasoned or spiced foods. Inflammation of the stomach may also accompany acute infectious diseases. Rarely, acute suppurative forms may occur. Symptoms include loss of appetite, nausea, vomiting, and varying degrees of indigestion and abdominal pain. Diarrhea is frequently present.

In treatment, food should be withheld as long as vomiting persists. If the latter is severe, gastric lavage with isotonic salt solution and rest in bed are indicated. After twelve to twenty-four hours of starvation, small amounts of liquids, such as milk, may be administered. If these are well tolerated, a bland diet is gradually instituted. Fluids rectally or parenterally may be necessary if dehydration develops. Morphine sulfate, 8 to 16 mg. (p. 399), may be indicated for relief of pain and restlessness.

Chronic gastritis is considered, perhaps not always with reason, to follow a great number of conditions, such as acute gastritis, focal infection, vitamin deficiencies, overindulgence in highly seasoned and coarse food, chronic alcoholism, the use of tobacco or certain drugs, and rapid eating as well as chronic cardiac failure, cirrhosis of the liver, and infected eroded cancer of the stomach. There is some doubt, moreover, as to whether indigestion, when it occurs, is due to the gastritis itself or to associated spasm. Gastroscopic examination may reveal localized or diffuse gastritis. Superficial, atrophic, and hypertrophic types are recognized. There is, however, no accepted correlation between gastroscopic, clinical, and gastric analysis findings, and many individuals with gastroscopic findings of gastritis have no symptoms. The gastroscopic findings of pernicious anemia disappear after specific therapy, but there is no return of free hydrochloric acid.

Treatment—The underlying cause should be treated when possible. If indigestion is present, therapy is in order as outlined on page 127. In the presence of anacidity, symptoms are sometimes relieved by the administration of acid, either as Diluted Hydrochloric Acid, U.S.P., 1 to 4 cc. diluted in a glass of water and sipped through a straw (p. 384), or as Pulvules 'Acidulin,' 2 to 4 at mealtime. Sometimes there is relief of symptoms and even improvement in the mucosal findings following oral administration of liver extract or liver-stomach concentrate (p. 369).

CANCER OF THE STOMACH

Cancer of the stomach is responsible for almost 30 percent of all cancer deaths. It occurs usually after the age of forty and is much more common in men than in women. Most of the lesions are near the pylorus, and they commonly follow chronic gastritis and anacidity. Indigestion of varying intensity may occur, but the disease may be asymptomatic until very late, then to be manifested indirectly through one of its complications, such as pyloric obstruction, acute hemorrhage, anemia due to chronic hemorrhage, or metastasis to the liver.

Cancer of the stomach should be suspected in anyone developing indigestion or symptoms referable to the stomach after the age of thirty-five, especially if accompanied by weight loss, pallor, and weakness. All such persons should have an x-ray examination of the stomach after a barium meal, and gastroscopy if the x-ray is inconclusive. These measures offer the only means of early diagnosis, and early diagnosis and treatment offer the only hope for cure. A tumor can seldom be palpated unless the growth has extended to the omentum, when a stony hard, nodular mass will be found in the epigastrium. Early in the disease there is sometimes difficulty in distinguishing benign from cancerous ulceration of the stomach.

The anemia of gastric cancer is usually hypochromic and microcytic, but occasionally it is macrocytic and hyperchromic. Gastric secretions are nearly always reduced and may be absent; usually the pH of gastric contents is between 3.5 and 7 (see p. 127).

Treatment—The only hope of cure is complete surgical extirpation of the growth. Unfortunately, patients seldom present themselves early enough to permit complete removal. In the later stages, operation may be indicated for relief of pyloric obstruction. Although medical treatment cannot affect the tumor, the patient's well-being may be much improved for considerable periods by symptomatic treatment and especially by the administration of liver extract (p. 369).

CONSTIPATION

The term "constipation" may refer to infrequent defecation or to passage of inspissated fecal material or both. Chronic constipation is probably the commonest complaint of individuals after middle life.

Although a regular daily bowel movement may be a convenience, it is not essential to health. The individual's bowel habit, his diet, and fluctuations in his nervous tension all influence the frequency of defecation and the duration of sojourn of food residues in the colon (this last period largely determines the degree of inspissation).

Headache, malaise, and nausea are often associated with constipation, and the idea is widely held that these symptoms are due to absorption of toxic substances from the colon. It has, however, been demonstrated that the symptoms are the result of reflexes from the distended rectum, since they can be reproduced in susceptible individuals by distending the rectum with cotton. Many other symptoms of ill health have been attributed to constipation. The relationship is exceedingly dubious; and if it exists, it is probably due not to constipation but to an excessive use of cathartics.

Constipation may result from obstruction arising from intrinsic or extrinsic tumors, or from adhesions, involving the colon. It may be due to hypothyroidism (p. 180) or to neurological disease such as spinal-cord injury or subacute combined degeneration (p. 173). However, constipation is most commonly a functional disturbance, the result of nervous tension, persistence of immature emotional attitudes toward authority or the sexual or excretory functions, inadequate or excessive bulk in the diet, neglect of the urge to defecation, or obesity.

Food residues normally require twelve to thirty-six hours to pass through the colon. Residues of different meals have been compared to individual freight cars pushed successively onto a railroad siding. Only when the siding is full will one be pushed off the other end of the siding onto the main line, that is, will the urge to defecate arise. When, for some reason, excessive peristaltic activity pushes several "freight cars" onto the main line at one time, no further such activity is to be expected until the siding has been filled up again. Even in those with extremely regular bowel habits, an occasional skipping of a day need cause no alarm. However, many people have been so thoroughly indoctrinated with the idea of the supreme importance of a daily movement that they take a laxative when they miss a day. The colon is still further emptied, and consequently there is no spontaneous movement on the day after the laxative "worked." Again a laxative is taken and a habit is built up. Actually, prolonged use of laxatives tends to aggravate rather than cure constipation when the latter condition actually exists.

The only physical sign associated with constipation is the occasional finding of a spastic, tender colon. Stools should be examined for evidence of inflammation or hemorrhage and to see if food has been properly chewed and digested. X-ray, particularly of the colon after barium enema, will help to rule out tumors, strictures, or important adhesions.

Treatment—The first element of treatment is correct diagnosis of the underlying cause. Considerable questioning may be necessary for correct evaluation of the complaint, particularly if the condition is chronic and the patient suffers from some of the widespread delusions about bowel function.

Organic causes of constipation should be treated directly. If the condition seems to be functional, it is necessary to convince the patient of the true facts of bowel function and to overcome the cathartic habit. It is explained that there is no toxic absorption in constipation and that a daily stool is not necessary. The habitual user of cathartics must not expect a bowel movement for several days after stopping the cathartics. The hyperirritable bowel must recover, and time must be allowed for the colon to fill before the defecation reflex can be initiated.

A definite regimen such as the following is usually helpful: a glass of water on arising and two or three glasses with each meal, a definite time schedule for going to stool (such as twenty minutes after breakfast), and increase or decrease in bulk of dietary residue (p. 585) as seems indicated. When spasm of the colon is a feature, treatment as for irritable colon (p. 135) may be useful.

If these measures do not suffice, they may be supplemented by use of methylcellulose, 1.5 to 4.5 Gm. two or three times daily (p. 386); agar, 10 to 40 Gm. daily (p. 386); or mineral oil, 15 to 45 cc. at night (p. 386). Glycerin Suppositories, U.S.P., may occasionally be necessary in those individuals requiring only slight stimulus to set the evacuation reflexes in motion. Olive or cottonseed-oil retention enemas, 180 cc., may be of benefit. Active laxatives should be avoided in chronic functional constipation.

If fecal impaction occurs, instillation of olive or cottonseed oil (100 to 200 cc.) to be retained overnight, followed by an enema of warm tap water or soapsuds in the morning, may relieve the condition, but often the impaction will have to be removed manually.

When chronic constipation seems to have deep psychological aspects, expert psychiatric handling is usually necessary for satisfactory results.

DIARRHEA

Although diarrhea is one of the most common manifestations of intestinal dysfunction, it is no more than a symptom indicating an increased gradient of excitability in the lower part of the intestinal tract. It may be due to inflammatory or other lesions in any part of the gastro-intestinal tract, to nervous and emotional tension, to reflexes arising in other parts of the body, or to a variety of systemic diseases of which hyperthyroidism may be taken as an example.

Acute Diarrhea—Acute enteritis (gastroenteritis, gastroenterocolitis, enterocolitis) is manifested by inflammation of the intestinal mucosa which may be due to infection, irritation, or intoxication. Food and drink are common sources. Local infections are most often due to the *Salmonella* group of organisms and to *Staphylococcus aureus*. Usually the food has been excessively handled and inadequately cooked and then improperly stored for six hours or more so that the contaminating organisms have had an opportunity to grow and produce their toxins. It is the toxins which cause the constitutional effects.

The attack is acute, beginning two to five hours after ingestion of the food, with nausea, vomiting, extreme prostration and collapse, abdominal cramps, and diarrhea which may be bloody. After six or eight hours there is generally gradual improvement, with recovery in twenty-four to forty-eight hours. When large groups of persons are involved, the diagnosis is readily made. Absence of eye symptoms differentiates the condition from botulism (p. 272).

Other infections which may be associated with acute diarrhea include bacillary dysentery (p. 4), amebic dysentery (p. 33), typhoid fever (p. 14), cholera, acute ulcerative colitis (p. 135), trichinosis (p. 41), brucellosis (p. 2), and malaria (p. 34).

Acute diarrhea with or without constitutional manifestations may be due to food poisoning (p. 271); ingestion of unripe fruit, large amounts of cellulose, or alcohol; acid food or drink which has been stored in containers of cadmium, zinc, or antimony; uremia (p. 223); heavy-metal poisoning; or arsenic poisoning.

Nervous tension must always be considered in differential diagnosis of acute diarrhea. The pre-examination diarrhea of college students is a well-known illustration.

Chronic Diarrhea may be associated with many types of disease, the most important of which are listed below. Frequently, the cause is extraintestinal and the gut is involved only symptomatically.

Disease of the stomach
   Anacidity (p. 126)
   Gastritis (p. 130)
   Cancer (p. 130)

Intestinal infection
   Bacillary dysentery (p. 4)
   Amebic dysentery (p. 33)
   Intestinal parasites (p. 37)
   Intestinal tuberculosis

Other intestinal disease
   Chronic ulcerative colitis (p. 135)
   Regional ileitis
   Cancer of colon (p. 136)
   Diverticulitis
   Megacolon with impaction
   Prolonged use of laxatives
   Fecal impaction
   Idiopathic steatorrhea

Other disease
   Deficiency states, including pernicious anemia (p. 96), sprue (p. 133), and pellagra (p. 488)
   Pancreatic insufficiency (p. 144)
   Diabetes mellitus (p. 173)
   Biliary tract disease (p. 139)
   Hyperthyroidism (p. 180)
   Amyloid disease
   Allergy (p. 264)
   Nervous and emotional states (p. 149)

Extensive study may be necessary for the correct diagnosis of the cause of chronic diarrhea. In addition to a full history and physical examination, the following special examinations may be in order: examination of stools and proctoscopic swabbings for pus, blood, mucus, ova, and parasites; stool culture for pathogenic organisms; proctoscopic examination; gastric analysis; x-ray studies of the entire gastro-intestinal tract.

Treatment—In either acute or chronic diarrhea, it is of first importance to discover and treat the underlying cause. If acute diarrhea is severe, immediate symptomatic treatment is also in order. It may include opium derivatives, preferably by mouth (p. 402). If oral medication can be retained, one or more of the following may be given at frequent intervals:

   bismuth subcarbonate, 0.6 to 2 Gm.
   paregoric, 4 to 8 cc.
   'Pectocel,' 1 to 2 tablespoonfuls

Dehydration is treated by parenteral fluids (p. 56).

No food is given as long as vomiting persists. After it has subsided and the diarrhea is less severe, a bland, low-residue diet (pp. 588 and 585) may be given in small quantities. A normal diet is resumed gradually as recovery progresses.

In chronic diarrhea, it is sometimes necessary to employ symptomatic treatment as above while the diagnosis is being made and specific therapy is begun. It is also essential to restore and maintain nutrition, assuring adequate protein, calories (3,000 is a satisfactory goal), minerals, and vitamins. Supplements of calcium, iron, and multiple vitamins are advisable, and parenteral administration of vitamins may be indicated. The diet should be bland and low in residue.

INTESTINAL COLIC

The term "colic" is applied to any severe paroxysmal pain occurring in a hollow viscus. Intestinal colic results from muscular spasm and distention of the intestines which may result from many causes.

During the first three months of life an infant is especially susceptible to development of colic. Aerophagia, excessive fat or carbohydrate in the diet, constipation, overfeeding, and allergic reaction to some food have been considered as precipitating factors. Colicky pains, however, are present in tabes dorsalis, lead and arsenic poisoning, appendicitis, intussusception, dysentery, colitis, and diverticulitis; following the ingestion of unripe fruit or foreign bodies; and in the presence of large numbers of round worms. In addition, reflex stimulation can produce the spasm and distention necessary for the production of colic.

Treatment—In young infants, colic due to aerophagia can be prevented by holding the infant erect after feeding to permit eructation. Obvious errors in feeding should be corrected. Small warm enemas may help relieve distention in the colon. Belladonna Tincture, 0.06 cc., may be given and repeated cautiously as indicated to relieve spasm of the intestinal tract.

Colicky pains in older children and adults should be treated according to the nature of the underlying cause.

FLATULENCE

Flatulence, or distention of the stomach and intestines with gas, is a common complaint for which there are many causes. In addition, many individuals under nervous tension complain of distention, especially after eating, when no excess of gas is present in the gastro-intestinal tract.

One of the commonest causes of actual abdominal distention after eating is conscious or subconscious aerophagia. The swallowed air may be belched or it may pass on into the intestine. In the intestine the oxygen is absorbed but the nitrogen is not. Some individuals habitually swallow air as a final part of the procedure of belching. Such persons thus always carry a supply of gas in the stomach and can belch whenever and as many times as it suits their purpose.

Hypermotility of the small intestine may cause abnormal amounts of starches to reach the colon before they are fully digested. Here the normal bacteria cause fermentation with gas formation. In addition, the hypermotility may decrease the amount of gases normally absorbed in the small intestine. Hypermotility of the small intestine can occur as a result of nervous and emotional disturbances, hyperthyroidism, allergic reactions to some foods, the habitual use of laxatives, and ingestion of excessive amounts of vitamin B complex.

Flatulence may also result from overeating, constipation, biliary tract disease, intestinal obstruction or paralytic ileus, decreased external secretions of the pancreas, sprue, and megacolon. Certain foods, such as onions or cooked cabbage, may cause excessive gas formation in some individuals.

Treatment should be directed to the cause of the symptom. Aerophagia requires explanation and re-education of the patient. A useful procedure for persistent belchers is insertion of an empty thread spool between the teeth whenever the impulse to belch arises. If the tongue is kept away from the spool, the airway maintained through the hole in the spool will prevent swallowing of air after the belch. The patient is thus deprived of further ammunition and the attack ceases. When aerophagia and belching provide emotional satisfaction, the patient is a candidate for expert psychiatric management.

SPRUE

Sprue (nontropical sprue, idiopathic steatorrhea, adult celiac disease, celiac disease, intestinal infantilism, Gee-Thaysen disease) is a chronic nutritional disease characterized by severe glossitis; diarrhea with foul, bulky, fatty stools; loss of weight; abdominal distention; anemia; steatorrhea; and disturbances of absorption from the gastro-intestinal tract resulting in hypocalcemia, hypophosphatemia, and hypoprothrombinemia, with tetany and hemorrhagic tendencies in some cases. The exact cause of sprue is unknown, but it is probable that folic acid deficiency is responsible for the major symptoms of the disease. There is usually a history of improperly balanced diet and poor hygiene.

Sprue occurring in the tropics is more apt to be characterized by acute exacerbations followed by remissions. The related forms known as nontropical sprue and celiac disease are more likely to show severe hypocalcemia, with tetany and osteoporosis. Bone deformities and pathological fractures may occur in the nontropical varieties. Infantilism usually occurs in celiac disease.

In sprue, as in pernicious anemia (p. 96), there is a generalized inflammation and atrophy of the mucous membrane of the gastro-intestinal tract. Gastric secretion is reduced or absent, with corresponding hypoacidity or anacidity. Poor absorption of calcium and vitamin D leads to hypocalcemia (p. 345); of vitamin K, to hypoprothrombinemia and hemorrhagic tendencies. Under x-ray, the small intestine shows the loss of normal feathering and the hypersegmentation characteristic of multiple vitamin deficiency.

The anemia of sprue is of the macrocytic hyperchromic type in adults, and the blood and bone marrow resemble those of pernicious anemia (Plate 33). In children, on the other hand, the anemia of sprue is of the iron-deficiency type.

The glucose tolerance curve is usually flat.

The stools are characteristic: gray in color, soft, full of gas bubbles, sour smelling, and abnormally voluminous. There is great excess of fatty acids and soaps. Muscle fibers may be present, but starch granules are absent.

The two diseases most often causing difficulty in differentiation are pancreatic steatorrhea and pernicious anemia. In pancreatic steatorrhea the stools contain a great excess of neutral fat as well as muscle fibers and starch granules. The glucose tolerance curve is normal or high, and there may be glycosuria. All patients having pernicious anemia have anacidity, and when diarrhea is present it is usually not fatty and voluminous. Combined symptom disease, so often seen in pernicious anemia, is rare in sprue.

Treatment—Folic acid (p. 371), 10 to 20 mg. daily, is probably the treatment of choice. In some cases, Liver Extract Solution, Crude, 10 to 20 units daily, may be of value. Highly purified liver preparations are often ineffective. Oral administration of liver extract, 1 or 2 units daily, is effective in some patients, but the poor absorption from the gastrointestinal tract makes parenteral therapy more reliable. Some cases apparently have responded to nicotinic acid, 500 mg. daily.

The diet should be high in protein and low in fat and carbohydrate. Fruit, especially banana, is usually well tolerated. Particular attention should be given to mineral and vitamin deficiencies. Calcium salts should be administered routinely (see p. 505). The treatment of tetany is described on page 195. In addition, vitamin D should be given in doses of 3,000 to 6,000 U.S.P. units daily. Iron deficiency will be relieved by ferrous sulfate, 0.3 Gm. three times daily. Hypoprothrombinemia and hemorrhagic tendencies should be treated with vitamin K (p. 499). Vitamin B complex in rather large doses is also generally indicated.

APPENDICITIS

Acute appendicitis (bacterial infection of the appendix) is one of the most common and most serious abdominal disorders. It occurs predominantly in young individuals, but no age is immune. Chronic appendicitis undoubtedly exists, but it is difficult to determine just what symptoms actually result from it. Certainly the diagnosis is less frequently made than formerly.

Acute appendicitis usually has a sudden onset, with nausea, vomiting, malaise, and diffuse abdominal distress and cramps. The patient is usually constipated and practically never has diarrhea. After a variable period of time, but usually within twelve to twenty-four hours, local peritoneal irritation has developed, and pain becomes localized in the right lower quadrant. Physical examination in the early stages often fails to yield positive findings in the right lower quadrant; but as soon as peritoneal irritation develops, there is slight tenderness and muscle spasm there, with slightly increased resistance to the examining hand. If rupture occurs, great tenderness and rigidity are noted locally or generally over the abdomen.

Body temperature is usually slightly elevated, and the pulse is nearly always increased. Polymorphonuclear leukocytosis is practically always present, but the white blood count is rarely over 20,000.

Occasionally acute appendicitis presents an atypical picture which may baffle the most experienced physician. In old people, gangrene and rupture may occur early and asymptomatically, the patient presenting himself some days later with generalized peritonitis or with a large and possibly obstructing inflammatory mass which suggests neoplasm. In any case the differential diagnosis may include gastro-intestinal upset, pelvic inflammatory disease, and urinary tract infection.

Treatment—Early excision of the appendix is the only safe treatment. Any reasonable suspicion of appendicitis justifies operation.

IRRITABLE COLON

The term "irritable colon" is one of many which are applied to functional disturbance of the colon. Other terms, representing different facets of the condition, include mucous colitis, colonic neurosis, emotional or nervous diarrhea, spastic colon, chronic colonic spasm, unstable colon, colon consciousness, and neurogenic hypermotility of the colon.

The condition involves derangement of the autonomic innervation of the colon, with usually a relative overactivity of the parasympathetic portion. Parallel autonomic disturbances often are present in other organs.

Irritable colon appears to result from chronic emotional tension. The particular pattern of response is often familial. In most patients the predominating disturbance is colonic spasm, and they suffer intermittent attacks of constipation and dull pain in the lower abdomen or rectum. Even though constipation is a major symptom, nearly all patients have diarrhea at times. In other patients the autonomic imbalance may result chiefly in hypersecretion, and the patient passes large quantities of clear mucus, free of pus or blood. In still other patients the gastrocolic reflex may be hyperactive, so that diarrhea occurs after nearly every meal and at times of emotional stress. Attacks in any of these forms may be precipitated by fatigue, normal or abnormal premenstrual changes in endocrine balance, or anything which increases emotional and nervous tension.

Organic disease of the colon must be ruled out by examination of stools for pus, blood, parasites, or pathogenic organisms, by sigmoidoscopic examination, and by barium enema.

Treatment should be directed primarily at the tension state. Sometimes explanation of the role of tension, with a regimen for its reduction, is sufficient; sometimes expert psychiatric handling is advisable.

For the immediate treatment of exacerbations a bland, low-residue diet (pp. 588 and 585) is helpful. The time-honored combination of belladonna and phenobarbital is often most useful in controlling spasm or hypermotility. Phenobarbital Elixir may be added to 15 to 30 cc. Belladonna Tincture in sufficient quantity to make 180 cc.; the usual dose is one teaspoonful two to four times a day with meals and at bedtime. Different mixtures of phenobarbital and Belladonna Extract are also available in tablet form; the usual dose is 1/4 to 1/2 grain of the former and 1/8 to 1/4 grain of the latter two to four times daily. Undue dryness of the mouth or impairment of visual accommodation is an indication for reducing the proportion of belladonna. One of the hydrophilic colloids, such as agar (p. 386), may help prevent inspissation of the feces in extreme spastic constipation.

When severe diarrhea is not relieved by belladonna and phenobarbital, it is sometimes advantageous to institute the regimen described on page 132. Patients having predominantly an excess of mucus respond less well to symptomatic treatment. It should again be emphasized that the most important therapeutic approach is neuropsychiatric.

ULCERATIVE COLITIS

Ulcerative colitis is a diffuse ulcerative inflammation of the colon with or without initial specific infection and conditioned by immunologic, allergic, nutritional, and nervous factors. The exact cause is not established. Some cases appear to be of infectious origin, but no single organism has been demonstrated in all or even a majority of patients. Allergic states, nutritional deficiencies, and emotional tension appear to be important factors in many cases, but there is disagreement as to whether they can be primary causes.

Ulcerative colitis usually occurs in the young or middle-aged. Onset may be that of any acute dysentery with severe diarrhea, abdominal cramps, tenesmus, prostration, and fever; but the usual onset is insidious and the course slow and prolonged with many acute exacerbations and remissions. Some patients eventually reach a state of extreme emaciation, severe anemia, and multiple vitamin deficiencies. There is usually fever, perhaps quite high during the acute attacks. Anemia is nearly always present. Stools contain pus, mucus, and blood but no amebae or dysentery bacilli. Proctoscopic examination reveals the diffuse small ulcerations in the rectum and sigmoid. Barium enema demonstrates the extent and severity of the lesions beyond the reach of the sigmoidoscope.

Treatment—There is no specific therapy or any uniformly effective treatment. Maintenance of good nutrition and prevention of vitamin deficiencies are of the utmost importance. The diet should be bland and low in roughage (pp. 588 and 585) but high in protein. It should contain at least 3,000 calories per day (p. 584). Supplementary amino acids (p. 260) by mouth or vein may induce great improvement in general condition. Multiple vitamin supplements should contain several times the minimum daily requirements. Liver extract (p. 369) seems to improve the general condition in some cases.

When infection is a factor in exacerbations, the sulfonamides (p. 293) appear to shorten the acute attack. Neither they nor the antibiotics have value against the chronic disease. Spasm and hypermotility are often allayed by belladonna and phenobarbital (see under Irritable Colon, p. 135). If diarrhea is troublesome, it is treated symptomatically (p. 132). Sometimes the adsorbents are helpful (p. 382). The anemia is treated with iron (p. 368), liver (p. 369), and blood transfusions if necessary. In some cases, early ileostomy or colostomy rests the colon and is followed by clinical improvement.

CANCER OF THE COLON

Cancer of the colon accounts for about 10 percent of deaths due to cancer. It occurs much more frequently in men than in women. Practically all the malignant lesions are adenocarcinomata and are usually slow-growing and of a relatively low grade of malignancy. Although 85 to 90 percent occur after forty years of age, about 5 percent occur before the age of thirty.

Cancer of the proximal half of the colon presents a different clinical picture from cancer of the distal half. Cancer of the proximal colon tends to be fungating and ulcerated. Except when secondary infection causes extreme inflammation, it tends to cause obstruction only late. Although there may be indigestion and mild right-lower-quadrant pain, very often the presenting picture is anemia of the iron-deficiency type, progressive weakness, loss of weight, and sometimes a change in bowel habit.

Cancer of the distal colon is more apt to be firm and fibrous, tending to encircle the bowel. The predominant symptoms are usually obstructive: change in bowel habit; progressive constipation with occasional diarrhea; some abdominal pain, usually in the left lower quadrant. There may be gross blood in the stools. Constitutional effects usually occur late.

The finding of an abdominal mass, blood in the stools, or a space-occupying lesion on barium enema tends to confirm the diagnosis. A very low lesion may be visible to the sigmoidoscope.

Treatment consists in surgical excision. Because the cancer usually grows and metastasizes slowly, prompt surgery offers an excellent chance of permanent cure. In inoperable cases, colostomy may have to be done to relieve obstruction.

Rectum and Anus

The endoderm of the gut joins the ectoderm of the anal canal at the pectinate line. Because the gut carries no ordinary pain fibers, lesions extending no lower than the rectum are likely to be painless and to give rise to symptoms only when they become ulcerated or affect motility in some way, as by producing obstruction. In contrast, lesions involving the anal canal are likely to be painful and to produce spasm of the sphincters.

Diagnosis of rectal and anal lesions should depend not only on the history but also on the results of digital and visual examination. Because of the symptomatic silence of the rectum, it should always be examined with the proctoscope in the presence of complaints referable to the anal canal.

HEMORRHOIDS

Hemorrhoids (piles) are protruding masses of tissue at the anal orifice or in the anal canal. They contain distended veins and are termed "internal" or "external," depending on whether they arise above or below the pectinate line. The venous distention which causes hemorrhoids may be produced in a number of ways: habitual straining at stool (the most common cause), frequent heavy lifting, pregnancy, portal obstruction due to cirrhosis of the liver or metastatic cancer, or local venous obstruction due to infiltration of cancer in or about the rectum or lower sigmoid.

External hemorrhoids are rarely troublesome until venous thrombosis occurs; then they may suddenly become excruciatingly painful. Enucleation of the thrombus or excision of the thrombosed section of the vein under local anesthesia usually gives prompt relief. Local heat may provide some amelioration.

Internal hemorrhoids may be complicated by bleeding, infection, ulceration, strangulation, or thrombosis. Immediate symptomatic treatment may include hot sitz baths and analgesic ointment or suppositories (p. 446). When symptoms are mild, their recurrence can usually be prevented by treating the constipation or whatever other factor is responsible for straining and increased venous pressure. More severe symptoms may require injection of the hemorrhoids with a sclerosing solution or excision. Internal hemorrhoids should not be obstructed or removed, however, until the physician has assured himself that the patient is not suffering from portal obstruction for which the hemorrhoids may be providing collateral circulation.

FISSURE-IN-ANO

The term "fissure-in-ano" is applied to a painful longitudinal ulcer of the anal canal. It commonly occurs at the posterior commissure and results from infection of a break in the anal skin caused by passage of a large, hard stool. It may be associated with a small "sentinel pile" or infected crypt (see Cryptitis below). Symptoms are pain and bleeding, the former great, the latter usually small.

The fissure may heal spontaneously, but frequently the pain during and following defecation is so severe that the patient postpones this function as long as possible, with a resulting vicious cycle of increasing constipation, trauma, and symptoms.

Application of an analgesic ointment (p. 446) facilitates examination; and in cases of brief duration, repeated application may relax sphincter spasm and allow the lesion to heal. Sometimes the prolonged relaxation which follows dilatation of the sphincter under anesthesia allows healing. Since fissure-in-ano is practically always secondary to constipation, this underlying factor should always be treated (p.130). Excision of the fissure and surrounding scar tissue are necessary in long-standing cases.

CRYPTITIS

Cryptitis is an infection of the crypts of Morgagni, usually secondary to trauma from a large, hard stool, foreign bodies in the stool, enema tubes, or frequent anal spasms in diarrhea. The infection may produce no symptoms until inflammation extends to the adjacent papillae, when pain and spasm occur.

Treatment should be conservative. Constipation and additional trauma are avoided, generally by a bland diet and mineral oil (p. 386). Local heat is helpful in the form of sitz baths or rectal irrigations with a pint of warm isotonic salt solution. Analgesic ointment may relieve pain and spasm. Deep ulceration may require surgical drainage.

ISCHIORECTAL ABSCESS

Ischiorectal abscess usually is the result of cryptitis (see above). Pain, tenderness, and swelling in the region of the anus make the diagnosis obvious in most cases. The treatment is radical incision, the wound being packed loosely with sulfonamide or penicillin powder. Many cases do not heal completely and require treatment for fistula (see below).

FISTULA-IN-ANO

Fistula-in-ano is usually a direct or indirect result of cryptitis (see above). It is a tubular drainage tract lined with infected granulation tissue, leading from a crypt to the skin surface at one side or the other of the anus. If there has been an ischiorectal abscess, the fistula extends through what remains of its cavity. The skin opening may heal and reopen repeatedly. Sometimes the fistulous tract is tortuous, and there may be several openings, some of them a considerable distance away from the anus. Occasionally the tubercle bacillus is the primary infecting agent.

Intermittent or sudden foul drainage from a skin opening near the anus is diagnostic. Treatment consists in incision or excision of the entire fistulous tract from infected crypt to all of the cutaneous openings.

POLYPS

Polyps may occur solely in the rectum or in various portions of the colon. When they ulcerate and bleed they may be mistaken for hemorrhoids. Because polyps are precancerous lesions, they should be excised.

PRURITUS ANI

Pruritus ani, or itching of the anal and perineal region, is a common and troublesome complaint. Many factors enter into its causation. They may be grouped as infectious, allergic, mechanical, and nervous-emotional.

Bacterial infection of the anal and perianal skin may have its source in the intestinal or vaginal flora, or it may be carried by the fingers. Fungus infection usually comes from the feet via the fingers. The major part of the skin reaction may represent allergy to the organisms rather than actual infection. Both bacterial and fungus growth are favored by the relative alkalinity and high protein and carbohydrate content of the sweat in the anogenital region, as well as by the lack of evaporation from the depths of the gluteal cleft. Uncontrolled diabetes mellitus also predisposes to bacterial and fungus growth by increasing the carbohydrate content of the skin and, in some cases, by adding sugar to the urine residue left about the vagina.

The patient may be allergic, not only to local or distant bacteria and fungi, but also to food, drugs (including laxatives) taken systemically, remedial agents (including resorcinol, metals, and local anesthetics) applied locally for relief of the itching or for hemorrhoids, and the sulfite in cheap toilet tissue.

The region of the anus provides abundant opportunity for the slight traumata that may precipitate itching syndromes: the stool, toilet tissue, rubbing or scratching with the fingers, walking, and even instrumentation. Irritation may also be induced by discharge from fistulas or infected crypts or by vaginal discharge.

Nervous tension and chronic anxiety may serve to perpetuate an otherwise brief period of itching by keeping the patient attentive and alert to sensations from the perianal region. Trauma from scratching or rubbing, and this awareness of the condition, may thus start a vicious cycle. Of paramount importance in some cases is anal fixation, which is an expression of deep emotional conflict and maladjustment with sexual implications.

Treatment requires attention to all the facets of the situation indicated above. Thorough inspection and digital and proctoscopic examination should be made, and contributing factors thus discovered should be corrected.

Systemic factors, such as diabetes mellitus and obesity, are to be treated. The latter predisposes probably by impeding evaporation from the perineal region. If allergy is thought to be a factor, an antihistaminic drug (p. 509) may be administered systemically or locally. If such a drug gives relief, the source of the allergy can be sought with more conviction than if it does not.

It is almost always advisable to alter the intestinal bacterial flora. The carbohydrate content of the diet should be reduced, and roughage should be largely eliminated. Some patients appear to benefit from hydrochloric acid by mouth (p. 384). Alcohol intake should be stopped or greatly reduced, partly because such a step may help unmask emotional maladjustment (see Chronic Alcoholism, p. 159) and partly because the vasodilation produced by alcohol may itself precipitate itching.

If the apocrine sweat mechanism (axillary, submammary, periumbilical, and anogenital regions)

is hyperactive, emotional and sex factors should be especially sought for (although tension states are almost always present in chronic itching). In some cases, simple explanation and re-education suffice; in others, psychiatric handling is advisable.

Acute pruritus can often be relieved by extremely hot or extremely cold wet applications or by alternate use of the two. A good source of cold is an ice cube wrapped in a thin handkerchief and inserted well into the anal ring, being supported there by a folded towel or pad.

In general, however, local applications or manipulations are to be avoided except for those which clear up sources of infection or other directly contributing factors in the pruritus. Soap, water, toilet paper, and rubbing are interdicted. After defecation, the anus is cleansed with a 1:4,000 aqueous solution of potassium permanganate which is mopped on gently with absorbent cotton. Analgesic agents and mercurial antiseptics are generally disapproved because of their tendency to produce allergy. However, when local irritation is a factor, topical application of 'Surfacaine' (p. 446) may help to break a vicious cycle by affording temporary relief from itching. If lubrication is necessary, mineral oil or Hydrophilic Petrolatum, U.S.P., (p. 479) can be applied.

Castellani's paint is advocated by some as being extremely effective in certain patients. To make it, add 10 parts of a saturated solution of basic fuchsin in alcohol to 100 parts of a 5 percent aqueous phenol solution. Filter this and add 1 part boric acid. Let stand two hours; then add 5 parts of acetone. After another two hours add 10 parts of resorcinol. At first, this preparation is diluted with three parts of water. Only gradually is it worked up to full strength. Although resorcinol in the preparation adds to the effectiveness, it will have to be omitted if the patient is or becomes allergic to it.

In stubborn cases the stools should be examined for parasites, and there should be cultures for bacteria and fungi from stools, the crypts of Morgagni, mucocutaneous junction, and perianal skin. Elimination diets should also be tried, particular attention being paid to the common foods such as milk and wheat.

X-ray therapy sometimes gives great relief, but it is not always permanent.

CANCER OF THE RECTUM

Carcinoma arises more frequently in the rectum than in any other part of the colon. It is adenomatous in character. Bleeding is the most common symptom, and the possibility of cancer should be considered in all cases of anal bleeding. Even if hemorrhoids are found, the proctoscope should always be extended further to rule out coincident malignancy. Change in bowel habit is another symptom.

The treatment is surgical removal.

Liver and Biliary Tract

The liver is one of the vital organs. Its importance is indicated by a listing of the principal functions which it is at present known to perform:

Secretion of bile.

Metabolism of foodstuffs: storage, chemical alteration, and regulation of blood level of amino acids, carbohydrate, and fat.

Storage of accessory foodstuffs and other substances, such as vitamins, iron, copper, and the intrinsic factor which is essential in the treatment of pernicious anemia.

Regulation of plasma protein level.

Synthesis of substances concerned with the coagulation of blood, including heparin, fibrinogen, and prothrombin.

"Detoxification," destruction, or conjugation (into a soluble form for excretion) of many endogenous and exogenous substances, such as:

Amino acids (nitrogenous portion converted to urea)

Steroid hormones (estrogens, androgens, progesterone)

Uric acid

Phenol and its derivatives

Benzoates

Many drugs, including:
Morphine
Barbiturates

The liver receives a relatively small arterial blood supply from the celiac axis by way of the hepatic artery and a very large venous blood supply from the portal vein which drains the spleen and the entire gastro-intestinal tract, including the gall bladder and the pancreas, from the cardiac end of the stomach to the lower border of the rectum. Thus, everything that is absorbed from the gastro-intestinal tract passes through the liver before it reaches the general circulation.

The liver has an amazingly great power of regeneration following injury or destruction. This power depends, however, on maintenance of portal blood flow. It has been demonstrated that the resistance of the liver to toxic injury varies with the diet, the maximal protective effect being exerted by one that is high in protein and carbohydrate and low in, but not entirely void of, fat.

The bile pigments, bilirubin and biliverdin, are formed in cells of the reticulo-endothelial system from the porphyrin fraction of hemoglobin. Most of these cells in man are found in the sinusoids of the liver (Kupffer cells). The liver cells proper (polygonal cells) remove the excess of bile pigment from the blood and excrete it in the bile. In the intestine the bilirubin is reduced to urobilinogen by the action of the bacteria. Some of this urobilinogen is excreted in the stool, but a portion is reabsorbed and returns through the portal vein to the liver, which normally re-excretes practically all of it. That which escapes removal is oxidized to urobilin and appears as such in the urine. This continuous cycle of urobilinogen transport has been termed the enterohepatic circulation of bile pigment. A similar circulation occurs with steroid hormones when they are presented to the liver in larger quantities than can be immediately conjugated.

JAUNDICE

Jaundice (icterus) is a yellowish staining of the skin, mucous membranes, and tissues due to bile pigment. When the blood level rises sufficiently, the pigment diffuses into the tissues. The staining is most readily recognized in the sclera viewed by north daylight. Pigment also appears in the urine and sweat but not in the saliva, milk, or cerebrospinal fluid (except in children).

Jaundice may be the result of inability on the part of a normal liver to excrete promptly an unusually large overproduction of pigment (hemolytic jaundice), or inability of a damaged or obstructed liver to excrete normal quantities of pigment (hepatic jaundice). Hepatic jaundice may be obstructive, due to blockage of the bile passages, or nonobstructive (hepatocellular or toxic), due to impaired function of the liver cells.

Bile pigment is normally present in the blood in concentrations of 0.2 to 0.8 mg. per 100 cc. of serum. The simplest measure of its relative concentration is the icterus index (p. 534). The icterus index has, however, the disadvantage of failing to distinguish bile pigment from other yellow substances, such as carotene. The quantitative van den Bergh test is free of this objection, but it is complicated and at best only approximate. The original van den Bergh unit represents 1 part of bilirubin in 200,000 parts of serum. Thus, 1 unit equals 0.5 mg. per 100 cc., 0.5 unit equals 0.25 mg. per 100 cc., and 4 units equal 2 mg. per 100 cc. The qualitative van den Bergh was at one time thought to be helpful in distinguishing between types of jaundice, but it is now generally considered of no value.

Although 0.8 mg. per 100 cc. is often given as the upper limit of normal for serum bilirubin (corresponding to an icterus index of 6), other authorities consider anything over 0.5 mg. abnormal. Jaundice is said to be latent when it is of insufficient degree to be noted on inspection of the patient. The pigment present in the blood in obstructive jaundice diffuses into the tissues more freely than does that in hemolytic jaundice. Therefore, obstructive jaundice is more obvious in that jaundice appears at a lower blood level of pigment than is the case in hemolytic jaundice. The level for discernible icterus in obstructive and hepatocellular jaundice is usually in the neighborhood of 1.6 mg. of bilirubin per 100 cc. of serum, corresponding to an icterus index of 16.

In purely obstructive jaundice (as from a stone in the common duct or from pressure of a tumor on the duct), the stools will be clay-colored from lack of bile pigment. Since the enterohepatic circulation of urobilinogen (p. 139) ceases, urobilin will be absent from the urine after a few days. When there is infection of the bile ducts, as in cholangitis or infectious hepatitis, however, small amounts of urobilinogen may be formed in the presence of complete obstruction and find their way to the kidneys, and the same is true when jaundice is so profound that bilirubin diffuses into the lumen of the intestine from the wall. In obstructive jaundice, bile acids as well as bile pigment are found in the blood and urine. Plasma phosphatase (alkaline) is increased. Prothrombin deficiency (p. 107) occurs, with prolonged coagulation time of the blood and a consequent bleeding tendency. Bradycardia and generalized itching of the skin may be present; their cause is unknown.

In purely hemolytic jaundice, urobilin will be found in the urine and urobilinogen in the feces. The hyperbilirubinemia will be higher in relation to the degree of icterus and bilirubinuria than would be the case in obstructive jaundice because of the less diffusible state of the bile pigment in hemolytic jaundice. There is no change in plasma phosphatase, and bile acids do not appear in the blood and urine.

Hepatocellular jaundice is usually accompanied by some degree of intrahepatic biliary obstruction (from inflammatory swelling or bile thrombi) and discontinuity of bile canaliculi. A mixed picture may therefore be present. Unless biliary obstruction is complete, urobilinogen is present in the stool and urobilin in the urine.

ACUTE HEPATITIS

Acute hepatitis may be due to infectious or toxic agents. It involves inflammation and necrosis of liver tissue. When jaundice occurs, it is of the hepatocellular type (see above). The clinical picture and course vary with the cause.

Infectious hepatitis may be due to a spirochete (see Weil's Disease, p. 15) or to one or more viruses. An epidemic type of virus hepatitis is likely to occur when young men are crowded together as in armies. After an incubation period of about thirty days there is an insidious onset, with fever, anorexia, prostration, and perhaps nausea, vomiting, and diarrhea. Jaundice appears after three to five days. There may be rapid hepatic failure, but usually the disease is mild. At the height of the jaundice the stools are usually acholic. The urine always contains urobilinogen and sometimes bile. The so-called catarrhal jaundice is apparently sporadic infectious hepatitis.

A form of infectious hepatitis, the so-called homologous serum jaundice, may follow the injection of human plasma or serum. Though the clinical picture resembles that of epidemic infectious hepatitis, the incubation period is longer (sixty to ninety days), and the viruses are apparently different. Homologous serum jaundice may follow injection of plasma or serum from donors who do not themselves have any evidence of hepatitis.

Hepatitis may occur without jaundice. After the prodromal symptoms appear, the liver becomes enlarged and tender; tests of liver function show impairment; but there is no jaundice. The patient may continue for many weeks to have gastrointestinal symptoms, weakness, fatigability, malaise, and pain and tenderness over the liver.

Most patients with infectious or presumably infectious hepatitis recover completely within thirty to sixty days, but tenderness over the liver, weakness, and malaise may persist for weeks, during which time liver function tests (p. 543) are also impaired. The great majority of these patients with prolonged illness also go on to complete recovery. However, some apparently enter a latent phase and after months or, usually, years develop cirrhosis (see below).

Agents which are toxic to the liver include phosphorus, chloroform, carbon tetrachloride, organic arsenicals (such as arsphenamine), trinitrophenol (picric acid), and cinchophen. Other toxic agents of unknown nature are present in such conditions as eclampsia (p.212). Depending on the dose and other factors, they produce necrosis of liver cells of greater or less extent. The clinical picture is similar to that of infectious hepatitis except for the absence of fever and other evidence of infection.

Sudden widespread necrosis of liver cells gives rise to the condition known as acute yellow atrophy of the liver. It may be due to infectious or toxic agents; sometimes the cause cannot be found. The onset is accompanied by violent gastro-intestinal upset, prostration, and sometimes severe abdominal pain. As hepatic insufficiency continues, characteristic toxic symptoms supervene: restlessness, delirium, later drowsiness and coma, progressive rise in temperature and pulse rate, fall in blood pressure, and hemorrhagic tendencies. The course may last five or six weeks. Recovery is rare.

Treatment—Since bodily activity is capable of prolonging or reactivating acute hepatitis, all patients should be placed on complete bed rest, regardless of how mild the disease appears. If an infectious origin is suspected, the patient should be isolated. Discoverable toxic causative factors should be removed.

The diet should be high in calories, protein, and carbohydrate (p. 584). The protein should be of high value (milk, meat). The fat content should be low, but fat should not be eliminated entirely. Between-meal feedings high in carbohydrate, such as candy, are recommended. Multivitamin supplements should be given in large doses. Liver extract (10 to 20 units per day intramuscularly) may be of benefit.

The patient should not be allowed to become active or to increase the fat content of the diet until the jaundice has disappeared and the icterus index has returned to normal. No alcohol should be ingested during six months following recovery.

The daily intravenous injection of 1,000 to 3,000 cc. of 5 percent dextrose is indicated in severe hepatitis and may even shorten the illness in mild cases.

The injection of purified globulin has been reported as an effective means of preventing and ameliorating homologous serum hepatitis.

CIRRHOSIS

Cirrhosis of the liver (chronic hepatitis, Laennec's cirrhosis) includes those conditions in which destruction of the liver parenchyma is followed by fibrosis which eventually leads to further changes in structure and impairment of function.

The cause of cirrhosis is unknown in the great majority of cases. Some represent the late effects of recognizable acute hepatitis (see above). Others may be the end product of prolonged subclinical hepatitis. In animals, a form of cirrhosis follows chronic deficiency of protein and vitamins of the B complex. The cirrhosis which is attributed to chronic alcoholism may actually be due to an associated nutritional deficiency, or the alcohol may diminish resistance to a subclinical infection. In some instances, cirrhosis may follow chronic intoxication with substances like arsphenamine. Any substance which damages the liver in such a way as to produce fatty infiltration may also produce cirrhosis.

Cirrhosis decreases liver function and obstructs the portal circulation. As back pressure increases in the portal system, collateral circulation develops through the following principal routes: (1) the coronary veins of the stomach to the esophageal veins (producing esophageal varices); (2) retroperitoneal veins (of Retzius); (3) parumbilical veins in the falciform ligament of the liver to the superficial abdominal veins (the enlarged abdominal and occasionally thoracic veins can sometimes be seen and more often photographed with an infrared plate); and (4) hemorrhoidal veins (sometimes producing hemorrhoids).

The symptoms of cirrhosis usually begin insidiously. Until late in the disease the portal obstructive symptoms predominate. The initial symptoms are often swelling of the abdomen from ascites, edema of the legs, hematemesis (from esophageal varices), or indigestion or diarrhea (the result of gastritis and congestion of the gastro-intestinal tract). Later there is loss of weight, weakness, malaise, anemia, slight jaundice, bleeding from the mucous membranes, and finally coma, perhaps with high fever, and death.

Physical examination may reveal fluid in the abdomen, edema of the lower extremities, dilated veins over the chest and abdominal wall, hemorrhoids, and the characteristic spider angiomata that are due to excess estrogen which the liver has failed to inactivate. The enlarged abdomen stands out in contrast to the emaciated chest and extremities. The liver is enlarged until late in the disease and can usually be felt as a hard, often nodular mass in the right upper quadrant. The spleen may also be enlarged. The anemia which is usually present is often macrocytic and hyperchromic in character. The serum proteins are usually low, and there may be hypoprothrombinemia. Late in the disease, fibrinogen formation is decreased. Liver function tests show varying degrees of decreased function. Secondary infections are prone to develop and are often the immediate cause of death.

Diagnosis can usually be made on physical findings and the subnormal liver function tests.

The biliary cirrhosis which develops after bile stasis and infection is usually associated with an enlarged liver. An inflammatory reaction with fibrosis and scarring surrounds the bile ducts. Recurrent and increasing jaundice and gradual decrease in function of the liver dominate the clinical picture. Portal obstructive symptoms occur late, if at all.

Treatment—The diagnosis of cirrhosis is seldom made until liver destruction is very extensive. Treatment can then at best only slow the inevitable process. In spite of the unfavorable ultimate prognosis, however, a great deal can be done in the way of prolonging the period of usefulness, reasonable well-being, and life itself. Naturally, the treatment will be more successful the earlier it is started.

As in acute hepatitis, the diet should be high in protein and carbohydrate and low in, but not void of, fat. Vitamin supplements should be given in generous dosage, along with liver extract, 1 to 2 units by mouth daily, or dried brewer's yeast, 6 Gm. or more daily. In addition, liver extract should be given by injection, 10 to 20 units daily. Choline, 0.5 to 2 Gm. three or four times daily by mouth, is considered beneficial by many. Some have recommended the daily injection of 1,000 to 2,000 cc. of 5 percent dextrose.

The ascites should be removed periodically by abdominal paracentesis. If the patient responds satisfactorily to dietary management, the paracenteses become progressively less frequent. The injection of blood plasma may help to raise the plasma protein level and assist in eliminating edema. Iron salts (p. 368) or transfusions of whole blood are useful in correcting the anemia. However, in connection with administration of blood or plasma, the possibility must be considered of superimposing homologous serum jaundice (p. 140) upon the existing disease.

CHOLELITHIASIS

Cholelithiasis is the occurrence of concretions in the gall bladder or bile passages. Gallstones are composed of constituents of the bile which have precipitated. They are classified into pure choles-terol, cholesterol-pigment-calcium, pure bilirubin, bilirubin-calcium, and calcium carbonate stones according to their composition. The cholesterol-pigment-calcium stones are the commonest variety. The so-called pure cholesterol stones are usually single and are probably the result of disturbances of cholesterol metabolism. The pure bilirubin stones tend to occur in conditions in which there is excessive hemolysis.

Most stones are found in the gall bladder, but they may form in the hepatic duct or even in the smaller ducts of the liver. The actual mechanism of their formation is unknown, but the following are considered as causes: (1) injury, especially infection, of the gall-bladder wall; (2) disturbance of cholesterol metabolism; (3) stasis of bile; and (4) altered pH of the bile. Whatever the cause, gallstones are found in 7 percent of all autopsies. Cholelithiasis is two to four times more common in women than men. There is a steady increase in incidence after thirty years of age.

Gallstones may exist for years without producing any symptom. Their presence may be associated with indigestion and particularly with vague discomfort in the epigastrium or right upper quadrant, often exaggerated after eating fatty food. There may be slight tenderness in the right upper quadrant. Characteristically, this type of indigestion associated with gallstones occurs in obese middle-aged women.

Biliary colic occurs when a stone becomes impacted in the neck of the cystic duct. This may occur frequently or rarely and at any time during the course of the disease. The attack usually starts suddenly at night and consists of severe deep-seated right-upper-quadrant pain, often radiating to the back and right shoulder. It is frequently associated with nausea and vomiting. The attack usually lasts several hours and then gradually subsides. Right-upper-quadrant discomfort and slight nausea often persist for one or two days.

Pain due to stone in the common duct is usually not so severe as that due to stone in the cystic duct. At some time during the attack it is usually associated with jaundice. Fever and leukocytosis occur if infection is present. Chills and fever (intermittent biliary fever of Charcot) may occur. Hydrops of the gall bladder may result if the stone remains in the cystic duct. If the cystic artery is compressed by the stone, necrosis and infection of the gall bladder (empyema of gall bladder) results, and rupture may occur, with peritonitis. Recurring obstruction of the common duct with infection may result in a biliary cirrhosis of the liver.

The diagnosis is made on history, age, sex, and habitus, occurrence of jaundice, and findings upon x-ray of the gall bladder after administration of a suitable dye.

Treatment—Many patients with gallstones can be maintained for many years on a diet of well-cooked simple food containing nothing that is highly seasoned. Cooked fats should be restricted, because they often produce symptoms. Constipation should be relieved. Bile salts (p. 387), 0.3 to 0.6 Gm. one to three times daily, often are of help against constipation, but they should not be administered if stones are present in the common duct. Obesity should be controlled by restriction of fats and carbohydrates in the diet.

Acute biliary colic must be relieved by injection, preferably intravenous, of morphine or a similar analgesic (p. 399). The addition of atropine sulfate (1/100 to 1/50 grain) is often helpful if the injection is subcutaneous. Heat over the right upper quadrant is often gratefully received. Following the disappearance of nausea and vomiting, a liquid diet should be prescribed for a day or two. Any indication of pyogenic infection after biliary colic requires surgery. Stone in the common duct is always a serious condition and should be treated surgically. A high-carbohydrate diet and vitamin K (see p. 499) should be administered preceding surgery.

CHOLECYSTITIS

Acute cholecystitis is usually secondary to stones, cancer, or other antecedent lesion. Rarely, infection with streptococci, staphylococci, or intestinal bacteria develops in apparently normal gall bladders. Symptoms of acute cholecystitis include fever, chills, sweats, prostration, nausea and vomiting, epigastric or abdominal pain, and tenderness with spasm or rigidity of the abdominal wall over the gall-bladder area. An enlarged, palpable gall bladder may be found. Jaundice may or may not be present. A polymorphonuclear leukocytosis occurs.

Chronic cholecystitis occurs, usually in patients having gallstones, but there is some question as to whether it causes many of the symptoms attributed to it. Indigestion characterized by epigastric distress, fullness, excess gas formation, and nausea and vomiting made worse by eating greasy or fatty foods has been considered as resulting from chronic cholecystitis. Such indigestion is often identical with that caused by many other conditions.

The diagnosis of chronic cholecystitis should be made with care unless stones can be demonstrated or the patient has experienced an unequivocal acute attack. The symptoms of indigestion are apt to persist following cholecystectomy in patients with presumed chronic cholecystitis who do not fulfill the above criteria.

Treatment—In most cases of acute cholecystitis, emergency surgery is not indicated. If a stone is present in the cystic duct and there is increasing evidence of infection, surgical interference must be instituted. Uncomplicated cases may subside in a day or so on general supportive measures (absolute bed rest, intravenous fluids, and application of ice bag to gall-bladder area). If the signs of infection do not begin to subside within that time, surgery should be considered.

Chronic cholecystitis should be treated the same as cholelithiasis (see above).

Pancreas *

ACUTE PANCREATITIS

Acute pancreatitis is a sudden necrosis of the gland caused by liberation into it of digestive enzymes. In about half the cases it is brought about when impaction of a gallstone at the ampulla of Vater causes bile, usually infected, to back up into the pancreatic duct system, where it activates the pancreatic enzymes. In a few cases an accessory pancreatic duct allows regurgitation of intestinal contents; in others the mechanism is not apparent.

The onset of an attack is usually sudden, with violent abdominal pain, nausea, vomiting, prostration, and generally rapid and extremely profound shock. After a few hours, signs of peritoneal irritation appear. The usual course is rapidly downhill, and death occurs from shock or peritonitis. Recovery is rare.

Because of the lack of localizing indications, the diagnosis is seldom obvious. It must be considered in any case of violent illness with sudden, extreme shock, particularly in a patient known to have gallstones. Differential diagnosis includes perforated peptic ulcer (p. 128), acute appendicitis (p. 134), acute intestinal obstruction, and coronary occlusion (p. 67). A helpful point is determination of serum amylase, which is greatly elevated in acute pancreatitis (as high as 200 to 3,000 Somogyi units against a normal of 60 to 180).

---

*For disturbances of internal secretion of the pancreas, see Diabetes Mellitus (p. 173) and Hyperinsulinism (p. 177).

Treatment is directed first toward combating shock (p. 90). To protect the liver it is well to give intravenously 5 percent dextrose in Ringer's or lactate-Ringer's solution to a total of 2,000 cc. daily, mixing with it 20 to 30 units of Insulin. If the patient does not improve after relief of shock or if there is indication of spreading peritonitis, the abdomen should be opened surgically, with drainage of the infected fluid and, in the presence of jaundice, decompression of the bile ducts. Chemotherapy may be helpful if there is bacterial infection. Fluids, and particularly base, must be given freely to compensate for drainage.

CHRONIC PANCREATITIS

Chronic pancreatitis may result from repeated entries of mildly infected bile into the pancreatic duct, or it may be due to incomplete obstruction of the ducts from syphilis, endarteritis, or arteriosclerosis. It may accompany chronic alcoholism. In the more common interlobar form, there is deposition of fibrous tissue between the lobules, with compression of the parenchyma. In this form, diabetes mellitus is rare. In the less common interacinar type, atrophy of the parenchyma (including the islet tissue) is primary. Diabetes is the rule.

The symptoms are similar to those of the chronic biliary disease with which it may be associated: bloating and belching, epigastric tenderness and distress, constipation or diarrhea, and occasionally jaundice. There may be acute episodes of continuous pain of varying intensity referred to the left or right upper quadrant of the abdomen or to the region of the second lumbar vertebra in the back. The lack of functioning acinar tissue and the loss of pancreatic enzymes cause large, fatty, foul stools. Duodenal drainage reveals decreased or absent pancreatic enzymes. Involvement of the islets of Langerhans results in associated diabetes mellitus. Carcinoma of the pancreas or stomach, and chronic biliary disorders, must be considered in the differential diagnosis.

Treatment includes administration of pancreatic extracts as a substitute for the decreased enzyme secretion (2 to 8 Gm. of pancreatin with each meal), avoidance of excess fat and protein in the diet, and treatment of diabetes if it is present. Foci of infection, especially those of the biliary system, should be removed surgically. More radical surgery, such as cholecystogastrostomy, may be required, especially when the disease cannot be differentiated from carcinoma.

Peritoneum

ACUTE PERITONITIS

Acute peritonitis is usually a secondary condition and may result from a variety of causes. It may arise from infection of some abdominal organ, from a more remote source, or, rarely, from a hematogenous source (usually pneumococcal).

Acute perforations of abdominal organs usually give rise to acute peritonitis of some degree. It may develop quickly following strangulation, obstruction, infarction, intussusception, or volvulus of the intestinal tract. Occasionally, aseptic peritonitis may result from mechanical injury or from extravasation of urine, bile, pancreatic juice, blood, or the contents of cysts. The disease may appear postoperatively, particularly after operations which involve opening the gastro-intestinal tract.

Symptomatology varies with the origin, location, causative organism, and resistance of the patient. Localized peritonitis is usually secondary to an intra-abdominal condition; rigidity of the abdominal muscles over the affected area may be the only sign not attributable to the underlying condition. Localized peritonitis may become generalized without warning. When generalized peritonitis arises suddenly, there is usually severe abdominal pain, and the patient lies rigidly in bed with flexed thighs and shallow respiration. Pain may not be severe when the onset is gradual. Vomiting is characteristic, resembling regurgitation, and is usually frequent but not copious. The abdomen is generally distended. Fever, tachycardia, and polymorphonuclear leukocytosis are present. Hiccup may develop early. Shock and evidence of severe toxemia may appear.

Peritonitis must be distinguished from, or recognized as a complication of, biliary colic, pleurisy (with or without pneumonia), and renal colic, in addition to the conditions listed in the first paragraph above.

Treatment is twofold: that of the primary condition, and that of the peritonitis itself. Against susceptible organisms, sulfonamides or antibiotics have great value both therapeutically and prophylactically. In the presence of generalized peritonitis, nothing should be given by mouth until peristalsis returns. Abdominal distention should be relieved by the Wangensteen or Miller-Abbott tube technics. Other essential phases of treatment include control of shock (p. 90), control of pain, adequate replacement of fluids and electrolytes (p. 56), and general good nursing care. The use of morphine should be cautious because of its tonic action on the intestinal tract.

CHRONIC PERITONITIS

Chronic peritonitis is usually regional and follows recovery from some acute peritoneal infection. The most common forms are tuberculous peritonitis and, in women, chronic pelvic peritonitis. A serofibrinous form of peritonitis also occurs. More rarely, other forms are seen, such as actinomycosis and Pick's syndrome.

The symptoms of chronic peritonitis are indefinite and depend to a large degree on the amount of ascites and on the effect of the adhesions on the gastro-intestinal tract. Adhesions may cause symptoms of obstruction. A recurrent colicky type of pain, nausea and vomiting, a vague sense of ill-being, constipation, signs of obstruction, and slight fever may be present.

If the symptoms are due to adhesions that cause obstruction or interfere with function, the treatment is surgical. However, surgery should be attempted only when there is evidence that the cause of the symptoms can be corrected.

The occurrence of chronic peritonitis and adhesions following abdominal operations can often be avoided by careful handling of tissues, strict aseptic technic, and avoidance of spillage. Aside from surgery, control of low-grade infections, paracentesis for large accumulations of ascites, regulation of the diet and bowels, and general supportive measures are helpful.

NERVOUS SYSTEM

Symptomatic Disorders

HEADACHE

Headache is a symptom rather than an entity in itself. Perhaps the most common cause of headache is muscle tension associated with anxiety and emotional strain. Other causes are febrile and toxic states, disease of the nose and paranasal sinuses, diseases of the eye, cranial-nerve neuralgias, concussional trauma, and temporal arteritis. Pathological processes in the neck, such as arthritis of the cervical spine, scalenus anterior syndrome, and cervical ribs, are less common causes of headache. Intracranial disease processes such as aneurysm, brain tumor, brain abscess, encephalitis, and meningitis may also cause headache.

In contrast to the conditions just mentioned, headache is an essential part of migraine (p. 161) and of histaminic cephalalgia.

Histaminic Cephalalgia presents a characteristic picture. Only adults are subject to it. The headache is hemicranial, following the distribution of the external carotid artery and its branches and involving the eye, temple, neck, and face. It usually starts at night, waking the patient after one or two hours' sleep. Although lasting less than an hour, the pain is excruciating and becomes intolerable if the patient lies down. It is of a constant, boring nature. There is profuse watering of the eye, and the eye and nose are congested. There is swelling of the temporal vessels and increase in skin temperature. Pressure on the temporal and carotid arteries gives temporary relief. In susceptible individuals, the pain is reproduced by subcutaneous or intravenous injection of 0.1 to 0.2 mg. of histamine. The mechanism of the syndrome appears to be vasodilation which is presumed to be due to sensitivity to histamine.

Treatment of symptomatic, or secondary, headache should be aimed primarily at the underlying cause. In the simpler headaches, analgesics (p. 405) may provide temporary relief.

In histaminic cephalalgia, hyposensitization may be carried out as follows, using histamine acid phosphate (p. 366) (note that 0.1 mg. histamine is contained in 0.275 mg. histamine acid phosphate): Histamine, 0.05 mg., is given subcutaneously twice each day for two consecutive days. The dose is increased on the third day to 0.066 mg. twice a day, and by the fifth day 0.1 mg. twice a day should be well tolerated by the patient. This amount (0.1 mg. twice a day) is continued for two to three weeks. If severe headaches follow, the dosage should be reduced and the treatment prolonged. To prevent future attacks, some patients require a proper maintenance dosage, which will consist of approximately 0.1 mg. histamine (0.275 mg. histamine acid phosphate) one to three times weekly. A few patients do not require a maintenance dosage.

Antihistaminics (p. 509) have been reported to give relief in histamine headaches.

INSOMNIA

Inability to sleep, or abnormal wakefulness, has been classified according to time of occurrence as (1) initial insomnia, or delayed onset of sleep; (2) intermittent insomnia, or restless sleep; and

(3) terminal insomnia, or early morning wakening. Initial insomnia, the commonest variety, results most frequently from anxiety and worry. Chronic insomnia of this type may become a major medical problem, for sleeplessness accentuates the nervous state of the patient and a cycle of sleeplessness, fear of sleeplessness, and increasing insomnia becomes established. Intermittent insomnia, or broken sleep, also occurs in connection with mental fatigue and worry and often is associated with dreams. Restlessness of this type may result from indiscretions in eating and drinking in the evening hours. Terminal insomnia is often the complaint of elderly people, who normally require less and less sleep with advancing age and who frequently may take naps during the day. Early morning wakening is a common complaint also in patients with hypertension, arteriosclerosis, and certain mental disorders. Insomnia of any or all types may occur in association with a variety of diseases, especially conditions in which pain and discomfort are prominent.

Treatment of insomnia should be individualized, with the major effort being directed toward correction of the underlying cause rather than toward symptomatic therapy with hypnotic drugs. Sources of worry, anxiety, and fear may be revealed in a thoughtfully elicited history (see p. 148), and careful physical examination may uncover previously unsuspected disorders such as heart disease, hyperthyroidism, or arteriosclerosis. Correction of habits regarding food and stimulants, or such simple measures as excluding noise and light from the bedroom, may offer a solution. Maximum bedtime comfort is desirable, with attention being paid to mattress and bedding. Use of a hot-water bottle or heating pad to avoid chilling may be helpful. A hot bath and back rub at bedtime often are relaxing, and a glass of hot milk may be soporific. Relief of insomnia associated with tension states has been reported to follow use of a low-sodium diet (p. 585). The limitation required by different patients varied from 2 to 0.5 Gm. daily.

When all known psychogenic and physical factors have had attention and insomnia continues to be intractable, use of a hypnotic may be considered. However, such drugs must be used only as a temporary measure because of possible growing dependence upon the drug, the necessity for increased dosage if tolerance grows, and ultimate "habituation" to hypnotic medication. Preferably, such preparations should be used intermittently, and the prescription should provide only enough to carry the patient until the next visit to the physician.

Because of several advantages, the barbiturates (p. 390) have become the most widely accepted hypnotic and sedative drugs. Usually barbiturate medication is well tolerated, and through proper selection of drug and dosage almost any degree of sedation or hypnosis may be obtained.

For initial insomnia, 'Seconal Sodium,' 3/4 grain or 1 1/2 grains (0.05 or 0.1 Gm.), provides a rapid onset of effect which results in prompt sleep. Usually, if the patient is undisturbed, normal sleep will continue past the time when the effect of this short-acting drug is dissipated.

For those patients who sleep well during the first part of the night but who are victims of insomnia during the early morning hours, 'Enseals' 'Seconal Sodium' may be prescribed. Because of their coating, these tablets release the barbiturate in the intestine after a period of four to six hours, so that a dose taken at bedtime becomes effective several hours later.

When prompt but more prolonged hypnotic effect is required, Tuinal may be prescribed. This combination of equal parts of 'Seconal Sodium' and 'Amytal Sodium' may be given in 1 1/2-grain doses.

The type of insomnia encountered or the physical disorder which may be associated with it may make necessary administration of a longer-acting barbiturate. In the order of increasing duration of action, 'Seconal Sodium' is followed by pentobarbital sodium, 'Amytal Sodium,' 'Amytal,' and phenobarbital. The longer-acting drugs act less rapidly and may be expected to leave some effects the next day. Particularly is this true of phenobarbital.

Of the other hypnotic drugs, the bromides, chloral hydrate, and paraldehyde should be mentioned. Bromides are not suitable as single-dose hypnotics, for continuous medication is necessary to attain sedative action. Chloral hydrate is an effective hypnotic, the usual adult dose being 0.5 to 1 Gm. It should not be given to patients with hepatic, renal, or cardiac disease and may be irritating to the stomach. An elixir containing potassium bromide, chloral hydrate, and hyoscyamus is a widely used combination.

Paraldehyde may be given orally in doses of 3 to 8 cc., but it has an objectionable taste and, because of excretion by the lungs, imparts a strong odor to the breath.

CONVULSIONS IN CHILDHOOD

Often the physician is called to see a child in whom the principal immediate manifestation of disease has been an unexpected generalized convulsion.

TABLE 14 — *Causes of Convulsions in Children of Different Ages**

	Percent Incidence in Entire Group	Percent Incidence in Different Age Groups				
		Birth to 1 mo.	1 mo. to 6 mos.	6 mos. to 3 yrs.	3 yrs. to 10 yrs.	10 yrs. to 16 yrs.
Percentage of Total Cases in Each Age Group	100	7.0	12.9	47.0	27.3	5.8
DISEASE						
Acute infection with fever	33.4	10.0	31.6	47.0	23.1	1.4
Idiopathic epilepsy	26.3	3.4	4.6	16.7	48.5	73.3
Cerebral birth injury or residue	14.2	69.3	18.3	10.4	7.0	2.7
Infantile tetany	7.4	2.8	18.9	10.2	——	——
Miscellaneous causes	13.1	7.4	13.3	10.9	17.5	21.2
Cause not established	5.6	6.8	13.3	4.8	3.9	1.4

*From data of Peterman covering 2,500 cases.

Table 14, which lists the causes of such convulsions, may be of some assistance in differential diagnosis.

It will be noted that in the series as a whole, about one-third of the convulsions were associated with fever due to acute infection. The maximum incidence of this association—in the age group of six months to three years—was almost 50 percent. It is Peterman's opinion that infections or fevers precipitate convulsions only in those children who have low convulsive thresholds.

Idiopathic epilepsy is the next most common cause of convulsions in childhood. Its relative frequency increases from about 3 percent in babies under one month of age to almost 75 percent in the ages of ten to sixteen years. In skilled hands, the electroencephalograph is the most useful means for the diagnosis of active or latent epilepsy (p. 170).

Birth injury or its residue was the next most frequent cause of convulsions among children. The only other cause which occurred sufficiently often to be singled out for the table was infantile tetany (p. 496), which was not observed beyond the age of three years. In the 2,500 cases, no instance was observed of convulsions due to hypoglycemia.

Treatment—Most convulsive seizures will have terminated before the physician arrives. In such instances the principal need is for diagnosis. For controlling convulsive seizures in the absence of anoxia, phenobarbital sodium is recommended. It is given intramuscularly or (cautiously!) intravenously according to the following dosage schedule:

Infants	15 to 30 mg.
Young children	30 to 60 mg.
Older children	60 to 100 mg.

If the convulsions have subsided, it is still in order to administer a barbiturate—under these circumstances either by mouth or in a capsule perforated at both ends by a pin and inserted into the rectum.

If the barbiturate is ineffective, tribromoethanol (Avertin), $CBr_3 \cdot CH_2OH$, may be given by rectum in a dose of 60 to 80 mg. per Kg. of body weight as a 2.5 percent solution in water. If convulsions still continue, chloroform or vinyl ether may be administered by inhalation as a final resort. If there is evidence of anoxia, inhalation anesthesia and oxygen should be given at once.

When fever is present, it should be reduced. Antipyretic drugs (p. 405) are given; and during the interval before they act, hydrotherapy is administered in the form of cool sponges, ice packs or ice bags, and cool enemas.

The treatment of the disease causing the convulsions will be found under the heading of the specific disease (see Index).

The Personality and Its Disturbances

The personality is, in a sense, the sum total of an individual's experience in life together with all of his inheritance. It is important to the physician for several reasons: (1) It is a determining factor in the patient's reaction to any situation in his life, including illness, and therefore has an important bearing on diagnosis, prognosis, and treatment; (2) disturbances of personality appear to be essential factors in the pathogenesis of a number of diseases the manifestations of which are primarily organic; and (3) disturbances of the personality may interfere with the patient's life and therefore require direct treatment.

Like his visible parts, the personality of an individual has structure ("anatomy") and function ("physiology"). However, the intangibility of the personality has made it difficult to study and comprehend. Viewed from one aspect, the personality is found to be divided into two parts: the subconscious (unconscious) and the conscious. The primary driving forces, the sources of an individual's life energy and instincts, reside in the subconscious.

Viewed from another aspect, the personality appears to be made up of three general areas. The first is inherited and comprises that part of the subconscious which is concerned with the primitive needs and impulses: security, hunger, sex, and raw aggression. This area has been termed the "id" (a use of the word totally unrelated to skin reactions [p. 268]).

During the first years of life, the conscious aspect of the personality begins to develop as the result of contact with the environment. The very young child fails to distinguish clearly between the environment (reality, fact) and his own desires and primitive drives (fantasy). He expects the environment to conform to his wants. When it fails to do so, he rejects the reality. As he gets older, he learns to accept reality and to distinguish fact from fantasy. In this way, there begins the development of the second area of the personality, the "ego." The ego is that part of the personality which (1) tests and accepts reality and (2) adjusts the primitive drives to the demands of reality (the environment). As the ego develops, it becomes able to work out compromises whereby the primitive drives are channeled into less directly gratifying activity which still satisfies them yet meets the demands of the environment. At this point there begins to develop the third area of the personality, the "superego," which sets standards for the ego and acts generally as a sense of ethics and moral standards (a conscience).

The type of compromise outlined above is the essence of adult behavior; the ability to make it is called "emotional maturity," and the individual is said to be "well integrated." The minimum qualities now considered essential to emotional maturity include *all* of the following:

1. Independence.
2. Ability to give love and be interested in others.
3. Absence of egocentrically competitive drive.
4. Possession of a social conscience.
5. Ability to channelize sexual desires into mating and the binding together of a family.
6. A realistic attitude toward life rendered possible by the ability to be independent of one's feelings.
7. Adaptability (absence of fixation of attitudes and reactions in childish patterns).
8. Freedom from hate and hostility, although able to be aggressive in defense and for constructive purposes.

The development of the personality is fraught with hazards. A pattern is undoubtedly inherited, but there is uncertainty as to the extent to which any inherited predisposition governs the details of personality development. The importance of environment is clear. The growth of a mature personality is favored by a childhood environment of affection and understanding, physical security, the presence of social unity in the family (giving the child a feeling of "belonging"), and absence of rigid attitudes and standards on the part of the parents. Development of the personality may be inadequate or distorted in the absence of affection and physical and psychological security, or if rigid and arbitrary standards (which he cannot understand) are imposed on the child. Under the term "arbitrary standards" must be included demands on the child for a more advanced type of behavior or a higher standard of performance than that of which he is capable. An example is premature and overinsistent attempts at toilet training.

The most important period for personality development is from birth through the first five or six years, and the earlier part of this period is probably more consequential than the later part. It is at this early age that there develop the more important of the scars and inadequacies that predispose to regression under stress in later years. It is possible to damage the personality in older children, but it is not so easy.

Conflict between different parts of the personality is always manifested by anxiety (see p. 149). When the conflict is resolved (by mature adjustment, neurotic conversion, or psychotic denial), the anxiety diminishes or disappears in proportion to the extent to which the adjustment is satisfactory to the personality. Anxiety is, therefore, a symptom of underlying, unresolved conflict.

Most of the presently recognized disturbances of the personality appear to be due largely to faulty development of the ego. When the ego cannot find a satisfactory compromise between the primitive drives and the environment, one of two solutions is adopted: (1) The primitive drive is suppressed and relegated to the subconscious, thereby laying the groundwork for a neurosis (p. 150); or (2) the reality of the environment is rejected, thus providing the basis for a psychosis (p. 152).

Evidence is accumulating to the effect that certain diseases of obscure origin and organic manifestations are found consistently in individuals with definite types of psychological maladjustments, and there is a growing opinion that the psychological tension is an important contributing if not primary factor in pathogenesis. Such diseases include hypertension, peptic ulcer, hyperthyroidism, certain types of asthma, certain dermatoses, migraine, and many cases of dysmenorrhea, backache, constipation, chronic diarrhea, mucous colitis, impotence, frigidity, chronic indigestion, effort syndrome, cardiac irregularities, anorexia nervosa, eyestrain, and other conditions. Regardless of the objective somatic development of these diseases, it would appear that, like the neuroses and functional psychoses, they may have their ultimate etiology in disturbances of the personality.

EVALUATING THE PERSONALITY

Since the personality plays such an important part in an individual's reaction to any situation, the physician will find it well worth while to evaluate the personality of any patient who consults him for more than a trivial difficulty. He should be particularly concerned with (1) the presence and extent of anxiety, (2) the discovery of childhood events and situations of an emotionally traumatic nature which might have left residual scars and points of weakness, and (3) an assessment of the degree of emotional maturity.

There is no simple formula for evaluation of the personality. The physician must realize that any person will show anxiety and neurotic symptoms if placed under sufficient pressure. On the other hand, many persons maintain a continuously neurotic adjustment (often accompanied by anxiety) under which they manage to get along and lead productive lives unless subjected to too much external pressure.

Two concomitant lines of investigation should be followed: The physician should make his own observations, and he should survey the patient's personal relationship to those about him. First, the physician must be relaxed, unhurried, and sympathetic in his own relationship to the patient if he is to gain significant information. Second, the physician must be all-observing and ready to interpret not only what the patient says but what he does not say, his behavior, mannerisms, and facial expressions. Third, the patient must be given a chance to tell his story without hurry, pressure, or prejudgment on the part of the physician. Since many points which are important to the physician will not be told by the patient spontaneously, the patient's story must be supplemented by answers to the physician's questions, which will include the patient's environment and the potential stress which it entails—the patient's tempo of life, pressures at

work and at home, economic problems, and his "gripes" of any nature.

A survey of personal relationships should include (1) his parents, and particularly his childhood relationship to them, which has such an important bearing on the development of his personality; (2) his husband or wife; (3) his children; and (4) his employer and other business associates. The physician should attempt to discover specific attachments or hostilities, resentments, and possible dependencies. The occupational record should be investigated from the point of view of the number of jobs and the patient's reaction to them. Frequent change of jobs suggests unsatisfactory personal relationships. The social interests and contacts can be investigated from the same point of view. The patient's health record may be revealing. An individual who has gone from one doctor to another has an excess of anxiety, and the history may suggest the time and circumstances of its onset.

In eliciting information, especially about relationships, the indirect approach is usually more revealing. Questions such as "Are you worried about anything?" and "Is your home life happy?" are likely to bring conventional answers. This is not because the patient is trying to withhold something but because long ago the major problems were submerged in the unconscious and the patient is no longer aware of the cause or nature of his conflicts. The physician therefore must seek for *evidence* of worry or an unhappy home life.

ANXIETY

Anxiety (tension, emotional tension, emotional stress) is an emotional state rather than a disease. However, it is sufficiently common and has enough significance to warrant a separate discussion.

One form of anxiety is related to events or objects in the immediate environment which evoke powerful emotional responses. Typical is the tension which precedes a threatening or challenging situation, such as a school examination, an athletic contest, or the entrance of soldiers into combat. The college student may suffer from anorexia, urinary frequency, or diarrhea as a manifestation of such tension. The soldier may have palpitation, pilomotor activity (goose flesh), vomiting, and incontinence of urine and feces. These tensions may be discharged by action against the environment, either (1) against the threatening condition itself or (2) in some nonspecific way, such as taking a walk, playing a game, or attacking someone or something physically or verbally. This kind of tension is generally recognized as normal, and the physician is seldom consulted about it.

The other form of anxiety is not related to external threats or challenges or to any actual danger of which the patient is aware. It is extremely important, however, because (1) it may be disabling of itself, and (2) it is a symptom of conflict in the personality and is therefore a manifestation of threatened or actual neurosis. It is expressed by restlessness, apprehensiveness, fearfulness, chronic fatigue, or a combination of these. In children, anxiety may be expressed by nail biting or, at an earlier age, by thumb-sucking (however, there are additional causes for thumb-sucking). The physician should always be alert to detect the presence of this type of anxiety and estimate its extent.

Because anxiety is a secondary manifestation, treatment can seldom be appropriately directed toward its control in a primary way. The attack is more properly made on the underlying emotional conflict.

THE NEUROSES

When the reality-testing function of the ego is well developed but the ego's skill in adjusting primitive drives to reality is inadequate, the personality is said to be "immature." Failure of adjustment leaves the subconscious primitive drives clamoring for satisfaction. The individual is in a quandary. On the one hand, he does not know how to handle the drive; and, in addition, either he is afraid of the drive or the superego disapproves of it in its unmodified form. On the other hand, the ego is too well developed to deny the existence of either the reality or the drive. Its solution is to repress the drive—a process of burial in the subconscious which is distinct from denial. However, repression is not an adequate solution, for the drive continues to demand expression. If the demand is so strong that control by the conscious personality is threatened, the conflict is manifested by anxiety.

If the conflict is not resolved, the personality may resort to some type of automatic defense (see Figure 2, p. 153). A frequent defense is to channel the drive into expression as a disturbance of cardiovascular or gastro-intestinal function, headache and other affections of sensory or motor or visceral function, unreasonable fears, or bizarre compulsive behavior. Such a form of release is known as "conversion" or "somatization," and the symptoms are said to be "neurotic." These neurotic symptoms represent a socially approved form of escape for the disapproved drive. They serve to drain the tension and to satisfy the drive in an acceptable way, and in so doing they diminish or entirely relieve the anxiety and provide a distorted form of gratification. At the same time, however, they are painful or uncomfortable and serve as a punishment inflicted on one part of the personality (the ego) by another (the superego) for permitting the escape of a forbidden impulse.

Such neurotic symptoms (defenses against repressed impulses) are manifested at times by everyone. In some individuals they may be present continuously without creating definite ill health; often they are conspicuous as eccentricities, strange mannerisms, unusual personal habits, or other odd forms of behavior. In the struggle between one part of such an individual and another part or between the individual and his environment, he may receive unseen support from some strange philosophy or a long-suffering husband, wife, son, or daughter. When the routine of such people is not seriously disturbed, they are not incapacitated.

When neurotic symptoms cause incapacity, a "neurotic reaction" is said to be present. The defenses may break down acutely under great emotional stress, even in previously well-integrated individuals. Very often, however, the decompensation is slow and cumulative, as seen in the chronic neurotic invalid.

In those individuals who progress to neurotic reaction, with incapacity, it will generally be found that there has been some disturbance of development of the personality in childhood. All adults carry in their personalities the scars of emotional injuries in childhood. Scars of particularly injurious events may be vulnerable to similar traumatic experiences in adult life. As is the case in all biological reactions, there are wide variations in the type and degree of response of different individuals to analogous situations; therefore, it should not be surprising that, under apparently similar circumstances, one person may have a neurotic reaction and another may not.

The essence of a neurosis is that the drives whose frustration forms its basis are wholly subconscious and therefore not subject to the patient's awareness. Although functional, the symptoms are real and are neither imaginary nor consciously motivated. A neurotic reaction is not in any way akin to malingering.

The diagnosis of neurosis has both negative and positive aspects. As in any case, the diagnosis must account for the signs and symptoms. Since most neurotic symptoms are nonspecific (that is, they may occur in several different disease conditions), it is necessary to consider all possible causes before coming to a final conclusion. On the negative side, the physician must rule out likely organic bases for the symptoms. A careful dietary history is particularly important because of the frequent similarity between symptoms due to neurosis or anxiety and those of subclinical vitamin deficiency (see p. 483). However, a purely negative approach may lead to serious errors. If the diagnosis of neurosis were made solely on the basis of lack of evidence of organic disease, many cases of cancer and brain tumor (to mention only two diseases) would be tragically misdiagnosed in their early stages.

For a proper diagnosis of neurosis, the physician should have evidence of anxiety or conflict within the personality or both. An immature personality, which forms the background of neurosis, is characterized (and may be recognized) by the following attributes: rigid attitudes, with a tendency to base attitudes and behavior on fixed rules or external authority of some kind (such as a parent, a parental symbol, or even an authoritarian government); excessive stubbornness, willfulness, and inability to compromise; egocentric competitive behavior; childish or adolescent attitudes, language, or behavior; impulsive behavior; and irrational anxieties and obsessions.

Treatment—Before the patient can be satisfactorily treated, the physician must have made up his own mind (after adequate study) as to the presence of mismanaged emotions and their relation to the patient's complaints. Often, or perhaps usually, the question is not whether the problem is *either* functional *or* organic, but rather *how much* of the problem is functional and how much organic. Sometimes a period of observation is necessary to collect the evidence in the form of the patient's reactions to different situations. Once sufficient evidence is at hand, the physician must have the courage to make up his mind and to act on his convictions. This courage and conviction on the part of the physician are essential to successful management of the patient.

Actually, the basic question in treatment is how to enable the patient to grasp and understand his real problem. If his maladjustment is not too deep and if he is truly eager to get well, the technics available to the general practitioner may suffice. If the difficulty is serious and deep-rooted, the specialized technics of the psychiatrist will be necessary. Regardless of his decision as to the necessity of specialized technics, the physician cannot escape responsibility for acquainting the patient with the nature of his illness, if only as a preliminary to referring him for specialized help. Unfortunately, medical training in the past has generally provided insufficient information in the field of functional disease, and the physician must usually supplement this by his own reading, postgraduate study, and evaluated experience.

The physician will be much more successful in explaining the situation if he has previously established good rapport by the exercise of patience, sympathy, and understanding in hearing the patient's story. If he has been impatient or unsympathetic, he is likely to meet antagonism and possibly rebellion. He must come to know the patient *as a human being* and must make the patient feel his impartial friendship. In no instance must he allow his personal feelings and prejudices to enter into his judgment of the patient and his problems.

The explanation should be in terms the patient can understand. When possible, the physician should use familiar illustrations of the effect of emotions on body function (e.g., blushing, sweating, increased heart rate, or nausea). He can then explain how a major part of the personality is likewise beyond conscious control and how it is possible unconsciously to channel unacceptable impulses to various organs. If the patient has organic disease with neurotic overtones, the physician should explain that the disability is out of proportion to the disease and that the unacceptable impulses are being channeled to the diseased organ. The patient should be made to understand that there is nothing reprehensible about illness of emotional origin and that, just as in organic disease, there are definite measures available for recovery, provided the patient is willing to apply them.

Sometimes it is better not to attempt explanation but to reassure and encourage, at the same time giving specific directions. Of course, the physician must be careful not to minimize the illness or to imply that because no physical basis was discovered there is "nothing wrong" with the patient. On the other hand, he must not undertake such further investigation or administer such treatment as may suggest to the patient that the organic component of his difficulty is greater than the physician has stated.

In some instances, the physician will be able to discover the nature of the patient's emotional conflict. In others, it will remain obscure. Nevertheless, if he is alert, he will in any case see factors in the environment or the patient's reaction to them that are aggravating the emotional disturbance, and he can make suggestions and help the patient map out a way of living which will be palliative if not curative. When the offending material is deeply submerged, it is necessary to resort to psychoanalysis to bring it out. The basic aim of psychoanalysis is the same as that of the treatment which the physician carries out in his office, namely, to bring up into consciousness the underlying repressed drives, thus making them susceptible of direction by the conscious part of the personality. Whether the physician can succeed by himself or must seek the help of the trained specialist depends partly on the physician's interest in, aptitude for, and knowledge of the field and partly on the extent of the patient's illness.

A most important part of the problem is prevention. The psychological environment, or emotional climate, of patients and physicians alike is as important for health as is the water supply and everyday sanitation. At present the world is full of the stresses of personal competition, prejudice, suspicion, and strife. These are added to the problems of personal or family insecurity of social, financial, intellectual, or emotional origin. Because of his situation as family counselor and his position in the community, the general practitioner is in a peculiarly strategic position to be a powerful influence for the local dissemination of good mental hygiene. The crucial years, psychiatrically speaking, are from birth through adolescence. If parents can be persuaded to give their children real affection and security, to allow them to develop gradually without forcing, and to help them learn to handle their impulses consciously and without undue rigid pressure from above, a healthier generation of adults will ensue and there will be less demand for authoritarian forms of government and social control.

THE PSYCHOSES

The psychoses are diseases of the mind which separate the individual from the real world around him. The cause of the mental illness may be (1) primary dysfunction of the mind itself, in which case the psychosis is termed "functional"; (2) organic pathological processes arising within the brain (either from local disease or secondary to primary disease elsewhere); the resulting psychosis is termed "organic"; or (3) secondary toxic effects upon the brain, the result of external toxic agents or of toxic products elaborated through metabolic defects; such conditions are termed "toxic psychoses." The most common causes of these three types of psychoses are outlined in Table 15.

TABLE 15 — *Classification of the Psychoses*

I. Functional
  A. Obsessive state } sometimes called
  B. Compulsive state } "psychoneuroses"
  C. Paranoid psychosis
  D. Manic-depressive psychosis
  E. Involutional melancholia
  F. Postpartum psychosis
  G. Schizophrenia (dementia praecox)
  H. Psychopathic personality
  I. Perversions

II. Organic
  A. Vascular disease
    1. Senile dementia
    2. Arteriosclerotic and hypertensive psychoses
    3. Huntington's chorea
  B. Syphilis
    1. Paresis (general paralysis of the insane)
  C. Epilepsy
  D. Brain tumor
  E. Traumatic brain lesions
    1. Mechanical
    2. Inflammatory
      a. Encephalitis
  F. Mental changes secondary to any organic central-nervous-system disease

III. Toxic
  A. Exogenous
    1. Alcoholism
    2. Drug intoxication
      a. Bromide
      b. Opium, morphine, cocaine
      c. Marijuana
      d. Lead
      e. Other drugs
    3. Infectious delirium
  B. Endogenous
    1. Hyperthyroidism
    2. Pellagra
    3. Cardiac decompensation
    4. Any disease interfering with metabolic support of the brain

The responsibility of the general practitioner in relation to the psychoses is essentially threefold:

1. He must be able to make at least a general diagnosis and to guide the patient to the proper type of psychiatric help. To do this, he must be sufficiently familiar with the different types of psychoses and the mechanisms of their production to recognize them and to understand the general nature of the problems which the patient faces.

2. He must be able to assist the family to an understanding of their problem in relation to the patient. This requires a general understanding not only of the nature of the disease afflicting the patient and the elements which contributed to its development but also of the prognosis and the rationale of therapy.

3. He must be able to give suitable preliminary or emergency therapy until more settled arrangements can be made. His ability to do this depends in large measure upon his understanding of the nature of the patient's illness.

Functional Psychoses—In the discussion of the neuroses (p. 150), it was brought out that in them the basic difficulty lies in faulty development of the ego (that part of the personality charged with correlating the primitive impulses with the civilizing demands of the environment). In the functional psychoses, the basic difficulty is in the same area of the personality. There is, in fact, a parallel development up to a point (see Figure 2). In both, the patient early recognizes (although he may not admit, even to himself) his inability to meet life realistically, and this causes him anxiety. The anxiety soon spreads beyond the particular problems he is endeavoring to meet, and there results the typical "anxiety neurosis." His anxiety is now precipitated by many factors apparently unrelated to the problems he is trying to solve so that he becomes subjected to so-called "free-floating anxiety," and many of the fears of early childhood dominate his life in the form of irrational phobias. At this point he is a candidate for the development of either typical neurotic manifestations or the beginnings of psychotic phenomena. The determining factor now resides in the quality of his ego. If his ego is strong but unadaptable, he keeps hold of the fact of reality and endeavors to deal with it by repressing the qualities within himself which he cannot adapt to the demands of reality. If, on the other hand, his ego is weak and he can neither repress his primitive drives nor adapt them to reality, he attempts a solution of his dilemma by a flight from reality; psychotic phenomena are the result. The psychotic, in other words, has no respect for reality, and he prefers to compromise with it or to dispense with it entirely rather than attempt to bring his own impulses into harmony with it. From the way the patient handles his impulses in relation to reality spring the different categories into which functional psychoses are divided. These will be summarized briefly below.

Obsessive State—In this condition, the patient has given up his effort to control his primitive im-

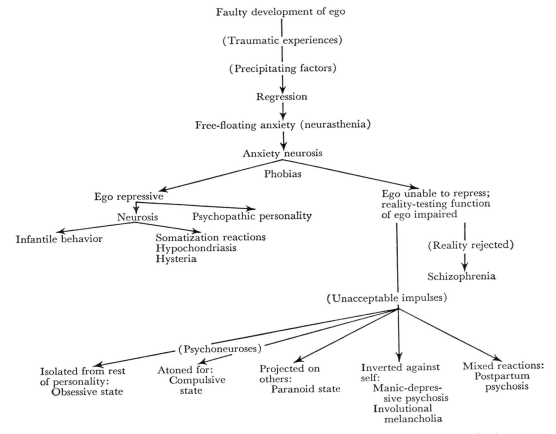

Figure 2—*Schematic Representation of the Development of the Neuroses and the Functional Psychoses*

pulses; he cannot, however, acknowledge their existence. His solution is to isolate them from the rest of his personality and thus deny all responsibility for them because they are, in his mind, no longer his. The obsessive state therefore manifests itself as sudden, primitive, asocial *ideas* such as assaults, murder, or incestuous ideas which appear to have no relation to the individual, who in his daily life is quiet, unemotional, usually intellectual, and often engaged in occupations involving abstract thinking. Rarely are the obsessive ideas translated into action.

COMPULSIVE STATE—This condition is closely allied to the above and often is an outgrowth of it. Here, the patient atones for his primitive ideas and impulses by elaborate ritualistic actions. These are frequently exaggerations of social behavior such as repeated hand washings, prolonged ceremonial baths, or exaggerated meticulousness in which shoes must be placed in exact symmetry with some part of the room; things must be touched or mentioned only in a certain order, and so on. Such a person is overcome by paralyzing doubt. He looks at things from all sides and finally cannot decide to do anything. Although he affects independence, he is very dependent on persons close to him: his parents, his wife, his professional superiors, or particular friends. The compulsive patient is hypermoralistic, punctilious, meticulous, truthful, conventional. He overdoes all this and can therefore allow himself to indulge in some prohibited fantasies. Thus the "good" and "bad" sides of his personality are in constant struggle, and his energies are so absorbed in preserving their equilibrium that no strength is left for constructive activity. Severe obsessive-compulsive psychoneuroses are among the most trying and difficult problems of psychiatry. The original trauma, which usually occurred in childhood, has become encrusted with so many layers of life experience that it is extremely difficult to uncover it.

PARANOID STATE—The paranoid patient denies the existence within himself of hostile impulses and projects them upon others. He is therefore the victim of delusions of various types. Such a person perceives accurately the existence of hostile or unacceptable impulses but locates them erroneously. In general, when the ego's reality-testing function is impaired, impulses of this kind are projected on others. The patient is unable to repress his impulses, and he cannot isolate them or atone for them as in obsessive-compulsive behavior; therefore he rids himself of them by attributing them to others. Paranoid tendencies occur as part of many psychotic states and share the prognosis of the basic difficulty. True "paranoia" is very rare, and the prognosis is nil.

MANIC-DEPRESSIVE PSYCHOSIS—The manic-depressive patient is aware of his own hostile impulses, and he is overwhelmed by a sense of guilt. Apparently the methods of handling the guilt as employed by the obsessive-compulsive and paranoid patients are, for some reason, not open to him. His solution is to invert his guilt—to turn it upon himself. This constitutes the beginning of the depressive phase, and the patient sinks into a deep depression. The psychological processes are retarded, interest in the environment is reduced, and there are profound tendencies toward self-criticism, self-depreciation, and self-destructiveness. Thus, the guilty conscience has imposed punishment, and the punishment is made an orgy of self-abasement. In so doing, the patient not only satisfies his conscience but goes further, feeling that he has overpaid for his sins and is now justified in defying the harsh and hated conscience. Now, therefore, there suddenly begins the manic rebellion, in which he gives license to all the base and primitive impulses which have been seeking expression. Consequently, the patient, who may be *normally* a warmhearted, convivial, friendly, and practical person, but who yesterday was lost in a deep, immobilizing, introverted gloom, is today suddenly a loud, licentious extrovert whose mental processes are so accelerated that there is often a "flight of ideas." The patient is now in an orgy of self-indulgence. His excess in this direction is ultimately checked by the returning sense of guilt, and the pendulum swings back to begin the cycle all over again.

INVOLUTIONAL MELANCHOLIA is a psychosis of many different manifestations which occurs in women three times as often as in men. The onset in women is most commonly in the age group of forty to fifty-five years; in men it usually begins about ten years later.

The most frequent manifestation of involutional melancholia is depression. In the depressed state the patient shows as much self-criticism, self-depreciation, and self-destructiveness as in manic-depressive psychosis. The motor retardation of the manic-depressive is, however, replaced in this affliction by motor overactivity ranging from restlessness to frenzied agitation. There are, in addition, many other types of manifestations, including paranoid trends, sadistic attitudes, and catatonic phenomena. It would appear, therefore, (1) that this disease represents a departure from reality induced by the stresses and strains of the climacteric or of middle age or both upon a vulnerable personality, and

(2) that the exact form the psychosis takes will be determined by the quality of the personality involved and the nature of the preceding experiences. The recovery rate is 23 to 40 percent.

POSTPARTUM PSYCHOSIS is a term applied to psychosis which is precipitated by childbirth. The condition is not a true entity any more than is involutional melancholia. Childbirth, like the menopause, is a period of great strain for the female personality. In the presence of a defect in the personality (usually having its origin during childhood), the problems associated with these two periods of life may prove greater than the personality can handle, even though all the previous vicissitudes of existence have been met satisfactorily. So-called "postpartum psychosis" may take any one of a number of different forms but is most frequently of the manic-depressive type. The prognosis is determined by the quality of the psychosis which supervenes.

SCHIZOPHRENIA (dementia praecox, split personality) is the most important of the psychoses because it is far more prevalent than any other single type. Furthermore, many early cases escape detection and pass through doctors' offices mistakenly diagnosed as cardiac disease, appendicitis, malingering, and, especially, neurosis. The earliest manifestations are usually evident in childhood; they go unrecognized because (1) in the majority of instances, the disease is of slow and insidious onset, and (2) only when it is well established are the manifestations sufficiently overt to be widely recognized. Sudden, acute onset occurs in only about 20 percent of cases.

The basic defect in schizophrenia is a severe impairment of the ego's reality-testing function (its ability to distinguish fact from fantasy). This function normally develops very early, and it forms the basis of the individual's acceptance of the external world. It is therefore assumed that the initial injury or defect in schizophrenia occurs or develops extremely early in life. Some investigators have held that, for the defect to appear so early, the individual must have been born with it. Others believe that significant environmental trauma can occur at a very early age. There is also disagreement over the possible presence of organic changes either in the brain or in the general metabolism which might be responsible for the mental changes. The majority of evidence, however, suggests that schizophrenia is a noninherited functional derangement of the personality.

All grades of severity of the disease are encountered. Thus, the affliction ranges all the way from those cases that never emerge from the incipient stage, through those who suffer serious illness but may recover, to the grossly deteriorated who appear to have lost all vestiges of adult behavior. Many close students of the disease hold that the prognosis is not as pessimistic as is generally believed and that the poor results reported have simply reflected the pessimistic attitude of the medical profession toward it. The important thing, according to the most modern point of view, is for the patient to gain or regain his belief in the desirability of reality. To do this, the environment must be made as congenial as possible and the persons who people it as understandable and convincing to the patient as possible. In the last analysis, the patient's re-acceptance of reality depends in large measure on what reality has to offer him in the way of security and opportunity.

The above remarks on the handling of schizophrenia are applicable only to early cases and imply a large measure of psychotherapy. This requires great patience, time, and expense but has been demonstrated to be effective in suitable cases. Insulin shock offers something in certain more advanced cases; electric shock is probably not a treatment of choice.

The chain of events in schizophrenia is briefly and schematically summarized in Figure 3 (p. 156). When the schizophrenic pattern is fully established, the patients show the following general types of symptoms:

Ideas of reference. Schizophrenic patients feel themselves to be the center of attention. They imagine that the words and actions of those around them are directed entirely toward *them*, usually with some insulting or persecutory connotation.

Ideas of influence. The uncomplimentary or ominous intentions of others are usually implemented in the mind of the schizophrenic by elaborate, highly technical, and often ingeniously conceived equipment such as "N" rays, radar, telepathy, and machinery of all kinds. Very often, bizarre notions exist concerning the functioning of his own body, such as "no stomach left" or "throat sealed off," and the sexual apparatus is often the imagined target of misuse by others.

Hallucinations. These are frequent, involving any one of the special senses, but particularly hearing.

Catatonia. This is a late manifestation in which the patient is mute, does not respond to pinpricks, maintains his limbs "moldable," and speaks a gibberish termed "dissociation of thought."

Deterioration of the emotions—a characteristic feature. At the same time that the patient manifests

Heredity (?)   Early trauma (?)

Initial defect (ego undeveloped; reality-testing function impaired)

Especially sensitive child (who says, in effect: "I do not like the world as I find it. I will substitute my own dream world.")

Early vague withdrawal (shyness; vague resistance to contacts with others)

> At this point, outcome might conceivably be averted by proper preventive therapy:
>   Keep child in contact with reality.
>   Make reality attractive.

Repeated ineffectual efforts to overcome obstacles

Repeated substitution of fantasy for success (earliest symptom is often a turning to pathological excuses for failure)

> Once more, outcome might be averted by proper preventive therapy:
>   Assist child to successful accomplishment so that he *experiences* success. Given strength from a sense of accomplishment, he may be able ultimately to acquire success by his own efforts.

Begins to live more within self (becomes more egocentric as he makes repeated unsatisfactory efforts to correlate wishes with reality)

Eventually abandons effort to correlate with reality (substitutes hallucinations of his own choosing for satisfactions of real life)

FIGURE 3 — *The Chain of Events in Schizophrenia*

any or all of the previously listed symptoms, he may be perfectly oriented with regard to events and surroundings. He seems, however, indifferent to all reality. Furthermore, his behavior is out of keeping with the emotions which he expresses. Thus, he may describe great injustices inflicted upon him; but as he does so, he shows no resentment. On the other hand, he may laugh inordinately over something about which he has expressed no amusement.

PSYCHOPATHIC PERSONALITY—The disturbance here termed "psychopathic personality" has been given many other names; among them are constitutional psychopathic inferiority, moral insanity,

neurotic character, and impulse-ridden personality. It is actually a form of neurosis rather than of psychosis (see Figure 2, p. 153). The basic defect is in the ego, which is unduly repressive, relegating to the subconscious a profound sense of guilt. The psychopathic personality is, however, essentially extroverted, and, instead of struggling to solve his problems alone in his own bedroom out of the sight of others as in the obsessive or compulsive state, he violently acts out his own agony, dragging with him many innocent people. For this reason, the psychopathic personality is one who typically performs acts involving risk to himself, thus satisfying his sense of guilt by the misfortune which usually befalls him. The psychopathic criminal is almost always apprehended because of the deliberate mistakes which he unconsciously makes. Punishment is essential for the expiation of his guilt. In this way he pays, with a comparatively minor offense, for the much greater guilt which he harbors within himself.

Psychopathic personalities tend to seek for themselves occupations involving risk and violent action. They are, therefore, found most frequently among gamblers, speculators, confidence men, sportsmen, and mountain climbers. Social position is an important factor in determining the form in which the neurosis may be expressed. Thus, a well-to-do person is more likely to express his difficulty in eccentricity, and the less privileged in delinquency. There are, therefore, many different types of personalities represented in this general group. All, however, have the following characteristics in common:

1. Irrationality.
2. Stereotyped repetition of behavior patterns, the recurring necessity of satisfying the hidden sense of guilt being the motivating force.
3. Self-destructiveness.

PERVERSIONS are pathological sexual behavior patterns resulting from the blocking of normal sexual development in childhood by insoluble emotional conflicts engendered through faulty family situations. Two types of perversions of the sexual instinct are recognizable: (1) perversions of the quality of sexual feeling (sadism, masochism, exhibitionism, voyeurism, transvestitism) and (2) perversions in the object of the sexual feeling (homosexuality, pedophilia, zoophilism).

In general, perversions represent fixations in early, immature forms of sexuality, the person involved never having reached mature sexual status in the emotional sense. Very occasionally, maturity has been reached but, because of scars sustained in early childhood, regression takes place, with loss of the mature reaction. In the normal person, the sexual impulse represents excess energy no longer needed in the process of growth and development. In perversion, much energy normally utilized in other ways is translated into sexual striving. Thus, in the masochist, punishment and suffering become a form of sexual gratification; and in the sadist, inflicting pain on others gives the same type of pleasure.

In childhood, excess energies which, because of the dependent position in society, are not needed for survival are frequently employed in an erotic manner. In perversions, these early erotic satisfactions continue to appeal because normal and mature sexual release is blocked. The causes for the block in normal sexual development vary in detail but are probably most frequently found in some variation of the Oedipus complex (a desire, fundamentally sexual, for the parent of opposite sex, with hostility toward the parent of the same sex and a desire to take his or her place). All human beings pass through this phase, but the majority leave it successfully behind. An example of how the distorted family relationship during this period, if exaggerated or arrested, may form the seed for later sexual perversions is as follows: A boy, in acting unconsciously under the temporary drive of the Oedipus complex, seeks his father's attention in an effort to divert him from the mother. If healthy possibilities for companionship between father and son are not available, the child may unconsciously try to attract the father by imitating what he senses as attractive to him in the mother. Feminine attitudes and behavior may thus become part of his personality and sow the seed for later homosexuality, particularly if they appear to meet with success at the early period.

Organic Psychoses—The organic psychoses are diseases in which the mental function is altered because of structural changes in the brain. The more common causes of organic psychoses are shown in Table 15 (p. 152). Regardless of cause, the changes in mental function and the consequent alteration in behavior fall into four general categories which are indicated in Table 16.

VASCULAR DISEASE—*Senile dementia* is the most prevalent organic psychosis. It is due to scattered areas of anoxic destruction of brain tissue secondary to deterioration of cerebral arteries and arterioles. The more common manifestations include loss of memory for recent events (with retention for remote happenings), insomnia with restlessness and

TABLE 16 — *Alterations in Mental Function and Behavior in Organic Psychoses*

I. Changes in mental capacity, as shown by
 A. Impairment of memory
 B. Defects in retention of facts
 C. Inadequacy of information
 D. Loss of orientation
 E. Impaired judgment

II. Loss of emotional stability, characterized by rapid and exaggerated shifts in mood

III. Changes in behavior, which most often include deterioration of personal habits, decline in ethical standards, and the commission of moral offenses

IV. Decreased tolerance to toxic agents, so that, for example, small amounts of alcohol or of drugs previously tolerated now produce confusion or delirium

increased motor activity, and deterioration of the emotions. Patients suffering from senile dementia become egocentric, with contraction of interests. They are often exceedingly stubborn and are the subjects of violent temper outbursts. Moral laxities are not uncommon, and indecent exposure, sexual assault on children, and the like are problems to be dealt with. Ethical veneer wears thin, and these unfortunate people are an easy target for "gold diggers," swindlers, and confidence men. In general, the symptomatology is determined by the previous personality, the symptoms representing an accentuation of previous personality traits.

The handling of patients suffering from senile dementia is first of all precautionary. The progress of the disease cannot be arrested, but the patient should be put into the best possible physical shape. This will permit better handling of the physical and emotional blows which are inevitable. Physical injuries occur frequently because of the patient's forgetfulness as well as his compulsion to wander about at night when failing eyesight and co-ordination are hazards. The family can do much in anticipating the patient's needs in the form of adequate food, proper clothing, personal cleanliness, fresh air, and sunshine. The physician may be called upon for a multiplicity of small services, such as treatment of skin ailments, hemorrhoids, bladder irritations, toothache, and so on. These should be supplied with great patience and consideration. On the sociological scale, the patient suffering from senile dementia is entitled to protection of his finances and his reputation.

Arteriosclerotic and hypertensive psychoses result in mental derangements essentially similar to those in senile dementia. The chief differentiating factor is the age of the patient at the onset of symptoms.

Huntington's chorea is a progressive degenerative disease of middle life entailing severe dementia. It is an inherited condition which is transmitted according to Mendelian pattern. The pathological process is one of degenerative destruction of scattered areas of the cortex. The early clinical signs are twitching and choreiform movements, followed years later by personality changes which are characterized by irritability and temper tantrums. The speech becomes slow and indistinct. There is extension of choreiform movements, with grimacing of the face. Ultimately, depression becomes profound, paranoid trends develop, and complete confusion and disorientation ensue. The prognosis is unfavorable.

SYPHILIS—*Paresis* (general paralysis of the insane) is a term given to the mental manifestations of late syphilis. The pathology is that of the syphilitic process involving the brain. It is typical and specific; for details, the reader is referred to textbooks dealing with syphilis. The diagnosis is made on the basis of the specific findings in blood and spinal fluid, the Wassermann being 4+ in both media, and the colloidal gold curve of the spinal fluid showing the specific steppage pattern. The incidence of paretic mental symptoms is approximately 10 percent among persons with untreated or inadequately treated syphilis. The most probable time for their development is ten or more years after the initial infection, and they are thus seen most often in the fourth and fifth decades. Men develop paresis more frequently than do women.

The earliest symptoms are memory lapse, defects of judgment, emotional lability, and character changes. These are associated with fatigability, either insomnia or somnolence, and weight loss. The patient at this stage is most often mistakenly diagnosed as a neurasthenic or hypochondriac. As time passes, the mental aberrations become more pronounced. In the late stages of the disease, the patients fall into the following general groups: dementing (40 percent), in which there is progressive organic dementia; depressed (25 percent); expansive (10 to 25 percent), with grandiose delusions, euphoria progressing to irritability, and great motor activity and aggressiveness; and agitated (10 to 15 percent), with excessive psychomotor activity and clouded consciousness. The last group may progress rapidly to exhaustion and death.

The treatment is that of the underlying infection (see p. 10), with additional measures as required by the patient's behavior. Institutional treatment is a necessity. Penicillin and, more recently, aureomycin appear to offer some hope of arresting the syphilitic process, but irreversible changes in the brain preclude any extensive rehabilitation.

EPILEPSY—The personality changes in epilepsy (for general discussion, see p. 170) are in part a reaction to the social ostracism imposed on victims of the disease; the form which they assume is determined, as in all psychoses, by the basic personality. The most common personality defects seen early in association with epilepsy are egotism, emotional instability, impulsive behavior, and sometimes pugnacious, cruel, irascible, or sadistic behavior. In advanced or severe epileptics, so-called epileptic equivalents begin to appear, and they may take the form of any one of the functional psychoses. Thus, all of the following have been observed: delirious confusion, hallucination, paranoid states, depression, or excitement. "Furor epilepticus" represents a manic phase in which the patient becomes maniacal, destructive, and sometimes horribly homicidal. Epileptic dementia may be profound, divesting the patient of almost every faculty that distinguishes him from the animal. The diagnosis is the diagnosis of epilepsy and is made on the basis of electroencephalographic changes.

The treatment is, as in all of the organic psychoses, primarily the treatment of the underlying disease (p. 171). If the epilepsy can be adequately controlled at its onset or soon thereafter, the chance that any of the epileptic equivalents will develop later is remote. Once these have supervened, however, it is better for the protection of the patient and the community that he be treated in an epileptic hospital.

BRAIN TUMOR is essentially a neurological problem rather than a psychiatric one. The diagnosis is made on the basis of the neurological signs, and where possible, the treatment is surgical. Secondary behavior and mental disorders may, of course, be profound and constitute a major problem in the handling of the patient, in which case he is best treated in a mental hospital. The nature of the behavior changes is determined by the location of the tumor.

TRAUMATIC BRAIN LESIONS—Injury to the brain may result from mechanical causes or from inflammation. Both may produce destruction of brain tissue and lead to changes in personality or behavior. Epidemic encephalitis (p. 164) is the most important cause of inflammatory brain injury. Any type of trauma to the brain is most disastrous in children, where distortions of brain pathways will lead to serious behavior difficulties. These follow a general pattern and account for a considerable proportion of delinquencies. The characteristic behavior problems are disobedience, lying, stealing, cruelty, sexual delinquencies, and criminality. The intellect is usually intact, but attention is limited and extreme restlessness is observed. In treatment, the physician must prepare a program of re-education early in convalescence from injury or illness. Such a program requires the intelligent co-operation of the parents, since it must be carried out patiently over a prolonged period. Punishment, which only makes things worse, must be circumvented by careful planning of the child's time so that it is constantly filled with interesting activities. Plenty of rest and nutritious food are essential.

Toxic Psychoses—Disturbance of mental processes or injury to the brain may result from ingested toxins, from toxic by-products of disease processes outside the brain, or from deficiencies or metabolic aberrations in other parts of the body.

ALCOHOLISM—Alcohol is the most frequently consumed of the exogenous substances toxic to the brain. The alcohol itself, however, is only incidental in the psychiatric problem of the alcoholic. The basic difficulty is a functional psychoneurosis arising from emotional immaturity. The trouble, as in all functional psychoses, began in childhood; the most frequent single factor in the early history of alcoholics is the presence of parental loving-dominance which unconsciously thwarted or blocked the attainment of emotional maturity. When the patient reached the age when society demanded maturity, he was unable to meet the demand. Failure induced a feeling of inferiority and an unconscious desire for regression to the childhood period of lessened responsibility, immaturity, and fantasy. A vulnerable individual of this type, as we have already seen, might have taken any one of a number of ways to effect regression. Alcohol, however, provides one of the easiest and quickest. It is readily available, and society at first applies little censure to its use. The emotionally immature patient is thus singularly susceptible to alcoholism. Under the effects of alcohol, he may, by the physiological fact of lowered inhibition secondary to its use, relieve his inferiority feelings through aggressive and licentious behavior not open to him normally. Unfortunately, however, indulgence of this type soon operates to initiate a guilt feeling which he is equally unprepared to handle. Once again he avoids reality by employing alcohol to relieve him of the new guilt emotion, and he is further submerged in his own difficulty.

Treatment, as it has been carried out in the past, has often served only to deepen the basic problem.

The measures of persuasion and threat, reward and punishment, as so frequently carried out by the family and physician, are geared to the patient's own immature level. Only if he can in some measure conquer his own immaturity will recovery be attained. Treatment should, therefore, be undertaken entirely outside the family, preferably by a psychiatrist, and it should deal only with the mature segment of the patient's personality in the hope of building it up. The patient must be required to make his own decisions, with no restrictions forced upon him. The psychological support of an organization like Alcoholics Anonymous is in many cases extremely helpful, even though it cannot offer the fundamental approach of the psychiatrist.

Certain late manifestations of alcoholism appear to be due largely to vitamin deficiency secondary to the substitution of alcohol for food: *delirium tremens*, in which the patient suffers from illusions and hallucinations, chiefly visual; *acute hallucinosis*, in which the hallucinations are primarily auditory; *Korsakoff's psychosis*, which is not solely alcoholic in origin but may occur in senile and other dementias, and in which the patient suffers memory loss, falsification of memory, and confabulation at the same time that he retains good appreciation of immediate impressions; and finally *chronic alcoholic hallucinosis*, in which the hallucinations are mostly sexual and a considerable latent homosexuality exists.

DRUG INTOXICATION—The mental symptoms in drug intoxications are the direct effect of the drug upon brain function, colored by the patient's personality. The drugs most frequently causing this complication include bromides, opium and its derivatives, cocaine, marijuana, and lead. Drug addiction is a different type of difficulty.

INFECTIOUS DELIRIUM—Any somatic illness may upset the mental stability; most frequently, however, the cause is a combination of fever plus infection. The symptoms are not specific to the particular infection but include the following: confusion, disorientation, illusions, and hallucinations, most frequently of a terrifying nature. The most constant mood displayed is fear, but this may shift into abject terror, anger, defiance, or rage. There is usually restlessness which may mount to frenzied agitation.

The general practitioner is more frequently called upon to treat this mental difficulty than perhaps any other. For discussion, see below.

ENDOGENOUS—Any process which significantly alters the metabolism of brain tissue will lead to concomitant changes in function. Thus, the mental agitation and occasional flight of ideas accompanying hyperthyroidism are familiar to all. The dementia of pellagra is an outstanding feature of the disease and is undoubtedly a direct result of the disturbance of cerebral metabolism induced by a deficiency of the B vitamins. Some of the confabulation of Korsakoff's psychosis may be on the same basis. The mental symptoms displayed by patients suffering persistent cardiac decompensation are probably due to altered cerebral metabolism secondary to inadequate blood supply. It is obvious that treatment in each instance is that of the underlying disease.

Treatment—Conventional medical practice is based on the assumption that the patient has a certain degree of contact with and respect for reality. The management of psychotic patients must obviously proceed from a different point of view. Effective active treatment of the functional psychoses is a highly specialized field, and all such cases (particularly schizophrenia) should be under the care of a psychiatrist and preferably in an institution. Likewise, the organic psychoses had best receive specialized and, if possible, institutional care. Nevertheless, the general practitioner will be required to manage acutely psychotic patients until psychiatric help can be secured; he will frequently have to handle toxic psychoses; and he must give at least temporary care to mental aberrations in the course of such diseases as syphilis and epilepsy.

EMERGENCY TREATMENT of psychotic patients may well embody the following suggestions:

Diagnose while allaying fear. The first problem which confronts the physician as he enters the patient's room is to ascertain what is wrong with the patient. This may be very difficult because the patient may be acutely disturbed (and consequently hard to approach), or he may be abnormally quiet, in which case he will communicate nothing. In either case, the physician's attitude is extremely important. Anxiety and fear attend the beginning of any psychosis, and they help to perpetuate it and determine its manifestations. A calm, reassuring attitude on the physician's part will help greatly. With an impersonal yet friendly approach and a little patience, actual force is seldom necessary.

In addition, it is often possible to obtain all the information necessary for a rough diagnosis without touching the patient. By *watching*, the physician can see whether he is paralyzed, is weak in any extremity, has suffered injury, and so on. By *listening*, one can detect aphasia, slurred speech, disorientation, confabulation, hallucinations, and the like. Allowing the patient to talk freely in a calm and friendly atmosphere may do much to allay his

fear, at least temporarily, and it will aid the physician in understanding him. One should not, however, appear to agree with false beliefs in order to humor the patient. The physician should be straightforward, accepting the patient as a sick person and explaining this fact kindly to him. Often the patient will be relieved to hear that his condition can be considered an illness.

Watch out for suicidal trends. Suicide is always a possibility in any psychiatric patient, and the physician must always proceed as though the attempt would be made. The patient must be *constantly attended for the full twenty-four-hour period.* All sharp instruments must be removed, even to such unlikely objects as the bottoms of tooth paste tubes and decks of cards. The most frequent times for suicide are the early morning, twilight, and shortly after midnight. It is important, therefore, that truly adequate sleep be secured to cover whatever wakeful period the patient characteristically has. This requires careful selection of the hypnotic drug and adequate doses.

Protect from fear. Fear is the major emotion to be combated in any psychosis, and it is especially prominent in the toxic deliriums (see p. 159). Certain simple measures will contribute greatly to the patient's feeling of security:

Have a member of the family near at hand (but select him or her carefully; family antagonisms will aggravate fear or excitement).
Keep the patient in familiar surroundings if possible.
Keep lights on in such a way that there are no shadows to frighten.
Watch out for flapping window shades or other unusual noises.
Keep the patient on the first floor if possible.

Provide rest. Battling the terrors of an acute psychosis is exhausting. It is essential to provide adequate rest, but it is important also not to contribute to the patient's confusion by injudicious or excessive use of sedatives. The tolerance for sedatives is high in the functional psychoses, but in others (notably senile dementia) it is very low. Paraldehyde (p. 398) is extremely useful in the psychoses, as are the barbiturates (p. 390). Supplementary measures such as warm tub baths may be helpful.

Provide nourishment. If the physician has established contact with the patient, he will probably succeed in coaxing him to eat and drink unless the patient has delusions about food. Otherwise, it is necessary to feed by stomach tube or vein. The physician must use his judgment as to whether the need for food and fluid outweighs the distress of the procedures to the patient.

SPECIALIZED CARE—If the above measures have been tried and the patient is still unmanageable, no psychiatrist is available, and a private psychiatric hospital is not a possibility, the patient should be transferred to a state hospital by one of the following steps:

1. In some states, the county health officer is empowered to issue a ten-day health office certificate which is not a commitment but which enables the superintendent of the state hospital to observe the patient for the stated period and arrive at his own decision.

2. In some states, it is possible for two qualified physicians to examine the patient and certify to the county judge that the patient should be sent to the state hospital for a period not to exceed thirty-five days. Within thirty days the superintendent and staff must report to the judge as to whether the patient should be discharged or retained further.

3. Finally, a lunacy or insanity warrant may be filed against the patient. The county judge then appoints two physicians to examine him and report, after which the judge may at his discretion commit the patient for an indefinite period.

The following technics may be useful when employed by trained and experienced personnel:

I. Radical technics.
  A. Shock therapies.
    1. Electroconvulsive therapy. This is helpful in acute functional psychoses except schizophrenia. The mortality approximates that from general anesthesia. Curare lessens attendant injuries but increases hazards slightly. It is a hospital procedure but may be employed on an outpatient basis with proper safeguards.
    2. Insulin shock therapy. This is employed almost exclusively in schizophrenia. It requires special handling and involves greater discomfort to the patient and more hazard than does electroconvulsive therapy.
  B. Continuous-sleep therapy. The treatment is hazardous and difficult and gives no better results than shock therapy.
  C. Frontal-lobe neurosurgery (leukotomy, lobotomy, topectomy). This treatment is employed for conversion of intractably agitated patients into placid individuals. It does not effect a return to normal and is reserved for near-hopeless cases.
  D. Intensive personality analysis (psychoanalysis and Myerian "distributive" analysis). These technics and their application in psychotic patients are still in process of evolution. The most important present factor is selection of an analyst congenial to the patient.
  E. Hypnosis. The aim of hypnosis is to circumvent conscious or preconscious resistance to psychotherapy. It is dangerous in the hands of those not psychiatrically trained; for if not properly handled, it may produce psychotic panic or involve the physician in the patient's delusional pattern. It is less effective than narcosis interviews.

II. Conservative analytic technics.
  A. "Nondirective" interviews. In these, the patient discovers his own trouble with direction from the analyst. The treatment is required for deep conflicts in which the patient must acquire his own insight.
  B. Narcosis interviews (narcodiagnosis, narcoanalysis, narcosynthesis). The aim of this technic is to by-pass conscious or near-conscious resistance and permit release of thoughts and feelings hitherto repressed. It is safer than hypnosis and is useful in discovering the underlying cause of a psychosis. It is strictly a hospital procedure; stimulants and assistance should be readily available when it is carried out.

Other Functional Disorders

MIGRAINE

Migraine is a syndrome of unknown etiology characterized by periodic attacks of unilateral headache of varying severity and duration which usually are accompanied by ocular and abdominal complaints. It occurs in intelligent, tense, nervous individuals with strong hereditary predisposition. They typically are rapid workers of the perfectionist type, have scintillating personalities, are hypersensitive to emotional strain, and are subject to episodes of undue mental and physical exhaustion.

Migraine is most common in women between the ages of twenty and thirty years. The first attack may occur with the onset of menstruation. It usually is absent during pregnancy and ceases after the menopause. In men, attacks are rare after the fifth or sixth decade. The estimated number of cases in the United States is two to eight million.

The disease has been related to a number of causes, such as allergy, endocrine dysfunction, hypertension, liver and gall-bladder disorders, and pelvic disease, but it is doubtful whether these are important etiological factors. Abnormal electroencephalograms occur in a significant percentage of victims and their relatives. Although there is disagreement about the basic pathological processes, it is generally accepted that the immediate mechanism involves vasoconstriction of the branches of the internal carotid artery. The resulting anoxemia causes the preheadache aura. This is followed by dilation of the intracranial branches of the external carotid artery, which gives rise to the throbbing headache. The third phase of severe, steady, more generalized pain is due to edema of the vessel walls and scalp. The pain is transmitted by the fifth, ninth, and tenth cranial and the first three cervical nerves.

The patient may be warned of an impending attack by malaise and minor gastro-intestinal symptoms for a day or two, or possibly by an unusually sound and restful sleep. In nearly every case, aurae immediately precede the acute attack by a few minutes. These arise mostly from disturbances of the special senses, are painless, and may include any of the following: bright scotomata, blurred vision, photophobia, hemianopsia, and diplopia; tinnitus, deafness, and vertigo; speech disorders; abnormal taste and smell; paroxysmal tachycardia; numbness or itching of the skin of the extremities; peripheral vasomotor instability; and mental confusion. Each patient has his own type of aura.

The second stage, or classical migraine, begins as an intense, throbbing, unilateral, localized headache lasting a few minutes or a few hours. It is commonly located in the right temple but, in contrast to most headaches of organic lesions, will appear on the left side at some time. The patient is prostrated and either irritable or depressed. Nausea, vomiting, retching, polyuria, pallor, and sweating occur. The pain is generally limited to the head but includes the face and neck. Photophobia and severe pain on moving the eyes are usually present. Hyperesthesia, especially of the scalp, may be present. The headache is intensified by lying down or shaking the head and, in some instances, is relieved by assuming the erect position. Pressure on the temporal, frontal, supraorbital, postauricular, occipital, and common carotid arteries may reduce the intensity. Migraine hardly ever disrupts sleep except for short periods. Slight elevation of temperature is common. Fever as high as $40\,^{\circ}$C. ($104\,^{\circ}$F.) may occur rarely as a substitute for an attack. Dilation of the retinal arteries and veins has been reported, but eye-ground examination usually is nonrevealing.

A third stage of steady, grinding pain, usually bilateral, is recognized. This results from edema of the artery walls, scalp, and underlying tissues which causes pressure on pain-carrying areas. Once it is established, vasoconstrictor drugs have no effect, and the pain may last for hours or days.

Attacks commonly terminate during sleep, and on waking the patient feels refreshed with a sense of buoyancy and well-being. There is complete freedom from headache between attacks.

Other conditions which may simulate migraine are brain tumor, cerebral aneurysm, cerebral thrombosis (p. 169), paranasal sinusitis (p. 111), histaminic cephalalgia (p. 145), and syphilis (p. 10).

Treatment—Identification and discussion of the factors which build up mental tension and bring on the psychic states conducive to attacks may help the patient to understand his own individual problem. Readjustment of the daily work to a slower tempo that is compatible with his fluctuating energy levels and mental processes should be attempted. Guidance in obtaining adequate rest and relaxation is an integral part of management. Hobbies, particularly those involving physical exercise not exceeding the point of moderate fatigue, are to be encouraged. Mild sedatives may be of some help during the early phase of readjustment but should not be used for extended periods or to compensate for lack of co-operation by the patient.

Attacks may be aborted occasionally with salicylates (p. 405). There is some evidence that nicotinic acid, amyl nitrite, acetylcholine, and other vasodilators (p. 362) may prevent migraine if given in therapeutic doses before the second stage begins, but these are not recommended for routine use. Ascorbic acid, 100 mg. three times daily, is said to prevent attacks in some patients.

Treatment of the acute attack with vasoconstrictor drugs should be instituted in the first or second stage. A high percentage of cases may be relieved with dihydroergotamine, ergotamine tartrate, or ergonovine maleate (p. 478).

Dihydroergotamine (DHE-45) is given intramuscularly, subcutaneously, or intravenously in single doses of 1 to 2 mg. If necessary, this may be repeated every half hour up to a total of 8 mg. Ergotamine tartrate, 0.25 mg. intravenously and 0.25 mg. intramuscularly or subcutaneously, is also effective but tends to produce nausea, vomiting, cramps in the extremities, paresthesias, and at times substernal oppression. DHE-45 is said to cause fewer untoward side-effects. Ergotamine tartrate may be given orally, but results are less satisfactory and doses of 5 mg. are required. A somewhat more rapid effect is obtained by crushing the tablets and allowing them to dissolve under the tongue, but often the taste is objectionable. Oral administration of larger amounts is sometimes possible by following the first dose of 5 mg. with 1 or 2 mg. every hour until a total of 9 to 11 mg. has been taken. With either preparation, simultaneous administration of caffeine citrate, 100 mg., is said to improve results. The drugs should not be employed on more than two days in any one week or six days per month. They should be withheld in the presence of obliterative vascular disease or septic states with intravascular foci.

Ergonovine provides relief in a smaller percentage of cases, but patients for whom it is effective usually prefer it because it is active when taken by mouth and produces few side-effects. Doses are the same as for ergotamine. Because of their oxytocic properties, ergonovine and ergotamine are contraindicated during pregnancy.

Atropine sulfate, 0.5 to 0.6 mg. (1/120 to 1/100 grain) orally or subcutaneously, may control the gastric components occurring during an attack or from administration of ergot compounds.

A number of other measures for management of the acute attack have been reported. Inhalation of pure oxygen, seven liters per minute for one-half to two hours, is said to give some degree of relief in 90 percent and complete relief in 40 percent of cases. Each of the following has been given intravenously with more or less success:

    25 to 50 cc. of 25 to 50 percent dextrose solution
    20 cc. of 10 percent sodium chloride solution
     1 Gm. of sodium thiosulfate
    10 cc. of 10 percent calcium gluconate
     2 to 5 cc. of 50 percent magnesium sulfate

Symptomatic therapy includes rest in a darkened room, cold compresses to the head, and administration of analgesics alone or combined with caffeine (p. 405). Codeine (p. 403) may be used with relative safety, but morphine or similar compounds may cause addiction and should not be given except in emergencies.

Prevention of attacks has been accomplished by intravenous administration of histamine (p. 366) or nicotinic acid (p. 366). Ascorbic acid, 500 to 1,000 mg., when added to the histamine solution, reduces the severity of flushing. Should excessive vasodilation occur, more ascorbic acid is added, the rate of administration is slowed, and ergotamine tartrate is administered. Estrogens, orally or intramuscularly (p. 463), may be tried in the occasional case in which there is a definite relationship between migraine attacks and menstruation. Migraine per se is not considered to be an indication for inducing menopause.

Thiamin chloride has been used prophylactically. Severe cases are given 100 mg. daily by intramuscular injection in conjunction with 50 mg. of nicotinic acid orally three times daily after meals. In addition, pyridoxine hydrochloride (15 mg. once daily) and a moderate therapeutic dose of vitamin B complex (two or three times daily by mouth) are employed. Doses are reduced proportionately for milder cases. For example, in a moderately severe case averaging one or two attacks a month with a total of three or four days of headache, the treatment consists in 100 mg. of thiamin chloride by intramuscular injection three times weekly, 25 mg. of nicotinic acid by mouth after each meal, and moderate doses of vitamin B complex. In some cases the pyridoxine is omitted. The treatment is continued for a minimum of four months; then, if results justify a reduction in dosage, the size and frequency of the doses are decreased gradually. If during this therapy the patient experiences a threat of impending migraine, he is given 100 mg. of thiamin chloride intramuscularly in addition to the regular dose and is instructed to increase the amount of nicotinic acid to 100 mg. after each meal on that day. If the symptoms persist for a second or third day, the extra doses are continued until the threatened attack has been averted.

TRIGEMINAL NEURALGIA

Trigeminal neuralgia (tic douloureux) is an affection of one or more of the three divisions of the trigeminal nerve and is characterized by spasmodic stabbing pain over the area supplied by the involved nerve. The cause of trigeminal neuralgia is unknown. It is a disorder of older age, and the vascular changes seen at this time of life have been regarded as a possible pathological basis. Aberrant blood vessels or tumors of the cerebellopontine angle which exert pressure on the nerve also have been mentioned as pathogenic factors.

The diagnosis usually is not difficult in a well-established case because of the typical paroxysmal pain which, without warning, strikes the temple, face, jaw, or teeth. The duration of pain is rarely more than a few seconds, and between attacks symptoms usually are completely lacking except for tenderness of the involved area. The frequency of attacks gradually increases, although there may be prolonged periods of complete freedom. Rarely is there bilateral involvement. The differential diagnosis should exclude intracranial lesions and such disorders as multiple sclerosis and tabes dorsalis, which sometimes may be responsible for facial pain.

Treatment—Medical management may be attempted but without optimism. As in neuritis, thiamin chloride (p. 483) has been used with some success in daily doses of 10 to 100 mg. intravenously. In conjunction with thiamin, concentrated liver extract (p. 369) containing 15 U.S.P. antipernicious-anemia units per cc. has been given intramuscularly in 1/2-cc. doses three times weekly along with a high-vitamin diet. Fever therapy with typhoid vaccine (p. 336) may help some patients.

Analgesics (p. 405) may aid in controlling pain, but opiates should be avoided because of the progressive nature of the ailment and the need for frequent medication. Trichloroethylene may be of value in controlling pain. Twenty drops are placed on gauze, and, while in a reclining position, the patient inhales the vapor until the odor has disappeared. This is repeated no more frequently than four times daily, and use of the drug should not be continued indefinitely.

Interruption of the branch or division of the trigeminal or of the entire nerve often is the only means of abolishing pain. This may be accomplished, usually only temporarily, by injection of alcohol into the nerve or, more permanently, by surgical resection of the involved nerve. Either procedure should be attempted only by the expert.

Attacks of pain which strike the teeth or sinus areas may result in unwarranted dental extractions or operations for sinus disease. These procedures are indicated only when there is demonstrable apical infection or sinus involvement, and they serve only to eradicate foci of infection.

Organic Diseases

THE ENCEPHALITIDES

"Encephalitis" means inflammation of the brain. The spinal cord also is usually involved either primarily or secondarily, and the word "encephalomyelitis" is often used instead of encephalitis. Encephalitis may be caused by physical means, chemicals, or infective agents or their toxins. The infective agents may be protozoa, fungi, bacteria, spirochetes, rickettsiae, or viruses. A virus causing encephalitis is referred to as being "neurotropic."

Virus Encephalitis—The encephalitides due to viruses may be divided into those that are epidemic and those that are nonepidemic. The more common epidemic encephalitides are poliomyelitis, encephalitis lethargica, Western and Eastern equine encephalitis, and Japanese B encephalitis. Encephalitides of the nonepidemic type include, among others, lymphocytic choriomeningitis, pseudolymphocytic choriomeningitis, and rabies (see p. 30). In addition, a number of rare types of encephalitis due to viruses, both of the epidemic and nonepidemic varieties, have been described and are not included in this discussion. Certain viruses have been isolated from mosquitoes which have not yet been isolated from the blood of man; it is considered possible that these viruses may eventually be shown to produce human encephalitis.

Although there is some variation in different kinds of encephalitis of virus etiology, the essential pathological process is an acute nonsuppurative inflammation of the central nervous system characterized by severe vascular congestion with occasional petechiae, cellular infiltration of the meninges with lymphocytes and monocytes, and degenerative changes and necrosis in the ganglion cells. In severe cases, cellular infiltration extends into the cerebral substance, with occasional small foci of necrosis.

The onset of virus encephalitis may be sudden, with fever, delirium, headache, or convulsions; involvement of the nervous system is manifested in such signs and symptoms as headache, drowsiness, ocular paralyses, excitement, stiff neck, mental

confusion, tremors, and choreiform or myoclonic movements. Any type of neurological syndrome can be simulated. Symptoms of brain-stem involvement, such as diplopia, facial weakness, or deafness, are common. In some instances the onset is slow, with mental deterioration or signs suggesting brain tumor. During epidemics, some patients may sustain infection without clinical manifestations, and the disease is not suspected until paralysis agitans appears.

In the acute stage the symptoms are extremely variable, the most common being paralysis of extraocular muscles and disturbances of the normal sleep rhythm. There may in addition be fever, headache and vague pains in other regions, delirium, pupillary disturbances, various cranial-nerve and upper-motor-neuron paralyses, and tremors and other motor disturbances.

The duration of active encephalitis varies from a few hours in severe cases to as long as two years. In the prolonged cases, sequelae usually appear before activity subsides. Encephalitis lethargica and St. Louis encephalitis generally have longer duration than other types, although, as in most types of encephalitis, those patients that recover usually do so in ten days to six weeks.

After recovery from the acute stage, there may be an intermediate phase characterized by fatigability, loss of memory, loss of ambition, and other apparently psychoneurotic manifestations. Many such patients are misdiagnosed as psychoneurotics because the acute phase may have been extremely mild or even absent. The chronic stage may be characterized by paralysis agitans (p. 172), behavioral changes, psychoses, and a variety of other organic nervous disturbances.

Encephalitis lethargica may have neurological and psychotic sequelae (including paralysis agitans) in 20 percent of cases.

In St. Louis encephalitis, 10 to 40 percent of children under six months show permanent damage to the central nervous system, such as mental retardation, hydrocephalus, and epilepsy; in adults, less than 5 percent have sequelae. Paralysis agitans is rare.

In Eastern equine encephalitis, it has been reported that as many as 60 percent of patients exhibit such sequelae as emotional instability, mental deterioration, and various types of paralysis.

Postinfectious Encephalitis (also called "demyelinating encephalitis") occurs not infrequently after virus infections, such as measles, influenza, mumps, varicella, variola, infectious hepatitis, dengue, and yellow fever. A virus etiology has not been established, and the cause of the encephalitis remains obscure. Clinically, postinfectious encephalitis is not unlike virus encephalitis. However, the course is usually rapid; in one or two weeks the patient either dies or recovers. The mortality rate is 30 to 50 percent. Recovery is usually complete. In a few instances permanent spastic paralysis, coarse tremors, mental deterioration, or transverse myelitis may result.

Diagnosis—Epidemiological considerations are of the utmost value in diagnosis. Encephalitis lethargica has a definite seasonal incidence and appears chiefly in the winter and early spring months. Its method of spread is not known but is probably not dependent on insects. Insect-borne encephalitis occurs during the summer months. Lymphocytic choriomeningitis tends to appear chiefly in winter, and a history of contact with mice is common. When the differential diagnosis of encephalitis is under consideration, attention should be paid to recent infectious diseases, vaccinations, or contacts with heavy metals.

Lumbar puncture may be of value in ascertaining the presence of an encephalitis, but it does not help in differentiating the types. Polymorphonuclear leukocytes may predominate in the spinal fluid in the first few days; they are replaced later by lymphocytes. The number of cells may be normal or increased. The pressure may or may not be elevated; the protein is normal or increased.

In the virus types, specific etiological determination requires serologic tests. For this purpose, whole blood drawn under strict aseptic precautions is necessary.

Treatment—There is no specific therapy. Any apparent causative factor should be treated. Otherwise, treatment is symptomatic.

MENINGITIS

Meningitis is an inflammation of the meninges, or coverings of the brain and spinal cord. The most common causes are listed in Table 17. The great majority of cases are of bacterial origin, the meningococcus, pneumococcus, tubercle bacillus, and *H. influenzae* being the most common agents.

The meningeal infection is preceded by an infection of the blood stream, the organisms passing through the choroid plexus to reach the cerebrospinal fluid. The onset of meningitis is usually sudden. General malaise and fever are evidence of

TABLE 17 — *Common Causes of Meningitis*

I. Infectious
  A. Bacteria
    Neisseria meningitidis (meningococcus)
    Diplococcus pneumoniae (pneumococcus)
    Hemophilus influenzae
    Staphylococcus (usually *aureus*)
    Streptococcus (usually *pyogenes*)
    Mycobacterium tuberculosis
    Other bacteria
  B. Viruses
    Mumps
    Lymphocytic choriomeningitis
  C. Spirochetes
    Treponema pallidum
  D. Fungi
    Torula
    Coccidioides immitis
    Streptothrix
II. Noninfectious
  A. Chemical
  B. Traumatic

systemic infection. Headache, vomiting, rigidity of the neck, apathy or restlessness, and positive Kernig, Brudzinski, and Babinski signs are indications of meningeal irritation. Convulsions and delirium are also seen.

Both the blood and the spinal fluid should be examined and cultured in every patient suspected of having meningitis. Spinal-fluid studies confirm the general diagnosis of meningitis and usually demonstrate the specific infecting organism. The findings characteristic of the different types of meningitis are listed in Table 18 (p. 166).

Meningococcus Meningitis—Meningococci may be present in the throats of well persons. For unknown reasons, they may invade the body and set up a meningococcemia. Sometimes the infection localizes no further, but in most cases the organism invades the meninges. Meningococcus infection may occur in epidemic form. The incubation period following invasion is usually short (one to four days), and chill, fever, headache, stiffness of the neck, and vomiting are the most common symptoms. In many cases a cutaneous eruption occurs —of petechial, purpuric, or maculopapular type. Early blood cultures, taken when only systemic symptoms are present, may reveal meningococci and permit specific treatment to be started before meningeal localization takes place.

Pneumococcus Meningitis occurs secondary to a focus of pneumococcus infection elsewhere in the body. Most commonly it follows pneumonia, but

TABLE 18—*Spinal-Fluid Changes in Meningeal Conditions*

	Appearance	Cells, Number per cc. and Predominant Type	Pressure	Sugar, mg. per 100 cc.	Protein, mg. per 100 cc.	Organisms
Normal	Colorless, no sediment	0–8 (lymphocytes)	3–8 mm. Hg	40–80	15–45	Absent
Transitory meningeal irritations (serous meningitis, meningismus)	Normal to clear-hazy	Normal or slightly increased	Increased↓	40–80	Normal or slightly increased	Absent
Meningitis Meningococcus	Cloudy sediment	500–20,000+ (polymorphonuclear)	Greatly increased	0–50	50–500	Present*
Other purulent infections	Cloudy sediment	50–20,000+ (polymorphonuclear)	Greatly increased	0–50	50–500	Present*
Tuberculosis	Clear-hazy	10–1,500 (young polymorphonuclear)	Increased	10–60	50–200	Present*
Syphilis	Clear-hazy	10–1,500 (lymphocytes)	Increased	10–60 or normal	50–500+	Usually absent†

* Organism to be determined by smear or culture or both.

† Wassermann, Kahn, and flocculation tests are positive in 90 percent of cases.

it may result from pneumococcus otitis media, mastoiditis, or endocarditis. Chemotherapy of the primary infection has greatly lowered the incidence of secondary meningitis.

Streptococcus and Staphylococcus Meningitis are also secondary infections, but they generally occur by direct extension from otitis media, mastoiditis, sinusitis, and osteomyelitis of the frontal bone rather than by transmission through the blood stream. Prompt diagnosis and chemotherapy of the primary infection will largely prevent the complication.

Tuberculous Meningitis is most common in children between the ages of two and ten years. It is usually the end stage of a preceding miliary tuberculosis which becomes disseminated by way of the blood. The base of the brain is the most frequent location for the infection, and there is usually an increase in intracranial pressure, with irritation and compression of cranial nerve roots in the area. The onset is insidious and may be obscured by symptoms of tuberculosis elsewhere in the body. Tuberculous meningitis should always be considered when signs of meningeal irritation appear in

a person exposed to or suffering from tuberculosis. When present, the most diagnostic signs and symptoms are headache, vomiting, convulsions, strabismus, and rigidity of the neck (sometimes of the entire back). The Kernig and Babinski signs are usually positive, and partial or complete paralysis of the cranial nerves may be present. The oculomotor, abducens, facial, and auditory nerves are most frequently affected.

H. Influenzae Meningitis—In this infection the organisms are transported from the throat or other parts of the respiratory tract to the meninges by way of the blood stream. *H. influenzae* is the third most frequent cause of meningitis in children, ranging behind the tubercle bacillus and the meningococcus. When patients of all ages are considered, the pneumococcus is the third most frequent cause of meningitis and *H. influenzae* the fourth. Vomiting, fever, headache, and stiffness of the neck are commonly encountered, as well as strabismus. In many cases, however, localizing symptoms do not appear until late. Slight fullness of the anterior fontanel may be present in infants. Culture of the throat yields the organism in 50 to 75 percent of cases.

Differential Diagnosis—In most cases the spinal-fluid examination will clarify the diagnosis of meningitis. In meningismus, in which neurological signs of meningitis are present, no pathological changes other than a slight lymphocytosis are found in the cerebrospinal fluid. Typhus, Rocky Mountain spotted fever, typhoid fever, purpura, drug rashes, bacterial endocarditis, and streptococcus bacteremia present petechial or purpuric rashes similar to that of meningitis. Anterior poliomyelitis, encephalitis, benign lymphocytic choriomeningitis, and syphilis of the central nervous system can produce symptoms similar to those encountered in meningitis. The spinal-fluid examination will decide the diagnosis. In all patients in whom coma is not explained with certainty, a lumbar puncture should be done to rule out meningitis.

Treatment of the meningitides is directed toward the systemic as well as the localized meningeal infection. The same general measures adopted in other infectious diseases should be used. If vomiting and signs of dehydration are present, parenteral administration of fluids is indicated (see p. 56). For sedation the barbiturates, chloral hydrate, and morphine can be used. Headache may be relieved by codeine or acetylsalicylic acid, or it may require morphine. Morphine increases the sugar content of the spinal fluid, and this should be taken into consideration in spinal-fluid tests of patients taking the drug. Although they are not always beneficial, lumbar punctures are sometimes advised for relief of the headache. They may be helpful, however, in controlling restlessness and delirium. Precautions should be taken to prevent decubitus ulcers, especially if the patient is incontinent. Eyes and mouth should be kept clean; and purpuric rashes must be watched, since they may become gangrenous.

The specific treatment is made with the sulfonamides and antibiotics. The drug to be used (see Table 31, p. 290) is determined by the etiological agent as disclosed by the spinal-fluid examination. Recovery is judged by a drop in temperature and pulse, reorientation, the disappearance of organisms from the spinal fluid, and the return of spinal-fluid dextrose values to normal. Treatment should not be discontinued until these manifestations have been normal for a week.

In meningococcus meningitis, sulfadiazine is the drug of choice, with sulfamerazine as an alternative. The sodium salt of sulfadiazine may be administered intravenously to start treatment in severe cases, but oral medication should be instituted as soon as the condition of the patient improves. Slow subcutaneous infusion and administration through an indwelling stomach tube are alternative modes of administration which may be adopted if oral medication is not possible. Penicillin is the second choice in meningococcus meningitis. Combined therapy may be advantageous in severe cases.

Penicillin is the drug of choice in meningitis due to the pneumococcus, streptococcus, or staphylococcus. Sulfadiazine is second choice. Combined therapy is advocated for severe infections. Even though penicillin does not diffuse easily from the blood into the spinal fluid, the intraspinal application of penicillin is not recommended for routine use because of the frequent occurrence of serious side-effects which include pleocytosis, arachnoiditis, myelitis, radiculitis, and subarachnoid block. To secure adequate concentrations of penicillin in the spinal fluid, it is therefore necessary to produce extremely high blood levels. This can be accomplished by two-hourly intramuscular injections of 1,000,000 units of crystalline penicillin. Comatose and delirious patients should receive one initial intrathecal dose of penicillin despite the risk of side-effects.

In the treatment of tuberculous meningitis, dihydrostreptomycin sulfate is the drug of choice. It should be given both intrathecally and intramuscularly. Para-aminosalicylic acid (p. 296) is commonly used at the same time. Dihydrostreptomycin sulfate can be administered intrathecally in doses of 20 mg. per day or 50 mg. every other day for the first three to five weeks, and at gradually increasing intervals up to twice weekly thereafter, for a total of three to four months. The intramuscular daily dose is 1 to 3 Gm., in divided doses, for the same period of time.

H. influenzae meningitis should be treated with dihydrostreptomycin sulfate following the schedule outlined for tuberculous meningitis, although not for the same length of time. A therapeutic program combining streptomycin with sulfadiazine affords the best results. Because the organisms are prone to become streptomycin-fast rather rapidly, successive streptomycin sensitivity tests are advisable. If the organism is or becomes resistant to more than 5 micrograms of streptomycin, it is best to give specific antiserum in addition.

A possible complication of streptomycin therapy is the development of meningitis or pneumonia due to *Staphylococcus aureus*; apparently this results from the inhibitory action of the antibiotic upon gram-negative organisms, which shifts the balance among the flora of the pharynx and allows the staphylococcus to multiply and spread. When such intercurrent infection is present, penicillin should also be given.

Prognosis—The prognosis of the meningeal infections was strikingly improved by the advent of chemotherapy. Before specific treatment was available, the fatality rate of *H. influenzae* meningitis, for example, approached 100 percent. With streptomycin and sulfadiazine, it was lowered to 15 to 25 percent.

In general, patients showing a high degree of neurological involvement and those delirious and in coma have poor prognoses. The spinal-fluid examination furnishes additional data of prognostic value: When a large number of organisms are found during microscopic examination, the case is always severe, for it indicates an overwhelming infection. Corollary to this, the dextrose content of the fluid is low on account of the utilization of this sugar as a source of nutrition by the infecting bacteria.

In meningococcus meningitis the mortality is higher (20 percent) in patients under one year of age, falls and remains low (5 to 10 percent) from one to thirty years, and then rises sharply (20 to 50 percent). In sulfonamide-treated patients, the over-all mortality is around 10 percent. The same is true in pneumococcus infections of the meninges, although the mortality rate is higher, the over-all death rate being about 30 to 40 percent in patients receiving sulfonamides and penicillin. The best results in pneumococcus meningitis are observed in those cases in which there is no discernible primary focus or when meningeal involvement follows otitis media or head injury. When pneumonia precedes the meningitis or when endocarditis is present, the mortality rate is considerably higher.

Since the introduction of the sulfonamides and penicillin, 30 to 40 percent of the cases of staphylococcus meningitis are expected to recover as against an almost 100 percent fatality in presulfonamide days. Streptococcus infections, however, are quite amenable to these drugs. From 95 percent the fatality rate dropped to around 30 percent with the sulfonamides, and penicillin is likely to lower it still further.

Tuberculous meningitis shows an extremely high mortality rate; only a small number of cases survive even after streptomycin therapy. In most cases in which recovery is observed, serious sequelae will be present.

Complications and Sequelae—The complications of meningitis may be divided into two groups, depending upon whether they affect the nervous system or other parts of the body. Paralyses of the cranial nerves are not uncommonly encountered, the facial, oculomotor, and acoustic nerves being the most commonly involved. Optic neuritis is present in a considerable number of cases of tuberculous meningitis; it causes narrowing of the ocular fields and sometimes total blindness.

Affection of the facial nerves leads to unilateral or bilateral loss of movement of the facial muscles. Hearing is affected either as a result of otitis media or of injury to the auditory nerve. Monoplegia, hemiplegia, and lesions of the peripheral nerves are rare.

The prognosis of the neurological complications varies considerably. In many cases of paralysis, recovery is observed by the time the cerebrospinal fluid has returned to normal. In others, completely normal function is not restored for weeks or months. In general, affections of the acoustic nerves are less prone to clear up completely than are those of other nerves. In children under eight years of age, complete deafness usually results in deaf-mutism.

Among the complications elsewhere than in the nervous system, arthritis and tenosynovitis are the most common. Conjunctivitis is present in some cases. Pneumonia occurs on occasion; more rarely, lung abscess, otitis media, thrombosis, gangrene of fingers and toes, endocarditis, pericarditis, epididymitis, orchitis, pleurisy, parotitis, and peritonitis are encountered.

Blocking of the foramina through which the cerebrospinal fluid circulates is followed by hydrocephalus. It is a serious complication which occurs especially in infants and causes pressure atrophy of portions of the brain. Since the advent of chemotherapy, hydrocephalus is rarely seen.

NEURITIS

Neuritis, or nerve inflammation, may involve a single nerve (as a localized, simple, or mononeuritis) or many nerves (as a polyneuritis or multiple neuritis). The inflammatory process may be accompanied by varying degrees of nerve degeneration. The causes of neuritis are numerous. Toxic neuritis may occur in such disorders as nephritis and diabetes mellitus and in infectious diseases, of which typhoid fever, diphtheria, and smallpox are examples. Neuritis may result from lead, mercury, or arsenic intoxication, and it is a common finding in deficiency states such as beriberi. Neuritis due to use of sulfonamide drugs has been reported. Other causes, usually producing localized neuritis, include trauma, exposure to cold, and extension of inflammation from tissues adjacent to a nerve.

Diagnosis of localized neuritis is made by consideration of symptoms, one of the most prominent being pain or tenderness over the course of the nerve. The pain is a distinctive, boring variety which is accentuated by movement of the affected member. Numbness, crawling, and tingling sensations also may be present. Multiple neuritis with its greater variety of signs and symptoms must be differentiated from other disorders of the nervous system which produce muscle pain, weakness, and paralysis. Among these are poliomyelitis, tabes dorsalis, and the muscular dystrophies.

Treatment of neuritis begins with removal of the etiological factors. Nerve compression from fracture, bony exostosis, ruptured intervertebral disk, or scar tissue often is amenable to surgical treatment. Following trauma which has resulted in nerve injury, surgery may be indicated, after which the affected part may be splinted to secure immobilization and to prevent contractures. Contact with the heavy metals should be eliminated, and use of alcohol or drugs which might be responsible for neuritis should be discontinued.

Application of moist heat and administration of analgesic drugs (p. 405) often aid in controlling pain. On an empirical basis, some have advocated intravenous administration of sodium iodide in 30-grain (2-Gm.) doses or a combination of sodium salicylate and sodium iodide with colchicine.

In polyneuritis resulting from deficiency of thiamin (p. 485), intravenous administration of the vitamin (50 to 150 mg. daily) may speed recovery. Oral therapy is substituted after improvement begins. Suspicion of multiple avitaminosis should prompt administration of the entire B complex (p. 483).

For treatment of the neuritis of lead poisoning, see page 558.

APOPLEXY

Apoplexy, or acute cerebral hemorrhage, occurs almost always in the presence of vascular disease, and particularly hypertension (p. 80) and arteriosclerosis (p. 74). A tendency toward hemorrhage (as in thrombocytopenia [p. 105], leukemia [p. 103], avitaminosis K [p. 501]) may be a contributing factor. A sudden rise in blood pressure seems to be the usual precipitating cause.

With or without preliminary cerebral symptoms, the patient suffers a partial or complete loss of consciousness, depending on the severity of the attack. There may be an initial convulsion. There is a partial or complete hemiplegia and temporary loss of sphincter control. Coma may continue up to several days.

Cerebral hemorrhage must be distinguished from the following:

1. Cerebral anemia. Brief episodes of clouding of consciousness, with or without hemiplegia, may be seen as a result of temporary cerebral anemia (presumably from local vascular spasm) in cerebral vascular disease, including that due to syphilis. The attack, though rapid in onset, is brief, and recovery is prompt (a day or two) and complete.

2. Cerebral embolism. Differential diagnosis may be difficult. However, embolism may occur at any age and in the absence of vascular disease. Usually an endocarditis or other infection involving bacteremia is present.

3. Cerebral thrombosis. Here, again, differentiation may be difficult. Thrombosis usually results from either sepsis or vascular disease, including that due to syphilis. Embolism usually has a rapid onset without premonitory symptoms. The latter are common in thrombosis, and the evolution of the full clinical picture proceeds more slowly than in embolism or hemorrhage. In addition, motor irritation (twitchings or Jacksonian seizures) is more common in thrombosis.

4. Cerebral tumor (primary or metastatic). Confusion in diagnosis is likely only when hemorrhage takes place into the tumor, in which case the clinical picture is likely to resemble cerebral thrombosis.

Patients with hypertension or arteriosclerosis of severe degree and patients showing a tendency toward spontaneous tissue hemorrhages not due to local causes should be warned against physical exercise and, especially, straining at stool or lifting.

Treatment—The patient should, of course, be put to bed and treated symptomatically. The head should be slightly elevated. If necessary, an airway or other device should be inserted to keep open the respiratory passages. The position should be changed at intervals to avoid decubitus and hypostatic pulmonary congestion. The bladder and bowel are emptied periodically if necessary. Flaccid limbs are supported in proper position to avoid contractures. Sedation is best avoided if possible.

Perhaps the most effective positive therapeutic measure is early block of the stellate ganglion with a local anesthetic. Block should be performed daily for about four days *on the side of the hemorrhage*. Details of treatment have not yet been standardized. Block of the opposite side, in addition, may be helpful in some cases. However, the opposite side should be injected not less than four hours after the ipsilateral block and only after the signs of Horner's syndrome from the latter (unilateral miosis, ptosis, vasodilation, and absence of perspiration over the face and head) have subsided. *Both sides should never be blocked simultaneously*. Following block, most patients show improved function within an hour, the less severe cases usually having the greatest relative improvement.

If (1) improvement following stellate ganglion block is not satisfactory or there has been no one available who is able to perform the block, (2) the patient is plethoric, and (3) the physician is certain of the diagnosis of hemorrhage, venesection of 500 to 700 cc. may be undertaken.

Beginning in the second week, the patient should receive gentle massage and passive exercise of the affected muscles. Mild faradic stimulation of the antagonists of contracted muscles may be given several times daily for a month or more. The patient should not try to walk until at least three weeks after the attack, and even then he should spend a great part of the day in bed for some time longer.

Especial precautionary measures should be taken (see above) to avoid a second attack.

EPILEPSY

Epilepsy is a syndrome characterized by repeated attacks of unconsciousness with or without convulsions. Attacks may take four different forms: the classical grand mal and petit mal, and the more recently recognized psychomotor and Jacksonian attacks.

Patients subject to grand mal may have premonitory symptoms such as migraine, tremors or muscular spasms, indigestion, pressure in the head, or noises in the ears; they may be irritable, be subject to outbursts of anger, or have other special personality traits. Directly before an attack they may experience various phenomena known as aurae, which may involve any aspect of sensory, motor, vasomotor, or psychic activity.

The epileptic attack itself is sudden and has several parts. In the first, or tonic, phase (lasting usually about half a minute), the body is rigid, with arms and legs extended, forearms pronated, and jaws closed. With the second, or clonic, phase, there is rapid transition to alternate contraction and relaxation of the limbs, jerking of the head, and vigorous thrashing about which sometimes causes fractures and dislocations. During this period, which lasts for two to five minutes, corneal and pupillary reflexes are lost and deep reflexes are diminished or absent. Toward the end of the phase or in the following phase, there is sometimes incontinence of urine or, less frequently, of feces. The attack terminates in a period of stupor or exhaustion, in which the patient drops into a deep sleep; he awakens from this without memory of the episode but often with headache.

In petit mal there is abrupt loss of consciousness, but usually there are no aurae. The patient seldom falls or has convulsions. He merely suffers a temporary lapse lasting a few seconds to half a minute. In this brief period he ceases activity and may be pale, with twitching of the eyelids, lips, tongue, face, or limbs or with sudden laughter or occasionally incontinence of urine. Following this period, he recovers without memory of the episode.

The patient with psychomotor attacks ("epileptic equivalent") performs some purposeless but co-ordinated act, such as running or talking, or he may suddenly display an irrelevant mood. His activities may be destructive. As in petit mal, the attack begins and ends suddenly, and the patient remembers nothing of the episode.

Jacksonian, or focal motor, attacks either are localized throughout or spread from a localized beginning. The parts involved are, in order of decreasing frequency: hand, face, tongue, foot, trunk. They are typically clonic in character but may be preceded by a brief tonic spasm.

The frequency of attacks varies considerably. In the so-called status epilepticus, attacks may succeed one another with such rapidity and intensity as to cause death, usually from anoxia. At the other extreme, patients may go for months or years between attacks. Patients may have only one form of attack or they may have more than one. Those who suffer from petit mal or psychomotor attacks usually have major seizures also.

Epilepsy may be due to pressure or to scar tissue which affects the motor cortex of the brain, and thus it may occur in connection with brain tumors, trauma, or thrombosis. It may also arise from localized areas of anoxic degeneration of brain tissue following minute vascular occlusions such as occur in the course of rheumatic fever and chorea. However, many cases are without known cause, and this type is sometimes termed "idiopathic" or "cryptogenic" epilepsy.

The fundamental cause and much of the pathological physiology are unknown. Most patients with the disease show definite and distinctive brain-wave patterns in the electroencephalogram. In grand mal, the rhythms are abnormally fast. In petit mal, they are alternately fast and slow. In the psychomotor attacks, they are slow. In some patients, electroencephalograms taken during sleep show abnormalities which are not present when the patient is awake. These abnormalities run in families and may be found in individuals who do not have epilepsy. A number of physiological and other alterations bring on or increase the frequency of epileptic attacks. They include sodium retention, water retention, alkalosis, the ingestion of alcohol, anoxia, and an inadequate amount of sleep.

Idiopathic epilepsy usually begins in childhood and almost always before the age of twenty-five. Its natural course is extremely variable. Some patients may have a few attacks, limited to childhood; others may have attacks for only a few years, without recurrence. In general, however, the earlier epilepsy starts, the graver is the prognosis. If the disease persists uncontrolled over a period of years, there is likely to be gradual mental deterioration.

The diagnosis of epilepsy is made partly by positive findings and partly by exclusion of other conditions known to cause convulsions. The latter phase is discussed under Convulsions in Childhood, page 146. Electroencephalographic abnormalities are strong evidence for epilepsy as the cause of convulsive seizures. X-rays of the skull should be taken for evidence of healed fracture. Pneumoencephalograms are also helpful. Electroencephalographic changes, or even seizures, may be brought on for diagnostic purposes by hyperventilation (producing alkalosis; see p. 61), by small doses of a cerebral stimulant such as Metrazol, or by administration of posterior pituitary extract (to induce water retention). The last test may be somewhat hazardous in older or debilitated patients, and all patients given it should be under continuous observation. For the test, the patient is kept on a salt-free and medication-free regimen. After a preliminary period of three or four days on the regimen, he drinks or is given through an indwelling stomach tube extra tap water at the rate of 75 to 100 cc. per Kg. (35 to 45 cc. per lb.) of body weight every three hours. At the same intervals he is given 6 to 12 pressor units (see p. 474) of posterior pituitary extract subcutaneously for its antidiuretic effect. The urine is collected every three hours, and the patient is weighed every six hours. The water and pituitary extract are continued until the patient has (1) had a seizure, (2) shown typical electroencephalographic abnormalities, or (3) gained in weight an amount equal to 5 percent of his initial weight.

The test is discontinued as soon as one of these possibilities is fulfilled. If it is one of the first two, the test is considered positive for epilepsy. If the patient gains 5 percent in weight without having a seizure or showing electroencephalographic abnormalities, he is considered not to have epilepsy.

The duration of the test is usually twelve to thirty-six hours. If there are repeated seizures after the test regimen is discontinued, the patient should be given 2 Gm. or more of sodium chloride. If the situation is urgent, it may be given slowly by vein as 1 liter of 2 percent solution.

Treatment—Since the cause and mechanism of idiopathic epilepsy are unknown, treatment is of necessity symptomatic. During attacks, steps should be taken to prevent self-injury. A wedge of soft wood wrapped with cloth or a wedge of some other material which will not break the teeth should be placed between the molar teeth on one side of the mouth. The clothing should be loosened. When the convulsions are over, the patient is allowed to rest and sleep. If convulsions are prolonged or if status epilepticus sets in, phenobarbital sodium is given intramuscularly, 5 to 7 mg. per Kg. (2 to 3 mg. per lb.) of body weight immediately and about half that dose every fifteen to twenty minutes until the convulsions stop, which is usually after the second or third injection. In those rare patients not controlled by phenobarbital sodium, general anesthesia, usually with chloroform or ether, may be effective. When cyanosis is present, oxygen therapy is indicated.

Patients with epilepsy should adopt a definite regimen. Obviously, they should not engage in any activity, such as driving an automobile, in which a lapse of consciousness may be dangerous to themselves or to others. At the same time, they need psychological handling which will enable them to overcome feelings of guilt, shame, or inadequacy. Advantage should be taken of any facilities for vocational habilitation.

Predisposing factors should be avoided (see above). The diet should have an acid ash. An excess of salt, or any actual or potential alkali (p. 352), should be avoided. The fluid intake should be low, alcohol should never be taken, and the patient should assure himself of plenty of sleep.

In children, the most effective method of specific treatment seems to be the ketogenic diet. Such a regimen is rather complicated and difficult to follow, but it has been reported that after two years of such a diet, gradual discontinuance may be followed by remissions of many years in about a third of the patients.

In contrast to the ketogenic diet, which offers hope of prolonged remission, drugs offer only symptomatic therapy, the effect of which rarely outlasts the period of administration. The most valuable of these seems to be phenobarbital, particularly in the treatment of grand mal. For dosage and administration, see page 414. Other drugs are discussed beginning on page 414.

In focal epilepsy, surgery for removal of the focus may be curative.

MULTIPLE SCLEROSIS

Multiple sclerosis (disseminated sclerosis) is a chronic disease of the central nervous system of unknown cause. It is characterized by degeneration of myelin sheaths in multiple areas, followed by sclerosis. Because of the apparently random number, size, and location of the affected areas, the clinical picture may be extremely varied. The occurrence of unpredictable remissions and exacerbations adds to the protean character of the disease.

The onset is usually insidious but may be sudden. The classical triad of Charcot—intention tremor, scanning speech, and nystagmus—is usually seen late and is commonly accompanied by pyramidal-tract signs, such as disturbance of reflexes and weakness. Disturbances of vision and of eye movements are common, along with various sensory changes, speech defects, and emotional instability. A later feature is temporal pallor of the optic disks. The duration of the disease is one to twenty-five years, the average being about ten.

Diagnosis may be extremely difficult in the early stages, and the disease is commonly mistaken for hysteria until the later changes occur.

Treatment—There is no known specific therapy. The most promising treatment consists in the daily intravenous administration of 2.75 mg. of histamine acid phosphate in 250 cc. of isotonic sodium chloride solution at the rate of 30 to 90 minims per minute, depending on the tolerance of the patient. The average patient receives forty to fifty such injections. In reports of patients treated, the minimal number of injections was thirteen and the maximal three hundred injections. As the patient's activity becomes limited, good nursing care is important.

PARALYSIS AGITANS

Paralysis agitans ("shaking palsy," the Parkinsonian syndrome) is a chronic, slowly progressive, organic disease characterized by muscular rigidity, tremor, slowness of movement, and impairment of certain so-called automatic movements. There is a primary essential form due to atrophy of the efferent striatal and pallidal systems of the corpus

striatum and a secondary, or symptomatic, form resulting from vascular, inflammatory, or neoplastic lesions. Juvenile, presenile, and senile types are described. In young patients it is a frequent sequel of encephalitis; when it begins in middle age, it is often associated with arteriosclerosis.

Diagnosis is ordinarily not difficult. Rhythmic tremors and the interosseous position of the hand and fingers produce the characteristic "pill-rolling" movement, which persists during rest but usually stops during voluntary movement. Rigidity, like the tremor, is of insidious onset and gradually becomes generalized and of a plastic quality, offering to passive movement a smooth resistance that is interrupted by rhythmic tremorlike oscillation (cogwheel symptom). The face becomes smooth and masklike, and the patient assumes an attitude of flexion and may sit motionless by the hour, even rarely blinking. Movements are slow and difficult to start. In walking, the arms hang motionless and rigid, and the body is thrown in advance of the feet (propulsion and festination). Sialorrhea is a frequent symptom. Purely reflex acts are not affected, and the tendon reflexes are not abolished. Intelligence as a rule is preserved.

Treatment is symptomatic. Physical therapy by a skilled attendant may do much to improve general health and strength. Most of the symptoms can be ameliorated to a greater or less extent by the administration of belladonna alkaloids (p. 420) as Belladonna Tincture, atropine sulfate, scopolamine hydrobromide, or Stramonium Extract or Tincture. Treatment is begun with small doses, which are increased until maximal improvement is obtained. Sometimes one preparation is more effective than another in a given patient, and usually very large doses are required. There seems to be no particular virtue in the Bulgarian variety of belladonna. Glaucoma is a contraindication to the use of the belladonna alkaloids.

A new and promising drug for symptomatic control is Artane Trihexyphenidyl (3-[1-piperidyl]-1-phenyl-1-cyclohexyl-1-propanol hydrochloride). It has antispasmodic properties, and it improves involuntary tremor, spasticity, and co-ordination. It is also a mild cerebral stimulant. It is equally effective in all types of paralysis agitans. For most patients, 6 to 10 mg. daily in divided doses are adequate. Some, and especially the postencephalitic group, may require 12 to 15 mg. Temporary blurring of vision or nausea may occur as a side-effect which requires discontinuation for a few days and later resumption at a lower dosage level.

Amphetamine sulfate (p. 429) in 10-mg. doses morning and noon also helps certain cases. Some observers report subjective improvement following administration of large doses of pyridoxine (p. 489) and other members of the B group.

SUBACUTE COMBINED DEGENERATION OF THE SPINAL CORD

Subacute combined degeneration of the spinal cord is usually seen as part of the disease process of pernicious anemia. Rarely, it may be associated with hypochromic anemia or with cachexia from any cause. However, it is not a consequence of anemia per se. It involves progressive degeneration of the posterior columns and pyramidal tracts of the spinal cord, leading to paresthesias, impairment of position sense and other proprioceptive sensations, loss of reflexes, ataxia, spastic muscular weakness, and, later, sphincter disturbances and girdle sensations.

Differential diagnosis includes tabes dorsalis, multiple neuritis, pellagra, multiple sclerosis, and spinal-cord tumor.

Treatment, when sufficiently vigorous, is usually effective in checking the progress of the disease. It consists in intensive treatment of the Addisonian anemia with liver extract or vitamin B₁₂ (p. 371). Folic acid is ineffective.

ENDOCRINE GLANDS

The organs generally classified as endocrine glands have in common two facts: The biological purpose of their secretions is to influence organs or tissues at a distance from the glands themselves, and the secretions are liberated into and transported by the blood stream. The group of endocrine glands is ordinarily considered to include the anterior and posterior pituitary, thyroid, parathyroids, adrenal cortices and medullae, islands of Langerhans, and gonads (ovaries and testes). Sometimes the thymus and pineal are added, although their function, if any, is unknown. The classification is somewhat arbitrary; on the one hand, internal secretions are produced by tissues (such as the duodenal mucosa) which are not included in the list, whereas, on the other hand, it seems probable that many cases of diabetes do not involve primarily a deranged secretion of insulin by the islands of Langerhans but rather a defective utilization.

The hormones of the gonads and adrenal cortex belong to the steroid family and are related to the vitamins D and the digitalis glycosides.* The other hormones are protein in nature. The hormones act either as growth stimulants or as regulators of metabolism. Some act on all cells, some on special tissues only. Some influence metabolism as a whole; others affect only particular phases; some of the hormones of the anterior pituitary gland have other endocrine glands as their specific target organs.

The various glands are discussed in the order of frequency and importance of the diseases affecting them.

Islands of Langerhans (Pancreas)

DIABETES MELLITUS

Diabetes mellitus is a hereditary disease characterized by impairment of the body's ability to utilize food. For an understanding of diabetes, it is necessary to be acquainted with the normal metabolism of food, which is discussed beginning on page 252.

The defect in diabetes appears to depend on either (1) an actual or relative deficiency of insulin resulting from a disturbance in the function of the islands of Langerhans of the pancreas, or (2) interference with the action of insulin in the tissues. Insulin is necessary for normal utilization of carbohydrate by the tissues and for deposition of glycogen in the liver. In diabetes there is faulty storage of sugar in the liver, overproduction of sugar by the liver, and, apparently, diminished utilization of sugar by the tissues. The result is an increased concentration of sugar in the blood and, subsequently, the appearance of sugar in the urine. When utilization of carbohydrate is sufficiently impaired, fat metabolism becomes disturbed in such a manner as to produce ketosis (the diabetic type of acidosis) and finally coma.

The onset of diabetes is usually indefinite. The most characteristic symptoms are the passage of large amounts of urine, increased thirst, and excessive appetite, accompanied by loss of weight and strength. Other commonly encountered complaints are skin disturbances, such as localized or generalized pruritus, furuncles, carbuncles, and slowly healing ulcers; disturbances of vision; numbness and tingling; and pain (neuritis), especially in the lower limbs. The patient's urine contains sugar and usually has a high specific gravity. Acetone

---

* Compare the following:
Figure 42, p. 461
Figure 43, p. 464
Figure 45, p. 470
Figure 53, p. 494
Figure 16, p. 354

and diacetic acid may also be present, indicating that acidosis exists. Examination of the blood discloses a sugar content above normal, especially after meals.

The diagnosis of diabetes is a simple matter in severe cases but may be difficult in instances in which glycosuria without symptoms is present. Sugar in the urine is presumptive evidence of diabetes until proved otherwise, but additional evidence should be actively sought if other symptoms are absent. Temporary glycosuria may occur in nondiabetic states and infections (meningitis), during or following anesthesia, following severe fractures, or after shock, accidents, and injuries involving especially the head.

To avoid confusion in diagnosis, Joslin's standard may well be adopted. Venous blood-sugar values of 170 mg. or more per 100 cc. (Folin-Wu technic, p. 531) obtained following meals are indicative of diabetes. If hyperthyroidism coexists, the postprandial level for diagnosis is raised from 170 to 200. Levels of 140 or above in persons who are in the fasting condition, without other evidence, arouse suspicion of diabetes and may call for a dextrose tolerance test (p. 533). The dextrose threshold for urinary excretion in health is approximately 170 to 180 mg. per 100 cc. of blood.

A simplified blood-sugar screening method has been described by Wilkerson and Heftmann, based on the Hagedorn-Jensen method which measures true blood dextrose. In screening large numbers of persons, it is not as essential to know the exact blood-sugar level as it is to determine whether a specified critical diagnostic level has been exceeded. Based on the surveys of Wilkerson and Heftmann, a true-dextrose level of 130 mg. percent has been chosen, and patients whose blood sugars are above this value postprandially are classified as cases of suspected diabetes and warrant further study if need be to establish a definite diagnosis.

Treatment is aimed at maintaining normal weight and well-being without glycosuria and, if possible, with normal blood sugar. In children, normal growth is an additional objective. Treatment involves control of the diet, in many cases the administration of Insulin, and always adequate check by patient and physician to be certain that diet and dosage of Insulin are optimal.

Education of a diabetic and his family is essential. Unless they are taught how to harmonize diet, the dose of Insulin, and exercise under various conditions of life, the whole structure of treatment is likely to collapse during even a minor emergency.

Most diabetics excrete sugar in the urine whenever the level of sugar in the venous blood rises much above 170 to 180 mg. per 100 cc., and urinalysis alone frequently is a satisfactory guide for routine diabetic control. The patient should be taught to use the Benedict test (p. 517) or the Urine Sugar Test, Sheftel (p. 518). The latter is a simple method of quantitative analysis; but if it is not available, a rough estimate can be made by recording the color changes of the Benedict test as red (4+), orange (3+), yellow (2+), or green (1+).

Urine specimens should be collected in four fractions daily: the urine voided (1) between breakfast and lunch, (2) between lunch and dinner, (3) between dinner and bedtime, and (4) between bedtime and breakfast. Each specimen should be examined separately and the results recorded to provide a basis for adjustment of the dose of Insulin. Thus, the presence of sugar in the fasting specimen and its absence from other specimens indicate that the dose of Protamine Zinc Insulin should be increased. If glycosuria occurs in the daytime (feeding hours), more Insulin is needed in relation to meals. During emergencies it is often convenient to administer Insulin every three to four hours, the dose being determined by the Benedict test: 4+ = 20 units; 3+ = 15 units; 2+ = 10 units; 1+ = 5 units.

Diet—The optimum diet for a diabetic patient is the one that will keep him well and strong, at the same time not permitting his weight to rise above the "ideal." Several requirements must be satisfactorily met: The diet should be palatable and satisfying both in quality and in quantity; it must supply the correct number of calories; it must contain proper proportions of carbohydrate, protein, and fat; and it must satisfy long-term nutritional requirements for vitamins and mineral salts in order to prevent the ultimate development of deficiency disease.

The general recommendation of allowing the adult diabetic 25 to 30 calories per Kg. (11 to 14 calories per lb.) of normal or ideal body weight is often made, and it is especially helpful as a guide in treatment. This amount should be reduced in the elderly or obese (or increased in young, active, and malnourished patients) to meet individual needs. Obviously, a latitude of a few hundred calories exists, and the *best guide for determining the maintenance caloric requirement is the general condition of the patient, especially as regards weight and strength and, in children, growth.* In patients who are grossly overweight, loss of weight should be accelerated by prescribing 20 to 30 percent fewer calories than the basal requirement. Vitamin and mineral deficiencies may be induced by such diets unless vitamin concentrates and calcium (p. 505) are prescribed.

The adult diabetic is usually given 1 to 1.5 Gm. of protein per Kg. (0.5 to 0.75 Gm. per lb.) of body weight; 1 Gm. per Kg. is a safe average. In diabetic children, it is especially important to supply enough protein to provide for growth, and an average allowance is approximately 3 Gm. per Kg. (1.5 Gm. per lb.) of body weight.

Good results have been obtained with diets containing widely varying amounts of carbohydrate, especially when slight undernutrition is imposed. There is little or no advantage in too rigorously restricting carbohydrate, nor does it appear desirable to go to the other extreme in a disease characterized by a defect in carbohydrate metabolism. At present, a ratio of approximately 2 Gm. carbohydrate to 1 Gm. fat seems most widely employed.

The amount of fat supplied in the diabetic diet need not differ radically from the quantity ordinarily taken in health; namely, from about 50 Gm. daily for young children to 100 Gm. for adults. It is rarely necessary to give more than 150 Gm. per day; an allowance less than this is usually possible and may be preferable.

It is a simple matter to prescribe a diet based on the above considerations. To obtain the total calories, multiply the ideal body weight in kilograms by 25 for basal conditions, by 30 if the patient is moderately active, or by 35 or more if the occupation is strenuous. The respective carbohydrate, protein, and fat components can then be calculated by supplying 40 percent of the allotment as carbohydrate, 15 percent as protein, and 45 percent as fat. For example:

```
Body weight.....................132 lb. =   60 Kg.
At rest......................25 Cal. × 60 = 1,500 Cal.
Carbohydrate...........40% × 1,500 Cal. =  600 Cal.
                  600 Cal. ÷ 4 Cal./Gm. =  150 Gm. C
Protein...............15% × 1,500 Cal. =  225 Cal.
                  225 Cal. ÷ 4 Cal./Gm. =   56 Gm. P
                                  (or approx. 1 Gm./Kg.)
Fat...................45% × 1,500 Cal. =  675 Cal.
                  675 Cal. ÷ 9 Cal./Gm. =   75 Gm. F
```

Conversion of the diet prescription into a menu is not difficult, and the patient soon learns to do it for himself. For the purpose, it is essential to have at hand a comprehensive food table, such as the Lilly *Diet Prescription*,* showing in percentage the

---
* The Lilly *Diet Prescription* (reprinted for convenience on pages 570 to 582 of this book) is separately available for distribution to the patient by his physician. Copies, including several blank pages for insertion of the individual diet, will gladly be sent upon request.

contents of carbohydrate, protein, and fat in various foods.

The usual practice has been to divide the total quantity for the day into three equal parts given at breakfast, lunch, and dinner or (in cases being treated with Protamine Zinc Insulin) into one-fifth, two-fifths, and two-fifths. Some clinicians provide small supplementary feedings between meals and at bedtime in order to distribute the metabolic load more evenly over a greater number of hours, lessen the amount of Insulin required, and thereby minimize danger of Insulin reactions. Supplementary feedings, particularly one given at bedtime, are especially valuable when Protamine Zinc Insulin is used; peak metabolic loads can thus be avoided.

The normal variability of foods and the inconstancy of the individual patient's requirements have led some clinicians to adopt a series of progressively larger diets based on a single standard diet which is suitable for instituting treatment in the average uncomplicated case. This simple procedure permits the application of the *ladder method* of treatment, which begins with a small diet that is increased by successive stages as improvement occurs or as is shown necessary by weighing the patient once or twice weekly and observing his general condition. If he gains weight excessively, the diet should be *lowered*; if he loses too much weight, the diet should be *increased*.

In uncomplicated cases of diabetes, a trial period of three or four days on a maintenance, basal, or low ladder-diet without the administration of Insulin may first be instituted in order to determine the patient's own metabolic capacity.

INSULIN THERAPY is indicated (1) always in diabetic children; (2) always during complications, such as infections, surgery, delivery, and diabetic coma; and (3) in all other cases that demonstrate inability to maintain normal weight and strength without hyperglycemia or glycosuria.

Insulin is available as:

Insulin, either amorphous or crystalline
Protamine Zinc Insulin
NPH Insulin
Globin Insulin

Treatment can also be carried out with mixtures of Insulin and modified forms. Insulin preparations and details of their dosage and use are discussed beginning on page 449.

Modified Insulins, such as Protamine Zinc Insulin and NPH Insulin, are regarded as basic in all cases, whereas unmodified Insulin (from either amorphous or crystalline sources) is employed as a supplement when a quick and short but powerful action is required. Unmodified Insulin is especially indicated in emergencies and during complications (in which the need for Insulin fluctuates rapidly), in very young children who are incapable of intelligently interpreting symptoms of hypoglycemia, and as a supplement to Protamine Zinc Insulin.

After stabilization of the previously untreated case without complications, NPH Insulin is preferable to unmodified Insulin, for treatment is easier and control is more effective. Severe diabetics, however, are usually in acidosis when first seen by the physician, and emergency treatment with unmodified Insulin will usually be necessary (see outline on p. 455).

Once the patient has been regulated and it is evident that either the total daily dose of Insulin exceeds about 30 units or both Insulin and Protamine Zinc Insulin are required, the necessity for multiple separate injections may be overcome by the employment of mixtures of regular Insulin and Protamine Zinc Insulin. The mixture found to be the most satisfactory has been one consisting of two parts of unmodified Insulin to one part Protamine Zinc Insulin. The preparation of extemporaneous mixtures can be avoided by the use of NPH Insulin, which has an effect similar to that of the 2:1 mixture (see p. 453).

HYPOGLYCEMIA—The dominant symptoms which follow overdoses of Insulin are acute hunger, sudden weakness, sweating, and nervousness with or without tremor. In patients taking Protamine Zinc Insulin, the characteristic early symptoms are more likely to be headache, drowsiness, and malaise. Later findings which follow an overdose of either preparation are emotional and mental disturbances such as anxiety, laughing or crying, confusion, aphasia, or delirium; muscle in-co-ordination with staggering, vertigo, diplopia, and convulsions; unconsciousness and, in neglected cases, death. At least part of the urine in the bladder may have accumulated before hypoglycemia developed, and the first urine specimen that is obtained may, therefore, disclose a "residual" glycosuria. The second specimen will be sugar-free.

The treatment of hypoglycemia is the same regardless of whether the patient has taken Insulin or Protamine Zinc Insulin. *The antidote is sugar.* Since a hypoglycemic reaction during treatment with Protamine Zinc Insulin may be not only prolonged but also recurrent in nature, it is advisable to give a soluble and, in addition, a slowly digestible carbohydrate in treating the patient (for example, corn syrup or honey with bread).

If it is temporarily impossible for carbohydrate to be given by mouth or if the patient is in a critical condition, from 10 to 20 Gm. of dextrose should be slowly administered intravenously, followed later by food or by repeated injections of dextrose as indicated by frequent laboratory estimation of the blood-sugar level. In severe and prolonged reactions, it may be necessary to give repeated injections of dextrose intravenously over periods of several hours.

Complications—ACIDOSIS AND COMA are the end results of uncontrolled diabetes. They are usually caused by too little (or sudden withdrawal of) Insulin or by infection (see below). Their diagnosis and treatment will be found on page 59.

ARTERIOSCLEROSIS—Diabetic persons are peculiarly subject to arteriosclerosis (p. 74). *Coronary sclerosis* is common, and in its presence a sudden lowering of blood-sugar level may be harmful, sometimes to the extent of precipitating coronary occlusion. However, judicious use of Insulin with an adequate supply of carbohydrate is beneficial and may even be followed by reduction in anginal pain and improvement in patients having coronary disease.

Gangrene is a direct result of arteriosclerosis of the blood vessels of the extremities. Not infrequently it is complicated by superimposed infection. The best treatment for gangrene is prevention by daily cleanliness and scrupulous protection of the feet from injury, however trivial. Prophylactic foot treatment should be a routine part of the management of diabetic patients. The physician should supervise it closely. Following is a suitable regimen:

1. Soak feet in a basin of warm, soapy water for five minutes each day.
2. Dry thoroughly with a turkish towel, using special care to dry between the toes.
3. Massage with alcohol.
4. Massage with lanolin (p. 479), especially the heels and those parts of the soles where calluses appear.
5. Do not wear circular garters or sit with knees crossed.
6. Wear shoes that fit and cause no localized pressure.
7. Avoid strong, irritating antiseptics. The physician should be consulted for even minor injuries to the feet.

Foot exercises may also be advisable. They should be practiced daily, or twice daily if the feet tend to be cold.

1. Sit on edge of bed. Point toes upward, then downward, repeating movement ten times.
2. Make a complete circle with the foot ten times.
3. Raise both legs to an angle of forty-five degrees, using as a support a chair placed on the bed with front down. Maintain position for three minutes.
4. Let legs hang over side of bed for three minutes.
5. Place legs flat on bed for three minutes, covering with blanket.
6. Repeat the exercises for a total of six times.

INFECTIONS are very serious in the diabetic, for they always increase the severity of the disease. In the presence of infection, the carbohydrate content of the diet should be 100 to 200 Gm., and the dose of Insulin must often be increased. If the patient is already taking Protamine Zinc Insulin, it should be continued as a basic dose, and fluctuations in requirements (which may occur in a few hours) are met by supplemental doses of regular Insulin. Insulin may be administered every few hours, the dose being regulated by the results of urine tests as in diabetic coma (p. 174).

SURGERY in the diabetic demands the combined services of the internist and surgeon for best results. Before operation, diabetes should be treated vigorously and the patient should be in as good a nutritional state as possible, with an adequate store of glycogen in the liver and abundant vitamin stores (especially of vitamin C, which is concerned with wound healing). Carbohydrate intake should be maintained by mouth or by vein, with sufficient Insulin to keep the urine sugar-free or nearly so.

Insulin permits use of practically any type of anesthesia. However, local, regional, or spinal anesthesia when possible, or ethylene or cyclopropane when general anesthesia is required, is probably the best choice. Chloroform should be especially avoided.

PREGNANCY—Diabetes having its onset during pregnancy may be difficult to recognize because other factors may influence sugar tolerance. Treatment follows the same principles as in the non-pregnant. Diabetic women are unusually susceptible to toxemia of pregnancy, premature labor, and death of the fetus. These conditions are discussed beginning on page 212. Delivery should be managed according to the principles for surgery (see above).

HYPERINSULINISM

Hyperinsulinism is a clinical entity originating in the pancreas and is due to overproduction of insulin as a result of overactive islet cells, hyperplasia of islet cells, or tumors (benign or malignant) of the islands of Langerhans. The term is not synonymous with spontaneous hypoglycemia (or functional hyperinsulinism); they must be carefully differentiated, since treatment of hyperinsulinism is essentially a surgical problem. It is the antithesis of diabetes mellitus.

The symptoms of hyperinsulinism are closely related to the central nervous system and are extremely variable, just as when induced by an overdose of Insulin. There may be sweating, flushing, pallor, numbness, nausea, hunger, tremor, weakness, palpitation, and syncope. Restlessness, speech disorders, diplegia, convulsions, and coma may appear. Psychiatric manifestations may be observed during mild, moderately severe, or severe attacks and include emotional instability, disorientation, amnesia, apprehension, negativism, mania, or coma.

Diagnosis is based on Whipple's essential triad of findings:

1. Attacks come on in the fasting condition in early morning or during severe effort when sugar reserves are low.

2. Blood-sugar levels during attacks are always below 50 mg. per 100 cc.

3. Symptoms are invariably and promptly relieved by the administration of sugar by mouth or by vein.

With true hyperinsulinism, food must be taken at least with usual regularity; if a meal is missed, an attack is likely to follow. The hypoglycemia of nervous origin is as a rule well tolerated. The "fast test" has greater diagnostic importance than the ordinary glucose tolerance curve, which is likely to be quite variable. Food is withheld under rigidly supervised conditions for as long as thirty hours, unless characteristic symptoms are provoked sooner.

Hypoglycemia is not always due to an overproduction of insulin. The maintenance of the normal blood-sugar level is the result of a dynamic balance between several organs, particularly the pancreas, liver, pituitary, adrenals, and thyroid. Obviously, in hypoglycemia a careful search is required for the cause of the low blood sugar. In cases due to liver lesions, the patients are usually gravely ill and show frank signs of liver damage. Patients having adrenal disturbances are usually seriously ill with Addison's disease or show signs of adrenal tumor. Low blood-sugar levels accompanying hypophyseal lesions are likely to be associated with tumors causing headaches, visual-field disturbances, and positive x-ray findings. In cases of hypoglycemia with hyperthyroidism, the basal metabolic rate is usually lower than is customary in Graves' disease, and such patients may exhibit a thyroid crisis after removal of an islet-cell tumor. Electroencephalograms may be the deciding factor in differentiating epileptiform attacks from those seen in hyperinsulinism.

Treatment of true hyperinsulinism is surgical. Excision of adenomas and questionably malignant tumors gives brilliant and lasting cures. The recurrence or persistence of hypoglycemia below 50 mg. per 100 cc. following a partial pancreatectomy is almost certain evidence that an islet-cell tumor has been overlooked.

If spontaneous hypoglycemia of the functional type can be identified and differentiated from the other organic conditions which cause hypoglycemia, considerable benefit may be obtained from diet therapy. The diet should be low in carbohydrate content, and rapidly assimilable carbohydrates such as sugar should be avoided in order to prevent an exaggerated secondary fall in blood-sugar level. The diet may contain large quantities of protein, because it can be transformed gradually into available dextrose for purposes of metabolism. Additional calories sufficient to maintain normal weight may be provided in the form of fat. The total quantity of food is usually divided into five or six small feedings per day. The diet is thus rather similar to the low-carbohydrate, high-fat diet generally employed in the treatment of diabetes several years ago.

Thyroid

The thyroid gland elaborates a secretion which stimulates the metabolism of all body cells. The form of the hormone which is stored in the gland is a globulin (see p. 456); the form which circulates in the blood is probably a polypeptide. The thyroid has a low rate of spontaneous function, and normally its activity is regulated by the amount of thyrotrophin which is liberated by the anterior pituitary gland (p. 473). Thyrotrophin has two actions on the thyroid: It stimulates hypertrophy and hyperplasia of the secretory epithelium, and it stimulates the synthesis and release of thyroid hormone. Synthesis, storage, and release of thyroid hormone appear to be separate processes; the factors influencing them are poorly understood. Iodine (p. 506) tends to increase the synthesis and storage of thyroglobulin and to inhibit the release of thyroid hormone into the blood. A high level of circulating thyroid hormone tends to inhibit (1) further release of thyroid hormone and (2) liberation of thyrotrophin from the anterior pituitary.

Since cell activity requires energy and energy is derived from oxidation, the rate of oxygen uptake by the organism is influenced by (among other things) the amount of circulating thyroid hormone. However, the number of factors which influence basal metabolism is so great that the B.M.R. is not an infallible guide to thyroid function. Further discussion of the B.M.R. begins on page 252.

SIMPLE GOITER

Simple, or colloid, goiter is due to an absolute or relative lack of iodine. It is common where the soil and water are deficient in this element. It is possibly aggravated, or brought on in the presence of borderline absolute deficiency, by the frequent inclusion in the diet of cabbage, Brussels sprouts, and related foods having a mild antithyroid action. In the same way, goiter may occur as a complication of thiocyanate therapy (p. 512). When iodine deficiency is mild, simple goiter is not accompanied by alteration of thyroid function.

The prevention and treatment of simple goiter are discussed under Iodine, page 506.

MYXEDEMA

"Myxedema" is the term applied to the condition of complete or almost complete absence of thyroid function. Myxedema can be produced by complete removal, destruction, or inhibition of the thyroid gland. Spontaneous myxedema is ordinarily due to atrophy of the gland of unknown etiology. Occasionally myxedema results from lack of secretion of thyrotrophin by the anterior pituitary gland (see also p. 193).

In myxedema, all body processes are slowed. The basal metabolic rate is low—generally −35 to −45 percent. Capillary permeability is increased, and there is an excess of interstitial fluid which is manifested by generalized nonpitting edema and accumulation of fluid in the serous cavities. Excess protein is stored in the tissues (this and the edema produce the characteristic thickening of the subcutaneous tissues which gave the condition its name), and the level of protein in the blood and cerebrospinal fluid is high. Cardiovascular function is poor, and blood flow is subnormal. Coronary sclerosis is not uncommon. Absorption from the gastro-intestinal tract proceeds slowly, and motility is reduced, giving rise to constipation. The mental processes are slow, as is nerve function in general. There may be anemia which after a time may become hyperchromic in type, leading to confusion with pernicious anemia (p. 96). In women there may be menstrual disturbances, especially functional uterine bleeding. The serum cholesterol level (p. 534) is high, usually 220 to 500 mg. per 100 cc.

The onset is usually slow and insidious, often escaping the patient's attention. The symptoms in order of diminishing frequency include, but are not limited to, weakness; lethargy; slowness of speech; dryness and coarseness of skin; edema of eyelids, face, and tongue; a sense of being cold most of the time; coarseness of hair and loss of hair (commonly involving the lateral portions of the eyebrows); constipation; menorrhagia, dysmenorrhea; deafness; slow pulse; and low arterial blood pressure (not too common). The patient may gain 10 to 15 pounds of fluid and protein but commonly loses actual tissue, so that there may be reduction in body weight. Myxedema is not accompanied by accumulation of fat. Poor cardiovascular function may lead to dyspnea, palpitation, and precordial pain. Some patients, in spite of mental slowness, suffer from nervousness and emotional instability.

Differential diagnosis includes nephritis (p. 218), pernicious anemia (p. 96), and Simmonds' disease (p. 192). The full, puffy face, the mental slowness, and the other characteristic physical findings and history usually make the diagnosis, which should be confirmed by the extremely low basal metabolic rate and the high serum cholesterol.

Juvenile Myxedema is essentially like that seen after maturity. It differs, however, in that retardation of body growth is an important and irremediable feature. Hence, it is of the utmost importance to recognize the condition early and treat it adequately.

Cretinism, or congenital myxedema, is common when the mother suffers from iodine deficiency, and it is occasionally seen otherwise. It is marked by slow development, including delayed ossification and union of epiphyses, delayed dentition, and hypoplasia of the brain.

Because the mother's thyroid hormone passes the placental barrier, the clinical onset seldom occurs before three months of age; even then it is insidious. The earliest indications are failure to nurse well and to cry normally and a tendency to sleep most of the time. After the condition is fully developed, all cretins look much alike; they become dwarfed and imbecile, with large head, short extremities, and protuberant abdomen with umbilical hernia. The features become heavy, giving a pig-like expression; the voice becomes deep and harsh; the tongue enlarges and protrudes from the open mouth, from which saliva drools. The diagnosis is by this time obvious. At any stage, it is confirmed by the high serum cholesterol and the delayed bone development as shown by x-ray. Differential diagnosis from Mongolism may be sufficiently difficult to justify a therapeutic trial of thyroid.

Early treatment is essential if permanent retardation is to be avoided, and it must be continued throughout the lifetime of the patient. The prognosis for recovery is almost nil in cases that have been long untreated; in fact, treatment *begun* in later childhood may serve only to make the patient unmanageable.

Treatment consists in oral administration of desiccated thyroid substance. The U.S.P. preparation is preferred. Initial dosage should be very small (see p. 457), and restoration of the patient to normal should be a gradual process taking not less than thirty days. The objective in the adult patient, which can be attained only by careful trial and close observation, is to maintain the patient on the *minimum* dosage which will keep him symptom-free. Adjustment of dosage should be based on clinical observation and not on the basal metabolic rate or any laboratory determination. Paradoxically, the more severe the myxedema, the smaller is the required dosage. Overdosage or overly rapid restoration is exceedingly dangerous. It may precipitate coronary occlusion or heart failure, or, in those patients with total pituitary failure in whom myxedema masks adrenal failure, it may bring on Addisonian crisis.

At the beginning of therapy, as adequate dosage is approached, there is diuresis and loss of 10 to 15 pounds of myxedema. The basal metabolism and basal pulse rates begin to rise. In another week or two, the appearance, behavior, and speech begin to change. The skin sheds as the patient literally grows a new one. The anemia is one of the last features to respond, sometimes remaining for several months.

Patients with myxedema should continue thyroid medication for life. It is important to follow them actively, for they tend to omit medication after they are well; and the return of myxedema may be so insidious that, when they realize what has happened, they no longer have the will to seek medical aid.

Because of the depression of all metabolic functions in myxedema, the tolerance to depressant drugs is reduced. Hypnotics and sedatives, or any drugs which tend to depress the central nervous system, should be avoided. One dose of 1/2 grain of codeine has been known to cause death.

As in adult myxedema, the dosage in cretinism and juvenile myxedema must be individualized. Since it varies greatly with age, the physician must be constantly alert for the need of change. During puberty, as much as 12 grains daily may be required. Adequacy of dosage is judged by (1) disappearance of signs and symptoms, (2) reduction of serum cholesterol to normal, and (3) maintenance of a normal growth rate. If any error is to be made, it should be on the side of overdosage. However, gross overdosage may produce irritability and behavior disturbances, sometimes culminating in psychotic episodes.

HYPOTHYROIDISM

In hypothyroidism there is depression rather than cessation of thyroid function. The severity grades from the very mildest down to myxedema. Hypothyroidism is probably overlooked more frequently than any other endocrine disturbance. The symptoms are of the same type as in myxedema, but they are less severe; and they may be vague and uncharacteristic, suggesting nervous exhaustion or psychoneurosis. Menopausal symptoms may mask the condition.

Hypothyroidism should be considered, and evidence of it sought, in any patient who complains of chronic fatigue, lethargy, weakness, cold hands and feet, low tolerance to external cold, constipation, or any menstrual disorder, including menopause. Some hypothyroid patients are nervous and irritable and suffer from insomnia, quite in contrast to beliefs current some years ago. Hypothyroidism is not related to obesity. When the two occur together, it is because the patient eats more calories than he burns; sometimes this comes about because he continues old eating habits during a period when energy expenditure is reduced. Many hypothyroid patients are so thin as to appear undernourished.

Just as the history may be inconclusive, so may the physical examination be negative. Likewise, the basal metabolic rate is an unreliable guide; some hypothyroid patients have rates that are within normal limits, and some individuals with low rates are not hypothyroid and do not respond to thyroid medication. The serum cholesterol may also be within normal limits in mild cases.

Probably the most reliable clinical features are chronic coldness of the hands and feet, intolerance to external cold, and fatigability; and the most difficult differential diagnosis is between hypothyroidism and psychoneurosis. If the physician can rule out other causes for the patient's symptoms, a therapeutic trial of thyroid is in order (see p. 457).

Despite the difficulty that frequently attends the diagnosis of hypothyroidism, the physician should be constantly on the alert for it. The results of treatment are sometimes spectacular in patients who have gone from one physician to another for years without being helped.

Treatment of hypothyroidism, as of myxedema, is oral administration of desiccated thyroid substance (p. 456). However, the dosage is larger than in myxedema, the tolerance to overdosage is greater, and the variability in requirements from one patient to another is wider.

Some hypothyroid patients require medication throughout life. In most, however, a period of six months to a year suffices to restore the endocrine balance. Therefore, in hypothyroidism, as contrasted with myxedema, thyroid should be gradually discontinued after six months of satisfactory maintenance, and the patient should be watched for recurrence. If symptoms return, medication is resumed. A patient requiring thyroid for as long as two or three years will probably need it for life.

Because the signs and symptoms of mild hypothyroidism are less extreme than in more severe cases, the response is less dramatic. A record of basal pulse rate, kept by the patient (see p. 457), is useful in judging whether an effect is being obtained and when the advisable limit of dosage has been reached.

HYPERTHYROIDISM

Hyperthyroidism is the condition brought about by overfunctioning of the thyroid gland. It may present a number of clinical pictures, as evidenced by the terms Graves' disease, Basedow's disease, exophthalmic goiter, toxic goiter, and toxic nodular goiter (toxic adenoma of the thyroid). The cause of hyperthyroidism is unknown. It has no especial geographical distribution, and it occurs at all ages. It is, however, more common in women than in men.

The excess of circulating thyroid hormone in hyperthyroidism is reflected in an elevated blood iodine level. The excess hormone increases the metabolic rate of all tissues, and there is a rise in (1) oxygen consumption, (2) basal metabolic rate (from +25 to +80 percent or more), (3) heat production, (4) caloric requirement, (5) protein catabolism, (6) vitamin requirements, (7) calcium excretion (with demineralization of the skeleton), and (8) blood flow and cardiac output. These activities place an abnormal strain on the heart and on the liver (which is the seat of much of the intermediary metabolism of foodstuffs). In addition, hyperthyroidism alters the functioning of the nervous system. In some cases there is exophthalmos which is due, at least in part, to an excess of circulating active thyrotrophin.

Hyperthyroid patients are sensitive to heat, just as hypothyroid patients are sensitive to cold. They need few clothes and little bedding. They prefer cold weather to hot. Their skin is warm and moist, and they perspire easily. Almost invariably, they have lost weight. Weakness, dyspnea, and palpitation are common complaints. The heart is overactive. The pulse rate is elevated, sometimes to an extreme degree. The systolic blood pressure is elevated; the diastolic is sometimes depressed. Gastro-intestinal motility is increased, and there may be diarrhea. In addition to being warm and moist, the skin becomes smooth and of fine texture. The hair becomes fine and silky.

Increased rapidity of mental processes, hyper-excitability, nervousness, and reduced need for sleep are the rule, especially in younger patients. There is a fine tremor, most noticeable in the tongue and extended fingers. In women, amenorrhea or oligomenorrhea is common. Osteoporosis may occur from demineralization of the skeleton. There is actual muscular weakness that may be severe enough to lead to muscle atrophy, which is often most easily noted in the temporal muscles and the interossei of the hands.

Hyperthyroidism that has been present for many years or that occurs acutely in severe form in older individuals may lead to auricular fibrillation, angina pectoris, or congestive heart failure. These may be the presenting symptoms; sometimes they are severe enough to mask the true underlying cause.

In some patients, the symptoms of hyperthyroidism may resemble those of chronic mild alcoholic intoxication, and the patient may resent bitterly any suggestion that he is ill in spite of unmistakable eye signs, goiter, and nervous phenomena.

At one extreme of the clinical picture is acute hyperthyroidism (Graves' disease), which tends to occur in young adults. The thyroid gland is usually slightly enlarged and smooth, and the glandular epithelium has undergone hypertrophy (from cuboidal to columnar shape) and hyperplasia, with infolding of the follicular walls and reduction in the amount of colloid. The high blood flow in the gland is evidenced by a systolic thrill and a bruit audible through the stethoscope. The symptoms may develop in the course of a few days, but more frequently they come on gradually over a period of weeks. The onset very often follows a severe emotional shock (especially in potentially neurotic pa-

tients), an acute infection, the beginning of pregnancy, or, curiously, a rapid reduction in weight. Some have thought the disease might be activated by an excessive intake of iodine. Acute hyperthyroidism may be mild or severe. The course is variable, unpredictable, and subject to unexplainable remissions and exacerbations.

At the other extreme is the picture of toxic nodular goiter (toxic adenoma), which is most commonly seen in middle-aged women. The thyroid is usually enlarged as a whole and contains one or more palpable nodules ranging from the size of a pea to that of a table-tennis ball or larger. A bruit is not common. Under the microscope, the gland shows areas of hyperactivity and often other areas of subnormal activity; the nodules may or may not be hyperactive. The patient may consult the physician because of an exacerbation of symptoms of hyperthyroidism, the onset of pressure symptoms from the enlarged gland, or a cardiac complication. A careful history will usually disclose the presence of symptoms of varying intensity over a period of many years, with perhaps such an insidious onset that the patient can hardly set the year. Enlargement of the thyroid may have been noted for a long period before symptoms occurred.

Between these two typical pictures, all variations may occur in such a way as to suggest that the extremes are no more than the ends of a spectrum of what is essentially a single disease process.

In a full-blown case, the diagnosis of hyperthyroidism may be obvious at a glance: the stare; the warm, moist, flushed skin; the alertness and tremor; the fullness in the neck. In less obvious cases, all aspects of the history and physical examination may have to be evaluated. The physical findings are more important than the history. The more significant signs are eye signs, if present (stare, widening of the palpebral fissure, lid lag, poor convergence, conjunctival edema, puffiness of the eyelids); firm enlargement of the thyroid (smooth or nodular), and especially the presence of thrill or bruit; fine tremor of the tongue and extremities; evidence of weight loss with history of good appetite; overactive heart with evidence of increased blood flow (see p. 65).

The basal metabolic rate is not especially helpful in diagnosis; for when it is extremely high, the diagnosis can usually be made without it, and when it is only moderately elevated, there are other conditions which might be responsible (see p. 253). A subnormal blood cholesterol level is of some weight, but a normal cholesterol is of no diagnostic significance. A high blood level of protein-bound iodine is pathognomonic; however, the determination is tedious and difficult, and the test is not generally available. In very difficult cases, a therapeutic trial of an antithyroid drug (p. 458) may be made, but with administration of a placebo for the first two or three weeks to distinguish psychotherapeutic effects.

Hyperthyroidism may have to be differentiated from neurosis or psychoneurosis (p. 150), colloid goiter with some complicating condition, cardiovascular disease, tuberculosis, and, because of the elevated basal metabolic rate, leukemia and polycythemia vera (erythremia).

Hyperthyroidism tends to be chronic and recurrent. Remissions and exacerbations, sometimes sudden and severe, occur without apparent cause. After many years of overactivity, the gland atrophies in some patients, and myxedema sets in. In other patients, hyperthyroidism and mild hypothyroidism may alternate. Still other patients develop cardiovascular disease and die of heart failure if the hyperthyroidism remains untreated.

Treatment—The therapy of hyperthyroidism is currently being revolutionized by the antithyroid drugs; and after a further period of experience, it may again be revolutionized by radioactive iodine.

For the past twenty-five years, the treatment of choice in hyperthyroidism has been subtotal thyroidectomy. Following such an operation, 90 to 95 percent of patients have no recurrence of hyperthyroidism, although a few develop hypothyroidism which requires continued administration of thyroid. It has been the custom to administer iodine for two to three weeks before operation. Given in this way, the iodine usually induces a partial remission, converting a moderate or severe case into a mild one.

The antithyroid drugs provide a more positive and a more prolonged control of hyperthyroidism than does iodine. They are, therefore, more satisfactory in preparing the patient for operation, and they have the possibility of acting as substitutes for operation. However, until more experience is gained, subtotal thyroidectomy must be considered the treatment of choice for those patients who can and will be operated on.

In mild hyperthyroidism without disability or prostration, the patient may continue moderate and nonstimulating activities while being prepared for operation. For more severe cases with disability, bed rest should be required, but it need not be complete if the patient dislikes it. Mild sedation (p. 390) should be employed in all cases. Since

hyperthyroidism depletes the body stores, the diet should be high in calories and protein (p. 584), and there should be a supplementary intake of calcium (p. 505) and of all the vitamins (p. 483), especially those of the B group.

Operation should be performed only after all manifestations of hyperthyroidism have disappeared and the patient has recuperated from them as fully as possible, especial attention being given to the state of the liver and the cardiovascular system. In acute hyperthyroidism in a young adult, the minimum period may be as short as five weeks. In complicated cases of long standing, preparation may require several months. Maximal recuperation is extremely important because it greatly reduces operative mortality and the incidence and severity of postoperative complications.

At present, propylthiouracil is the antithyroid drug of choice in a field where new developments may take place quickly. Its dosage and administration are discussed beginning on page 459. For the last two to three weeks before operation, the patient should be given iodine; 6 to 10 mg. per day are adequate (see p. 506 for dosage forms). The iodine makes the gland easier to handle at operation.

Antithyroid drugs may be employed as medical treatment in those patients who (1) cannot be brought into proper condition for operation; (2) have recurrent hyperthyroidism following thyroidectomy; or (3) refuse operative treatment. For details, see page 459.

In some patients, exophthalmos may be associated with extreme edema of the orbit, conjunctivae, and lids. The patient may have impairment of vision and severe discomfort, if not pain. Such a condition, known as malignant exophthalmos, requires special treatment. The patient should be given thyroid as well as an antithyroid drug; and operation should be postponed until the condition is greatly improved, for it is frequently exacerbated by thyroidectomy.

Radioactive iodine, properly administered, provides localized radiation therapy which has been successful in controlling hyperthyroidism by destroying a portion of the thyroid gland. The treatment is still experimental, however, and will probably remain so for a considerable period because (1) too little is yet known of the late effects; (2) unless properly handled, radioactive iodine is extremely dangerous to the attending personnel as well as to the patient (only a few micrograms are required for complete destruction of the thyroid gland); and (3) radioactive iodine is at present available (from the U. S. Government plant at Oak Ridge, Tennessee) only in small quantities and to properly accredited research institutions.

Adrenal Cortex

The adrenal glands are small paired organs lying just cephalad to the kidneys. Their cortices are capable of producing a variety of steroid substances; some twenty-eight different steroid compounds have been extracted from them. Most of these are or are closely related to substances having principally estrogenic, androgenic, or progestational activity. However, six have activity that is considered to be peculiar to extracts of the adrenal cortex, and these may be considered as adrenocortical hormones proper. Actually, most of the activity resides in the amorphous fraction of adrenocortical extracts after the known crystalline hormones have been removed. The nature of the principles in the amorphous fraction is unknown.

Exact classification of the properties of the adrenocortical hormones is at present impossible. Two types of action are clear: one on carbohydrate metabolism (gluco-corticoid activity) and one on sodium and potassium metabolism (mineralo-corticoid activity).

These are shared in varying proportions by a number of compounds; in general, the actions are mutually somewhat antagonistic. A third important action of adrenal hormones is anabolic and androgenic (see Testosterone, p. 469). The principal compound secreted by the adrenals that has this property is adrenosterone, which differs chemically from testosterone (Figure 45, p. 470) only in having an oxygen atom (keto group) at the eleventh carbon atom and a keto group instead of a hydroxyl group at the seventeenth carbon atom. It appears, however, that the adrenal androgens act particularly on axillary and pubic hair growth and have possibly less effect on the penis or clitoris or on libido and sexual potency. The adrenals are the source of practically all androgen in women and about two-thirds of the androgen in men, the remainder in the latter being supplied by the testes. In addition, adrenal function is essential for the development of resistance to certain forms of stress; this type of activity is associated with gluco-corticoid properties. The actions of the adrenocortical hormones are discussed in more detail beginning on page 460.

The functional activity of the adrenal cortices is regulated by the anterior pituitary gland through secretion of adrenocorticotrophic hormone (ACTH; see p. 473). Disturbances of adrenal function may therefore be of either pituitary or adrenal origin.

ADDISON'S DISEASE

Addison's disease (hypoadrenalism, adrenal insufficiency) is a syndrome due to deficient production of adrenocortical steroids. It may be secondary to hypopituitarism (p. 193), or, more commonly, it results from disease of the adrenal glands themselves. Typically, Addison's disease is a chronic condition of insidious onset. It is usually caused by either bilateral tuberculosis of the adrenal glands or disappearance of adrenal tissue (with atrophy of the gland) of unknown origin. Uncommonly, Addison's disease may be due to destruction of both adrenals by other diseases such as syphilis, metastatic malignant tumors, or thrombosis of the adrenal blood vessels.

Lack of mineralo-corticoid hormones causes a deficiency of sodium, with resultant inability of the tissues to retain water; there is reduction in blood volume and arterial blood pressure. Deficiency of gluco-corticoids results in a lack of physical energy and a tendency toward hypoglycemia. The combined deficiency leads to the usual symptoms of Addison's disease: fatigability; lack of energy; weakness; tendency toward dizziness, syncopal attacks, and circulatory failure; gastro-intestinal disturbances, such as anorexia, hiccups, nausea, vomiting, and constipation or diarrhea; attacks of mild or severe epigastric pain (solar crises); psychic and emotional disturbances; changes in hearing and vision; and weight loss.

In many but not all cases, the skin gradually assumes a peculiar smoky, brownish color which may progress almost to black. The pigmentation, which is due to an abnormal amount of the normal pigment, melanin, is deepest in those areas most exposed to light, pressure, or friction (e.g., the face, neck, backs of the hands, thighs and knees). The mucous and serous membranes (and even the retina) may also become pigmented. In the mouth, the pigmentation is usually in the form of bluish or grayish-black spots on the lips, tongue, gums, and buccal mucosa.

In well-developed cases, the patient is listless and apathetic. The heart is small and feeble in action. The systolic blood pressure is less than 100 mm. Hg and may be less than 80. The lymphoid tissue (lymph glands, tonsils, thymus) tends to be enlarged. Axillary and pubic hair growth is sparse or absent. Body temperature tends to be low. The basal metabolism is often moderately subnormal.

The fasting blood sugar is low (60 to 70 mg. per 100 cc.), there is increased dextrose tolerance (see p. 533), and there is extreme sensitivity to Insulin. The plasma levels of sodium and chloride are reduced, whereas that of potassium is increased. There is often a mild hyperchromic anemia and sometimes lymphocytosis.

Diagnosis—In early or mild cases, the diagnosis of Addison's disease may be difficult. A number of laboratory procedures have been proposed as diagnostic aids. In the "water test" of Robinson, Power, and Kepler, the patient eats three ordinary meals the day before the test but takes no extra salt. After 6 p.m. he eats and drinks nothing. At 10:30 p.m., he empties his bladder and discards the urine. All urine passed during the night is saved, as is that from a special voiding at 7:30 a.m. The volume of night urine is measured, and it is saved for possible chemical examination.

The patient eats no breakfast, and he remains in bed except when he arises to empty his bladder. At 8:30 he voids again, and he is at once given a volume of water equal to 20 cc. per Kg. (9 cc. per lb.) of body weight, which he is to drink within the following forty-five minutes. If possible, he voids also at 9:30, 10:30, 11:30, and 12:30. Each specimen is kept in a separate container, and the volume of the largest voiding is measured. If the patient cannot void every hour, a maximum hourly volume is calculated from a two-hour specimen.

If the volume of any single hourly specimen voided during the morning is larger than the entire volume passed during the night, the response to the test is said to be negative, and the chances are great that the patient has normal adrenal cortical function. If the volume of the largest hourly specimen is less than the night volume, the test is considered positive, and a second procedure is indicated.

For the second procedure, blood is drawn (preferably under oil) while the patient is still fasting, and the plasma content of urea and chloride is determined. The night urine specimen is also analyzed for these constituents. These values and the results of the urine volume determinations are then substituted in the following equation:

$$A = \frac{\text{urea in night urine (mg./100 cc.)}}{\text{urea in plasma (mg./100 cc.)}} \times$$
$$\frac{\text{chloride in plasma (mg./100 cc.)}}{\text{chloride in night urine (mg./100 cc.)}} \times$$
$$\frac{\text{maximum hourly vol. day urine (cc.)}}{\text{entire vol. night urine (cc.)}}$$

If the numerical value of A is greater than 30, the patient probably has normal adrenal cortical function. If the value of A is less than 25, the patient probably has Addison's disease, provided that nephritis can be excluded. If the value of A is between 25 and 30 or if the procedures are negative in the face of strong clinical evidence of Addison's disease, the more reliable potassium-resistance test of Cutler, Power, and Wilder (J. A. M. A., 111: 117, 1938) may be employed. However, the potassium-resistance test carries a definite risk to the patient with Addison's disease, and the physician undertaking it must be prepared to treat an Addisonian crisis.

Another possible diagnostic measure is administration of adrenocorticotrophic hormone. No food is eaten after 8 p.m. the night before the test. Water is taken as desired. On the day of the test, 200 cc. of water are ingested at 6 a.m., 8 a.m., and 10 a.m. The patient empties his bladder at 6 and at 8 a.m.; the second voiding is saved. Immediately after the voiding at 8 a.m., venous blood is drawn for an eosinophil count, oxalate being used as anticoagulant, and the patient is given 25 mg. of purified adrenocorticotrophic hormone intramuscularly. The patient voids again at 9 a.m. and at 12 m., and the second specimen is saved. Blood is taken at noon for a second eosinophil count.

The two urine specimens are analyzed for uric acid and creatinine, and the change in uric-acid-creatinine ratio is calculated. The oxalated blood is drawn into a white-cell-counting pipette as for a white cell count, but a special diluting fluid is employed which contains 5 percent of a 2 percent aqueous eosin solution and 5 percent acetone (v/v) in distilled water. The mixture is filtered and stored under refrigeration. The pipette is shaken not too vigorously. A Levy counting chamber is employed, and the count is made after the fluid has stood in the chamber for three minutes to allow staining. With this procedure, the eosinophils appear dark red against a pink background; the other white cells are colorless. From eosinophil counts of the two blood specimens, the percent decrease is calculated.

If the eosinophil count increases or remains the same or falls less than 20 percent, the patient has no adrenal cortical reserve, and Addison's disease is present. The normal fall is 50 to 100 percent. In normal individuals, the uric-acid-creatinine ratio increases 60 percent or more (average, 100 percent) after administration of 25 mg. adrenocorticotrophic hormone. Increases of less than normal reflect diminutions in the adrenal cortical reserve. It is important to remember that, even in normal individuals, acute stresses may call into action the full reserve power of the adrenal cortices. Under these circumstances, no additional function is possible as a response to the injected pituitary hormone. Such temporary depletions of adrenal reserve must be differentiated from the chronic depletion of Addison's disease. Clinical observation will usually distinguish such situations; they can also be suspected from unusually high initial uric-acid-creatinine ratios (above 0.55 in men and 0.7 in women).

A third test for Addison's disease is a trial of adrenocortical therapy. A great improvement in clinical and laboratory manifestations is positive evidence. Purely subjective improvement is not.

Untreated Addison's disease is ultimately fatal, but the course is subject to remissions and exacerbations. A striking feature is inability of the organism to meet the stresses of trauma, excessive exertion, infection, solar and roentgen irradiation, intoxications of various sorts, malnutrition, extremes of temperature, and drugs (see p. 462). Addisonian patients are particularly susceptible to thyroid substance, sedatives such as barbiturates, morphine and its analogues, cathartics, and Insulin; and these drugs should be employed very cautiously in patients having inadequate adrenal cortical function. Surgical operations are to be avoided insofar as possible. In Addison's disease, stresses such as the above are likely to precipitate crises which may prove fatal unless immediately and vigorously treated. During such crises, all manifestations are greatly increased, although one or another phase may be most prominent. Patients may die of hypoglycemia, renal insufficiency, or dehydration.

Secondary hypoadrenalism may occur in otherwise normal individuals as a result of the stresses listed above, especially burns and severe infections. Severe acute adrenal insufficiency is most often seen in fulminating meningococcic septicemia, in which it is often termed the "Waterhouse-Friderichsen syndrome." There are usually hemorrhages into the adrenals, but their significance is controversial. The disease was formerly fatal, but some patients have recovered following vigorous chemotherapy and adrenocortical replacement therapy.

The prognosis in Addison's disease is always uncertain because of several unpredictable factors: (1) the difficulty in meeting the fluctuating body needs, (2) the danger of sudden overwhelming crisis, and (3) the underlying disease (e.g., tuberculosis), which may be resistant to treatment.

Treatment—The aim of treatment in Addison's disease is restoration of normal body function by regulating the intake of sodium, potassium, and carbohydrate and by supplying the deficient hormones. Of course, any underlying disease should be treated.

Mild cases can be controlled fairly satisfactorily by regulation of the diet plus administration of sodium salts. The intake of potassium should be low (foods highest in potassium include meat, fish, meat extract [meat soups], potatoes, nuts, legumes, greens [including lettuce], bananas, cereals, cocoa, lemons, limes, mushrooms, molasses, and honey). Sodium salts should be taken in amounts of 5 to 20 Gm. daily—as enteric-coated tablets of sodium chloride, as sodium bicarbonate, as sodium chloride and sodium citrate in lemonade, or as a combination of these. The diet should be high in carbohydrate, and there should be frequent feedings. A bedtime feeding is especially important as a protection against nocturnal hypoglycemia.

For more complete control and in those more severe cases in which regulation of mineral intake is grossly inadequate, hormonal replacement is in order. Potent adrenocortical extracts are available, or the physician may administer desoxycorticosterone. The use of these preparations is described on pages 463 and 460. Theoretically, the combination of desoxycorticosterone and a gluco-corticoid such as cortisone (p. 462) should be extremely effective. However, there is some difference of opinion as to the value of cortisone which will doubtless be resolved by further study.

Many men with Addison's disease show evidence of hypogonadism as well as hypoadrenalism. Even after adequate adrenal therapy, the secondary sexual characteristics may be deficient and the patient may lack normal vigor and well-being. In such cases, the administration of testosterone usually results in more improvement than is obtained from adrenal therapy alone. It also allows reduction in dosage of desoxycorticosterone or adrenocortical extract. The dosage of testosterone is the same as for primary hypogonadism (p. 191). Testosterone therapy may be of value in women also, although in smaller doses.

In spite of the best treatment now possible, Addisonian patients must be protected against physical stresses of all kinds (for enumeration, see p. 462). They are "brittle" and are easily thrown into crisis by stress.

The patient in crisis should be kept warm and at absolute rest in bed. Until improvement occurs, he should receive 20 to 100 cc. of a potent adrenocortical extract intravenously every three or four hours and 1 to 2 liters of 5 percent dextrose in isotonic sodium chloride solution by the same route every eight to twelve hours. As his condition improves, the dosage of extract is reduced and it is given intramuscularly, and sodium and carbohydrate are given by mouth. Desoxycorticosterone alone is of less value in crisis than is extract, because it is slower in action and has no effect on carbohydrate metabolism. However, a single intramuscular dose of 10 to 20 mg. in oil is usually given at the beginning of the treatment of crisis as a supplement to extract, and smaller doses may be given daily thereafter. When surgical operation is necessary, the patient is fortified with sodium and extract for several days before and after.

CUSHING'S SYNDROME

The rare condition now known as Cushing's syndrome has long been recognized; only recently is it beginning to be understood. Its immediate cause appears to be an oversupply of the gluco-corticoid hormones of the adrenal cortex; this oversupply may be the result of primary adrenal overactivity or of adrenal hypersecretion secondary to excessive pituitary output of ACTH. Attention was focused on the syndrome by Harvey Cushing, who attributed it to basophilic adenoma of the anterior pituitary gland. When it is associated with either basophilic or mixed pituitary tumor, it is known as Cushing's disease. The same clinical picture may, however, also be associated with tumors of the adrenal cortex or thymus or with lesions of the hypothalamus, or it may occur without apparent associations. There is disagreement as to whether the associated pituitary tumors are causes or effects of the adrenal cortical hyperactivity.

Cushing's syndrome is characterized by profound disturbances of protein, fat, carbohydrate, and calcium metabolism. The skeleton becomes demineralized, the vertebrae collapse, and the spine loses its lumbar lordosis and develops a thoracic kyphosis. The resultant shortening of the neck and trunk makes the neck thicker; the ribs are elevated, producing a barrel chest; and the abdomen protrudes and is often striated from the relatively rapid increase in circumference. The face becomes round and fat (moonface), whereas the extremities usually become or remain thin (from muscle atrophy due to deficient protein anabolism). The result is the so-called buffalo appearance.

The sugar tolerance in Cushing's syndrome is low, and the blood sugar is high. In some cases

diabetes mellitus develops; when it does, it is usually Insulin-resistant. A few patients are obese, but most have subnormal fat deposits. The tendency toward excessive conversion of protein to carbohydrate (the result of the oversupply of gluco-corticoids) results in muscular atrophy and fatigability. Other common features are polycythemia (with plethora), hypertension (possibly secondary to increased blood volume due to the polycythemia), cardiac enlargement, tendency toward ecchymosis, and hypogonadism (amenorrhea or impotence). Either the gluco-corticoids themselves or an associated oversupply of adrenal androgens (for the unusual properties of which, see p. 183) leads to hirsutism and acne vulgaris (p. 231). At the same time there is hypogonadism (amenorrhea or loss of libido and potency). Often there is overproduction of mineralo-corticoids as well as gluco-corticoids. Sometimes the patient presents a mixed picture of Cushing's syndrome and acromegaly (p. 193). Hyperthyroidism is a frequent complication.

Cushing's syndrome tends to run a chronic course with spontaneous remissions. Death is commonly due to the complications of hypertensive cardiovascular disease, diabetes mellitus, or intercurrent infection.

Treatment—No certain method of control is known. In some cases, x-ray therapy of the pituitary region leads to considerable improvement. When adrenal tumors are present, their removal may be followed by prolonged or even permanent remission. Sometimes bilateral partial resection of hyperplastic adrenal glands is beneficial. Testosterone may lead to symptomatic improvement, but its ultimate usefulness has not been established.

ADRENOGENITAL SYNDROME

The adrenogenital syndrome (adrenal virilism) appears to result from overproduction of adreno-cortical steroids, particularly androgens. It tends to run in families and is more common in women (5:1) than in men. The ultimate cause is unknown in most instances. The pathological changes in the adrenal cortex include simple hyperplasia, adenoma (often in the form of multiple small tumors), or primary carcinoma. Sometimes the changes occur in accessory adrenocortical tissue, as in the so-called hypernephroma of the ovary. There may be associated pituitary adenomata (usually basophilic).

The clinical picture in adrenogenital syndrome depends to a certain extent on the age at onset. When it begins during fetal life, it is likely to produce pseudohermaphroditism in girls. When it begins during childhood, there is precocious puberty; girls may or may not develop pseudohermaphroditism (depending apparently on the relative supply of androgen and estrogen); boys do not. In adult women, pseudohermaphroditism is common; it may occur in men but is rare. Naturally, the degree of sexual change is greatest when the onset is early. In a few instances, adrenal carcinoma may secrete mostly estrogen. Such tumors lead to pseudohermaphroditism in men.

In addition to the sexual changes, the adrenogenital syndrome is characterized by the features of Cushing's syndrome, with the difference that there is a greater tendency to obesity in the former. In children, there is likely to be precocious bodily as well as sexual development.

The diagnosis is based on the clinical manifestations, evidence of a lesion in the adrenal region (palpable tumor or x-ray visualization of adrenal hypertrophy by injection of air into the renal capsule), and detection of an excess of adrenocortical hormones in the urine (at present a research-laboratory procedure). The disease must be distinguished from arrhenoblastoma, ovarian hypernephroma, luteomas and Leydig-cell tumors of the ovary, Cushing's syndrome, and tumors of the hypothalamus, pineal body, and thymus.

Treatment—If a tumor can be demonstrated or even suspected in the adrenal region, exploratory operation should be performed, and both adrenals should be inspected. The prognosis of malignant tumors depends in large part on the promptness of their removal. The surgeon is, of course, more reluctant to operate when the symptoms are mild or of long duration or when the onset is in adult life. In the presence of a single hyperfunctioning adenoma or an early carcinoma, removal of the tumor or of the involved adrenal may be curative. In the absence of tumors or in the presence of multiple benign adenomata, adrenal resection is of little value. Bilateral adrenalectomy appears to be inadvisable under any circumstances.

The patient should be given intensive adrenal therapy for a few days before operation in the same way as if he had Addison's disease (p. 183). If a tumor or one adrenal is removed, adrenal therapy should be continued postoperatively. In such cases, the uninvolved adrenal is usually so atrophic that it cannot resume normal function at once, and lack of pretreatment may be followed by an Addisonian crisis.

Aside from surgery, treatment is symptomatic. Pseudohermaphroditism presents a difficult psychic problem. Usually the best total results are achieved by whatever plastic or hormonal therapy may be of assistance in making the patient conform physically and hormonally to the sex to which he had previously thought he belonged.

Adrenal Medulla

The adrenal medullae are small paired organs, each of which is enfolded within an adrenal cortex lying just cephalad to the kidney. Embryologically and functionally, they are part of the autonomic nervous system. They are innervated by preganglionic adrenergic (sympathetic) fibers from the great splanchnic nerves, and their cells correspond to those found in paravertebral ganglia. The function of the adrenal medulla is to secrete epinephrine under adrenergic stimulation, with the apparent biological purpose of reinforcing the effect of general adrenergic stimulation. The release of epinephrine normally occurs only during emotional stress, as in fear or anger. Epinephrine does not circulate constantly and is not a factor in the normal regulation of blood pressure; its actions are discussed on page 422.

PHEOCHROMOCYTOMA

Pheochromocytoma is a tumor composed of the characteristic chromaffin cells of the adrenal medulla (the term means literally "a tumor composed of cells which stain dark"). It may occur in the adrenal medulla or in association with a sympathetic ganglion (when it is called a "paraganglioma"). It may appear at any age but is most common between twenty and forty. Tumors vary from 1 to 12 cm. or more in diameter; they are commonly multiple, and 10 percent are malignant. They may contain extremely large amounts of epinephrine which is suddenly released into the blood by physical pressure on the tumor or through unknown mechanisms. In the case of tumors located in the adrenal, epinephrine may be liberated by massage from repeated deep breathing, bending over, or even palpation of the abdomen by the physician.

The characteristic clinical feature of pheochromocytoma is attacks of paroxysmal hypertension associated with pounding headache, hyperglycemia (and sometimes glycosuria), tremor, palpitation, hyperhidrosis, and, in extreme cases, convulsions or collapse. An attack is, of course, due to sudden release into the circulation of large quantities of epinephrine. In some cases epinephrine is liberated continuously, producing sustained hypertension.

This occurs most often in children and late in the course of previously undiagnosed cases in adults. The clinical picture may resemble hyperthyroidism (p. 180), including elevation of basal metabolic rate and mild exophthalmos.

Unless the physician is aware of the clinical picture in pheochromocytoma, the diagnosis will be missed. The disease should be ruled out in any case of hypertension or of paroxysmal attacks with suggestive symptomatology. The diagnosis is based on two types of procedures: reproduction of an attack by mechanical means, and termination by administration of an adrenergic blocking agent. Sometimes the patient will have discovered a maneuver or a posture which precipitates an attack; if not, the physician may try massage of each flank separately and of the paravertebral areas deep in the abdomen. Of course, these attempts will fail if the tumor is a thoracic paraganglioma. Benodaine is probably at present the drug of choice for termination of an attack (see p. 432 for details); tetraethylammonium compounds (p. 433) may also be employed.

If the tumor or tumors are in the adrenal glands, they can often be visualized by means of x-ray. Sometimes it is necessary to inject air into the adipose capsule of each kidney (but not at the same session); this is a specialized and somewhat hazardous procedure.

Pheochromocytoma must be distinguished from glomerulonephritis and coarctation of the aorta (especially in children), hypertension, hyperthyroidism, diabetes mellitus, anxiety states, tabetic crises, and, if convulsions occur, from epilepsy, brain tumor, and eclampsia (see also p. 212).

Treatment of pheochromocytoma consists in surgical removal of the tumors. Special precautions are necessary to minimize squeezing of the tumors, and expert employment of vasodilator or antiadrenergic drugs may control blood pressure during the operation. However, the blood pressure may fall to dangerously low levels as soon as the last tumor has been removed, and large amounts of systemic vasoconstrictors (p. 362) may be required to raise it, particularly if antiadrenergic drugs have previously been given. The first two or three postoperative days may be stormy.

Ovary

The ovaries (the female gonads) are paired organs attached to the upper and outer corners of the broad ligaments in the pelvis. They occur only in females and have the dual function of producing ova and secreting estrogens (p. 463) and progesterone (p. 468). They apparently secrete small and rather constant amounts of estrogens until the age of eight, when estrogen production begins to increase gradually. About a year and a half before the onset of menstruation, production becomes cyclic, with gradual increase in When estrogen withdrawal at the er becomes sufficiently rapid and exte bleeding takes place, and the mena rived. After a variable number of cycles (see p. 202), ovulation and cor formation begin. The mechanism of th cycle is discussed on page 202. The av the menarche is thirteen to fourteen years, but the normal range includes ten to sixteen or possibly eighteen years. Development of the female reproductive tract and secondary sexual characteristics is dependent on the supply of estrogen from the ovaries.

Ovarian function takes place only under stimulation by the gonadotrophic hormones of the anterior pituitary gland. When these are not released, or if they are released in inappropriate quantities or at inopportune intervals, ovarian function will be absent or abnormal. Ovarian hyperfunction has never been recognized as a clinical entity. Various types of hypofunction occur; they are discussed below and also under Menstrual Disturbances (p. 202).

Obviously, ovarian insufficiency may be due to lack of pituitary stimulation or to intrinsic ovarian failure. Eventually, the ovaries of all women become refractory to gonadotrophic stimulation and ovarian function ceases (for discussion, see Menopause, p. 206).

OVARIAN AGENESIS

Sometimes ovarian tissue fails to develop in the fetus, and the ovaries are consequently absent. This uncommon condition is known as ovarian agenesis. Typically, the patient of adult years is short (average height, 4 ft., 9 in.) and has a juvenile body contour, with complete lack of breast development and only scanty axillary and pubic hair. There is primary amenorrhea (see p. 205).

The condition is to be distinguished from cretinism or juvenile myxedema (by normal mentality), from other types of dwarfism (in which sexual development may be normal), and from primary pituitary failure (by the presence of relatively large quantities of gonadotrophins in the urine). Ovarian agenesis may be associated with the following congenital anomalies, in which case it is known as Turner's syndrome: webbed neck, genu valgum, and increase in the carrying angle at the elbow.

Treatment consists in administration of estrogen for the purpose of stimulating further skeletal growth (if the epiphyses of the long bones have not closed, as determined by x-ray), causing maturation of the sexual organs and secondary sexual characteristics, and keeping the patient in proper nitrogen balance. Initially, rather large doses are required, such as 5 mg. of diethylstilbestrol daily by mouth. After satisfactory growth and sexual maturation have occurred (usually after six to eight months), the dose is reduced to about 0.5 mg. daily. Estrogen administration should be continued until forty or forty-five years of age, when discontinuation will mimic the natural climacteric. Of course, estrogen therapy is not likely to cause periodic flow simulating menstruation. If the patient is extremely desirous of experiencing cyclic uterine bleeding, estrogen and progesterone can be administered as outlined under Amenorrhea (p. 205).

HYPOGONADISM (FEMALE)

When it is not due to ovarian agenesis, hypogonadism in women is usually caused by failure of gonadotrophin secretion. The effects of hypogonadism depend on whether the condition begins before or after puberty. *Postpuberal* hypogonadism results in menstrual disturbances. Mild degrees may produce functional uterine bleeding; more severe degrees cause amenorrhea (p. 205). *Prepuberal* hypogonadotrophic hypogonadism disturbs both growth and sexual development. Sexual development is deficient or may be absent as in ovarian agenesis. In contrast to patients with ovarian agenesis, however, individuals with prepuberal hypogonadotrophic hypogonadism are usually tall and have a boyish (eunuchoid) rather than a childlike configuration. Urinary gonadotrophin excretion is subnormal (an important diagnostic point). The ovaries are present but are unstimulated.

Treatment should theoretically be administration of anterior pituitary gonadotrophins. These rarely give satisfactory results (for discussion, see p. 472), and it is usually necessary to rely on estrogen substitution therapy, as in ovarian agenesis. In contrast to the latter condition, estrogen usually causes prompt closure of epiphyses in patients of adult age with prepuberal hypogonadotrophic hypogonadism.

Testis

The testes are paired organs which are suspended in the scrotum, apparently for the purpose of allowing them to function at a temperature somewhat lower than that of the rest of the body. It has been demonstrated that raising the temperature of the testes inhibits their function. The testes have two functions: the production of androgen (p. 469) by the Leydig cells and the formation of spermatozoa by the germinal epithelium of the seminiferous tubules.

Before adolescence, androgen production is at a low level and spermatozoa are not formed. At the beginning of puberty, the testes respond to gonadotrophic hormones; follicle-stimulating hormone causes sperm formation, and luteinizing hormone stimulates androgen production. Development of the male reproductive tract and secondary sexual characteristics and sexual potency are dependent on a supply of androgen normally provided by the testes.

Testicular hyperfunction is extremely rare; it may be part of the picture of hyperpituitarism (see Pituitary Gigantism, p. 193, and Acromegaly, p. 193), or it may be due to Leydig-cell tumor or to unknown causes. Testicular hypofunction (male hypogonadism) is well known; it may be due to lack of pituitary stimulation or to intrinsic testicular failure.

HYPOGONADISM (MALE)

The male hypogonadal syndromes may be classified as to (1) whether they begin before or after puberty and (2) whether gonadal failure is primary in the testes or is secondary to pituitary failure.

Prepuberal Testicular Failure may be due to aplasia, castration, or destruction of both testes by disease. It is characterized by eunuchism or eunuchoidism (incomplete eunuchism). In severe prepuberal hypogonadism, sexual development does not take place. The genitalia remain small. Libido and potentia are lacking. Spermatogenesis does not occur. There is delay in epiphyseal closure, and the limb bones grow to extraordinary length, producing a disproportion between trunk and limbs and sometimes unusual height (eunuchoid gigantism). The general body proportions, lack of muscular development, and, in those cases that are obese, distribution of fat to hips and breasts resemble those of childhood or may carry a suggestion of femininity. The voice retains a high pitch, and the thyroid cartilage of the larynx lacks the size and prominence characteristic of the adult male. The skin is dry and fine in texture; the beard is composed only of fine hair; pubic and axillary hair are absent or scanty; and the scalp hairline fails to recede in adult years.

The condition is distinguished from other forms of eunuchoidism by (1) lack of testes in the scrotum, (2) gynecomastia (gross or microscopic), (3) a high titer of gonadotrophin in the urine, and (4) failure of response to chorionic gonadotrophin (see below).

The most common form of prepuberal hypogonadism (known as Klinefelter's syndrome) involves failure principally in function of the seminiferous tubules. It often goes unrecognized because it is accompanied by minimal or only moderate degrees of eunuchoidism. Diagnosis is based on (1) atrophic testes (often as small as Lima beans), (2) gynecomastia (gross or microscopic), (3) high urinary gonadotrophin excretion, and (4) presence of some (although incomplete) sexual development and maturation.

Prepuberal Hypogonadotrophic Hypogonadism is due to lack of pituitary gonadotrophin secretion (p. 472). Puberty fails to occur, and the patient presents the features of eunuchoidism (see above). The following points serve to distinguish this type from other forms: (1) The testes are present in the scrotum but are smaller than normal although larger than in Klinefelter's syndrome (see above); (2) urinary gonadotrophin excretion is subnormal; (3) there is no gross or microscopic evidence of gynecomastia; and (4) there is favorable response to a therapeutic test with chorionic gonadotrophin.

For the therapeutic test, chorionic gonadotrophin (p. 472) is given intramuscularly in doses of 750 International Units twice daily for three weeks. If maturation is initiated (increase in size of the testes, penis, and scrotum and slight pubic hair development), the patient is a hypogonadotrophic eunuchoid. If no change occurs, it may be assumed that the testes are unresponsive.

Delayed Puberty in Boys—When puberty seems merely to be delayed—that is, when development has appeared to progress normally to the threshold of puberty and when there is no obvious damage to the testes—several considerations are pertinent. There is no uniform age for the onset of puberty, and there is as yet no sure means of foretelling which boys will mature late but fully and which ones will never mature properly. Against premature

or unnecessary treatment are the observations that (1) a large percentage of boys with a less than average degree of sexual maturation do eventually mature; (2) large amounts of androgens may induce premature closure of the epiphyses and thus limit height; and (3) administration of androgen tends to diminish testicular function, and administration of chorionic gonadotrophin tends to reduce gonadotrophin secretion by the anterior pituitary—both of which actions are undesirable when pituitary-gonadal function is on the low side of normal.

The only defects in hypogonadism which become irreversible with the passage of time are those of the skeleton. It would thus seem wise to withhold endocrine treatment until perhaps the age of sixteen unless it becomes evident earlier that sexual development will be so delayed as to result in skeletal abnormalities. Only rarely should the psychological problem of physical difference from the patient's associates force the issue.

Adult Testicular Failure—Complete testicular failure beginning in adult life is usually due to bilateral destruction of the testes by trauma or disease (such as mumps or syphilis) or to surgical removal. The resulting eunuchism is not accompanied by changes in the skeleton (as distinguished from the effects of prepuberal hypogonadism), because the epiphyses are already closed. The secondary sexual characteristics show regression, but the larynx and genitalia do not diminish in size, except for the scrotum, which tends to shrink and to lose its pigment. The voice retains its adult character, and a more or less limited degree of sexual desire and ability may remain, with considerable variation among patients. The skin becomes soft and of a pasty color because of loss of cutaneous pigment, and it tans less easily on exposure to ultraviolet radiation. In older men, it contains many fine wrinkles. In most areas of the skin, blood flow is diminished. Hot flushes, lack of energy, weakness, and emotional disturbances may occur, similar to those in some menopausal women.

There is controversy over the existence of a climacteric in men corresponding to the menopause in women. If such a syndrome occurs in men, it certainly is not physiological, as it is in women; for decline in testicular function (as evidenced by increased urinary gonadotrophins, reduced androgen excretion, and histological changes in the testes) does not generally begin until the seventh decade of life, and there is no evidence of an abrupt decline at any certain age range which would in any way be analogous to the menopause.

Series of cases have been reported in which men patients presented symptoms falling into the following categories: sexual—diminution of libido and potentia; constitutional—weakness, fatigue, muscle pains or cramps, arthralgia, various gastro-intestinal and abdominal complaints, and weight loss; vasomotor—hot flushes, sweating, chilliness, palpitation, and headache; psychic—nervousness, irritability, depression, inability to concentrate, paresthesias, pruritus, and so on; and urinary—decreased force and size of stream, frequency, and hesitancy. It is clear that these symptoms go well beyond those commonly associated with complete cessation of testicular function, as by castration. Furthermore, many such patients have evidence of normal testicular function (normal gonadotrophin excretion and testicular biopsy). Evidently the syndrome which has been termed "the male climacteric" may in some patients be associated with hypogonadism, whereas in others it is not. In the latter instances, it is presumably of neurotic origin. In the absence of facilities for urinary gonadotrophin assay, presumptive diagnosis can be made by a careful history plus a therapeutic test. The important points are as follows:

1. Character of symptoms. Hypogonadal men tend to have hot flushes (although 40 percent do not) and a symptomatology similar to that of the menopause, whereas those with normal testicular function tend to have symptoms more suggestive of neurosis (see p. 150).

2. Mode of onset. Hypogonadism is strongly suggested by a normal past history, with onset of impotence, hot flushes, and nervousness occurring almost simultaneously over a period of a month or two. Presence of symptoms throughout adult life or their precipitation by psychic trauma suggests neurosis.

Therapeutic tests must always be applied and interpreted with caution because of the strong psychotherapeutic element inseparable from any form of treatment. In cases with history suggesting hypogonadism rather than psychoneurosis, 25 mg. of testosterone propionate may be injected intramuscularly five times weekly for two weeks. If symptoms and sexual potency are unimproved at the end of this period, it may be concluded that further androgen therapy will be ineffectual. If symptoms and sexual potency *are* improved, the next and most important parts of the test are undertaken. First, the injections are discontinued, but the patient continues to report at intervals. If symptoms do not return, no further treatment is needed, and one may conclude that the patient was not hypogonadal. If symptoms return, injections are resumed *but with a placebo.* If symptoms are relieved, it is clear that hypogonadism is not present. If symptoms are not relieved in two or

three weeks, testosterone propionate is substituted for the placebo without the patient's knowledge. Prompt relief after this change is rather strong evidence of hypogonadism and of the validity of androgenic therapy.

Adult Hypogonadotrophic Hypogonadism seldom occurs as an entity in itself; it is usually part of the picture of multiple pituitary deficiency. The features are the same as those of adult testicular failure, with the following exceptions: (1) urinary gonadotrophins are decreased rather than increased, and (2) hot flushes and other climacteric symptoms are lacking.

Treatment—In *prepuberal hypogonadotrophic hypogonadism*, if the therapeutic test with chorionic gonadotrophin is positive (see p. 190), that preparation may be continued in the same dosage (750 International Units intramuscularly twice daily) for an additional two months. For the following four months, the same individual doses may be continued once daily. A six months' rest period is then allowed, during which the patient is followed to ascertain whether maturation progresses spontaneously. If it does, no further treatment is needed. If it does not, courses may be repeated as may be necessary. In *adult hypogonadotrophic hypogonadism*, chorionic gonadotrophin may be tried, and in a few instances it may restore or improve fertility. In many patients, however, androgen therapy (p. 469) may prove more satisfactory.

In *primary testicular failure*, either prepuberal or adult, gonadotrophin administration is useless. Androgens should be administered, as set forth on page 470.

Anterior Pituitary

The anterior pituitary gland (adenohypophysis, anterior hypophysis) occupies the anterior part of the sella turcica of the sphenoid bone at the base of the skull. It secretes a number of hormones; those which are known are listed below. It will be noted that, with the exception of the growth and lactogenic hormones, all of them have other endocrine glands as their sole target organs.

1. Growth (somatotrophic hormone, STH)
2. Follicle-stimulating gonadotrophic (FSH, thylakentrin)
3. Luteinizing gonadotrophic (LH, interstitial-cell-stimulating hormone, ICSH, metakentrin)
4. Luteotrophic gonadotrophic (LTH, lactogenic hormone, prolactin)
5. Thyrotrophic (TTH, TSH)
6. Adrenocorticotrophic (ACTH)

These hormones are discussed beginning on page 471. In man, the epithelial cells of the anterior pituitary are of three types:

1. Acidophil cells (oxyphil cells, alpha cells), which contain acidophilic granules in their cytoplasm. They comprise about 37 percent of the total epithelial cells and are believed to secrete the growth hormone and possibly one of the gonadotrophins.

2. Basophil cells (beta cells), which contain basophilic cytoplasmic granules. They constitute about 11 percent of the epithelial cells and are believed to secrete adrenocorticotrophin and some of the gonadotrophins.

3. Chromophobe cells (chief cells), which stain with difficulty. They comprise about 50 percent of the epithelial cells and are thought to be precursors of the other two types.

The mechanism by which the anterior pituitary is stimulated to release its hormones is not understood. It has, however, been established that the secretion of ACTH in response to stress occurs by way of certain regions of the hypothalamus which release a hormone or hormones which in turn cause the pituitary to release ACTH. It appears likely that similar complex mechanisms exist for other pituitary factors.

The clinical features of disturbed anterior pituitary function may be extremely varied because of the relative independence of the secretion of the different hormones. The clinical picture depends not only on the age of the patient at onset but also on which hormones are deficient and which are being produced in excess.

PITUITARY DWARFISM

Pituitary dwarfism (prepuberal panhypopituitarism, Lorain-Levi syndrome) is characterized by lack of growth, sexual infantilism, low basal metabolic rate, low blood pressure, hypoglycemia, low resistance to stress—in short, by what would be expected when the growth, gonadotrophic, thyrotrophic, and adrenocorticotrophic hormones of the anterior pituitary are deficient during childhood.

Treatment is not uniformly satisfactory. A trial of growth-hormone preparations (p. 471) is worth while. Growth as well as maturation may be accelerated by administration of chorionic gonadotrophin (p. 472) in boys and an estrogen (p. 463) in girls (a suitable dose of diethylstilbestrol is 0.5 to 1 mg. daily by mouth). Thyrotrophic hormone (p. 473) may be tried, but usually growth and body metabolism are more easily accelerated by administration of thyroid as in juvenile hypothyroidism (see p. 457). In instances in which adrenal failure becomes a problem, adrenocorticotrophic hormone (p. 473) may be employed, or the patient may be treated as for Addison's disease (p. 183).

SIMMONDS' DISEASE

Simmonds' disease (adult panhypopituitarism, hypophyseal cachexia) is due to destruction of most or all of the anterior pituitary gland. It is the adult analogue of pituitary dwarfism (see above). The condition is characterized by a combination of symptoms due to secondary failure of the various target organs of the anterior pituitary hormones. Perhaps the commonest cause of Simmonds' disease is anoxic necrosis of the pituitary during shock, particularly the shock of severe postpartum hemorrhage. Less commonly, it is caused by tumors, emboli, thrombi, cysts, or inflammatory lesions of the pituitary.

The symptoms are weight loss, asthenia (sometimes of late onset), amenorrhea in women (an early occurrence), loss of libido and potency in men, psychic changes (apathy, dullness, drowsiness, confusion or disorientation, and depression), and anorexia (frequent but not universal). The physical findings include emaciation, premature senility (in about half), loss of axillary or pubic hair or both (in 80 percent), genital atrophy or infantilism (in about half), loss of hair of eyebrows, scalp, and beard (in about half), and subnormal body temperature (not universal). The basal metabolic rate is low (−20 to −45 percent), the fasting blood sugar is low, and there is often slight anemia.

Differential diagnosis may be difficult. Other causes of cachexia (except gross undernutrition) are not commonly associated with a low basal metabolism. Addison's disease (p. 183) or myxedema (p. 178) may appear somewhat similar. If the usual diagnostic criteria of these diseases do not suffice, a therapeutic trial of desoxycorticosterone or thyroid substance is usually definitive; neither one alone causes any improvement in Simmonds' disease, and the patient may be made worse temporarily.

Anorexia nervosa may present a very similar picture. The diagnosis of Simmonds' disease is favored by an onset postpartum or following a severe infection, alteration in the x-ray appearance of the sella turcica (in about 40 percent of cases of Simmonds' disease), atrophy of the breasts, loss of axillary and pubic hair, premature senility, and pallor. In addition, very few patients with Simmonds' disease improve under therapy; most patients with anorexia nervosa do. Anorexia nervosa almost never occurs in men, and the women who have it are usually young; Simmonds' disease generally occurs in older individuals. Psychopathic disturbances are more common in anorexia nervosa.

Treatment of Simmonds' disease is seldom satisfactory. Combined replacement therapy with thyroid, adrenocortical substances, and androgen may be tried and in a few cases has appeared to be beneficial. Most patients eventually die of the cachexia.

MILD HYPOPITUITARISM

Mild hypopituitarism most commonly results from adenoma of the chromophobe cells (see p. 192). The early symptoms are usually amenorrhea in women and impotence in men (secondary gonadal failure). Climacteric symptoms are rare. Later, there may be a waxy pallor and smooth whitening of the skin, loss of body hair, weakness, and intolerance to cold. The basal metabolic rate and fasting blood sugar are usually low.

As the tumor grows out of the sella turcica, it encroaches on the suprasellar structures and produces visual disturbances and symptoms (obesity, somnolence) referable to the diencephalic structures.

The condition may have to be distinguished from myxedema (p. 178) or pernicious anemia (p. 96) in its early stages. Repeated x-rays will eventually show distortion of the sella turcica.

When a tumor can be diagnosed, x-ray therapy may be given if there are no visual symptoms. Surgery is advisable if vision is disturbed. Replacement therapy, as in Simmonds' disease (see above), is generally unsatisfactory.

PITUITARY GIGANTISM

Pituitary gigantism is a disturbance of anterior pituitary function involving principally oversecretion of growth factor. When the excessive secretion begins during or continues into adult years, the result is acromegaly (see below); when the onset occurs before the epiphyses have closed, pituitary gigantism is produced. Often there is excessive production of some pituitary hormones and deficient production of others, which gives rise to a confusing clinical picture that, in addition, may change from time to time. The usual cause is an adenoma or carcinoma of the anterior pituitary involving the eosinophilic cells or a mixture of pituitary cells.

There is a generalized, symmetrical overgrowth of the skeleton and soft tissues, the individual commonly being more than seven feet tall and sometimes more than eight feet. The body proportions are normal, in contrast to eunuchoid gigantism (see p. 189). The individual is usually physically strong, alert, and intelligent. Libido and sexual

potency are generally above normal. Sometimes, however, there is deficiency of gonadotrophins, with genital hypoplasia. Occasionally, pituitary gigantism is associated with hyperthyroidism or hypothyroidism. When hypersecretion of growth hormone continues past the time when the epiphyses close, acromegaly develops (see below), and the result is an acromegalic giant.

When the cause of pituitary gigantism is a tumor, the patient is liable to suffer headaches, visual defects, dizziness, and sometimes fainting spells. In many patients, the neoplastic tissue eventually breaks down, and the picture of hypopituitarism supervenes.

Pituitary gigantism may be difficult to distinguish from the so-called primordial gigantism, apparently a hereditary functional hyperactivity without tumor. If a hypophyseal tumor can be demonstrated, the patient is considered to have pituitary rather than primordial gigantism.

X-ray treatment of the pituitary region is generally considered the best treatment. If the tumor is large enough to threaten vision, operation may be undertaken. However, the technical difficulties are usually great.

ACROMEGALY

Acromegaly is a rare disease due to hypersecretion of the growth factor of the anterior pituitary which begins or continues after the epiphyses have closed. It is thus a form of hyperpituitarism and is the adult analogue of pituitary gigantism (see above). As in pituitary gigantism, the usual cause of acromegaly is an adenoma or carcinoma of the anterior pituitary involving the eosinophilic cells or a mixture of pituitary cells. About half of the cases of acromegaly have their onset during the third decade; however, the full clinical picture may not appear before the fifth decade.

Following closure of the epiphyses, the bones cannot increase in length, and growth hormone causes appositional bone growth, particularly at the ends of the body (the "acra"), such as the jaw, nose, supraorbital ridge, hands, and feet. The soft tissues increase in bulk, too, especially the viscera and the tissues of the face, hands, and feet. The skin becomes thick and wrinkled, notably over the "acra." With the onset of acromegaly, the first thing that comes to the notice of the patient is usually that larger gloves and shoes are necessary. The hands, for instance, are not only large; they become broad (spade hands), and the fingers become thick and blunt (sausage fingers). The terminal phalanges may become "tufted." The appearance of the face is characteristic: prominent supraorbital ridges, large thick nose, heavy features with deep skin folds, large lips and tongue, and long jaw. The chin tends to turn up, and the jaw lengthens as the angle of the jaw straightens; the result is often a severe prognathism and separation of the teeth. The paranasal (especially the frontal) sinuses become greatly enlarged.

X-rays usually reveal an enlarged sella turcica. All the bones, including those of the skull, are thickened. The bodies of the vertebrae increase in anteroposterior dimensions and develop exostoses; at the same time they undergo degenerative changes which may lead to severe kyphosis.

The pituitary tumors which cause acromegaly tend to be relatively large (up to two inches in diameter), and consequently signs of increased intracranial pressure and encroachment on the optic nerves and diencephalon are common. During the period of tumor expansion, most acromegalics suffer from headaches. There may also be visual disturbances, choked optic disks, dizziness, and fainting spells. During this period there may be an increase in muscular strength and endurance and sexual potency, suggesting an overproduction of gonadotrophins. Disturbances of carbohydrate metabolism are common and may include diabetes mellitus, often in Insulin-resistant form. Pituitary hyperthyroidism may occur. Sometimes adrenocorticotrophic hormone is present in excess and leads to a mixed picture of acromegaly and Cushing's syndrome (p. 186). The pressure of the tumor may impede function of the posterior pituitary and give rise to diabetes insipidus (see below). Later in the course of acromegaly, the tumor may undergo degeneration, and hyperpituitarism is followed by hypopituitarism (p. 193).

Patients with acromegaly frequently survive thirty to fifty years without great incapacity. Sometimes the neoplasm becomes malignant and causes death through invasion and compression of the brain. More commonly, the cause of death is (1) intercurrent infection or cachexia occurring during the later hypopituitary phase, (2) diabetic coma, (3) hyperthyroidism, or (4) congestive heart failure.

As in pituitary gigantism, x-ray treatment of the pituitary region is considered the best therapy. In very large tumors which threaten vision, operation may be indicated in spite of the great technical difficulties. In the hypopituitary phase, replacement therapy may be attempted, as in Simmonds' disease (p. 192), but without optimism.

Posterior Pituitary

The posterior pituitary gland, like the adrenal medulla, is an extension of the central nervous system. It occupies the posterior portion of the sella turcica and is connected to the brain by many nerve fibers. Its function is intimately associated with that of certain portions of the hypothalamus. The posterior pituitary body and its stalk are collectively known as the neurohypophysis.

Posterior pituitary extracts possess three types of activity: vasopressor, antidiuretic, and oxytocic. These are discussed beginning on page 473. It has been established that the antidiuretic action is part of the renal mechanism for controlling salt and water balance. However, a physiological role for the vasopressor and oxytocic effects has not yet been demonstrated with certainty, even though cases have been reported in which individuals with diabetes insipidus (see below) have suffered from extreme uterine inertia during parturition.

DIABETES INSIPIDUS

Diabetes insipidus is the only disturbance of body function known to result from deficiency of posterior pituitary hormone. Sometimes it occurs without apparent cause. Other cases are secondary to injury or disease involving the hypothalamus or hypophysis. Any lesion which destroys the posterior pituitary body itself, its stalk, the tuber cinereum, or the supraoptic nuclei is followed by degeneration of the other structures mentioned; diabetes insipidus results, provided there is some degree of anterior pituitary function. It appears that total destruction of the hypophysis does not produce diabetes insipidus. The mechanism involved is unknown. Possible causative lesions in diabetes insipidus include basal skull fractures, pituitary or suprasellar tumors, chronic encephalitis, and basilar meningitis. The disease may be transient when it is secondary to infectious disease or trauma. Usually it is permanent.

The essential clinical feature of diabetes insipidus is polyuria (usually four to thirty liters daily). The urine is of low specific gravity, generally 1.005 to 1.007. In secondary diabetes insipidus, other manifestations of the primary lesion may be seen, such as acromegaly or Cushing's disease in pituitary tumor, and somnolence, hypothermia, and obesity in hypothalamic lesions. Some, but not all, women with diabetes insipidus have uterine inertia during parturition; this presumably results from lack of posterior pituitary hormone.

Differential diagnosis may involve diabetes mellitus (distinguished by the presence of glycosuria), hyperparathyroidism (p. 197), and hysterical polydipsia and polyuria. In the last, the polydipsia is primary; in diabetes insipidus, the polyuria is primary. The relatively simple test of Brown and Rynearson will usually make the distinction. The patient goes as long as possible without taking fluids. When he feels that he has reached the limit of his tolerance and can abstain no longer, a urine specimen is collected. If the specific gravity is above 1.010, diabetes insipidus is extremely unlikely.

Treatment—Except for extremely rare cases, administration of posterior pituitary extract is specific therapy (see p. 473). The most satisfactory method is intranasal insufflation of Posterior Pituitary, U.S.P., which is a powder. Administration is simple and is suitable for prolonged therapy, and the nasal route eliminates the systemic reactions which may occur with injected extract. The usual dose is 40 to 50 mg. three or four times daily. Doses are measured for a time, but patients soon learn to judge the necessary quantity without the need for accurate measurement. Some employ powder blowers, but many find that the powder can be inhaled satisfactorily from the palm of the hand, from between the thumb and finger, or from the "anatomical snuffbox." Others place the powder on a small square of paper and roll the paper up into a narrow enough cylinder so that one end can be inserted into one side of the nose. The head is then tilted back, and the powder is inhaled.

Rarely, the powder proves irritating, and injection is necessary. The aqueous extract may be employed in doses of 1 to 10 units two or three times daily, or Pitressin Tannate may be given in doses of 3 to 5 pressor units every thirty-six to forty-eight hours.

Parathyroids

There are usually four parathyroid glands, and these are normally situated on the posterior edge of the lateral thyroid lobes. However, glands are occasionally found dependent from pedicles in the mediastinum or between the trachea and the esophagus, an important consideration in connection with the diagnosis and treatment of hyperparathyroidism.

The chief function of the parathyroid hormone is to control the level of calcium ions in the blood. This is apparently achieved indirectly as follows. The hormone acts directly on the renal tubules to diminish the reabsorption of phosphate. The following successive readjustments then take place:

The serum level of phosphate is automatically decreased, which leads to mobilization of inorganic phosphates from the bones. Since this phosphate is present in the bones as calcium salts, a rise in blood calcium results. This is not the only action of the parathyroid hormone, however, for it is able to decalcify bone in nephrectomized animals. Moreover, the parathyroid hormone is not the only factor influencing blood calcium (see p. 345). The stimulus to parathyroid secretion is apparently a low level of calcium ions in the blood.

HYPOPARATHYROIDISM

Hypoparathyroidism is most commonly due to accidental removal or injury of one or more parathyroid glands during thyroidectomy. Postoperative hypoparathyroidism may have an acute or insidious onset; the severity may be great or mild; and the remaining parathyroid tissue may regenerate sufficiently to carry on normal function, or it may degenerate to produce complete parathyroid failure. Hypoparathyroidism may also occur spontaneously.

The principal symptoms of hypoparathyroidism stem from the increased neuromuscular excitability induced by the low level of calcium ions in the blood and tissue fluids (p. 345). The syndrome is called *tetany*. It may present varied aspects. In the full-blown picture there are tonic and clonic spasms (usually painful) of various groups of skeletal muscles and sometimes of smooth muscle such as the urinary bladder or gastro-intestinal tract. The hands and feet usually assume characteristic positions; the hands show flexion of the wrists and proximal phalanges, extension of the distal phalanges, and adduction of the fingers and thumb ("obstetrician's hand"). Sometimes there are other positions of the extremities.

When the hyperexcitability is less extreme, tetany may remain latent, attacks being brought on by alkalosis due to overbreathing or other causes, or by emotion or other factors. Latent tetany may be demonstrated by the following signs, which are more easily elicited if the patient overbreathes for a few minutes:

1. Motor hyperexcitability as shown by the strength of the galvanic stimulus necessary to produce a muscular response. This test is potentially the most reliable, but only in experienced hands and with accurate apparatus.

2. Strong contraction or spasm of the facial muscles on gentle tapping over the facial nerve (Chvostek's sign).

3. Characteristic spasm of the hand within six minutes after inflation of a blood pressure cuff above the systolic arterial pressure (Trousseau's sign).

4. Painful spasm of the leg muscles on flexion of the thigh with the leg extended (Pool-Schlesinger's sign).

In addition to tetany, hypoparathyroidism may lead to psychosis or, in chronic cases, symmetrical cerebral calcifications (particularly of the basal ganglia), lenticular cataracts, dystrophy of the nails, alopecia, and dermatitis. The bones are denser than normal.

The causes of tetany are listed in Table 19. All must be considered in a differential diagnosis. The most frequent nonparathyroid causes for hypocalcemic tetany are rickets, osteomalacia, and renal insufficiency with phosphate retention. In addition, hypoparathyroidism must be distinguished from epilepsy and other diseases of the nervous system, neurosis, and hypothyroidism.

The diagnosis of post-thyroidectomy hypoparathyroidism is seldom difficult; in chronic idiopathic cases, five criteria must be fulfilled before the diagnosis can be considered as established: low serum calcium, high serum phosphate, normal bone *texture* by x-ray, absence of renal insufficiency, and response to parathyroid extract. The last qualification is necessary because of the existence of pseudo-hypoparathyroidism, which has the clinical picture of true hypoparathyroidism but which is due not to deficiency of the hormone but to unresponsiveness to it. Those patients so far reported as having the pseudo disease have been of stocky build with round faces.

TABLE 19 — *Causes of Tetany*

I. Alkalosis
   A. Overbreathing
      1. Emotional disturbance
      2. Fever
      3. Low partial pressure of oxygen in inspired air (high altitudes)
   B. Disturbed acid-base balance in blood
      1. Persistent loss of acid gastric juice (from vomiting or tube drainage)
      2. Excess ingestion of alkali, as during treatment of peptic ulcer

II. Low level of ionizable calcium in the blood
   A. Deficient calcium intake
   B. Defective calcium absorption
      1. Persistently alkaline upper-intestinal contents
      2. High phosphate intake
      3. Disturbed fat absorption (sprue, celiac disease)
      4. Vitamin D deficiency (rickets, osteomalacia)
      5. Diarrhea
   C. Excessive demand for calcium
      1. Late pregnancy
      2. Lactation
   D. High level of serum inorganic phosphate (renal insufficiency with phosphate retention)
   E. Hypoparathyroidism

Treatment has for its object the establishment and maintenance of a normal or slightly subnormal level of blood calcium. The most rapid means of elevating blood calcium is by intravenous administration of calcium salts, a procedure which is necessary only in acute tetany with laryngeal spasm. For dosage and precautions, see page 345. In acute tetany, one may also be justified in giving parathyroid extract (see p. 475). For maintenance therapy or in cases that are not of emergency nature, it is best to administer by mouth one of the activated sterols, such as calciferol (vitamin D_2) or dihydrotachysterol.

The dosage of parathyroid extract or of the activated sterols depends in part on the severity of the hypoparathyroidism and in part on the intake and absorption of calcium and phosphorus. A high-calcium, low-phosphorus diet enables the dosage to be held to a minimum. Milk, cheese, eggs, and meat are the richest dietary sources of phosphorus, with nuts, legumes, and whole-grain cereals also furnishing large quantities. Because a diet lacking these foods is quite uninteresting, their restriction is usually relaxed after control is established.

A high calcium intake is achieved by administering calcium salts by mouth (p. 505) rather than by including in the diet foods rich in calcium. The reason for this is that foods high in calcium are also high in phosphorus. The daily dose of calcium itself should be 2 to 4 Gm., but it need not be too exact.

Initial dosage of calciferol (p. 494) is ordinarily 3 to 10 mg. (120,000 to 400,000 U.S.P. Units) daily; maintenance dosage, 1 to 10 mg. (40,000 to 400,000 U.S.P. Units) daily. Although these doses are very large compared with those employed in rickets, they have not proved toxic in patients with hypoparathyroidism (for manifestations of overdosage, see p. 495). It is better to use pure calciferol rather than mixtures of the various vitamin D fractions, for hypercalcemic action does not always parallel antirachitic effect, and it is the latter property only which is measured by the U.S.P. Unit. If dihydrotachysterol is used, initial dosage is 2.5 to 12.5 mg. daily, and maintenance dosage 1.25 to 5.5 mg. by mouth once or twice a week.

Since hypercalcemia is even more harmful than hypocalcemia, it is absolutely necessary to control the effects of hypercalcemic agents by objective tests of calcium metabolism. Of greatest value is a series of determinations of serum calcium, serum phosphate, and plasma or serum protein (see p. 345). For most patients, the frequency of blood tests can be minimized by regular checking of calcium excretion in the urine with the Sulko-witch reagent (p. 523). The serum calcium should not be allowed to exceed 12 mg. per 100 cc. (provided serum protein is normal). It must be remembered that several days elapse between ingestion of activated sterols and their maximum effect on blood calcium.

HYPERPARATHYROIDISM

Hyperparathyroidism may accompany adenoma or diffuse hypertrophy of the cells of the parathyroid glands, or it may be secondary to a disturbance of calcium or phosphate metabolism of other origin, in which case it represents a compensatory mechanism. The excessive quantity of circulating parathyroid hormone results in hypercalcemia (p. 345), hypophosphatemia (p. 347), increased renal excretion of calcium and phosphate, and demineralization of the bones, with formation of characteristic bone tumors.

The effects of hypercalcemia as such are described on page 345. Demineralization of the bones may produce bone tenderness. The excessive urinary calcium may be precipitated and result in milky urine, gravel, or even stones, which may in turn cause dysuria, hematuria, and proteinuria. There is usually polyuria and polydipsia. There may be calcium deposits in the renal pyramids (nephrocalcinosis) which impair renal function and have a characteristic x-ray appearance.

The high blood calcium also gives rise to tissue calcifications, particularly in the walls of arteries and bronchi. If the calcium intake is low, there will be demineralization of the bones, with increase in serum alkaline phosphatase, pathological fractures, skeletal deformities, or the formation of cysts and giant-cell tumors (osteitis fibrosa cystica generalisata).

The early symptoms of hyperparathyroidism are often vague and do not of themselves direct attention to the parathyroids. Studies of serum calcium, phosphate, and protein should be carried out on all patients with urinary calculi, renal colic, polydipsia and polyuria not associated with glycosuria, or appropriate bone changes, and in those with unexplained ill health which includes any of the symptoms listed in previous paragraphs. The repeated finding of high serum calcium and low serum inorganic phosphate in the presence of normal serum protein (or the finding of normal serum calcium in the presence of low serum protein; see p. 345) leads one to suspect hyperparathyroidism. Until proved by operation or response to treatment, the diagnosis is presumptive only.

The bone changes of primary hyperparathyroidism must be distinguished from osteoporosis, osteomalacia, Paget's disease, polyostotic fibrous dysplasia, multiple myeloma, metastatic malignant neoplasm, and a number of less common bone disturbances. The differential diagnosis of hyperparathyroidism also includes glomerulonephritis, diabetes insipidus, myasthenia gravis, and psychoneurosis. Secondary hyperparathyroidism may result from deficiency of vitamin D (rickets and osteomalacia) and chronic renal insufficiency (from phosphate retention).

Even mild hyperparathyroidism (with almost normal serum calcium) is a serious matter, for such patients are "brittle" and succumb easily to mild infection or other intercurrent disease.

Treatment—If hyperparathyroidism is secondary, one treats the primary cause. The treatment of primary hyperparathyroidism is surgical removal of parathyroid tissue and for best results requires special experience in the operation itself and in pre and postoperative management. Operative problems include finding aberrant adenomatous glands and determining the amount of parathyroid tissue to leave behind. When a patient with severe hyperparathyroidism is first seen, fluids should be forced and milk should be withdrawn from the diet to prevent further nephrocalcinosis. A high-calcium diet should be avoided because of the dangers associated with extreme hypercalcemia (p. 345).

In patients with extreme bone disease and high serum phosphatase (20 Bodansky units or more), complete removal of an adenoma may be followed by severe hypocalcemia and tetany because of the sudden shift of balance between bone destruction and bone formation. The only satisfactory treatment of this hypocalcemia is continuous intravenous administration of calcium (p. 345), possibly supplemented by administration of parathyroid extract (p. 475).

FEMALE GENITAL SYSTEM

LEUKORRHEA

Leukorrhea, or vaginal discharge, is one of the most frequent complaints of adult female patients. A certain amount of vaginal secretion results from the action of estrogen, either that from the patient's ovaries or estrogenic substances therapeutically administered. An excess of secretion or a purulent discharge is a symptom of congestion or inflammation in the genital tract and may be due to a number of causes. Outstanding among these are gonorrheal infection (p. 6), *Trichomonas vaginalis* vaginitis (see below), and cervicitis (p. 200).

Infection with *Candida* (*Monilia*) *albicans* may be responsible for leukorrhea, particularly in pregnant women. Characteristic patches of thrush are usually visible on the vaginal walls, and the organism can be demonstrated in a fresh hanging drop prepared from the secretion or in a gram-stained smear. Vaginal moniliasis usually responds promptly to thorough cleansing followed by painting of the vaginal walls with 1 percent aqueous solution of gentian violet.

In severe infections in which continued use of gentian violet may prove irritating, it may be well to change after one or two days to a 1 or 2 percent solution of thymol in olive oil. A tampon is saturated with the thymol-olive oil preparation and inserted into the vagina, where it is left for a period of six hours. This is repeated on four or five successive days. If the labia or perineum or both are involved, the inner surface of a perineal pad should be coated with the solution, applied, and left in place for the periods specified.

Strong Iodine Solution, U.S.P., (Lugol's solution) and stronger preparations of iodine also have been applied topically in some instances.

The leukorrhea which results from senile vaginitis responds to treatment with estrogens (see p.199).

TRICHOMONAS VAGINALIS VAGINITIS

Vaginitis associated with itching, inflammation, and purulent vaginal discharge may be produced by the flagellate *Trichomonas vaginalis*. The source of the invader is not known. The occasional recovery of *T. vaginalis* from the urinary tract in the male suggests a possible source of infection for the female. The Skene and Bartholin glands are capable of harboring the parasite. Vaginal inoculation with the organism while bathing in contaminated water is considered a likely possibility.

T. vaginalis is present in the vaginal discharges of a high percentage of women with persistent leukorrhea, but its consistent pathogenicity in such individuals has been questioned. In inoculation experiments, it has not been possible to produce the infection in every subject; on the other hand, the organism has frequently been isolated from the vagina of women who have no symptoms of the disease. Examination of vaginal secretions in large groups of maternity patients has revealed presence of the flagellate in from 4 to 13 percent of white fe-

males and in as high as 33 percent of colored women.

Presence of *T. vaginalis* should be suspected in women who complain of irritating leukorrhea which has a disagreeable odor and which produces a variable degree of genital pruritus. Dyspareunia is a frequent complaint in such patients, whereas urinary tract symptoms are uncommon. On examination, the cervical and vaginal mucosa is red, and the vaginal vault contains a yellowish discharge often permeated with minute air bubbles which give a foamy appearance. Diagnosis is strengthened by finding the parasite microscopically. A small portion of secretion may be placed on a hanging-drop slide, where it is diluted with warm physiological salt solution and examined with the high dry lens. The protozoa are seen in constant motion among pus cells and debris.

Treatment—Success sometimes follows such simple measures as acid or alkaline douches or cleansing of the vagina with green soap and water followed by thorough drying. The importance of general measures for improving the patient's general health has been emphasized. More often, however, a satisfactory result depends upon local therapy, for which a great variety of technics and remedies has been suggested. In the past there has been, in general, a persistence or recurrence rate of 10 to 20 percent despite varied and aggressive therapy. In many cases it seems probable that cure was achieved but that reinfection took place during sexual intercourse; for the parasite may be harbored for long periods in the prostate gland without producing symptoms. Unfailing use of a condom during intercourse will prevent reinfection of the woman in most such cases.

Many chemical substances are capable of promptly killing the trichomonad on contact. Among them are gentian violet, 1:1,000; glycerin, 50 percent; lactic acid, 2 percent; mercuric chloride, 1:5,000; potassium permanganate, 1:1,000; liniment of soft soap, 10 percent; silver nitrate, 2 percent; and 'Merthiolate' solution, 1:2,000 (p. 307). In applying these, a suitable vaginal speculum is introduced; and after the vagina has been thoroughly dried with gauze or cotton, the entire mucosa is sponged with the chosen solution. A medicated vaginal tampon then may be put in place. The tampon is removed by the patient the following morning, and a douche is taken each day until office treatment again is applied. If 'Merthiolate' is the chosen remedy, nightly insertion of a vaginal suppository may be prescribed for the intervals between office visits.

Among the arsenical preparations having extensive use is carbarsone (p. 314) in suppository form. For home treatment, the patient is instructed to insert one suppository into the vagina at the time of retiring each night for two weeks. A sodium bicarbonate douche is permitted once each week if desired. In office treatment with carbarsone suppositories, the vagina is thoroughly cleansed and dried and two 2-grain (0.13-Gm.) suppositories are inserted, followed by a tampon which the patient removes the following morning. Treatment is repeated twice a week; on the days between treatments, the patient may douche with a solution of green soap.

In use of carbarsone, as with all arsenical drugs, caution should be used, particularly in patients with kidney or liver disease. Individuals with such disorders or with a history of previous intolerance to arsenicals should be carefully observed during therapy.

'Negatan' has also proved effective. Details of use will be found on page 513.

LEUKOPLAKIA OF THE VULVA

Leukoplakic vulvitis is a disease of the female external genitalia characterized by atrophy, keratinization, and blanching of the skin. Loss of elasticity, dehydration, and cracking of the tissues are common. The cause is unknown, but the usual occurrence after the menopause suggests a factor of hormonal imbalance. Vaginal discharge and trauma from scratching are aggravating influences.

Pathologically there is proliferation and keratinization of the epithelium, with edema, round-cell infiltration, and vascular proliferation in the subcutaneous tissue. If untreated, about 50 percent of cases become malignant.

The most common symptom is intense itching. Coitus may be painful or impossible. The characteristic patches of white, brittle, cracked skin make the diagnosis.

Treatment—In patients past the menopause, estrogens should be given in physiological dosage (p. 463 *et seq.*). Local application of Hydrophilic Petrolatum or a similar preparation (p. 479) is soothing and helps allay itching, particularly in early cases. X-ray therapy may prove beneficial early in the course, but it should be used cautiously, for it is not without hazard.

In advanced cases without malignancy, vulvectomy may be indicated. In the presence of cancer, the excision should be radical and should include regional lymph nodes; it may be followed by x-ray therapy to the primary site and the regional lymph nodes. Radon seeds may be implanted if there is local recurrence. X-ray is contraindicated as a preoperative measure in demonstrated or suspected malignancy because of the amount of local reaction which may follow.

SENILE VAGINITIS

The term "senile vaginitis" is applied to a condition of vaginal irritation, ulceration, or infection which is secondary to the vaginal atrophy that follows withdrawal of estrogen supply. It is seen during the menopause and after irradiation or excision of the ovaries. The usual symptoms are vaginal discharge, itching, and irritation, sometimes with slight bleeding or pelvic pain. Adhesions between the vaginal walls are common.

The characteristic symptoms and the finding of a somewhat irritated, atrophic vaginal mucosa, with an atrophic smear, make the diagnosis. One must, however, rule out the concomitant presence of uterine cancer or of primary vaginal infection, particularly with the gonococcus or *Trichomonas*.

Treatment consists primarily in estrogen replacement therapy. The most direct approach is by vaginal administration. However, both local and systemic effects will result from either local or systemic administration. A regimen which is usually satisfactory is as follows:

1. Vinegar douches (4 or 5 tablespoonfuls to the quart of water) twice daily.

2. Following each douche, the vulva is gently bathed with mild soap and warm water. The suds are rinsed off with warm water, and the skin is dried by patting (not rubbing) with a soft towel.

3. After washing and drying, Hydrophilic Petrolatum or a similar preparation (p. 479) is applied to the vulva.

4. Scratching is prohibited. Gloves should be worn at night while itching persists. 'Surfacaine' cream or lotion (p. 446) may be applied at night during this period.

5. Sedation (phenobarbital or 'Amytal,' 1/4 grain three times daily, and 'Seconal Sodium,' 1 1/2 grains at bedtime; the bedtime medication is discontinued [usually within a week] as soon as nocturnal itching ceases).

6. Vitamin B complex and vitamin C in liberal dosage (see pp. 483 and 490).

7. Estrogen (p. 463), systemically or by vaginal suppository (such as diethylstilbestrol, 0.5 to 1 mg. daily by mouth or a 0.5-mg. suppository at bedtime).

After a month, all measures can usually be discontinued except the last two. The extra vitamins had best be continued at least an additional month. The dosage of estrogen can usually be reduced, but administration may have to be continued indefinitely to prevent recurrence. Continued douching not more frequently than once daily is optional; it may add to the patient's comfort, especially during the summer months or in warm climates.

CERVICITIS

Cervicitis, or inflammation of the uterine cervix, is most often due to infection with the gonococcus, staphylococcus, streptococcus, or colon bacillus. It is frequently initiated by the trauma of childbirth and often is found in association with lacerations and erosions of the cervix. Because of the deep branching of the racemose glands in the cervix, infections of this part are apt to become chronic. Also, cystic disease of the cervix often is present because of obstruction of nabothian gland ducts with retention of secretions and superimposed infection. Polyps may develop, and stenosis of the cervix may be an etiological factor in the inflammatory process. The presence of cervical lesions, particularly leukoplakia, calls for consideration of possible cancerous changes.

In the majority of patients, leukorrhea is the major complaint resulting from cervicitis. Others mentioned less frequently are disturbance of menstruation, dyspareunia, and backache. The differential diagnosis of cervicitis should exclude such specific causes of vaginal discharge as *Trichomonas vaginalis* vaginitis (see above), gonorrhea (p. 6), and other infections in the vagina which may be responsible for leukorrhea (p. 197).

Treatment of cervicitis is directed toward eradication of infection and correction of structural abnormalities. Mild infections associated with superficial lacerations or erosions sometimes can be eliminated with bactericidal agents topically applied. Among these are Iodine Tincture, U.S.P., 'Negatan' (see p. 513), and silver preparations such as silver nitrate solution, 10 percent. 'Merthiolate' may be applied as the tincture directly to the lesion by applicator, or vaginal suppositories may be prescribed. Sulfonamide suppositories may be helpful if organisms are involved which are susceptible to the drug topically applied. Lactose is used in the vagina to lower the pH of vaginal secretions, encouraging growth of acid flora and inhibiting pyogenic organisms. Douches with vinegar solution, four or five tablespoonfuls to the quart of water, provide another means of acidification.

Deeper cervical infection usually requires coagulation treatment or cauterization. These steps should not be taken in the presence of acute infection. If lacerations are extensive trachelorrhaphy (or occasionally more radical surgery) may be needed.

ACUTE MASTITIS

Acute mastitis is the result of bacterial invasion of the breast. Clinically, it resembles local infection elsewhere in the body, but during lactation it tends to develop rapidly and in severe form

Treatment is along the lines of other local infections (see Abscess, p. 1). During lactation, the child should be removed from the breast. Engorgement can usually be greatly reduced by administering diethylstilbestrol (p. 467), 5 mg. orally, three times daily for two or three days.

When given early, roentgen irradiation is frequently of value. If incision is necessary, it should be radial to the nipple to avoid unnecessary severing of mammary ducts.

CHRONIC MASTITIS

The term "chronic mastitis" is used to describe certain noninfectious fibrotic and cystic changes in the female breast which are of uncertain etiology. Distinguishable at one extreme is adenofibrosis, in which the essential lesion is a fibrosis that is relatively diffused throughout the breast. Pure adenofibrosis is almost never followed by malignancy. At the other extreme is pure cystic disease, in which there is a solitary-appearing cystic mass of the breast, usually in an elderly woman. Long-continued relative excess of estrogen over progesterone is believed to be a factor in the production of cystic disease. The incidence of cancer in such cases is estimated as 2 to 4 percent. Cole distinguishes two other intergrading types of change—benign parenchymatous hyperplasia and precancerous hyperplasia. In the latter, the incidence of cancer may be 20 to 30 percent. Clinically, a distinction may be difficult; it is sometimes possible only after careful microscopic study of removed tissue. Uncommonly, all four types of change may coexist in the same breast, but usually one predominates.

Although the masses of chronic mastitis are usually tender, the condition does not cause extreme pain.

Treatment depends on classification, with malignancy the primary consideration. Skin retraction, in the absence of a history of previous inflammation, is a rather reliable sign of malignancy. In young women, it is considered safe to observe the lesion and treat it medically as long as indications of malignancy are absent (see below). When nodulation of the breast is of brief duration, it may subside spontaneously. Adequate support to the breasts is indicated for relief of pain. Heat therapy may be beneficial. Pregnancy and lactation usually lead to regression.

In cases of several months' or years' duration, progesterone (p. 468) may be given twice weekly for the last two weeks of one or two consecutive menstrual cycles. Such courses may have to be repeated at intervals of twelve to eighteen months. Estrogens are probably contraindicated.

As women pass forty years, the danger of malignancy becomes much greater; and even in the absence of indications of malignancy, if the mass has been present for more than a few months, local excision, including all masses and considerable normal surrounding tissue, may be done. The removed tissue is subjected to careful microscopic study. Of course, any indication of actual malignancy demands immediate surgery. If precancerous tissue is found, complete mastectomy is advised; perhaps radical mastectomy should be considered in view of recent reports of the finding of metastatic breast cancer in axillary lymph nodes, without evidence of primary lesions in the breast.

CANCER OF THE BREAST

Cancer is the most common neoplasm of the female breast; it occurs rarely in the male breast. In women, its incidence is second only to that of uterine cancer. In some instances, the growth induces very little reaction in the normal tissues; it then has a predominantly cellular character and is termed *medullary carcinoma*. In other cases, there is a pronounced fibrous tissue reaction, and the growth is termed *scirrhous carcinoma*. All possible gradations between the two are seen. Scirrhous carcinoma presents a hard mass; growth is usually slow; and the degree of malignancy may be less than in the medullary type. If there is a semblance of gland formation, the growth may be called *adenocarcinoma*. Chronic cystic mastitis is a common forerunner of adenocarcinoma.

Metastasis is usually by infiltration through lymphatics and is often retrograde. The axillary lymph nodes are most commonly involved; other frequent sites include the pleura and lungs, liver, skeleton, and brain.

The early development of breast cancer is insidious—a single small lump which is hard but has indistinct outlines; it is movable, irregularly rounded, and quite insensitive, and is usually found in the upper outer quadrant. If it is superficial, there may be dimpling of the skin over it, either spontaneously or on moving the breast or trying to separate the tumor from the skin. There are many late signs due to local or metastatic spread of the tumor, necrosis of tumor cells, development of fibrous tissue, or blockage of lymphatic drainage.

The frequency of breast cancer is such that any tumor of the breast in a woman of middle age or older must be considered to be cancer until proved otherwise. The features set forth in the previous paragraph may be helpful in diagnosis. Perhaps the most confusing differentiation is from papillary cystadenoma and chronic cystic disease (see Chronic Mastitis above).

The course of untreated breast cancer is extremely variable. The average survival after discovery is one and one-half to three years, but the range is from a very few months to twenty years or more.

Treatment—The only hope of cure is by operative removal of the breast, pectoral muscles, axillary contents, an extensive area of deep fascia, and a wide margin of apparently sound skin and subcutaneous tissue. Under average conditions, about 30 percent of patients so treated can be expected to survive for five years. The duration of survival and the incidence of actual cure are vastly increased by early diagnosis and operation; hence the great emphasis on prompt discovery of lumps in the breast. However, before a patient is subjected to such an operation, an x-ray of the chest for metastasis should be made routinely, and other metastases should be sought; their presence makes removal of the primary growth futile.

When the diagnosis is in doubt, exploratory operation should be done. If incision into the growth leaves any uncertainty as to its nature, a specimen is removed with the electrocautery and subjected to immediate examination by a pathologist. The operation should always be planned and undertaken in such a way that the exploration can be turned into a radical procedure if the tumor proves to be malignant.

Radiation may be useful in several ways. Inoperable lesions may be held in check, sometimes for long periods, by repeated implantation of radium needles. Preoperative x-ray therapy may reduce the vitality of cancer cells and diminish the possibility of operative spread. Postoperative radiation may destroy cancer cells that have escaped removal.

Androgens and estrogens are sometimes capable of producing temporary regression of breast cancer or symptomatic improvement or both. This form of treatment should, however, be reserved for those patients in whom operation and irradiation either cannot be applied or have proved unsuccessful. Experience is still too limited to permit final conclusions, but the following tentative statements seem warranted.

Testosterone propionate may be expected to cause objective improvement in both osseous and soft-tissue metastases in about 20 percent of cases and subjective improvement (relief of pain, feeling of well-being, and increased appetite) in about 60 percent. Age does not affect response. About one-third of those with soft-tissue lesions who respond to androgen do so within two months; the rest require a longer period. Of patients with painful osseous lesions, about 80 percent have some degree of relief within a month. The duration of improvement has not been adequately determined, but in about 20 percent it can be expected to exceed nine months.

The effective dosage of testosterone propionate is 50 to 100 mg. intramuscularly three times weekly. A total of at least 3 Gm. should be given. Side-effects are common and sometimes unpleasant (see p. 471).

The administration of estrogen in breast cancer should be limited to patients who are at least five years past the menopause. About 60 percent of patients receiving estrogen are likely to show subjective improvement; and about 50 percent, objective improvement of soft-tissue lesions. Data on the response of osseous lesions are inadequate for conclusions. More patients respond symptomatically after two months than before; objective response usually requires at least five months. The duration of improvement is still unsettled, but about 25 percent maintain it for nine months or longer.

Diethylstilbestrol is most commonly employed. The usual dosage is 5 mg. three times daily. The total dose should be no less than 2 Gm. Side-effects are common and include nausea, vomiting, uterine bleeding (especially on withdrawal), and edema (see also p. 465).

Menstrual Disturbances

Menstruation represents the terminal event in the normal ovarian cycle. This cycle begins with the liberation from the anterior pituitary gland into the blood of gonadotrophin of the follicle-stimulating type (FSH). The ovaries take up the FSH, and under its influence one (only occasionally more in man) of the primary follicles begins to develop further, with antrum formation. At this stage, lu-

teinizing hormone (LH) is secreted in small amounts by the anterior pituitary, and under the combined influence of FSH and LH, estrogen is secreted by the growing follicle. The LH also causes differentiation of the theca interna of the follicle, and the estrogen causes differentiation of the granulosa. The final maturation and rupture of the follicle, with release of the ovum, is the result of further combined action of FSH and LH in the proper proportions.

Following ovulation, LH stimulates the development of the corpus luteum. Progesterone secretion seems to depend on the presence of a third pituitary secretion, the luteotrophic hormone. Many investigators consider the luteotrophic hormone to be identical with prolactin (p. 472). Actually, progesterone production may begin a few hours before ovulation and before a corpus luteum is present. The latter is, however, necessary for continued progesterone secretion.

The estrogen formed in the developing follicle and the corpus luteum has many actions (p. 463). In connection with menstruation, three are important: development of the proliferative phase of the endometrium, an early stimulation of formation and release of LH and luteotrophic hormone by the anterior pituitary, and a later inhibition (in association with progesterone) of release of FSH and LH. Progesterone (p. 468) converts the endometrium from the proliferative to the progestational phase and acts with estrogen to inhibit release of FSH and LH.

As a result of the cessation of gonadotrophic stimulation, ovarian production of estrogen and progesterone stops. Menstruation is the result of the sudden withdrawal of estrogen and progesterone. Since menstrual flow almost always begins on the fourteenth day following ovulation, it is apparent that variations in total length of *ovulatory* cycles are due to differences in duration of the preovulatory phase. Menstrual function is influenced by many accessory factors: endocrine, nutritional, and emotional. The limits of normal for hormone production, time of ovulation (which determines length of cycle), and duration and volume of flow are not clearly defined.

An important type of abnormal cycle is the anovulatory one, in which ovulation fails to occur. No corpus luteum is formed, and there is no progesterone secretion. Uterine bleeding takes place, often after a normal interval, but from a proliferative endometrium and as a result of estrogen withdrawal. The unruptured follicle may continue for a time as a simple follicular cyst.

It is often of importance to determine when or if ovulation takes place. A simple method which is reliable in careful hands involves only the daily recording and interpretation of waking body temperature. It depends on the observation that estrogen depresses body temperature, whereas progesterone elevates it. A sustained production of progesterone does not occur in the absence of ovulation, and, ordinarily, sufficient progesterone is produced to cause a significant elevation of body temperature at about the time of ovulation or within twenty-four hours of that time. Of course, there are many factors that influence body temperature, but the cyclic fluctuations recorded on successive mornings have proved a reliable guide to ovulation in most women when suitable precautions are taken and the curve is carefully interpreted.

Sample temperature curves for ovulatory cycles, anovulatory cycles of the same duration, and total lack of ovarian function are shown in Figure 4. The most probable day of ovulation is marked by "O." The "A" indicates an adventitious rise due to an upper respiratory infection. There are intermediate types of curves, the interpretation of which cannot be dealt with here. Oral temperatures may be taken instead of rectal; the former will average 1°F. lower than the latter.

Not all women are able to obtain temperature records which permit satisfactory interpretation. The quality of the records can, however, be held to a maximum by the application of a few simple principles and rules.

First, the patient must be given sufficient explanation of the purpose of the procedure so that she becomes actively interested in obtaining a faithful and accurate record. Second, she must be thoroughly instructed in *every* step of the procedure, including which end of the thermometer is to be inserted and exactly where and how far. The following rules should be observed by her:

Always use the same thermometer. If it is broken and has to be replaced, a notation should be made on the record. Shake the thermometer down at night; place it within easy reach and have a watch or clock within easy sight. Waking temperatures are to be taken immediately on awakening and before sitting up, eating, drinking, smoking, or any activity. The thermometer is always to be left in for the same length of time by the clock. The temperature is to be recorded at once on a pad or chart which, with a pencil, is kept at the bedside. The patient is also to record the menstrual days and any unusual occurrence or symptom, illness, coitus, or special medication. Great variation in the daily routine makes for irregular curves.

ABNORMAL UTERINE BLEEDING

Before uterine bleeding can be considered abnormal, the following must be ruled out:

1. Menstrual bleeding.

2. Implantation bleeding, which occurs about two weeks after conception and may involve an external show of blood.

3. Preovulatory bleeding associated with hyperemia (uncommon).

The usual causes of abnormal genital bleeding are listed in Table 20. Most functional uterine

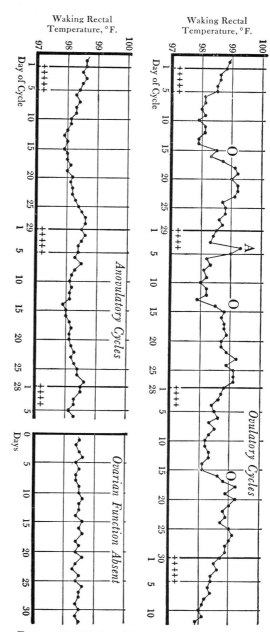

FIGURE 4 — *Typical Waking Temperature Records in Various States of Ovarian Function*

bleeding is anovulatory (see above). A record of
waking body temperature (see above) or a series of
endometrial biopsies, or both, may be helpful in determining the extent and rhythm of ovarian activity.

Treatment—First the physician must assure himself that the bleeding is actually from the uterus or
higher and that it is abnormal. Anatomical causes
must be looked for and treated according to their
nature. The diagnosis of functional uterine bleeding
is always tentative and must not be made until
anatomical causes are eliminated.

If blood loss from the uterus is so severe as to
require its prompt cessation, one may undertake
either uterine curettage or the administration of
large quantities of estrogens. The latter are usually
effective. Diethylstilbestrol (p. 467) may be given
by mouth, 5 mg. every four to six hours, until
bleeding ceases. The patient is, of course, put to
bed. After cessation of estrogen therapy, withdrawal bleeding may occur, but this usually resembles normal menstruation. After acute bleeding
is controlled, one searches carefully for its cause.

When the bleeding is apparently functional, one
looks for evidence of nervous and emotional factors,
hypothyroidism, and disturbances of the blood and
its clotting mechanism, as outlined in Table 20.
If other factors can be eliminated and the bleeding
seems to be due to a pituitary-ovarian disturbance
of unknown cause, several considerations must be
weighed. Functional uterine bleeding often cor-
rects itself in time, especially in adolescents. Therapy may not be needed unless blood loss is excessive,
the condition is a source of undue worry or incon-
venience, or a desired fertility seems to be impaired.

In the premenopausal group, radiation of the
ovaries sufficient to stop their function permanently
is often satisfactory. In younger women, a regimen
of adequate nutrition (with especial attention to
protein and vitamins) and adequate physical and
mental rest may be all that is needed.

When more specific therapy is desired, one may
give any of the following:

DIETHYLSTILBESTROL (p. 467) or other estrogens.
To stop continued bleeding one gives 5 mg. diethylstilbestrol by mouth every four to six hours. When
bleeding is regular but excessive, the following
schedule may be followed:

1 mg. daily for seven days, then
5 mg. daily for seven days, then
0.3 mg. daily for ten days or until bleeding recurs

Usually one such course suffices.

PROGESTERONE (p. 468) by intramuscular injection, 30 mg. or more subdivided into four to eight

TABLE 20—*Causes of Abnormal Genital Bleeding*

I. Anatomical (exclusive of late pregnancy)
   Carcinoma
     Cervix of uterus
     Fundus of uterus
     Uterine tube
     Ovary (through functional mechanism)
   Sarcoma of cervix or corpus of uterus
   Pregnancy, early
     Tubal pregnancy
     Abortion
     Hydatid mole
     Chorionepithelioma
   After delivery or abortion
     Retained fragment of placenta or membranes
     Lacerations (especially following curettage)
     Subinvolution
   Infection
     Endometritis
     Salpingitis
     Oophoritis (through functional mechanism)
   Vaginal or cervical ulceration
   Senile vaginitis
   Ill-fitting or neglected pessary
   Prolapse of uterus
   Endometrial polyps
   Submucous fibroids
   Acquired stenosis of cervix

II. Functional
   Imbalance between estrogen and progesterone
     Altered ovarian and pituitary function, includ-
       ing anovulatory cycles
   Hypothyroidism (p. 180)
   Disturbances of clotting of blood
     Leukemia (p. 103)
     Thrombocytopenia (p. 105)
     Aplastic anemia (p. 97)
     Hypoprothrombinemia (p. 107)
   Altered sensitivity of coiled arterioles of endo-
     metrium
   Of emotional origin (?)

daily doses. If the bleeding is regular but excessive,
the course may be started three weeks after the
onset of the last previous flow. In about a third of
the cases, normal cycles can be expected to follow
treatment; in another third, abnormal bleeding
will recur within four months; and in the remaining third, amenorrhea will follow, either at once
or after one or two cycles.

ANDROGENS, such as testosterone propionate or
methyltestosterone (p. 469). If bleeding is severe,
one may give 25 mg. testosterone propionate intramuscularly three times weekly (or about 35 mg.
methyltestosterone daily by mouth or 20 mg. per
day sublingually). During the period of therapy at
this dosage level, it is most important to study
vaginal smears twice weekly. At the first sign of
regression in the smear, treatment is discontinued;
otherwise overdosage may occur (see p. 471). If

there is little or no symptomatic improvement during the menstrual period following the beginning of treatment, the course is repeated. If there has been moderate improvement, testosterone is given the following month in half the original dosage. If the period following the first course is about normal, a second course is given at one-third the original dosage level.

When the bleeding is of moderate degree, 25 mg. testosterone propionate may be administered every three or four days for the first month (total monthly dosage—150 to 200 mg.), or 15 to 25 mg. methyltestosterone may be given daily by mouth. During the following month, a second course is given with half the dosage.

If there is recurrence after several months of normal menses, 25 mg. testosterone propionate once a week or 10 mg. methyltestosterone daily for four to six weeks are usually adequate for a further period of several months.

If menstruation is suppressed or delayed and the vaginal smear shows estrogen deficiency, testosterone therapy should be discontinued. Acne is not considered a serious deterrent to further therapy, but voice changes or facial hirsutism are indications for immediate discontinuation of androgenic therapy.

Excellent results have been reported from combined therapy—25 mg. testosterone propionate and 10 mg. progesterone daily for four or five days. The flow often stops on the first or second day. The amenorrhea lasts two to four days, after which there is progesterone withdrawal bleeding. Progesterone is given (or, if withdrawal bleeding is excessive from progesterone alone, progesterone and testosterone are administered together) in subsequent courses for several months, beginning twenty-one to thirty days after previous bleeding has stopped.

CHORIONIC GONADOTROPHIN (p. 472) has been used, but present evidence suggests that its action is to stop ovarian function, and therefore it would seem to be contraindicated except in premenopausal bleeding.

AMENORRHEA

Amenorrhea is the result of failure of function somewhere in the pituitary-ovarian-endometrial mechanism. The fault may lie in one of these organs, or failure may result from the action of outside influences.

If menstruation has never occurred, one must ascertain if a uterus is present, and if so, whether an imperforate hymen or other complete obstruc-tion exists. If the genital passage is clear but the secondary sexual characteristics are undeveloped, then one presumes that amenorrhea is a part of hypogonadism (p. 189) and treats it as such. If sexual development is normal, the ovaries must have some degree of function. A record of waking body temperature (p. 203) or a series of endometrial biopsies or both over a period of one or two months may help to determine the extent of failure. Occasionally, cyclic ovulation may be associated with fluctuations in hormone level which are inadequate to precipitate menstruation, or the spiral arteries of the endometrium may for some reason be unresponsive.

Treatment—Before amenorrhea is treated, the three physiological causes—pregnancy, preadolescence, and menopause—must be ruled out. When sexual development is normal, certain general measures should first be taken. Emotional disturbances (p. 147) and either obesity (p. 260) or undernutrition are important factors in amenorrhea and must be corrected. The patient should be assured ample physical and mental rest.

Since amenorrhea of itself is quite harmless, more specific therapy is hard to justify unless the patient desires a fertility that has been demonstrated to be lacking or she or her family is unduly distressed by the condition. Thyroid (p. 456) is probably the most useful endocrine preparation and should always be given if there is evidence of hypothyroidism; in the absence of such evidence, its value is in dispute.

Withdrawal bleeding simulating menstruation can be produced by administration of estrogens (p. 463) and progesterone (p. 468): 0.5 to 1 mg. diethylstilbestrol daily by mouth for three weeks out of every four, with or without 5 mg. progesterone given daily by injection for the last five days of estrogenic therapy. However, neither ovarian function nor fertility is apparently increased by such a regimen.

The gonadotrophins are seldom of value.

DYSMENORRHEA

There are, in general, two types of dysmenorrhea. The "secondary" type is characterized by dull aching and is due to pelvic congestion, usually from a pelvic lesion. The "primary" type is manifested by sharp cramplike pains and is probably related to an abnormal type or intensity of uterine contraction. "Primary" dysmenorrhea does not occur in the absence of progesterone, and there is some evidence that it may be associated with a relative, but not absolute, deficiency of this hormone. However, psychic and emotional factors are extremely important. A record of waking body temperature (p. 203) may be helpful in that primary dysmenorrhea occurs only during ovulatory cycles; lower abdominal cramps at the end of an anovulatory cycle cannot be due to dysmenorrhea.

Treatment is not entirely satisfactory. It is important to evaluate carefully and eliminate insofar as possible the factors of physical fatigue or disability, emotional tension, unfortunate attitudes toward menstruation and other sexual functions, and improper diet and habits. Systematic athletic activity is often very helpful, especially during adolescence.

A full-term pregnancy is usually curative, and sustained relief often follows dilatation and curettage. Presacral neurectomy is a radical measure, but in skilled hands it has achieved permanent relief.

Dysmenorrhea can be averted for the current cycle by preventing ovulation through the administration of estrogen during the first half of the cycle. Diethylstilbestrol (p. 467) may be given, usually 2 mg. daily by mouth for ten days, beginning at least twenty-one days before the expected period. The advisability and safety of such treatment when repeated over long periods are subject to question.

Relief during the current cycle may also be achieved, but in a smaller percentage of cases, by progesterone (p. 468), 1 to 5 mg. by injection daily or on alternate days for a week preceding the onset of flow, or by testosterone propionate (p. 469), 10 mg., given on a similar schedule. Thyroid (p. 456) is sometimes helpful.

Palliative therapy may consist in the application of heat or in the administration of a great variety of analgesics (p. 405). The uterine contractions may be modified by a combination of atropine sulfate, 1/150 to 1/100 grain (0.4 to 0.6 mg.), and papaverine hydrochloride, 1 to 2 grains (65 to 130 mg.), given hypodermically or by mouth.

In some instances, dysmenorrhea has been relieved by antihistaminic drugs (p. 509). Since histamine causes uterine contraction in experimental animals, it is possible, but not as yet proved, that allergy may be a factor in these cases.

MENOPAUSE

The immediate mechanism of the "natural" menopause is the development of a refractory condition of the ovaries whereby they no longer respond to gonadotrophic stimulation. The cessation of ovarian function may progress slowly or rapidly. Very often corpus luteum function fails before estrogen production, resulting in a relative excess of estrogen. In "surgical" menopause, the cessation of function is immediate and complete.

With cessation of estrogen production, there is atrophy of the genital structures dependent on estrogenic stimulation. The so-called "senile vaginitis" is the result of irritation, ulceration, or infection of the atrophic vaginal mucosa (see p. 199). There is an excess of gonadotrophin in the blood and urine.

The majority of women pass through the menopause without difficulty. Approximately 10 percent have one or more of the following complaints: hot flushes, headaches, giddiness, obesity, nervous instability, "rheumatic" pains, uterine hemorrhage, pain in the breasts. Psychic and emotional factors have great influence on both the incidence and severity of symptoms.

Certain complications of the menopause may arise. Abnormal uterine bleeding (p. 203) is common and requires immediate attention because of the possibility that it may be due to genital malignancy. Arthralgia or arthritis may be related to the menopause, in which case it usually responds to estrogens. The relation of neuroses and psychoses, particularly involutional melancholia, to the menopause is still in dispute, as is the response to estrogenic therapy. Disturbances of thyroid function (p. 178) are common, and their diagnosis is easily missed unless they are sought for. They should be treated. Hypertension is probably not related to the menopause.

Treatment—The menopause as such is a physiological state which does not require treatment in the absence of symptoms. Since none of the symptoms occurs exclusively in the menopause, the physician should rule out other disease before attributing them to the menopause. Many patients with menopausal symptoms need no more than an explanation of the condition and a measure of reassurance. Others will benefit by general supervision and mild sedation, as with phenobarbital (p. 390), 1/4 to 1/2 grain (0.016 to 0.032 Gm.), twice daily. The shorter-acting barbiturates (p. 392) may be useful in addition, in doses of 3/4 to 3 grains (0.05 to 0.2 Gm.) at bedtime, to assure restful nights.

For the minority in whom the above measures do not suffice, estrogens (p. 463) should be prescribed. With diethylstilbestrol administered by mouth, starting doses may be 0.1 to 0.25 mg. daily.

Maintenance doses, which should be no larger than needed, usually do not exceed 0.5 mg. daily. For dosage of other estrogens, see page 467. After six or eight months of estrogenic therapy, a rest period should be given. If symptoms do not return, no further treatment is needed. If they do, it can be resumed.

During the period of treatment and after the maintenance dose has been approximated, there are many advantages to cyclic administration which mimics the estrogen levels of the menstrual cycle. The patient may take, for example, 0.25 mg. daily the first week, 0.5 mg. daily the second week, 0.25 mg. daily the third week, and none the fourth week. To avoid confusion, the patient should mark the dosage for each week on a calendar. For possible complications of estrogen therapy, see page 465.

Androgens provide an alternative therapeutic agent. They are generally less effective than estrogens against menopause symptoms. In a sense they are contraphysiological, and women receiving them must be watched carefully for masculinizing effects (see p. 471). Nevertheless, they may be tried (1) when women with menopausal symptoms are still menstruating or have functional uterine bleeding; (2) when menopausal symptoms are only partially relieved by estrogens (in which cases androgen is given as a supplement to estrogen); and (3) in those patients in whom even careful estrogenic therapy results in uterine bleeding. Average dosage is 10 to 25 mg. of testosterone propionate three times weekly or an equivalent amount of methyltestosterone by mouth.

Pregnancy and Parturition

PHYSIOLOGY OF PREGNANCY

Following ovulation (p. 202), the ovum normally passes into the uterine tube. Unless it is fertilized, it dies—probably within twenty-four hours. Fertilization, when it occurs, usually takes place in the outer third of the uterine tube, the spermatozoa having traveled by their own motility from the vagina by way of the uterine cavity. The fertilized egg is carried slowly down the uterine tube, segmenting and dividing as it goes. About nine or ten days after fertilization it implants itself in the uterine wall, nidation being accomplished with the aid of enzymes that digest locally the surface of the endometrium, which is then in the secretory phase because of the action of progesterone from the corpus luteum.

At about this time the ovum begins the secretion of chorionic gonadotrophin, a hormone which is absorbed by the mother. Chorionic gonadotrophin not only prevents regression of the corpus luteum following withdrawal of the gonadotrophins of the anterior pituitary; it also stimulates additional growth of the corpus luteum and continued secretion of estrogen and progesterone. Estrogen and progesterone, or certain products of their metabolism, are necessary for the maintenance of pregnancy. The exact relationships are not established.

During the last part of the second and the first part of the third month of pregnancy, the placenta takes over the production of estrogen and progesterone. At the same time the output of chorionic gonadotrophin diminishes. From this point on, the corpus luteum is no longer indispensable. After the third month, estrogen and progesterone are secreted in constantly increasing amounts which reach a maximum one to four weeks (average, two weeks) before term. Although there are great individual variations within the limits of normal, the average maximum excretion in milligrams per twenty-four hours is of the order of: estradiol, 0.2; estrone, 1.6; estriol, 35; progesterone (as pregnanediol), 95.

After the maxima are reached, formation of estrogen and progesterone progressively diminishes until delivery, when detachment of the placenta abruptly ends its production of these hormones. There is some evidence that the altered metabolism of estrogen due to the diminished progesterone supply may be an important factor in bringing on labor.

DIAGNOSIS OF PREGNANCY

Tests Depending on Chorionic Gonadotrophin— The most extensively used laboratory tests for pregnancy depend on the excretion in the urine of chorionic gonadotrophin. When injected into certain animals, this substance stimulates ovarian function, and the evidence of this induced ovarian function forms the basis for interpretation of the tests. Since the production of chorionic gonadotrophin by the ovum does not begin until about ten days after ovulation and fertilization, it is clear that these tests cannot be expected to become positive in any case much before the time of the first missed period. In practice, of course, such tests are not performed until a period is delayed. Positive tests have been obtained as early as three days after the expected onset of menstruation. Ordinarily, however, the period should be at least two weeks overdue before a positive test can reasonably be expected. It should be emphasized that none of the tests is infallible. Some women go through pregnancy without ever excreting sufficient chorionic gonadotrophin for a positive test. In some individuals, false positive tests may be obtained in other conditions than pregnancy. Very high titers are the rule in hydatidiform mole and chorionepithelioma.

Although many animals and technics have been suggested, only three will be described.

HOGBEN TEST—This test, probably the most accurate of the group, makes use of the South African clawed frog (*Xenopus laevis*). A morning urine specimen is concentrated, and in the late afternoon a portion is injected into the dorsal lymph sac of a female frog which has been isolated from males. The next morning the frog case is inspected for the presence of eggs, which constitutes a positive test. The Hogben test is simple and highly accurate, giving very few false negatives and, it has been claimed, no false positives. One of its great advantages is that it distinguishes between chorionic and anterior pituitary gonadotrophin, being unresponsive to the latter. It thus does not give false positives in those conditions listed under the Friedman test (see below). A further advantage is that the same animals can be used repeatedly. The only drawback is the difficulty of maintaining the frog aquarium. A careful feeding regimen is necessary; the temperature of the water must be closely controlled; and extreme care is necessary in the choice of animals, for certain of the females do not produce eggs at all times of the year and under all conditions.

ASCHHEIM-ZONDEK TEST—This, the oldest of the tests utilizing chorionic gonadotrophin, employs the immature female white mouse. The concentrate of morning urine or, preferably, a quantity of the patient's blood serum is injected subcutaneously into five such mice over a period of two days. Four or five days after the first injection the mice are killed, and the ovaries are examined. A positive reaction is indicated by the presence of corpora lutea or hemorrhagic follicles or both. In some series, erroneous results have been obtained in as many as 5 percent; but it now appears that careful attention to technical detail can reduce the errors to less than 1 percent, exclusive of distinctions which are beyond the capacity of the test (see below).

The test has several disadvantages. It takes almost a week to perform. Several animals must be sacrificed, and a constantly renewed supply must be available. Only in the most experienced hands will the test distinguish the amenorrhea of pregnancy from that of the menopause.

FRIEDMAN TEST—This test uses mature virgin female rabbits which have been isolated for a period of four weeks. The concentrate of morning urine is injected intravenously, and sixteen to twenty-four hours later the rabbit is killed and the ovaries are examined. Ruptured, hemorrhagic follicles indicate a positive test.

The Friedman test has the advantage over the Aschheim-Zondek test that a report is available more promptly. It shares with the A-Z test the disadvantage of sacrificing the animals. It fails completely to distinguish chorionic from pituitary gonadotrophin, and false positive tests may therefore be obtained in the menopause, primary deficient ovarian function in younger women, pituitary dysfunction (including tumor and acromegaly), adrenogenital syndrome, benign or malignant tumors of the adrenal cortex, hypothyroidism, hyperthyroidism, diabetes mellitus, functional and organic diseases of the nervous system (such as psychosis, psychoneurosis, anorexia nervosa, epilepsy), and miscellaneous conditions which include essential hypertension, progressive myopia, keratoconus, and alopecia areata.

In men, positive tests may be obtained in those conditions listed above which are not necessarily confined to women, and also in primary testicular deficiency and in some testicular tumors.

The Engle modification of the Friedman test utilizes blood serum instead of urine as the source of chorionic gonadotrophin. Blood serum probably gives more accurate results.

Tests Depending on Responsiveness of Endometrial Vascular Bed—The altered hormonal status during even very early pregnancy affects the responsiveness of the endometrial blood vessels. This change has been utilized in a test for pregnancy.

NEOSTIGMINE TEST—To perform this test, the patient is given 2 cc. of a 1:2,000 solution of neostigmine methylsulfate by subcutaneous injection on each of three successive days. Failure to have vaginal bleeding within seventy-two hours of the last injection is considered a positive result. Bleeding constitutes a negative result. If bleeding follows the first or second injection, no additional injections are given.

The advantage of the neostigmine test is its simplicity. Its disadvantage is its lack of specificity. As with the Aschheim-Zondek and Friedman tests, positive neostigmine tests are obtained not only in the amenorrhea of pregnancy but also in amenorrhea due to endocrine disturbance, including menopause. In addition, false positives (that is, failure to induce bleeding) may occur in the presence of organic pelvic disease in nonpregnant women. False negatives (i.e., bleeding) have been reported in uterine and tubal pregnancies.

Tests Depending on Progesterone—The ability of progesterone to raise body temperature and the excretion of progesterone as pregnanediol glucuronidate have been used as indices of the increased progesterone secretion which accompanies pregnancy.

BODY TEMPERATURE—Perhaps the earliest reliable indication of pregnancy is the maintenance of a high waking body temperature instead of the normal premenstrual fall. This is the only test which can be depended on to indicate pregnancy before the first period is missed. However, it is useful only in women who have been taking their morning temperatures regularly, and a small minority are unable to obtain readings which are sufficiently consistent to be interpretable. The determination and interpretation of waking body temperature are discussed on page 203.

GUTERMAN TEST—This test involves the isolation and colorimetric determination of pregnanediol from morning urine. Normally, pregnanediol appears in the urine from about the ninth day of the menstrual cycle until one to four days before the onset of bleeding. At the beginning of normal pregnancy, pregnanediol excretion continues at or above the maximum premenstrual level.

The test thus depends on the finding of a normal substance at a time which is abnormal in the nonpregnant. Obviously, positive results will be obtained during progesterone therapy and in the presence of a corpus luteum cyst. False positive results may also occur when menstruation is late because of delayed ovulation. Under these circumstances, the urine specimen may be collected during the luteal phase of a delayed but otherwise normal cycle. Thus, the test is of no value during progesterone therapy and has its maximum reliability only during actual amenorrhea in a woman whose menstrual function is customarily regular.

The test is quicker and less expensive than those utilizing chorionic gonadotrophin, although the technic appears to be rather exacting. The test has the additional advantage that false positive results are unlikely in hydatidiform mole or chorionepithelioma and are never caused by those conditions outside of pregnancy in which excretion of pituitary gonadotrophin occurs (p. 208).

Because of its newness, there are still differences of opinion regarding the reliability of the Guterman test as a criterion of pregnancy, and its reported accuracy varies from about 75 percent to 98 percent. There can be no doubt about the value of serial determinations as a prognostic aid in threatened abortion (p. 211).

Anatomical Evidence of Pregnancy—One of the earliest physical evidences of pregnancy is persistence of, and even increase in, the premenstrual breast tenderness. In an intelligent woman of regular menstrual function, a missed menstrual period with unusual breast tenderness is strongly suggestive of pregnancy.

Purely objective anatomical criteria appear later. In about the sixth week after the beginning of the last menstrual period, the lower uterine segment becomes softened and ballotable (Hegar's sign). By the end of the second month, the uterus is soft and globular and about the size of a goose egg. The vagina has taken on a bluish hue (Chadwick's sign). The breasts have become more full and turgid, the areolae are darker, and the nipples are more erectile. Colostrum may be present.

In experienced hands, pregnancy can be diagnosed with considerable probability on the basis of physical examination by the end of the second month. However, pregnancy cannot be established with absolute certainty except by one of the following: hearing and counting of the fetal heart, outlining the fetus, perception of active and passive movements, or recognition of the fetal skeleton by means of x-ray.

MANAGEMENT OF NORMAL PREGNANCY

Medical Care—Medical supervision during pregnancy has the dual purpose of assisting the patient to meet the needs of normal pregnancy and anticipating, if possible, the development of complications. The physician should, therefore, obtain a full medical history, including details of menstrual function and previous pregnancies, and perform a thorough physical examination. The pelvic examination should include internal and external pelvic measurements.

The patient should see the physician every three or four weeks during the first six months of pregnancy, every two weeks during the seventh and eighth months, and once a week during the final month. She should bring a specimen of the first morning urine each time, and at each visit the following should be recorded: weight, blood pressure, height of the fundus, and rate of fetal heart. Questioning should be especially directed toward gastro-intestinal symptoms, abdominal pain, edema, visual disturbances, fetal movements, and vaginal bleeding.

During the last week or two before term, the patient should take a vitamin K preparation (p. 499) daily to prevent hemorrhagic disease in the newborn. If labor begins without this treatment, single large doses are effective if given a few hours before delivery. If even this is not possible, the child may be given an injectable preparation on delivery, but such late treatment is not so effective as administration to the mother an adequate interval before birth.

Dietary Needs—The diet is especially important during pregnancy, for it affects the welfare of both mother and child. The total caloric intake should increase about 20 percent in the second and third trimesters, but weight gain should be limited to 15 or, at most, 20 pounds above the "ideal" weight (p. 568) for the individual patient (see below for the role of fluid retention in weight gain). The protein intake in the latter half of pregnancy should be at least 1 Gm. per Kg. of body weight, with a minimum of 85 Gm. During lactation it should be 100 Gm. A quart of milk should be taken daily, plus liberal quantities of meat, eggs, and cheese.

The National Research Council has recommended the following daily intakes:

	Pregnancy (Latter Half)	Lactation
Calcium, Gm.	1.5	2
Iron, mg.	15	15
Vit. A, I.U.	6,000	8,000
Thiamin, mg.	1.5	1.5
Riboflavin, mg.	2.5	3
Niacin, mg.	15	15
Vit. C, mg.	100	150
Vit. D, I.U.	400	400

More than half of otherwise normal pregnancies are accompanied by some degree of generalized edema. Although this edema in itself seems to do no harm, it appears to predispose to toxemia, and it obscures tissue weight gain. It is therefore advised that sodium intake be restricted in pregnant women who show generalized edema (in distinction to edema limited to the lower extremities in late pregnancy) or who gain suddenly or excessively in weight. Low-sodium diets will be found on page 585. Restriction to 1.5 Gm. of sodium chloride daily should be adequate in most cases.

Restriction of sodium intake during the last six weeks of pregnancy appears to shorten and facilitate labor, and some obstetricians limit sodium intake as a routine matter over this period.

Minor Complications—One of the first complaints is likely to be frequency of urination. This is due to impingement of the expanding uterus on the bladder, and it may be accompanied by mild inflammation of the trigone. Urinary tract infection (p. 224) should be ruled out. Usually an explanation will satisfy the patient. If frequency is very disturbing, a tight lower-abdominal binder may be worn, or the patient may assume the knee-chest posture for a few minutes several times a day. Sometimes mild sedation or one of the "urinary antiseptics" (pp. 305 and 310) is helpful.

One-half to two-thirds of pregnant women have some degree of anemia. Characteristically it is mild and of the hypochromic, microcytic type (p. 95). Response to iron (p. 368) or to liver (p. 369) and iron is usually prompt. Anemia from other causes, coincidental to pregnancy, must not be overlooked.

Pains in the back, head, or extremities are common during pregnancy. Back pain and "sciatica" may be postural. Numbness and tingling of the extremities may be due to impairment of the circulation from increased intra-abdominal pressure, anemia, or early toxemia. Severe pain may be a symptom of toxemia. Neuritis (p. 168) may occur; it is treated by vitamin B complex, salicylates, and adequate rest.

Insomnia is a frequent complaint. Awareness of the physiological changes of pregnancy (such as increased intra-abdominal pressure, changes in gastro-intestinal motility, and fullness of the breasts) may be a factor, as well as the emotional impact of pregnancy itself. Regulation of diet, adequate exercise, and mild sedation are usually effective.

Heartburn, sour eructations, and other manifestations of indigestion are common. In their presence, fat and carbohydrate intake should be reduced. Antacids (p. 382) may be employed, but soda should be taken sparingly or, better, avoided because of its systemic alkalizing effect. For treatment of flatulence, see page 133. Constipation may be especially troublesome. In many cases the taking of a glass of hot water containing 1/2 teaspoonful of table salt half an hour before breakfast will help to establish regularity. For additional treatment of constipation, see page 130. Enemas are best avoided during pregnancy.

Abdominal discomfort, especially late in pregnancy, is due to the weight of the gravid uterus. Constipation, faulty shoes, and inadequate or improper abdominal support may be complicating factors and should be corrected.

Leukorrhea is a frequent complaint. The natural increase in cervical secretion and vaginal moisture due to estrogen and progesterone during pregnancy must be distinguished from pathological causes of leukorrhea (see p. 197). Coitus during pregnancy probably increases the natural secretion. In the presence of vaginal infection, active treatment may be carried out until the seventh month of pregnancy. When leukorrhea is profuse in the absence of infection, cleansing douches may be employed up to the seventh month.

In order to prevent reflex pelvic congestion, the patient should dress warmly when out in cold weather. Full-length stockings should be worn, and these should preferably be heavy rather than sheer.

ABORTION

Abortion threatens at one time or another in at least 16 percent of all pregnancies, and spontaneous abortion occurs in about 10 percent. This means that without treatment six out of sixteen (or about 40 percent) of threatened abortions do not abort, whereas without treatment ten out of sixteen (or 60 percent) do abort. In about two-thirds of spontaneous abortions, the product of conception is defective or has died before the onset of abortion or for some other reason probably could not have been saved; but it is estimated that one-third of spontaneous abortions are theoretically salvageable at the time the patient is first seen by the physician. Thus, under treatment, there is potential salvage of not only the 40 percent of threatened abortions that would have continued to term without treatment, but also of the 20 percent (one-third of the 60 percent that aborted) considered salvageable by treatment.

The maintenance of pregnancy appears to depend primarily on a continued supply of estrogen and progesterone secreted by the placenta or by the corpus luteum of pregnancy under stimulation by chorionic gonadotrophin formed in the fertilized ovum or placenta. Death of the ovum, embryo, or fetus leads to cessation of estrogen and progesterone production. There may be a dangerous drop in hormone output during the twelfth to sixteenth week, when chorionic gonadotrophin production is diminishing and estrogen and progesterone production by the placenta is not yet fully under way. In spite of normal hormone production, the uterus may be stimulated to empty itself by extrinsic factors or by abnormal conditions of the endometrium or decidua. Maternal factors include low implantation of the placenta, uterine abnormalities (e.g., fixed retroversion, fibroid tumors), febrile and inflammatory disease, hypothyroidism, toxemia of pregnancy, and trauma.

An abortion is termed "missed" when the fetus is dead but abortion has not occurred within a few days. It is "incomplete" when fragments of the products of conception remain in the uterine cavity. It is "threatened" when vaginal bleeding or uterine cramps or both indicate that the membranes have begun to separate from the decidua or strong uterine contractions have begun, or both. It is "imminent" when these manifestations are so severe that the abortion can probably not be prevented. "Habitual abortion" is the term applied when the occurrence of two or more consecutive spontaneous abortions suggests that there is a high probability that succeeding pregnancies will end in the same way.

Abortion is sometimes undertaken therapeutically when continuation of pregnancy involves grave risk to the life or health of the mother. Curettage of the uterus in the first trimester, abdominal or anterior vaginal hysterotomy in the second trimester, and induction of labor or cesarean section in the third trimester constitute the only safe and accepted methods for therapeutic abortion. There is no known medication that will induce abortion except as a secondary effect of serious intoxication.

Treatment—When abortion threatens, the first principle is to keep the patient and her uterus quiet. She is put to bed, and sedatives (p. 390) or analgesics (p. 405) or both are administered as indicated. There should be no abdominal or vaginal manipulation, and laxatives and enemas are withheld.

Recent evidence indicates that the percentage of cases salvaged can be considerably increased by oral administration of diethylstilbestrol (p. 467). Dosage is not entirely settled, but an effective schedule seems to be 25 mg. as soon as the diagnosis is made, followed by 5 mg. every fifteen minutes or 25 mg. every hour until bleeding or cramps or both have ceased. After this, 5 mg. are given three times daily. It is difficult to determine when the drug can be safely discontinued. There is no harm in continuing it through the thirty-sixth week. If threatening symptoms recur, the original schedule is repeated.

Progesterone (p. 468) has been used in threatened abortion, but the amount required (at least 10 mg. daily) is large and it does not seem to be as effective as diethylstilbestrol.

If abortion actually occurs (as indicated by passage of membranes or fetus or both), diethylstilbestrol is discontinued and oxytocics (p. 476) are given, preferably ergonovine maleate, 0.2 to 0.4

mg. every six hours until bleeding ceases or for a maximum of two days. If incomplete abortion is not completed within two days (as shown by careful examination of expelled material) or if bleeding persists or is profuse, curettage should be performed. At its completion, ergonovine maleate may be administered intravenously. Infection, which contraindicates curettage, should be treated with systemic anti-infective agents (p. 286).

The treatment of habitual abortion should preferably start before conception with correction of all demonstrable endocrine and nutritional disturbances in both prospective mother and father. In particular, thyroid (p. 456) is advocated when there is any evidence of hypothyroidism (p. 180).

In the absence of hypothyroidism, probably the most effective agent is diethylstilbestrol. Its administration should be begun after pregnancy occurs but well before the expected threat of abortion. The dosage may be the same as that given during the corresponding week of pregnancy as prophylaxis against toxemia of pregnancy (see below).

Progesterone has been advocated (for dosage and administration, see p. 468), but it is apparently less effective than diethylstilbestrol. Administration of vitamin E (p. 497) has been proposed, but the results are hard to evaluate.

In the presence of retroversion, a pessary should be worn until the uterus has risen well out of the pelvis.

NAUSEA AND VOMITING OF PREGNANCY

One-half to two-thirds of women have some degree of nausea and vomiting during the first trimester of pregnancy. It usually begins about the sixth week and may last as long as two or three months. The cause has not been definitely established, but several lines of evidence point to an allergic mechanism. As in other forms of allergy, emotional and psychic factors may be extremely important.

In some patients the vomiting is severe enough to lead to serious dehydration (hyperemesis gravidarum). Possible causes outside of pregnancy should always be considered.

Many types of treatment have been advocated in the past. The most effective now seems to be an antihistaminic drug (p. 509). The dosage may have to be large (e.g., 50 to 100 mg. of 'Histadyl' three or four times daily), and sometimes better results are obtained if pyridoxine hydrochloride (p. 489) is added in doses of 50 to 100 mg. or more daily. In severe cases, initial doses should be intravenous. After relief has been obtained, the oral route may

be used, and the dose and frequency of administration can often be reduced. In very mild cases the oral route may be effective from the beginning. In very resistant cases, concomitant administration of 50 to 100 mg. of thiamin chloride (p. 484) is often of value. However, intravenous administration of thiamin chloride is not recommended because of the possible development of sensitivity following repeated doses by this route.

If drug therapy is relatively ineffective, the physician should investigate the emotional factors. Particular attention should be directed toward the possibility that the pregnancy is not desired or that there has been undue mother attachment or difficulties in the sexual field.

Traditional measures which are sometimes helpful include frequent small feedings of solid food, avoidance of fluids within an hour before or after meals, taking of dry crackers or toast before arising (in cases of morning nausea), and mild sedation.

If the patient is able to retain little or no food or liquid, she should be hospitalized promptly. Extragenital causes and genital causes outside the pregnancy (such as retroflexed uterus or ovarian cyst) should be ruled out. Special nursing care is provided, and all visitors, including the husband, are barred. Nothing but a small quantity of cracked ice is allowed by mouth, and the patient is treated as for dehydration (p. 56). Adequate psychotherapy should be undertaken.

If there is considerable improvement after two days, solid foods may be given while parenteral fluids are continued. A general diet and fluids by mouth are gradually resumed as tolerated. If improvement does not occur, fluids, vitamins, and carbohydrate are given by duodenal tube. If, in spite of treatment, the condition becomes worse, consultation should be sought with a view to emptying the uterus. Indications for therapeutic abortion in hyperemesis gravidarum include persistent tachycardia, jaundice, fever, hypotension, psychosis, or loss of twenty pounds' weight. Local or regional anesthesia should be employed.

TOXEMIA OF PREGNANCY

Toxemia of pregnancy (eclampsia and pre-eclampsia) is the third largest cause of maternal mortality. It is a specific condition peculiar to pregnancy. Its onset is limited to the latter half of pregnancy, and typically it recedes completely prior to or shortly after delivery. Its manifestations include one or more of the following: hypertension, proteinuria, generalized edema. In full-blown cases there may be headache, vomiting, visual disturbances, convulsions, coma, heart failure, pulmonary edema, and death.

The cause of toxemia of pregnancy is unknown. The geographic incidence varies considerably, being highest in southern United States. Predisposing factors include the presence of hypertension before pregnancy, generalized edema during pregnancy, primiparity, diabetes mellitus, twin pregnancies, and hydatidiform mole.

Toxemia of pregnancy is characterized by a hormonal disturbance which has been most closely studied in diabetic women. In them, there begins ten weeks or more before the development of toxemia an increased excretion of estrogen and progesterone such as normally occurs in the first half of the last month of pregnancy. In some cases a rise in blood level of chorionic gonadotrophin may occur about five weeks later. Somewhat before the onset of toxemia the level of estrogen and progesterone excretion falls below normal. With the onset of clinical manifestations, the excretion pattern changes: progesterone output becomes very low, and the estrogen fraction contains little or no estrone but a relatively high percentage of estradiol.

Treatment—As in many other conditions, the best treatment of toxemia of pregnancy is prevention. In early pregnancy, or even before pregnancy, the physician should recognize those women who are predisposed to toxemia because of pre-existing hypertensive or renal disease. The patient's weight is followed closely, and she is instructed to report promptly the occurrence of edema, headache, visual disturbance, or other possible manifestation. Rapid weight gain or frank edema should lead to a low-sodium regimen. In place of sodium bicarbonate or other sodium compounds for gastrointestinal symptoms such as heartburn, the patient should employ milk of magnesia, magnesium trisilicate (p. 383), or aluminum hydroxide (p. 382). It may be advisable to administer ammonium or potassium chloride in doses of 2 to 12 Gm. daily.

Proteinuria and rise in blood pressure should be watched for. Either one is an indication for bed rest at home or in hospital, with daily checks of weight, blood pressure, urine, edema, and symptoms. Fluids are allowed freely, but sodium intake is limited to 0.5 Gm. daily (p. 585). If manifestations subside promptly, limited activity may be resumed cautiously; but sodium restriction should be continued, and excessive caloric intake should be avoided. If the condition does not improve, bed rest is continued, sedation is prescribed, and

sodium and water elimination is pursued more vigorously.

In the past, treatment of eclampsia (convulsions or coma) and severe pre-eclampsia (very high blood pressure and an extreme degree of such symptoms as headache, visual disturbances, edema of hands or face, nausea and vomiting, epigastric pain with liver tenderness, or jaundice) has been largely symptomatic and has included intravenous administration of magnesium sulfate, oxygen therapy, and, as a last resort, evacuation of the uterus. The mortality remained relatively high. Recently it has been demonstrated that eclampsia or severe pre-eclampsia can be fully controlled in almost all cases by prolonged high spinal or epidural anesthesia (p. 439). These procedures do not, of course, attack the cause, but they prevent the effects, apparently by blocking a sufficiently large proportion of the sympathetic nervous system. The success of these measures adds considerable support to the idea that the effects of eclampsia are due to vasoconstriction. If labor begins or cesarean section is undertaken, the caudal or spinal anesthesia suffices for these events.

In the past few years a number of workers have been able to prevent toxemia of pregnancy in predisposed women by treatment with diethylstilbestrol, either alone or combined with progesterone. Most of the studies have been on diabetic women. In them, diethylstilbestrol has greatly reduced the incidence of toxemia and of premature delivery and has increased severalfold the percentage of live babies. Recommended dosage is given in Table 21 (p. 214). When progesterone is employed in addition, the average daily dose is 15 mg. by intramuscular injection.

PARTURITION

Duration of Pregnancy—The average interval between the first day of the last menstruation and delivery of a living child is 280 days. A table for calculation of dates based on this interval appears on page 589. About half of all such deliveries can be expected to occur within seven days of the calculated date.

Induction of Labor—Labor is sometimes induced for conditions which threaten the welfare of mother or baby or in those few cases in which the baby is truly postmature. Probably the most effective method is rupture of the membranes under sterile precautions. However, this procedure should be carried out only by an experienced person, for a definite indication, and only if the head is the

TABLE 21 — *Dosage Schedule for Oral Administration of Diethylstilbestrol in Prevention of Accidents of Pregnancy*

Week of Pregnancy, Dating from First Day of Last Menstrual Period	Daily Dose
7th and 8th	5 mg.
9th and 10th	10 mg.
11th and 12th	15 mg.
13th and 14th	20 mg.
15th	25 mg.
16th	30 mg.
17th	35 mg.
18th	40 mg.
19th	45 mg.
20th	50 mg.
21st	55 mg.
22d	60 mg.
23d	65 mg.
24th	70 mg.
25th	75 mg.
26th	80 mg.
27th	85 mg.
28th	90 mg.
29th	95 mg.
30th	100 mg.
31st	105 mg.
32d	110 mg.
33d	115 mg.
34th	120 mg.
35th	125 mg.
36th	Drug discontinued

presenting part and is well engaged and the cervix is already partly effaced and dilated.

Medical induction is less frequently successful, but it avoids vaginal entry and artificial breach of the membranes. The myometrium may be made more responsive by administering diethylstilbestrol (p. 467) on the day before induction (10 or 15 mg. once an hour by mouth for ten doses). On the day of induction the following schedule may be carried out:

6 a.m.—castor oil, 2 oz.

8 a.m.—hot soapsuds enema

10 a.m.—posterior pituitary extract, 2 U.S.P. Units hypodermically or intranasally (p. 474)

If labor does not set in, the posterior pituitary is repeated at half-hour intervals for a total of four doses. If no labor results, the patient is given another hot soapsuds enema at seven in the evening, and posterior pituitary is again given for no more than four doses at half-hour intervals.

Quinine was formerly used, but its advisability has been questioned because it apparently may cause deafness in some of the babies. Posterior pituitary should not be given to a patient with toxemia of pregnancy or severe hypertension.

Pain Relief—It has been demonstrated that judicious pain relief during labor and delivery results not only in greater comfort for the mother but also in lower mortality rates for both mother and baby. There is, however, still considerable controversy among obstetricians as to the relative merits of the different means of providing pain relief.

The need for pain relief varies greatly among women. In general, there is discomfort beginning with the actual onset of labor. The most that is needed during this period is mild sedation. Women who are not apprehensive need nothing. Sooner or later the discomfort progresses to the point where relief is justified. Here one can employ systemic narcotic or hypnotic drugs which produce analgesia or amnesia or both, or one can administer regional nerve block. Toward the end of the second stage of labor a much greater degree of relief is usually necessary, and one may add to previous measures inhalation or intravenous anesthesia or regional or spinal nerve block.

Agents and methods commonly employed are listed below. They are discussed and their use outlined in the cross references given.

General inhalation anesthetics
  Volatile agents
    Ether (p. 411)
    Chloroform (p. 412)
  Gaseous agents
    Nitrous oxide (p. 412)
    Ethylene (p. 412)
    Cyclopropane (p. 413)
Systemic analgesic agents
  Narcotic and amnesic agents
    Morphine and opium (p. 399)
    Synthetic morphine-like drugs (p. 404)
    Scopolamine (p. 421)
  Hypnotic agents
    Barbiturates (p. 394)
Drugs given intravenously
  Barbiturates (Pentothal Sodium) (p. 394)
Drugs given rectally
  Ether (p. 411)
  Paraldehyde (p. 398)
  Barbiturates (p. 394)
Regional anesthesia (p. 437 *et seq.*)
  Infiltration of perineum
  Pudendal block
  Continuous caudal anesthesia
  Terminal caudal block
  Continuous lumbar epidural anesthesia
  Continuous spinal anesthesia
  Terminal spinal anesthesia, including saddle block

THE PUERPERIUM

The puerperium extends technically from the end of the third stage of labor until uterine involution is complete, the endometrium has entirely regenerated, and all the reversible effects of pregnancy have disappeared.

There is a growing advocacy of early rising in the puerperium, the patient being allowed, in the absence of complications, to get up for the toilet on the day following delivery. Additional graduated activity is allowed beginning on the third or fourth day. However, full home responsibility had best not be assumed for at least two weeks. Many obstetricians routinely prescribe ergonovine maleate (p. 476), 0.2 to 0.4 mg. two or three times daily by mouth, for the first two weeks postpartum, for maintenance of firm uterine contraction and prevention of late hemorrhage.

Uterine involution probably results, at least in part, from withdrawal of the estrogen circulating during pregnancy. Oxytocics and maintenance of uterine contraction apparently do not influence uterine involution, but the incidence of subinvolution appears to be less after caudal anesthesia than after systemic analgesia.

Hemorrhage—Postpartum hemorrhage is the leading cause of maternal mortality. Furthermore, hemorrhage predisposes to puerperal infection, which is the second cause of maternal death. Blood loss is not generally termed hemorrhage unless it exceeds 500 cc. It is obvious, however, that damage does not start suddenly as that figure is reached, and it is reasonable to believe that all reductions in blood loss are beneficial to the mother.

Postpartum blood loss comes from two sources: from the decidua and placental site, and from lacerations or episiotomy incisions. Lacerations may involve the introitus, the vagina, the cervix, or the uterine wall itself (rupture of the uterus). Bleeding from the decidua and placental site may be due to uterine atony or retention of secundines, including all or part of the placenta. Uterine atony may be due to exhaustion from prolonged labor, overdistention of the uterus (multiple pregnancy, hydramnios), sedative or general anesthetic drugs, or unknown causes. Blood dyscrasias affecting coagulation (p. 107) may increase blood loss.

TREATMENT—The best treatment is prevention. Lacerations may be avoided or minimized by employing regional anesthesia which induces relaxation of the cervix and perineum, by not forcing dilatation of the birth canal, and by employing episiotomy to replace an uncontrollable tear with a clean controlled incision. Immediately after delivery of the child, the vulva, perineum, and lower vagina should be inspected carefully, and bleeding arteries should be secured. Continuous or excessive venous bleeding or the appearance of any bright arterial blood should lead to exposure and inspection of the upper vagina and cervix for lacerations.

Uterine atony will be minimized by the avoidance of general anesthetic agents (including ether) or large doses of sedatives and by such a management of labor as will prevent uterine exhaustion. Caudal or spinal anesthesia leads to a maintenance of uterine tone which materially reduces blood loss from the denuded surface of the uterus.

It is almost universal practice to administer an oxytocic agent at the end of either the second or the third stage of labor as a prophylactic against uterine atony. Posterior pituitary extract is a traditional agent, but ergonovine maleate is more potent and more enduring and carries less chance of adverse reaction. The dosage and use of these preparations are discussed beginning on page 476.

In the presence of sudden severe hemorrhage, the physician can stop all blood flow to the uterus temporarily by compressing through the abdominal wall the abdominal aorta just above its bifurcation. While pressure is thus maintained, the cause of the bleeding is sought. If it cannot be corrected, alternatives are packing of the uterus with gauze or, as a last resort, hysterectomy.

Often a relaxed uterus can be induced to contract by skillful massage, repeated as necessary. If this is not quickly effective (it is assumed that oxytocics have already been given), intravenous administration of calcium salts may produce sudden and dramatic contraction (see p. 344 for dosage and precautions). Packing of the uterus may be helpful but is less used than formerly.

If retained secundines are a factor in postpartum hemorrhage, they should be removed. Whole-blood transfusions should be given in the presence of excessive blood loss.

Infection is the second most important cause of maternal mortality. Postpartum uterine infection does not differ fundamentally from infection elsewhere. The commonest infecting organisms are streptococci (usually anaerobic) and staphylococci; less frequently present are pneumococci, gonococci, colon bacilli, and the anaerobic spore bearers. Predisposing and causative factors include hemorrhage, uterine trauma, a long labor (permitting entry of organisms from vagina), uterine atony, excessive manipulation or instrumentation, and faulty aseptic technic. Such factors should obviously be prevented when possible. Once infection has developed, it should be vigorously treated with systemic anti-infective agents (p. 286). Whole-blood transfusions may be of great value, especially if blood loss has been excessive.

Painful Engorgement of the Breasts is most likely to occur when lactation is beginning or ending. Contrary to the general view, the engorgement is not due to colostrum or milk but is vascular and lymphatic.

Estrogenic therapy is capable of preventing post-partum breast engorgement in a high percentage of cases; it will relieve a somewhat smaller percentage, once engorgement is present. Although lactation is not inhibited by such treatment, the onset is delayed and the volume is temporarily diminished. The percentage of children requiring bottle feeding is increased, and the value of estrogenic therapy would therefore seem to be greatest when the mother is not to nurse her baby.

A total dose of 30 mg. diethylstilbestrol or its equivalent (p. 467) is usually adequate. It may be given as 5 mg. three times daily for two days or as 5 mg. once daily for six days. Failures in treatment are usually due to inadequate dosage.

Androgens may be given as alternative therapy (p. 469), the average dosage being three injections of 10 mg. of testosterone propionate at daily intervals or 150 to 200 mg. of methyltestosterone by mouth distributed over a two-day period.

Mild recurrence of engorgement with watery secretion may occur about a week after cessation of therapy. This is ordinarily controlled by a second course of the drug in the same dosage.

MALE GENITAL SYSTEM *

ORCHITIS

Acute orchitis, or inflammation of the testis, is usually the result of trauma or of infection with mumps (p. 26). Rarely it may accompany other systemic infections. The swollen and inflamed testis is exquisitely tender. Suppuration or gangrene is occasionally seen. Atrophy of the testis is a common sequel, with spermatogenesis much more affected than androgen production (p. 189). Chronic orchitis is usually due to syphilis or tuberculosis.

Treatment—In acute orchitis the patient should remain in bed with the scrotum elevated and im-

mobilized. Cold applications and sedation are usually gratefully received. Extreme swelling may be treated by multiple incisions of the tunica albuginea. For treatment of mumps orchitis, see page 28.

EPIDIDYMITIS

Acute epididymitis is usually secondary to infection of the posterior urethra, prostate, or seminal vesicle on that side and is most commonly due to the gonococcus (p. 6). Mild trauma predisposes to the complication. Treatment is similar to that for orchitis.

PROSTATITIS

Infection of the prostate gland, like that of the epididymides and testes, is usually secondary to infection elsewhere; but after the gland is once infected, it may itself be a factor in disturbances, if not infections, elsewhere, such as arthritis, neuritis, and iritis. Acute prostatitis in younger men is usually due to the gonococcus (p. 6). Chronic prostatitis, particularly in older men, is seldom directly associated with this organism; although it may have had its origin in acute gonorrheal infection, the gonococci have been displaced by other organisms.

When prostatitis causes symptoms, these may include urethral discharge, urinary frequency, burning, nocturia, urgency, pyuria, dribbling, hematuria, straining, and so on. There may also be loss of libido, weakness or loss of erections, nocturnal erections, premature ejaculation, painful ejaculation, sterility, or prostatorrhea.

Treatment of prostatitis includes (1) systemic anti-infectives, such as penicillin or the sulfonamides; (2) prostatic massage; (3) rectal application of heat to the prostate; and (4) appropriate variations in diet.

The choice and use of anti-infective agents depend upon the susceptibility of the causative organism. Gonococci and staphylococci are usually susceptible to either penicillin or a sulfonamide (for dosage, see pp. 288 and 293). Improvement caused by these drugs is usually apparent within a week. The so-called urinary antiseptics, which do not penetrate tissues, are valueless in prostatitis.

Local therapy is also of considerable importance. Prostatic massage is employed in chronic (but *not* in acute) prostatitis for the purpose of emptying

———
* For endocrine aspects, see page 189.

the gland of purulent material and stimulating the local circulation. It must always be gentle; it is usually repeated twice a week until the prostatic strippings are free of pus and there is evidence of recovery otherwise. Local heat is applied, usually in chronic prostatitis, by the use of sitz baths, hot rectal irrigations, or special forms of apparatus using hot water or the electric current.

Attention should also be directed toward the infection to which the prostatitis is secondary. Constipation (p. 130) must be prevented, and condiments and alcoholic beverages should be avoided.

BENIGN PROSTATIC HYPERTROPHY

About 30 percent of men past sixty years of age have some degree of prostatic hypertrophy, and a third of these have symptoms. The cause of the hypertrophy is unknown. Connective-tissue and smooth-muscle elements of the gland undergo progressive hyperplasia which may be limited to one lobe or may involve several.

The most common symptoms are due to urinary obstruction. They include urinary frequency (especially nocturnal), diminution in force and size of the stream, difficulty in starting the stream, urgency, and painful urination. Other possible manifestations are hematuria, discomfort or mild pain referred to the perineum, back, rectum, or suprapubic region, rectal symptoms (from disturbed hemorrhoidal circulation or bulging of the enlarged prostate into the rectum), and disturbance of sexual powers (early increase and later loss). As the condition progresses, there may be incomplete emptying of the bladder, urinary tract infection (p. 224), or hydronephrosis and uremia (p. 222).

Diagnosis depends on the finding of smooth, firm, but not hard, enlargement of the prostate gland on rectal examination, or a characteristic picture of deformity of the posterior urethra or base of the bladder on cystoscopy, or both. Differential diagnosis includes prostatic calculus, tuberculosis, thick-walled abscess, cancer and other neoplasms, and neurogenic bladder.

Treatment—If symptoms are troublesome or there is objective evidence of a significant degree of urinary obstruction (slight trabeculation of the bladder and thickening of the trigone, residual urine, slight hydronephrosis, or elevation of the blood urea or nonprotein nitrogen level), operation is indicated; it may take the form of transurethral resection or perineal or suprapubic prostatectomy,

depending on the location of the hypertrophy and other considerations. Special examinations or surgical procedures should be undertaken only after a careful survey of general health, with particular attention to cardiovascular and renal function. The presence of acute urinary retention requires catheterization, which should always be accompanied by the most rigid aseptic precautions.

Various forms of medical therapy have been proposed, but none is helpful in a high percentage of cases. Androgens may provide temporary symptomatic improvement by increasing muscle tone of the bladder, but they do not affect the underlying cause. Estrogens appear to lessen the degree of obstruction in some cases, but the mechanism of such action is unknown, and the ultimate effect is uncertain.

IMPOTENCE

Sexual potency in men depends on psychic, functional and organic nervous, and endocrine factors. Androgens are necessary for the development of sexual potency; but once the normal adult state has been established, subsequent androgen deficiency is not always accompanied by impotence (see p. 190). Temporary impotence may be due to fatigue, nervous tension, or toxemia. Interference with the autonomic nervous system (as exemplified by the operation of sympathectomy) may result in permanent loss of sexual capacity.

Prolonged impotence in normally developed young men is almost always due to psychic and emotional factors. In older men it is commonly due to similar forces. Chronic prostatitis and benign prostatic hypertrophy may be contributory factors but are rarely primary causes.

Unless impotence is due to demonstrable lack of testicular function, it is not relieved by androgen therapy except insofar as this may constitute psychotherapy. The usual case of impotence requires unraveling and correction of the emotional factors.

PROSTATIC CANCER

Latent cancer is present in the prostate glands of almost half of men beyond the age of fifty. About 10 percent of these neoplasms become active, so that the incidence of clinical cancer of the prostate in men over fifty is 4 to 5 percent.

The cancer arises in the glandular epithelial cells, and ordinarily in the posterior lobe. Once activated, it spreads slowly and insidiously, often metastasizing before it is large enough to cause symptoms of urinary obstruction. Metastasis is by way of the lymphatics; and the lower vertebral column, sacrum, pelvic bones, and femurs are common sites. Carcinomatous lymph nodes may be palpated in the pelvis, over the promontory of the sacrum, along the spine, or in the supraclavicular fossae. Metastasis may occur to any structure of the body.

Early diagnosis is usually accidental, and incident to rectal palpation of the prostate. Prostatic cancer has a characteristic "stony" feel to the trained finger. Most cases are not diagnosed until metastases form visible or palpable tumors or cause pressure symptoms somewhere.

Metastatic prostatic cancer cells, particularly when in bone, liberate into the blood large quantities of the enzyme, acid phosphatase. The normal serum level is not more than 5 King-Armstrong units per 100 cc. A level of 10 units or more is indicative of active metastatic cancer of the prostate.

Treatment—Before treatment is decided upon, a survey for metastases should be undertaken. In the absence of suggestive symptoms or positive findings on complete physical examination, an x-ray including the lower spine, pelvis, and upper halves of the femurs should certainly be made, and probably one of the chest as well, for both bony and pulmonary metastases. If no metastases can be found and the growth seems still to be confined within the capsule of the prostate gland, immediate radical prostatectomy is indicated in an attempt at complete removal of the growth. In the presence of metastases, operation is indicated only for control of urinary obstruction.

In many cases of prostatic cancer, the epithelial cells, even though malignant, still require androgen for proliferation, and withdrawal of androgen causes regression of both primary growth and metastases for considerable periods of time. Such androgen withdrawal may be accomplished either by castration or by administration of an estrogen such as diethylstilbestrol (p. 467). There appears to be a longer average period of survival if the two methods are combined. At present the usual initial dosage of diethylstilbestrol is 3 mg. daily, with reduction to an average of 1 mg. daily after the condition is fully under control.

The response to androgen withdrawal is often very dramatic. In a few days the patient is free of pain, and he rapidly gains in weight and well-being. Hemoglobin and red cell count return to normal. In the course of many months x-ray evidence of metastases may disappear, and the pri-mary growth regresses. Not all patients respond so completely, and some do not respond at all. As time goes on there is an increasing incidence of relapse, so that the treatment is definitely palliative rather than curative.

Serial determinations of serum acid phosphatase are of value in following progress; for if there has been a high level which returns to normal under treatment, maintenance of the normal level seems to afford assurance of continued inactivity of the neoplasm. If relapse occurs under a single form of treatment, the other may be tried, but in this situation the percentage of success is not high. For complications of estrogen therapy, see page 465.

Administration of androgens, such as testosterone, reactivates prostatic cancer and is therefore absolutely contraindicated. The role of androgen in activating latent prostatic cancer has not yet been determined.

URINARY TRACT

The kidneys have as their major function the maintenance of the "internal environment"—the tissue-fluid medium in which the body cells actually live. They regulate the composition of the blood—and therefore of the "internal environment"—with respect to practically all its constituents except oxygen and carbon dioxide, the levels of which are controlled by the lungs.

Regulation of the internal environment by the kidneys involves three processes:

1. Removal by filtration of a portion of the blood plasma water with its dissolved substances;

2. Selective reabsorption for the most part of substances needed to maintain the internal environment; and

3. Secretory excretion of certain waste and foreign substances.

The daily volume of glomerular filtrate is normally about 190 liters. All but about twenty-one liters is *passively* reabsorbed by osmotic action in the proximal convoluted tubule and loop of Henle, leaving to the distal tubule the *active* reabsorption and concentration which determine the volume and specific gravity of the urine. Much of this distal tubular activity is under hormonal control by the posterior pituitary gland (p. 194).

GLOMERULONEPHRITIS

Glomerulonephritis, or hemorrhagic Bright's disease, is one of a group of bilateral nonsuppurative diseases of the kidney. The essential renal lesion is glomerular inflammation, and the most significant clinical feature is microscopic hematuria.

Glomerulonephritis may have an acute stage, often subsequent to infectious disease, characterized by diastolic hypertension, generalized edema, and oliguria which may progress to anuria. The urine contains abnormal quantities of red blood cells, protein, and casts (see Addis Count of Urine Sediment, p. 520). The edema of acute glomerulonephritis is typically "hard" and nonpitting, in contrast to the "soft," pitting edema of chronic glomerulonephritis, nephrosis (p. 220), and cardiac failure (p. 63).

Although the patient may die in the acute stage of glomerulonephritis, or more often recover completely, the disease may progress to a chronic stage in which the rate of progress is slow (so-called latent phase) or rapid (subacute). Microscopic hematuria and usually proteinuria persist, and their measurements form perhaps the best indices to the rate of progression or regression of the renal lesion (hence the importance of serial Addis counts). The extent of the renal lesion is revealed by the urea clearance and urine concentration tests (p. 520). The terminal stage is said to be reached when urea clearance has been reduced to 20 percent of normal.

Perhaps the majority of cases of chronic glomerulonephritis arise not as sequelae of acute nephritis, but insidiously without detectable antecedents, the first symptom usually being unexplained edema. Diagnosis is often impossible without the Addis count of the urine sediment. Diagnosis and the following of the course of the disease may be facilitated by tests of urea clearance, concentrating ability, and plasma protein content. The prognosis of this form of the disease is poor.

Treatment depends on the stage of the disease. In acute glomerulonephritis the first principle is bed rest. Bathroom privileges should be denied. It is important to keep the patient warm. The diet is as nearly sodium-free as possible (p. 585). If there is nausea or vomiting, give 10 percent dextrose in distilled water by vein or 5 percent by hypodermoclysis (saline or Ringer's Solution is to be avoided). When food can be taken by mouth, the daily protein intake (for adults) should be restricted at first to about 45 Gm., but carbohydrate and fat should be given to the patient's comfortable capacity in order to spare endogenous protein. As the acute stage subsides, protein intake for the adult is raised to about 75 Gm. daily (3 Gm. per pound of "ideal" body weight for a child). A liberal vitamin intake should be assured.

Total fluid intake must be adequate (see p. 52). Additional water beyond the basic requirement should be given as a diuretic. Provided sodium intake is restricted, water is a potent and safe diuretic. If a diuretic response is seen following an excess of one-half to one liter of water, the intake may be safely increased. In the absence of diuretic response, more water may be harmful. Unfortunately, the criteria for water intake are not definite. Other diuretics are to be avoided in the acute stage.

Penicillin (p. 288) and the sulfonamides (p. 293) appear to have curative value in those cases of acute glomerulonephritis which are related to infection with beta-hemolytic streptococci. However, certain precautions are imperative. The disease must have had an acute onset, and treatment should be begun as soon as possible—certainly not more than two months after onset. Renal damage from the sulfonamides is especially to be avoided. Dosage should be controlled by determinations of blood level (p. 537), and the urine should be kept alkaline (with *potassium*, not sodium, salts) and of adequate volume so that the specific gravity is below the maximum of which the kidneys are capable but at the same time not below 1.010. The occurrence of sulfonamide crystals or increased protein in the urine is cause for redoubling precautions. The presence of renal insufficiency or urinary obstruction should be evaluated before treatment is begun.

Other treatment of the acute stage is symptomatic. Convulsions may occur, especially in children, and usually in association with hypertension. They may be controlled by barbiturates (p. 390) given intravenously or, preferably, intramuscularly in doses corresponding to 0.25 to 0.5 Gm. (3 3/4 to 7 1/2 grains) for an adult. A wedge of soft wood or a tongue blade wrapped with cloth should be inserted between the teeth to prevent laceration of the tongue. If the blood pressure is very high, venesection of 500 to 700 cc. may be helpful. Magnesium sulfate (as $MgSO_4 \cdot 7H_2O$; p. 346) is often of great value and may be given intravenously as 20 cc. of 10 percent solution, or as 500 cc. of 2 percent solution during a thirty to sixty-minute period. A second or third injection may be given in a few hours if convulsions or twitchings persist. When magnesium sulfate is given, the knee jerks must be tested frequently (p. 347). Calcium salts (p. 344) given intravenously are antidotes for overdoses of magnesium.

Cardiac failure should be treated in the usual manner (p. 63), with venesection and digitalis. Diuretics other than water are to be avoided.

Anuria is a serious complication. It is important to catheterize the patient to rule out mechanical obstruction. In anuria without obstruction, 50 percent dextrose solution (p. 353) should be given by vein. A hot bath lasting at least thirty minutes may be tried, 400 to 500 cc. of fruit juice being administered at the same time. If acidosis is present, sodium lactate (p. 349) should be given by vein. This constitutes an exception to the rule against sodium.

The combination of vomiting, drowsiness, severe headache, and hypertension should be treated with magnesium sulfate, as outlined above for convulsions.

For constipation, milk of magnesia may be given. Soda bicarbonate and saline laxatives containing sodium are to be avoided.

Bed rest should be maintained until the Addis count of the urine is normal, even though several months may be required. Cure obtained in this way is usually permanent; early cessation of treatment seems more likely to be followed by a chronic nephritis.

CHRONIC GLOMERULONEPHRITIS—Because of the poor ultimate prognosis, the aim of treatment is limited to the maintenance of adequate nutrition and slowing of the destructive process. The diet of an adult should contain 50 to 70 Gm. of protein daily; that of a child, about 3 Gm. per kilogram of "ideal" body weight. As in all wasting diseases, the vitamin intake should be in excess of estimated minimum needs. Underfeeding may be harmful. Both dehydration and acidosis (p. 56) should be avoided, since either may precipitate uremia prematurely. Periodic determinations should be made of the carbon-dioxide combining power of the blood (p. 535). The patient should be protected from contact with infection, which may reactivate the disease process. Edema of the nephrotic type may occur and require treatment (for which see below).

In terminal nephritis, salt loss may become excessive because of defective tubular reabsorption, and, in contrast to earlier stages, it may be necessary to supplement the salt intake to maintain blood chlorides at a normal level. (See also Uremia, p. 223.)

NEPHROSIS

Nephrosis, or degenerative Bright's disease, may appear as a stage of chronic glomerulonephritis. It may also occur independently in the presence of toxic agents. Light and transient forms may accompany infectious fevers, jaundice, diabetic acidosis, and mild poisoning with various drugs and chemicals. A more severe form may accompany amyloi-

dosis and poisoning by heavy metals. A distinctive type of rare occurrence is the so-called "genuine," or "lipoid," nephrosis.

The essential renal lesion is degeneration of the tubular epithelium, which may vary from simple cloudy swelling to complete necrosis. The striking clinical feature of severe or chronic nephrosis is generalized edema associated with a low level of serum albumin. The urine typically contains large quantities of protein, fat, and casts; an increased red cell content indicates the presence of glomerulonephritis. Concentrating power (p. 520) is impaired, but urea clearance is occasionally greater than normal. In chronic nephrosis, as distinct from chronic glomerulonephritis, patients often recover.

Treatment—The mild and acute forms usually recover spontaneously. Treatment of chronic nephrosis rests on the following principles:

1. Discovery and eradication of underlying chronic infections or intoxications.

2. Limitation of edema. The diet must be as nearly sodium-free as possible (p. 585), and it should contain 75 to 150 Gm. protein daily (3 Gm. per pound of "ideal" body weight for children) and provide ample calories and vitamins.

Water should *not* be withheld. Edema depends on retention of sodium, not water; retention of water is secondary. The damaged kidney, with impaired concentrating power, requires even more water than normal for a given excretion of sodium. The specific gravity of the urine is the key to the daily volume of water to be administered. The volume should be sufficient to maintain the specific gravity of the mixed daily urine under the maximum concentrating power of the kidneys as determined by the urine concentration test (p. 520), or at a specific gravity of about 1.012.

If an adequate water intake together with restricted sodium intake does not control the edema, diuretic salts (p. 350) should be given, but not in the presence of extreme oliguria or anuria or nitrogen retention. Potassium nitrate is the most powerful diuretic salt and is best given as 'Enseals,' 3 Gm. (6 'Enseals') three times daily. Ammonium chloride is also used. In severe and unresponsive cases, blood plasma or its albumin fraction (p. 352) is employed intravenously. If diuresis does not result, blood chlorides and carbon-dioxide combining power (p. 535) should be determined and, if necessary, brought to normal levels. If anemia is present, transfusion of whole blood may be helpful.

3. Thyroid administration. Although opinion is divided on the subject, many clinicians find thyroid

of great value. Doses of 0.2 to 0.4 Gm. (3 to 6 grains) a day are usually well tolerated (p. 456). More, up to 1 Gm. (15 grains) daily, may be required.

4. Prevention and treatment of intercurrent infections. This includes prevention of contact with potential sources of respiratory infections, as well as care of the mouth and protection of the skin against excoriations and decubital ulcers.

NEPHROSCLEROSIS

Nephrosclerosis is a term applied to the lesions of the renal arterioles occurring in the course of hypertensive disease (p. 80). It is not a clinical entity. The alternate term, arteriosclerotic Bright's disease, is an even greater misnomer, since the condition is merely the renal aspect of a generalized vascular disturbance. It is not related to the common senile sclerosis of the medium or large arteries.

The symptomatology and course are usually dominated by those of the general disorder. The disease process in the kidneys is marked by gradual destruction of renal tissue as the blood supply is progressively cut off by arteriolar lesions and the resulting scar tissue. Changes in the urine depend on the extent of renal destruction and the presence of other factors such as passive vascular congestion due to cardiac decompensation. Slight proteinuria and an increase in the number of hyaline casts are common (p. 520). Constant microscopic hematuria, as in chronic glomerulonephritis, does not occur, but there may be showers of red cells from minute renal infarcts or following rupture of small mucosal vessels in the urinary passages.

Although some aspects of renal function may remain normal for long periods, concentrating power (p. 520) may be early impaired. Death from heart failure or cardiovascular accident commonly occurs before urea clearance is fatally reduced.

Treatment is that of the underlying disease (p. 83). (See also Uremia, p. 223.)

PYELONEPHRITIS

Chronic pyelonephritis is a polymorphic disease resulting from infection of the interstitial tissue of the kidneys. Acute pyelonephritis of greater or less severity is believed to accompany almost every case of pyelitis (p. 224). The parenchymal lesions may heal, leaving scar tissue, or they may persist and become chronic after clinical recovery of the urinary passages. Acute attacks may recur.

Some clinicians believe that even in the absence of persistent or recurrent infection, the scar tissue may continue to contract, disturbing local renal circulation and setting up a progressive vicious cycle of parenchymal destruction, scarring, circulatory deficiency, and further destruction. In a small percentage of cases, local nutritional disturbances become sufficient to cause hypertension (p. 80), often of extreme degree, probably by activating the renal pressor system. Thus, in the late stages, pyelonephritis may resemble chronic glomerulonephritis or malignant hypertension both clinically and histologically. Pyelonephritis beginning in childhood is usually responsible for so-called "contracted kidneys" and "renal rickets."

Death may be due to uremia (p. 223) or to cardiovascular disturbances secondary to the hypertension. The disease may be unilateral, in which case early removal of the affected kidney may be curative.

Diagnosis often is difficult. The acute form should be suspected in every case of upper-urinary-tract infection. Presence of the healed or chronic forms can often be inferred from a history of single or recurrent "pyelitis," the finding of otherwise unexplained hypertension, and small or poorly functioning kidneys or both. Pyuria and bacteriuria may be present, but their absence is without significance. Diagnostic measures include careful history; repeated study and culture of the urine; excretion pyelograms for kidney size, as well as retrograde pyelograms; and studies of renal function (p. 520).

Treatment—All upper-urinary-tract infections should receive early and vigorous systemic anti-infective therapy (p. 286). The so-called "urinary antiseptics" should not be relied upon since they do not affect the parenchymal infection, which, although silent, may be more important than the infection of the urinary passages. Every effort should be made to stop the infection before the stage is reached at which the cycle of chronic disease becomes self-perpetuating.

In the chronic stage, one should try to determine whether the disease is bilateral or unilateral. This may be difficult, involving systematic study of the size and physiological state of both kidneys and the urinary passages. Truly unilateral disease is cured by surgical removal of the affected kidney. The indication for nephrectomy should be surgical rather than the presence of hypertension.

In bilateral chronic pyelonephritis, the treatment is the same as that for chronic glomerulonephritis (p. 220) or hypertensive disease (p. 83).

CRUSH SYNDROME

The term "crush syndrome" has been applied to a type of renal failure which results from extensive crushing injury in those species, such as man, whose muscles contain large amounts of myoglobin. The condition has also been called "lower nephron nephrosis." The genesis of the renal failure has been demonstrated by experiments on the rat, the muscles of which contain little myoglobin. Neither crushing injury nor the intravenous administration of myoglobin separately produces more than minor and transient renal damage in the rat, whereas the combination produces severe renal failure with extensive renal-tubule degeneration and precipitation of heme pigment similar to that following crushing injury in man.

Renal failure similar to that of crush syndrome occurs in a wide variety of situations: not only (1) following crushing injury, but (2) subsequent to shock from any cause, such as other trauma, hemorrhage, severe infection, burns, or excessive vomiting; (3) after sudden destruction of red blood cells, as in severe malaria or following transfusion of incompatible blood; and (4) in the course of poisoning by many types of substances, including the sulfonamides, carbon tetrachloride, and certain heavy metals. All of the conditions mentioned above are accompanied by renal tubule degeneration and evidence of renal vasoconstrictive ischemia; most of them involve precipitation of heme pigment in the distal convoluted and collecting tubules. The exact mechanisms have not been demonstrated.

In renal failure of the crush syndrome type, oliguria, which may progress to anuria, usually begins in the first twenty-four hours. Such urine as is passed is of low specific gravity, tending to become fixed at 1.010 and indicating complete loss of concentrating power. The urine may be highly acid at first but later becomes fixed at a slight acidity. The urine sediment resembles that of acute nephritis (p. 219), and there is usually a positive benzidine test (p. 522).

The blood pressure, which may have been at or near shock levels the first day, is usually normal the second day and moderately elevated (150/90) on the third and succeeding days. The level of blood urea or nonprotein nitrogen increases rapidly and may exceed 150 mg. per 100 cc. by the third day. After crushing injury, the potassium and phosphate content of the blood serum rises because of liberation of these ions from traumatized muscle. Other electrolyte disturbances are those expected to result from the original trauma or disease.

The mortality from crush syndrome is high. Death may result from either the primary condition or uremia; once the cardinal manifestations of the latter have appeared, the mortality rate approximates 90 percent. Most of the deaths occur between the third and twelfth days.

Treatment is centered on prevention. Shock from any cause must be treated promptly and effectively (see p. 90). During sulfonamide administration, sufficient fluid and alkali should be given to prevent the urine from becoming concentrated and acid. The occurrence of any other condition which may lead to crush syndrome also calls for administration of fluid and alkali, since precipitation of heme pigment is likewise favored by a concentrated acid urine. However, after crush syndrome develops, alkali therapy must not be overdone, for the kidneys are then unable to secrete basic ions selectively, and alkalosis may easily be produced.

It seems probable that both neural and humoral factors are involved in the renal vasoconstriction. The neural factor can be overcome by sympathetic block, which is best achieved by maintaining high caudal or spinal anesthesia. The efficacy of this measure is currently being assessed.

During anuria, only the insensible water loss should be replaced (see p. 51). If the patient survives this phase and enters a stage of extreme diuresis, large quantities of sodium may have to be administered because of the great loss in the urine.

HYDRONEPHROSIS

Hydronephrosis is a dilatation of the pelvis and calyxes of the kidney, resulting from obstruction and leading eventually to pressure atrophy of kidney substance. Sudden or gradual prolonged obstruction of the urinary tract will result in hydronephrosis. Causes of obstruction include stones, stricture, spasm, foreign body, and tumor within the tract, and neoplasms, adhesions, operative trauma, or aberrant blood vessels acting from without.

Hydronephrosis may be mistaken for kidney tumor, neoplasm of the retroperitoneal glands, encysted ascites, enlarged gall bladder, and, in the female, an ovarian cyst. Accurate diagnosis of hydronephrosis depends upon pyelography, either retrograde or intravenous.

Treatment—Obstruction should be removed, if possible. This may necessitate dilatation of ureteral stricture, removal of a calculus, or fixation of a movable kidney. If useful function of the kidney has been destroyed, it is usually thought better to remove the hydronephrotic kidney, but one had best be certain of normal function in the other kidney.

UREMIA

Death in renal failure is due to uremia, a syndrome which follows accumulation of metabolites in the internal environment as the result of inadequate renal function. To the extent that scar tissue acts, directly or indirectly, to reduce renal function, the loss cannot be restored. Frequently, however, uremia is precipitated by reversible factors such as:

Heart failure (p. 63)
Urinary tract obstruction (see Hydronephrosis above)
Dehydration (p. 56)
Sodium deficiency (p. 342)
Acidosis (p. 59)

Attention to these factors can sometimes prevent or postpone uremia or, less frequently, relieve it once it has developed.

The damaged kidney, with impaired concentrating power, requires more water than normal for a given excretion of metabolites. If water is inadequately supplied, filtration fails and uremia results. Therefore, if nitrogen or other retention is present, the need of the kidneys is for water to carry away the retained substances. Water administered intravenously (as dextrose solution, p. 349) is often more effective in increasing nitrogen excretion than the same quantity taken by mouth. For specific criteria of adequate water intake, see the paragraph on water under treatment of nephrosis, page 220.

The diet should be relatively low in protein (not more than 50 Gm. daily) and high in carbohydrate (because of its protein-sparing action).

Nitrogen retention is often paradoxically accompanied by excessive loss of electrolytes, especially of sodium and chloride. Normally, the tubule cells reabsorb most of the filtered electrolyte while actively excreting some metabolites and reabsorbing relatively little of others. When renal failure is advanced, excretion of the two types of substances may be oppositely affected, nitrogen being retained because of deficient filtration and electrolytes being lost because of tubular inadequacy. Thus, in terminal nephritis, a moderate salt intake may postpone uremia by preventing hypochloremia, whereas at an earlier stage a low salt intake may have been necessary to prevent edema. To this end, 2 to 10 Gm. of sodium chloride may be given daily, the

dose being governed by (1) absence of edema and (2) appearance in the urine of most of the extra salt.

Acute uremia, such as may occur in acute glomerulonephritis, often presents a clinical picture resembling that of eclampsia (p. 212). Chronic uremia, occurring typically late in chronic glomerulonephritis, presents the symptomatology of a cumulative intoxication. There is progressive general depression, fatigue, asthenia, and cachexia. Headache, extreme anorexia, and generalized itching are common. Nausea and vomiting are frequent. Acidosis develops, and, if the uremic state is prolonged, there may be anemia. Drowsiness, disorientation, delirium, stupor, and coma may precede death. In some uremic patients, the blood potassium level rises and the symptoms of hyperpotassemia develop (see p. 342). These are usually added to other manifestations not attributable to excess potassium.

Aside from the considerations discussed above, the treatment of uremia is largely symptomatic. If there is persistent vomiting, fluids must, of course, be given parenterally. It is especially important to maintain an adequate vitamin intake, particularly the B complex and C, in such patients by parenteral administration.

URINARY CALCULUS

Urinary calculus is a stonelike formation which may be found anywhere from the collecting tubules of the kidney to the urethra. Calculi may be single or multiple and may vary in size from microscopic to the capacity of the renal pelvis or urinary bladder.

Many causes have been suggested; their very number is evidence that there is no single etiology. Possible factors, which perhaps act in combination, have included vitamin A deficiency (p. 493), geographic and climatic influences, parathyroid disease (p. 197), bone lesions, faulty calcium metabolism, and obstruction of, injury to, or infection of the urinary tract.

Pain, due to distention or spasm of the urinary tract, is the most prominent and characteristic symptom. It may be dull or, more commonly, intermittent and cramp-like. It is often extremely severe. The area to which the pain is referred ranges from the upper lumbar and abdominal region, across the lower abdomen, to the inguinal region, genitals, and upper part of the thigh. Hematuria is also common; it is due to trauma of the urinary passages by the stone.

Tentative diagnosis can be made in practically all cases on the character of the pain and the area to which it is referred. Confirmation is obtained by visualization of the calculus in x-ray plates of the urinary tract. Often the diagnosis can be confirmed by the patient's actually passing the stone or some associated gravel. When renal calculus is suspected, the patient should be instructed to screen all urine through several layers of cheesecloth and save the cloth. Frequently the physician can find calcareous matter when a calculus is present.

Treatment is usually first directed to controlling pain. Morphine sulfate, 1/6 grain (0.01 Gm.) or more (p. 399), or papaverine hydrochloride, 1 grain (0.065 Gm.) or more (p. 363), may be given, preferably intravenously, but they should not be used together. Papaverine tends to relieve the spasm. Morphine acts by dulling sensitivity to pain, at the same time tending to increase the spasm and overriding any relaxing effect of papaverine. If a stone is too large to pass through the ureter, it may cause chronic obstruction and hydronephrosis (p. 222). Such a stone should be removed surgically. Occasionally stones can be removed through the cystoscope. Sometimes it is desirable to inject oil just below the stone through a ureteral catheter, in the hope that lubrication will facilitate passage. Recurrences are common.

Efforts at prevention may be directed toward controlling the causative factors, if they can be determined. In any case, fluid intake should be at least three liters daily, the intake of calcium should be limited (not more than one pint of milk or its equivalent daily), and the urine should be maintained acid (by administration of ammonium chloride if necessary). In experimental animals, vitamin A has proved effective in preventing urinary calculi. Vitamin A in doses several times the optimal human requirements (p. 252) has been advocated for clinical use, but its value is not clearly established.

URINARY TRACT INFECTION

Pyelitis is infection involving primarily the mucosa of the renal pelvis and ureter. The organism may be blood-borne, or the infection may ascend from the bladder. Obstruction and stasis are important predisposing and aggravating factors. Pyelitis is usually accompanied by some degree of acute pyelonephritis (p. 221), the treatment of which is even more important than that of the pyelitis.

The usual organism is *Esch. coli*. Less frequent causes are staphylococci, streptococci, diplococci,

pneumococci, *H. influenzae*, *B. proteus* (producing alkaline urine), *E. typhosa*, *S. paratyphi*, *Pseudomonas aeruginosa* (*B. pyocyaneus*), and others.

Symptoms are systemic (chills, fever, malaise, prostration) and often local (referred pain, frequent urination). The urine usually contains an excess of leukocytes, and the causative organism can be cultured from it unless complete obstruction prevents drainage. Pyelitis should be suspected whenever general symptoms of infection occur without obvious cause.

Cystitis may be secondary to infection of the urethra, prostate, or seminal vesicles in the male, or the bacteria may pass up the urethra from the outside in the female without causing demonstrable urethritis. Infection may be introduced by instrumentation or catheterization. The organism may come from the blood stream by way of the kidneys and urine, or it may travel from adjacent structures by way of lymphatics. Incomplete emptying of the bladder, as in prostatic hypertrophy, and overdistention, such as may occur during various forms of anesthesia, predispose to infection.

The organisms responsible for cystitis are the same as those which cause pyelitis. The gonococcus may be added as an occasional offender.

The symptoms are predominantly local: lower abdominal and perineal pain, urinary frequency, burning, and tenesmus. The urine contains pus and the causative organisms.

Urethritis is usually due to the gonococcus (p. 6). Other possible causes include syphilis with intraurethral chancre, trichomoniasis, chancroid, common organisms such as the staphylococcus, trauma, and irritant substances which may be introduced from outside or carried in the urine.

Early gonococcal urethritis in men is ordinarily limited to the terminal portion, but it may later extend to the posterior urethra. Chronic gonococcal urethritis usually involves the prostate as well. The mucopurulent discharge which characterizes it may be intermittent. Scar tissue may lead to stricture.

Treatment—Contributing factors of obstruction and stasis should be removed. Systemic anti-infective therapy is used to eradicate the infection. Because the latter is in the tissues about the urinary passages, it is not sufficient merely to render the urine sterile. Therefore, the sulfonamides (p. 293) and antibiotics (p. 287) are the most effective agents provided the causative organism is susceptible to them.

For organisms resistant to the sulfonamides and antibiotics, mandelic acid (p. 305) is usually the next choice. However, mandelic acid does not act on deep mucosal infection or on the parenchymal element in pyelonephritis. Adults usually require 6 to 12 Gm. of mandelic acid daily. This can be prescribed as 4 to 10 'Enseals' Mandelic Acid and Ammonium Chloride repeated four times daily, or as a tablespoonful of Elixir Mandelic Acid three or four times daily. Children under two years of age require 2 to 4 teaspoonfuls of the elixir daily. The urine must be kept at a pH of 5.5 or less by giving additional ammonium chloride or other acidifying agents (p. 352). Methyl red (p. 521) is a useful test substance. In adults, the daily urine output should not exceed 1,200 cc.

Methenamine (p. 310) is sometimes helpful if the previously discussed agents fail. Again, the urine must be kept acid—at pH 6.5 or less—and the daily volume at less than 1,200 cc. The effective dose is usually 4 to 5 Gm. (60 to 75 grains) daily subdivided into four equally spaced doses. The acidifying salts (p. 352) are given at the mid-intervals between doses of methenamine.

For local irrigation in cystitis, a number of solutions may be used:

potassium permanganate, 1:5,000
'Merthiolate,' 1:5,000 or 1:10,000
Mild Silver Protein, N.F., 10 to 25 percent

ENURESIS

Enuresis, or repeated involuntary urination, becomes a clinical entity when it occurs after the age of two and one-half to three years. The majority of children attain day control of the bladder before they are two years old, and most are able to remain dry at night a few months later. Enuresis may begin after bladder control has been accomplished, but as a rule it develops insidiously as a continuation of nocturnal incontinence from infancy. Diurnal enuresis frequently accompanies nocturnal enuresis, but the diurnal form rarely occurs alone. The condition usually disappears spontaneously during adolescence, particularly in girls. Most adult cases represent continuation of the condition from childhood. Those who have had long periods of freedom respond more readily to treatment.

The condition is to be distinguished from the urinary incontinence due to gross organic or infectious lesions of the urogenital and nervous systems. Minor local conditions, such as balanitis, phimosis, and adherent prepuce, probably are of no etiological significance. Cures following correction of these lesions may be explained on a psychic rather than a physiological basis. There are numerous theories of pathogenesis, including anatomical lesions, improper habit training, personality disorders (particularly when associated with emotional stress), and hereditary dysfunction of the urinary bladder. Enuresis may be part of a general disorder, such as epilepsy, diabetes mellitus, multiple sclerosis, or diabetes insipidus. It sometimes develops following a severe illness in children previously continent. The drinking of large amounts of water before retiring may lead to bed-wetting. Premature institution of training, before the nervous system is adequately developed and before the bladder capacity is large enough, may cause psychological conflict and enuresis. Neither the pH of the urine nor abnormality in fusion of the spinal vertebrae is a factor in pathogenesis. Enuresis is commonly associated with pronounced mental deficiency but not necessarily with moderate mental retardation.

Wetting generally occurs every night and usually once or twice a night. Some wet within an hour after going to sleep; with others this does not occur until the early morning hours. Urgency and frequency during the day are present in a large majority of cases. These are highly sensitive to stimuli such as cold, damp weather, and excitement, any of which may increase bladder irritability.

Treatment—The multiplicity of treatments is evidence of the difficulty of the problem. The success of many remedies undoubtedly is due to the psychotherapy which accompanies their administration, whether or not this is recognized as such.

Preventive treatment, consisting of habit training for bladder control, should be started at about one year of age. The diaper is not worn during waking hours of the day. The infant is placed on his toilet and encouraged to urinate at regular intervals—on awakening, after each meal, and at intermediate intervals of every three hours at first and less often as bladder capacity and control permit. It is important that the training does not become a disagreeable ordeal, nor should it become a time for participating in unusually pleasant play. By the age of two years most children will notify attendants of their desire to urinate. At this time the diaper may be removed during daytime naps with appropriate encouragement to the child to remain dry. When the child has an occasional dry night, he should be awakened four or five hours after going to bed and placed on the toilet. If wetting occurs later in the night, it may be necessary to repeat this about half an hour before it usually happens. Moderate praise for dry nights and no comment about failures are an important part of the program.

Active treatment is primarily psychological. The parents should be urged to assume an unemotional attitude toward the condition. Great concern, severe censure, punishments, threats, and shaming must be avoided. The parents should be told that the child is not primarily at fault and that the abnormality probably was inherited from one of them. Conversations with the child are directed toward reducing nervous tension, promoting self-confidence, and correcting feelings of hopelessness, shame, and guilt. A system of rewards sometimes is effective. A chart may be devised on which the dry and wet nights are designated by colored stickers or other means.

Fluid intake may be reduced in the late afternoon and a dry supper given provided that the child's co-operation can be obtained willingly. Depending upon the frequency of wetting, the child is fully awakened one or more times during the night to urinate. Administration of 5 Gm. of salt immediately before bedtime tends to reduce the volume of urine but in some instances causes undue discomfort from excessive thirst. Tea, coffee, and soft drinks containing caffeine should not be allowed at any time.

The belladonna alkaloids (p. 420) tend to inhibit the action of the detrusor muscle of the bladder and may be of benefit in some cases. The medication is given orally, three or four times daily, in gradually increasing amounts until the enuresis is relieved or until flushing of the skin, dry mouth, or mydriasis is produced. Treatment is continued for about two months after voluntary control is established. The starting dose of atropine sulfate may be 0.1 mg. (1/600 grain) under the age of six years, 0.15 mg. (1/400 grain) at six to ten years, and 0.2 mg. (1/300 grain) beyond the age of ten.

Ephedrine (p. 426) may be helpful by increasing the tone of the bladder sphincter. It is given at bedtime as the sulfate or hydrochloride, beginning with 15 to 30 mg. (1/4 to 1/2 grain) and increasing up to tolerance. Older children have been given as much as 0.3 Gm. (5 grains). If stimulation of the central nervous system is excessive, barbiturates (p. 390) should be used to obtain sleep. Amphetamine (p. 429), 5 to 25 mg. daily at bedtime, is of value in some cases.

Should psychological and medical treatment fail, detailed urologic examination, including cystometry, is in order. Many patients will respond to repeated treatments with the cystometer.

DISEASES INVOLVING MAINLY THE SKIN AND ITS APPENDAGES

COMMON INFLAMMATIONS OF THE SKIN: GENERAL PRINCIPLES OF LOCAL TREATMENT

The skin may respond with an inflammatory reaction to many types of irritant or toxic substances of bacterial or other origin. Often some time is required to determine the exact cause of the inflammation. Fortunately, it is the nature and stage of the lesion and not the diagnosis which determine the type of therapy for the early phases. Specific treatment of acute dermatitis should be withheld until acute inflammation has subsided and the nature of the primary lesion becomes apparent.

Common inflammations of the skin respond to mild, conservative treatment. Initial therapy should be carried out with mild drugs and low concentrations. Irritating treatment is the most frequent cause of spreading dermatitis.

Acute Weeping and Pustular Eruptions, regardless of origin, should be treated with wet dressings using Aluminum Acetate Solution, U.S.P., (Burow's Solution) diluted 1 to 30 with water; potassium permanganate solution, 1:10,000; or 10 percent magnesium sulfate solution. Old, washed muslin sheeting is better than gauze as compress material. Warm dressings should be used in the presence of obvious infection or suppuration; otherwise, cold is most desirable. Dressings may be applied continuously the first forty-eight hours, and for one hour four to five times daily thereafter. A bland preparation, such as cold cream or a plain hydrophilic ointment (p. 479), may be used in the interval. In eruptions covering large areas of the body, baths with a potassium permanganate solution, 1:12,000, or starch (p. 479) may be required.

Acute Nonweeping Eruptions—Wet dressings as above may be used until swelling and erythema have subsided. In mild cases a shake lotion may be employed, such as plain Calamine Lotion or one made as follows:

```
zinc oxide . . . . . . . . . . . . . . . . . . . . . . . . . . . . . . . .20
talc . . . . . . . . . . . . . . . . . . . . . . . . . . . . . . . . . . . . .20
glycerin . . . . . . . . . . . . . . . . . . . . . . . . . . . . . . . . .15
water . . . . . . . . . . . . . . . . . . . . . . . . . . . . . . . . . . . .60
```

These should be applied generously several times daily and removed with a soapless detergent (p. 481) if caking or stiffness develops.

Dry Hyperkeratotic Skins—Bland oils or greases, such as mineral oil and olive oil in equal parts, Hydrous Wool Fat, or Hydrophilic Petrolatum (p. 479), can be safely used for long periods of time. When prolonged use is contemplated, it is better to avoid the inclusion of active chemicals of any kind because of the danger of sensitization and irritation.

Follicular and Papular Eruptions, such as folliculitis and heat rash—whether localized or widespread—do not as a rule tolerate ointments or oily solutions. It is better to use powdery lotions such as Calamine Lotion or the zinc oxide-talc lotion noted above. If infection is present, use germicidal tinctures, such as Tincture 'Merthiolate,' or alcohol sponges.

Erythemas—Local treatment is of little value in the erythema group of eruptions, including erythema nodosum and multiforme, and the exanthemata, such as measles and scarlet fever, and serves no purpose except to relieve itching. A powdery lotion may be used in the acute stages and a simple cream (see above) if desquamation is present.

General Reminders

1. Do not use ointments on weeping lesions unless they are hydrophilic.

2. Do not use soap and water on acute dermatitis.

3. Do not use strong drugs, bactericides, or fungicides in the presence of acute dermatitis.

4. For control of pruritus, burning, or pain, employ cold wet dressings (see above) and systemic sedation. Local anesthetics, including phenol and menthol, produce temporary relief but are potential irritants and are not recommended for acute dermatitis.

CUTANEOUS REACTIONS TO DRUGS

The great majority of drugs, for both local and systemic use, are capable of producing cutaneous reactions. These may be the result of primary irritation, epidermal sensitization, or toxic and sensitization injury to the vascular system of the skin.

Discussion here will be limited to eruptions resulting from drugs that reach the systemic circulation, regardless of how administered. Eruptions due to *local* action of drugs on the skin are discussed under Contact Dermatitis (p. 228).

Skin reactions produced are (1) the erythemas, which include simple erythema, scarlatiniform and morbilliform erythema, erythema nodosum and multiforme (including vesicular and bullous types), and the nondescript toxic erythemas; (2) eczema, erythroderma, and exfoliative dermatitis (hereafter referred to as "dermatitis-eczema"); (3) urticaria and angioneurotic edema; (4) acneform eruptions; (5) papular eruptions resembling lichen planus or pityriasis rosea; (6) keratoses; (7) pigmentation; (8) fixed eruptions (discrete patches recurring in previously affected skin); (9) purpura; (10) light sensitivity.

Most drugs are capable of producing several different types of eruptions, and it is usually impossible to identify the offending drug with certainty from the morphology of the eruption. Furthermore, with few exceptions, it is impossible to identify the eruption as being definitely caused by drugs until a history is taken. For example, erythema nodosum, urticaria, and scarlatiniform erythema due to drugs are morphologically indistinguishable from those due to infection. In the presence of any lesion of the type listed above, drugs should always be considered as a possible cause.

Space does not permit a listing of all drugs and the reactions they may cause or of all reactions and the drugs which cause them. It can be stated that most organic and many inorganic drugs may cause cutaneous reactions. The more important drugs commonly causing skin reactions, and the common cutaneous reactions to drugs, are cross-listed below.

Drugs in Common Use and the Reactions They Frequently Cause

ARSENIC (usually organic)—Dermatitis-eczema, exfoliative dermatitis, the erythemas, fixed eruption, the papular eruptions, purpura, urticaria.

ASPIRIN (and the coal-tar derivatives)—Fixed eruption, urticaria, the erythemas, purpura.

BARBITURATES—The erythemas, vesicular and bullous eruptions.

BROMIDES—Acneform eruptions, fungating granulomas, the erythemas.

GOLD—Dermatitis-eczema, exfoliative dermatitis, the papular eruptions (especially those resembling lichen planus).

IODIDES—Acneform, vesicular, and bullous eruptions, granulomas, purpura.

MERCURY—Dermatitis-eczema, the erythemas, stomatitis (see Plate 26).

PENICILLIN—Urticaria and angioneurotic edema, dermatitis-eczema, vesicular and papular erythemas.

PHENOLPHTHALEIN—Fixed eruption, the erythemas (see Plate 20).

QUININE—Dermatitis-eczema, the erythemas (especially scarlatiniform).

SULFONAMIDES—The erythemas, urticaria, dermatitis-eczema, vesicular and bullous eruptions, light sensitivity (see Plate 21).

Common Drug Eruptions and the Drugs Which Frequently Cause Them

ACNEFORM—Iodides, bromides.

DERMATITIS-ECZEMA—Arsenic, gold, mercury, penicillin, quinine, sulfonamides.

ERYTHEMAS—Arsenic, aspirin and coal-tar derivatives, barbiturates, bromides, mercury, phenolphthalein, quinine, sulfonamides (see Plates 20 and 22).

EXFOLIATIVE DERMATITIS—Arsenic, gold.

FIXED ERUPTION—Arsenic, aspirin and coal-tar derivatives, gold, phenolphthalein (see Plate 20).

FUNGATING GRANULOMAS—Bromides, iodides.

LIGHT SENSITIVITY—Sulfonamides.

PAPULAR ERUPTIONS—Arsenic, gold.

PURPURA—Arsenic, aspirin and coal-tar derivatives, iodides.

URTICARIA AND ANGIONEUROTIC EDEMA—Arsenic, aspirin and coal-tar derivatives, penicillin, sulfonamides.

VESICULAR AND BULLOUS ERUPTIONS—Barbiturates, iodides, penicillin, sulfonamides (see Plate 26).

Treatment—There are relatively few specifics. Most reactions will subside with prompt discontinuance of the offending drug. Local treatment is of little value except in the presence of weeping dermatitis. General supportive treatment and large amounts of fluid are useful in toxic patients.

Antihistaminic drugs (p. 509) are usually effective against urticaria, angioneurotic edema, and the erythema group of eruptions. They are worth trying against any type of skin reaction to a drug. However, they may in some instances accentuate the leukopenia which frequently accompanies a drug eruption.

Dimercaprol is a specific antidote for arsenic and mercury reactions and may be of value in gold reactions (see p. 515).

Reactions to iodides and bromides are treated the same as iodide or bromide poisoning (pp. 508 and 398). In the granulomas due to these drugs, local treatment is also necessary (bactericides and x-ray). Large doses of vitamin C (p. 490) and of parenteral calcium (p. 344) may be of value in sulfonamide reactions and in most of the exudative eruptions.

CONTACT DERMATITIS

Contact dermatitis (dermatitis venenata) is an all-inclusive concept covering eruptions resulting from sensitization to agents reaching the skin or mucous membranes externally. It does not include dermatitis from direct irritation due to caustics, heat, and so on. Contact dermatitis may be due to plants, occupational exposures, cosmetics, local medication, clothing, and innumerable other agents. It is probably the most common dermatosis of modern life. The skin eruption is generally nonspecific in type, a variety of causes producing the same clinical reaction. Determination of etiology depends on history, patch tests, and common sense.

The reaction may vary from ill-defined erythema to edematous, papular, vesicular, and bullous eruptions, depending on degree of sensitization and concentration of inciting agent. (See Plates 23 and 26.) Although exposed areas are most commonly involved, any part of the skin or mucous membrane may be affected. The reaction may continue for days or weeks after the inciting agent has been removed.

Treatment consists in identifying and avoiding the inciting agent, and the use of simple soothing and protective measures. See page 226 for therapy of acute inflammation of the skin. Unless secondary infection and suppuration are predominant, bactericides have no place in treatment.

A careful history will often identify the offending agent or will at least limit the possibilities to a relatively small number of substances, with which patch tests can then be carried out (see below).

Although desensitization to contactants may apparently occur spontaneously, success is infrequent when the procedure is attempted therapeutically. An exception is the case of poison oak and ivy (*Rhus*) extracts, which may be useful prophylactically. They are valueless in treatment.

Patch Tests—The patch test is performed by applying to the skin surface a substance suspected of being the cause of a dermatitis. It should be designed to simulate closely the conditions under which the patient may have been exposed to the offending agent. Provided (1) the substance does not cause reaction in nonsensitive individuals and (2) the concentration is too low to produce primary irritation, a positive reaction indicates hypersensitivity. The reaction may progress through erythema and edema to vesiculation, depending on the degree of sensitivity.

The actual procedure consists in applying the substance to an area of normal skin by means of a small (1 cm. square) piece of linen or muslin covered by a piece of cellophane and sealed to the skin with adhesive tape; the air is excluded. The patch should be left in place for forty-eight hours unless there is severe reaction as indicated by burning and pain. The site should be inspected not only when the patch is removed but also on the third, seventh, and fourteenth days, since delayed reactions may occur.

Substances should be put into solution when possible. Insoluble material should be moistened slightly when applied. Generally, concentrations simulating natural exposure are chosen. However, if high sensitivity is expected, much lower concentrations should be used. Tests should not be done during the active phases of a dermatitis, since a patch test may on occasion produce severe exacerbation of the disease. Routine patch testing with a long standard list of substances is not recommended and may actually be harmful. Selection of substances to be used should be based upon the history of exposure to them by contact, inhalation, or ingestion. In addition, it should be remembered that the demonstration of hypersensitivity to a given substance has no diagnostic significance unless it can be proved that the individual has had an opportunity to be exposed to it.

Because there are many details and precautions regarding choice and concentration of individual testing materials, it is recommended that the physician consult textbooks on allergy or dermatology before undertaking patch tests.

VESICULAR ERUPTIONS OF THE HANDS

Vesicular eruptions of the hands, especially of the fingers and palms, are common. They may be due to various factors, including emotional and other influences acting through the nervous system, contact irritants and sensitizers, fungus infections (either primary of the hands or acting allergically from a distant site), and systemic toxic and sensitization reactions to drugs, bacterial infection, and so on.

Unfortunately, since the various causes may produce the same type of skin reaction, it is frequently not possible to determine the etiology merely by looking at the lesions. On a statistical basis, nervous system influences and contact factors are the most common causes in present-day practice, and it seems quite certain that fungus infection is not as frequent a factor as was formerly thought. Furthermore, when fungus infection of the hands is present, the lesions in most instances will show the characteristic features of fungus infection, i.e., grouping of vesicles and development of marginated patches (see p. 230). Lesions of the hands due to allergic "id" reaction to fungus infection (of the feet, for example) are relatively uncommon; but when they occur, they present a nonspecific picture.

Because of the thickness of the stratum corneum on the palmar aspect, contact dermatitis in this location is uncommon; almost always it involves primarily the dorsa of the hands. The clinical picture varies from what has been called "pompholyx-dyshidrosis" to severe inflammatory exudative patches of dermatitis or eczema. The morphologic types are briefly described below.

Pompholyx-Dyshidrosis presents discrete, relatively noninflammatory, deep-set vesicles which have no tendency toward grouping; they are distributed on the sides and palmar aspects of fingers and hands and are almost invariably bilateral. Burning and itching often precede and accompany the eruption. Excessive perspiration is common; it suggests but does not prove that the cause is nervous-autonomic in nature. The vesicles tend to remain discrete and rupture only after several days, or they may not open at all; if not, the contents are reabsorbed and the overlying epidermis is shed as a dry brownish callus-like plate. Occasionally two or three vesicles will merge to form a multilocular bulla. The fluid may become turbid and purulent, since secondary bacterial infection is not uncommon. Lymphangitis may occur.

Vesicular Exudative Dermatitis—The morphologic picture of pompholyx may be thought of as the stage of mildest degree. Increasing severity will produce eruptions progressively characterized as follows: erythema; coalescence of vesicles; early rupture of vesicles; edema; formation of nonmarginated exudative patches of nonspecific dermatitis. When the dorsa of the hands and fingers are involved, the vesicles rupture early and the exudation may be more severe because the stratum corneum is thinner.

Treatment should be planned on the basis of etiology (when this can be determined) and carried on as recommended in the corresponding sections of this book. However, a general recommendation would be to avoid the local use of strong drugs, especially fungicides and bactericides, unless specific signs of infection are present. Bland local medication (p. 227), systemic sedation, and antihistaminic drugs are good initial treatment until the etiology is established.

FUNGUS INFECTIONS OF THE SKIN

Tinea Capitis is the most common cause of patchy alopecia in children before the age of puberty. Clinically, the appearance varies from a simple noninflammatory patch of alopecia, with short, brittle, lusterless, broken hairs, to a deep dusky-red, boggy, swollen area called "kerion Celsi." The high and increasing incidence of this disease and consequent loss of school attendance make it a condition of major importance.

The disease is acquired by mediate or immediate contact with animals (cats, dogs, sheep) and with other children. The diagnosis is made by:

1. Microscopic examination of spore-laden hairs in a 10 percent potassium hydroxide mount.

2. Wood's light (ultraviolet lamp with Wood's filter) examination.* Hairs infected by *Microsporum* fluoresce brilliant green.

3. Culture on Sabouraud's medium.

Determination of the causative species, of great prognostic importance, can be made only by culture. Under the treatment outlined below, *Microsporum lanosum* and *M. fulvum* infections usually clear between six weeks and four months and may clear spontaneously in a longer period; on the other hand, *M. audouini* infections without treatment may last until puberty and, when treated, rarely clear within six months. *Trichophyton* infections of the scalp, which are rare and relatively unimportant, respond well to treatment, but in the absence of therapy will persist until the adolescent period.

TREATMENT involves the following procedures:

1. Clip the hair to a distance of one-half inch around each lesion.

2. Shampoo three times weekly.

3. Manually remove infected hairs. Five to fifteen minutes a day should be spent at home in this procedure under a safe source of filtered ultraviolet radiation.* This may be augmented by similar treatment in the office.

4. Apply fungicidal preparations (see page 310).

5. Have the child wear at all times a close-fitting, tightly woven cap to prevent possible infection of other children.

The patient is considered cured only when no fluorescent hairs can be found on three consecutive weekly examinations under Wood's light.

The Superficial Dermatomycoses—Superficial fungus infections of the skin are of common occurrence. Except for those due to *Microsporum* (see Tinea Capitis above and Trunk, Extremities, and Face below), they are not considered to be "communicable diseases" in the usual sense; for simple exposure is not sufficient to cause them, and it is generally impossible to determine the time and source of infection.

---

* A "Purple-X" bulb may be employed, or an RS-type sun lamp with a Wood's filter to shut off the visible spectrum.

The superficial dermatomycoses are best classified for practical purposes according to the region involved. A few general characteristics are common to all. The fungi live in the superficial epidermis. The lesions spread peripherally (central clearing may occur), and the greatest activity is at the margins. Uncomplicated fungus infection is usually of relatively low-grade inflammatory character; severe inflammation and exudation are almost invariably due to secondary bacterial infection or to chemical irritation from treatment. The typical lesions are circinate scaly patches with miliary vesicles in the active border. Sensitization and subsequent eczematization or distant toxic "id" lesions may result spontaneously or after irritating treatment.

Laboratory aids in diagnosis are frequently of great value:

1. Direct microscopic examination of scrapings of epidermis in 10 percent sodium or potassium hydroxide will often reveal fungus elements.

2. Culture on Sabouraud's medium, especially in scalp infections in children and any doubtful case.

3. Filtered ultraviolet (Wood's light) to demonstrate fluorescent hair.

4. Intradermal testing with fungus extract (p. 339). This test is analogous to the tuberculin test in that (1) a positive reaction does not appear for one or two days (although an immediate urticarial reaction may occur within the first half hour and subside rapidly); and (2) a positive test may be related to a previous infection and therefore does not establish the mycotic nature of an existing eruption. Thus, like the tuberculin test, the test is more informative when it is negative than when it is positive.

FEET AND HANDS—The characteristic lesions are circinate scaly patches or grouped miliary vesicles located on the plantar aspects of the feet or the palmar aspects of the hands and fingers. The common causative organisms are *Trichophyton mentagrophytes* (*gypseum*), *T. purpureum*, and *Candida* (*Monilia*) *albicans*. Allergic ("id") reactions (p. 268) on the hands are not as common as was formerly thought. Many other dermatoses (e.g., contact dermatitis [p. 228], neurodermatitis [p. 235], and bacterial infection) also occur on the hands and feet and must be differentiated.

The interdigital spaces of the feet are a common site for fungus infections of intertriginous nature, producing the so-called "athlete's foot." However, it is erroneous to consider all intertriginous lesions in this location to be due to fungi unless the organisms are demonstrated, for a similar appearance may be produced by simple maceration or bacterial infection. Furthermore, secondary bacterial infection is usually present in fungus infection about the toes and must be considered in planning treatment.

There has been much interest in the communicability of fungus infection of the feet. Studies have failed to demonstrate that barefoot walking in barracks, gymnasiums, shower rooms, and swimming pools is of importance in spreading the disease. The value of fungicidal foot baths is equivocal. Rather, the important factors in the development of clinical infection are poor foot hygiene, insufficient aeration of the feet, maceration of the skin, local bacterial action, and lack of systemic immunity.

Acutely inflamed, weeping, crusted lesions should be treated with wet dressings (p. 226). After acute inflammation has subsided, mild bactericidal and fungicidal agents can be applied (p. 310). The prolonged use of mild agents is the desirable course rather than potent drugs for quick results. Ammoniated mercury, 1 percent, or bacitracin (p. 292) in a water-miscible ointment base (p. 479) is effective for the bacterial phases; undecylenic acid and its salts or 2 percent sulfur and salicylic acid (p. 482) are the fungicidal preparations of choice. They may be applied twice daily. Four to six weeks may be required to cure the average case.

INGUINAL, PERINEAL, AND PERIANAL REGIONS— Fungus infection of these regions is common and is usually caused by *Epidermophyton inguinale*, *Trichophyton mentagrophytes* (*gypseum*), or *Candida* (*Monilia*) *albicans*. The uncomplicated case is characteristic in appearance: circinate, marginated, inflammatory areas in the inguinal and crural areas. These are usually dry and scaly except when irritated, when secondarily infected, or when due to *C. albicans* (the latter infections are characteristically moist and have a mucoid surface).

Wet dressings are needed in acutely inflamed and secondarily infected cases. Thereafter, fungicides should be used in ointment form at night and in lotion or powder form during the day. The choice of drugs is the same as for the feet.

TRUNK, EXTREMITIES, AND FACE—The classical "ringworm" is found on the trunk and extremities and, less commonly, on the face. The lesion is round, discrete, and scaly, with a clearing center and an active margin in which may be found miliary vesicles. The commonest cause is *Microsporum lanosum* and the source usually an animal (kitten). Multiple lesions are common, develop rapidly, and are pruritic. Scalp involvement is a frequent complication in children (see Tinea Capitis, p. 229).

Lesions of the glabrous skin are ordinarily treated without difficulty, since secondary infection and eczematization are uncommon. The average lesion can be cured in ten to twenty days by applications twice daily of (1) sulfur, 2 percent, and salicylic acid, 2 percent, in water-miscible ointment; (2) undecylenic acid preparations; or (3) a mixture of equal parts of Iodine Tincture and glycerin.

Tinea Versicolor (pityriasis versicolor, chromophytosis) is a relatively common superficial fungus infection due to *Malassezia* (*Microsporon*) *furfur*. The lesions are yellow or light-brown, scaly, rounded macules involving most commonly the upper chest and back and, in extensive cases, the arms and entire trunk. They are extremely superficial, cause no inflammation, and often coalesce to form large areas of brown discoloration. The condition may persist for many years and is usually symptomless or may produce mild pruritus. If the patient has been exposed to sunlight, the affected areas will often fail to pigment normally, giving the appearance of a loss of pigment by contrast with the pigmented, nonaffected parts. This must be kept in mind in the diagnosis of vitiligo and other conditions characterized by loss of pigment. The diagnosis is readily made clinically and can be proved by the finding of grapelike clusters of spores in scrapings immersed in potassium hydroxide solution.

TREATMENT—The condition usually responds readily to treatment with daily applications of a fungicidal ointment for seven to ten days (p. 310). The patient should be examined in good light before being pronounced cured, since redissemination of the eruption will occur if a few patches are overlooked.

ACNE VULGARIS

Acne vulgaris is essentially a disturbance of sebaceous glands, having its onset most frequently in adolescence and usually terminating early in the third decade. Endocrine factors (including relative excess of androgen) are the most important underlying cause, secondary factors being associated disturbances of carbohydrate and fat metabolism (including fat-soluble vitamins), local infection, and foreign-body reaction. The face, shoulders, chest, and back are sites of predilection.

The primary and essential lesion is the comedo (blackhead), and unless it is present, the diagnosis is not acne vulgaris. Inflammatory papules and nodules, suppuration, cyst formation, and scarring are frequent sequelae. The disease must be differentiated from iodide and bromide eruptions, simple folliculitis, syphilis, tuberculids, and eruptions due to external agents such as oils, chlorine, and other contactants.

Treatment is directed at controlling secondary factors (listed above) and minimizing permanent damage to the skin. Systemic measures consist in correcting existing anemia; administering thyroid substance (p. 456); taking a diet low in fat and carbohydrate and eliminating chocolate, nuts, and highly seasoned, spicy foods; and maintaining proper bowel and gall-bladder function. Large doses of vitamin A (150,000 units daily) for five or six months should be routine. In cases characterized by severe suppuration, aureomycin (p. 291) is of value; it is generally given in two courses of four or five days each, with a rest period of ten days or two weeks between. The seborrheic dermatitis which almost invariably accompanies acne vulgaris should receive attention (see p. 237). In some instances among both boys and girls, improvement follows estrogenic therapy. Dosage is not entirely agreed upon but is apparently in the range of 0.5 to 1 mg. daily in the case of diethylstilbestrol.

Local Treatment—The most beneficial medicinal agent for local use is sulfur, which may be employed in any of several forms (p. 482). These should be used at intervals of every other day to several times daily to produce mild peeling without erythema or irritation. Their application should follow thorough cleansing of the affected area with soap and warm water. Gentle mechanical removal of comedones (with comedo extractor) and drainage of suppurating cystic lesions through a very small incision should be the limit of surgical measures.

Fractional x-ray (38 r unfiltered) treatments once weekly for twelve to sixteen weeks are highly useful in experienced hands. However, x-ray is an adjunct and should never be relied upon as the sole treatment.

ALOPECIA

Alopecia (loss of hair) may be transient or permanent. There are many causes and many types. Two common types, premature alopecia and alopecia areata, are discussed here.

Premature Alopecia occurs commonly in men, follows a hereditary predisposition, and probably depends on circulation of androgens. Loss begins at the frontal and temporal hairline, at the vertex,

or at both. Seborrheic dermatitis of the scalp (p. 237) is an important contributing factor when present. Aside from control of this sometime accessory factor, there is no treatment.

Alopecia Areata is characterized by sudden hair loss in marginated patches, usually on scalp and beard. The patches are white and smooth, all the hair in the involved area having fallen at the same time. This condition frequently follows nervous shock or prolonged nervous tension and exhaustion. In other cases no apparent cause can be demonstrated.

Regrowth of hair usually occurs spontaneously in periods of weeks or months. Its return may be speeded by mildly stimulating local measures, such as ultraviolet radiation in erythema doses or a 3 percent tincture of iodine once daily. Large doses of vitamin B complex are advisable. Existing systemic disturbances should be corrected. In patchy alopecia, fungus infection must always be ruled out.

DECUBITUS

Decubitus, or bedsore, is a local necrosis of the skin and subcutaneous tissue due to pressure. Areas over bony prominences such as the sacrum, greater tuberosity of femur, crest of ilium, heels, and malleoli of ankles are commonly involved. Diseases impairing peripheral circulation and sensation are predisposing causes.

Prevention is most important. Patients who are extremely ill or who have nerve lesions or local circulatory disturbances should have especial attention to areas of pressure. Such patients should be turned and moved frequently. Bedding should be kept smooth and the skin clean and dry. Mildly antiseptic powder is useful. Pressure can be reduced by the use of loosely inflated rubber rings.

Treatment consists principally in accentuating preventive measures. High protein and ascorbic acid intake is important. Cod liver oil ointment or bacitracin ointment (p. 292) and mild sunlight exposure are useful locally.

FURUNCLES AND CARBUNCLES

Furuncles and carbuncles are related lesions which differ principally with regard to size and depth. They are acute infections, usually due to *Staphylococcus aureus*, which start in hair follicles and produce tender, painful swellings that proceed to necrosis and suppuration in several days. A furuncle is relatively small and is largely limited to the skin. A carbuncle is larger and extends deeply below the skin. Typically, carbuncles occur on the back, back of the neck, upper lip, and hairy dorsa of the fingers and hands. In these regions the skin is thick and tough and is underlain by the adipose columns of Warren, which easily carry infection down to the fascia. This anatomical arrangement accounts for the burrowing and multiple openings characteristic of carbuncles.

The term "boil" is used by some to describe large furuncles and by others to describe small carbuncles.

Particularly in the case of furuncles, new lesions may develop from surface spread of the organisms. In recurrent cases, one looks for a source of infection in the patient or his family.

Carbuncles produce systemic evidence of sepsis (fever, malaise). The prognosis is grave in the aged or debilitated. Death may result from septicemia or septic emboli.

Systemic factors, such as hyperglycemia and other disturbances of carbohydrate metabolism, anemia, and debilitation, undoubtedly predispose to pyogenic infection and should always be considered in severe, persistent, or recurring infection.

Hidradenitis suppurativa (p. 234) should be ruled out in multiple "boils" in the axillae.

Treatment—Predisposing systemic factors should be corrected, and the patient should be placed on a low-carbohydrate diet with large doses of vitamin B complex (p. 483).

In *furunculosis*, proper management of individual lesions, careful disposal of discharges, and adequate skin disinfection will control the average case. Trauma with fingers, or premature incision, is dangerous and may lead to cellulitis and sepsis, especially in lesions about the face. Local heat is the most useful method for accelerating softening and suppuration. When "pointing" has occurred, the pus may be drained through a small incision at the apex. This should be a bloodless, painless procedure which is properly delayed until only a very thin skin remains covering the abscess (incisions cutting across the inflammatory border of the lesion are dangerous). The necrotic plug should be given several days to soften and drain spontaneously, encouraged by continuation of heat. Mechanical removal is usually unnecessary and undesirable.

During the period of drainage, great care should be taken to prevent contamination of normal skin.

Dressings should be changed several times daily. Adhesive tape should not be used on adjacent skin.

The skin immediately surrounding the lesions should be painted with an antiseptic tincture (p. 307) twice daily. Bactericides applied to the lesion itself are of little value. In the absence of fever or other systemic evidence of sepsis, the local or systemic use of sulfonamides is not recommended.

In chronic and recurring furunculosis, cases with multiple lesions, and those which have not responded to simpler measures, autogenous or stock vaccines (p. 326), bacteriophage, or anti-infective agents (p. 286) should be used.

Carbuncles, especially in the presence of systemic symptoms, should be treated by prompt administration of systemic anti-infective agents (p. 286). If the lesion is open, healing is usually hastened by scattering in it 200,000 to 500,000 units of crystalline penicillin—G. A covering of gauze impregnated with petrolatum helps conserve the penicillin. Isolated pockets of pus should be drained surgically.

HEAT RASH

Heat rash (prickly heat, miliaria rubra) is a common, acute inflammation of the skin characterized by the sudden appearance of small, discrete red papules and vesicles accompanied by intense itching and burning. The lesions are the result of sweating when the sweat ducts are plugged because of hyperkeratosis. Superficial secondary bacterial infection is common. Miliaria usually occurs in hot weather but may develop in patients with fever.

Excessive or too-warm clothing, exercise, the use of alcoholic beverages, and drugs (such as the salicylates) which cause profuse perspiration may initiate the condition and should be avoided.

Cleanliness is paramount. For symptomatic relief, the parts may be sponged frequently with starch or bran water and dried gently, and soothing lotions or dusting powders (p. 480) may be applied. Tanning of the skin by sunlight or ultraviolet radiation is extremely effective in both treatment and prophylaxis.

Recent studies suggest that fat depletion of the skin may be a contributing factor in development of the keratin plugs found in the orifices of the sweat ducts and that replacement of the fat of the skin surface may be very helpful in treatment. Such replacement may be effected by local applications containing animal fats. Lanolin is the animal fat most commonly employed. It is generally applied as such; but it may be incorporated into a bland emollient preparation (p. 479).

HIDRADENITIS SUPPURATIVA

Hidradenitis suppurativa is characterized by multiple tender inflammatory dome-shaped nodules occurring in the axillae and inguinal areas. It is a disorder of apocrine glands and is extremely resistant to treatment. Systemic anti-infective therapy (p. 286) is useful. Estrogens are of value in some cases.

INTERTRIGO

Intertrigo (erythema intertrigo, chafing, diaper rash) is an inflammatory disorder of skin surfaces which are in constant apposition; e.g., skin of axillae, intergluteal cleft, under female breast, inguinal and crural areas, interdigital webs of toes, and so on. Friction, heat, accumulations of secretions and debris, and superimposed bacterial, fungus, or yeast infections are essential factors in causation. Systemic factors, particularly disorders of carbohydrate metabolism and obesity, are important.

Intertrigo may present the picture of specific infection, seborrheic dermatitis (see p. 237 and Plate 25), or simple inflammation (p. 226), and treatment should be planned accordingly. Cleanliness and dryness are essential. Solutions, powders, or powdery lotions (p. 480) with or without active medicinal agents are preferable to ointments. Existing systemic disturbances should be corrected.

LICHEN PLANUS

Lichen planus is an inflammatory process in which the essential lesion is a shiny, flat-topped, angular papule of violaceous color, usually involving the flexor aspect of wrists and forearms, anterior aspect of legs, and genitalia. The lesions may coalesce to form patches. The buccal mucosa is frequently involved, showing retiform white areas. In severe acute cases, distribution is generalized. Pruritus is a prominent symptom. Etiology has not been established, but there is some evidence implicating the nervous system and virus infection. The disease may last months or years, spontaneous involution being slow.

Treatment consists of general tonic measures, large doses of vitamin B complex (p. 483), crude liver extract (p. 369) twice weekly, and systemic mild air-cooled ultraviolet or sunlight exposure. Mild sedation such as phenobarbital, 1/2 grain three times daily, is valuable. Simple antipruritic lotions (p. 480) and fractional (38 to 75 r) x-ray treatments once weekly are of value locally.

LUPUS ERYTHEMATOSUS

Lupus erythematosus is a systemic disease characterized by a disturbance of small blood vessels and collagen. It is probably similar in nature to rheumatic fever and periarteritis nodosa. Skin lesions are often the most obvious clinical manifestation. Pathogenesis is not fully established, but past or present systemic bacterial infections (particularly streptococcal or tuberculous) plus local trauma (such as cold and sunlight) are known to precipitate, if not actually cause, the disease.

Chronic, subacute, and acute forms are seen. The commonest appears as chronic discoid skin lesions on the face or other exposed areas without systemic symptoms (see Plate 24). The lesions are distinctive when fully developed; they are erythematous, sharply marginated, round or oval patches and show scanty, adherent, white, dry scales, dilatation of sebaceous orifices, telangiectasia, and atrophy. The nose, cheeks, scalp, ears, and dorsa of hands are the most common locations. Involvement of the scalp results in hair loss in the lesion. This form of the disease may persist and progress for many years, become subacute or acute, or undergo spontaneous remission.

The subacute form may or may not arise from a previously existing chronic discoid form. It is characterized by erythematous plaques which appear not only on exposed surfaces but on the trunk and extremities. It is accompanied by low-grade fever, leukopenia, joint pains, and microscopic hematuria. This is a much more serious form and may end fatally after a number of remissions and exacerbations, or it may change into the acute form, with rapid death.

The acute form is a rapidly fatal febrile disease, with suddenly appearing inflammation of the face spreading to the trunk and extremities, prostration, leukopenia, nephritis, and terminal bronchopneumonia. The skin lesions resemble erysipelas or toxic erythema. Occasionally the patient may die before the skin lesions are fully developed.

Treatment—No specific therapy is known. Cortisone (p. 462) or ACTH (p. 473) may produce a temporary remission, but their ultimate value and safety are not established. In addition to general supportive care, patients may be given crude liver extract intramuscularly (p. 369) and adequate rest. Some appear to improve when taking para-aminobenzoic acid, 2 Gm. daily by mouth in divided doses, along with salicylates (p. 405).

Individuals with the subacute disseminated form

should be kept in bed until afebrile and until the disseminated lesions have become inactive. They should be studied carefully for evidence of diffuse vascular disease (p. 74), which should be treated if present.

Excessive exposure to actinic rays, such as sunlight or ultraviolet radiation, may initiate the disease or cause the chronic form to become disseminated in the acute or subacute forms. For this reason, *known or suspected cases should never be exposed to ultraviolet radiation*, and exposure to sunlight should be minimal. X-ray is probably also deleterious.

Although active foci of infection may be considered to play a role in production of the disease, surgical interference should be undertaken with the greatest caution and only after the case has become relatively quiescent. Preparation with systemic anti-infective agents (p. 286) for several days prior to surgery is advisable, even though these drugs appear to be of no value in the treatment of the active lesions.

NEURODERMATITIS DISSEMINATA

The cutaneous inflammation which is called "neurodermatitis disseminata" by dermatologists is termed "atopic dermatitis," "allergic eczema," or "atopic eczema" by allergists. In support of the latter terminology, the condition usually occurs in those who are susceptible to other types of allergy (see Allergy, p. 264) or in those who have a family history of allergy; and some cases, mostly infants, respond to desensitization to or avoidance of presumptive antigens. On the other hand, the appellation "neurodermatitis" is favored by the observation that in many cases there is no apparent connection with allergy and the patient does not respond to the therapeutic measures employed in treating allergy; at the same time, a close correlation can be demonstrated between the state of the patient's skin and the amount of nervous and emotional tension which he is undergoing. The mechanism of production of the lesions is unknown.

The condition occurs at all ages and results in acute, subacute, or chronic diffuse inflammation of the skin. The sites of predilection are the face, neck, and antecubital and popliteal fossae; but any area may be affected, and in severe cases almost the entire body surface may be involved. The well-developed case shows thickened, lichenified, excoriated skin which may weep and become crusted, and sometimes undergoes secondary infection (see Plate 28). The skin is extremely sensitive to nervous and emotional states and to many external agents. The disease may persist for years with remissions and exacerbations. Nocturnal pruritus, which at times becomes uncontrollable, is the outstanding symptom.

Treatment—A careful history regarding possible allergens, skin tests, and desensitization to or avoidance of presumptive allergens (see p. 264 ff.) is effective in some patients, mostly infants, but in perhaps the majority of adult cases the results are unsatisfactory. More fruitful in adults is the psychotherapeutic approach. In some patients a simple explanation of the relationship to tension and a discussion of the possible sources of tension will pave the way for remission. In many, however, expert psychiatric handling will be necessary.

Local treatment should consist of bland greases, such as Hydrophilic Petrolatum or one of the vegetable or hydrocarbon oils (p. 479). All local irritants, such as active drugs, wool, and silk, should be avoided. Starch baths (p. 479), barbiturates (p. 390), and antihistaminic drugs (p. 509) may help control pruritus.

PITYRIASIS ROSEA

Pityriasis rosea is important because it may be confused with secondary syphilis. It is characterized by an acute inflammatory eruption of oval maculopapular lesions which have a pale pink-yellowish color, crinkly scaly center, and reddish border. The long axis of the lesion is parallel to the lines of cleavage of the skin. The disease is self-limited, the duration usually being from several weeks to two or three months. An initial lesion ("the herald patch") resembling tinea circinata frequently appears seven to twelve days prior to the onset of the eruption, which involves the trunk, upper arms, and thighs. The face, forearms, hands, legs, and feet are usually free. Itching may be a prominent symptom.

Treatment consists of starch baths (p. 479), bland shake lotions (p. 479) (ointments are not well tolerated), and bland diet. Mild erythema, produced by air-cooled ultraviolet radiation or sunlight, early in the course of the disease may shorten the duration. All local irritants should be avoided.

PRURITUS

Pruritus (itching) is a feature of a great variety of disorders of the skin and a number of systemic disturbances. Discussion here will be limited to those conditions in which there is no obvious skin lesion to account for the itching (essential pruritus) or in which the only skin lesions are excoriations.

Common local causes are animal parasites that inhabit clothing, environment, or skin; contact with plants or volatile chemical irritants; wind; sunlight; excessive use of soap and water; temperature changes; clothing (especially silk, rayon, and wool); accumulation of secretions (sebum and sweat); and senile atrophic skin.

Common systemic causes are diabetes mellitus, hepatic disturbances (especially jaundice), vitamin deficiency (especially A and B), gout, uremia, lymphoblastoma, drug ingestion (especially morphine and quinacrine), organic lesions of the nervous system, emotional tension, and menopausal syndrome.

Pruritus ani or vulvae in the absence of obvious local or systemic disease is an important example of essential pruritus. It is most often psychogenic in nature. (For further discussion of pruritus ani, see p. 137.)

Treatment—The most important phase of treatment is the search for and elimination of the factors listed above.

With regard to symptomatic control, since itching is essentially a central phenomenon (probably thalamic), systemic measures are usually more effective than local applications to the skin. Barbiturate sedation (p. 390), starch baths (p. 479), bland creams, and cold wet dressings and sponges of Aluminum Acetate Solution, U.S.P., (Burow's Solution) are recommended. Antihistaminic drugs (p. 509) may be useful. Local application of active drugs and particularly of anesthetics should be avoided because of the possibility of sensitization dermatitis.

PSORIASIS

Psoriasis is a chronic inflammatory disease characterized by red, dry, scaly papules which coalesce to form discrete oval or irregular-shaped patches. The scales are characteristically dry and white and flake off readily, sometimes leaving bleeding points. The scalp, elbows, knees, and fingernails are typical locations, but lesions may occur anywhere except on the mucous membranes. Etiology is unknown. Although psoriasis is essentially chronic and recurrent, its course may be erratic. The disease is usually asymptomatic, but itching may be present in acute cases.

Treatment is generally unsatisfactory. A low-fat, low-cholesterol diet (p. 587) may be of value. Small

doses of thyroid (p.456) and large doses of vitamin A (p. 492) are recommended.

The most useful local treatment seems to be a combination of ultraviolet radiation and the crude coal-tar ointment of C. J. White (p. 482). The air-cooled mercury-vapor ultraviolet lamp is used rather than the cold quartz. A suberythema dose is given as often as once daily or as infrequently as twice weekly. Overtreatment is harmful. For those who must work, the ointment is applied at night after the ultraviolet therapy. It is to be rubbed into the lesions vigorously with a smooth tongue blade (for precautions, see p. 482). In the morning it is removed with warm mineral oil. Those who can remain at home should reapply the ointment after cleansing the skin. The morning application is removed before the ultraviolet treatment in the evening.

Other local applications sometimes employed are ointments containing (1) ammoniated mercury, 5 percent, and salicylic acid, 3 percent; (2) sulfur, 2 percent, and salicylic acid, 2 percent; or (3) Anthralin, 0.25 percent.

PYODERMA

Pyoderma is a term covering several conditions characterized by purulent superficial lesions of the skin.

Impetigo is a superficial cutaneous infection that is usually due to staphylococcus and streptococcus, singly or together. The lesions are discrete, with narrow erythematous halo, and are covered by yellowish crusts or flaccid vesicopustules. They occur most commonly on the face, neck, and hands, but any part of the body may be involved. New lesions are produced by autoinoculation, and the disease is transmissible by direct contact and through fomites.

Ecthyma is similar, but the lesions are deeper and may produce ulcers and scarring. It is more resistant to treatment and is often associated with systemic disorders such as anemia, malnutrition, and debilitating disease.

Treatment is according to the following steps: (1) correction of systemic factors such as anemia or disorders of carbohydrate metabolism; (2) daily cleansing of normal skin with rubbing alcohol; (3) application of bacitracin ointment (p. 292) or 3 percent sulfadiazine ointment (for not more than five days), or 3 percent ammoniated mercury ointment, several times daily, the crusts being removed with warm saline solution beforehand (persistent and extensive cases should be treated with penicillin, 300,000 units intramuscularly each day for three to five days; the local use of penicillin is not recommended because of the possibility of sensitization); (4) men with infection in bearded areas should shave every forty-eight hours.

Infectious Eczematoid Dermatitis is an acute or subacute dermatitis which arises in and spreads from localized lesions such as impetigo, a draining middle ear or osteomyelitis sinus tract, stasis ulcer, or fungus infection of the feet. It is caused by sensitization to bacterial products probably conjugated with tissue protein. The occurrence is promoted by improper, irritating treatment of simple skin infections. The lesions tend to marginate and pustulate.

Treatment should be as for acute dermatitis (see p. 226) until the acute weeping stage has subsided. Since the condition is due to bacterial products rather than to living bacteria, bactericidal agents used locally are of no value and often aggravate the condition. Systemic penicillin should be used for three to five days, or longer if obvious suppuration is present. After the lesions have become dry, ichthammol or crude coal tar (p. 482) in 1 to 2 percent concentration in a water-miscible base (p. 479) may be tried cautiously. Iodochlorhydroxyquin (Vioform, p. 315), 3 percent in a water-miscible base, is frequently effective. Fractional superficial x-ray treatment is useful in expert hands.

Many of these cases occur in "seborrheic" individuals, and the general measures recommended for this condition should be instituted (see below).

SCABIES

Scabies is an infestation of the skin by the *Acarus scabiei*, acquired by more or less prolonged contact with an infected individual, his clothes, or his bedding. The eruption consists of minute papules which are not inflammatory unless scratched or secondarily infected (Plate 27). Itching is usually severe, especially when the infected individual is warm. The typical locations are the genitalia, finger webs, buttocks, flexor aspect of wrists, abdomen, and (in women) breasts. The acarus or its eggs can often be found in the epidermis cut from a papule and examined in 10 percent sodium hydroxide solution under a high dry objective.

Treatment consists in a single application of (1) 'Topocide' (p. 317) or (2) Kwell, a preparation containing 1 percent gamma hexachlorocyclohexane in a vanishing-cream base; or two successive daily applications of (3) 10 percent sulfur ointment or (4) 25 percent emulsion of benzyl benzoate. Thereafter, only plain calamine lotion should be used, even though itching and skin lesions may continue for several days. Patients should not be re-treated unless persistence of infection is proved.

SEBORRHEIC DERMATITIS

Seborrheic dermatitis is a subacute or chronic inflammation of the skin which produces discrete or ill-defined erythematous patches, usually covered by greasy scales. The common locations are the scalp, eyebrows, external ear, nasolabial folds, sternal and interscapular regions, and the intertriginous areas, including the perineal region (see p. 137 and Plate 25). In intertriginous areas the lesions are often moist, raw, and weeping.

Seborrheic dermatitis is essentially an infection in a skin predisposed by certain poorly understood systemic factors ("seborrheic diathesis") and by excessive intake of carbohydrates, excessive sebaceous secretion, or any combination of these. The infection may be due to bacteria, fungi, or yeasts, singly or in combination.

Treatment — Limitation of carbohydrate intake, control of active or latent diabetes mellitus, and large doses of vitamin B complex (p. 483) and crude liver extract (p. 369) over a period of many months are necessary to control active attacks of dermatitis and to prevent recurrence. Topical application of 3 percent Vioform cream (p. 315) may be of value.

Local treatment will vary with the location and type of lesions. Generally, sulfur is the most effective agent in the usual lesion. It is used in a water-miscible ointment base in 2 percent strength, with salicylic acid, 2 percent. Intertriginous lesions require lotions and wet dressings, the active drug to be incorporated depending upon whether the local infection appears to be bacterial, fungus, or yeast (see appropriate section). Copper sulfate, 1 percent, plus zinc sulfate, 2 percent, in Camphor Water, diluted 1:20, is particularly useful as cold wet dressings.

SYCOSIS VULGARIS

Sycosis vulgaris (coccogenous) is a subacute and chronic inflammatory disorder of hair follicles caused by pyogenic bacteria, usually staphylococci. The bearded area of men is the most common site, but any hairy region may become affected.

The typical lesion is an indolent inflammatory follicular papule or nodule, often topped by a pustule. Coalescence of lesions or irritating local treatment results in boggy, indurated, crusted, exudative plaques. Scarring and irregular hair loss may develop in cases of long duration. It is curable with proper treatment and must be differentiated from infection due to fungi (p. 229).

Treatment—Seborrheic dermatitis of the scalp and chronic systemic diseases such as anemia and diabetes mellitus may be background factors; sources of virulent organisms, such as active infection of sinus, teeth, middle ear, etc., may be local causes for relapse and recurrence. Correction of these is the first step in treatment.

Acutely inflamed stages should be treated by systemic administration of aureomycin (p. 291). The patient's comfort may be increased by lukewarm wet dressings of 3 percent boric acid solution for an hour four times daily, 3 percent Vioform ointment (p. 315) to be used in the intervals. When the acute stages have subsided, 3 to 5 percent ammoniated mercury ointment may be applied twice daily. Ointments containing either chlorohydroxyquinoline (Quinolor), 0.5 percent, or bacitracin (p. 292) are useful in chronic stages but may not be tolerated by all patients. Sulfonamides and penicillin are not recommended either locally or systemically. Autogenous and stock vaccines of toxoid type are of value. Patients should shave at least every forty-eight hours.

Attention to systemic factors and persistence with nonirritating local treatment will produce good results in the majority of cases.

VERRUCA

A verruca (wart) is a benign, usually small, circumscribed, autoinoculable epithelial tumor. It is contagious and due to a filtrable virus. Warts disappear spontaneously in days, weeks, or years. In view of this fact, treatment methods which leave large scars or are dangerous are not justified.

Treatment is nonspecific, and the results are unpredictable and generally unsatisfactory. Psychotherapy (suggestion) probably accounts for whatever success attends many methods of treatment. Disturbance of circulation or induction of inflammation (regardless of how produced) at the base of the wart is often effective. Ten percent salicylic acid in collodion applied once daily, or superficial electrodesiccation, may afford good results. X-ray therapy, especially of painful plantar warts, has many serious disadvantages and should be done only by experts.

XANTHOMATOSIS

The xanthomatoses are a heterogeneous group of systemic and local conditions having in common the presence of yellowish-red papules, tumors, or plaques in which lipid-containing foam (xanthoma) cells are found. Different members of the group have different prognoses and require different treatment. The classification employed here is based largely on the work of Thannhauser and Magendantz.

Appearance and distribution of skin lesions are not helpful in diagnosis of the type of xanthoma because there is no close correlation between the form of skin eruption and systemic findings. Eventual classification of the individual case will depend on full clinical study of the patient, including plasma cholesterol determination (p. 534), total plasma lipids, and biopsy of a skin lesion.

Local treatment is of little value except for plaques of the eyelids or in cases in which only very few nodules are present. Local application of trichloroacetic acid may produce satisfactory results in the former, and lesions elsewhere may be excised. However, recurrence of lesions is not uncommon.

Essential Hypercholesteremic Xanthomatosis (xanthoma tuberosum) is often familial and is characterized by (1) hypercholesteremia, which may be the only sign of the condition. The high blood cholesterol is believed to be due to excessive formation or inadequate removal of cholesterol by the liver. Other manifestations may include (2) xanthomatous lesions of the skin which are usually large nodules found on the extensor surfaces (flat lesions on the eyelids are common and may be the only symptom); (3) xanthomata on tendons; (4) xanthomata of blood vessels; and (5) xanthomatous biliary cirrhosis (occurring late in the course of the disease). Cardiovascular disease is a common cause of death.

Treatment is not often satisfactory, but a low-cholesterol diet (p. 587) that is also low in animal fat should always be tried. Response is good in some cases.

Essential Normocholesteremic Xanthomatosis (xanthoma disseminatum) is associated with a normal level of plasma cholesterol. Apparently the cholesterol in the lesions is produced in or accumulated by the large reticulo-endothelial (foam) cells which are present. Findings may vary from a few small yellow papules or plaques in the flexures of the extremities to the severe generalized form known as Hand-Schüller-Christian disease. Occasionally xanthomatous infiltrations in special places produce special results: in the posterior pituitary gland, diabetes insipidus; in the orbit, exophthalmos.

There is no known treatment. In adults, the course of the disease may be benign, but in children it is usually fatal in a few years.

Secondary Hypercholesteremic Xanthomatosis is due to hyperlipemia and hypercholesteremia which occur as a result of other known disease, such as uncontrolled diabetes mellitus (p. 173), chronic pancreatitis (p. 144), nephrosis (p. 220), hypothyroidism (p. 180), glycogen storage disease, and idiopathic (familial) hyperlipemia with hepatosplenomegaly. The skin lesions often appear in eruptive form. They usually regress when blood lipid levels are reduced. Obviously, prognosis and treatment in this group are those of the primary disease.

Localized Xanthomata are due to phagocytosis by reticulum cells of cholesterol released by traumatic or toxic destruction of tissue. Included in this group are inflammatory xanthoma of the breast, necrobiosis lipoidica diabeticorum, and nevoxanthoendothelioma.

Xanthoma palpebrarum (xanthelasma) and juvenile xanthoma are not entities. The former refers to a mild form, with lesions involving especially the eyelids, of any of the systemic xanthomatoses—most commonly the essential hypercholesteremic type. Juvenile xanthoma is xanthoma of any type occurring in childhood.

EYE

BLEPHARITIS

Blepharitis is an inflammation of the eyelids. It frequently consists of a chronic inflammation of the hair follicles and sebaceous glands of the margins of the eyelids and may be ulcerative or nonulcerative. In the nonulcerative form, the lid margins are red and there are dry whitish scales on the lids where the lashes emerge. The lashes may fall out but are replaced.

In the ulcerative form, there is some degree of destruction of the hair follicles. Yellowish crusts form on the lids. If these crusts are removed, small bleeding ulcers are seen underneath. Since the hair follicles are damaged, the lashes may fall out and are either not replaced or are replaced in a distorted form.

A common cause of ulcerative blepharitis is failure to treat or to remove the causes of nonulcerative blepharitis. The causes of the latter are numerous and include refractive errors, muscular disturbances, allergy affecting the lids, exposure of the eyes to dust or other irritants, lacrimal obstruction, and various infections such as measles, tuberculosis, congenital syphilis, nasal infection, or trichophytosis of the eyelids.

Treatment consists primarily in removing the cause. If the ulcerative form is infected, it may be desirable to apply an ointment or solution containing bacitracin (p. 292) or 5 percent sulfonamide (p. 293). Ophthalmic Ointment Zinc Sulfate, 0.5 percent, may be desirable in some cases. Removal of the crusts must be gentle and may be aided by warm 5 percent sodium bicarbonate solution.

HORDEOLUM

Hordeolum (sty) is an infection, usually by a staphylococcus, of small glands, particularly sebaceous glands, on the free edge of the eyelids. The lid becomes red, swollen, and tender. Later pus appears. Styes may be associated with blepharitis and are frequently seen in persons with anemia, malnutrition, and uncorrected errors of refraction.

Treatment—Cold compresses are frequently applied in the early stages in the hope of aborting the lesion. At other times, hot compresses are applied to hasten the appearance of pus. When this stage is reached, the pus is evacuated cautiously, and one may apply bacitracin (p. 292) as ophthalmic ointment or solution, or Ophthalmic Ointment Sulfathiazole or Sulfadiazine, 5 percent. When styes continue to appear, errors of refraction are corrected, if present, and the general health and nutrition are improved. Immunization with staphylococcus toxoid or vaccine may prevent further attacks.

CHALAZION

A chalazion is a small tumor of the eyelid due to distention of a meibomian gland by secretion. The meibomian glands are sebaceous organs which lie embedded in the tarsal plates. Obstruction of their ducts along the lid margin gives rise to the meibomian cyst, or chalazion. The cyst may grow slowly for weeks or months until it reaches the size of a pea and is quite noticeable. Occasionally the cyst ruptures through the conjunctiva and disappears. The contents may become infected, resulting in a collection of pus known as an internal sty.

Treatment may be sought by the patient in uninfected cases merely because of the disfigurement. When the tumor is small, it may sometimes be made to disappear by the application to the lid margin of ointment of yellow oxide of mercury or of ammoniated mercury, followed by hot compresses and gentle massage of the lid. When the tumor is larger, it is removed surgically, usually through the conjunctiva.

DACRYOCYSTITIS

Dacryocystitis is inflammation of the tear sac, usually secondary to obstruction of the tear duct. In the acute case there is distention of the lacrimal sac, with a resultant small swelling at the inner canthus and redness and tenderness in the surrounding tissues. In the chronic case the swelling is still to be seen but the inflammation is less apparent. The lacrimal duct may become occluded by disease in the nose, and infection by pyogenic organisms may give rise to inflammation.

Treatment consists in attempting first to overcome active infection and next to reopen the duct. Correction of deformity or inflammation in the nose is often a necessary preliminary. Irrigations of the lacrimal sac with physiological salt solution may be tried. If the duct remains occluded, the ophthalmologist may find it necessary to probe the canal. If strictures are present, repeated probing may be necessary. Extirpation of the lacrimal sac is a last resort in long-standing cases in which all other treatment has failed.

CONJUNCTIVITIS

The conjunctiva is the membrane that lines the eyelids and covers the anterior portion of the eyeball. Conjunctivitis may be caused by bacteria, allergic sensitivity, or irritation from various substances. The most common cause is bacterial infection, and the most common bacteria are the Koch-Weeks bacillus, the Morax-Axenfeld diplobacillus, pneumococci, gonococci, staphylococci, and *M. catarrhalis*. Other organisms include various gram-positive cocci, *Esch. coli*, *B. subtilis*, *Pseudo-*

monas aeruginosa (*B. pyocyaneus*), *B. mucosus capsulatus* (Friedländer's bacillus), *B. proteus*, and others.

The Koch-Weeks bacillus is thought by many to be identical with *H. influenzae*. The diplobacillus of Morax-Axenfeld causes mild catarrh of the eye with inflamed canthi. Possible complications are corneal ulcer and iritis. Pneumococcal conjunctivitis may run a severe course of a week or ten days and be associated with pneumococcal bacteremia. Gonococcal conjunctivitis may be seen in newborn infants if the mother has gonorrhea, or in adults with gonorrhea. Meningococcal conjunctivitis may accompany meningitis due to this organism.

Allergic conjunctivitis may accompany hay fever when both the conjunctiva and nasal mucosa are hypersensitive to the same pollen. When only the conjunctiva is hypersensitive, the presence of conjunctivitis without other signs of allergy makes the diagnosis difficult. The finding of eosinophils in stained smears of conjunctival fluid supports the diagnosis.

Conjunctivitis sometimes results from late hours, alcoholism, dust, smoke, and exophthalmos which unduly exposes the eye to irritation.

Treatment—Ophthalmic Ointment Sulfathiazole or Sulfadiazine is often effective in conjunctivitis due to Koch-Weeks bacillus, pneumococcus, streptococcus, staphylococcus, gonococcus, meningococcus, *Esch. coli*, and some other organisms. It is said to be ineffective against the Morax-Axenfeld organism. Ophthalmic Ointment 'Merthiolate' may be more effective than a sulfonamide in some forms of infective conjunctivitis and less effective in others. Bacitracin (p. 292) may be applied in isotonic salt solution or ophthalmic ointment containing 500 units per cc. or Gm. Penicillin is effective in gonococcal ophthalmia when given systemically; it is ineffective against gram-negative bacilli such as *Esch. coli* or Koch-Weeks bacillus.

In allergic conjunctivitis, the most important procedure is to identify the substance to which the eye is allergic and avoid it. The offending substance is not always a pollen. It may be a food, drug, or other substance. Symptomatic treatment is the same as in hay fever (p. 264).

KERATITIS AND CORNEAL ULCER

Infection or inflammation of the cornea may accompany conjunctivitis (keratoconjunctivitis) or may occur alone (keratitis). Lesions of the cornea are dreaded because of the danger of opacities.

Purulent keratitis is due to invasion of the cornea by pyogenic organisms. Corneal ulcer means loss of tissue and some degree of opacity. In nonulcerative keratitis, transparency of the cornea is usually restored after the infection. In interstitial keratitis, small vascular loops extend from the margin into the corneal tissue. These vessels disappear partially or completely after resolution of the keratitis. Phlyctenular conjunctivitis begins with the appearance of a millet-seed-sized phlyctenule, usually at the margin of the cornea. Keratitis arising from a phlyctenule, if neglected, leads to astigmatic irregularity.

Epidemic keratoconjunctivitis appeared in the shipyards of western United States in 1942. It was thought to be due to a virus. Many cases resisted local sulfonamide therapy; in other cases it appeared that 'Thizodrin' diluted with saline 2:5 or 1:3 might be helpful.

A form of keratitis may develop because of deficiency of riboflavin (p. 487). Vascularization of the cornea may be seen with the slit lamp. In severe cases, interstitial opacities and corneal ulcers may appear.

Treatment—All forms of keratitis call for improvement of the nutrition and health of the individual, with treatment of any vitamin deficiencies or anemia. For suppurative keratitis, local application of ophthalmic ointment containing a sulfonamide (p. 293), 'Merthiolate,' or bacitracin (p. 292) is in order. Atropine, 'Metycaine Hydrochloride,' or phenacaine is useful. Corneal ulcers should be protected from dust. In ulcer, especially when complicated by a collection of pus in the anterior chamber, a solution of penicillin is helpful. Temporary applications of dry heat are sometimes beneficial, whereas cold applications or continuous moist heat may be harmful. The wearing of dark glasses adds to the patient's comfort.

IRITIS

Iritis is inflammation of the iris. Because of the intimate association of the iris with the other portions of the uveal tract—the ciliary body and the choroid—iritis is frequently associated with cyclitis and sometimes with choroiditis. Iritis and iridocyclitis may be due to trauma, tuberculosis, syphilis, or various bacteria or their toxins.

Iritis must be distinguished from conjunctivitis (p. 240) on the one hand and from glaucoma (see below) on the other. In iritis, the iris is swollen, dull, and discolored; in conjunctivitis it is not. In iritis the pupil is small, gray, and sluggish and is irregular after the application of atropine; in acute glaucoma the pupil is dilated, oval, and immobile. In further distinction from iritis, one finds in glaucoma a shallowness of the anterior chamber and occasional turbidity of the aqueous humor, and a steamy appearance and insensitivity of the cornea. A normal intraocular pressure excludes acute glaucoma, but an increased tension does not exclude iritis. The distinction is important because the proper treatment for iritis would be disastrous in glaucoma.

Treatment has two aspects: discovery and elimination of the causative agent, and the care of the eye itself. When the infection is local rather than systemic and the organism is penicillin-susceptible, penicillin may be given subconjunctivally.

The first essential for the eye is rest and the prevention of adhesions. The patient is put to bed, and the eyes are protected from light. Prolonged mydriasis and cycloplegia are induced, atropine being the most effective agent (p. 420). A 1 or 2 percent solution or ophthalmic ointment of atropine sulfate is instilled into the conjunctival sac to keep the pupil widely dilated (every two hours at first; later three or four times a day). For technic and precautions, see page 436. Ethylmorphine (Dionin) has been applied traditionally for analgesic and local stimulating effect—one or two drops of 1 or 2 percent solution or ointment. Continued use may lead to loss of effectiveness.

Hot compresses for several hours daily may reduce pain and inflammation. In traumatic iritis, cold compresses may be substituted for the first two days. Nonspecific therapy with intramuscular injections of sterilized milk, 5 to 10 cc. (1 to 3 dr.), or intravenous injections of typhoid vaccine (p. 336) twice weekly may be of service in severe cases.

GLAUCOMA

Primary glaucoma is a disease of unknown etiology which occurs mainly after the age of fifty years and is characterized by increased intraocular tension due, in part, to defective absorption of intraocular fluid into the canal of Schlemm at the angle of the iris.

Acute glaucoma may be preceded by attacks of dim and foggy vision with rainbowlike rings seen about sources of light. Then suddenly there is rapid failure of sight, with contraction of the visual field, especially on the nasal side, scotomata, severe pain in the eye, and severe headache. Acute glaucoma must be differentiated from iritis and conjunctivitis, as discussed under Iritis above.

Chronic glaucoma may come on insidiously without congestive attacks or pain but with progressive increase in intraocular pressure and loss of vision. Primary optic atrophy is distinguished from glaucoma by normal tension and a shallower and more gradual excavation of the optic disk. Sometimes the greenish discoloration of the lens in glaucoma is mistaken for cataract, leading to delay in proper treatment.

Glaucoma may be secondary to ocular injury or disease causing obstruction of the canal of Schlemm. The treatment is that of primary glaucoma, plus elimination of the cause.

Treatment is most effective when begun early. Most cases require operation on the eye to preserve sight. Nonoperative treatment consists principally in the maintenance of miosis by physostigmine or pilocarpine (p. 436).

During an acute attack, hot compresses may be helpful. Epinephrine hydrochloride, 1:1,000, may be applied to a cotton pledget which is left for a few minutes in the upper conjunctival cul-de-sac. Ethylmorphine (Dionin) may be used as in iritis.

Atropine is absolutely contraindicated in glaucoma.

EAR

OTITIS MEDIA

Infection usually reaches the middle ear from the nasopharynx by way of the eustachian tube. Virulent organisms may exist in the nose and throat in the absence of clinical infection. They may be forced through the eustachian tube when the nose is blown with the nares partially occluded, when atomizers are used which occlude the nostrils, as a result of swimming, or when infants with upper respiratory infection are allowed to lie on their backs for long periods. Among the more common agents in acute purulent cases are streptococci, staphylococci, pneumococci, and influenza bacilli.

Acute Purulent Otitis Media may produce the following symptoms: impairment of hearing, a feeling of fullness in the ear, ringing in the ear, and pain. Infants may present no recognizable symptoms; head rolling is sometimes a manifestation. Fever plus congestion or bulging of the tympanum is usually present. Possible complications include

mastoiditis, chronic otitis media, unhealed perforation of the drum, paralysis of the facial nerve, meningitis, and encephalitis.

Chronic Purulent Otitis Media may result from failure of an acute case to recover or from frequent reinfections. It is more severe when associated with diabetes mellitus, tuberculosis, or syphilis. Unhealed perforation of the drum may cause chronic otitis media or keep it active. Extension of epidermis into the middle ear, with its characteristic exfoliation of epithelial cells, leads to cholesteatoma.

Acute Nonpurulent Otitis Media results from occlusion of the eustachian tube. Swelling of the mucous membrane of the nasopharynx resulting from pharyngitis, adenoiditis, tonsillitis, allergic reactions, and the like may be sufficient to close the orifice of the eustachian tube. Unless air is constantly supplied to the middle ear, a partial vacuum results and gives rise to engorgement of the blood vessels and filling of the middle ear with a serous exudate. This causes pain and impairment of hearing. During the partial vacuum the tympanic membrane may be retracted; but after exudation has occurred, it may show a fluid level, bulging, congestion, and even spontaneous rupture.

Chronic Nonpurulent Otitis Media is usually due to chronic obstruction of the eustachian tube. Long-continued infiltration may lead to proliferation of connective tissue and eventually to atrophy.

Treatment—In *acute purulent* otitis media, the early and adequate administration of anti-infective agents (p. 286) may abort the condition. These drugs are also valuable adjuncts to surgical treatment but should never be considered a substitute for surgery when definite indications for drainage are present. Paracentesis of the drum should be performed if pain, fever, and bulging of the drum are present. Paracentesis is urgently indicated by pain and tenderness over the mastoid or symptoms suggestive of meningitis (p. 165).

Following myringotomy, the causative organism should be identified from the discharge, and the therapeutic agent should be changed, if necessary, to the one which is most effective against that organism. In appropriate cases the anti-infective agent may be administered locally as well as systemically, in conjunction with a vasoconstrictor if there is excessive congestion. It may be introduced in solution from the external ear after myringotomy by alternate suction and pressure.

Certain problems may arise in connection with anti-infective therapy of otitis media. The drug may mask symptoms. If discharge has persisted longer than two weeks, then the slightest symptom—slight rise in temperature or leukocyte count, transient headache or earache, slight mastoid tenderness, increase in discharge—may be indicative of a serious complication. It is well to stop the drug until the situation is clear. Systemic reactions to sulfonamides (p. 295) may be difficult to distinguish from complications of the infection, such as mastoiditis and meningitis.

Early in the course of otitis media, analgesia may be obtained by instilling into the external canal warmed anhydrous glycerin, possibly containing phenol (3 to 5 percent) or some other analgesic agent. Systemic analgesics and antipyretics (p. 405) may be useful.

In *chronic purulent* otitis media, all persistent foci of infection in the nose and throat should be eradicated. Local treatment consists essentially in keeping the middle ear clean and dry, usually by the use of cotton wicks two or three times daily, followed by insufflation of a dusting powder. When the infectious agent is susceptible to an antibiotic that can be employed topically, application of an appropriate solution may be helpful. Zinc iontophoresis has been recommended.

When the infection has produced considerable necrosis of mucous membrane and bone in the middle ear, the condition is much more serious, and specialized treatment is usually necessary.

In *acute nonpurulent* otitis media, anhydrous glycerin containing phenol (5 percent) may be instilled in the external auditory canal for analgesic and mild antiseptic effect, provided the drum is intact. In *chronic nonpurulent* cases, an effort should be made to reopen the eustachian tube and restore it to normal function. Tonsillectomy and adenoidectomy are often necessary.

MASTOIDITIS

Almost all cases of purulent otitis media are complicated by some degree of inflammation of the mastoid antrum and cells. If myringotomy is done promptly or if the otitis media heals because of some other treatment, this early mastoidism usually clears up also. Continued presence of pus in the middle ear is very likely to be followed by accumulation of pus in the mastoid cavity. The symptoms include those of purulent otitis media, with the addition of pain and tenderness over the mastoid process and possibly retroauricular swelling.

Treatment of acute mastoiditis is surgical; but unless the course is fulminating, operation is usually delayed for several days to allow localization.

In very seriously ill patients, the use of systemic anti-infectives may precede mastoidectomy and thus overcome the general septic condition before surgery is begun. Postoperatively, bacitracin (p. 292) may be applied locally through a rubber tube left in place at the time of operation and kept closed except during aspiration of discharge and instillation of bacitracin solution at intervals of four to six hours. Some prefer to implant powdered sulfonamide in the wound and then close without drainage.

OTITIS EXTERNA

Otitis externa is an anatomic diagnosis, not an etiological one. It is most often applied to seborrheic dermatitis (p. 237) or bacterial dermatitis of the external ear, usually beginning in the meatus or in the retroauricular fold. Recent studies have indicated that *Pseudomonas aeruginosa* and streptococci are frequently responsible for these lesions. Fungi found in cerumen are saprophytic types and have never been proved to have etiological significance; thus otomycosis is either a misnomer or a rarity. Other diseases commonly involving the external ear are psoriasis (p. 236), discoid lupus erythematosus (p. 234), and contact dermatitis (p. 228).

Treatment obviously cannot be the same for all dermatitis involving the external ear; it must be guided by the type of the lesion. An attempt should be made to ascertain the cause and to treat accordingly.

AERO-OTITIS EXTERNA

Aero-otitis externa is a syndrome consisting of hyperemia, petechial or ecchymotic hemorrhages, or large hemorrhagic bullae involving the soft tissues of the external auditory canal and tympanic membrane. The condition results from the use of imperforate or inadequately perforated ear plugs or other protective devices for the ears during descent from altitude, usually in aircraft. The mechanism of injury is similar to that in aero-otitis media (see below). The degree of injury varies from mild hyperemia and congestion of the canal walls, and redness of the tympanic membrane, to hemorrhagic bullae involving the canal and tympanic membrane.

Treatment is usually not required in mild and moderate cases. If hemorrhagic bullae are present in the canal, however, they should be incised, the clot wiped away, and a cotton wick saturated with a nonirritating antiseptic agent (p. 304) inserted for twenty-four hours. At the end of this period, the wick should be removed, the canal cleaned with 3 percent hydrogen peroxide solution and 70 percent alcohol, and a dry cotton plug placed in the concha. Complete healing requires seven to ten days. Secondary infection seldom occurs.

Individuals should be warned to avoid complete occlusion of the external auditory canals by imperforate or partially perforate ear plugs during flight. Cotton plugs are equally satisfactory for reduction of noise, and they cause no difficulty.

AERO-OTITIS MEDIA

Aero-otitis media is an acute, recurrent or chronic traumatic inflammation of the middle ear caused by a relative negative pressure of air in the middle ear as compared with the pressure of the surrounding atmosphere.

Etiologically, aero-otitis media is dependent upon two factors: (1) inadequate ventilation of the cavity of the middle ear, and (2) a relatively great (and usually rapid) increase of the environmental atmospheric pressure. It usually occurs during descent from altitude while flying but may occur in mountain travelers, caisson workers, and the like. On ascent, as air in the middle ear expands, an increase of 30 mm. Hg pressure will usually open the eustachian tube automatically; on descent, however, the middle ear must be ventilated to equalize the pressure. This is usually done by swallowing, but may require yawning, thrusting the jaws forward and producing a roaring sound in the ears, or holding nose and mouth closed and puffing out the cheeks. If the pressure in the middle ear becomes 80 to 100 mm. Hg lower than atmospheric, such ventilation may be impossible. Acute upper-respiratory infection is the most frequent cause of inability to ventilate the middle ear. Other occasional causes are blocking of the canal by lymphoid tissue, lack of voluntary ventilation (as in sleep or unconsciousness), and swelling of the tubal membrane.

Subjectively, the symptoms are bilateral in approximately 50 percent of cases. The most frequent complaint is loss of hearing followed by pain (immediate or delayed and varying in intensity), tinnitus, and occasionally vertigo. Objectively, the tympanic membrane is retracted, hyperemic, and congested and contains interstitial hemorrhages varying from petechiae to blebs. There may be serosanguineous effusion into the middle ear, and in the most severe cases the membrane may rupture. The disease must be differentiated from purulent otitis media and external aero-otitis.

Treatment is directed at equalizing the pressure in the middle ear with that outside. Usually the nasal mucosa is first shrunk with a vasoconstrictor, and nasal secretions are removed by suction. Then, while one nostril and the mouth are closed, air is forced into the other nostril under a pressure of one pound per square inch by means of a nasal tip. The patient swallows several times while the pressure is being applied. The effectiveness of the treatment may be judged by observing the shape of the tympanic membrane. The process may be repeated six to nine times at ten-minute intervals. A large rubber bulb may be used as a source of compressed air, but a tank with accurately measured pressure is more satisfactory. In unusually severe cases, it may be necessary to catheterize the eustachian tubes. External heat, analgesics, and sedatives may be useful adjuncts.

The disease can be avoided by proper prophylaxis, that is, maintaining middle ear ventilation during descent. Nasal vasoconstrictors may assist.

MÉNIÈRE'S DISEASE

Ménière's disease, or endolymphatic hydrops, is characterized by recurrent, paroxysmal attacks of vertigo with nystagmus, pallor, nausea, and usually vomiting. Between attacks, there is fluctuating tinnitus and progressive deafness in the involved ear or ears.

The etiology has not been established. The acute attacks appear to be caused by increased fluid pressure in the semicircular canals of the inner ear, and it has been postulated that physical or intrinsic allergy (in contrast to the antigen-antibody type) provides the pathogenesis. According to this hypothesis, a physical or emotional stimulus affects the autonomic nervous system, causing decreased capillary circulation, cell injury, and release of histamine; the resulting alteration in cell permeability disturbs fluid and electrolyte balance and leads to fluid accumulation in the endolymphatic system. Others believe the disease to be the result of a general disorder of water metabolism. It is possible that a variety of factors may be responsible for the sudden increase in endolymphatic pressure. It is unlikely that lesions of the eustachian tube or middle ear are involved. There is no evidence that there are disturbances in the trunk of the eighth nerve or central nervous system; consequently, treatment by surgical division of the eighth nerve is not justified.

The disease occurs in either sex with about the same incidence and is most frequent between the ages of thirty and sixty years. The clinical manifestations vary considerably in intensity and in order of appearance. The paroxysmal attacks appear suddenly at any time of day or night. They have no apparent cause and are not related to any physical or mental activity. Tinnitus may increase to high intensity or change in quality just before onset of the vertigo, or the two symptoms may appear simultaneously. The tinnitus may be unilateral or bilateral and often is louder on one side. As a rule, it persists throughout the attack and subsides soon after the vertigo stops.

With the onset of vertigo, the patient feels that objects are revolving about him when the eyes are open; when they are closed, he feels that he himself is revolving. The disturbance may be so severe that the erect posture cannot be maintained, and, when prone, the patient must brace himself to keep from turning or falling off the bed. At other times the vertigo is mild, and balance can be maintained by grasping or leaning against some solid object. Nystagmus is nearly always present, with the quick component directed toward the least involved ear. Consciousness is maintained, and the patient may have sufficient presence of mind and muscular control to stop an automobile or to gain seclusion by walking short distances. On the other hand, he may suddenly become completely helpless. When attacks continue to recur at short intervals, consciousness may be lost from exhaustion.

Along with the vertigo there is pallor, profuse sweating, increased intestinal peristalsis, and abdominal distress. Headache and sensations of fullness in the ears are sometimes noted. Nausea is nearly always present and usually is accompanied by severe retching and vomiting. After recovery the patient is weak, mentally depressed, and, if undisturbed, will sleep for several hours. Attacks may last for a few seconds or a few hours and often occur in quick succession. The interval between major episodes is irregular and may be a matter of hours, days, months, or even years.

Between attacks, the patient enjoys good health except for the tinnitus and deafness. Dizziness (but not vertigo) of varying intensity comes and goes. The suddenness of attacks and their occurrence at any time of day or night are likely to create a tension state from fear of future episodes. This may lead to voluntary social isolation and personality changes.

In Ménière's disease there is true vertigo, which must be differentiated from dizziness and in-coordination. In addition to endolymphatic hydrops, vertigo may be caused by tumors of the eighth nerve, multiple sclerosis, tumors of the brain stem, epilepsy, intracranial vascular accidents, inflammatory processes within the labyrinth, obstruction of the eustachian tubes, and otitis media. Ocular vertigo, from paralysis of the extraocular muscles or from looking at moving objects, is readily differentiated. Special tests for hearing and labyrinth function may be required for diagnosis.

Treatment—Medical treatment consists in administering vasodilators such as nicotinic acid (p. 366) or histamine (p. 366), which give more consistent results than attempts to control water and electrolyte metabolism with potassium chloride (p. 342) or low-sodium diet (p. 585).

Combination of these measures may be employed to advantage. Sodium intake is limited (to 0.5 Gm. daily at first; see pp. 341 and 586), and potassium chloride in enteric-coated tablets is administered in doses of 6 to 9 Gm. daily. The total fluid intake is generally limited to 3,000 cc. per day. Nicotinic acid may be given as described on page 366, or this may be modified by subcutaneous injections of 25 mg. which are gradually increased, depending upon the degree of vasodilation, to an average of 100 mg. one or more times daily. Suitable oral doses may be used for maintenance. Intravenous histamine injections (p. 366) may be substituted for nicotinic acid and are believed by some to give better results. There is evidence that antihistaminic drugs (p. 509) give relief in some cases. In addition, psychotherapy is required to allay the patient's fears and to obtain his co-operation during the therapeutic regimen.

Control of the acute attacks may be obtained with a few minims of epinephrine solution injected intravenously or by subcutaneous administration of atropine in doses of 0.6 to 1 mg. (1/100 to 1/60 grain).

Surgical treatment may be necessary for severe cases when medical measures fail. Fenestration of the labyrinth with destruction of the membranous labyrinth is in current favor. The operation results in deafness of the operated ear and usually some difficulty in maintaining equilibrium, particularly following sudden movement of the head.

BONE

OSTEOMYELITIS

Osteomyelitis is an infection of bone caused by pyogenic organisms, usually *Staphylococcus aureus.*

The bacteria may be introduced by open trauma to the bone, or they may be carried by the blood or by direct extension from a focus in an adjacent area. The hematogenous route is the most common. The primary lesion is in any case nearly always in the metaphysis of a long bone (particularly the tibia), where the vascular pattern and slowing of the blood stream favor the clustering of organisms. The infection may be acute or chronic, localized or diffuse; and symptoms may be severe or mild. Osteomyelitis occurs most frequently in children, particularly at the age level of eight to twelve years, when injuries are frequent and when boils and other skin infections may more easily escape attention or receive inadequate treatment. However, since the advent of chemotherapy, the frequency and severity of osteomyelitis have been diminished materially. Chemotherapy in compound fractures has reduced the incidence of the disease from this source to the vanishing point.

Early symptoms are abrupt, with pain and loss of function in the affected limb and often chill and fever. The patient may give a history of previous trauma, and there may be local evidence of inflammation. However, it is usually not until twelve or fifteen hours following the onset that an area of localized tenderness can be identified on deep pressure. This is usually found at one end of the bone, near the epiphysis. The pain is increased by application of heat.

Diagnosis is usually not difficult if the patient is seen during the first day or two following onset. Localized pain, high fever, leukocytosis, and especially the finding of an area of exquisite tenderness over the shaft of the bone near the epiphyseal line are all suggestive. During the early stages, the x-ray is of no service in diagnosis; however, about seven days after onset, the pathological changes which the bone undergoes will show as a haziness in the metaphysis, with thickening due to subperiosteal bone formation. Because osteomyelitis is usually localized near the end of a bone, it may be confused with acute rheumatic fever. In the latter, the onset is less abrupt, the temperature is lower, and the leukocyte count is less. Also, in acute rheumatic fever the pain is in the joints, whereas in osteomyelitis the pain and tenderness are at the end of the shaft. In rheumatism the joints are swollen from the onset; in osteomyelitis this symptom is delayed two or three days. Salicylates will relieve pain in rheumatism but not in osteomyelitis. In more severe cases it may be necessary to rule out typhoid fever, meningitis, or pneumonia, for often the local signs of bone involvement may be superseded by acute symptoms simulating these diseases.

Untreated osteomyelitis may become chronic, especially if the infected region covers a wide area. Constitutional symptoms of infection increase as the infection spreads. The patient suffers from stiffness of the joints and muscle atrophy and, in long-standing cases, becomes emaciated and anemic. Other bones may become involved metastatically, and multiple sinuses may develop which at first drain to the surface but later may become blocked as the openings narrow. Sudden acute exacerbations are not uncommon. When the infection intensifies, the resultant severe toxemia may terminate fatally, although this usually takes place only when the patient suffers a severe infection from the onset.

Treatment of osteomyelitis has been greatly influenced by the advent of chemotherapy. Prior to that, much depended on the patient's resistance, and surgical intervention was nearly always indicated. The Orr method has been generally preferred; it involves immobilization, drainage of the infected area, protection of the wound, enclosure of the affected part, and infrequent postoperative dressings. However, it is now generally agreed that if treatment is begun within two or three days of the onset, especially before circulation has been so impaired that chemotherapeutic agents cannot reach the infected parts, recovery will sometimes occur without recourse to surgery. Depending on the infecting organism, one of the antibiotics or the sulfonamides should be administered systemically (see Table 31, p. 290, for choice of drug). In chronic conditions, in which chemotherapy is of less value, surgery is usually indicated, with chemotherapy as an adjunct. Because of the poor blood supply to bone, chemotherapy may have to be intensive and long-continued.

Competent surgical and orthopedic consultation is always necessary, even though most cases remain in the hands of the medical therapist.

LOCOMOTOR SYSTEM
The Rheumatic Diseases

Among disorders of the locomotor system, the rheumatic diseases are the most frequent. Under this general classification are included the disturbances that produce stiffness, soreness, and pain in some part of the musculoskeletal system. In addition to the conditions discussed below, rheumatic fever (for which, see p. 46) and the rare disorders lupus erythematosus (p. 234), periarteritis nodosa (p. 77), dermatomyositis, and scleroderma may properly be included among the rheumatic diseases because they are all characterized pathologically by a type of fibrinoid degeneration of collagen which is similar to that seen in rheumatoid arthritis.

Of the rheumatic disorders, rheumatic fever and the various types of arthritis are of greatest clinical importance. A brief classification of arthritis includes (1) arthritis due to specific infection, (2) rheumatoid arthritis, (3) arthritis due to gout, and (4) degenerative joint disease.

ARTHRITIS DUE TO SPECIFIC INFECTION

Arthritis may result from invasion of a joint by a specific organism. Although a penetrating wound may occasionally infect the area, transmission by way of the blood stream from a site of infection elsewhere in the body is the usual mechanism. Most often, specific infectious arthritis is due to the gonococcus, streptococcus, staphylococcus, or pneumococcus. The first is most prevalent and here serves as an example of treatment.

Gonorrheal Arthritis occurs in patients with a gonorrheal infection (urethritis or cervicitis) which has been present for one to three weeks. It occurs most often in men, and in most cases there is multiple joint involvement at the outset, with mild to acute discomfort. Later, a single joint may be the major point of attack (often a knee, wrist, or ankle), with redness, swelling, and severe pain on motion. A positive urethral smear is a substantial aid in diagnosis, and a positive gonococcus complement-fixation test of the blood is helpful if the urogenital manifestations of gonorrhea are not present. Aspirated synovial fluid will show an increased number of cells and decreased sugar content. Special technics are described for culturing the organism from joint fluid. The disease should be distinguished from other varieties of infectious arthritis, rheumatoid arthritis, and rheumatic fever.

When untreated, gonorrheal arthritis may be exceedingly destructive, often progressing to ankylosis. With early diagnosis and modern therapy, the process can be reversed and permanent damage avoided. Penicillin is first choice in therapy, and usually the infection is eliminated after seven to ten days of treatment with 300,000 units daily. If a resistant organism is encountered, the sulfonamides (p. 293) or streptomycin (p. 289) may be used. Occasionally it may be necessary to intro-

duce penicillin directly into the joint. Rest of the affected member is an important part of treatment; it should be held by splints or other supports in such a position as to prevent deformity. Analgesic drugs and occasionally opiates may be administered to control pain.

RHEUMATOID ARTHRITIS

Rheumatoid arthritis (atrophic arthritis) is a systemic disease of unknown etiology. Through the years, many theories as to cause have been considered. It has been regarded as an infectious disease, a deficiency disorder, and a manifestation of hypersensitivity; and in later years it has been included in a group of diseases characterized by alteration of the interfibrillar substances of connective tissue.

Almost all body tissues may be involved in this disease, but the main site of attack is in the joints. Here, the synovial membrane becomes inflamed and thickened, and, as the process continues, the cartilage is invaded by connective-tissue panniculus. Ultimately, all joint motion may be lost through fibrous and, later, bony ankylosis. Other important pathological changes occur in bone, muscles, tendons, and nerves, and lesions may appear in the visceral organs.

Rheumatoid arthritis occurs most often in asthenic individuals sometime between the ages of twenty and fifty years. However, Still's disease, now thought to be rheumatoid arthritis in children, makes up about 6 percent of cases, and the disorder may appear in elderly persons. Women are more often the victims, the ratio to men being about three to one.

The onset is usually slow, beginning with vague complaints of discomfort in the extremities, loss of weight and appetite, and fatigue and slight fever. As joint involvement becomes more definite, pain, stiffness, and swelling with local heat are outstanding symptoms. At the outset, the hands, feet, and wrists are most often attacked; the fusiform, or spindle-shaped, fingers due to involvement of the proximal interphalangeal joints are characteristic. The knee, elbow, ankle, and shoulder are common sites; the hip, temporomandibular, and sternoclavicular joints are less often involved. Distribution tends to be symmetrical. Rheumatoid spondylitis may occur with or without involvement of peripheral joints, particularly in young men. Muscle atrophy may be extreme, and subcutaneous nodules appear (often on the dorsa of the forearms) in 10 to 20 percent of cases.

A greatly elevated blood sedimentation rate is

found quite consistently, but other common laboratory procedures are not particularly helpful in diagnosis. The x-ray appearance of the joints is not altered in early stages of the disease, but after the destructive process is under way, changes in cartilage and bone may be evident; generalized osteoporosis is usually the first abnormality. In very severe cases, differentiation from acute rheumatic fever may be difficult.

The course of rheumatoid arthritis often is erratic. Perhaps one out of four patients will go into a more or less permanent remission, whereas another 25 percent progress steadily to invalidism. Others continue along without much change in their disease, sometimes quite disabled and sometimes relatively free of symptoms. Constantly progressing rheumatoid arthritis with multiple joint involvement is likely to result in contracted, ankylosed extremities, extreme muscle wasting, and a state of complete incapacity.

Treatment of rheumatoid arthritis has always been unsatisfactory; but with the recent dramatic relief of symptoms through use of cortisone (Compound E) and pituitary adrenocorticotrophic hormone, there is some hope that a practical therapy can be developed. Until this is accomplished, however, the older and often inadequate measures should be used.

Of first importance are rest of the affected joints and rest for the patient. Hospitalization often is desirable to change environment, provide rest, and make available such measures as splinting (to prevent deformity), physical therapy, and close medical supervision. Constant attention should be given to passive and later active motion to avoid fixation and muscle atrophy. This is best utilized in conjunction with heat therapy and massage. The acute joint should be put through its full range of motion twice daily to prevent ankylosis.

Acetylsalicylic acid in doses of 0.3 to 1 Gm. (5 to 15 grains) given at three or four-hour intervals may be employed regularly to control pain. Use of narcotics in this chronic disease is inadvisable because of the possibility of addiction. Blood transfusions are often helpful. X-ray therapy is of little value in disease of peripheral joints, but in rheumatoid spondylitis great improvement often follows its use over the spine. Intramuscular injection of gold salts (p. 515) has many proponents; however, others are convinced that the conservative type of treatment described above is equally helpful and carries much less hazard. Vaccines, foreign proteins, sulfur, and vitamin D are therapeutic agents of questionable value.

GOUT

Gout is a disorder resulting from abnormal uric acid metabolism. It is characterized almost invariably by an increased uric acid concentration in the blood. Hyperuricemia appears to originate in a disturbed metabolism of purines, but the mechanism is not clear; nor is the process known which brings about deposit of sodium urate crystals in the articular, periarticular, subcutaneous, and certain other tissues. It is these urate deposits which are responsible for the symptoms of the disease.

Gout is hereditary and occurs almost exclusively in men, usually after the age of thirty. A predisposed individual may carry an elevated uric acid concentration for some time without symptoms of gout, but eventually he develops the typical acute attacks of joint pain which are characteristic of the disease. Years after the first attack, the chronic form of gout may appear gradually, and severe disability ultimately may result.

The first indication of gout often is an acute attack of joint pain coming on very suddenly, with rapid appearance of swelling and redness of the overlying skin. One of the metatarsophalangeal joints, often the great toe, is commonly involved. The extent of the inflammatory change is greater than is seen in other types of joint disease. The acute attack may last from two days to as long as two weeks. It usually subsides without treatment. Subsequent attacks of similar nature in the same or another joint are to be expected, but the interval between attacks is unpredictable. Usually within two years or less, the disease again becomes manifest, and again there is complete restoration of function. The frequency of bouts increases as the years go by, but the monarticular pattern remains the same in almost all cases. Finally, in the chronic form of gout, pain in one or several of the small joints is more or less continuous, deformity appears, and extensive disability results.

Palpable subcutaneous deposits of sodium urate (tophi) ultimately appear in 25 to 50 percent of cases. They are found most often on the ear but may develop in the bursae of the elbow and knee and in the tendons of the hands and feet. Deposits also occur in bones, particularly near the epiphyseal lines. These appear in the x-ray as punched-out areas. Uric acid stones or accumulations of urate in the kidneys may be responsible for severe renal disease in advanced gout.

Recognition of gout is usually not difficult, provided the physician is conscious of the possibility, since the sex distribution and age of onset are so definite, the acute attack is so typical, and the laboratory finding of increased blood uric acid is so diagnostic. Early cases may, however, be confused with arthritis if gout is not considered. In the well-established case, tophi may be confused with the nodules of rheumatoid arthritis or the Heberden's nodes of degenerative joint disease.

Treatment of the acute attack begins with bed rest and protection of the affected joint through use of splinting or a cradle to carry the weight of bedclothes. Colchicine (p. 409) is begun immediately, since it is almost specific in its effect. The drug is given orally in doses of 0.65 mg. (1/100 grain) every hour until there is relief from pain or until evidence of toxicity appears in the form of nausea, vomiting, or diarrhea. If pain persists after gastrointestinal complaints develop, the dose may be given at four-hour intervals, but usually no more than ten doses are needed to abort an attack. While the effect of colchicine is becoming established, use of analgesic drugs or even opiates may be necessary.

After the acute attack is terminated, a program to prevent or at least postpone a subsequent attack should be developed. A strict diet, high in carbohydrate but low in purine and fat, should be followed indefinitely. Foods high in purine include liver, sweetbreads, kidney, sardines, beans, peas, and spinach. Alcohol should be avoided. Continuation of a daily dose of 0.65 mg. of colchicine may be desirable, or 3 to 6 Gm. (45 to 90 grains) of sodium salicylate may be given per day for two or three days each week for a prolonged period of time to aid in eliminating uric acid. Small doses of cinchophen or neocinchophen have been employed for similar effect, but the toxic action of these drugs on the liver is such that they are now little used.

DEGENERATIVE JOINT DISEASE

Degenerative joint disease (osteoarthritis, hypertrophic arthritis) is a disorder most often affecting the terminal interphalangeal joints of the fingers and the weight-bearing joints during middle and old age. It appears to result, at least in part, from long-continued trauma within the joint and, except for the consequences of mechanical irritation, is not of inflammatory nature. The pathological changes in joint cartilage are those of wear, varying from roughening of the surfaces to complete erosion through to the subchondral bone. As the disease advances, bony proliferations develop at the joint margins and may be visualized in x-rays as lipping or spurring. The synovial villi may be increased in numbers and

size and may become calcified and break off to become loose bodies within the joint (joint mice).

Slight or moderately advanced degenerative joint disease may produce few symptoms; but as the roughened articular surfaces are further damaged, motion becomes painful. Although complete inability to move the joint is seen rarely, the wearing-through of the cartilage to the underlying bone may result in extensive disability due to pain. Loose bodies within the joint may be a further source of discomfort, sometimes becoming wedged between the articular surfaces and "locking" the joint until it is freed by cautious motion.

Degenerative joint disease should be considered when the complaint is pain or crepitus on motion of one or more weight-bearing joints in overweight patients past fifty years of age or in younger individuals in whom the joints have been subjected to unusual trauma. Often the disorder may become evident as painful terminal interphalangeal joints which ultimately develop characteristic Heberden's nodes. The pain is not so intense as in well-established rheumatoid arthritis or gout and usually disappears with rest. Resumption of motion may produce accentuated discomfort which decreases as activity continues. There may be joint enlargement, but there is seldom local heat on palpation. Particularly in the knees, crepitus may be very noticeable when the joint is moved. The fingers, knees, hips, spine, and shoulders are the usual sites; the feet, wrists, and elbows rarely are involved. Joint effusions are uncommon, and rarely does ankylosis occur. Although victims may be somewhat incapacitated, actual crippling seldom is seen except with extensive hip-joint involvement.

There are no particularly helpful laboratory aids in diagnosis, the red blood cell sedimentation rate being normal in contrast to the elevated values seen in rheumatoid arthritis. In the well-established case, x-ray of the joint will show characteristic narrowing of the joint space, lipping at the joint margins, and increased density of adjoining bone. Differentiation from other types of arthritis usually is not difficult because of the noninflammatory character of degenerative joint disease.

Treatment of degenerative joint disease should begin by reassuring the patient concerning the noncrippling nature of the disease and by explaining its chronic and incurable nature. Therapeutic measures are nonspecific, but much can be done to slow the progress of joint damage and to provide greater comfort. Rest of the affected joints is a primary aim. When the knees or hips are involved, weight bearing should be interrupted by periods of rest several times daily. Reduction in body weight is essential in the obese. Application of heat to the joint should be routine several times daily. This may be accomplished with the inexpensive infrared light globes now available, with an electric heating pad, or with hot wet fomentations. Gentle massage should follow. Exercise of the limb is necessary to prevent muscle atrophy. Painful hands may be exercised and heat-treated at the same time by having the patient squeeze a sponge immersed in hot water for short periods once or twice daily.

Mild analgesic drugs such as acetylsalicylic acid and acetophenetidin should be used freely in dosage adequate to control discomfort. Local injection of a few cc. of 1 percent procaine or 0.5 percent 'Metycaine Hydrochloride' into the joint and surrounding tissue may be helpful temporarily.

In the unusual case in which pain in the hip joints prevents walking and in which conservative therapy has failed to provide relief, surgical aid may be sought to fix the joint in painless ankylosis or to reconstruct functioning articular surfaces. Surgery also may be necessary to remove loose bodies, particularly in the knee.

FIBROSITIS

Fibrositis is a poorly understood inflammatory condition which may affect fibrous tissue, fascia, and tendons anywhere in the body. The associated muscles may also be involved, but in true fibrositis the joints are not affected. The most common types are intramuscular (muscular rheumatism or myositis) and periarticular (capsular rheumatism). Different localizations may produce torticollis (wryneck, cervical myalgia), pleurodynia (intercostal myalgia), abdominal myalgia, lumbago, and so on. Other types are tendinous (producing Dupuytren's contracture when the palmar fascia is involved), perineural (some cases of sciatica), bursal (producing bursitis), and pannicular (causing panniculitis, or fibrositis of subcutaneous fibrous tissue).

The causes of fibrositis are not established. However, acute attacks may follow exposure to cold and dampness, barometric changes, muscular strain, overwork, trauma, and various generalized or localized infections. The lesions occur in white fibrous tissue. In the early stages there is localized serofibrinous inflammatory exudate. If this inflammatory exudate persists, it becomes organized, and the resultant scar tissue may cause obstruction of lymphatic channels, adhesions, and contractures. The lesions are of nonspecific character.

The symptoms are localized pain and disability and, later, contractures in some cases. The great variety of possible localizations of the process makes for a varied clinical picture which is easily confused with other inflammatory conditions, and at present the diagnosis is made largely by exclusion. For that reason, a diagnosis of fibrositis should always be considered as tentative, and the physician should remain alert to other possibilities.

Treatment should begin with a consideration of possible associated factors. Faulty posture, frequent chilling, muscle strain, general or local (focal) infections, improper diet, and unhygienic habits should be sought and corrected. Rest (general and to the part, sometimes involving taping or splinting) and local heat often provide relief and may speed recovery from acute attacks. Systemic analgesics are often prescribed. Massage and counterirritation may be helpful. Great and sometimes prolonged relief may follow local injection of solutions of local anesthetics into areas of tenderness; starting at the point of maximum soreness, the injection is extended until all tenderness and pain are abolished. In the "muscular rheumatism" type, improvement has been reported to follow oral administration of 100 to 300 mg. of vitamin E daily (p. 497).

Myasthenia Gravis

Myasthenia gravis is a disease of unknown origin which is characterized by extreme fatigability of the skeletal muscles, particularly those of the eyes, face, tongue, throat, and neck. It is believed to be a disturbance involving acetylcholine or cholinesterase or both at the myoneural junctions (see p. 416). The disease rarely occurs before the age of ten or after seventy, and the incidence is higher from ten to twenty and from forty to fifty than in other decades.

The onset may be insidious. In mild cases there may be no signs of disability in the morning after a night's rest, but as the day passes, muscular weakness sets in and eventually paralysis. There may be difficulty in chewing, swallowing, and speaking; ptosis of the eyelids, diplopia, and strabismus; inability to hold up the head; and weakness of other muscles as they are used. Sensory changes are rare, although paresthesias of the extremities may occur. The course is unpredictable, and periods of remission may last months or years. On the other hand, patients may become worse rapidly and, if untreated, die of respiratory paralysis.

There is frequently a persistence or hyperplasia of the thymus in myasthenia gravis, with lymphoid infiltrations (called "lymphorrhages") in various parts of the body. Their meaning is uncertain.

The diagnosis of myasthenia gravis can often be made from the history and from observation of the characteristic distribution and onset of weakness. In questionable cases, a test injection (subcutaneous) of 1.5 mg. of Prostigmine Methylsulfate and 0.6 mg. of atropine sulfate is usually decisive; in myasthenia gravis, the weakness rapidly disappears. It is especially important to note the effect on three types of movement which are commonly affected in myasthenia gravis: (1) ability to move the eyes and facial muscles and chew, swallow, and talk; (2) ability to hold up the head and lift the arms above the shoulders with arms and fingers fully outstretched; and (3) ability to cross the legs while sitting.

In distinguishing myasthenia gravis from bulbar palsy, it is of value to study with the fluoroscope the act of swallowing a thin barium mixture. Atropine is given in the diagnostic test to prevent the effects of the Prostigmine on smooth muscle (pallor, sweating, intestinal peristalsis, diarrhea, constricting sensations in the chest, or even collapse). Sometimes an additional injection of atropine alone is necessary.

Treatment—Prostigmine (p. 419) is the drug of choice in treatment of myasthenia gravis. It is given in such a way as to maintain a level of the drug commensurate with the amount of physical exertion to be expected during the various portions of the day. Prostigmine Bromide, taken by mouth, is preferred when it is effective. When more powerful action is required, Prostigmine Methylsulfate is given by subcutaneous or intramuscular injection.

Some patients are maintained by 15 mg. of the bromide taken orally in two divided doses. The average dose is about 165 mg. daily; a maintenance dose of 375 mg. daily has been reported. The distribution of the total dose throughout the day is also of importance. This is worked out with the patient on the basis of trial and experience. Four

administrations per day usually suffice. The drug should be taken with a small amount of food to diminish the unpleasant symptoms of smooth-muscle stimulation (see above).

Because weakness of the respiratory muscles may come on suddenly, all patients should have a small supply of the injectable drug at home with a letter of instruction, so that any physician or nurse can give the injection without previous experience with the disease. Some patients need an injection a half hour before each meal in order to be able to eat adequate amounts of food. More severe cases may have to be maintained by injection. Usually 0.5 mg. of the methylsulfate by injection is about equal to 15 mg. of the bromide by mouth.

Ephedrine sulfate (p. 426) has about 10 to 15 percent of the effectiveness of Prostigmine. A few patients can be maintained on it. In others, the dosage of Prostigmine can be reduced by giving 25 mg. of ephedrine sulfate two or three times daily by mouth. If the last dose is given at noon, insomnia will be infrequent.

Potassium chloride (p. 342) has a mild effect on myasthenia gravis when taken in single oral doses of 12 Gm. or doses of 4 to 6 Gm. six times daily. Most patients, however, find it of more trouble than value. It is given as an adjunct to Prostigmine.

Guanidine is an effective drug, but it is little used because it tends to produce disagreeable paresthesias around the mouth and at the finger tips.

The operation of thymectomy has in many instances reduced the severity of myasthenia gravis. Its status is unsettled, however, and the operation must still be considered as somewhat experimental. Younger patients with consistently severe manifestations which do not respond well to drugs are considered the most suitable candidates.

Curare (p. 447) and quinine aggravate the weakness of myasthenia gravis and are therefore contraindicated in the presence of the disease. However, curare may be given very cautiously as a diagnostic measure in questionable cases.

NUTRITION *

There is probably no other single factor with greater influence on health than nutrition. As the subject came under scientific study, the concept was developed of the "adequate" diet as one which would permit relatively normal growth, development, and function and at the same time prevent clinically recognizable nutritional disease. In recent years it has been appreciated that beyond the "adequate" diet

is an "optimal" diet with additional advantages to the organism. The Food and Nutrition Board of the National Research Council has surveyed existing evidence, from which recommendations for optimal daily allowances of essential nutrients have been made. These are shown in Table 22 (p. 252).

* Vitamins and their deficiencies are discussed beginning on page 483; minerals, on page 505.

TABLE 22 — *Optimal Daily Dietary Allowances* (*Food and Nutrition Board, National Research Council, 1948*)

	Calories (Suggested Average)	Protein, in Gm.	Calcium, in Gm.	Iron, in mg.	Vitamins					
					A, in I. U.	Thiamin, in mg.	Riboflavin, in mg.	Niacin, in mg.	C, in mg.	D, in I. U.
Man (154 lb., 70 Kg.)										
Sedentary	2,400	70	1	12	5,000	1.2	1.8	12	75	*
Physically active	3,000	70	1	12	5,000	1.5	1.8	15	75	*
Heavy work	4,500	70	1	12	5,000	1.8	1.8	18	75	*
Woman (123 lb., 56 Kg.)										
Sedentary	2,000	60	1	12	5,000	1.0	1.5	10	70	*
Moderately active	2,400	60	1	12	5,000	1.2	1.5	12	70	*
Very active	3,000	60	1	12	5,000	1.5	1.5	15	70	*
Pregnancy (latter half)	2,400	85	1.5	15	6,000	1.5	2.5	15	100	400
Lactation	3,000	100	2.0	15	8,000	1.5	3.0	15	150	400
Children up to 12 yrs.										
Under 1 yr.	50/lb.	1.6/lb.	1.0	6	1,500	0.4	0.6	4	30	400
1-3 yrs. (27 lb., 12 Kg.)	1,200	40	1.0	7	2,000	0.6	0.9	6	35	400
4-6 yrs. (42 lb., 19 Kg.)	1,600	50	1.0	8	2,500	0.8	1.2	8	50	400
7-9 yrs. (58 lb., 26 Kg.)	2,000	60	1.0	10	3,500	1.0	1.5	10	60	400
10-12 yrs. (78 lb., 35 Kg.)	2,500	70	1.2	12	4,500	1.2	1.8	12	75	400
Children over 12 yrs.										
Boys										
13-15 yrs. (108 lb., 49 Kg.)	3,200	85	1.4	15	5,000	1.5	2.0	15	90	400
16-20 yrs. (141 lb., 64 Kg.)	3,800	100	1.4	15	6,000	1.7	2.5	17	100	400
Girls										
13-15 yrs. (108 lb., 49 Kg.)	2,600	80	1.3	15	5,000	1.3	2.0	13	80	400
16-20 yrs. (122 lb., 55 Kg.)	2,400	75	1.0	15	5,000	1.2	1.8	12	80	400

* Normal adults having a reasonable exposure to sunlight apparently need little or no supplemental vitamin D. A small intake is desirable for persons working at night and those whose habits shield them from sunlight.

PROTEIN AND CALORIES

Normal Physiology

ENERGY METABOLISM

Work and heat production in the body are made possible by combustion of food. The number of calories (Kg. calories) produced varies with the type of food burned, fat giving 9.3, carbohydrate 4, and protein 4 calories per Gm. These are average values but are sufficiently accurate for calculation of the available energy in ordinary mixed diets. The energy requirements of man are determined by his basal or minimal caloric needs plus the number of calories required for performing physical work plus the increase in metabolism above the basal rate caused by the specific dynamic action of food.

Basal Metabolism is the minimum heat production of the body at mental and physical rest twelve to fourteen hours after the last meal. Basal metabolic rate (B.M.R.) usually is determined indirectly with a spirometer which measures the oxygen consumption per minute under standard conditions.

The caloric output per square meter of body surface per hour can then be calculated. The basal metabolic rate is expressed as the plus or minus percentage deviation of the actual caloric output from the predicted normal.

Certain technical difficulties are inherent in the B.M.R. determination. It is unreliable in the presence of cardiac failure or dyspnea from any cause. The judgment and opinion of the operator are involved in deciding the exact slope of the oxygen-uptake graph. A leak in the spirometer system or around the face mask causes the determination to err on the high side. Quite apart from technical variations and errors, there is wide latitude in the limits of normal. Certainly anything between +15 percent and −15 percent in adults must be considered entirely normal, and even +20 or −20 cannot be regarded as definitely abnormal (most bio-assays have an accepted tolerance of ±20 percent). It has been difficult to establish normal standards for infants, children, and adolescents because of the great influence of growth and stage of development on basal metabolism. In addition, it is often impossible to maintain basal conditions in children younger than eight years. Pronounced abnormalities in physical development introduce considerable error when currently available standards are applied.

Basal metabolism is definitely altered by a number of physiological conditions, of which age is one of the most important. Premature infants have extremely low levels during the first ten days of life (as little as 46 to 92 calories in twenty-four hours). As the premature develops, metabolism increases but does not equal that of the mature infant of the same postpartum age until height and weight are equal. The average basal heat production of mature newborn infants is about 43 calories per Kg. per day. This doubles in a few weeks and continues to increase until the age of five years. From five to ten years the rate declines and then rises slightly at puberty. From puberty to twenty years of age there is another decline, after which there is a very gradual fall throughout the rest of life. After the second year of life, females have lower basal metabolic rates than do males. Climate and race have been said to affect heat production but probably are of slight importance. Pregnancy causes little change except possibly for a slight rise during the last three months. Elevation of the basal metabolic rate is caused by such drugs as caffeine, epinephrine, and amphetamine and by androgens, such as testosterone. Sedatives and narcotics tend to reduce it slightly.

The basal metabolic rate is usually *below* normal in the following conditions:

Starvation or undernutrition
Shock
Obesity
Hypothyroidism
Myxedema, cretinism (usually —35 to —45 percent)
Adrenal cortical insufficiency (Addison's disease)
Hypopituitarism, Simmonds' disease (usually —25 to —35 percent in complete absence of anterior pituitary function)
Hypothalamic disorders
Nephrosis

It is usually *above* normal in the following disorders:

Fever (about 13 percent for each degree centigrade or 7 percent for each degree Fahrenheit)
Hyperthyroidism
Cardiac failure (up to +50 percent)
Severe anemia
Erythremia
Leukemia
Diabetes insipidus
Hyperpituitarism
Acromegaly
Cushing's syndrome
Poisoning with thyroid substance or dinitrophenol
Diabetic pseudodwarfism

Specific Dynamic Action of Food is the term applied to the increase in metabolism above the basal rate which follows the absorption of food. For the most part, it takes place in the liver. Its cause is uncertain. The effect begins within an hour after eating and increases to a peak over a period of about three hours. The amount of increase varies with the type of food consumed: protein, about 30 percent; carbohydrate, 6 percent; and fat, 4 percent. From another point of view, it may be considered that part of the available energy from each of the foods is expended as the cost of preparing the ingested food for use by the body. The specific dynamic action uses up more than 10 percent of the fuel value of protein, about 5 percent of that of carbohydrate, and about 2.5 percent of that of fat. Since this energy is not available for satisfying the needs of the body (except under unusual conditions of great heat loss, when the heat generated by the specific dynamic action of food may spare other heat-generating mechanisms, such as shivering), it is sometimes necessary to allow for it when calculating dietary requirements. For a mixed maintenance diet, 5 or 6 percent may be added to the total calories; 2 to 5 percent more is needed for a diet below caloric needs. A liberal diet with more than one-eighth of the calories derived from protein should be increased by 6 to 8 percent; for high protein intakes, two or three times this much will be needed.

Physical Activity—The amount of energy required for different degrees of physical activity has been measured. Light exercise such as sitting or standing raises metabolism 25 to 60 percent above the basal level; moderate exercise raises it 100 to 200 percent; and heavy labor or strenuous sports may increase it as much as eight to fifteen times.

Although it is possible to design a diet which will supply the caloric requirements of an individual, there are many variables (such as food quality, amount eaten, and efficiency of digestion) which may change the caloric intake. Table 22 may be used as a rough guide, but certain nutrition surveys and metabolic studies suggest that the recommended caloric intakes are too high. It is emphasized that the best means for determining the caloric adequacy of a given diet is the gain, loss, or equilibrium of weight during the course of its consumption.

CARBOHYDRATE

Carbohydrates, together with fats, are the chief source of energy. In the average diet, carbohydrates supply one-half and sometimes more of the total caloric intake. In contrast to fats, carbohydrates are indispensable to the tissues but are stored in relatively small amounts. In the presence of a deficiency, protein and fat can be converted into carbohydrate in order to supply the constant demand of the tissues for immediately available fuel. However, this process is inefficient, for it requires the expenditure of energy and places a strain upon the metabolic mechanism. When the total caloric intake is for some reason less than the output, it is wise to provide at least 100 Gm. of carbohydrate daily (parenterally, if necessary). Such an amount reduces the catabolism of protein, prevents ketosis, and reduces the fluid intake which is necessary to prevent dehydration.

The important dietary carbohydrates are (1) the monosaccharides (simple sugars) dextrose (glucose) and fructose (for structural formulas, see Figure 5), which are found in fruits, vegetables, and animal tissues; (2) the disaccharides—sucrose (in fruits, beets, and cane), lactose (milk), and maltose (starches); and (3) the polysaccharide starch, which is available from vegetable food-

stuffs. Cellulose is a polysaccharide which cannot be utilized by man, even though it contributes to the energy requirements of ruminants. It is found in the structural elements of plants and, when present in the diet in moderate amounts, appears to stimulate intestinal peristalsis.

Digestion—Carbohydrate digestion begins in the mouth, where the enzyme ptyalin in saliva rapidly breaks down boiled starch to dextrins and eventually to maltose. Ptyalin has very little effect on raw starch and does not act upon the simpler carbohydrates. Salivary digestion continues in the stomach until stopped by the action of hydrochloric acid. Digestion of disaccharides by acid hydrolysis starts in the stomach. The enzymes of the pancreas and intestinal mucosa are the most important in digestion of carbohydrates. Amylase in pancreatic juice completes the hydrolysis of raw and cooked starches to maltose. Three intestinal enzymes, maltase, sucrase, and lactase, bring about the breakdown of disaccharides to their respective hexoses, dextrose, fructose, and galactose.

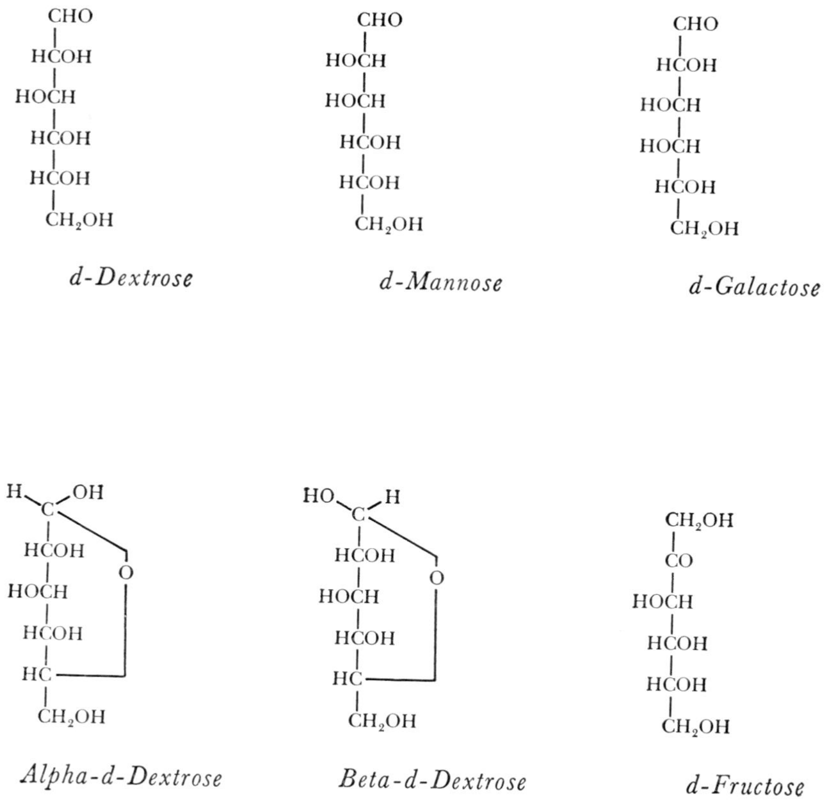

FIGURE 5—*Structural Formulas of Some Hexoses*

Absorption—Normally all assimilable carbohydrates are absorbed by the time they reach the ileocecal valve. The exact mechanism is not clear. Simple diffusion is known to occur; but selective absorption, probably by phosphorylation in the intestinal wall, is also important. The rate of absorption varies with the composition of the diet; it is greatest with a high carbohydrate and lowest with a high fat intake. Diarrhea and inflammation of the intestines impair absorption. Other retarding factors are prolonged starvation, vitamin deficiencies (particularly of the vitamin B complex), infections, and thyroid deficiency.

Utilization—After absorption, the three hexoses dextrose, fructose, and galactose are carried to the liver by the portal circulation. Some enter the general circulation and are carried to the tissues for immediate oxidation. Others may be transformed to fat. The liver converts a portion to the polysaccharide glycogen, which is stored to provide the principal source of blood dextrose. Muscle tissue converts a large part to glycogen, which it stores to supply energy for muscle contraction. Unlike liver glycogen, that present in muscle is not directly available for energy requirements elsewhere. Other tissues synthesize small amounts of glycogen. Thus, the glycogen of general tissues serves as a local fuel supply, whereas liver glycogen is used primarily for maintaining blood sugar. The central nervous system is unable to convert glycogen to dextrose, nor can it utilize protein or fat for energy. Consequently, nervous tissue is entirely dependent upon the circulating blood for its dextrose requirements.

The absorbed sugars are not the only source of glycogen. As mentioned previously, carbohydrate may be derived from protein. This is accomplished by the breakdown of certain amino acids to pyruvic acid and lactic acid, both of which can be converted to glycogen. In addition, the glycerol fraction of fats may yield dextrose.

The production of energy from glycogen is accomplished by a complex series of chemical reactions involving enzyme systems. In the liver dextrose is produced, but in muscle the reaction does not proceed this far; this accounts for the fact that muscle glycogen does not directly influence the blood-sugar level. The end product of muscle metabolism is lactic acid, which may be further decomposed to carbon dioxide and water or may be carried by the blood stream to the liver, where it is reconverted to glycogen.

Under normal conditions, the liver alone regulates the level of sugar in the blood. Endocrine imbalance alters the ability of the liver to produce or withhold dextrose from the blood. Insulin deficiency leads to hyperglycemia. The secretions of the anterior pituitary gland tend to change the blood-sugar level in the opposite direction; thus, in hypopituitarism there is a hypoglycemia, and in hyperpituitarism, hyperglycemia. Deficiency of adrenal gluco-corticoid hormones lowers and an excess raises blood sugar in a similar manner. To a lesser extent this is also true of the thyroid. In addition, there is an emergency mechanism for combating sudden and profound hypoglycemia, namely, the secretion of epinephrine by the adrenal medulla in response to sympathetic stimulation. The epinephrine causes a breakdown of liver glycogen and liberation of dextrose into the blood.

Parenteral administration of carbohydrate (in the form of dextrose solution) is a common therapeutic procedure. It is an excellent means of supplying water free of electrolyte (see p. 341), and it has value for its own sake (see first paragraph under Carbohydrate, p. 253) in patients who are unable to take adequate quantities by mouth. However, parenteral administration of carbohydrate is not a practical means of supplying full caloric needs over a prolonged period. Details of administration are discussed on page 349.

FAT

Fat is an important component of the diet because of its high fuel value. In addition, it adds to the palatability of food, serves as a vehicle for the fat-soluble vitamins, retards digestion (thereby increasing the "staying power" of a meal), and, after absorption and deposit, provides a large internal reservoir of food for the body, serves as a protective cushion for internal organs, and insulates against temperature changes.

The National Research Council recommends that fat be included in the diet of the average individual to the extent of at least 20 to 25 percent of the total calories. For very active persons requiring as many as 4,500 calories and for children and adolescents, it should make up 30 to 35 percent of the caloric intake. At least 1 percent of the total calories should be supplied by the "essential fatty acids" (see Item 6 below). Foods such as meat, milk, cheese, and nuts or nut products (e.g., peanut butter) usually contribute from one-half to two-thirds of the dietary fat; the remainder is generally supplied by butter, oleomargarine, and shortenings.

The term "lipid" includes the true fats, or triglycerides, as well as other substances which are related to fats on the basis of common physical or chemical properties. They may be classified as follows:

1. Triglycerides (neutral fats), which make up the greater part of the lipids in the diet and are the typical constituents of animal fats.
2. Waxes, which include the cholesterol esters in blood and body tissues; they have no nutritional value.
3. Phospholipids, which are present in all animal and vegetable cell protoplasm and include lecithin, cephalin, and sphingomyelin; they are highly concentrated in the myelinated portions of the nervous system.
4. Glycolipids (cerebrosides), found mostly in the white matter of the brain and the medullary sheaths of nerves.
5. Steroids, including cholesterol, hormones of the gonads and the adrenal cortex, the bile acids, vitamin D, and the digitalis glycosides.
6. Fatty acids, which are the form in which fat is oxidized in the body. They are mostly derived from triglycerides but to a lesser extent from phospholipids and esters of cholesterol. There are more than twenty-two fatty acids available in food, and they are classified according to the degree of saturation (with hydrogen). Body fats are composed chiefly of the glycerides of palmitic, stearic (both saturated), and oleic (unsaturated) acids. They may contain small amounts of myristic (saturated), linoleic, and arachidonic (both unsaturated) acids. The unsaturated fatty acids linoleic, linolenic, and arachidonic cannot be synthesized by animals, and they have therefore been termed "essential." However, their exact physiological role is not known, and their essentiality in man has not been proved.

Digestion—Very little change in dietary fat takes place in the stomach. A few fatty acids are liberated from lipid-protein complexes by hydrochloric acid, and gastric lipase exerts some hydrolytic action on the highly emulsified fats of milk and egg yolk. After entering the small intestine, fats are emulsified in the alkaline medium by the bile salts with the aid of the motility of the intestines and possibly by a small amount of soap formed from fatty acids. Emulsification is necessary because the fat-splitting enzymes of pancreatic juice and succus entericus are water-soluble and therefore can act only on the surface of fat globules. The pancreatic lipase, steapsin, rapidly hydrolyzes emulsified fats to glycerol and fatty acids. Fats passing on from the upper intestine are digested by lipases of the succus entericus. Colonic bacteria also split fats, but fatty acids liberated in the colon are not absorbed. It was formerly believed that vegetable fats were digested and utilized less efficiently than those of animal origin, but this has been disproved.

Absorption of fats is considerably slower than that of other foods. The exact mechanisms have not been identified. Glycerol diffuses directly into the intestinal mucosa and, unless used to re-form fats there, passes to the liver, where it is converted to

glycogen. Water-soluble complexes of bile salts and fatty acids form and diffuse into the mucosa, where they are broken down to re-form neutral fat. Some fatty acids combine with cholesterol before absorption. The major portion of resynthesized fat passes into the lacteals of the intestinal villi and is carried by the lymph through the thoracic duct into the systemic circulation. The blood lipids reach a maximum level five or six hours after a fatty meal and return to normal values in about nine hours.

Methods for determination of plasma lipids are available; but, with the exception of those for cholesterol (p. 534), they are not practical for the average clinical laboratory. There is disagreement about normal values for adults, as indicated in Table 23.

TABLE 23 — *Normal Values for Plasma Lipids in Adults, as Suggested by Two Authorities*

	Plasma Level, in mg. per 100 cc.	
Total lipids	530 ± 74*	720 ± 200†
Neutral fat	142 ± 60	225 ± 140
Total fatty acid	316 ± 85	———
Total cholesterol	152 ± 24	200 ± 50
Free cholesterol	46 ± 8	55 ± 15
Combined cholesterol	106 ± 25	145 ± 35
Phospholipid	165 ± 28	200 ± 40

Utilization—A portion of the blood lipids is carried to fat depots for storage. Some is oxidized within the tissue cells of the body for the production of heat and energy. These reactions have not been identified, although it is known that during utilization the liver produces intermediary compounds (the ketone bodies beta-hydroxybutyric acid, acetoacetic [diacetic] acid, and acetone) which are in turn distributed to the tissue cells and oxidized. When liver glycogen is diminished, fatty-acid oxidation increases, with resultant acceleration of ketone-body formation. If the capacity of the body to oxidize ketones is exceeded, they accumulate and ketosis develops (see Diabetic Acidosis, p. 59). However, if the need for lipid oxidation is removed by administration of carbohydrate in starvation or Insulin in diabetes, then ketone production declines and ketosis is eliminated. Thus, carbohydrate is antiketogenic rather than ketolytic.

* White, A., in Diseases of Metabolism, edited by Duncan, G. G., Ed. 2, p. 167. Philadelphia: W. B. Saunders Company, 1947.
† Everett, M. R.: Medical Biochemistry, Ed. 2, p. 215. New York: Paul B. Hoeber, Inc., 1946.

PROTEIN

Proteins are complex biological compounds occurring in all living tissue. They are the sole dietary source of nitrogen. They are essential constituents of protoplasm and cell nuclei; make up a large portion of the muscle and glandular tissue of the body; contribute to the structure of enzymes, hormones, and antibodies; and are important in regulating the osmotic relations between intracellular and extracellular fluid. Plants and a few microorganisms can synthesize proteins from the inorganic elements of soil and atmosphere, but animals are unable to do this and must ingest ready-made proteins obtained from vegetable sources and from other animals. Since such sources provide proteins distinctive to the species of origin, they must be broken down in the body of the recipient and resynthesized to compounds suitable for utilization.

The structural units of protein molecules are amino acids, of which twenty-one or more have been identified. These are joined by peptide linkages to form various patterns which govern the chemical, physical, and biological properties of each protein. Certain amino acids are indispensable because they cannot be synthesized by animals; consequently, the nutritional value of an individual protein varies according to the concentrations of these essential units. The proteins of eggs, meat, and milk have superior biological value, whereas many of cereal and vegetable origin are deficient in essential amino acids and will not maintain nitrogen equilibrium or support growth. Table 24 lists the known amino acids of natural origin. Their chemical structures are shown in Table 24 and Figure 6 (p. 258). Cystine and tyrosine have been termed "valuable" for the reason that omission from the diet may result in protein deficiency because their synthesis in the body is too slow to meet normal requirements. The dispensable compounds are needed for optimal nutrition; inadequate supply may impair growth by causing less efficient utilization of proteins generally.

Digestion—The digestion of proteins begins in the stomach, where the enzyme pepsin starts degradation in the presence of hydrochloric acid. Peptic digestion may produce free amino acids but usually is terminated earlier by gastric emptying at the proteose or peptide stage. Rennin, the other proteolytic enzyme found in gastric juice, acts only on casein, the protein of milk. It probably aids in the digestion of milk by infants, but its importance in adults is negligible and is overshadowed by the

TABLE 24 — *The Amino Acids of Natural Origin*

Indispensable

Lysine,
$NH_2 \cdot (CH_2)_4 \cdot CH(NH_2) \cdot COOH$
Tryptophane (formula in Figure 6)
Phenylalanine (formula in Figure 6)
Leucine,
$(CH_3)_2 : CH \cdot CH_2 \cdot CH(NH_2) \cdot COOH$
Isoleucine,
$CH_3 \cdot CH_2 \cdot CH(CH_3) \cdot CH(NH_2) \cdot COOH$
Threonine,
$CH_3 \cdot CHOH \cdot CH(NH_2) \cdot COOH$
Methionine,
$CH_3 \cdot S \cdot CH_2 \cdot CH_2 \cdot CH(NH_2) \cdot COOH$
Valine,
$(CH_3)_2 : CH \cdot CH(NH_2) \cdot COOH$
Arginine,
$NH_2 \cdot C(:NH) \cdot NH \cdot (CH_2)_3 \cdot CH(NH_2) \cdot COOH$
Histidine (formula in Figure 6)

Dispensable

Glycine,
$CH_2(NH)_2 \cdot COOH$
Alanine,
$CH_3 \cdot CH(NH_2) \cdot COOH$
Serine,
$CH_2OH \cdot CH(NH_2) \cdot COOH$
Norleucine,
$CH_3 \cdot (CH_2)_3 \cdot CH(NH_2) \cdot COOH$
Aspartic acid,
$HOOC \cdot CH_2 \cdot CH(NH_2) \cdot COOH$
Glutamic acid,
$HOOC \cdot CH_2 \cdot CH_2 \cdot CH(NH_2) \cdot COOH$
Hydroxyglutamic acid,
$HOOC \cdot CH_2 \cdot CHOH \cdot CH(NH_2) \cdot COOH$
Proline (formula in Figure 6)
Hydroxyproline (formula in Figure 6)
Tyrosine (formula in Figure 6)
Cystine, $\begin{array}{l} S \cdot CH_2 \cdot CH(NH_2) \cdot COOH \\ | \\ S \cdot CH_2 \cdot CH(NH_2) \cdot COOH \end{array}$

rennin effect of the chymotrypsins from the pancreas. The gastric phase of protein digestion is usually terminated in three or four hours.

Digestion of the partially hydrolyzed proteins proceeds rapidly in the duodenum. Pancreatic juice contains trypsinogen, which is inactive in itself but becomes activated to trypsin in the presence of enterokinase from the intestinal juice. Trypsin rapidly converts the partially digested proteins to peptides and amino acids and can slowly digest native proteins. Chymotrypsins also are supplied by pancreatic juice; they act similarly to trypsin but also have a strong rennin-like action. In addition, the pancreas supplies enzymes for digestion of nuclear proteins. The intestinal mucosa and succus entericus contain peptidases such as aminopeptidase

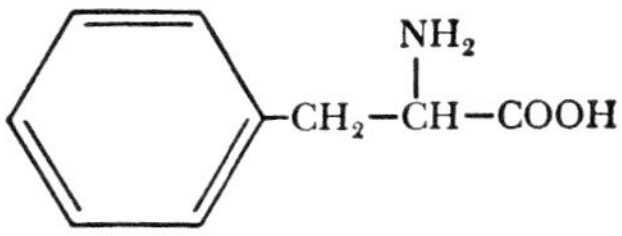

Phenylalanine

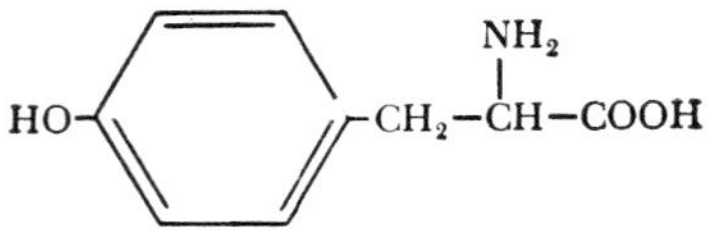

Tyrosine

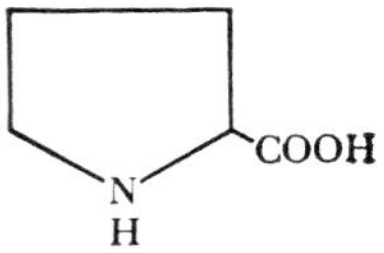

Proline

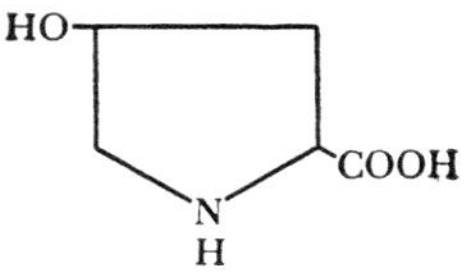

Hydroxyproline

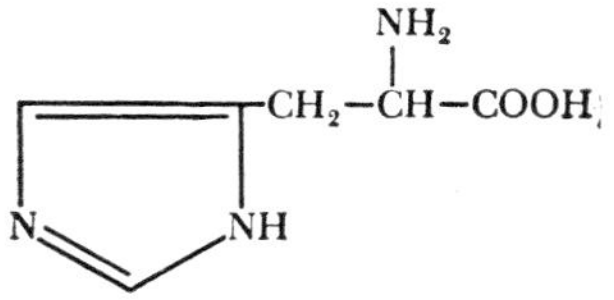

Histidine

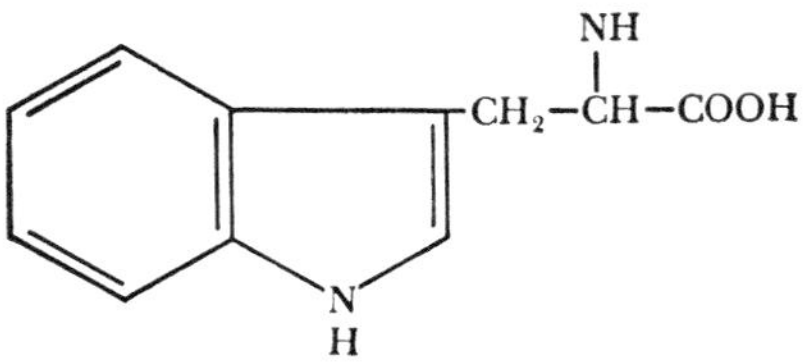

Tryptophane

FIGURE 6 — *Structural Formulas of Some Amino Acids*

and dipeptidase, which are sometimes termed "erepsin." These do not require activation by enterokinase but act directly on peptides and complete the digestion to amino acids. Peptidases in the intestinal mucosa tend to prevent absorption of polypeptides and peptones.

Absorption—There is little or no absorption of protein or its split products from the stomach under normal conditions. Absorption of protein digestion-products is most rapid in the duodenum and usually is completed in six to nine hours, by which time the intestinal contents generally have reached the ileocecal valve. On the whole, the amino acids are absorbed rapidly by simple diffusion, but the rate varies with their chemical complexity.

Small amounts of intermediate protein compounds and even native proteins may be absorbed intact. Undigested egg-white proteins are quite readily absorbed by infants and by adults with damaged or abnormally permeable intestinal mucosa. Under these circumstances, specific protein sensitization may develop which is manifested clinically by food idiosyncrasies or more serious allergic reactions.

Amino acids which pass the ileocecal valve and those administered in nutrient enemas are partially absorbed from the large intestine. Here, unabsorbed proteins undergo more or less putrefaction, the reaction being governed by the amount of protein present, the length of time it is retained, and the type and number of putrefactive bacteria. Depending upon the kinds of amino acids present, putrefaction gives rise to a variety of amines and phenols, such as histamine, isoamylamine, putrescine, cadaverine, skatole, indole, and others. Absorption of such cleavage products has been said to give rise to numerous clinical manifestations sometimes termed "autointoxication." Even though many of these compounds are extremely toxic when given orally or parenterally, the amounts required are much greater than could possibly be obtained from colonic putrefaction if their absorption were complete, which it is not.

Utilization—After passage through the intestinal wall, most of the amino acids are transported to the liver by the portal circulation. Small amounts find their way into the lymph of the thoracic duct. Normally, the circulating amino acids are assimilated very rapidly, the liver being particularly active. There is no permanent storage, although excessive amounts may be retained temporarily. There is a constant exchange of amino acids between tissues and cells, so that a dynamic equilibrium exists. Synthesis of proteins from amino acids takes place through the medium of enzymes, reducing agents, and energy derived from carbohydrates. Amino acids not required for protein synthesis are deaminated, chiefly in the liver, with the formation of carbohydrate and nonprotein nitrogenous products. The latter are excreted in the urine. The liver is the chief source of the plasma proteins albumin, fibrinogen, and prothrombin. It also supplies the major portion of globulin.

The healthy adult is in a state of nitrogen equilibrium, in which the nitrogen excretion equals the intake. Excessive excretion causes a negative nitrogen balance; this is found in starvation, shock, dehydration, fevers, acidosis, malnutrition, wasting diseases, hyperthyroidism, and fractures of large bones. The protein-sparing effect of carbohydrate and the administration of Insulin aid in correcting a negative balance. Growth and convalescence produce a positive nitrogen balance because of accelerated protein synthesis. Nitrogen equilibrium is maintained on high-protein diets, but an excessively high intake causes a negative balance because of exaggeration of the specific dynamic action and depletion of thiamin and other essential elements.

Protein Requirements—The recommended protein allowances of the National Research Council (Table 22, p. 252) represent amounts that are desirable in the diet from the standpoint of optimal nutrition. They are definitely not minimal requirements. During growth, high-quality proteins from animal sources should supply from one-third to one-half of the total; somewhat less will suffice for adults. The recommendations for adults are based on Sherman's standard of 1 Gm. of protein for each Kg. of body weight; those for children are on the basis of 3.5 to 4 Gm. per Kg. of body weight during the first two years, 2.5 to 3 Gm. from two to six years, and 1.5 to 2 Gm. from six years through adolescence.

In many pathological conditions, protein requirements are increased considerably. Rapid losses are common following surgery, trauma, hemorrhage, shock, and during the course of severe infections. Convalescence may be shortened considerably by preventing or correcting protein deficiency and thus promoting wound healing and resistance to infection. In cases of thyrotoxicosis, the protein need is great because of increase in the metabolic rate. Burns and fractures cause toxic destruction of protein, loss of serum protein in

exudates, and impaired liver function. Patients with liver disease often are unable to maintain nitrogen equilibrium. Considerable loss may occur in pleural or peritoneal exudates. Gastro-intestinal malfunctions such as vomiting, peptic ulcer, ulcerative colitis, enteritis, chronic pancreatic disease, diarrheas, and draining fistulas are important factors. Enforced immobility and long confinement to bed may be complicated by trophic ulcers from protein depletion. Chronic infections, such as tuberculosis and rheumatic fever, increase protein requirements.

Disturbances of Protein and Caloric Balance

PROTEIN DEFICIENCY

Protein deficiency may be acute, subacute, or chronic. The clinical manifestations vary with the severity and duration. There are no suitable laboratory methods for detecting a specific amino acid deficiency, although a number of clinical and laboratory procedures may be utilized to determine an over-all protein deficiency. The dietary history is very important and will disclose whether there is a quantitative or qualitative lack or, in the presence of an adequate diet, whether the difficulty lies in increased nutritive requirements or in impaired digestion, absorption, and utilization. Dependent edema of a constant or transitory nature is usually the first clinical sign. Other findings of pallor, anemia, and weakness sometimes appear later. Determination of the plasma or serum protein concentration may reveal abnormally low levels, although significant alteration may be lacking. Quantitative analysis for albumin and globulin is of more importance than mere determination of the albumin-globulin ratio. Blood volume should be measured simultaneously, since this may be reduced and so obscure changes in the total protein content.

The normal concentration of total protein in plasma is from 6.2 to 8.5 percent; of albumin, 4.3 to 5.7 percent; and of globulin, 1.4 to 3 percent. Children over two years of age have about the same blood protein concentrations as do adults. Low levels of plasma protein may of themselves induce edema, or they may be merely contributing factors (see under Edema, p. 55).

Treatment—Protein for oral administration may be supplied by a proper selection of natural foods or, when specially indicated, as amino acid mixtures. In feeding sick, convalescent, starved, or growing individuals, the object is to supply not only sufficient protein to maintain nitrogen equilibrium but additional amounts for tissue synthesis. Daily intakes of 2 to 4 Gm. of protein per Kg. of normal body weight (1 to 2 Gm. per lb.) are needed for rapid recovery of depleted persons.

Selection of protein foods for a given dietary depends upon a quantitative and qualitative evaluation. Little is known of the amino acid content of natural foods; in order to obtain adequate amounts of the essential amino acids, current practice directs that one-half of the protein be from such animal sources as milk, eggs, meat, poultry, fish, and cheese. Less complete but fairly good-quality proteins are obtained from beans, soybeans, oats, yeast, almonds, and peanuts. Milled wheat, corn, and rice are poor sources. When individual diets are arranged, the basic protein foods (see p. 582) may be fitted into the daily dietary. By proper modification, varying protein intakes can be provided.

Synthetic amino acids are available in crystalline form, but their use is impractical at the present time because of high cost. However, protein hydrolysates which are inexpensive and are suitable for oral or parenteral administration can be prepared by acid or enzyme digestion. These products may contain as much as 4 percent sodium chloride. In preparations produced by enzymatic hydrolysis, about 70 percent of the nitrogen is present as amino acids; most of the remainder consists of peptides. Although acid hydrolysis converts nearly all of the protein to free amino acids, tryptophane is destroyed in the process and must be added to the mixture.

Oral administration of amino acids obviates the necessity of protein digestion and is indicated when (1) natural protein is not tolerated, (2) protein intake is inadequate, or (3) digestion is impaired. Patients with severe protein allergy, particularly infants, can frequently be relieved and their nutrition restored to normal. Amino acids have been used to good advantage during the diagnostic period in food allergy. In peptic ulcer, the use of amino acid mixtures by mouth appears to hasten recovery.

The taste of some preparations is unpleasant and sometimes cannot be disguised successfully. Protein hydrolysates may be dissolved in water, milk, or juices. Daily oral intake of 200 to 300 Gm. may be accomplished by frequent administration of a suspension of the powder in a small amount of water followed by 20 cc. of syrup. Another method is to dissolve the preparation in hot water, allow to cool, and then serve cold after mixing with plain milk, malted milk, or fruit juice.

Parenteral administration of amino acids is necessary in severe gastro-intestinal disease or in persistent vomiting from any cause. It is particularly valuable in the preoperative and postoperative care of gastro-intestinal carcinoma and other chronic conditions characterized by severe malnutrition. Sterile preparations containing all of the essential amino acids are available. Ordinarily, they are given in 5 or 6 percent concentration in either 5 percent dextrose or isotonic electrolyte solution. The rate of intravenous injection should be somewhat slower than that for dextrose solution alone. The drip technic is appropriate. Too-rapid administration may cause flushing, abdominal pain, or nausea and vomiting. Amino acids may be given subcutaneously if in isotonic solution. For this, the 5 percent protein hydrolysate in 5 percent dextrose solution (the combination is hypertonic) is diluted with an equal volume of sterile distilled water. Stronger solutions are absorbed poorly and tend to produce local inflammation.

The parenteral administration of amino acids should be correlated with administration of fluid. Fluid requirements are discussed under Treatment of Dehydration (p. 57). For patients in nitrogen equilibrium, 50 Gm. of protein hydrolysate are considered an adequate daily ration. This quantity is contained in 1,000 cc. of 5 percent hydrolysate in 5 percent dextrose, which provides, in addition, 50 Gm. of carbohydrate, from none to 20 Gm. of electrolyte (depending on the product), and 1 liter of fluid. In moderate protein depletion, twice this quantity may be given; it is best to administer half in the morning and half in the afternoon. Severe protein deficiency may require 3 liters of solution daily, or 150 Gm. of protein derivative.

In many instances the caloric requirements need not be met completely, since energy can safely be derived from body fat for short periods. In severe malnutrition, however, the body's reserve is depleted and cannot be relied upon. Fat emulsions for intravenous feeding are being developed and may eventually become a standard part of parenteral feeding regimens. Vitamins, particularly those of the B complex and vitamin C, should be given separately (p. 483).

OBESITY

Obesity is defined as an excess of adipose tissue. Whether or not the quantity is excessive in a given instance is still essentially a matter of judgment.

"Normal" weight is a function of sex, height, and body build. In children, age is also a factor, whereas in adults there is considerable evidence for the view that increases in weight after the age of about thirty are not physiological. Tables are available (p. 568) giving average "normal" weight for sex, age, and height; but only in children has the factor of body build been given statistical attention. Therefore, in dealing with adults, the clinician must use his own judgment in allowing for this factor.

Obesity is extremely common. The milder grades are often considered normal. In fact, it is probably the inclusion of cases of mild obesity in data for tables of "normal" weight that is responsible for the increase of "normal" weight with age in such tables. Even mild obesity places the individual at a biological disadvantage. After the age of forty years, mortality rates are higher for the obese than for those of normal weight. Dublin and Lotka demonstrated that in the age range of forty-five to fifty years there is approximately a 1 percent increase in mortality rate for each pound of excess weight. For older groups, mortality increases even more sharply. The obese are more susceptible to hypertension and other cardiovascular diseases, diabetes mellitus, biliary disease, osteoarthritis, and even cancer than are those of normal or less than normal weight.

All obesity is due ultimately to a disparity between the caloric intake and the energy output. Painstaking investigation of obese persons has failed to reveal either an unusually high absorption of energy from their food or any abnormal process in utilization of that energy which could account for the accumulation of fat. Because of their large size, obese people actually have a higher total basal metabolism than normal people, and the energy expenditure is higher for a given amount of work. They must, therefore, eat more than normal people simply to avoid losing weight.

Careful investigation has also established that obesity is not the result of endocrine disturbance. Patients with myxedema seldom lose more than fifteen pounds under thyroid therapy, and this loss leaves them, on the average, somewhat below normal weight. Pituitary disease, likewise, is not related to obesity. However, both in human beings and in animals, lesions of certain portions of the hypothalamus are associated with obesity. Pressure on, or extension to, the hypothalamus from tumors and other lesions of the near-by pituitary has apparently been responsible for the obesity observed in pituitary disease. The role of the hypothalamus in ordinary obesity remains to be established. Sta-tistical studies have yielded no evidence that obesity (as distinct from body build) is inherited, although eating habits may be passed from one generation to the next by example and training.

Obesity, then, is due to overeating. The patient's history on this subject is notoriously unreliable and may be disregarded. Newburgh has listed the following proximate causes which, in some persons, lead to overeating: (1) overemphasis by a parent of the importance of food in a child's upbringing; (2) gratification obtained from the flavors of foods; (3) the feeling of repose and comfort produced by a full stomach; (4) the temporary respite from anguish caused by intellectual, social, or sexual failure; (5) the food habits of youth which are carried over into middle age, even though the need for food is diminished; and (6) disabling disease with its lessened energy requirement which is compensated for by indulgence in food.

Prevention is a matter of education: (1) as to the nature, causes, and consequences of obesity; and (2) as to dietary needs and food values.

Treatment is a matter of dietary restriction to the point where caloric intake is less than caloric output. The co-operation of the patient (and with children, of the parents also) is obviously essential. Such co-operation is more often promised than given. The patient must be convinced of the hazards of obesity and of the impossibility of weight reduction without dietary restriction. When, as is frequently the case, the overeating is serving some emotional purpose—and these are not always easy to discover—the purpose must be unmasked. Sometimes expert psychiatric handling is necessary.

Obesity in children is often the result of emotional maladjustment in one or both parents. In such cases, readjustment on the part of the parents is a prerequisite to satisfactory therapy of the child.

The most desirable total caloric intake cannot always be determined in advance. It must be governed by the progress in weight reduction. If this is too slow, the patient may become discouraged. Newburgh advocates a total daily caloric intake of 450 calories, with 60 Gm. of protein (see pp. 582 to 583). A pint of whole milk should be allowed per 1,000 calories. Meat or meat substitutes should be taken twice daily, lean cuts preferred. Unlimited quantities of green vegetables are allowed, cooked by steaming, baking, or boiling in salted water (but use no oil!) or taken raw in salad (but without oil dressings!). Low-sugar fruits may be taken liberally. Sometimes their use between meals helps dull appetite. Potatoes, bread, and other ordinary foods are given in sufficient quantity to complete the caloric allowance. Concentrated sweets and fat foods are interdicted, as are most soft drinks. Supplementary vitamins and minerals may be indicated in some cases.

In children, actual weight reduction will be necessary only in extreme obesity. It usually suffices if further weight gain is prevented until other aspects of development have come into balance. In judgment of this point, the Wetzel grid* may be of great value. Children should receive, as a minimum, 3/4 Gm. of protein per pound of "ideal" weight; and, as an optimum, perhaps 1.5 Gm. During periods of submaintenance caloric intake, this may be increased to 3 Gm. per pound. Supplementary vitamins and minerals are especially important when the quantity of food is limited.

It may be very helpful to have the patient spend the first two or three weeks of the treatment period in hospital. Old habits are more easily broken there, the patient becomes more quickly educated in the new regimen, and cheating is more difficult. Positive initial accomplishment in the form of weight reduction is a great stimulus to continued adherence to directions. After two or three months, new habits are usually well established and relapse is less likely.

---

* Obtainable through N E A Service, Inc., 1200 West Third Street, Cleveland, Ohio.

Certain of the sympathomimetic amines, particularly amphetamine, have been suggested as aids in dulling appetite, but the ultimate value and wisdom of such therapy is as yet undetermined.

If endocrine disease is present, it should be treated, but for its own sake and not in the expectation of weight reduction. In the absence of demonstrable endocrine disturbance, endocrine therapy, including the administration of thyroid or pituitary preparations, should be avoided: first, because it will be ineffective; and second, because it may lead the patient to underestimate the importance of dietary restriction.

Exercise will, of course, use up energy, but it is impractical as an aid to weight reduction. First, a 250-pound man must walk thirty-six miles to rid himself of one pound of adipose tissue. Second, the stimulation of appetite usually more than makes up for the fat destroyed. Many obese patients lose weight fastest on a regimen of bed rest.

Since a loss of adipose tissue is often accompanied by temporary retention of water, periods of even two or three weeks on a submaintenance diet may pass with no apparent reduction in scale weight. Such a period is usually followed by a very rapid loss of the excess water, after which scale weight again reflects for a time the loss of fat. The patient should be made to understand these fluctuations and delays in change of scale weight; otherwise they may confuse and discourage him.

AGE AS A FACTOR IN TREATMENT

When a physician thinks in a general way of disease and its treatment, he is likely to visualize a patient in his twenties or thirties. However, age has a definite effect on body function, and it seems worth while to discuss the variations in therapeutic approach which are made necessary by considerations of age.

INFANCY AND CHILDHOOD

In addition to the obvious differences in size and proportions, infants and children vary significantly from adults in (1) their increased nutritional requirement due to high basal metabolism and to growth, (2) the rapidity and violence of their reaction to disease or injury and the rapidity of recuperation and repair, and (3) their greater susceptibility to infection.

In infancy, many body functions are yet poorly developed. It is several months before the digestive tract is equipped to handle more than very small amounts of cellulose. The kidneys do not have great concentrating power; consequently, disturbances in water balance, such as dehydration, are easily produced (p. 56). For the first few months of life the infant is protected against many infectious diseases by passive immunity from the mother (see p. 319). After the first year, however, this wears off and an increased susceptibility is the rule. Infections of the respiratory system account for about one-half of the illnesses of childhood. Chronic nasal infection may persist for months or even years. Often the patient becomes allergic to the infecting bacteria, and a slight residual infection may thus lead to symptoms of a troublesome nature. The nervous system and gastro-intestinal tract often react violently to infections of any type, with convulsions, vomiting, and diarrhea marking the onset of infections not directly involving these systems.

In the treatment of children, special consideration must be given to the dosage of drugs. The most common general rule is that of Clark, by which the child's weight in pounds is divided by 150 (or the weight in kilograms by 70), and the resulting fraction of the adult dose is given. Under this rule, an infant weighing 10 lb. would receive 1/15 of an adult dose, and a child weighing 45 lb. would receive 3/10. It should be emphasized that any such rule is of limited value. Children are relatively more susceptible than adults to some drugs and relatively more resistant to others. If the physician is not familiar with the action of a given drug in children, dosage should be very cautious until he gains experience; it is easier to repeat administration than to attempt to remove a drug after alarming symptoms have appeared. Initial dosage of powerful drugs should always be conservative because of the great range of response in different children.

In contrast to former ideas, it is now considered entirely appropriate to administer analgesics and sedatives to children. Considerable caution and discrimination are, however, necessary with hypnotics. Morphine is especially depressing to infants and children. Some of the newer synthetic hypnotic agents, such as methadon, are not unduly so.

MIDDLE AND OLD AGE

Perhaps the most striking characteristic as individuals grow older is the slowing down of the processes of recuperation and repair. Stieglitz has said that "for every five years of life, it takes twenty-four hours longer for repair after a given injury." Older people may show only slight reaction to injury and disease. For example, pneumonia can exist without fever. Complications may arise quickly and silently; e.g., coronary occlusion may be superimposed on a mild infection, or a cold or influenza may progress rapidly to pneumonia, without great change in symptoms. An infection in one part of the body may cause symptoms elsewhere, such as an apoplectiform onset of pneumonia manifested by mental confusion, stupor and unconsciousness, unilateral weakness, and other signs simulating a cerebral accident. In acute appendicitis, rupture may occur early almost without symptoms.

The most important bodily changes due to age are commonly seen in the cardiovascular system; and even in the absence of symptoms, the physician should appraise the cardiovascular system of all patients of middle age or older. The myocardium tends to require a progressively longer portion of diastole to recover from the preceding systole. Its reserve capacity is thus diminished. The sensitivity of the sinus node is decreased, and the heart rate tends to become slower and relatively fixed. Arteriosclerosis is common.

The aging skin tends to undergo changes which are either involutional or progressive. The involutional changes include the common atrophy or glossy thinning of the skin, wrinkling due to loss of subcutaneous fat, atrophy of hair follicles, diminution in the amount of sweat and oil, and the appearance of a special type of freckle called "lentigo." The progressive changes include telangiectasia, small angiomas, cutaneous tags, seborrheic keratoses, senile keratoses, and thickening of the nails due to excessive amounts of keratin. Other conditions which may remain silent for long periods, but which should be looked for in all middle-aged or older persons, include pulmonary emphysema, gallstones, prostatic hypertrophy in men, and cancer —particularly of the stomach and colon, of the prostate in men, and of the breasts and uterus in women.

Faulty diet is believed to be a factor in inducing the degenerative changes of old age. Once these have begun, an improvement in the diet will not erase them. However, such improvement may be expected to slow down the rate of change. Obesity (p. 260) is particularly to be avoided after the age of forty. Digestion and absorption may become impaired, so that there may be an increased requirement for protein, minerals, and vitamins. The energy requirements become less, but caloric undernutrition may be as serious as overnutrition. As physical endurance and speed of recuperation diminish, there should be an appropriate reduction in physical exertion. This frequently necessitates a revision of the patient's pattern of life which is not easy to accomplish. If it could be more generally carried out, it would doubtless prevent or postpone many vascular accidents and other incapacitating events.

Older individuals tend to turn their interests more upon themselves and less upon the outside world. Neuroses and psychoneuroses become increasingly common with age and are likely to include anxiety states and hypochondria. As children grow up and leave the home, it is natural for a mother to feel that her usefulness is ended, particularly if she has recently passed through the menopause. Similarly, retirement from active work or business life may produce in men a feeling of insecurity because they no longer seem needed. It is well to anticipate attitudes of this kind and try to develop in patients hobbies or outside interests which will give them a feeling of usefulness when they retire or when the children leave home. Sympathy and an understanding of the person as an individual will often solve problems which appear to the patient to be concerned with a single organ or group of organs.

Older persons require the stimulus of a certain amount of physical activity to maintain normal body function. Complete or prolonged bed rest may produce rapid physical and psychological deterioration. It is therefore of the utmost importance to avoid or minimize a period of complete immobility, whether for treatment of a medical condition such as coronary occlusion or a surgical condition such as a fracture. One is often justified in modifying traditional attitudes toward the importance of complete bed rest or immobilization when caring for older patients.

ALLERGY

Allergy is a form of hypersensitivity which may affect various tissues. As the result of exposure to a substance termed the "allergen," there is developed in the cells of the allergic tissues a substance or substances termed collectively "reagin." Subsequent contact of the cell with the allergen leads to a reaction between allergen and reagin that is thought to liberate histamine (p. 366) and related substances ("H-substances") which, in turn, mediate the allergic response. Most, but not all, allergens are protein. Each allergen and each reagin is highly specific. It is obvious that, up to the point of the allergic response, there is a close analogy between allergy and immunity (p. 319).

The fundamental cause of allergy is unknown, but there is much evidence for hereditary predisposition. The occurrence and intensity of allergic reactions, and possibly the development of allergy itself, are very much affected by climatic, nervous, endocrine, and metabolic factors.

The nature of the allergic response depends on the exact tissue or "shock organ" which contains the specific reagin as follows:

Hay fever—tissues of nasal mucosa

Asthma—bronchial smooth muscle, glands, and mucosa

Urticaria, neurodermatitis, prurigo, infantile dermatitis—blood vessels of dermis

Angioneurotic edema—blood vessels of subcutaneous tissue

Contact eczema—epidermis

Search for the allergen or allergens to which the patient is sensitive may be difficult. A careful history is most important. With respect to inhalants and contactants, skin tests are usually helpful. For ingestants, however, skin tests may be unreliable, and elimination diets may be necessary for diagnosis as well as treatment.

There are four general principles in the treatment of allergy:

1. Avoidance of contact with the offending allergen.

2. Correction of contributory factors.

3. Hyposensitization if the first principle cannot be effected and the second is not successful in preventing attacks. One gives, usually by injection, extracts containing the allergen—at first in extremely minute doses, which are gradually increased according to the tolerance of the patient as judged by local, focal, and systemic reactions.

4. Symptomatic control by antihistaminic (p. 509), adrenergic (p. 422), spasmolytic (p. 434), and anticholinergic (p. 419) drugs when the preceding principles cannot be carried out or are incompletely successful.

HAY FEVER

In hay fever (pollinosis) and other forms of nasal allergy such as perennial vasomotor rhinitis, the nasal mucosa is the shock organ. The symptoms are rhinorrhea, nasal blocking, sneezing, and other manifestations of nasal irritation. Conjunctivitis and bronchial symptoms may occur simultaneously. The nasal discharge is usually watery but may in the course of time become viscid and contain many eosinophils.

Allergic rhinopathy due to inhalation of dust, animal emanations, orrisroot powder, and numerous other substances can occur at any season of the year. Attacks are frequently misdiagnosed as infectious "colds." Seasonal allergic rhinopathy is due to inhalation of mold spores or the pollens of trees, bushes, grasses, and weeds. It is often called "hay fever"; but since it is not always due to the pollen of hay and is not usually complicated by fever, the term "pollinosis" is to be preferred. The commonest and, as a rule, most severe form is that due to ragweed pollen, the liberation of which begins in late summer and continues until frost. In the United States, ragweed does not grow in significant amounts in the most northern, western, and southern parts of the country; but there are other pollens, particularly in the West and South, which cause "hay fever." Next in importance as a cause of pollinosis are the grasses, such as timothy, redtop, and the like. These appear earlier in the year. Still earlier are the pollens of a number of trees.

In regions where atmospheric pollen counts of ragweed pollen have been made, the symptoms of pollinosis in patients of that vicinity vary roughly in proportion to the count. The count may be decreased by rain. It can be increased by a dry wind blowing from a section where ragweed is pollinating in abundance.

Treatment—Identification of the offending pollen or mold is accomplished in part by the history and in part by skin tests. The latter should include not only molds and the pollens of weeds, grasses, trees, and shrubs but also various animal emanations and other inhalants. Moreover, it is desirable also to determine whether or not allergy to foods and to various ingestants and contactants exists.

When the offending pollen is identified, it is in order to attempt to "desensitize" the patient by administering the allergen in a series of subreaction doses which are gradually increased as the tolerance of the patient increases. The aim is to build the dose up to the point where the patient can tolerate the exposure which he is likely to undergo. Injections are given at intervals of three to seven days, and the dose is gradually increased as long as reactions do not occur and until what is considered a satisfactory maintenance dose is reached. When a reaction occurs, the next dose is smaller and the rate of increase is reduced. For treatment of systemic reactions, see page 269.

When the patient does not present himself for desensitization until the hay-fever season is beginning, the treatment is termed *coseasonal*. The value of coseasonal treatment is questioned by many. When it is given, daily injections are preferred, subreaction doses being increased until the patient shows improvement. It is advocated by some that the dose not be increased further during the season.

Better results are obtained if *preseasonal* treatment is started well in advance of the season. Injections are begun eight to twelve weeks before the expected onset, with the aim of reaching the peak dose just before the season begins. Because one cannot predict the patient's tolerance to increasing doses, more satisfactory results may be obtained from *perennial* treatment. Patients sensitive only to ragweed or other strictly seasonal allergens may be treated no more frequently than every three or four weeks during the winter season. Others are treated once a week. When more than ten days have elapsed since the last injection of a given allergen, the dose is not increased. Under the perennial method, weekly increasing injections are begun earlier than with the preseasonal method and the increase is more gradual, so that there is greater assurance of reaching a proper peak at the onset of the season.

Extracts for testing and treatment may be dry or they may be in an aqueous medium containing buffer salts, glycerin, or dextrose. In recent years, Rockwell has given whole pollen orally in pulvules (see 'Panoral,' p. 337).

When hyposensitization is incompletely successful, symptomatic treatment may give considerable relief. The antihistaminic drugs (p. 509) are of great value in controlling the nasal and ocular symptoms. Ephedrine or other vasoconstrictors (p. 426) taken internally or, in some instances, applied to the nasal mucosa are of recognized value in controlling nasal congestion. Internal administration of a combination of an antihistaminic drug and a vasoconstrictor has in many cases of hay fever proved more desirable than either drug alone.

In some instances, control of nasal and ocular discomfort and nasal obstruction by the above drugs may not be accompanied by complete cessation of the watery nasal discharge. Control of this phase can then usually be accomplished by the addition of atropine sulfate or belladonna (p. 420), the average dose of the former being 0.3 to 0.4 mg. (1/200 to 1/150 grain). The dosage and frequency of administration of the belladonna drugs must be individualized to find the level which, in conjunction with the vasoconstrictor, controls nasal discharge without drying the mouth unduly or affecting vision.

ASTHMA

The term "asthma" is applied to a syndrome characterized by recurrent attacks of paroxysmal dyspnea with wheezing, cough, and a sense of constriction in the chest. Allergic asthma must be distinguished from cardiac asthma (p. 64), chronic bronchitis (p.114), and bronchial obstruction due to foreign bodies or tumors. In allergic asthma the bronchi are the shock organs for the allergic reaction, and the attack is characterized by bronchoconstriction, edema of the mucosa, and often by a viscid mucous secretion containing eosinophils and sometimes Curschmann's spirals. The dyspnea is mainly expiratory.

The causative allergens may be exogenous (pollens, dust, mold spores, animal emanations, foods, drugs) or endogenous (products of chronic bacterial infection to which the patient has become sensitized).

Treatment—Some measure of symptomatic relief is afforded by drugs having adrenergic, anticholinergic, spasmolytic, or antihistaminic actions. Such preparations may be given by mouth, sublingually, by inhalation, by rectum, or by subcutaneous or intravenous injection, depending on the nature of the agent and the urgency of the situation. To be most effective, treatment should begin as early in the attack as possible.

Apparently the most effective preparation for administration during asthmatic attacks is 'Aerolin' (p. 426). 'Aerolin' is an aqueous solution containing aludrine sulfate, 'Clopane Hydrochloride,' atropine sulfate, procaine hydrochloride, and propylene glycol. It is inhaled from a special nebulizer which yields a very fine spray. Proper technic is imperative for success, and the patient must inhale deeply as the bulb is squeezed. In most patients, inhalation of 'Aerolin' seems to give more complete relief than any other measure; it has been effective in patients who had become unresponsive to epinephrine and aminophylline. Six inhalations often bring adequate relief; however, more may be taken if necessary. When attacks are infrequent, the patient may be told to repeat the treatment only as an attack occurs. In status asthmaticus or in chronic asthma, he may be directed to repeat the series of inhalations often enough to prevent reappearance of symptoms. Usually he should be cautioned to continue a series of inhalations for no longer than a three-minute period and to allow no less than fifteen minutes between successive periods of inhalation. However, in severe cases when the life of the patient may be at stake, the above restriction may be waived, provided the pulse rate is followed carefully during and between periods of treatment. Actually, side-effects are rare.

Until the advent of 'Aerolin,' one of the simplest and most satisfactory measures for relief of all but the severest paroxysms was inhalation of epinephrine hydrochloride, 1:100 (see p. 424). The same type of nebulizer and the same technic are necessary for successful use. Another simple form of treatment is sublingual administration of aludrine hydrochloride, 10 mg. However, aludrine administered in this form is less effective than is inhalation of 'Aerolin' (of which aludrine is a principal ingredient).

For the prevention of attacks or for relief of mild ones, one may employ oral administration of ephedrine sulfate (p. 426), 25 to 50 mg. (3/8 to 3/4 grain), or aminophylline or 'Monotheamin' (p. 359), 0.1 to 0.3 Gm. (1 1/2 to 5 grains). A combination may be employed (see Pulvules Amesec, p. 608). These drugs are usually given three or four times daily. Because they may produce in some individuals central-nervous-system stimulation, they are often combined with barbiturates. In addition, sedation of itself may be helpful in those cases marked by anxiety.

In order to continue the action of any of these drugs throughout the night, they may be given as 'Enseals' (p. 282) along with the regular dose in capsule or tablet form. The effect of the 'Enseals' usually begins as that of the capsules or tablets is wearing off.

Iodides (p. 506), particularly potassium iodide, may be valuable, especially in long-standing cases and when secretion is excessive. For adults, 0.5 Gm. (7 1/2 grains) may be given every two hours during the day for a few days, and then every four hours. In children, Hydriodic Acid Syrup, U.S.P., is a useful dosage form.

For relief of severe paroxysms, it was formerly standard practice to inject (1) epinephrine hydrochloride, 1:1,000 (Epinephrine Injection, U.S.P.), hypodermically or (2) aminophylline or 'Monotheamin' intravenously. If aludrine or 'Aerolin' is used, parenteral medication will rarely be needed. The usual intravenous dose of aminophylline or 'Monotheamin' is 0.25 to 0.5 Gm. (3 3/4 to 7 1/2 grains) in 2.5 percent solution. Both drugs must be given very slowly, with avoidance of leakage into the tissues. They may be repeated as needed. Like aludrine and 'Aerolin,' they retain their full effectiveness for patients who have become unresponsive to epinephrine.

In patients who have not become tolerant to it, the initial dose of Epinephrine Injection should be small—0.2 to 0.3 cc. (3 to 5 min.). If no relief is obtained in five minutes, the site of injection is massaged. If another five-minute period passes without effect, the dose is repeated. Seldom are more than three such doses required. Excessive dosage results in tremor, pallor, severe nervousness, palpitation, and precordial distress. Children must receive proportionately smaller doses, special precautions being taken against overdosage.

Search for the causative allergens and hyposensitization follow the same general lines as in hay fever (p. 264). Bacterial allergy is not uncommon as a factor in asthma. Chronic sinusitis and other chronic infections must be searched for and eliminated.

Frequent and severe attacks may develop into status asthmaticus, a condition more easily prevented than treated. Every effort must be made to recognize and check the condition at its onset, and so prevent the loss of sleep and the fear, anxiety, fatigue, and discouragement which later complicate the situation. The patient should be hospitalized, in a dust-free, conditioned atmosphere if possible. Often epinephrine will already have been given in large doses, and resort should be had, first, to 'Aerolin' by inhalation and, second, to aminophylline or 'Monotheamin,' 0.5 Gm. (7 1/2 grains), administered intravenously in 500 cc. of 10 percent dextrose solution. Sedatives may be required in large doses to provide necessary sleep. A barbiturate (p. 390) or paraldehyde (p. 398) is effective. However, neither morphine nor any other drug which depresses the respiratory center should ever be administered during an attack of asthma, and sedation should never be pushed to the point of dulling the patient's will to recover.

After the patient awakes, it is well to repeat the above medication, whether or not the asthma persists. A soapsuds enema is given in the presence of abdominal distention, for the purpose of reducing upward pressure on the diaphragm.

If the patient is overly fatigued or cyanotic or if the above measures fail, oxygen therapy is instituted; an oxygen tent is preferred, with the oxygen concentration kept at 40 percent. Especially valuable is an atmosphere of 20 percent oxygen and 80 percent helium. Removal from such an atmosphere should be attempted only when the patient is considerably improved.

In intractable status asthmaticus, it may be necessary to resort to anesthesia with ether, 150 to 200 cc. (5 to 7 oz.) in four parts of olive oil, given by rectum.

When bacterial allergy seems to play a part in status asthmaticus, relief may sometimes be obtained from a course of antibiotic therapy (p. 287).

URTICARIA

Urticaria, otherwise known as hives, is characterized by the sudden appearance of smooth, elevated, itching wheals in the skin, which are due to extravasation of fluid in the corium, or dermis. The epidermis is unaltered.

Urticaria may be acute or chronic. Acute urticaria may be due to an allergen which is (1) ingested or injected as a food or drug, (2) deposited in the skin during the bite of an insect, or (3) inhaled. Sometimes it is caused by physical agents such as cold or by mechanical stimulation of the skin as in dermographia. It may be psychogenic. The condition may persist for days or weeks after elimination of the causative agent.

Chronic urticaria may be psychogenic, or it may be due to chronic infection or to frequent ingestion of drugs or foods to which the patient is sensitive. Often the cause is obscure.

Lesions of urticaria may occur on mucous membranes in various parts of the body, causing symptoms referable to the organ involved. Urticaria of the larynx, glottis, pharynx, or tongue may obstruct respiration to the extent that tracheotomy must be performed if epinephrine is not promptly effective.

Treatment has two aspects: elimination of the causative agent and control of the itching and other symptoms. Inquiry is made regarding medication, with particular attention to coal-tar analgesics (such as antipyrine or acetophenetidin), phenolphthalein, salicylates (including acetylsalicylic acid), sulfonamides, barbiturates, morphine and codeine, and quinine. Commonly offending foods include milk or substances transmitted in milk, wheat, eggs, shellfish, strawberries, nuts, pork, and chocolate. A search may be made for other allergens.

The best symptomatic treatment of urticaria is the internal administration of antihistaminic drugs (p. 509). When the lesions are extensive, local treatment may take the form of colloidal starch baths (see p. 479).

Chronic urticaria is a more difficult problem. Possible allergens are sought. Any drug or other substance that the patient has been taking regularly should be discontinued temporarily until it is ruled out as the cause. The diet should be studied with a view to eliminating those foods suspected of causing the symptoms. If the suffering due to pruritus is great, temporary relief may be obtained by adequate doses of antihistaminics. If there is reason to suspect vitamin C deficiency, this vitamin should be given in large doses (1,000 mg. daily).

Hyposensitization with histamine (p. 366) may be attempted. A strength of 0.1 mg. per cc. (1:10,000) is used at first, and 0.05 cc. is injected twice daily. After the first day, the dose is gradually increased in size and decreased in frequency so that by the twenty-fourth dose 0.3 cc. of 1:1,000 is being given every third day. Ten or more injections may be necessary before improvement begins. If benefit is to result, it is usually manifest by the twentieth treatment.

If chronic infection in the paranasal sinuses, prostate, or elsewhere is suspected as the causative agent, hyposensitization with appropriate vaccines may be attempted.

ANGIONEUROTIC EDEMA

Angioneurotic edema—also called giant urticaria, Quincke's disease, or urticaria oedematosa—is characterized by localized transient edematous swellings. The lesions differ from those of urticaria in occurring below rather than in the dermis. Itching may therefore be absent, whereas the degree of swelling is much greater because of the greater distensibility of the subcutaneous tissues. Otherwise, angioneurotic edema and urticaria have much in common, both as to etiology and to treatment. Distribution of the lesions tends to be different, however, since angioneurotic edema very frequently involves the lips and eyelids. As with urticaria, angioneurotic edema of the larynx, glottis, pharynx, or tongue may obstruct respiration.

Treatment is basically similar to that of urticaria. For angioneurotic edema obstructing respiration, epinephrine hydrochloride (p. 422) should be given as a spray (1:100) by inhalation or as a 1:1,000 solution by hypodermic injection. Antihistaminic therapy should be commenced promptly and in emergency should be given intravenously. If these measures are ineffective within five to ten minutes, tracheotomy may be required for serious obstruction.

Other systemic treatment and the search for possible causative agents are the same as for urticaria (see above). In angioneurotic edema, local therapy is, of course, ineffective because of the depth of the lesion.

ECZEMA

The word "eczema" is a general term which has been applied to a considerable number of dermatitides, most cases of which can now be diagnosed more exactly. One which has been so included is contact dermatitis (see p. 228), which results from sensitization to agents reaching the skin or mucous membranes externally. Another subgroup includes those conditions which allergists call "atopic dermatitis," "allergic eczema," or "atopic eczema," and which dermatologists call "neurodermatitis disseminata." Many cases appear to result primarily from sensitization to agents that enter the body through the respiratory or alimentary tracts. Other cases appear to be primarily psychogenic. The condition is discussed on page 235.

"Id" reactions are worthy of special mention. They are eruptions which represent allergic responses in one part of the body to infection elsewhere. The site of the id reaction itself contains no organisms. Id reactions can occur in response to many types of infection. Hyposensitization may reduce the tissue reaction both at the primary focus and in the id reaction.

SERUM SICKNESS

Serum sickness is an allergic reaction resulting from the parenteral administration of a foreign serum. It is characterized, after an incubation period of eight to twelve days, by skin eruptions, enlarged lymph nodes, fever, edema, and polyarthritis. Antibodies capable of giving rise to the reaction are found in the blood of patients suffering or recovering from serum sickness. After two or more treatments with the same type of foreign serum, the patient may exhibit an accelerated reaction occurring in less than eight days, or even an immediate reaction occurring within a half hour after injection.

Treatment—Serum sickness should be treated energetically by antihistaminic compounds. If asthmatic episodes occur, the patient should receive inhalations of 'Clopalene' (p. 426), sublingual tablets of aludrine (p. 425), or subcutaneous injections of epinephrine hydrochloride, 1:1,000 (Epinephrine Injection, U.S.P.), 0.2 to 0.3 cc.

Prophylaxis of serum sickness is more important. The use of toxoids (which contain no serum) to develop and maintain active immunity makes the use of the corresponding serums unnecessary.

The patient who requires serum therapy should be questioned regarding previous serum injections and any symptoms that followed. He should be asked whether he or some blood relative has asthma or other evidence of allergy. Excessive "natural" hypersensitivity to horse dander (as in "horse asthmatics") is reason for not giving serum.

Sensitization tests should be made. The intracutaneous test can be done by injecting 0.1 cc. of a 1:10 dilution of horse serum in physiological saline. The development of a large wheal within ten to twenty minutes is an indication of hypersensitiveness. Moderate reactions may be seen in persons who will have little or no serum sickness. On the other hand, severe serum sickness may occasionally occur even when both the ophthalmic and intracutaneous tests have been negative.

For the ophthalmic test, a drop of a 1:10 dilution of serum is instilled into the patient's conjunctival sac. A positive reaction may occur in ten to twenty minutes in the form of a diffuse reddening of the conjunctiva with watery discharge. When the reaction has developed, it should be controlled by the instillation into the eye of Epinephrine Injection. A positive eye test contraindicates serum therapy unless its use is mandatory as a lifesaving measure.

The desensitization technic may be used when serum must be given to a person who is moderately sensitive to it. The initial dose is 0.1 cc. of the serum subcutaneously. (In a highly sensitive patient, the serum must be diluted.) If this results in no symptoms other than a moderate local hyperemia, 0.2 cc. is given at the end of the next half hour, and the dose is doubled again each half hour thereafter. If moderate symptoms appear after any dose, repeat it every half hour until symptoms diminish. If no symptoms occur, continue the gradually increasing injections until the full dose has been given. If an intravenous dose is to be given, continue the subcutaneous injections until 1 cc. has been tolerated. Then dilute 0.1 cc. of the serum with 2 cc. of sterile physiological saline and inject slowly by vein. If no reaction occurs, double this dose every half hour until the necessary amount has been given.

ANAPHYLACTIC SHOCK

Serum or protein shock is an immediate, shocklike, sometimes fatal reaction which occurs in individuals who are unusually hypersensitive to a serum or other protein-containing preparation which has been administered. In many ways it is similar to anaphylactic shock seen in animals. The symptoms include vomiting, colonic spasm with diarrhea, abrupt fall in blood pressure, subnormal temperature, pallor, cyanosis, thready pulse, and loss of consciousness.

Treatment—Unless the injection has been intravenous, a tourniquet is applied to the extremity between the site of injection and the trunk. A subcutaneous dose of 0.2 to 0.5 cc. (3 to 8 min.) of Epinephrine Injection, U.S.P., is then given hypodermically into the opposite arm, the size of the dose depending on the severity of the reaction. When the reaction begins to subside, the tourniquet may be released for a few seconds, thus permitting a little of the serum to escape into the general circulation. More epinephrine is given from time to time as required; and as time goes on, the tourniquet can be released for longer intervals. A sphygmomanometer is preferable to a tourniquet because (in the case of an arm) it permits one to follow the blood pressure and to determine when epinephrine injections are required. Epinephrine may be given intravenously in very severe cases. Ether anesthesia may be useful for control of spasms.

DISEASES DUE TO PHYSICAL AND TOXIC AGENTS

ALCOHOLISM

Alcohol affects almost all body tissues but especially the nervous system, for which it is a primary and continuous depressant. The apparent stimulating effect of alcohol is in reality a depression of inhibitory influences, corresponding to the excitement phase of general anesthesia.

Chronic alcoholism is now generally considered an emotional disorder in which the effects of alcohol on the central nervous system provide an escape from emotional conflicts (see p. 159). Although chronic alcoholics often suffer from chronic gastritis and sometimes from cirrhosis of the liver and other disorders, there is some question as to relative etiological importance, in these disorders, of alcohol itself, of impurities in alcoholic beverages, and of nutritional deficiency. Certainly polyneuritis and alcoholic pellagra, and possibly delirium tremens and other psychotic manifestations, are due to vitamin deficiency from substitution of alcohol for food as a source of energy.

Treatment of Acute Alcoholism—The patient is put to bed and kept warm. The stomach is washed out by tube. Apomorphine as an emetic is avoided because of its later central-depressant effect. Recovery is reported to be greatly speeded by the slow intravenous injection of 50 cc. of 50 percent dextrose solution containing 15 units of Insulin, 50 mg. thiamin chloride, and 50 mg. nicotinamide. The inhalation of a carbon-dioxide-oxygen mixture may be helpful, particularly if respiration is depressed.

Caffeine is an effective antagonist to alcohol. Caffeine and sodium benzoate, 0.5 Gm. (7 1/2 grains), may be given hypodermically, or 8 ounces of strong coffee may be administered rectally. Ephedrine sulfate, 0.05 Gm. (3/4 grain), intramuscularly may be similarly useful. For deep coma, one of the stronger cerebral stimulants, such as Metrazol (p. 389), may be used cautiously.

If the patient is violent, sedation is in order. Paraldehyde (p. 398) is useful in doses of 1 to 4 drams (4 to 15 cc.), the more chronic alcoholics requiring the larger doses. It may be given orally mixed with cracked ice as a "cocktail," or rectally as a small retention enema followed by a few ounces of water. Barbiturates (p. 390) are also effective.

For postalcoholic headache, analgesics (p. 405) may be helpful. For the treatment of alcoholic gastritis, see Acute Gastritis, page 130.

Treatment of Chronic Alcoholism—The chief problem in chronic alcoholism is the psychiatric one of removing permanently the emotional disturbance from which alcohol provides a temporary escape (see discussion on p. 159). Institutional treatment is often essential. Second is the maintenance of proper protein and vitamin intake. Delirium tremens is reported to respond promptly in most cases to 5 to 150 mg. thiamin chloride daily by injection. Some believe that even better results are obtained with the dextrose-Insulin-thiamin-nicotinamide solution advocated for acute alcoholism.

THERMAL BURNS

Thermal burns are produced by excessive heat applied to the body. They may result from hot water, hot oil, steam, mechanical friction, flames, and contact with hot surfaces. Sunburn, due to overexposure to the ultraviolet radiation of the sun, is not a thermal burn and usually is not of clinical importance except for pain, possible dehydration, and heat stroke (p. 273).

Thermal burns may be divided into three degrees according to the severity of the injury: first degree—hyperemia and erythema; second degree—moderate to severe coagulation and necrosis, with vesiculation, involving the outer layers of the skin but not its entire thickness; third degree—necrosis of all layers of the skin and frequently subcutaneous fat and even fascia. The area involved may be estimated if it is remembered that the lower extremities comprise 38 percent, the thorax and neck 38 percent, the upper extremities 18 percent, and the head 6 percent of the body surface.

The subjective symptoms of thermal burns are usually pain, thirst, and sometimes chilliness. The systemic manifestations of severe burns include shock (p. 90), "toxemia" as evidenced by high fever, increasing coma, irrational behavior, irregular respirations, suppression of urine, and sometimes duodenal ulcer (see "alarm reaction," p. 462).

Laboratory findings in extensive burns include evidence of hemoconcentration, with red blood cell counts as high as 8 million; leukocytosis as high as 20,000 but sometimes even higher (a bad prognostic sign); hypoproteinemia; elevated nonprotein nitrogen; acidosis; and anemia which develops within several days.

Treatment of first and second-degree burns of small area need be only local. It is not necessary that the burned region be cleansed unless there is a strong possibility of bacterial contamination. Petrolatum, or a plain cream or ointment containing a local anesthetic such as 'Surfacaine,' may be applied. These are covered with a dry dressing and bandaged snugly but not tightly. Blisters are left intact; if accidentally broken, they should be trimmed away with a knife or scissors. Aseptic technic is used throughout, and the area is subsequently protected from contamination.

In more severe or extensive burns, treatment should be directed first toward the prevention of shock or to its relief if present (see p. 90). Pain may be relieved by the administration of small doses of morphine sulfate, not to exceed 32 mg. (1/2 grain). During this time and until shock is relieved, specific treatment should be limited to placing the patient in a sterile bed and covering the burned areas with sterile drapes.

Once shock is relieved, specific therapy may be begun. Burned clothing should be removed—by cutting the cloth if necessary rather than, for example, dragging a burned arm or leg through a coat sleeve or pant leg. The therapy of burns has varied from time to time, and a great number of therapeutic substances have been recommended which, in the hands of their advocates, usually have been successful. However, the experiences of the Coconut Grove fire and World War II have demonstrated the efficacy and superiority of relatively simple therapeutic measures and substances.

Scrupulous maintenance of aseptic technic is essential. Masks should be worn by the patient and all those who come in contact with him until the burns have been cleansed and covered. The burned areas may be cleansed carefully with soap and water and then débrided. An anesthetic may be employed if necessary but with care not to aggravate or precipitate shock. Blisters are best left unopened; but, if opened accidentally, the blister should be removed by sharp dissection. Good success has been obtained without this preliminary cleansing. Whether to cleanse or not probably depends upon the possibility of contamination prior to the time the burn is seen.

As soon as possible, the burned area should be covered. The dressing may consist merely of dry gauze or other fabric (preferably fine meshed), or the burned area may be first covered with a simple ointment. Petrolatum is a very satisfactory substance, and petrolatum gauze is excellent. This in turn may then be covered with a dry dressing. Where possible, the dressing should be enclosed by elastic compression carefully applied to exert sufficient pressure to produce a therapeutic effect (minimization of edema and loss of plasma into the tissues) but not so much as to constrict circulation. It is imperative that the dressings extend well beyond the apparent burned areas and that the edge of the dressings be applied firmly to the skin to avoid contamination. Properly prepared and applied, the dressings should not be disturbed for a week or more unless pain occurs or evidence of impaired circulation is noted. The matter of infrequent dressings should be explained to the patient lest he think he is being neglected.

Heat, such as is provided by cradles, probably is best avoided. Saline packs may be utilized to loosen adherent dressing and dried exudate. Later in the course of therapy, saline immersions may prove of comfort to the patient and should be alternated with periods of exposure to the air, great care being taken to prevent contamination of the burned surfaces. It is imperative that every effort be made to keep the nutritional level high. The anemia which accompanies severe burns must be watched for; it is best treated by transfusion. Adequate fluids, first by vein, later by mouth, are essential (see p. 56). A urine volume of 1,500 to 1,800 cc. per day is desirable.

In properly treated severe cases, grafting of skin to repair defects should be performed as early as possible. Successful treatment should provide an ideal grafting surface, free of infection, in a matter of days or weeks.

Infection is an ever-present menace in thermal burn cases. The development of infection results in the usual systemic manifestations of suppuration. This is best combated by systemic anti-infective therapy (p. 286). No attempt should be made to place grafts on infected burned surfaces.

CHEMICAL BURNS

Chemical burns may result from caustics, acids, or alkalies. It is imperative that the causative agent be removed completely and as promptly as possible. For this purpose, applications of copious quantities of water are probably best, most efficacious, and least likely to result in additional damage. Once the chemical agent is removed, the therapy for thermal burns may be followed (see above).

FOOD POISONING

The ingestion of food may produce many injurious effects. In medical usage, the term "food poisoning" is generally reserved for the following conditions:

1. Food infection.
2. The effects of poisons occurring naturally in a few foods (particularly mushrooms).
3. Food intoxication from the toxin of *Clostridium botulinum*.

Food Infection is most commonly due to organisms of the *Salmonella* group or to *Staphylococcus aureus*. The latter occurs especially in food containing cream or other milk products which has been kept without refrigeration.

Mushroom Poisoning—The most common type of mushroom poisoning is from the species *Amanita phalloides*. The nature of the toxin is unknown. Symptoms usually develop eight to twelve hours after eating the fungus and are characterized by severe abdominal cramping, nausea, vomiting, and violent diarrhea. Stools are usually choleric and may contain undigested food, mucus, or blood. Jaundice and cyanosis may develop within forty-eight hours, the patient rapidly becoming comatose and the whole episode ending in death. Convulsions are frequently seen in children, but in adults they are rare except in fatal cases.

The active agent in the species *Amanita muscaria* is the cholinergic substance muscarine (p. 418). The onset of symptoms is more rapid than in *A. phalloides* poisoning, usually beginning in two to three hours. Initially, there is stimulation of the salivary and lacrimal glands, accompanied by profuse perspiration, violent nausea, and vomiting. There is irregular pulse, increased respiratory rate, mental confusion, and contraction and fixation of the pupils.

For poisoning with *A. phalloides*, treatment is symptomatic. For *A. muscaria*, atropine (p. 420) provides specific therapy. It is given to the point of neutralizing the symptoms.

Other Food Poisoning—Illness has been reported following the ingestion of sprouting potatoes, certain kinds of fish, and other foods. Many of these cases are probably infections from micro-organisms contained in the food. The signs and symptoms are usually those of a severe gastroenteritis, with sudden onset preceded by chilliness and headache. There are usually severe griping abdominal pains, intense nausea, persistent vomiting, and diarrhea. Prostration may be extreme, and nervous disorders, such as muscular twitchings, restlessness, emotional outbursts, or even delirium, are not uncommon. There may be a sharp rise in temperature.

Diagnosis of the isolated case may be extremely difficult. Food poisonings are more prevalent in hot weather and usually involve a group of individuals who have attended a banquet or picnic. The occurrence of several similar gastro-intestinal upsets in individuals eating the same foods is an important helpful point in diagnosis. Because the condition is of such an acute nature, stool cultures are rarely, if ever, of any value.

Treatment is nonspecific, except that of botulism, which is discussed below. The measures employed in the treatment of acute gastritis (p. 130) and diarrhea (p. 132) are used. If the patient is seen early, gastric lavage with plain warm water or normal saline will remove any remnants of contaminated food from the stomach. Frequently it is advisable, in order to clear the intestinal tract, to administer a cathartic, such as magnesium sulfate (15 cc. of a saturated solution), castor oil (15 cc.), or Magnesium Citrate Solution, U.S.P. (360 cc., or 12 ounces). A plain warm-water enema, 1/2 to 1 pint, may be used at once to evacuate the large bowel. Rarely is morphine indicated for pain. After the

enema and the cathartic have cleared the gastro-intestinal tract, 1 dram (4 cc.) of paregoric (p. 402) may be given after each bowel movement to stop the abnormal peristalsis. Once the peristalsis has been controlled, the abdominal pain and cramping will subside. All food should be withheld until the acute attack is over. If there is dehydration, fluids should be administered. If there is no nausea and fluids are retained by mouth, strong or weak tea, water, milk, or any other bland liquid the patient desires may be used.

The diet should be gradually built up after the acute attack; it sometimes requires several days before the patient is able to take a full normal diet.

Botulism is a form of intoxication resulting from ingestion of food containing the toxin produced by *Clostridium botulinum*. This is one of the most potent bacterial toxins and, so far as is known, the only one concerned in food poisoning. It is found mostly in improperly canned or inadequately cooked food, in which the organism has escaped sterilization and has then been under anaerobic conditions. Home-canned food should be well heated before being served, for the toxin is destroyed in ten minutes at 75°C. It does not occur in fresh food.

The toxin has an affinity for nerve tissue. The initial acute gastro-intestinal disturbances are nausea, vomiting, and diarrhea. They are probably the result of local irritation from spoiled food. They appear early, last for twelve to thirty-six hours, and usually disappear with the onset of the typical symptoms of botulism.

The characteristic symptoms of botulism are decrease, complete arrest, or abnormal increase in secretion of saliva; mydriasis, paralysis of accommodation, diplopia, and internal strabismus; and dysphagia, aphonia, obstinate constipation, and retention of urine. There is a general weakness of all voluntary muscles. Fever is usually absent. There are no sensory or mental disturbances. There may be bulbar paralysis resulting in respiratory and circulatory disturbances which may cause death.

Differential diagnosis should include careful consideration of epidemic encephalitis, acute poliomyelitis, cerebrospinal syphilis, methyl alcohol intoxication, and drug poisoning, especially with belladonna.

Rapid diagnosis is essential if therapy is to be successful. It has been reported that the injection of guinea pigs or white mice, using three animals injected respectively with 1 cc., 0.5 cc., and 0.1 cc. of the suspected food, is a rapid method of diagnosis. There should be three sets of three animals, one animal in each set to be first inoculated with type A antitoxin and one with type B antitoxin, and one to be uninoculated. Laboratory tests have indicated that results would be swift enough to be of material assistance, both in establishing a diagnosis and in determining the type of toxin.

TREATMENT must be instituted before the onset of objective signs if it is to be successful. Bivalent botulinus antitoxin is given in doses of 10,000 to 20,000 units subcutaneously or intravenously (with caution) every two to four hours.

Treatment of the ordinary gastro-intestinal signs and symptoms is the same as in food poisoning, but all attention should be given to the treatment of the botulism.

HEAT PROSTRATION

Heat prostration is the result of elevation of body temperature, dehydration, and salt depletion due to inadequate dissipation of body heat in a hot, humid atmosphere. It occurs the more readily with increased physical work. Body heat is ordinarily dissipated by radiation, conduction, and the evaporation of moisture from the skin. As the atmosphere becomes warmer, radiation and conduction diminish and cease, and sweating begins and increases. As humidity increases, evaporation decreases, and finally body temperature rises because heat is generated faster than it can be dissipated. Sweating becomes increasingly active and may result in depletion of body water and salt (see Dehydration, p. 56).

Mild heat retention (body temperature of 102° or 103°F.) causes restlessness, headache, throbbing, dizziness, dyspnea, and tachycardia. Sweating, which has been excessive, may diminish. Later the patient may collapse, with weakness, dilation of the pupils, weak pulse, and cold, clammy skin in spite of elevated rectal temperature.

When salt loss has been relatively great, there may be muscular twitchings followed by cramps of the trunk and extremities. Nausea and vomiting may be severe. There may be oliguria or anuria and hemoconcentration.

Heat stroke is usually marked by sudden collapse and rapid, extreme rise in body temperature. The skin is dry and very hot. The pulse is extremely rapid; the respiration is deep and labored and later of the Cheyne-Stokes type. There may be muscular flaccidity, or twitchings and spasms.

Prevention—Avoidance of physical work in hot and humid surroundings is an obvious measure.

When such work is necessary, the administration of vitamin C, 100 mg. daily, plus liberal amounts of salt (up to 1 Gm. sodium chloride per hour) and water (up to 4 quarts per hour) will virtually eliminate the occurrence of heat prostration. Use of a 0.1 percent salt solution as drinking water is recommended. Ingestion of water alone without salt may precipitate or intensify muscle spasms.

Treatment—In the mildest forms, rest and removal to cooler surroundings may suffice. Water, salt, and vitamin C should be given. For heat cramps, give salt solution and employ rest, warm baths, and perhaps massage.

Heat stroke has a high mortality. Treatment must be prompt. Fever must be reduced at once, preferably by spraying the patient with cool water in a draft (use fans). Circulation should be maintained in the skin by constant rubbing. When muscle spasm of the diaphragm interferes with respiration, artificial respiration may be indicated. Reduction of temperature should be discontinued at 102°F., lest subnormal temperature develop.

At the same time, the patient should receive an intravenous infusion of isotonic sodium chloride solution to which have been added dextrose to the extent of 5 percent and 500 mg. vitamin C. After heat stroke, relapse is common, and headache and other mental and nervous symptoms may persist.

INJURY DUE TO COLD

Exposure to different degrees of cold and moisture produces immersion foot, trench foot, frostbite, and high-altitude frostbite. The body normally reacts to cold by vasoconstriction. Local damage from cold itself is thus augmented by damage from ischemia. The most susceptible tissue is the endothelium of capillaries, arterioles, and venules. With mild degrees of injury the vessels may subsequently dilate, causing redness, swelling, and burning sensations or actual pain. More severe damage leads to multiple thromboses of the very small vessels, with tissue necrosis. The tendency toward thrombosis is augmented by the fact that cold itself causes white blood cells to disintegrate.

Immersion foot and immersion hand follow immersion of the extremities in cold water. Because of the relatively slight degree of cold, prolonged exposure (usually days) is required to produce clinical disturbances. Similarly, trench foot follows prolonged standing in cold, wet places (freezing temperatures are not necessary). Lack of movement of the limb and tightness of the clothing predispose by impairing circulation, and wetness of the skin increases the rate of heat loss.

Frostbite is due to actual freezing of tissues. High-altitude frostbite is distinguished by the extreme cold and the usual presence of some degree of general anoxia at the time of exposure.

Early symptoms are local coldness, pallor, numbness, and sometimes cyanosis. In frostbite the tissues are frozen hard. The exact clinical picture depends on the severity of injury. Within a few days there may develop vesiculation, edema, or trophic changes including gangrene.

Late sequelae are common. They fall into three categories: sensory disturbances, vasomotor instability, and pain.

Treatment—Certain principles of early treatment are clear:

1. Prevention of further damage and infection. Injury to the local circulation is greater than to other local tissues. Undue warming of the part increases the metabolic requirements of the cells. Cooling serves to minimize oxygen and other needs until the circulation improves. Careful padding and change of position will minimize localized pressure. When a break in the skin is present or imminent, sterile dressings should be applied. Sulfonamides or antibiotics should be given when infection is a possibility.

2. Relief of pain. Cooling has an analgesic as well as protective effect.

3. Protection against toxemia. Amputation is indicated when it becomes clear that the tissues will not heal or when toxemia demands it.

There is disagreement regarding the *early* use of sympathetic block and anticoagulants and about details of treatment. During convalescence, massage and graded exercise may be helpful.

Late sensory disturbances (such as cutaneous hyperesthesia and hyperirritability with, in the more severe cases, adjacent hypesthesia or anesthesia) are almost always abolished by sympathetic nerve block (p. 440). Late vasomotor instability (as manifested by hyperhidrosis, local coldness, pallor or cyanosis, or intermittent claudication) tends to regress spontaneously. If it persists or if the skin begins to atrophy within three months, sympathectomy is indicated; it is almost always helpful.

Deep-seated aching pain on use of the extremity, seeming to the patient to come from the bones and joints, is usually the principal disabling factor. It appears to be due to the presence of fibrous tissue. No satisfactory treatment is known.

ALTITUDE SICKNESS

Altitude sickness is a condition resulting from oxygen want (hypoxia) while at altitude. Acute and chronic phases have been distinguished.

Acute altitude sickness is seen during single high plane flights. Table 25 gives the symptoms in their usual order of frequency. The higher the altitude, the shorter the time necessary for their development. Hypoxia also produces respiratory and cardiovascular alterations, increased output of urine, symptoms referable to the gastro-intestinal tract, dulling of vision and perhaps of hearing, loss of sense of touch and pain, progressive deterioration of voluntary muscular control, and changes in behavior. The individual may progress to collapse and unconsciousness, and death may follow if the blood oxygen level falls sufficiently low.

When high altitudes are reached more gradually (as during mountain ascents) or when acute exposure is recurrent (as in repeated plane flights at altitude), a chronic form of altitude sickness develops. Some of the symptoms of the acute phase may be present; headache, nausea, and weakness are common. There are also chemical changes in the blood and tissues, the full nature of which is imperfectly understood.

Treatment consists in increasing the partial pressure of oxygen in the inspired air, either by inhalation of pure oxygen or by a return to lower altitudes, or both. Tolerance to anoxia varies in different individuals. Altitude sickness is usually prevented by maintaining the partial pressure of oxygen in the inspired air at least equal to that found at 10,000 feet altitude.

TABLE 25—*Symptoms of Acute Altitude Sickness in Their Usual Order of Frequency*

(Data from Armstrong, Harry G. [Maj. Gen., M.C., U.S.A.]: *Principles and Practice of Aviation Medicine.* Baltimore: Williams & Wilkins Company, 1939)

Altitude, in Feet		
12,000	14,000	16,000
Sleepiness	Headache	Headache
Headache	Altered	Altered
Altered	respiration	respiration
respiration	Sleepiness	Psychological
Lassitude	Psychological	impairment
Fatigue	impairment	Euphoria
Psychological	Lassitude	Sleepiness
impairment	Fatigue	Lassitude
Euphoria	Euphoria	Fatigue

The only active treatment required in mild cases of chronic altitude sickness is rest of two to five days' duration under more normal atmospheric conditions. In the more severe cases, an extended rest period under similar circumstances is indicated.

MOTION SICKNESS

Motion sickness embraces a symptom complex in susceptible persons which results from the movements of a vehicle (ship, train, airplane, car, or other conveyance). Symptoms consist primarily in epigastric awareness (which may progress to nausea), increased salivation, muscular weakness, tremor, dizziness (vertigo), pallor, and sweating. Vomiting may ensue, with prostration if the stimulus continues, until the individual feels utterly wretched. Motion sickness is a response to an abnormal environment. In the case of airplane travel, it should not be confused with "altitude sickness."

Headache seldom develops, and no consistent, noteworthy changes in blood pressure, pulse rate, or respiration are observed as a rule. The act of vomiting may temporarily relieve the majority of symptoms. The resulting feeling of well-being soon may be engulfed in another cycle of similar symptoms leading to temporary disability. All difficulties usually subside without aftereffects as soon as rolling, pitching, yawing, or other motions are eliminated.

Treatment is prophylactic and symptomatic. Susceptible individuals should consume only small amounts of liquid and food before a journey. Greasy foods are to be avoided. People who, by virtue of debility, age, or illness, may become sick (and thereby possibly aggravate existing conditions if vomiting and straining occur) should not travel except when absolutely necessary. An untroubled mind, the absence of odors, and avoidance of stale, stuffy air are helpful. Assumption of a reclining position while traveling, adequate ventilation, use of cotton ear plugs to reduce noise, and a cushion to absorb vibration are indicated.

Many, many drugs have been employed but none are one hundred percent effective. However, during World War II, considerable study was given to the drug treatment of motion sickness; of the large number of remedies investigated, a few emerged as having definite value. A combination of 1 grain 'Amytal Sodium,' 1/300 grain hyoscine hydrobromide, and 1/400 grain atropine sulfate seemed particularly effective when taken about one-half hour before travel began; it may be repeated in four hours if necessary (adult dose).

'Seconal Sodium' in small doses of 3/4 grain or less may be used for children, the amount depending upon the age of the child.

Hyoscine (scopolamine) camphorate, 1/300 grain, plus hyoscyamine camphorate, 1/80 grain, taken one to two hours before departure and repeated in three to four hours, is reported to be beneficial. Dosage for children is one-half of the above for those between the ages of seven and fourteen. Nicotinamide, 100 mg., has been added to this combination.

Hyoscine alone (1/100 grain) has been used, as well as phenobarbital (1/2 grain) and a mixture of Belladonna Tincture and Phenobarbital Elixir (1:10) in amounts of 1 to 2 drams before travel. Other drugs and combinations of drugs have been tried. By and large, the afore-mentioned trio of 'Amytal Sodium,' hyoscine hydrobromide, and atropine sulfate is at least as effective as other drugs and does not produce undesirable side-effects.

As in the case of all barbiturates and drugs combined with them, repeated dosage must be tempered with reason. Adequate instruction to prospective travelers should suffice.

Recently, chemical combinations of antihistaminic drugs with 8-chlorotheophylline have been investigated in motion sickness. Some are effective, but their comparative worth has not been fully evaluated. Their action against motion sickness is not due to any antihistaminic effect.

SNAKE BITE

Poisonous snakes encountered in the United States include the rattlesnake, copperhead, moccasin, and coral snake. Snake venom usually contains two types of toxin in varying proportion from one species to another: a hemotoxin which produces hemolysis of erythrocytes, extravasation of blood, local destruction of tissue, and extreme edema; and a neurotoxin which affects principally the respiratory center. Venom of rattlesnakes, copperheads, and moccasins contains relatively more hemotoxin; that of the coral snake, relatively more neurotoxin.

Treatment consists most importantly in preventing absorption of the toxins. If an extremity is bitten, a tourniquet (a garter, necktie, handkerchief, shoelace, or even a vine or weed) is applied between the bite and the trunk. It should be tight enough to prevent venous and lymphatic flow but not arterial flow. Right-angle incisions are made through the fang marks to the depth of probable penetration of the fangs, and suction is applied either with the mouth or with a special cup and bulb. Every five minutes the wound may be washed out with sterile, or even clean, water if available. The tourniquet should be loosened for a few moments every ten or fifteen minutes. When local swellings occur, crossed incisions are made into each area, and suction is applied. Such treatment should be continued for an hour or more. After the above treatment has been instituted, the patient should be transported to a hospital if possible, but not by walking.

If antivenin is available, it should be given as soon as possible. The average dose is 10 cc., which may be repeated as indicated in the directions. However, the use of antivenin is merely supplementary to the drainage outlined above; it cannot be considered a substitute.

In connection with snake bite, certain things are definitely *contraindicated*. The victim should remain quiet; walking or running stimulates the circulation and speeds absorption of the toxins. In spite of tradition, alcohol should be avoided. Potassium permanganate and strong acids or other cauterizing agents should be avoided; they are of no value.

Shock should be treated by fluids, electrolytes, and plasma; anemia, by transfusion.

UNCLASSIFIED DISEASES

CANCER

Cancer* is a disturbance of cellular growth characterized by an autonomous, unlimited, invasive growth of tissue capable of metastasis and, if unchecked, destruction of the host. A variety of factors, varying with the location of the cancer, apparently predispose to its development. Although cancer may appear in any tissue of the body, it is more commonly seen in certain ones. Next to heart disease, it is the most frequent cause of death in the United States.

There is no specific treatment and no specific preventive; but if it is diagnosed and removed or destroyed early enough, cancer is curable. There is general agreement that the early diagnosis of cancer is primarily the responsibility of the family physician and that upon his knowledge, alertness, and judgment the hope of the control of cancer will rest for many years to come.

Etiology—A vast amount of research is under way in an effort to determine the cause of cancer. Results to date suggest that at least three general types of factors are involved:

1. The fundamental physiological disturbance.
2. A group of determining factors which, in a variety of combinations, form the background from which the disturbed physiology develops.
3. The local precipitating factors.

The basic disturbance in cancer appears to be in the factors which limit and regulate normal growth. Much research effort is, therefore, being devoted to a study of these factors in the hope that, when the normal processes are fully understood, it will be possible to determine what has gone wrong in cancer. The importance of this type of research is pointed up by the fact that, whereas cancer was at one time thought to spring only from embryonal or abnormal cells, it now appears that normal cells subjected to certain adverse conditions may also develop the characteristics of malignancy. A further important observation is that, once malignancy is established, an apparently typical metabolic pattern evolves regardless of the location or original source of the malignant cells. This suggests that when the metabolic pattern of malignancy is thoroughly understood, a way may be found to block it without interfering with the metabolism of normal cells. Chemotherapy offers an analogy; namely, the blocking of bacterial metabolism through the interposition of metabolically inert compounds.

A variety of determining factors have been identified which, acting together, may influence the initial development of malignancy. The role which each plays appears to vary with the location of the cancer. In fact, the variables entering into the initiation of cancer are so many that, at its inception, cancer can be regarded as a group of separate diseases in spite of the ultimate metabolic similarity of the fully developed malignant processes. Some

* In addition to the general discussion which appears here, the clinical features of cancer of certain organs are described in other parts of the book:

Esophagus (p. 126)   Rectum (p. 138)
Stomach (p. 130)   Breast (p. 201)
Colon (p. 136)   Prostate (p. 217)

of the determining factors now identified, together with their known role in a few cancers, are listed in Table 26.

TABLE 26 — *Known Determining Factors in the Genesis of Malignancy*

I. Genetic constitution. Heredity appears to play a determining role in some types of carcinoma in that a certain genetic pattern must be present for the neoplasm to develop.

II. Viruslike agent. Notably in mammary cancer in mice, a transmissible, filtrable agent appears capable of determining the development of cancer in the presence of other suitable conditions. Viruslike agents have not been demonstrated in human cancer.

III. Hormonal factors. The presence or absence of hormones may be *one* of the determining factors in development of cancer of the breast, prostate, testis, and adrenal gland.

IV. Immune factors. Whereas there is no evidence of host immunity to its own cancer, immunity has been observed to cancer transplanted experimentally from one species to another. Together with the fact that certain tissues (striated muscle, heart muscle, kidney, spleen) seem to have a relative natural immunity, this suggests that immune factors may play a role in certain instances.

V. Diet. The role of diet as a determining factor has not been extensively explored; but in view of the specific dietary factors required for the maintenance, growth, and reproduction of normal cells, it is regarded as an important field for further research.

Given the proper combination of determining factors, the shift from the normal to the malignant process probably still does not take place without the local action of precipitating factors, known as carcinogenic agents. Some 250 different substances are known to be capable of inducing tumors experimentally, and there are undoubtedly many more which may so function in daily life. A few of the common carcinogenic agents are listed in Table 27.

For any agent to act as a carcinogen, however, either it must act as a source of repeated mild irritation over a prolonged period or it must produce chronic infection over a prolonged period. It is thus evident that repeated small applications of the carcinogenic agent are necessary to produce the mild irritation or chronic infection which, *after a long time* and only in the presence of the proper combination of determining factors, will ultimately lead to the malignant changes. Variation in a person's daily habits is, therefore, desirable when feasible to avoid the unconscious continued application of unsuspected carcinogens.

On this basis, one might do well to avoid too-rigid diets, continuous and repeated exposure to sunshine (such as that to which farmers and seamen are subject), and excessively prolonged medication with coal tar and its derivatives, estrogens, and azo dyes. Industrial personnel should be protected from the substances listed in Table 27. It is probably impossible to avoid all potential carcinogens, but adherence to the above principles will be helpful.

Types of Neoplasms—There are two general types of neoplasms: the carcinomas and the sarcomas. Both display all the essential features of malignancy and are differentiated mainly on the basis of their point of origin. The carcinomas are far more numerous than the sarcomas. They are divided into epidermoid carcinoma and adenocarcinoma. The epidermoid carcinomas spring from epithelial tissue and are, therefore, found in such locations as the skin, lip, penis, vulva, cervix, and so on. Adenocarcinomas, as the name implies, spring from glandular structures and are, therefore, found in such localities as the stomach, intestine, endometrium, and the like. Sarcomas arise from the mesoderm (muscle, connective tissue, fibrous tissue, fat, bone) and derive their name from their parent tissue: fibrosarcoma, liposarcoma, rhabdomyosarcoma, etc. In general, sarcomas tend to appear at an earlier age and to have a more rapid rate of growth than carcinomas. Both types of tumors are graded by number (I to III or I to IV in different clinics) on the basis of the rapidity of their growth. Grade I represents the more slowly

TABLE 27 — *A Partial List of Substances Known Frequently to Act as Precipitating Factors (Carcinogenic Agents) under Certain Conditions*

Foodstuffs
  Browned fats
  Condiments
  Alcohol
  Other unidentified substances
Coal tar and coal-tar derivatives
Azo dyes and related compounds
Fission products
Plutonium
Certain hydrocarbons
Decayed teeth
Abuse of tobacco
X-ray
Ultraviolet radiation
Parasites
Syphilis
Tuberculosis of the skin
Estrogens

growing tumors which tend to retain many of the characteristics of the parent tissue, whereas the higher grades indicate greater rapidity of growth, less differentiation into cells of recognizable function, greater invasiveness, and greater tendency to metastasize.

Occurrence and Clinical Course—The incidence of neoplasms in various areas of the body is correlated with age and sex. In males, the most common malignant tumor between the ages of twenty-five and twenty-nine is testicular, from thirty to fifty-four years carcinoma of the skin, fifty-five to sixty-nine years carcinoma of the stomach, and seventy to eighty-four years carcinoma of the prostate. In females, carcinoma of the cervix is the most frequent malignant tumor between the ages of thirty and thirty-four, whereas carcinoma of the breast is the most common form of cancer after thirty-five. In both sexes, leukemia is the most common neoplastic disease below nine years.

Although varying in different localities, the incidence of malignant disease in the general population was approximately an average of 218 new cases of cancer per year per 100,000 population in 1947, the incidence being higher in the female by about 0.5 percent. These cases are primarily in the age group above fifty, as indicated by the fact that not until that age does the incidence reach 5 per 100,000 per year. Approximately one out of every eight deaths in this country each year is due to cancer. At present, out of every four patients with cancer, one is being cured by present therapy, one is dying needlessly because of delayed and inadequate therapy, and two are doomed to die unless new knowledge and methods are obtained through research.

As already indicated, the rate of growth and spread of neoplasms is variable. A tumor may be slow-growing or may increase rapidly in size. A malignant growth may directly invade contiguous organs, or, without increasing locally, it may rapidly spread to distant organs by way of the lymphatics and veins. Chance can play a pertinent role. A very small tumor accidentally breaking into a large blood vessel may result in widespread metastases, whereas another may reach a huge size and still remain confined within its capsule. Malignant tumors are rarely the direct cause of death but kill indirectly by pressure on or destruction of vital organs.

Diagnosis—In spite of all the advances in our understanding of the fundamental nature of cancer, in spite of progress in tissue chemistry and physiology pointing toward the ultimate possibility of diagnostic tests for the presence of cancer, and in spite of the vast amount of effort going into the study of the disease as a whole, it is the opinion of students of the field that for many years to come the clinical acumen of the general practitioner will continue to stand as the greatest potential bulwark against the inroads of cancer. The late James Ewing, dean of cancer specialists, said, "Until the practicing physician learns to keep the suspicion of cancer constantly in mind, knows the early manifestations of the disease and pursues, *as an invariable routine*, the following up of all danger signs, there will be no great increase in the cures of cancer."

Even with the aid of alertness and thoroughness, the diagnosis of cancer may be difficult because of the following characteristics of the disease:

1. Inaccessible carcinomas outnumber those which can be felt or can be seen either by the unaided eye or by endoscopy.

2. The manifestations of cancer do not fit into a pattern of any one kind; hence it is impossible to outline the clinical changes which one may expect *invariably* to accompany a cancer in *any* location. The appearance of complete well-being displayed by some patients with advanced cancer is, for example, highly misleading.

3. Some of the early teachings about the characteristic clinical manifestations of cancer were inaccurate but still persist and hinder early diagnosis. For example:

a. "Tumor" meant "a lump" in early teaching; and by extension of that concept, the presence of a cancer was thought to mean an increase in size of the organ involved. It is now known that lethal cancers may exist without either sign; e.g., duct carcinoma of the breast, in which there is no lump and the organ actually decreases in size.

b. Cancer was synonymous with pain. Actually, most early cancers are painless with the exception of bone sarcoma. When pain develops, the cancer has usually spread beyond control.

c. Age was thought a limiting factor. No age is exempt.

4. Training of medical students in the diagnosis of early cancer has generally been inadequate. Students should have careful training in all the new knowledge of tumor pathology so that they may be equipped to handle the protean manifestations of this disease.

The basic requirements on the part of the physician for the successful diagnosis of early cancer may be summarized as follows:

1. He must constantly entertain the *possibility* and therefore the suspicion of cancer.

2. He must have a thorough knowledge of precancerous lesions (Table 28) so that he may recognize a potentially dangerous lesion promptly.

3. He must exert good clinical judgment in estimating the significance of early symptoms.

4. Suspicious symptoms or signs must be studied promptly and thoroughly until the presence of cancer can be positively ruled out. It has been suggested that the slogan "look and see" be adopted rather than the cautious "wait and see" attitude. The extreme importance of this admonition is conveyed in

TABLE 28 — *Common Precancerous Lesions*

SKIN
Keratoses	Tuberculosis
Moles	X-ray burns
Chronic ulcers	Syphilis

MOUTH
Leukoplakia	Ill-fitting dentures
Chronic glossitis	Syphilis
Stomatitis	

GASTRO-INTESTINAL TRACT
Gastric ulcer	Polyps { gastric
Chronic gastritis	{ intestinal

BREAST
Chronic cystic mastitis

CERVIX
Cervical lacerations with chronic infection

recently compiled figures on carcinoma of the rectum, which show an average lapse of 9 1/2 months from the first symptom until the diagnosis was made, 4 1/2 of these months having been spent in the doctor's office. The relative curability of early lesions as compared with late cannot be overemphasized (Table 29). In view of these considerations, it can be said that the fate of the cancer patient first rests upon the knowledge and judgment of the general practitioner as it later does on the skill of the radiologist and the surgeon.

5. The physical examination of the patient must be complete and periodic. Careless, incomplete, or perfunctory examinations lead to oversight of precancerous lesions. Suspicious lesions should be handled gently because careless manipulation can dislodge malignant cells and hasten metastasis. The minimum components of a complete examination, insofar as cancer is concerned, may be listed as follows:

a. Careful history.
b. Routine blood count, urinalysis, and serologic tests.
c. X-ray of the chest.
d. Careful scrutiny of the skin of exposed surfaces.
e. Careful nose and throat examination, including lips and tongue.
f. Examination of the breasts: bimanual and in sitting as well as supine position.
g. Examination of chest, abdomen, and extremities, including the skin of each.
h. Palpation of lymph nodes: neck, axillae, and groins.
i. Pelvic examination in good light with visualization of the cervix.
j. Rectal examination.

6. Once the diagnosis is made, treatment should be prompt but not hasty (see below).

TABLE 29 — *Curability of Early Cancerous Lesions Compared with Late in Certain Areas*

Location	Early	Moderate	Late
Lip	95%	25%	Very small
Breast	75%	25%	Very small
Uterus	75%	15-25%	Very small

Special procedures available to aid in the diagnosis include the following:

1. Diagnostic x-ray. For successful interpretation of x-ray findings, the roentgenologist, practitioner, pathologist, and surgeon should be in close touch.

2. Endoscopy. Here again, close co-operation between the specialist and the practitioner is essential.

3. Biopsy. There is controversy over the place of biopsy in the diagnosis of cancer. The best opinion probably is that it should be used only as a last resort. The reasons for this are (1) that in unskilled hands it may disseminate the tumor (as in the removal of portions of breast cancer) and (2) that accurate histological diagnosis is extremely difficult and, unless done by a person with extensive experience, may give false information.

4. Histological diagnosis. This is a developing specialty to which a pathologist may devote his full time. By this means it is possible to identify the nature, origin, and grade of malignancy of the tumor and estimate its radiosensitivity. Because such specialized service is not generally available, tissue-diagnosis services have been set up in several states whereby tissue may be mailed to the diagnostic center for study. Although performing a useful service, these have the drawback of being remote from the patient, whereas ideally the pathologist should be close to the individual he is studying so that he can become familiar with the history, symptoms, and physical signs.

5. Cancer detection centers. In 1946, the American Cancer Society in conjunction with the American College of Surgeons initiated plans for the promulgation and standardization of Cancer Detection Centers throughout the country. The local county medical societies must approve these centers, and they must conform with the local regulations of medical practice. The purpose of these centers is "to provide a complete, thorough, physical examination for an apparently well person; to detect sooner than would otherwise be discovered early cancer, precancerous lesions, areas of chronic irritation or abnormal physiological conditions which might lead to cancer. . . . " In the opinion of some, better than isolated centers of this type are tumor clinics located in general hospitals staffed by men with special interests in this field. In such clinics, which are already established in many of the large hospitals, it is possible to secure the services of experts in a variety of aspects of the disease who are able to work in close co-operation with one another and with other members of the hospital staff.

6. Diagnostic tests. A number of different tests have been devised for the detection of early cancer. Success has been attained (1) with those tests depending on local changes, such as the vaginal smear for the detection of preclinical cancer of the uterus; or (2) when there is excessive excretion of a particular hormone, as in testicular or adrenal cortical cancer or chorionepithelioma. Attempts to secure a reliable single early diagnostic test for cancer anywhere in the body are, in the opinion of most students of the disease, not likely to succeed. Such tests must depend on alterations in cellular ferments or cellular metabolic products or in certain physical properties of the serum, all of which changes are likely to be so small as to defy detection when they result from the presence in the body of a few abnormal cells.

Treatment—Before instituting any form of treatment for a proved cancerous lesion, the practitioner should do two things:

1. Determine, if possible, the presence or absence of metastases. To do so effectively requires a knowledge of the characteristic sites of metastasis of the lesion in question. Thus, it may be an x-ray of the chest, the skull, or the bones which is indicated; or it may mean careful palpation for lymph nodes in the characteristic drainage area. Whatever is required, the physician's responsibility is to carry it out before therapy is begun, since it is not proper from any point of view to subject a patient in a hopeless situation to radical treatment.

2. Consult with the radiologist and the surgeon before deciding upon any action. Precipitate institution of one kind of treatment may rule out other types or combinations which might have been preferred if a comprehensive plan based on consultation had been evolved at the outset.

The three types of therapy available are surgical, radiological, and medical. Details of treatment are best considered in conjunction with a discussion of individual cancers. Only a brief consideration will be given here to certain problems connected with each type of therapy, together with a brief review of the new trends in therapeutic research.

SURGERY approaches the ideal therapy for relatively small localized growths, and it is unlikely that any method will soon replace surgical removal in this group. However, with every necessity of increasing the field of operation, surgical treatment becomes less satisfactory. Some surgeons have questioned the ultimate value of such radical operations as complete resection of all lymph-node-bearing areas on each side of the neck for cancer of the lip and the Wertheim operation for uterine cancer.

RADIATION is the best method for palliation in advanced cases and is curative in many forms of localized disease. There is a real art in the application of radiation therapy, and it is extremely important that the radiotherapist be a highly trained person. He must have a thorough understanding of the physical and biological forces with which he is dealing; he must have good clinical judgment in selecting dosage in relation not only to the radiosensitivity of the tissue he is treating but to the patient's general clinical condition; and he must be a skillful technician.

The dangers inherent in the use of x-ray, radium, or other radioactive substances are generally well known. They are summarized below:

1. Radiation sickness. The nature of this reaction is unknown. It can be avoided to some extent by the spacing of exposures and greater protection of the body surfaces not under exposure. The use of antihistaminic drugs, pyridoxine, and thiamin has been found empirically helpful.

2. Persistent functional disturbances. Disorders of this type seem to represent a more deep-seated and general reaction than radiation sickness; and in considering x-ray therapy in old people or in advanced carcinoma, the possibility of their occurrence must be weighed. Sometimes a rapid downward course begins in such persons the day radiation is started.

3. Specific effect on the hematopoietic system. The leukocytes are the most radiosensitive of all tissues. Sometimes severe granulocytopenia follows even moderate therapy (see Agranulocytosis, p. 102).

4. Untoward local reactions may be encountered. These are epilation, erythema, edema, epidermitis, ulcers, and cancer. The latter, of course, follows only repeated exposure and was seen frequently in physicians and technicians before adequate protective technics were instituted. In general, proper dosage and application circumvent all of the above.

MEDICAL THERAPY—There is as yet no medical treatment which is curative, but several procedures recently developed have had remarkable effects in reducing incapacity and prolonging life:

1. The use of androgen or estrogen in the treatment of breast carcinoma and estrogen in prostatic cancer. These are discussed on pages 201 and 218.

2. Radioisotopes. These are elements that have the same atomic structure as the stable, naturally occurring elements except for the nucleus, which, because of previous bombardment by small atomic particles, has too many neutrons in relation to protons. This situation renders the nucleus unstable, and it emits radiations composed of beta rays (high-speed electrons) or gamma rays (extremely high frequency x-rays) or both. Except for this property, the element behaves in every way like its stable isotope, and the body for the most part does not distinguish between the two. This means that it is possible to use radioisotopes both to deliver radiation to a desired point and also to serve as tracer substances, since their presence is readily detected by the Geiger counter. A number of different radioisotopes have already been investigated as therapeutic agents. Their usefulness is at present limited because (1) in general, neoplastic tissue has not been found to attract enough of the material for it to deliver an effective radiation dose, and (2) the toxicity is high. The Atomic Energy Commission is, however, preparing more than one hundred new isotopes, and it is hoped that among these may be substances with high affinities for different types of neoplastic tissue. At present, radioactive phosphorus is of considerable effectiveness in the treatment of erythremia, and it and radioactive gold, sodium, and manganese are all moderately successful in advanced Hodgkin's disease and in certain leukemias. Radioactive iodine has proved only moderately effective in cancer of the thyroid. Therapy with radioisotopes is still experimental and must remain so for some time.

3. Nitrogen mustards (certain chlorinated amines) are used chiefly in Hodgkin's disease. For discussion, see page 107.

In connection with interpretation of the effects of any newly proclaimed therapeutic agent, it should be remembered that many cancer processes are delicately balanced in relation to their environment, particularly from a nutrition standpoint; therefore, the injection of almost any alien substance may cause temporary cessation of growth and amelioration of symptoms. Furthermore, there is always a small proportion of apparently hopeless cases that show temporary improvement as the result of rest, improved appetite and nutrition, relief from irritation, and so on.

TRENDS IN RESEARCH—A great deal of research effort is being expended to uncover a therapeutic agent capable of attacking cancer cells generally. The hope for finding such an agent is based on the differences in metabolism between cancer cells and normal cells. At present, the greatest attention is being directed toward four types of substances: chemical agents, antibiotics, analogues of essential metabolites, and antiserums.

DRUGS

Drugs – Actions and Uses

INTRODUCTION

Definition and Sources—Perhaps the broadest definition of a drug is "any chemical agent which affects living protoplasm." Drugs are used in medical practice to modify body function, locally or generally, for the purpose of preserving or restoring health. The first drugs were obtained from plants, animals, or minerals. Today, an increasing number of active medicinal agents which were formerly extracted from natural sources are being made synthetically, and there is a rapidly growing list of valuable agents that are synthetic in both origin and production.

Potency and Assay—Drugs which can be obtained in pure form are prescribed in terms of weight. Such drugs are usually either crystalline or crystallizable. However, crystalline form is not of itself a guarantee of purity, for many mixtures will crystallize. To take an extreme example, Insulin is amorphous and can be made to crystallize only by the addition of a small quantity of zinc or certain other metals. Some active principles which are not obtained in pure form can nevertheless be assayed chemically. The potency of desiccated thyroid, for example, can be determined by assaying its content of organic iodine.

Certain other active principles, however, can be neither isolated nor assayed chemically, and for their standardization one must resort to bio-assay, which is usually carried out in animals. Of the two alternatives, chemical or biological assay, the latter is less desirable for two reasons: The action in animals does not always parallel the desired therapeutic effects in man, and the results are usually more variable because of the number of extraneous and uncontrollable factors which influence biological response. In fact, in most types of bio-assay, an allowance of plus or minus 20 percent is made; and the highest acceptable figure, 120 percent of the theoretical, is actually half again as large as the smallest acceptable figure, 80 percent of the theoretical.

The potency of drugs which are assayed biologically is stated in terms of *units*. A unit is the amount of drug required to produce a certain arbitrarily determined quantitative response in the test animal. Many types of units have been made official in the U.S.P., and some of them have been the subject of international agreement. To reduce the margin of difference between laboratories, a preparation of each drug is chosen as the standard and is used as the basis for comparison. In addition, the procedure of the test is made as exact as possible, with a view to controlling all relevant factors which are susceptible of control.

Stability—The stability of different drugs and drug preparations varies considerably. The most destructive agents are heat, light, air (oxygen), and moisture. Thus, dry preparations such as tablets are, in general, more stable than solutions, and sealed ampoules are more stable than open bottles. It is a wise precaution to avoid warm places, such as warming cabinets or the vicinity of radiators, for the storage of drugs.

When preparations are subject to significant deterioration even under reasonably careful storage, an expiration date is stamped on the package label. Such a date is that prior to which the contents can be expected, beyond reasonable doubt, to exert their specific effects. Naturally, deterioration does not begin and go to completion on the exact date specified; rather, it is a gradual process depending for its speed on the amount of exposure to the deleterious influences mentioned above. In determining expiration dates, the expected conditions of storage are considered. Some preparations which are customarily kept under refrigeration deteriorate slowly even when cold but very rapidly when at room temperature. Others which remain fully potent indefinitely under refrigeration are dated because they are customarily stored at room temperature. On pages 625 and 626 will be found lists of Lilly products which (1) are dated, (2) must be stored under refrigeration, or (3) are damaged by freezing.

Administration—Drugs may be administered for either local or systemic effect. For local application they may be incorporated into powders, solutions, suspensions, creams, jellies, ointments, pastes, lotions, or liniments (see Drugs Acting Locally on Skin and Mucous Membranes, p. 479). Special forms may be appropriate for particular regions: lozenges or troches for the mouth and pharynx; suppositories for rectal, vaginal, or urethral administration; nebulized liquids or very fine powders to be taken by inhalation for the bronchial tract.

The intact skin is an oily membrane. Consequently, aqueous solutions and oil-in-water emulsions act on the superficial layers only. For penetrating action an oil solution or a water-in-oil emulsion should be employed (see p. 481). In contrast, damaged skin, like mucous membrane, acts as an aqueous membrane, on which oil solutions and water-in-oil emulsions have a superficial action, whereas aqueous solutions and oil-in-water emulsions are more easily absorbed.

It is sometimes hard to draw a line between local and systemic action; for in some situations drugs are given systemically for local effect, the drug being transported to the intended area by the blood, whereas if locally applied medication is absorbed with sufficient rapidity, systemic effects will be obtained. Oil-soluble agents, such as the steroid hormones, are efficiently absorbed from the

skin, but the percutaneous route is little employed because of the difficulty of controlling dosage.

Most commonly, systemic effects are achieved by systemic administration, that is, by the enteral or parenteral routes. There are three possibilities for enteral administration: The medication may be swallowed, inserted into the rectum, or placed under the tongue (sublingual administration) or between the cheek and the lower gum (buccal administration) for direct absorption into the blood.

ORAL AND RECTAL—The simplest and most convenient of the enteral procedures is to swallow the drug, and this is what is commonly meant by the term "oral administration." Dosage forms intended to be swallowed include tablets, capsules, sealed capsules (such as elastic filled capsules or gelseals), powders, suspensions, liquids and solutions, and sweetened and otherwise flavored solutions such as elixirs and syrups.

When drugs either irritate the stomach or are destroyed by gastric juice, they may be ingested in "enteric-coated" tablets which are expected to delay release of the medication until there is a probability that the stomach will have been passed. Salol and other coatings which depend on pH for dissolution are unreliable, for the supposedly acid stomach is frequently neutral or even alkaline in reaction because of regurgitation of intestinal contents, and the intestine may be neutral or slightly acid for several feet because of reception of acid gastric contents. The most reliable coating appears to be one (such as 'Enseals') which disintegrates in a given interval after wetting, regardless of the reaction of the liquid in which it is immersed.

Some drugs which are irritating to stomach and small intestine alike may be administered rectally without producing symptoms. Liquids and solutions are given by tube with the patient prone or on his left side. For solid medication a rectal suppository is most frequently used, but a capsule is satisfactory if it is punctured at each end with a pin before insertion. Because of its less favorable shape, a capsule may have to be inserted farther than a suppository in order to insure retention and absorption.

The rapidity of absorption of drugs from the gastro-intestinal tract varies with the nature of the drug, its solubility, whether or not it is introduced in solution, its concentration (if in solution), its coating (if a tablet), the state of the gastro-intestinal tract (including the presence of other matter such as food), the state (and particularly the adequacy) of the local and general circulation, and systemic factors (e.g., the level of thyroid function).

SUBLINGUAL AND BUCCAL—The third mode of enteral administration, namely, direct absorption into the blood stream from the oral cavity, in which the drug is placed beneath the tongue (sublingually) or between cheek and lower gum (buccally), has a limited but distinct usefulness. Drugs so absorbed are not exposed to the gastric and intestinal digestive juices; and they also by-pass the liver, through which must pass all substances absorbed from the stomach and intestine and most of what is absorbed from the rectum.

Hypodermic tablets (of nitroglycerin, morphine sulfate, atropine sulfate, and apomorphine hydrochloride in particular), when administered sublingually or buccally, are usually as promptly and fully effective as after hypodermic injection. Powdering the tablet hastens absorption. Aludrine has a *more* satisfactory action when given by this route than when injected or swallowed. Some of the steroid hormones, e.g., testosterone propionate, methyltestosterone, and desoxycorticosterone acetate, are also efficiently absorbed, and the by-passing of the liver makes them almost as active by this route as by intramuscular injection.

Sublingual and buccal administrations have their disadvantages also. If saliva containing the drug is swallowed, the administration becomes to that extent peroral, and the especial virtues of the sublingual or buccal route are lost. Patients must learn the technic of administration in order to avoid (1) sucking on the tablet, (2) swallowing prior to complete solution of the tablet, and (3) a nervously conditioned excessive salivation initiated by the presence of the drug in the mouth.

Another simple route for systemic administration which employs a body surface is the intranasal. It is employed particularly for posterior pituitary extract; the solution is used in obstetrics (see p. 473), and the powder for treatment of diabetes insipidus (p. 194).

PARENTERAL—"Parenteral administration" ordinarily refers to subcutaneous, intramuscular, or intravenous injection, but it also includes intradermal injection, which has a special usefulness for certain vaccines and other antigens. The parenteral route is indicated in the presence of one or more of the conditions listed in Table 30. However, not all medications are suitable for parenteral administration. The requirements for the three parenteral routes differ considerably, but all injected medications must be sterile, and the skin should be cleansed well before a needle is inserted.

HYPODERMIC, or subcutaneous, administration is employed for two different types of medication:

active drugs which are given in small doses, and electrolyte and dextrose solutions which are given in large volumes. The latter type of injection is termed an infusion or a hypodermoclysis. Medication for subcutaneous injection must be in aqueous solution (sparingly soluble, nondiffusible, or colloidal substances are very slowly absorbed from subcutaneous tissue), close to neutrality in reaction, as nearly isotonic as possible, and relatively nonirritant. The volume for injection, as contrasted with infusion, is seldom less than 0.5 cc. and should not exceed 2 cc.

The less sensitive areas are chosen for injection— most commonly the outer aspects of the arms and thighs. In the case of antigens or drugs which may produce acute systemic reactions, it is well to choose a site far enough from the shoulder or hip so that a tourniquet can be applied proximal to the injection, should a reaction develop. Such a tourniquet can be released periodically for a few minutes to make systemic absorption slow enough to avoid serious consequences. If for any reason a hastening of absorption is desired, the site may be massaged, or heat may be applied.

Hypodermic injection of unsuitable material may lead to inflammation, necrosis, or abscess formation. Even with appropriate medication, the dan-

TABLE 30—*Indications for Parenteral Administration of Drugs*

I. The drug cannot be given by the enteral route because
   A. It is poorly absorbed from all three sites (stomach and intestine, rectum, and mouth).
   B. It is irritating to those sites from which it is absorbed.
   C. In the case of oral administration, the drug is destroyed by the digestive juices.
   D. In the case of rectal administration, there is diarrhea or local disease of the rectum.
   E. The patient can take nothing by mouth, and the drug is contraindicated by the other enteral routes for one of the reasons given above.

II. The action of the drug is needed more quickly than can be expected after oral, rectal, or sublingual administration.

III. Special effects are desired which do not follow enteral administration (such as elevation of blood calcium level with calcium salts [p. 344]).

IV. It is important that the physician be assured the patient has taken the medication.

gers of infection and intravenous injection are still present. Infection is avoided by the use of sterile needles, syringes, and medications, thorough cleansing of the skin, avoidance of areas in which there is already infection of the skin or subcutaneous tissue, and avoidance of contamination during preparation and administration of the drug.

Inadvertent injection of a potent drug into a vein may produce highly undesirable effects. It can be avoided by (1) choosing areas not well supplied with veins, such as the outer and posterior surfaces of the arms and the outer and anterior surfaces of the thighs; (2) avoiding visible veins; and (3) drawing back on the plunger for a few seconds after insertion of the needle and before injection of the drug (if blood appears in the syringe, the needle is withdrawn and reinserted at a different site).

SUBCUTANEOUS INFUSION (hypodermoclysis) is employed to introduce relatively large volumes (500 to 2,000 cc.) of electrolyte or dextrose solutions. Even greater precautions than for hypodermic injection must be taken to avoid infection or irritation of the tissues. Isotonicity is especially important. Dextrose solutions should be mixed with equal volumes of electrolyte solutions, for even isotonic dextrose solution is somewhat irritating when given alone.

The most common sites for subcutaneous infusion are the anterolateral surfaces of the thighs and the lateral thoracic areas (just lateral to the pectoral muscles). Flow is controlled by gravity, and the height of the container is adjusted so that flow is maintained without undue distention of the tissues. Gestures are commonly made toward warming the infused solution. Actually, proper warming is difficult to maintain, and its advantage is questionable. The enzyme hyaluronidase increases the rate of absorption when added to the injected solution; as yet, however, its use has not been extensive. In general, no more than 1,000 cc. of infusion should be introduced per hour.

The popularity of subcutaneous infusion has been greatly diminished by improvements in the technic of intravenous drip. It is now used principally as an alternative when a patient must receive large quantities of parenteral fluid over a long period.

INTRAMUSCULAR injection has a different usefulness from that of hypodermic. Injected material is more rapidly absorbed because of the greater vascularity of muscle and the absence of restricting tissue. More-irritant material is tolerated; it is possible to give intramuscularly oils, suspensions, and other preparations which are either too irritant

for subcutaneous injection or physically unsuitable for intravenous injection. As much as 5 cc. may be introduced at one site, although volumes of 1 to 2 cc. are better tolerated.

On the other hand, intramuscular injection requires more skillful technic and carries slightly more danger to the patient. The vascularity of muscle makes for a greater likelihood of intravenous or even intra-arterial injection, and more care must be taken to avoid them. Precautions are especially important in the case of suspensions, oil vehicles, or any other preparations which are insoluble in plasma, contain particulate matter, or lead to aggregation or precipitation in the blood stream. Material must be fairly accurately deposited. Too superficial an injection may be subcutaneous; too deep an injection may be so close to bone as to cause periosteal irritation; deposition in the vicinity of nerve trunks may lead to prolonged pain.

The upper outer quadrant of the buttock is the most favorable site for intramuscular injection, and to receive it the patient should be prone on a table. The deltoid is satisfactory for small and infrequent injections, but it is not suited for large injections or for repeated deposits of suspensions, oil, or other material which is slowly absorbed. The paravertebral muscles may also be used, and, especially in children, the vastus lateralis.

Local reactions to intramuscular injection are fundamentally similar to those which may follow hypodermic injection. Tenderness may be more troublesome because of the greater mobility of muscle. Inadvertent intra-arterial injection may lead to a local arterial spasm or thromboarteritis which may cause extensive necrosis.

INTRAVENOUS—The intravenous route is a very popular one because of its accessibility and its dramatic character. However, it always carries a certain amount of risk and should be employed only when the advantages over other routes distinctly outweigh its disadvantages and hazards. The advantages include the following:

1. Effects can often be obtained which are not possible by other routes, e.g., fever following typhoid vaccine, elevation of blood calcium from administration of calcium salts, osmotic effects from hypertonic solutions.

2. It provides the quickest means of distributing medication throughout the body.

3. Material too irritant for subcutaneous, intramuscular, or even oral or rectal administration can often be diluted and given by vein without local reaction.

4. The volume which can be given is limited

only by the capacity of the patient's circulatory system to accommodate it without disturbance.

The intravenous is the route of choice for increasing blood or plasma volume quickly, as in shock or after hemorrhage. It is preferred for prolonged administration of large volumes of fluid, as in parenteral nutrition with electrolyte, dextrose, and amino acid solutions.

The disadvantages and dangers of intravenous therapy include the following:

1. Collapse, shock, and even death may follow too-rapid injection of almost any material which differs greatly from plasma in composition; the danger of such "speed shock" is particularly great with active drugs.

2. Heart failure may result from too-rapid introduction of large volumes of fluid, regardless of composition.

3. Chill and fever may follow administration of fluids containing pyrogens (oral, subcutaneous, or intramuscular administration of pyrogens has no such effect).

4. Embolism or chill and fever may be a sequel to introduction of air, insoluble matter, or substances which precipitate constituents of the plasma or which agglutinate or lake red blood cells.

5. Anaphylaxis may be caused by injection of a substance to which the patient is allergic.

6. Accidentally introduced bacteria are disseminated, whereas on subcutaneous or intramuscular injection the body defenses have an opportunity to localize them.

Large volumes are contraindicated in the presence of heart failure, severe anemia, or pulmonary edema and are seldom advisable in edematous patients. Inquiry should always be made regarding allergy in general and sensitivity to the proposed medication in particular before intravenous injection is undertaken.

Perhaps the most frequent adverse general reaction to intravenous injection is some degree of speed shock following relatively rapid administration of concentrated solutions of potent drugs. A drug for intravenous injection should always be adequately diluted in as nearly an isotonic medium as possible (except when departure from isotonicity is made purposely to obtain osmotic effects); the injection itself should always be timed with a watch or clock to avoid the common tendency toward rapid administration.

Local reactions following intravenous injection include the following:

1. Hematoma from transfixion of the vein.

2. Local perivenous inflammation or necrosis following inadvertent paravenous injection of irritating substances.

3. Thrombosis of the vein or phlebitis.

The antecubital veins are the most accessible for intravenous administration because of their size and location. The veins of the dorsum of the hand are also useful, especially in patients under anesthesia, but they must not be used for irritating solutions. The veins of the leg or foot can also be employed. The external jugulars should be avoided because of the danger of injuring near-by vital structures and because, their internal pressure often being less than that of the atmosphere, entry into them may be followed by massive air embolism. The longitudinal sinus is sometimes utilized in infants under emergency conditions, but it is dangerous. Dextrose, electrolyte, and amino acid solutions, plasma, and even whole blood, which would be given intravenously to adults and older children, are often injected into the peritoneal cavity in infants.

Intravenous injections can be subdivided into two groups on the basis of volume. The smaller quantities—1 to 20 cc. or, occasionally, 50 cc.— are given from a syringe and generally contain a potent drug. It is these small volumes that offer the greatest temptation toward dangerously rapid injection. Larger volumes are administered from a reservoir by means of rubber or plastic tubing. A special drip bulb in the tubing is an aid in gauging rate of flow, except when the rate must be very rapid, as in shock. For administration over a period of hours or days, a cannula of metal or plastic tubing is often used in the vein in place of a needle. Flow from the reservoir should be by gravity; positive-pressure bottles should be avoided because of the danger of air embolism. Likewise, a loop of tubing should dip well below the level of the chest, especially in dyspneic patients, to prevent the possibility of aspiration of air into the vein after the reservoir is empty.

Materials for intravenous injection *must* meet the following requirements. They must be:

1. In aqueous solution.

2. Clear and free from
   a. Pyrogens.
   b. Particulate matter, including colloidal suspensions (except in the case of blood).
   c. Substances capable of forming a precipitate with constituents of the plasma.
   d. Substances capable of agglutinating or laking the recipient's red blood cells.

3. Sufficiently dilute to avoid undue irritation of the vein into which they are introduced.

In addition, protein material should be given intravenously with great caution and only after inquiry and preliminary testing (see p. 334) for evidence of sensitivity.

Pyrogens are substances which induce fever. Pyrogens are likely to develop in water (even distilled water) unless it is sealed into a container and then sterilized promptly after distillation. The pyrogens are thought to be produced by nonpathogenic bacteria which are carried on dust particles. Only freshly distilled water should be employed in making up solutions which are intended for intravenous use. In commercial production, ampoules are filled and sterilized promptly, and each lot is tested for pyrogens by intravenous injection into rabbits before release. Pyrogens almost never produce fever when given intramuscularly or subcutaneously unless they are present in very large amounts.

Many drugs must be given intravenously at a very slow rate and with great caution, not only to avoid speed shock but also to avoid undesirable special effects observed only on intravenous injection. An example is calcium salts (p. 344).

OTHER ROUTES—Intracutaneous injection is employed for administration of certain types of antigens: (1) diagnostic antigens (see p. 338), and (2) boosting doses for patients already having a primary immunity (see p. 320). In infants, large volumes of nonirritant solutions (blood, plasma, electrolyte, dextrose, amino acids) which in older individuals would be given intravenously can be injected intraperitoneally or into the sternal bone marrow.

Dosage—Medication is ordinarily given to produce a certain physiological effect. The proper dose is the quantity which just achieves that effect. Because of the great variation in the response of different patients, each administration of a drug is in fact a clinical experiment. It is useful, however, to have dosage statements which can serve as points of departure for determination of the optimum dose for a given patient.

Dosage is influenced by many factors. Two of the most important are rate and completeness of absorption and rate of excretion and destruction. In myxedema, for example, absorption from the gastro-intestinal tract is abnormally slow, and drugs taken by mouth cannot be expected to act as quickly as in normal individuals. Likewise, in shock, absorption from subcutaneous tissue may practically cease, and consequently in that condition it is useless to give medication hypodermically. Many drugs are destroyed in the liver; they will therefore have a prolonged action in the presence of severe impairment of hepatic function, and, accordingly, maintenance dosage should be less than average. Other drugs leave the body primarily by way of the kidneys, and they must be given conservatively when renal function is impaired.

The frequency of administration should be related to the rate of destruction and excretion. Drugs which are rapidly disposed of, such as crystalline penicillin and propylthiouracil, must be given every few hours for sustained effect. Digitalis, with a more prolonged action, need be given only once daily for maintenance, and even then the effects tend to be cumulative. Extremely long-acting substances, such as thyroid, are ordinarily given once daily as a matter of practical convenience; however, the fact that the full effect of a given dose of thyroid is not manifested until a week after administration (1) makes it necessary to be somewhat cautious regarding initial dosage, and (2) necessitates delay in judging the effect of a given dosage level.

The influence of age on dosage is discussed beginning on page 262.

SYSTEMIC ANTI-INFECTIVE AGENTS

Systemic anti-infective agents are substances that kill or prevent the reproduction of micro-organisms without damaging the host. A considerable number of these agents are now available for clinical use in combating the various infections to which man is subject.

Chemotherapeutic agents are those synthesized by the chemist and include sulfonamides, arsphenamines, para-aminosalicylic acid, and quinacrine.

Antibiotics are metabolic products of micro-organisms which are capable of inhibiting or destroying other micro-organisms. A great number of antibiotics have been isolated. Many are too toxic to the host for systemic use, but some of these toxic ones have proved themselves satisfactory for local application. Penicillin is perhaps the best example of an antibiotic which is also a systemic anti-infective. It is possible that all antibiotics can eventually be termed chemotherapeutic agents as methods of chemical synthesis are discovered.

Other systemic anti-infectives which cannot readily be classed as either chemotherapeutic or antibiotic agents include quinine and chaulmoogra oil. These are metabolic products of plant life which inhibit or destroy pathogens and which are active in vivo in dosages that can be given systemically.

ANTIBIOTICS

In recent years, efforts have been made to identify as many antibiotics as possible and to determine which of them might be of value as local or systemic anti-infectives. Not all antibiotics are capable of being used as anti-infectives. Some act against certain nonpathogenic organisms but are inactive against pathogens; others are effective in vitro but not in vivo. The clinical value of some very potent antibiotics is likewise limited by their extreme toxicity at therapeutic blood concentrations.

The antibiotics are thought to act upon the anabolic, protein-synthetic phases of metabolism. This theory as to their mechanism of action is supported by two fundamental properties shared by these substances: They act only upon growing cells, and they do not inhibit the respiration of resting organisms or the combustion of added substrates in the absence of growth.

The practical aim of antibiotic therapy is to establish at the focus of infection that concentration of the systemic anti-infective agent which has been found to be optimal in in-vitro tests against the infecting organism. There are two conflicting schools of thought, however, as to the maintenance of that concentration. One thinks it is better to hold the level continuously above the effective in-vitro sensitivity of the organism until the infection is eradicated. The other believes that the concentration of antibiotic should be allowed to fall periodically in order to enable the bacteria to undergo brief episodes of growth during which they would again be subject to the bactericidal action of the drug. Evidence in the matter is conflicting, and the situation is complicated by the difficulty of determining antibiotic concentrations at the site of human infection.

The most feasible measurement is the blood level. Its relation to tissue concentration is also controversial, although it is certain that there is great variation in different types of tissue, the highest tissue levels being found in the kidneys and the lowest in the brain, spinal cord, and nerves. In view of all these uncertainties, it is not surprising to find sharp divergence of opinion regarding both the interpretation and the management of blood levels. Nevertheless, subject as it is to controversy, the blood level remains as the only indication of the probable drug concentration in the infected tissues.

The establishment and maintenance of an effective blood level for an antibiotic depend upon the following factors: dosage and frequency of administration; rate of absorption from the drug depot, wherever established; rate of drug inactivation, if any, within the body; extent of binding to plasma and other tissue proteins; and rate of excretion. In regard to penicillin, most work has been done on developing intramuscular preparations that decrease the rate of absorption from the muscle depot. This may be accomplished by the following methods: suspension of crystalline penicillin in vehicles that are slowly absorbed; use of a water-insoluble form of penicillin, e.g., procaine penicillin; alteration of the particle size of the penicillin crystals (large particles slowly absorbed, small particles rapidly absorbed); and coating of the individual penicillin crystals with water-repellent substances, e.g., aluminum monostearate gels.

Another approach to maintenance of constant plasma levels of antibiotics has been methods to slow renal excretion. Benzoates (which are excreted as hippurates), para-aminohippurates, caronamide, and certain other substances containing ring structures block the excretion of penicillin by the renal tubules and thus, when present in sufficient amount, increase the average plasma level of penicillin.

Toxicity to antibiotics is of two kinds: One bears a definite relationship to dosage; the other falls into the category of sensitivity phenomena, whose incidence and severity do not strictly depend upon the amount of the antibiotic administered. Penicillin is a unique therapeutic agent in that no toxic effects of the dose-related type have been reported; however, sensitivity reactions occur in approximately 5 percent of patients. Streptomycin, unfortunately, exhibits toxic effects of the dose-related type and also sensitivity reactions. The former toxicity involves the eighth cranial nerve and vestibular apparatus.

In antibiotic therapy, the development of resistant strains of micro-organisms through mutation has presented a major problem. This is especially true in the treatment of tuberculous infections with streptomycin. It is generally conceded that the development of resistance is quite independent of the host, and there is no sure method of avoiding this drug fastness. At present, there appear to be two methods of combating the resistance problem —initial maximal dosage continued until the infection is thoroughly eradicated, or combined medication with two or more antibiotics or chemotherapeutics. By the latter method, the few variants resistant to one agent can be controlled by the others before selective reproduction makes them the predominant type.

PENICILLIN

The term "penicillin" was first applied by Fleming to a then-unknown antibiotic substance which he inferred was present in filtrates of broth cultures of the mold *Penicillium notatum*. It is now used to signify any of several known antibiotic substances (penicillin—G, penicillin—F, penicillin—X, etc.), whether they are produced by the growth of *P. notatum* or *P. chrysogenum*. The accepted formula for penicillin is shown in Figure 7. It may be thought of as a ring condensation of two amino acids— alanine and beta-dimethylcysteine. The various penicillins (G, X, F, K, and other biosynthetic penicillins) differ in the substituent acid group

coupled to the alanine amino group (upper left corner of the formula in Figure 7; as shown, the substituent in penicillin—G is a phenacetyl group). The penicillins are moderately strong acids whose sodium, potassium, calcium, and other salts may be used therapeutically. The penicillins and their sodium and potassium salts are freely soluble in water, but they are unstable in its presence. Aqueous solutions deteriorate seriously within twenty-four hours at room temperature but retain a reasonable degree of potency for five to seven days under refrigeration. However, they are best when freshly prepared.

Procaine base (see p. 442) combines with penicillin to form a compound which is almost insoluble in either water or oil. Procaine penicillin can therefore be prepared as a suspension in oil or water suitable for intramuscular injection. A depot is thus established from which absorption is prolonged. Suitably buffered aqueous suspensions of procaine penicillin retain their stability for months if refrigerated.

Penicillin—G, which will hereafter be meant

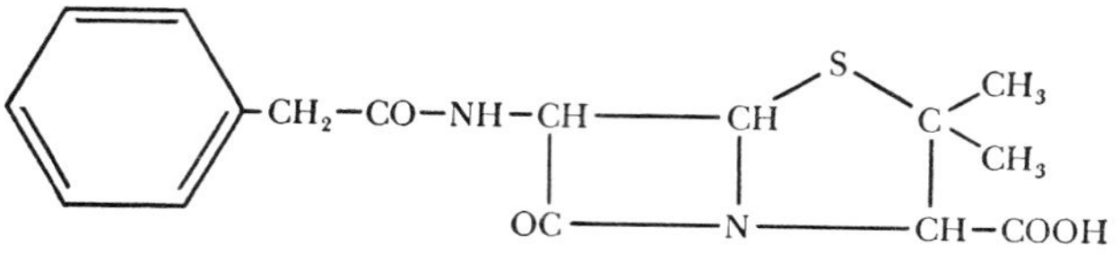

Penicillin—G

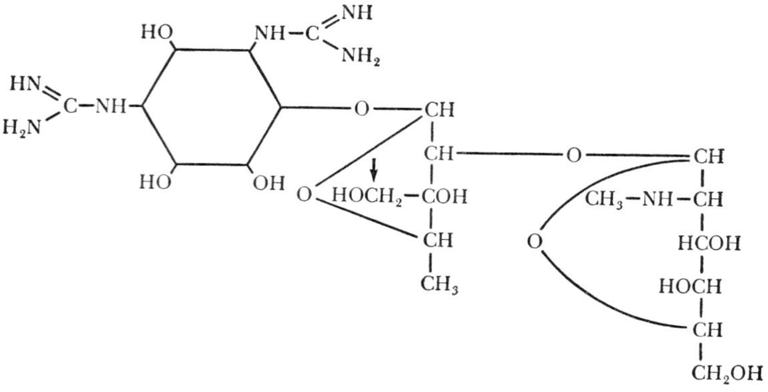

Dihydrostreptomycin

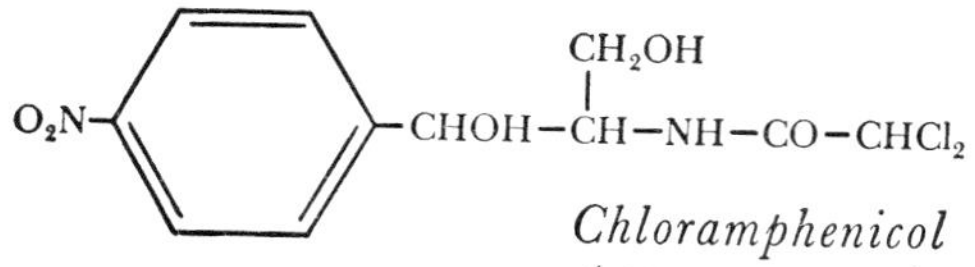

Chloramphenicol
(Chloromycetin)

FIGURE 7—*Structural Formulas of Antibiotics*

when the term "penicillin" is used, is the form which is generally available on the market. Actually it is slightly less potent than penicillin—X (which differs from it in having a hydroxyl group in the para position of the benzene ring); but the spectrum of activity is qualitatively the same, and penicillin—G is more easily produced on a large scale. Pure penicillin—G has an activity of $1,666\frac{2}{3}$ units per mg. The unit of activity is biologically determined on the basis of inhibition of bacterial growth in vitro under standard conditions. Unfortunately, no agreement has yet been reached as to the most suitable test organism; the Food and Drug Administration employs *Staphylococcus aureus* (F.D.A. Strain 209-P).

Penicillin is bacteriostatic in threshold concentrations and bactericidal in higher concentrations, but neither effect is observed unless cells are growing; and the more rapid the growth, the greater is the antibiotic effect. The rate of killing is also proportional to the concentration of agent up to a certain maximal point. A few species of bacteria are capable of producing an enzyme, penicillinase, which destroys the drug.

Clinically, penicillin is of great value in the treatment of all streptococcus and staphylococcus infections with or without bacteremia; treponemal diseases, including syphilis, pinta, and yaws; gonococcus infections; pneumococcus pneumonia and meningitis; and all meningococcus infections which have failed to respond to sulfonamides. Penicillin is likewise a valuable adjunct to other procedures in the therapy of many diseases which are included in Table 31 (p. 290).

The antibiotic is rapidly absorbed from intramuscular and subcutaneous depots but is poorly absorbed from the gastro-intestinal tract. It readily permeates most tissues except brain, cornea, and lens. In order to achieve therapeutic levels in the cerebrospinal fluid and vitreous humor, doses as large as 1,000,000 units every two hours must be administered. Such massive systemic dosage schedules eliminate the need for intrathecal therapy, which may be harmful. Intrathecal administration of penicillin should be restricted to desperate cases in which the possible benefits to be obtained by this route outweigh the risk of the grave neurotoxic complications that may ensue.

Approximately 60 percent of parenterally administered penicillin is excreted in the urine. High concentrations are likewise found in the bile, indicating excretion from this source.

Penicillin is available for intravenous, intramuscular, oral, and topical administration. Dosage by any route depends upon the severity of the infection and must be necessarily at the discretion of the physician. The average daily dose of penicillin for most infections is 300,000 to 600,000 units intramuscularly, which may be given as one injection of slow-absorbing penicillin or as several divided doses of crystalline penicillin at intervals of three to six hours.

When penicillin is administered orally, the dosage should be three to five times that by intramuscular injection. The oral preparations should be given in divided amounts every three to four hours. If an infection does not respond promptly to oral administration of penicillin, the intramuscular or intravenous routes should be employed.

There are various preparations of penicillin available for local application. These include nose drops which contain added vasoconstrictor substances; sublingual tablets; ointments for local and ophthalmic use; powders for dusting surgical wounds; troches and chewing gum for oral infections; and penicillin dust for inhalation therapy. These preparations are made in various concentrations, depending upon their application.

Penicillin aerosol therapy is valuable in tracheobronchitis (p. 112) and infection secondary to bronchiectasis (p. 115) when these are due to penicillin-sensitive organisms. Penicillin in amounts of 25,000 to 50,000 units is dissolved in 1 to 2 cc. of isotonic salt solution or distilled water and inhaled as a fine mist every three to six hours.

Special dosage schedules and technics are necessary in treating certain specific infections. They are discussed under the diseases: subacute bacterial endocarditis (p. 73), meningitis (p. 165), syphilis (p. 10), empyema (p. 122), actinomycosis (p. 42).

Penicillin may be given in dosages of millions of units without toxic effects. Reactions due to allergic hypersensitivity occur in about 5 percent of patients following the intravenous or intramuscular injection of the antibiotic. Symptoms of hypersensitivity include urticaria, contact dermatitis, drug fever, gastro-intestinal reactions, and conditions similar to serum sickness. Penicillin may be continued despite the above-mentioned symptoms provided they can be controlled by appropriate therapy. The antihistaminic drugs (see p. 509) are of value in these allergic reactions.

STREPTOMYCIN AND DIHYDROSTREPTOMYCIN

Streptomycin is a basic glycoside with antibiotic properties which is produced by the moldlike or-

TABLE 31 — *Use of Antibiotics in Infections*

Infection or Disease	Penicillin	Streptomycin or Dihydrostreptomycin	Aureomycin	Chloramphenicol	Bacitracin	Sulfonamides
Actinomycosis	1					
Anthrax	1					2
Brucellosis		2	1	1		
Chancroid			2	2		1
Cholera						1
Diphtheria (carriers)	1					
Dysentery, bacillary		2	?	?		1
Endocarditis, subacute bacterial						
(a) Alpha streptococcus	1					
(b) *Str. faecalis* D	1 ———— 1 ———— 1 ———— combined therapy					
(c) Staphylococcus	1					
(d) Gram-negative bacilli		1 ———— 1 ———— 1 —— combined therapy				
Glanders						1
Gonorrhea	1		2	2		2
Granuloma inguinale		1	2	2		
Lymphogranuloma venereum		2	1	1		2
Meningitis, *H. influenzae*		1 ———] 2 [—— combined therapy —— 1				
Meningococcus infections	1 ———————— combined therapy ———————— 1					
Paratyphoid fevers				1		
Peritonitis	1 ———— 1 ———— combined therapy ———— 1					
Plague		1				2
Pneumonia, Friedländer's		1	1			
Pneumonia, pneumococcus	1					2
Pyogenic infections	1				1	
Ratbite fever						
(a) *Spirillum minus*	1		2	U		
(b) *Streptobacillus moniliformis*	1		U	U		
Rheumatic fever (prophylaxis)	1					1
Surgical conditions of the bowel, preoperative and postoperative		1	1	U		1
Syphilis	1					
Tetanus-gas gangrene	1 —— (combined, as adjunct to serum therapy) —— 1					
Trachoma				U	U	1
Tuberculosis		1				
Tularemia		1	2			
Typhoid fever				1		
Typhus and related fevers			1	1		
Urinary tract infections						
(a) *Escherichia coli*		2	1	1		
(b) *Aerobacter*		2	1	1		1
(c) *Proteus vulgaris*		2		1		1
(d) *Pseudomonas*		1	1	1		
Vincent's angina	1					
Whooping cough			1	1		

The numbers indicate the order of choice of the various drugs, 1 indicating first choice. When the activity of a given antibiotic is unknown, the symbol "U" is employed.

ganism *Streptomyces griseus.* It can be changed by hydrogenation to dihydrostreptomycin, the structural formula of which is shown in Figure 7. The arrow in the figure points to the portion of the molecule to which the hydrogen has been added. The result in dihydrostreptomycin is an alcohol group, as shown; the corresponding group in streptomycin is an aldehyde (CHO·). The rest of the molecule is the same in both compounds. The two substances appear to have the same therapeutic properties and to differ only in their toxicity. Because of its lower toxicity, dihydrostreptomycin will be principally mentioned.

Dihydrostreptomycin is employed as the sulfate or hydrochloride. These salts are stable in dry form and also in aqueous solution if kept sterile. It is recommended, however, that solutions be stored under refrigeration.

Streptomycin and dihydrostreptomycin are active against a number of gram-negative bacteria. They are of definite value in the treatment of tularemia, infections with *Hemophilus influenzae,* pneumonia due to *Klebsiella pneumoniae* (Friedländer's bacillus), and urinary tract infections, bacteremia, and wound infections due to gram-negative organisms sensitive to the antibiotic. They are effective as adjuncts in the treatment of certain phases of tuberculosis, particularly when given with para-aminosalicylic acid (p. 296). When combined with sulfadiazine, aureomycin, and chloramphenicol, they are of value in the therapy of acute undulant fever. For a complete list of the diseases in which streptomycin and dihydrostreptomycin may be indicated, see Table 31.

Therapeutic blood concentrations of the two substances are easily obtained by subcutaneous or intramuscular injection of the material. Oral administration results in the appearance of little or no drug in the blood, but it is not destroyed in the gastro-intestinal tract and does exert a bactericidal action on the intestinal flora. After injection, about 50 percent is excreted in the urine. The drugs penetrate the peritoneal cavity after systemic administration but do not reach empyema cavities or spinal fluid in therapeutic amounts. Streptomycin and dihydrostreptomycin are bactericidal for growing cells, and the killing rate of the compounds increases as their concentration is raised. The potency of the antibiotics is likewise increased as the pH increases.

Streptomycin displays a serious toxic effect on the eighth nerve and vestibular apparatus. The relative infrequency of this injury in the therapy of acute infections indicates that duration of therapy or total dose of the antibiotic is the crucial factor. After prolonged streptomycin therapy, a significant number of patients will notice vertigo, tinnitus, and eighth-nerve deafness which may be irreversible. Dihydrostreptomycin has much less tendency to affect hearing and the vestibular apparatus. Either compound may induce sensitivity reactions, including contact dermatitis among personnel handling the drug; however, the incidence is lower with dihydrostreptomycin.

Both drugs are available for intramuscular, oral, and topical administration. The average daily dose when administered systemically is 1 to 2 Gm. However, as with any antibiotic, dosage must be regulated according to severity of infection and sensitivity of infecting organism. The crystalline material is dissolved in isotonic salt solution or distilled water and is given intramuscularly.

For oral administration (for local effect in the gastro-intestinal tract only), 2 to 3 Gm. dissolved in fruit juices, milk, or other suitable vehicle are administered three to six times daily. Twenty-five or 50 mg. of the dry material in 1 to 2 cc. of distilled water may be used as aerosol therapy against respiratory infections caused by sensitive organisms.

Solutions containing 0.25 to 0.5 mg. per cc. may be used in treating wound and eye infections. Intrathecal injections of 20 mg. of dihydrostreptomycin in 8 to 10 cc. of isotonic salt solution have been used in the treatment of influenzal and tuberculous meningitis (see p. 166).

AUREOMYCIN

Aureomycin is an antibiotic derived from cultures of *Streptomyces aureofaciens.* It has not been crystallized, but it is known to be a weakly basic, organic compound containing both nitrogen and nonionic chloride and having a molecular weight of not less than 508. It is unstable in an alkaline medium and when in contact with serum or water.

In vitro, aureomycin possesses bacteriostatic and, in higher concentrations, bactericidal properties. Determinations of minimal inhibitory concentrations are difficult because of its instability in solution at incubator temperature. In low concentrations it inhibits the growth of most gram-negative organisms, but on a weight basis it is considerably less active than penicillin against most gram-positive organisms. Large doses of the drug (up to 100 mg. per Kg. per day) have been given to individuals for periods of as long as seven weeks without evidence of hematological, renal, or hepatic damage.

Aureomycin is indicated in the treatment of resistant gram-negative urinary tract infections, rickettsial diseases (p. 16), virus pneumonia (p. 117), and brucellosis (p. 2). Its value in the treatment of other diseases has not been fully evaluated (see Table 31, p. 290).

Aureomycin appears to be rapidly absorbed when administered orally or intramuscularly. Intramuscular use of the drug is limited because of pain and the development of erythematous and tender areas at the sites of repeated injections. Small amounts of aureomycin appear in the cerebrospinal, pleural, and ascitic fluids following administration. The concentration in bile is from eight to sixteen times that in the serum. Renal excretion is rapid.

The need for parenteral therapy with aureomycin is limited, and in most cases oral use gives satisfactory results. The initial dose of 10 mg. per Kg. (4.5 mg. per lb.) of body weight is divided into three or four parts and given at hourly intervals. In severe infections the initial dose may be increased by half. The total daily maintenance dose is calculated on the basis of 25 to 50 mg. per Kg. (11 to 22 mg. per lb.) of body weight and given in divided amounts at four to six-hour intervals until the infection is controlled. In emergency, aureomycin may be given intravenously. Doses of 3 to 5 mg. per Kg. (1.4 to 2.2 mg. per lb.) of body weight are dissolved in dextrose or isotonic salt solution and are given by drip. Administration may be repeated every eight to twelve hours until the drug can be taken by mouth. Inflammatory reactions are occasionally seen in the vein.

Untoward reactions to aureomycin are mild and consist mainly in nausea, vomiting, and diarrhea. When doses of 50 mg. per Kg. are maintained for a long period of time, emotional symptoms resembling mild depression have been noted; these disappear promptly when the dosage of the antibiotic is reduced or medication is discontinued.

CHLORAMPHENICOL

Chloramphenicol (Chloromycetin) was originally obtained from cultures of *Streptomyces venezuelae*, but chemical synthesis is now possible. The structural formula is shown in Figure 7, page 288. It is of considerable interest to the chemist because of the rarity in nature of aromatic nitro compounds and derivatives of dichloroacetic acid. The compound is a neutral substance of bitter taste, stable in solution over a pH range of 2 to 9 and unaffected by boiling in distilled water. At room temperatures it is soluble to the extent of 0.25 percent in water and 15 percent in propylene glycol.

The antibiotic is indicated in the treatment of typhoid fever (p. 14), the rickettsial diseases (typhus, p. 17; Rocky Mountain spotted fever, p. 18; scrub typhus, p. 18), and certain gram-negative urinary tract infections. It is of some value in the treatment of brucellosis when given in combination with streptomycin (p. 290), but its usefulness in the treatment of virus infections, cholera, whooping cough, relapsing fever, and bacillary dysentery has not been thoroughly established.

Assays in experimental animals and man show that chloramphenicol is rapidly and almost completely absorbed from the gastro-intestinal tract; blood concentrations of the active form of the drug reach a peak within two hours after ingestion. The amounts of chloramphenicol in the bile are comparable to those in the blood, but cerebrospinal fluid levels are lower and are reached more slowly. The antibiotic is excreted largely in the urine, the amounts normally reaching 200 to 700 micrograms per cc. two hours after 1 and 2-Gm. doses.

Chloramphenicol should be given by mouth, for intravenous and intramuscular administration produce local reactions and undesirable side-effects. In treating moderate or severe infections, a large initial quantity should be administered to establish effective blood concentrations promptly. The first dose (60 mg. per Kg. [27.5 mg. per lb.] of body weight) is divided into three or four doses which are given at hourly intervals. The daily maintenance dose of 30 to 60 mg. per Kg. of body weight is given in divided doses every four to six hours.

There are few toxic reactions to chloramphenicol administered orally. An occasional patient may develop nausea, vomiting, or diarrhea.

BACITRACIN

Bacitracin is an antibiotic obtained from an aerobic strain of *Bacillus subtilis*. Its chemical structure is not known, but it appears to be a protein. The material is a light powder that is freely soluble in water, neutral in reaction, and stable in the dry state at room temperature. When in solution, bacitracin retains its potency for three weeks at room temperature.

Experimental work and clinical usage demonstrate that bacitracin has a range of activity which parallels that of penicillin, and experience indicates that (1) bacitracin rarely induces sensitization, and (2) there is no cross sensitivity to the two antibiotics. The clinical usefulness of bacitracin has been limited, however, because of its toxic action on the kidneys when administered parenterally.

It is possible that further refinement may produce a form which can be given systemically. Oral administration is without hazard because the drug is not absorbed from the gastro-intestinal tract.

Bacitracin is now employed in two ways: by topical application in local infections and by oral administration in gastro-intestinal infections. The oral dosage is 100,000 to 200,000 units daily in divided quantities. In the local treatment of pyogenic skin infections, surgical infections, localized abscesses of the skin and subcutaneous tissues, and external pyogenic ocular infections, it is applied in a strength of 500 units per Gm. or cc. in the form of ointment or solution; or 0.2 to 5 cc. of such a concentration in sterile isotonic salt solution may be injected locally into the base of a pyogenic lesion. The antibiotic is also available in combination with a vasoconstrictor for intranasal administration and as a lozenge for local oral therapy.

Even though it is not administered clinically by this route, bacitracin is readily absorbed following intramuscular injection and reaches a maximum blood concentration in two hours. It is distributed to pleural and ascitic fluids, but only traces are found in pericardial and cerebrospinal fluids. A considerable amount of systemically administered bacitracin is either retained or metabolized in the body, for only 9 to 30 percent appears in the urine over a twenty-four-hour period.

TYROTHRICIN

Tyrothricin is an antibiotic obtained from cultures of *Bacillus brevis* and consists of two active principles, gramicidin and tyrocidine. The material is insoluble in water and body fluids. It is rapidly destroyed by gastric juice but remains active in the presence of serum, pus, or urine.

Tyrothricin is toxic when injected intramuscularly or intravenously. In experimental animals, the reactions are those of a hemolytic effect, with death due to respiratory failure.

Clinically, tyrothricin is of value in the topical therapy of leg ulcer and chronic skin infections. Since one of the active principles (tyrocidine) is effective against both gram-negative and gram-positive infections, the material can be used in treating contaminated wounds. Unfortunately, sensitization is not uncommon.

Tyrothricin is available (usual concentration, 0.5 mg. per Gm. or cc.) in the form of ointments, in solutions containing a vasoconstrictor, and also as tablets (containing 1 mg.) for local oral therapy. It should not be administered systemically.

TERRAMYCIN

Terramycin is a new antibiotic obtained from cultures of *Streptomyces rimosus*. It is a crystalline amphoteric substance that forms crystalline salts with either acids or bases. It is sparingly soluble in water, but its solutions are reasonably stable. A unit of terramycin has been defined as 1 microgram of the pure compound.

The antibiotic has in-vitro and in-vivo activity against a wide variety of both gram-positive and gram-negative bacteria. As of this writing, it is undergoing intensive clinical investigation.

SULFONAMIDES

To the chemist, the term "sulfonamide" designates only an amide of a sulfonic acid. In medicine, the term is applied to a group of substances consisting of para-aminobenzenesulfonamide (sulfanilamide) and its derivatives. Several thousand such sulfonamides have been prepared; relatively few have found wide use in medicine. The more important compounds are shown in Figure 8 (p. 294). Sulfapyridine and sulfaguanidine are not shown because they are very little used. Sulfanilamide itself has also been largely superseded by more effective and less toxic derivatives.

It will be noted that in the first six formulas after sulfanilamide itself the substitution is entirely in the amido group (N_1) which is attached to the sulfone radical. These substances are readily absorbed after oral or parenteral administration. The last two formulas contain substitutions in the amino group (N_4) which is attached directly to the benzene ring. These compounds are poorly absorbed from the gastro-intestinal tract and are employed only for treatment of gastro-intestinal infections. All of the sulfonamides shown in Figure 8 are white crystalline substances which are sparingly soluble in water. Their solubility increases as the *p*H or temperature of the medium is raised.

The sulfonamides are capable of preventing the growth and reproduction of certain types of bacteria, and under especially favorable conditions the organisms are killed outright. The most susceptible types include streptococci, staphylococci, pneumococci, gonococci, meningococci, *Escherichia coli*, *Hemophilus influenzae*, *Aerobacter aerogenes* (*B. aerogenes*), and *Proteus vulgaris*. Much less susceptible are *Salmonella typhimurium*, *Lactobacillus acidophilus* (*B. acidophilus*), and *Pseudomonas aeruginosa* (*B. pyocyaneus*), which are frequent causes of urinary tract infection.

The antibacterial action of the sulfonamides ap-

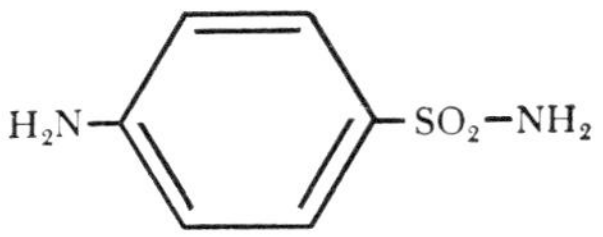

Sulfanilamide

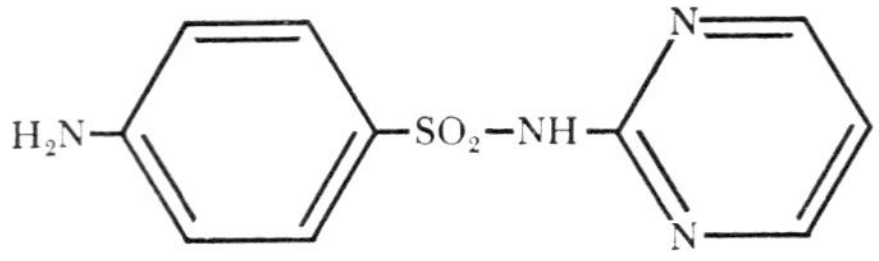

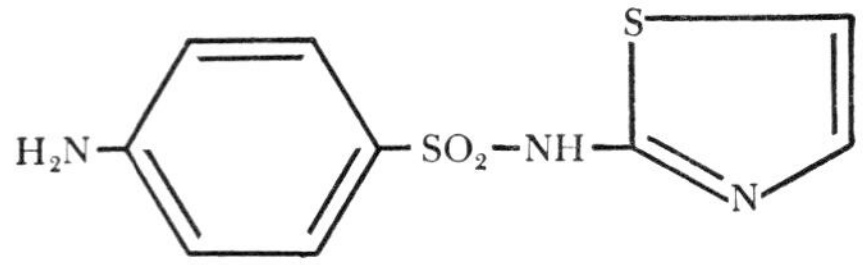

Sulfathiazole

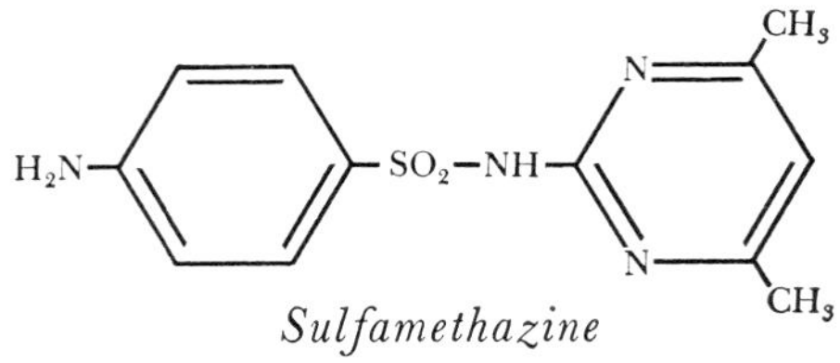

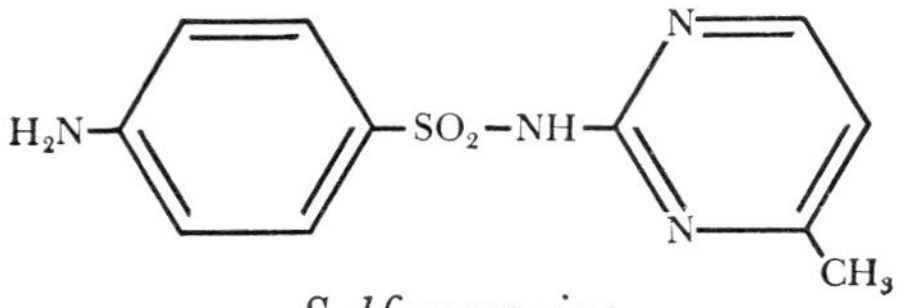

Sulfadiazine

Sulfamerazine

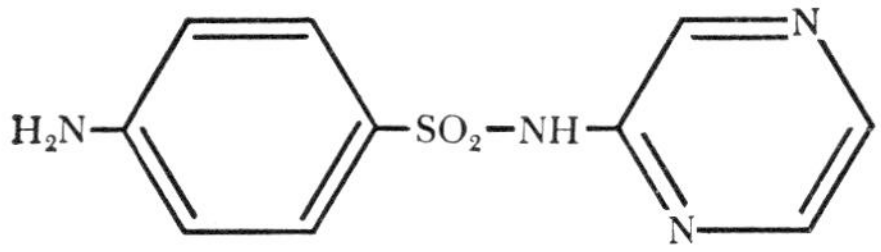

Sulfamethazine

Sulfapyrazine

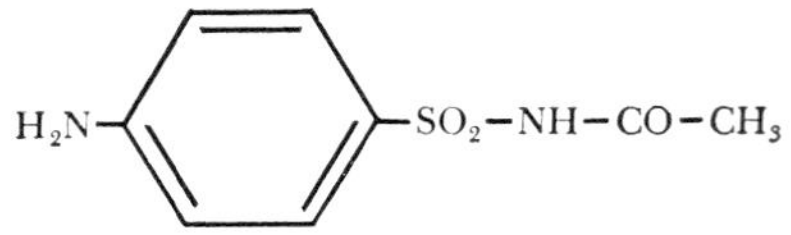

Sulfacetimide

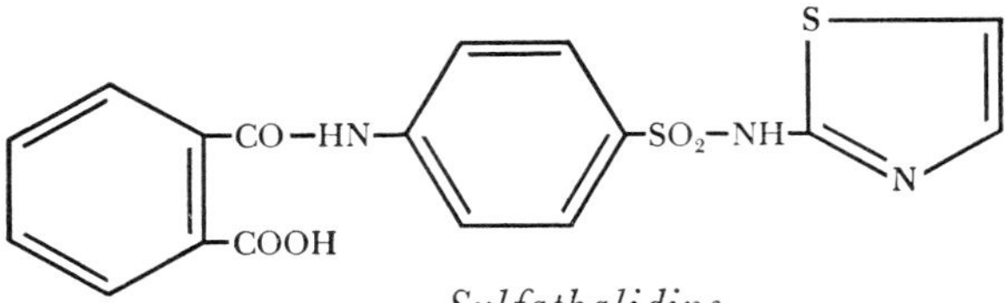

Sulfathalidine
(*Phthalylsulfathiazole*)

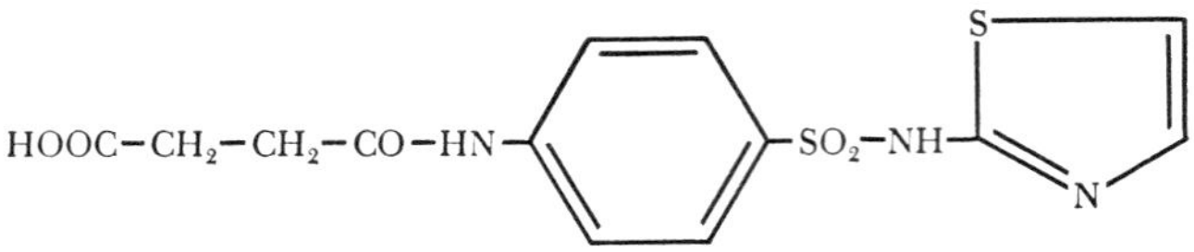

Sulfasuxidine
(*Succinylsulfathiazole*)

FIGURE 8—*Structural Formulas of Sulfonamides*

pears to depend on competition with para-amino-benzoic acid, $H_2N \cdot C_6H_4 \cdot COOH$, for a place in the enzyme system of the micro-organism. It would seem that when a sufficient number of para-amino-benzoic acid groups have been replaced by sulfon-amide groups, the bacterium is unable to grow or to multiply. This explanation is in accord with the actual observation that the antibacterial action of the sulfonamides is prevented by unnaturally high concentrations of para-aminobenzoic acid and by procaine and other substances which liberate para-aminobenzoic acid in the body. The effectiveness of the sulfonamides is also impaired by the presence of pus or other products of tissue breakdown which presumably liberate para-aminobenzoic acid.

From the qualitative point of view, there is apparently little difference in the action of the various sulfonamides. The more recently developed compounds (sulfathiazole, sulfadiazine, sulfamerazine, sulfamethazine, and sulfapyrazine) have practically the same degree of effectiveness. There are, however, differences in solubility, absorption, penetration, metabolism, and rate of excretion.

After absorption into the blood stream, a portion of the sulfonamide is bound to plasma protein and rendered inactive. Another portion is conjugated with other groups, especially the acetyl group, $CH_3 \cdot CO \cdot$. It is the N_4 amino group (which is directly attached to the benzene ring) that is acetylated (see Figure 8), forming, in the case of sulfanilamide, N_4-acetylsulfanilamide, $CH_3 \cdot CO \cdot NH \cdot C_6H_4 \cdot SO_2 \cdot NH_2$. Other sulfonamides form analogous compounds. The conjugation takes place mainly in the liver, and the conjugated forms are therapeutically inactive. Acetylated sulfanilamide (N_4) must be distinguished from N_1-acetylsulfanilamide (sulfacetimide, see Figure 8), which is therapeutically active.

For the drugs in the absorbable group, the rate of absorption is rapid, blood concentrations from a single oral dose reaching their peak in one to six hours. Among the more commonly used compounds, absorption is most rapid for sulfathiazole, followed by sulfamerazine, sulfadiazine, sulfapyrazine, and sulfamethazine. In clinical use, these differences are not important. When the sodium salt of a sulfonamide is used intravenously, immediate passage of the drugs to the different tissues is secured.

The absorbable sulfonamides are diffused throughout the various organs and fluids of the body, their penetration being influenced by their degree of combination with plasma proteins, which do not normally pass out of the blood vessels. Sulfadiazine combines in relatively small percentage with plasma proteins, and, accordingly, its concentration in the spinal fluid averages 75 percent of that in the blood. The corresponding percentages for other drugs are sulfanilamide and sulfamerazine, 50 percent; sulfathiazole, 30 percent.

The sulfonamides are excreted in the urine to the extent of 80 to 90 percent of the quantity administered. Sulfanilamide and sulfathiazole escape most rapidly and sulfamerazine most slowly. The percentage which is in acetylated form varies with the drug and with the patient.

With sulfanilamide and sulfapyridine, the side-effects of dizziness, headache, mental confusion, cyanosis (methemoglobinemia), and acidosis were commonly observed; less frequently, there was thrombocytopenic purpura or hemolytic anemia. These effects are very rare with the newer sulfonamides. There may be occasional instances of gastric intolerance; allergic skin reactions occur in 1 to 4 percent of patients receiving the drugs; and leukocytolysis and leukopenia are seen in less than 1 percent.

The possible side-effect of the presently used sulfonamides that merits the greatest consideration is precipitation of the drug in the renal tubules, which may be associated with hematuria, tubular degeneration, and tubular obstruction. The solubility of the sulfonamides and their N_4-acetyl derivatives is somewhat low in urine, as it is in water. It is diminished by acidity and increased by alkalinity. Since on most diets and during starvation there is a net balance of acid to be excreted by the kidneys, a reduction in total daily urine volume causes an increase in the concentration of acid (decrease of pH) in that urine, and an augmentation of urine volume lessens the concentration of acid. It is for this reason that *all patients under sulfonamide therapy should take a sufficient quantity of fluid to maintain an adequate urine volume* (1,500 cc. daily for adults) *and should receive alkalizing therapy* (p. 352) *whenever the urinary pH falls below* 5.5.

The danger of sulfonamide precipitation in the kidneys can be still further reduced by the administration of sulfonamide mixtures. The solubility of each of the sulfonamides is independent of the presence of the others, and the use of mixtures maintains the therapeutic effect while reducing very greatly the chance of precipitation. Since they are of approximately equal potency, the administration of 2 Gm. each of sulfathiazole, sulfadiazine, and sulfamerazine, for example, has the same therapeutic action as 6 Gm. of one of the three, but the amount to be excreted is the equivalent of only 2 Gm.

If, in spite of precautions, renal complications should occur, the drug is discontinued, and adequate quantities of fluid and alkali are administered (see under Crush Syndrome, p. 222).

When the well-absorbed sulfonamides are given for systemic effect, the oral route is preferred. Sulfathiazole, sulfadiazine, sulfamerazine, sulfamethazine, and sulfapyrazine can be used more or less interchangeably, and preferably in mixtures. In order to establish a high concentration in the body, the initial dose should be large—3 to 6 Gm. in adults, and one-half the calculated twenty-four-hour maintenance dose in children. The maintenance dosage for adults is 1 Gm. every four hours; infants and children should receive 1 to 2 grains (0.06 to 0.12 Gm.) per pound of body weight per day, divided into six equally spaced doses. If the drug must be administered by stomach tube, it is dissolved in tap water. It may also be given rectally in 2 percent solution.

In case of necessity, the sulfonamides can be given intravenously or by hypodermoclysis. The sodium salts are employed in the same doses as the free sulfonamides by mouth. One-sixth-molar sodium lactate solution (p. 349) is the best solvent, although isotonic sodium chloride solution is permissible. Strengths up to 5 percent may be given by vein, and 0.5 to 0.8 percent subcutaneously.

For local action, the sulfonamides in powder form may be sprinkled into open wounds. They have also been incorporated into ointments (5 to 20 percent), lozenges, chewing gum, and dental cones. Sulfacetimide (Sulamyd) is more soluble than the preparations named above; it is, however, much less potent and, since much of it is converted into sulfanilamide in the body, shares the disadvantages of sulfanilamide for systemic administration. It is of value for local application in conjunctival infections.

The soluble but poorly absorbed sulfonamides, Sulfasuxidine (succinylsulfathiazole) and Sulfathalidine (phthalylsulfathiazole), are useful in treatment of gram-negative infections within the intestine and for preparation of patients for intestinal surgery. They provide a high concentration of drug in the bowel and a low concentration in the blood and tissues. Sulfasuxidine is effective against bacillary dysentery (p. 4); Sulfathalidine is not recommended for this purpose. The daily dose of Sulfasuxidine is 0.25 Gm. per Kg. (0.1 Gm. per lb.) of body weight, subdivided into six equally spaced administrations. A total daily quantity should be given as an initial dose. Sulfathalidine is given in an initial dose of 0.125 Gm. per Kg. (0.05 Gm. per lb.) and in maintenance doses of 3 to 7 Gm., subdivided as for Sulfasuxidine. The maintenance dose for children is 0.05 to 0.1 Gm. per Kg. (0.025 to 0.05 Gm. per lb.).

PARA-AMINOSALICYLIC ACID

Para-aminosalicylic acid (also known as PAS or PASA), $H_2N \cdot C_6H_3(OH)(COOH)$, is not a sulfonamide, but it is closely related to this group of drugs. It is a white crystalline substance which is only slightly soluble in water but is readily soluble in alkali. It is decomposed by heat, light, and excessive moisture. As a chemical compound, para-aminosalicylic acid has long been known, but only recently has it found use in medicine. The substance was discovered to increase the oxygen consumption and carbon-dioxide production of the tubercle bacillus, and it was considered possible that this stimulant action on the metabolism of the organism might make the latter more susceptible to the antibacterial effect of antibiotics.

Clinical investigation has shown that para-aminosalicylic acid is of definite value as an adjunct to streptomycin and dihydrostreptomycin in the treatment of tuberculosis. Not only does para-aminosalicylic acid appear to potentiate the effects of the antibiotics, but the emergence of organisms resistant to the latter drugs is inhibited or significantly delayed. Recently developed, exudative pulmonary lesions seem to respond most favorably. Renal and gastro-intestinal lesions and tuberculous peritonitis are also benefited. Less improvement has been obtained in chronic fibroid lesions in the lungs. The results in other types of the disease are currently being studied.

Following oral administration, the absorption of para-aminosalicylic acid shows large individual variations. After a single dose, the blood concentration of the drug reaches a maximum in one to three hours, and renal excretion is practically complete in ten to twelve hours. The drug is distributed widely in the tissue fluids, in which there is apparently no storage of the material after it disappears from the blood. It is extremely soluble in the urine, more so as the pH increases.

As an adjunct to streptomycin and dihydrostreptomycin in the treatment of tuberculosis, para-aminosalicylic acid is administered by mouth in quantities of 10 to 15 Gm. daily. The total amount is subdivided into four or more individual doses spread over the waking period. It appears to have some value when given alone. The side-effects of nausea, vomiting, and diarrhea are not uncommon. They tend to disappear as treatment is continued for a few days, and they can be minimized or prevented by administration of the drug in enteric coating. In an occasional case, proteinuria, hematuria, or allergic reactions have been observed; they disappeared promptly on cessation of therapy.

ANTISYPHILITIC DRUGS

The first synthetic chemotherapeutic drugs—the arsenicals investigated by Ehrlich—were intended for the treatment of syphilis. Since that time, steady progress has been made toward Ehrlich's goal of a *therapia sterilisans*, and it is just possible that with the advent of penicillin the goal is in sight.

PENICILLIN

It is, of course, recognized that syphilis is a disease of chronicity and latency (see p. 10) and that years of observation are required to evaluate fully a new form of treatment. Nevertheless, it seems likely that penicillin has displaced all other antisyphilitic drugs. The dosage of penicillin in syphilis is given on page 11. The general properties and uses of penicillin are discussed beginning on page 288.

ORGANIC ARSENICALS

Until the advent of penicillin, the organic arsenicals were the most active antisyphilitic agents. All of them are potentially toxic drugs which must be employed intelligently if best results are to be obtained. Only the barest principles of their use can be given here, and it is suggested that standard textbooks on syphilis be consulted for additional discussion.

The organic arsenicals are capable of producing several types of systemic side-effects: The Jarisch-Herxheimer reaction, also known as therapeutic shock, may occur with any active treponemicidal drug. It consists of a general response (fever and malaise) and a focal response (intensification of the inflammatory or exudative process in the lesions of the disease). It is analogous to the reaction which may occur when a patient with active tuberculosis is given tuberculin subcutaneously. It follows the first injection only and is believed to be due to toxic products released from the bodies of large numbers of spirochetes which are killed almost simultaneously. It is especially dangerous to patients with tertiary syphilis of the cardiovascular system, larynx, or central nervous system, in whom focal reactions may have serious consequences. Jarisch-Herxheimer reactions are avoided by (1) preliminary treatment with bismuth before the arsenical is begun and (2) small initial dosage of the arsenical.

Other reactions include speed shock (nitritoid reaction), which is discussed on page 285; angioneurotic edema; vomiting, diarrhea, headache, and malaise beginning four to twelve hours after injection and lasting sometimes as long as several days; various forms of skin eruption, the most severe of which is exfoliative dermatitis; blood dyscrasias, including thrombocytopenia, agranulo-cytosis, and aplastic anemia; polyneuritis; and hemorrhagic encephalitis. The reactions involving the skin, bone marrow, and central nervous system are apparently allergic. They can usually be controlled with dimercaprol (see p. 514). Serious reactions contraindicate further arsenical therapy.

Arsphenamine (606) was the first organic arsenical to be used successfully in the treatment of syphilis. It is a basic substance, the structural formula of which is shown in Figure 9. Because of the instability of the base, it is marketed as the dihydrochloride acid salt, which is an amorphous yellow powder. Before injection, the drug must be carefully alkalinized to form the disodium salt. The difficulty in preparation and administration makes this drug of little use to the general practitioner.

Neoarsphenamine is a derivative of arsphenamine containing 19 to 22 percent arsenic in trivalent form and having the formula shown in Figure 9. It is a yellow powder which dissolves in water to produce a neutral solution. Neoarsphenamine is useful when a vigorous antitreponemal activity is desired. It has, therefore, been used in primary and secondary syphilis and, after a preliminary course of a less vigorous agent such as bismuth, in latent and tertiary syphilis, including neurosyphilis.

The drug is contraindicated in patients who have an idiosyncrasy to arsenic and in the presence of cachexia or of severe disease of the cardiovascular or central nervous system unless these are due to syphilis.

Neoarsphenamine is given intravenously in courses of ten to twenty injections. In early syphilis, treatment is continuous; in late syphilis a rest period of four to six weeks is allowed after five to ten weeks of treatment, during which interval a bismuth compound is administered. In early syphilis, injections are usually given twice weekly; in late syphilis the period may be extended to once weekly. The size of the individual dose depends in large part on the patient's weight; one rule is to allow 0.1 to 0.15 Gm. for each 25 lb. of body weight for both men and women (except during pregnancy). The initial dose should never exceed half this quantity, but the full dose should be reached by the third or fourth injection. In general, the frequency of treatment varies inversely with the size of the individual dose, with preference for frequent small doses.

Neoarsphenamine deteriorates rapidly on exposure to air, and consequently rigid precautions must be taken in preparing solutions for injection.

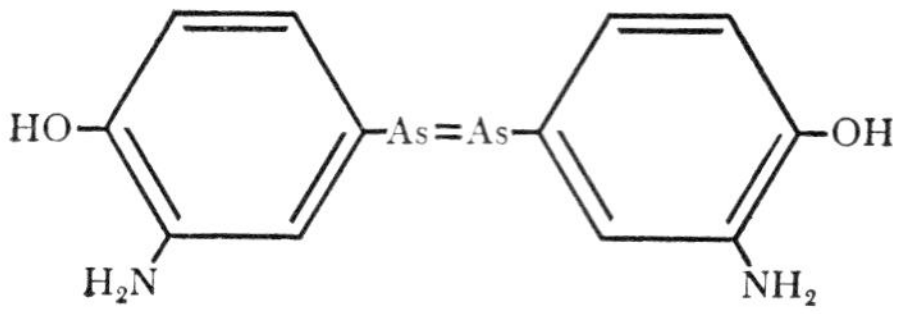

Arsphenamine

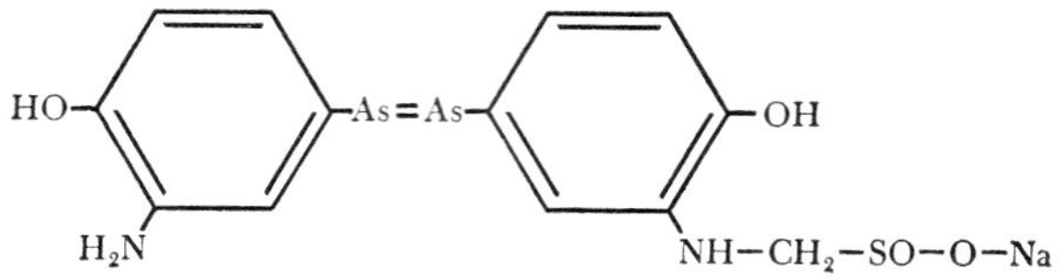

Neoarsphenamine

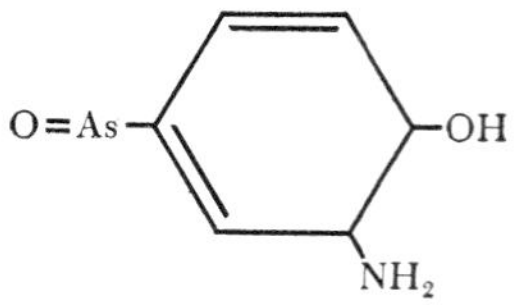

Oxophenarsine
(Arsenoxide, Mapharsen)

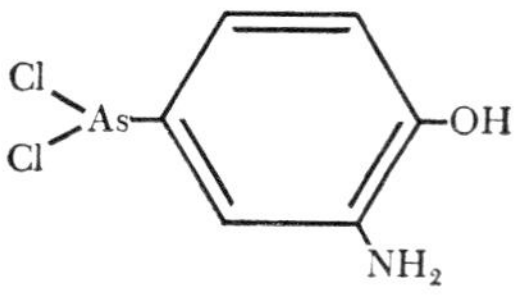

Dichlorophenarsine
(Clorarsen)

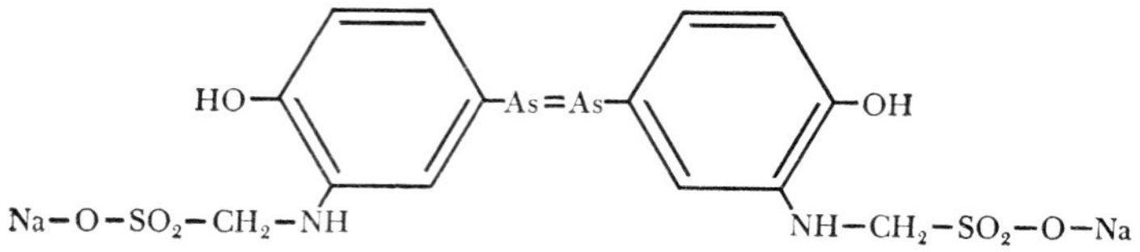

Sulfarsphenamine

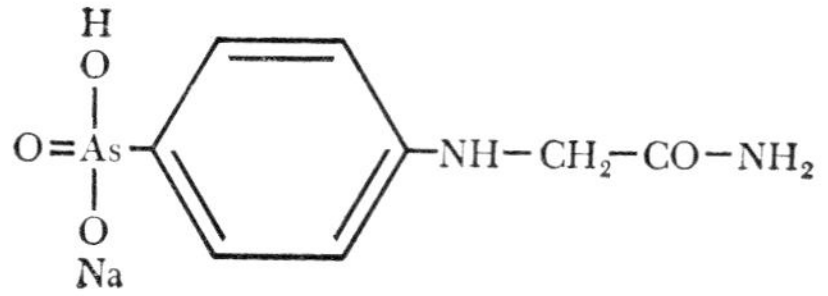

Tryparsamide

FIGURE 9—*Structural Formulas of Antisyphilitic Drugs*

The ampoule containing the drug is immersed in alcohol for the detection of possible cracks. If the powder does not become wet, the outside of the ampoule is dried and the neck is filed and broken. The contents are sprinkled on the surface of 10 cc. of *cool* sterile distilled water and are allowed to dissolve *without shaking*. If the contents do not dissolve completely, they are discarded. The solution is injected, without warming, immediately after preparation. It must not be allowed to stand.

Intravenous injection must be *slow*. It should be timed with a watch, and the rate should not exceed 0.1 Gm. of drug each thirty seconds. In some patients it must be slower if speed shock (nitritoid reaction) is to be avoided (p. 285). Care must be taken to avoid paravenous injection, for the drug is very irritating to the subcutaneous tissues and may produce necrosis and sloughing. If extravasation takes place, the region should be promptly infiltrated with a large quantity of an isotonic electrolyte solution (such as Ringer's) containing a local anesthetic agent. The arsenical is thus diluted at the same time that the pain is relieved. Solutions of neoarsphenamine may also produce thrombophlebitis.

Oxophenarsine (arsenoxide, Mapharsen) is a partial oxidation product of arsphenamine (for structural formula, see Figure 9). It contains 29 percent trivalent arsenic. Oxophenarsine has two principal advantages over the arsphenamines: It and its solutions are stable, and it produces fewer skin reactions and a negligible incidence of nitritoid reactions. In efficacy it is apparently the equal, or nearly the equal, of neoarsphenamine.

Administration is intravenous and should be *rapid*, in contrast to that of neoarsphenamine. The drug is given in courses in the same way as neoarsphenamine. Individual doses average 6 to 7 mg. per 25 lb. of body weight, with a maximum single dose of 60 mg. Oxophenarsine is usually well tolerated but should not be given to patients who have any form of arsenical sensitivity.

Dichlorophenarsine (Clorarsen) is closely related chemically to oxophenarsine (see Figure 9). It contains about 26 percent trivalent arsenic. The ampoules as marketed contain an alkaline buffer; on the addition of water a reaction occurs, and oxophenarsine is believed to be formed. It is thought that the latter substance is the therapeutically active agent.

Dichlorophenarsine is used in the same way as oxophenarsine, and it has the same therapeutic properties. The dosage is about 10 percent greater than that of oxophenarsine, corresponding to the smaller arsenic content.

Sulfarsphenamine has the formula shown in Figure 9. It contains 19 percent trivalent arsenic. It is a light-yellow powder which is stable in dry form and for many hours in solution. Sulfarsphenamine is used almost exclusively for the treatment of congenital syphilis in infants and young children. It should not be given to adults because of the frequency of serious reactions in them. It is administered in courses of six to eight injections of 10 to 25 mg. per Kg. (4.5 to 10 mg. per lb.) of body weight (maximum single dose, 400 to 500 mg.), alternating with bismuth. In contradistinction to other arsphenamine derivatives, it is injected intramuscularly rather than intravenously.

Bismarsen (bismuth arsphenamine sulfonate) contains about 13 percent arsenic and 24 percent bismuth. Its exact structural formula is unknown. It is a brownish-yellow powder that is readily soluble in water and oxidizes slowly in air. Bismarsen is the slowest acting of the arsphenamine derivatives, and it tends to cause local pain after injection. It is administered intramuscularly. The usual initial dose is 0.1 Gm., and succeeding doses are 0.2 Gm. A local anesthetic agent is usually employed as a solvent. A course is made up of twenty injections given once a week at first and, later, twice a week.

Tryparsamide contains about 25 percent of pentavalent arsenic (see Figure 9 for structural formula). It is used in the treatment of syphilis only when the central nervous system is involved; it does not affect syphilis in other tissues. It has a specific toxic action on the optic nerves which necessitates extreme caution in its use. Visual fields must be carefully mapped before and at weekly intervals during treatment. Contraindications are any contraction of the fields or other evidence of optic damage or atrophy.

Administration is intravenous, and the dosage for adults varies from 1 to 3 Gm. dissolved in 10 to 20 cc. of sterile distilled water. A course usually consists in ten to twelve weekly injections.

BISMUTH COMPOUNDS

Bismuth compounds have an interesting place in the treatment of syphilis. Bismuth is less actively treponemicidal than the arsphenamines and also less toxic. Its mode of action is unknown. Clinically, it is an excellent supplement to the arsphenamines early and late in the management of syphilis.

Bismuth is useful in latent, asymptomatic syphilis, in which it provides an adequate and safe therapy without disturbing the body's resistance and defense mechanism. It is effective as preparatory treatment for the arsenicals, averting the reactions and unsatisfactory results which may accompany the sudden exhibition of arsenic. It is also recommended as a "finishing" treatment with which to "taper off" a course of arsenical.

Bismuth is valuable in late syphilis with minor manifestations; in this situation it averts the risks of the arsenicals. It has good symptomatic effect in late neurosyphilis; it is invaluable in patients who are resistant or intolerant to the arsphenamines or who for some other reason should not receive arsenic; and it is useful in old age and in patients with renal disease.

On the other hand, bismuth should not be relied upon to the exclusion of the arsphenamines, particularly in early syphilis. Even though Jarisch-Herxheimer reactions are uncommon with bismuth, they may occur, especially when tertiary syphilis has involved the liver or the cardiovascular system.

After absorption, bismuth is stored in the tissues, from which it is released and excreted slowly over a long period of time. Excretion is mainly in the urine, but a significant amount appears in the feces, even after parenteral administration. After intramuscular injection, salts of the metal appear in the urine within a day and continue to appear for twenty to thirty days. Massage of the injection site speeds absorption. The more quickly absorbed compounds are excreted more rapidly.

In clinical use, bismuth compounds may be given in courses alternating with the arsphenamines, or they may be given concurrently. When used together, the dose of both the bismuth compound and the arsenical may be reduced. Bismuth preparations are classified as to solubility: Water-soluble or water-miscible compounds act quickly and must be given frequently; oil solutions act somewhat more slowly; suspensions of insoluble compounds act most slowly but eventually have the most sustained effect.

The number of bismuth compounds which are available is very large. With slowly absorbed compounds which are to be given for a long period, an average dosage level should contain about 0.5 mg. of *bismuth metal* per Kg. of body weight per day. When water-soluble compounds are to be given for rapid effect over a short period, the dosage in terms of *bismuth metal* should be about 0.7 mg. per Kg. per day.

All injections should be intramuscular, and the site should be well massaged afterward. An air bubble left in the syringe during preparation and injected after the medication, cleans the needle and minimizes the chance of depositing the drug along the needle track in the subcutaneous tissues. Before each injection, the site of the last previous injection should be palpated. Induration or tenderness is an indication of poor tolerance to the preparation employed; if the technic of injection has been adequate, repeated evidence of intolerance should lead to a change in bismuth preparation.

Compounds given in water solution include:

Bismuth sodium tartrate (about 73 percent Bi), given three times weekly.
Bismuth sodium thioglycollate (Thio-Bismol; about 38 percent Bi), given twice weekly.
Sodium iodobismuthite (Iodobismitol; about 21 percent Bi), given twice weekly.

Preparations injected as oil solutions include:

Bismuth camphocarboxylate (Bismo-Cymol; about 38 percent Bi), given every five to seven days.
Bismuth ethylcamphorate, given every five to seven days.

Compounds given as suspensions include:

Bismuth subsalicylate in oil (about 57 percent Bi), given once weekly.
Bismuth potassium tartrate in oil (about 62 percent Bi), given once weekly.

In the form of Sobisminol Mass, a complex organic product, bismuth is effective by the oral route, but it is relatively little used in this form because of uncertainty in the physician's mind as to the faithfulness with which the medication is being taken.

Bismuth has relatively low toxicity, and side-effects are very infrequent except after injudicious use, as exemplified by overdosage or intravenous administration. Intoxication may cause anorexia; vomiting; diarrhea; black deposits of bismuth sulfide in the mucous membranes, and particularly near the margins of the gums; stomatitis with ulceration of the tongue, gums, and buccal mucosa; weakness; slowness and in-co-ordination of movement; and, in especially severe cases, tetanic convulsions, paralysis, and even death.

MERCURY

Mercury exerts a mild and relatively weak antisyphilitic effect. At present its use is limited to difficult therapeutic situations in which Jarisch-Herxheimer reactions would have serious consequences, such as advanced and badly damaged cases of cardiovascular, hepatic, or neurosyphilis. The standard textbooks on syphilis should be consulted for principles and details of administration and dosage.

ANTIMALARIAL DRUGS

World War II stimulated a tremendous amount of research in the treatment of malaria, which resulted in the introduction of several new drugs. These differ in their therapeutic indications as shown in Table 32 and in several other respects as described below. Against specific stages and species of *Plasmodium* they may have prophylactic, suppressive, or curative action or some combination or modification of these. When the drug attacks the pre-erythrocytic stage of the parasite, causal *prophylaxis* is achieved which, if complete, permanently prevents infection. In those cases in which the drug attacks the asexual, erythrocytic parasites, *suppressive* action is gained which lasts as long as the drug is continued. When persistent, fixed-tissue forms of the parasite are attacked, the drug will have a *curative* effect.

Chloroquine (see Figure 10 for structural formula) acts principally on the asexual, erythrocytic parasites. It stops acute attacks of malaria in two or three days. Falciparum infections are usually cured, but relapses from vivax malaria are common one to three months after treatment is stopped. It does not affect the gametocytes of *P. falciparum*. Chloroquine appears to be superior to quinacrine and is believed to be the best drug at present available in the control of paroxysms once they have developed. It is also of value in amebic hepatitis or liver abscess (p. 33).

The recommended therapeutic dosage is 1 Gm. of the diphosphate (0.6 Gm. of the base) followed by an additional 0.5 Gm. in six to eight hours, with

TABLE 32 — *Actions of Antimalarial Drugs*

Drug	Suppressive	Prophylactic	Curative
Chloroquine	++++	0	++++
Quinacrine	+++	0	+++
Chlorguanide	++	+++	++
Primaquine	0	0	++++ (with quinine)
Pentaquine	0	0	++++ (with quinine)
Plasmoquine	0	0	+ (with quinine)
Quinine	++++	0	++

a single dose of 0.5 Gm. on each of the two following days. The suppressive dose is 0.5 Gm. every seven days. The hydrochloride salt has been used for intramuscular administration in doses of 0.225 to 0.335 Gm. (0.2 to 0.3 Gm. of the base).

Side-effects of chloroquine are usually mild, the most common being blurring of vision, pruritus, mild headache, and gastro-intestinal complaints, which subside when the drug is discontinued. Suppressive doses appear to be innocuous.

Quinacrine (Atabrine) is a bright-yellow crystalline powder, the structural formula of which is shown in Figure 10. It acts similarly to chloroquine and does not affect the exoerythrocytic stages of the parasites. If continued long enough, it will permanently prevent *P. falciparum*, but *P. vivax* malaria recurs when the drug is withdrawn.

Dosage of quinacrine dihydrochloride for suppressive purposes is 0.1 Gm. per day. For acute malaria, doses are 0.2 Gm. every six hours for five doses, followed by 0.1 Gm. three times daily for six days, making a total of 2.8 Gm. in seven days. Quinacrine may be given intramuscularly in doses of 0.2 Gm. dissolved in 5 cc. of sterile distilled water. If necessary, injections may be repeated one or two times at six to eight-hour intervals.

Quinacrine is toxic to about the same extent as chloroquine and in similar ways. The principal objection to quinacrine has been that its use discolors the skin. A lichen-planus type of skin eruption has complicated suppressive medication in some areas, but absolute proof of etiology has not been established.

Chlorguanide* (chloroguanide, Paludrine) has a different type of structure from other antimalarial compounds (see Figure 10). The drug will cure *P. falciparum* infection and relieve the clinical manifestations caused by *P. vivax*, although in the latter relapses will occur. Its therapeutic action is somewhat slower than that of the 4-aminoquinoline compounds (such as chloroquine).

Optimal doses of 'Guanatol Hydrochloride' (Chlorguanide Hydrochloride, Lilly) for prevention, suppression, or treatment of malaria will vary in different localities, depending upon the susceptibility of the local strains of organisms to the drug, the immune status of the individual, and the duration and intensity of the infection.

Prevention of falciparum and suppression of vivax malaria have been achieved by oral admin-

---

* Chlorguanide hydrochloride is marketed by Eli Lilly and Company as 'Guanatol Hydrochloride.'

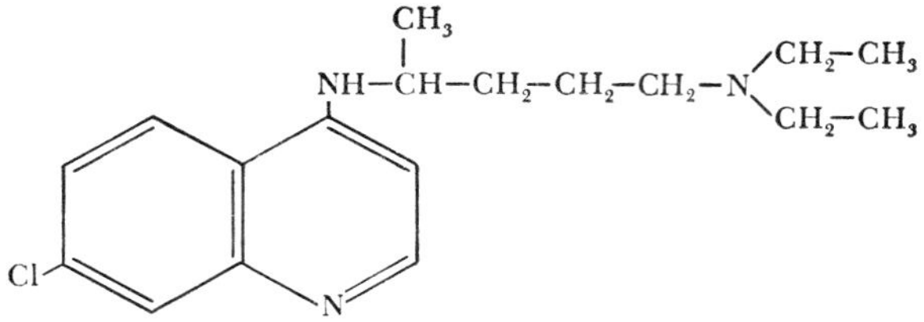

Chloroquine

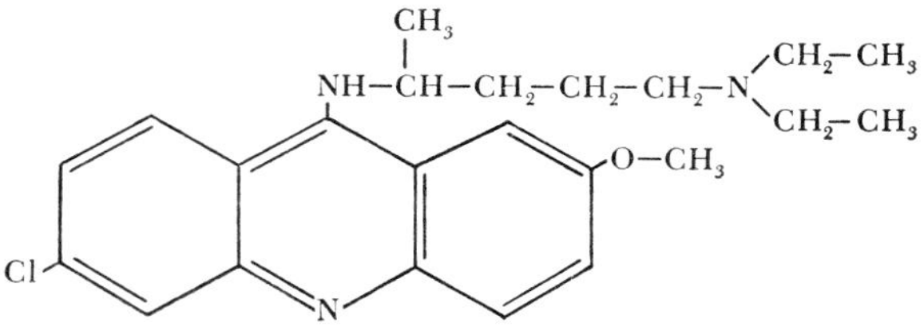

Quinacrine
(Atabrine)

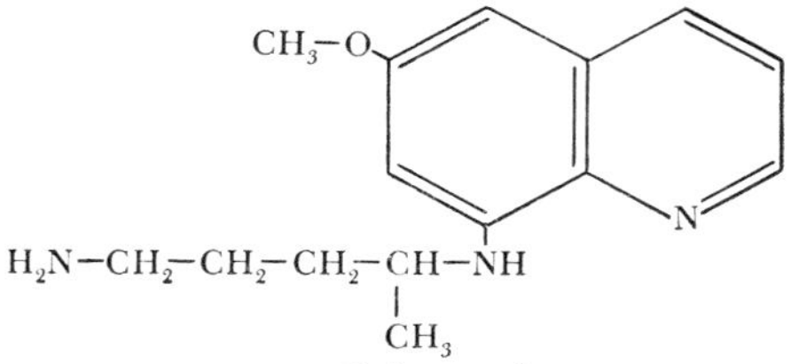

Primaquine

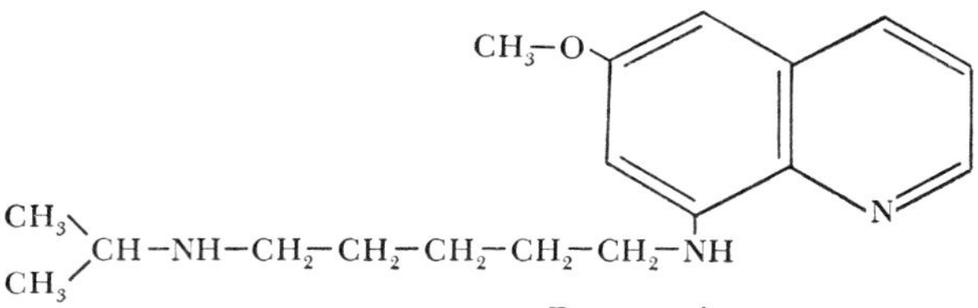

Pentaquine

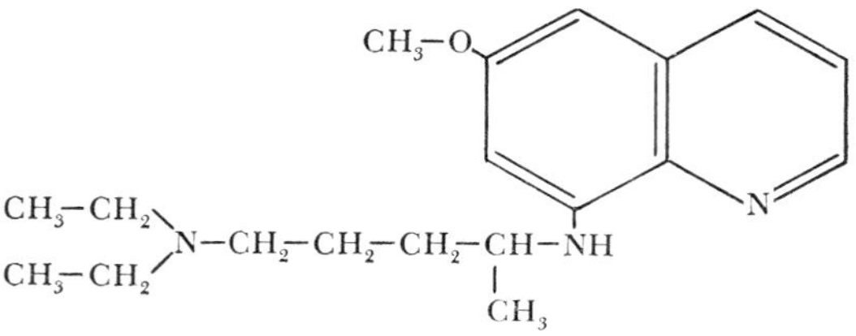

Plasmoquine
(Plasmochin, Pamaquine)

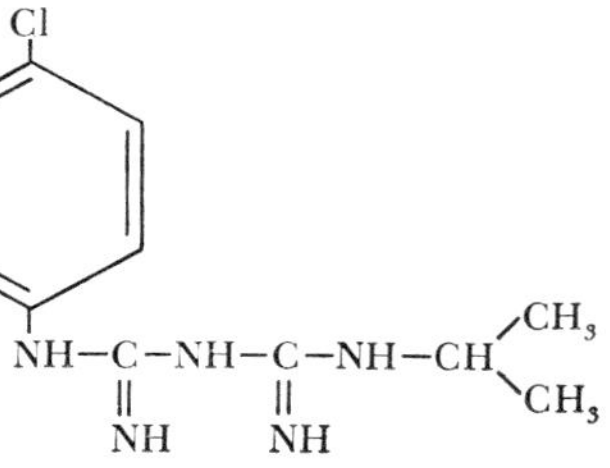

Chlorguanide*
(Paludrine)

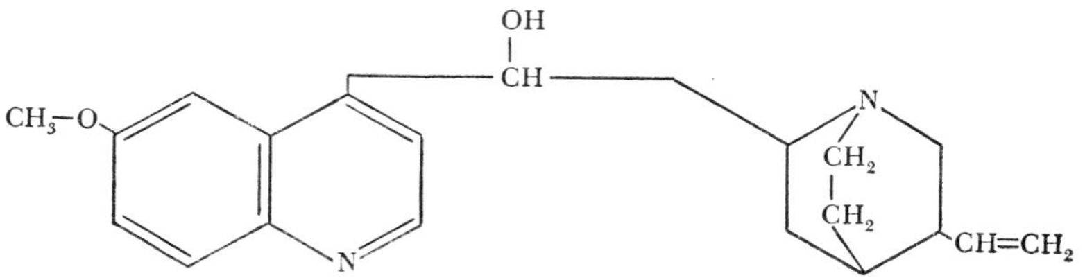

Quinine

FIGURE 10—*Structural Formulas of Antimalarial Compounds*

*The hydrochloride of chlorguanide is marketed by Eli Lilly and Company under the trade-mark 'Guanatol Hydrochloride.'

istration of 100 mg. once weekly. However, a semiweekly dose of 100 mg. given every three or four days will give more consistent results. Resistant strains may require weekly or semiweekly administration of 300 to 500 mg., and occasionally doses of 100 mg. or more per day may be needed.

Control of the acute paroxysms of falciparum infection is obtained with 300 mg. given two or three times on the first day of treatment. The infection may then be eradicated by administration of 300 mg. once or twice daily for an additional nine days. The fever of vivax malaria usually responds to a single dose of 300 to 500 mg. Relapse may be prevented by continued treatment with suppressive doses as outlined previously.

The following individual doses for administration according to the above schedules are recommended:

Infants (under two years)..............10 to 25 mg.
Children:
 Two to five years....................25 to 50 mg.
 Five to ten years....................50 to 100 mg.
 Ten years or more................... Adult doses

Side-effects from the recommended suppressive and therapeutic doses are notably lacking. When the drug is used as a suppressant, some acquired resistance has been reported.

Primaquine, a derivative of 8-aminoquinoline, is less toxic than plasmoquine or pentaquine (see below). Its structural formula is shown in Figure 10. Primaquine is indicated for radical cure of relapsing vivax malaria in individuals who have left endemic areas and wish to discontinue suppressive drugs. Single daily doses of 22.5 mg. of the base (37 mg. of the diphosphate salt) for fourteen days have eradicated vivax infections in nonimmune subjects. Probably smaller doses will be effective in individuals who have had malaria for some time. Toxicity has not developed with therapeutic doses.

Pentaquine is also a derivative of 8-aminoquinoline (for structural formula, see Figure 10). It is indicated only for radical cure of relapsing vivax malaria. Its toxicity precludes use as a suppressant. Patients receiving full therapeutic doses should be hospitalized during treatment. Quinine, 2 Gm. per day, should be given in combination, since this potentiates antimalarial action and reduces the toxicity to some extent. Therapeutic doses are 90 mg. of the phosphate (60 mg. of the base), or 45 mg. of the phosphate (30 mg. of the base) concurrently with 2 Gm. of quinine, per day for fourteen days.

Side-effects of severe abdominal cramps, methemoglobinemia, anorexia, postural hypotension,

nausea, and vomiting are not uncommon but disappear when the drug is stopped. Leukopenia develops occasionally, and, rarely, serious hemolytic anemia may complicate therapy.

Plasmoquine (Plasmochin, pamaquine), another drug of the 8-aminoquinoline group (see Figure 10), was the only drug available before World War II which was effective against the gametocytes of *P. falciparum* when combined with quinine. It also has been used in this combination against the relapses of vivax malaria.

The incidence of toxic symptoms is so great with this drug (principally methemoglobinemia) that it has been replaced by other 8-aminoquinoline derivatives.

Quinine was for many years the only available antimalarial drug. With the development of new agents, it is now little used except in combination to reduce toxicity and potentiate action of the 8-aminoquinoline group (see above).

Quinine has the structural formula shown in Figure 10; the asymmetric carbon atom of the secondary alcohol group which links the two rings has a levo configuration. The compound having a dextro configuration of this carbon atom is quinidine, which is discussed on page 360. Quinine may be said to be a general protoplasmic poison which stimulates in low concentrations and depresses in higher concentrations. In addition to its effect in malaria, it has the following important properties: It is a local irritant, but in slightly higher concentrations it induces prolonged local anesthesia as well as irritation. It is antipyretic and analgesic, but less so than the salicylates. It is a cardiac depressant but is little used for this purpose because its isomer, quinidine, is more potent in this respect. It tends to stimulate uterine contraction, but too unreliably for clinical usefulness. It increases the contractile response of skeletal muscle and is effective in treatment of myotonia congenita; at the same time it potentiates the action of curare (p. 447) and opposes that of neostigmine (p. 419). When quinine is given alone for treatment of acute attacks of malaria, the dosage is 2 Gm. per day for seven days. In emergencies, the bisulfate or dihydrochloride may be given intravenously in doses not exceeding 0.6 Gm. Slow injection of a dilute solution is necessary. Intramuscular administration is painful and may cause muscle necrosis.

Side-effects (cinchonism) are tinnitus, vertigo, partial deafness, visual disturbances, headache, mental depression, fullness in the head, and nausea.

LOCAL ANTI-INFECTIVE AND ANTIPARASITIC AGENTS

ANTISEPTICS

The term *antiseptics* is a general one for substances which inhibit the growth or reproduction of bacteria, with special reference to the surface of the skin or mucous membranes. *Germicides* are substances that destroy micro-organisms, with the connotation of very strong action which might injure animal or human tissues. By definition, *bactericides* destroy micro-organisms, but the term carries the connotation of a gentler action which is not injurious to tissues. *Bacteriostatic* agents, also by definition, prevent the growth or reproduction of bacteria; however, the term is not precise because of uncertainty regarding the exact conditions under which bacterial growth and reproduction are inhibited.

At present there is wide variation in thought concerning the field of antiseptics, and many aspects of the subject must be considered as controversial. One of the most striking of the newer developments is the demonstration that certain agents formerly considered bactericidal do not actually destroy bacteria, for the addition of certain substances is capable of reviving cultures which were "dead" by all previously employed criteria. The question of what constitutes death in bacteria is apparently an open one.

Another increasingly supported concept is that bacteriostatic and bactericidal activity overlap. As the concentration of most antiseptic agents is gradually increased, starting with very high dilutions, the first action on bacteria is one of stimulation of growth and reproduction. As higher concentrations are reached, growth and reproduction are progressively slowed and may finally be stopped altogether. As the duration of this bacteriostasis continues, a progressively smaller number of bacteria may resume growth when the antiseptic agent is neutralized, inhibited, or diluted out; in other words, bacteriostatic activity has become bactericidal. It is evident that concentration is all-important in determining the action of an antiseptic.

There is still much disagreement over the criteria by which the effectiveness of antiseptic agents is to be judged. The advent of systemic chemotherapy has narrowed the use of antiseptics almost entirely to the skin. Clinical experience appears to be the only tangible way of judging efficacy. In-vitro tests

are helpful insofar as they approximate the conditions of clinical use. The ideal antiseptic should meet the following requirements:

1. Nontoxicity to tissues.
2. Effectiveness against relatively high concentrations of pathogenic organisms.
3. Effectiveness against the more virulent strains of pathogenic organisms.
4. Effectiveness in the presence of serum and tissue fluids.
5. Effectiveness in the presence of soap, alcohol, and other substances commonly used in the operating room.
6. Effectiveness in a wide range of dilutions (this is a safety measure).
7. Effectiveness which is both quick and lasting.

Although few, if any, of the available agents meet all these specifications, all should be considered in evaluating a given compound. The goal of irrevocable destruction of 100 percent of the bacteria on and in the human skin is not attainable with any known agent which does not also injure the skin. The most that can be expected of present-day antiseptics is a reduction of 98 or 99 percent in the number of viable organisms as determined by available laboratory methods.

The commonly used antiseptic agents are grouped for discussion into the following chemical categories: phenol derivatives, alcohols, oxidizing agents, mercurials, silver compounds, detergents, triphenylmethane dyes, acridine dyes, and miscellaneous.

Phenol Derivatives

Phenol (hydroxybenzene), C_6H_5OH, itself is sometimes added to biological products as a preservative, but it is now little used as a clinical antiseptic. In adequate concentrations it is both bactericidal and fungicidal, but it is also a general protoplasmic poison. In high concentrations the compound is a protein precipitant; in dilute solutions it denatures protein without precipitation (coagulation). It has a severe toxic action on tissues and will even affect the unabraded skin. Spores and viruses are very resistant to phenol, and its bactericidal efficacy is greatly reduced by cold and an alkaline medium.

Applied locally, phenol penetrates to the sensory nerve endings and consequently has a local anesthetic action. A 5 percent solution applied to tissues or mucous membranes precipitates the proteins, is irritating, and may cause extensive tissue necrosis. Therapeutically, phenol may be used to cauterize small wounds, and it is commonly employed as an antipruritic in 1 to 2 percent concentration in lotions or ointments.

Cresols are methyl derivatives of phenol. They are available as a mixture of the three isomers. Because this mixture is soluble in water to the extent of only one part in sixty, it is commonly used in the form of Saponated Cresol Solution, N.F., (compound cresol solution) which is fully miscible with water. The toxic properties of cresol are almost identical with those of phenol, and poisoning may result from the use of cresol compounds. Cresol is a fairly efficient bactericide against common pathogenic bacilli and is slightly less active against cocci. The compound solution is used for disinfecting inanimate objects. In 2 percent solutions it is sometimes used as a handwash.

Mandelic Acid, $C_6H_5 \cdot CHOH \cdot COOH$, has been used as a "urinary antiseptic." It is a relatively nontoxic compound which is excreted unchanged in the urine, where it exerts bacteriostatic and bactericidal effects on most of the pathogenic organisms encountered in pyelitis and cystitis. However, it should be employed only against organisms not susceptible to systemic anti-infectives.

For mandelic acid to be effective, the urine must be acid (preferably pH 5.3 or less), and it is best to limit urine output to 1,200 cc. daily. If necessary to maintain urine acidity, ammonium chloride or other acidifying agent (p. 352) is given in whatever dosage is necessary.

Mandelic acid is given in courses of five days each. Sometimes the ketogenic diet is a valuable supplement, the ketone bodies (to which mandelic acid is related chemically) reinforcing the bacteriostatic action. During treatment, the urine should be examined frequently for casts and red blood cells. Their appearance requires temporary discontinuation of the drug. Mandelic acid is contraindicated when kidney function is impaired or when mild acidosis is undesirable. Transient nausea and, occasionally, diarrhea are seen as side-effects. Idiosyncrasy, with tinnitus, deafness, muscular pains, and urticaria, is rare.

Preparations and average doses are as follows:

'Enseals' Mandelic Acid and Ammonium Chloride, 4 to 10 every six hours.
Elixir Mandelic Acid, 1 tablespoonful every six to eight hours (children under two years of age, 1/2 to 1 teaspoonful).

Resorcinol (meta-dihydroxybenzene) is both bactericidal and fungicidal but only about one-third as active as phenol. It is also a protein precipitant, and after absorption the compound resembles phenol in its systemic actions. Therapeutically, resorcinol is used in the treatment of such conditions as ringworm, eczema, psoriasis, and seborrheic dermatitis as an ointment or a lotion varying in strength from 1 to 10 percent.

Thymol (methyl-isopropyl-phenol) possesses some bactericidal and fungicidal properties, being more active than phenol against pathogenic cocci but less active against gram-negative bacteria. Thymol has been used in the treatment of dermatophytosis, either as a 1 percent alcoholic solution or incorporated in a dusting powder. It is said to be effective in the treatment of actinomycosis and is used both locally and orally. The oral dose is 1.5 Gm. daily in divided doses given two out of three days.

Alcohols

The aliphatic alcohols are germicidal in varying degree, those of higher molecular weight being more active but also more toxic.

Ethyl Alcohol, $CH_3 \cdot CH_2OH$, is the most widely used for its antiseptic action. It is often ineffective, especially against spores. The optimal concentration is 70 percent by weight (approximately 77 percent by volume at 15°C.). Slight variations from the optimal in either direction reduce the effectiveness very greatly, the ordinary 70 percent alcohol by volume being almost useless. Since ethyl alcohol is extremely irritant to tissues and mucous membranes, its clinical use is limited to disinfection of the skin and inanimate objects.

Isopropyl Alcohol, $(CH_3)_2:CHOH$, is similar in properties to ethyl alcohol but is slightly more potent and twice as toxic. It is not potable and is used chiefly to disinfect needles, syringes, and instruments. The optimal concentration is about 45 percent.

Oxidizing Agents

Certain oxidizing agents are capable of destroying micro-organisms. However, organic substances not part of living cells are more susceptible to their attack, and since the oxidizing agents are used up in the process of destroying either living or dead organic matter, the oxidizing agents are relatively ineffective in the presence of blood, serum, discharge, or other organic matter.

Three types of oxidizing agents are discussed below; they liberate respectively iodine, chlorine, and oxygen itself, probably in nascent form.

IODINE

Iodine is a powerful germicide, an effective fungicide, a potent amebicide, and a moderately active virucide. Presumably it acts by iodizing and oxidizing portions of the protoplasm of these organisms. Only free iodine is antiseptic. The great chemical activity of iodine and its ineffectiveness in combined form make it of little value in the presence of organic matter. This fact, combined with its corrosive action on tissues, has limited its usefulness chiefly to disinfection of the skin.

The U.S.P. Iodine Tincture has been reduced in strength from 7 percent to 2 percent free iodine (it also contains 2.4 percent sodium iodide in 49 percent alcohol [v/v]). The new strength is considered to be less irritant and no less effective. When stronger solutions are used, the excess should be removed from the skin with alcohol.

Official aqueous preparations include Iodine Solution, N.F., containing 2 percent iodine and 2.4 percent sodium iodide in water, and Strong Iodine Solution, U.S.P., (Lugol's solution) containing 5 percent iodine and 10 percent potassium iodide in water.

CHLORINE

Elemental chlorine is one of the most potent germicides, and it has virucidal and amebicidal properties as well. However, its efficacy is diminished by a number of factors, chief among which is the presence of organic matter, with which it reacts. Its activity is also influenced by temperature and pH, it is more potent at higher temperatures, and a shift of pH from 9 to 6 increases the effectiveness tenfold.

A number of preparations are available which release elemental chlorine slowly. They are used in surgery and for disinfection of inanimate objects. All are somewhat irritating to the skin.

Chloramine-T, N.F., has the following formula. $CH_3 \cdot C_6H_4 \cdot SO_2 \cdot N(Cl) \cdot Na \cdot 3H_2O$. It contains about 13 percent chlorine, all of it available. Chloramine-T is employed for the irrigation and dressing of wounds in 1 or 2 percent concentration, and on mucous membranes in 0.1 to 0.2 percent solution.

Dichloramine-T, N.F., $CH_3 \cdot C_6H_4 \cdot SO_2 \cdot N(Cl)_2$, is almost insoluble in water but soluble in oils. It is applied in solution in chlorinated paraffin, in which form it is more irritant, more solvent, and longer lasting than Chloramine-T. A 5 percent solution

is used for wounds, a 1 or 2 percent solution, for mucous membranes.

OXYGEN

Nascent oxygen is most powerfully antiseptic against gram-positive bacteria and certain spirochetes and trypanosomes. As with other oxidizing agents, organic matter greatly diminishes its effectiveness. The following substances owe their antiseptic properties to their oxidizing effect.

Permanganates—Potassium permanganate, although used less extensively than in the past, is still of service in some ways. In persistent urinary infections, irrigation of the bladder with a solution of 1:5,000 is helpful. A 1:10,000 solution is employed as a wet dressing in the vesicular stage of dermatitis-eczema, and a 1 percent solution can be used in Vincent's angina. Permanganate, 1:5,000, is also used as a gastric lavage. Zinc permanganate, 1:4,000, is employed as a urethral douche in urethritis.

Hydrogen Peroxide—Although its bactericidal action is weak and of brief duration, the effervescence of hydrogen peroxide makes it useful for the cleansing of wounds and, as an adjuvant to penicillin, as a mouthwash in Vincent's angina.

Metallic Peroxides—Sodium peroxide readily releases oxygen in solution, leaving a residue of sodium hydroxide. The usefulness of this compound is limited principally to the treatment of acne and the removal of comedones.

Sodium Perborate is principally used in a 2 percent solution in oral infections. It has also been incorporated into tooth pastes. Because boron is a chronic poison, prolonged use of sodium perborate is not recommended, particularly in children, who are likely to swallow anything placed in the mouth.

Mercurials

INORGANIC COMPOUNDS

Inorganic mercury compounds have a bactericidal action much lower than was originally supposed. They depend for their action on release of the mercuric ion, which has an affinity for and a precipitant action on protein. This effect is not selective for bacterial protoplasm, and therefore inorganic mercury compounds are very irritant to tissue, have poor penetrability, and lose much of their germicidal potency in the presence of extraneous protein. Spores are very resistant to their action. The inorganic mercurials are extremely toxic after absorption.

Mercuric Chloride (bichloride of mercury, corrosive sublimate), $HgCl_2$, is the most commonly used inorganic mercury compound. It is employed as a handwash in a concentration of 1:2,000. It is also used in a 1:1,000 solution for the sterilization of surgical instruments which may be harmed by boiling.

Mercuric Cyanide, $Hg(CN)_2$, is reported to be as effective as mercuric chloride and less irritant. Any superiority is probably not great.

Mercuric Oxide (Yellow Mercuric Oxide, U.S.P.), HgO, is an insoluble powder which is mildly antiseptic. It is used almost exclusively as an ointment, usually 1 percent, for local application to the conjunctiva.

Ammoniated Mercury, $NH_2 \cdot Hg \cdot Cl$, is a white, insoluble powder which has been used in the form of ointment for treatment of superficial skin and conjunctival infections, particularly impetigo (p. 236). A 5 or 10 percent ointment is applied to the skin, and a 3 percent ointment to the eye.

ORGANIC MERCURY ANTISEPTICS

The organic mercurials are compounds in which mercury is present in complex organic combination. As a group they are more bactericidal, less irritating, and less toxic than the inorganic mercurial salts. They are ineffective against spores.

Mercurochrome was the first of the organic mercurials. It is a red compound which is relatively nonirritating but possesses inadequate penetrability for living tissue, and its activity is reduced by organic matter and change in pH. Its activity is greatly reduced at the pH of body fluids.

'Merthiolate' (Thimerosal, Lilly) is sodium ethyl mercuri thiosalicylate. It is a white solid that contains approximately 49 percent mercury in organic combination. It is readily soluble in water or physiological salt solution, and the resulting solutions are stable under ordinary conditions of light and temperature. 'Merthiolate' is incompatible with acids, the salts of heavy metals, and iodine and

should not be used in combination with or immediately following their application. It may be used with or following soaps or sulfonamides. It is compatible with serum and body fluids. It has both bacteriostatic and bactericidal properties in relatively high dilutions. Either an aqueous solution (colorless) or an alcohol-acetone-water solution (colored with eosin) can be used as a skin antiseptic in dilutions of 1:1,000, and both forms can be used on the abraded skin. The aqueous solution can be applied to mucous membranes and has been introduced into the pleural cavity. 'Merthiolate' is incorporated in jelly and ointment bases for use in dressings and in ophthalmic ointments.

Metaphen is an organic mercurial antiseptic with properties similar to those of 'Merthiolate.' Weight for weight, however, it is not as effective as some of the other organic mercurials, since it requires a 1:200 solution as compared with 1:1,000 of others.

Phenylmercuric Nitrate is available as a molecular compound or mixture of phenylmercuric nitrate and phenylmercuric hydroxide, the chemical composition of which may be represented by the formula $C_6H_5HgOH \cdot C_6H_5HgNO_3$. It is a stable substance, the bactericidal and fungicidal properties of which are not diminished in the presence of tissues. It is applied in the following strengths: on skin, 1:1,500, on mucous membranes, 1:15,000 to 1:24,000.

Silver Compounds

The silver ion is directly toxic to micro-organisms; it has a protein-precipitant action that includes protein of the bacterial protoplasm. Active silver compounds exert the same action on body tissues and are so destructive that the simple silver compounds such as the nitrate must be classified as caustics and corrosives. In colloidal silver preparations, the silver is present for the most part in a nonionized form, and they are noncorrosive, nonirritant, and nonastringent. However, the only organism against which they are highly effective is the gonococcus. The antiseptic activity of colloidal silver preparations is not related to the total content of silver, but rather is a function of the concentration of free silver ions.

The colloidal silver preparations may be divided into the strong and the mild types, represented by Strong Silver Protein, N.F., and Mild Silver Protein, N.F. The former contains about 8 percent silver; the latter, about 21 percent. In spite of having a lower silver content, the Strong Silver

Protein liberates the higher concentration of silver ions and is therefore more powerful and more irritant. The colloidal silver preparations are used almost entirely on mucous membranes—the Strong Silver Protein usually in 0.5 to 10 percent solution, and the Mild Silver Protein ordinarily in 10 to 25 percent solution.

Detergents

ANIONIC DETERGENTS

Detergents are cleansing agents which hold foreign matter in suspension or emulsion. Anionic detergents are those in which the active portion of the molecule is an acidic ion.

Soaps, the sodium and potassium salts of fatty acids, are typical anionic detergents (see also p. 481). Although their antiseptic action is largely a matter of mechanical removal of the organisms, they have a certain amount of direct antibacterial action, particularly against spirochetes, gonococci, meningococci, and diphtheria, dysentery, and influenza bacilli. Streptococci are moderately resistant, and staphylococci and typhoid bacilli are extremely so. Serum and other protein materials interfere with the antibacterial action of soaps.

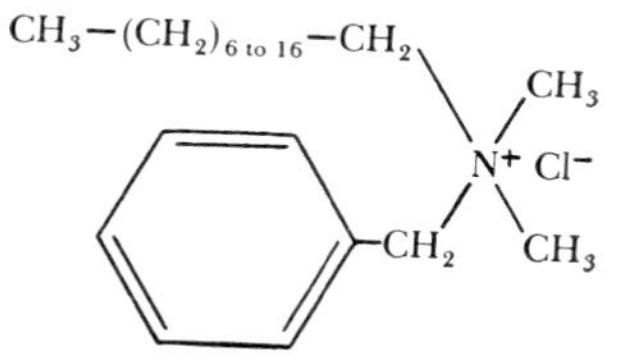
CH3—(CH2)6 to 16—CH2
CH3
N+ Cl−
CH2
CH3

Benzalkonium Chloride (Zephiran Chloride)
(Benzalkonium chloride represents a mixture of compounds with alkyl groups ranging from 8 to 18 in number of carbon atoms.)

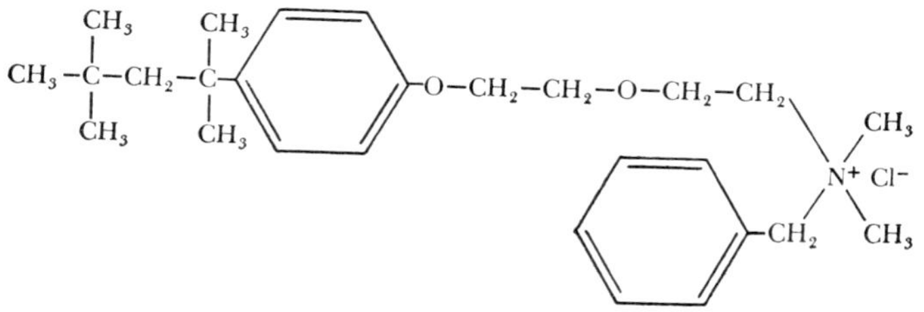
CH3 CH3
CH3—C—CH2—C—
CH3 CH3
—O—CH2—CH2—O—CH2—CH2
CH3
N+ Cl−
CH2
CH3

Benzethonium Chloride (Phemerol Chloride)

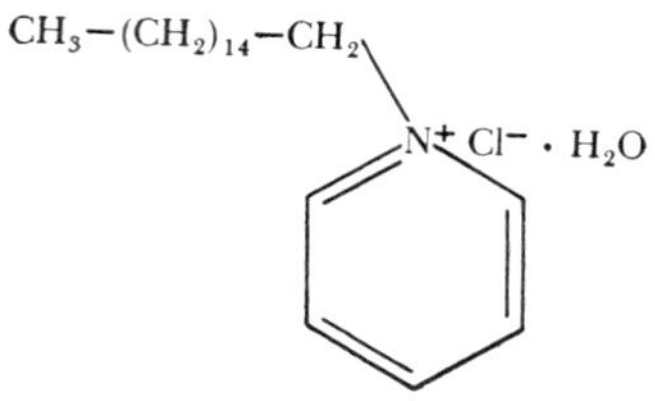
CH3—(CH2)14—CH2
N+ Cl− · H2O

Cetylpyridinium Chloride (Ceepryn Chloride)

FIGURE 11—*Structural Formulas of Cationic Detergents*

CATIONIC DETERGENTS

Cationic detergents are cleansing agents in which the active part of the molecule is a basic ion. Most of them are quaternary ammonium salts. As cleansing agents they are inferior to the anionic detergents, but they are superior as wetting agents and as antiseptics.

The quaternary ammonium compounds form an imperceptible film on the skin which may persist as long as three hours under favorable circumstances. This film is antiseptic on the outer surface but not on the inner, and bacteria on the skin beneath the film may remain viable. The film is resistant to ordinary trauma, brief dips in water or blood, and exposure to tissues, but it is disintegrated by fifteen to thirty seconds' exposure to running water or by continuous dips in water, physiological salt solution, blood or other body fluids, or strong alcohol. Their antiseptic activity is greatly reduced by the presence of even small quantities (0.1 percent) of soap; if soap is used in preparing the skin, it should be rinsed off thoroughly with water and then with alcohol before a cationic detergent is applied.

Benzalkonium Chloride (Zephiran Chloride) is a mixture of quaternary ammonium compounds which may be represented by the structural formula shown in Figure 11. It is used for prophylactic disinfection of the intact skin (tincture or aqueous solution, 1:1,000) or mucous membranes (aqueous solution, 1:2,000 to 1:10,000), in treatment of superficial injuries and infected wounds (1:2,000 to 1:10,000), and for irrigation of deep wounds or body cavities (1:5,000 to 1:40,000).

Benzethonium Chloride (Phemerol Chloride) is a quaternary ammonium compound having the structural formula shown in Figure 11. Its use is similar to that of benzalkonium chloride. The tincture (1:500) or aqueous solution (1:1,000) is used full strength except in the nose and eye; on these surfaces a 1:5,000 aqueous solution is employed.

Cetylpyridinium Chloride (Ceepryn Chloride) is also a quaternary ammonium compound, in which the nitrogen is part of a pyridine ring (see Figure 11). Its properties are similar to those of other cationic detergents. On intact skin the tincture (1:500 or 1:1,000) is suitable, or the surface may be scrubbed for five to ten minutes with a 1:100 aqueous solution. For mucous membranes and abraded skin, an aqueous solution (1:1,000 to 1:10,000) may be employed.

Triphenylmethane Dyes

Pararosaniline Chloride—A number of highly colored derivatives of triphenylmethane have selective antiseptic properties. The simplest of these is pararosaniline chloride (fuchsin), a red dye which has the formula shown in Figure 12. Fuchsin, phenol, and resorcinol are important ingredients of Castellani's paint, which is employed for topical application to fungus infections of the skin. It stains clothing.

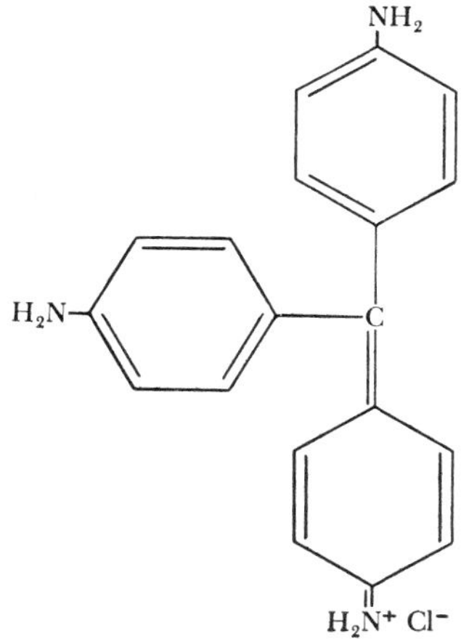

FIGURE 12—*Structural Formula of Pararosaniline Chloride (Fuchsin)*

Methylrosaniline Chloride—Substitution of methyl groups for the hydrogen atoms in the amino groups of pararosaniline chloride changes the color of the compound through green to violet. In *brilliant green* there are four methyl groups; *methyl violet* consists mostly of the pentamethyl derivative; and *crystal violet* is a relatively pure form of the hexamethyl substitution product. Methylrosaniline Chloride, N.F., (*gentian violet*) consists mostly of the hexamethyl derivative with an admixture of the other two. All stain clothing.

The three derivatives and their mixtures have similar antiseptic properties. They are bactericidal to gram-positive organisms in dilutions of about 1:1,000,000 and are particularly effective against staphylococci, *Corynebacterium diphtheriae*, *Pseudomonas aeruginosa* (*B. pyocyaneus*), *Candida* (*Monilia*) *albicans*, and the *Trichophyton* and *Epidermophyton* genera. For application to skin and mucous membranes, a 1 percent solution is generally employed. For direct contact with tissues, a 0.1 or 0.2 percent solution is used. For instillation into wounds or body cavities, the concentration should not exceed 0.01 percent (1:10,000). The methylrosaniline dyes combine with necrotic tissue to form an eschar, and this property was at one time employed in the local treatment of burns. If they are used, these dyes should not be applied to ulcerative lesions of the face because of the possibility of tattooing.

Gentian violet is an effective vermifuge in strongyloidiasis and in oxyuriasis (pinworm, *Enterobius vermicularis* infection). For dosage and administration, see page 311.

Acridine Dyes

Certain amino derivatives of acridine have antiseptic activity, particularly against the gonococcus and gram-positive organisms. They are more effective in an alkaline medium. Because of their yellow color, they are called "flavines." *Acriflavine* (acriflavine base, neutral acriflavine) is a mixture of 2,8-diamino-10-methylacridinium chloride (shown in Figure 13) and 2,8-diaminoacridine. *Acriflavine hydrochloride* is a monohydrochloride salt of acriflavine; it is more soluble than acriflavine but also more irritating because of its acidity. *Proflavine sulfate* is the monohydrogen sulfate monohydrate salt of 2,8-diaminoacridine. *Proflavine dihydrochloride* is the analogous dihydrochloride salt.

The acriflavine preparations are similar in activity. They are applied to open wounds as 1:1,000 solutions or 1 percent ointments. For mucous membranes, solutions of 1:1,000 to 1:10,000 may be used, depending on the area to be included. For the middle ear, a 0.2 percent solution in 50 percent alcohol has been employed. Solutions should be stored in dark bottles and should not be kept more than a week. The acriflavine drugs were formerly administered by mouth as urinary antiseptics, but the antibiotics and sulfonamides are much more effective.

Miscellaneous

Methenamine (hexamethylenamine, Urotropin), $N_4(CH_2)_6$, is a condensation product of formaldehyde and ammonia. It was formerly much used as a "urinary antiseptic." The sulfonamides and antibiotics are more effective, however, and methenamine is now indicated only when they and such agents as mandelic acid have failed because the infecting organism is insusceptible.

The antiseptic action of methenamine is due to formaldehyde, which is liberated when methena-

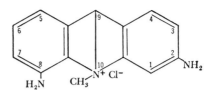

FIGURE 13—*Structural Formula of One of the Components of Acriflavine Base*

mine comes into contact with acids. Obviously, methenamine is ineffectual in neutral or alkaline urine. The drug is given by mouth. The effective dose is usually 60 to 90 grains (4 to 6 Gm.) daily, subdivided into four or six equally spaced doses. Acidifying salts (p. 352) are given at the mid-intervals between doses of methenamine in sufficient quantity to maintain the urine at pH 6.3 or less (p. 521).

Side reactions occasionally seen include renal irritation (casts and red blood cells in the urine), bladder irritation, gastro-intestinal upsets, and skin rashes.

FUNGICIDES

Certain general principles apply to the choice and use of drugs for local application to fungus infections of the skin:

1. The drugs should be nonirritating and nonsensitizing. Irritating and sensitizing drugs may themselves induce dermatitis.
2. Better final results will usually be obtained from three to six weeks of persistent mild treatment than from efforts to eradicate the disease more quickly with stronger agents.
3. Any drug should be immediately discontinued which seems to increase the degree of inflammation.
4. To be of value, preparations must be rubbed thoroughly into the affected areas. Patients should be carefully instructed on this point.
5. Infections of the feet, hands, and scalp are likely to be more resistant than those involving only the trunk.

Fatty Acids are at present the most satisfactory agents for treating all types of superficial fungus infection. They combine high fungicidal activity with very low irritant and sensitizing properties. They are also moderately effective against the secondary bacterial infection which is usually present. The ointments may be applied once or twice daily and should be rubbed in well. The powder is preferred for prophylaxis and for use during the day in warm weather.

UNDECYLENIC ACID, an unsaturated straight-chain fatty acid, $CH_3 \cdot CH:CH \cdot (CH_2)_7 \cdot COOH$, apparently has the greatest fungicidal activity. It is ordinarily used with its zinc salt, which is slightly astringent. It is available in the following forms:

Desenex Ointment, containing 5 percent undecylenic acid and 20 percent zinc undecylenate in a vanishing cream (buffered with triethanolamine).

Compound Undecylenic Acid Ointment, N.F., containing 5 percent undecylenic acid and 20 percent zinc undecylenate in an ointment base of Polyethylene Glycol 4000, U.S.P., and Polyethylene Glycol 400, U.S.P.

Desenex Powder, which contains 2 percent undecylenic acid and 20 percent zinc undecylenate in talc.

PROPIONIC ACID, $CH_3 \cdot CH_2 \cdot COOH$, and CAPRYLIC ACID, $CH_3 \cdot (CH_2)_6 \cdot COOH$, are natural constituents of sweat and sebum which are claimed to be even less irritating than undecylenic acid. Available forms include:

Sopronol Ointment (Improved), consisting of:

sodium propionate	12.3%
propionic acid	2.7%
sodium caprylate	10.0%
zinc caprylate	5.0%
dioctyl sodium sulfosuccinate	0.1%

in a water-soluble base containing *n*-propyl alcohol, polyethylene glycols, stearyl alcohol, and diethylene glycol monoethyl ether. A powder and solution of essentially similar composition may also be obtained.

Other Preparations—T-CAP (trimethylcetylammonium pentachlorphenate), having the formula $C_6Cl_5 \cdot O \cdot N(CH_3)_3 \cdot (CH_2)_{15} \cdot CH_3$, is an active fungicidal agent which has similar clinical properties to the fatty acids. It is available as T-CAP Cream—an oil-in-water emulsion containing 2.2 percent T-CAP and 1 percent undecylenic acid.

Salicylanilide, $C_6H_4(OH) \cdot CO \cdot NH \cdot C_6H_5$, has fungicidal properties which make it of value in treatment of tinea capitis (p. 229). It is generally applied as a 5 percent ointment or cream.

When scaling and hyperkeratosis are present in fungus infections of the hands and feet, a water-miscible ointment (p. 479) containing precipitated sulfur and salicylic acid, 20 percent of each, may be applied twice daily.

For acutely inflamed infections of the extremities and inguinal-crural areas, a solution of 1 percent cupric sulfate and 2 percent zinc sulfate in camphor water may be diluted 1:20 with cold water and applied as wet dressings.

For fungus infections of the scalp, in addition to the fatty acid, T-CAP, and salicylanilide preparations, a mixture of equal parts of glycerin and Iodine Tincture may be beneficial. When secondary bacterial infection is troublesome, 5 percent ammoniated mercury ointment may be helpful. Mercury and iodine preparations must not be used at the same time.

ANTHELMINTICS

METHYLROSANILINE

Gentian Violet Medicinal (Methylrosaniline Chloride, N.F.) is a methylamino derivative of triphenylmethane. Its chemistry and use as an antiseptic are discussed on page 309.

Gentian violet is the drug of choice for treatment of strongyloidiasis (p. 39) and oxyuriasis (pinworm, *Enterobius vermicularis* infection; p. 39). It is nontoxic on oral administration; in fact, it is not absorbed. The drug is, however, somewhat irritating to the gastro-intestinal tract as evidenced by the occurrence of nausea, vomiting, mild abdominal pain, and, infrequently, diarrhea, headache, dizziness, or lassitude. These symptoms usually respond to temporary withdrawal of the drug.

Contraindications to systemic administration of gentian violet have not been fully defined. It should possibly not be given to patients with moderate or severe cardiac, hepatic, renal, or gastro-intestinal disease. Alcohol should not be taken during treatment.

To avert gastric irritation, gentian violet should be given in enteric-coated tablets. For oxyuriasis, the coating should be timed to release the drug in about four hours. The dosage for adults is 1 grain three times daily one hour before meals. Those under seventeen years of age are given 3/20 grain daily for each year of apparent (rather than actual) age, the total dose being subdivided and administered before meals. Table 33 outlines the average

TABLE 33 — *Average Daily Dose of Gentian Violet in Oxyuriasis According to Age and Tablet Size*

Age in Years	3/20-Grain Tablets	1/2-Grain Tablets
3	2 to 3	
4	3 to 4	
5	3 to 5	
6	4 to 6	
7	5 to 7	
8	6 to 8	
9	7 to	3
10	8 to	3+
11		3 to 3+
12		3+ to 4
13		3+ to 4+
14		4 to 5
15		4+ to 5+
16		4+ to 6

dosage according to age. The drug should be given in two courses of eight days each, with a seven-day rest period between courses. It is important to treat all infected members of a household simultaneously.

Treatment of young children and infants who are unable to swallow tablets may sometimes be accomplished by manually placing the medication in the oral pharynx. Because of the danger of aspiration, this must be attempted only by those experienced in the technic. Otherwise, it may be necessary to crush the tablets in jelly or syrup. Nausea and vomiting are then more likely to occur, although this very young group is often quite tolerant to the dye.

In some instances gastro-intestinal upsets develop, but they usually do not reappear if medication is interrupted for a day or two or if the dose is temporarily reduced. Children generally tolerate treatment better than adults.

For strongyloidiasis the same dosage is recommended. Enteric coatings which release the dye in one and one-half hours have been recommended by some in order that greater concentrations of the dye will be available in the upper intestine where the parasite is found. However, unless gastric emptying is unusually fast, such a preparation would be expected to release considerable quantities of the dye in the stomach and might cause nausea and vomiting. In refractory cases, 25 cc. of a 1 percent aqueous solution of gentian violet may be introduced by tube directly into the duodenum.

In pulmonary strongyloidiasis, the dye is sometimes given (to hospitalized patients only) by intravenous injection, 25 cc. of a sterile 0.5 percent aqueous solution being used. This dose is repeated every other day for not more than five doses. Injections should be given very slowly, for alarming shocklike reactions are occasionally seen. The dye sometimes produces a temporary bluish discoloration of the skin which resembles cyanosis.

HEXYLRESORCINOL

Hexylresorcinol (1,3-hydroxy-4-*n*-hexylbenzene), $C_6H_{13} \cdot C_6H_3(OH_2)$, is a pale-yellow, crystalline substance having a slight pungent odor and an acrid astringent taste. It is freely soluble in organic solvents but sparingly so in water (1:2,000). It is the drug of choice for treatment of ascariasis and mixed infections with *Ascaris lumbricoides* and hookworm, but it is less effective against pinworms, whipworms, and dwarf tapeworms. Because of its relatively low toxicity, the drug may be used in

debilitated individuals and children when more active compounds are contraindicated.

After oral administration, about one-third of the dose is absorbed from the intestinal tract and excreted in conjugated, inactive form by the kidneys. The remainder is eliminated in the feces unchanged. Hexylresorcinol is a local irritant and will cause superficial erosion of the oral mucosa if permitted to escape from the hard gelatin capsules. The gastric mucosa is rarely affected. No evidence of systemic toxicity follows the administration of single therapeutic doses in man, although a few individuals may develop itching and swelling of the buccal mucosa or epigastric discomfort.

When used as an anthelmintic, hexylresorcinol should be administered in the form of hard gelatin capsules, care being taken that they are swallowed intact. In young children who are unable to do this, it is necessary manually to place the medication far back on the tongue so that it will be swallowed automatically. Because of the danger of aspiration, this should be carried out only by one skilled in the procedure.

The effectiveness of the drug is greatly reduced by the presence of food in the intestinal tract. Therefore, it is desirable, but not essential, that the evening meal preceding treatment be light and be followed by a saline purgative, preferably with sodium sulfate (p. 386). The desired dose is given in the morning on an empty stomach, after which food and drink are withheld for five hours. A saline purge immediately after treatment is not necessary but may be given twenty-four hours later. Patients may remain ambulatory.

The dose is the same for all infections. Adults and children past ten years of age receive 1 Gm.; children below ten years, 0.1 Gm. for each year of apparent (not chronological) age. Treatment may be repeated in three days.

TETRACHLOROETHYLENE

Tetrachloroethylene (ethylene tetrachloride, perchloroethylene), $Cl_2C:CCl_2$, is an unsaturated halogenated hydrocarbon which occurs as a clear, colorless, mobile, noninflammable liquid having a characteristic ethereal odor. It is slowly decomposed by light, and by various metals if moisture is present. It is relatively insoluble in water (1:10,000) but is miscible with alcohol, ether, chloroform, benzene, and petroleum benzine.

Tetrachloroethylene is the drug of choice for the treatment of hookworm infection due to *Necator americanus*, but it is less effective against *Ancylos-*

toma duodenale. If ascariasis is also present, treatment with tetrachloroethylene should be postponed until the ascarides have been removed. In the absence of fats or alcohol in the intestinal tract, the drug is not absorbed to an appreciable extent and consequently is practically nontoxic. This is well exemplified by the lack of serious reactions in reports of clinical studies on many thousands of individuals. Some absorption does occur and may result in vertigo, headache, nausea, and drowsiness.

Contraindications are ascariasis, alcoholism, gastro-intestinal inflammation, concurrent arsenical therapy, severe anemia, and marked debilitation.

When tetrachloroethylene is to be given, all fats and alcohol should be eliminated from the diet for one or two days. The night before treatment, a light or liquid evening meal is allowed, which is followed by a saline purgative, preferably of sodium sulfate. Tetrachloroethylene is administered the following morning on an empty stomach. Two hours later the saline purgative is repeated. Food is withheld until the bowels have moved freely. Fats and alcohol are best omitted from the diet for the next twenty-four hours. Bed rest is advisable but not essential during the treatment period.

Tetrachloroethylene is usually given in gelatin capsules but may be administered mixed with watery vehicles or dropped on sugar. Inhalation of concentrated vapors should be avoided. The average adult dose is 3 to 5 cc. Children are given 0.2 cc. (3 minims) for each year of age up to the adult maximum.

ASPIDIUM

Aspidium Oleoresin, U.S.P., (extract of male fern, filix-mas) is an ether extract of the dried rhizomes of *Dryopteris filix-mas.* It contains several methyl derivatives of phloroglucin, of which filicic acid is the most important.

Aspidium is generally considered to be the drug of choice for treatment of intestinal tapeworm infection. It is of no value in other types of helminthiasis.

Aspidium is a local irritant and, when given undiluted, causes nausea, vomiting, abdominal cramps, and diarrhea. If used during late pregnancy, abortion may occur as a result of reflex stimulation of the uterus. The anthelmintic action of the drug is believed to be directly upon the musculature of the parasite and, therefore, is dependent upon the degree of local concentration. Absorption from the intestinal tract is not desirable but does occur even with therapeutic doses. The amount absorbed is not directly proportional to the dose. Individual susceptibility varies, but toxic manifestations from involvement of the central nervous system, liver, kidneys, and heart may occur. Aspidium should not be prescribed if disease of these parts is present or if there exist ulcerative lesions in the gastro-intestinal tract.

Mild toxic symptoms include vertigo, headache, nausea, vomiting, diarrhea, icterus, and increased reflex excitability. Severe poisoning is manifested by amblyopia, yellow vision, blindness which sometimes is permanent, muscle cramps, tonic convulsions, coma, and circulatory and respiratory depression or collapse.

For two or three days preceding treatment, the diet should be high in carbohydrate, adequate in protein, and low in fat. Alcohol should be avoided. On the day before treatment, the noon and evening meals are limited to low-residue foods; or, if the condition of the patient permits, food is omitted entirely. Fluids should be taken in liberal amounts. A saline purgative, preferably sodium sulfate (p. 386), is given in the evening. Castor oil or other oily preparations should not be used, because they favor absorption of aspidium. The following morning the patient should remain in bed, and the diet should be restricted to black coffee or plain tea.

The maximum and usual adult dose of the oleoresin of aspidium is 5 Gm., although as much as 8 Gm. and even 12 Gm. has been recommended. Children under ten years of age are given 0.5 Gm. for each year of apparent (not chronological) age up to the adult maximum. The total dose is divided into two, or preferably three, fractions and administered at half-hour intervals starting at seven or eight o'clock in the morning. Two hours after the last dose a saline purgative is given. Since aspidium has a disagreeable taste, it should be prescribed in capsules or in a suitable vehicle. Food is permitted after there have been one or two copious bowel movements. If toxic symptoms appear, treatment should be stopped and a saline purgative administered immediately.

All stools should be collected for the next forty-eight hours and examined carefully for the head of the worm. Treatment should not be considered successful unless the head has been found and identified. A warm, soap-water enema may facilitate passage of the worm. Traction on the parasite should be avoided. In case of failure, treatment should not be repeated for at least seven to ten days or, better, until segments reappear in the stools.

An alternate method for administration of aspidium to children is sometimes preferred. The patient is prepared in the same manner, and on the morning of treatment a duodenal tube is passed. When in the proper location, as ascertained by fluoroscopic examination, a mixture containing the estimated dose of the oleoresin, 30 cc. of gum acacia, an appropriate amount of saline purgative, and 30 cc. of water is then slowly intubated. No further purgation is necessary.

AMEBICIDES

ARSENICALS

Carbarsone (*p*-carbamino phenyl-arsonic acid), $NH_2 \cdot CO \cdot NH \cdot C_6H_4 \cdot AsO:(OH)_2$, is the arsenical of choice in intestinal amebiasis. It may also be useful in treating vaginitis due to *Trichomonas vaginalis*.

Carbarsone is a white crystalline solid which is almost insoluble in water but which dissolves in carbonate or bicarbonate solutions. It is the least toxic of those arsenicals which act on amebae.

In amebiasis, carbarsone kills *Endamoeba histolytica* in the intestinal contents, on the surface of the mucosa, and within the intestinal wall. It is of no value in amebic hepatitis or liver abscess. It is given in courses of ten days each, with rest periods of ten to fourteen days between courses. One course is often sufficient. In children, the total dosage per course is about 75 mg. per Kg. (34 mg. per lb.) of body weight; this is subdivided and taken two or three times daily. A simpler schedule which is both safe and effective is to have children from two to four years old take about 65 mg. three times daily, or a total of 2 Gm.; those from five to eight take 0.1 Gm. three times daily for a total of 3 Gm.; and children over eight and adults take 0.25 Gm. twice daily for a total of 5 Gm. per course. In resistant cases in adults, three doses can be given daily, making a total of 7.5 Gm. In children it is necessary to divide the contents of the pulvule and administer the medication in half a glass of milk or orange juice, in jelly, in a small volume of 1 percent sodium bicarbonate solution, or in food. The taste is not objectionable.

In adults who do not tolerate the drug by mouth, or when there is severe colonic ulceration, the drug may be given as a retention enema; 2 Gm. of medication are dissolved in 20 cc. of warm 2 percent solution of sodium bicarbonate and instilled following a cleansing enema. Such doses are administered every other night for a maximum of five times. Oral medication is omitted during the period of rectal therapy.

In vaginitis due to *Trichomonas vaginalis*, carbarsone is administered as 2-grain (0.13-Gm.) vaginal suppositories, usually one each night for two weeks. A rest period of two weeks is then allowed. Many different regimens have been employed, some with douches, some without. For discussion, see page 198.

As with any arsenical preparation, toxic manifestations must be watched for. The drug should not be administered (1) in amebic hepatitis, (2) in the presence of any type of liver or kidney damage, or (3) to any patient with contracted visual or color fields or a history of intolerance to arsenical preparations. Possible toxic signs include sore throat, edema, splenomegaly, icterus, pruritus, skin eruptions, gastro-intestinal irritation, neuritis, and visual disturbances.

Stovarsol (acetarsone, *m*-acetylamido-*p*-hydroxyphenylarsonic acid) and **Treparsol** (a mixture of the above and the *m*-formylamido compound) are as effective as carbarsone in amebiasis, but their toxicity is such that they are little used.

EMETINE

Emetine, one of the alkaloids of ipecac, is useful in certain phases of amebiasis. It is a complex chemical compound with the empirical formula $C_{29}H_{40}N_2O_4$. It is employed as the hydrochloride, which is a white or slightly yellowish crystalline powder, unstable to light. It is freely soluble in water.

Emetine is highly effective against amebae in the tissues and is the drug of choice in amebic hepatitis and liver abscess. It is relatively ineffective against cysts. For this reason and because it is extremely irritating to the gastro-intestinal tract, it is not given by mouth and is not useful in intestinal amebiasis except when there is severe diarrhea.

The drug is a general protoplasmic poison, producing hyperemia, cloudy swelling, and cellular degeneration in the heart, kidneys, liver, and skeletal muscles. It is particularly toxic to the heart, causing arrhythmias and myocardial degeneration which may produce sudden heart failure and death. Other toxic manifestations include muscular weakness, tremors, and pains; nausea, vomiting, and bloody diarrhea; vertigo; purpura; and hemoptysis. Emetine is contraindicated in the presence of cardiac or renal disease. It should not be given to children except when there is severe diarrhea which has not yielded to carbarsone. It is best avoided during pregnancy.

The maximum dose of emetine hydrochloride is

60 mg. daily, which may be given as a single injection or subdivided into two injections. The subcutaneous route is generally preferred over the intramuscular. Local pain and swelling are common. The drug should not be given intravenously. A course of treatment should last no more than ten days, with a maximum total dose of 0.6 Gm. For children, a daily dosage of 1 mg. per Kg. (0.45 mg. per lb.) of body weight should not be exceeded.

Emetine therapy should be discontinued as soon as symptoms have disappeared, which is usually within three or four days. Courses should not be repeated oftener than every six weeks. The patient should remain in bed under careful observation during the course of therapy and for several days afterward. The blood pressure should be taken twice daily. The drug should be stopped on any evidence of toxicity.

OXYQUINOLINE DRUGS

A group of compounds containing iodine, oxyquinoline, and sulfonic acid radicals are effective against amebae in the lumen of the intestine. However, they do not kill amebae in the intestinal wall, and their usefulness is limited to interim therapy during rest periods from carbarsone. All are nontoxic in therapeutic doses.

Chiniofon, U.S.P., (Anayodin, Yatren) is a mixture of 7-iodo-8-hydroxyquinoline-5-sulfonic acid (see Figure 14 for structural formula), its sodium salt, and sodium bicarbonate, containing not less than 26.5 percent and not more than 29 percent iodine. It is given as enteric-coated tablets, starting with 0.5 Gm. three times daily for adults and increasing to 0.75 to 1 Gm. three times daily. A course of chiniofon therapy lasts eight to twelve days. A rest period should follow.

Large initial doses may induce diarrhea. Diarrhea may also occur as full dosage is reached, but the drug should be stopped only if the diarrhea is severe or lasts more than two or three days.

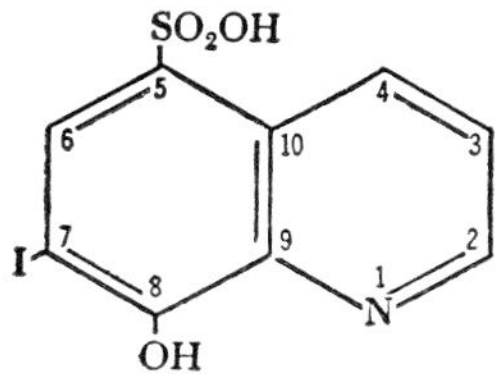

FIGURE 14—*Structural Formula of the Active Principle of Chiniofon*

Chiniofon is contraindicated in the presence of liver damage. Because of its iodine content, it should be used cautiously in patients with hyperthyroidism or idiosyncrasy to iodine.

Vioform (iodochlorhydroxyquin) is similar chemically to chiniofon except that it has a chlorine atom at the 5 position in place of a sulfonic acid group. The iodine content is 37.5 to 41.5 percent. The adult dose is 0.25 Gm. three or four times daily, and ten days constitute a course. A rest period of seven to ten days should follow. Vioform is more irritating locally than chiniofon and is more inclined to produce gastric distress than diarrhea. It has the same contraindications as chiniofon.

INSECTICIDES AND INSECT REPELLENTS

Control of biting and nonbiting arthropods is important from the standpoint of health and comfort. Many are vectors of serious diseases, and most of those attacking man cause painful skin lesions by biting or burrowing. There are now available a number of efficient chemicals which may be classified as insecticides (poisons) or repellents. The distinction is not absolute, since a few compounds are both.

INSECTICIDES

There are three types of insect poisons: contact, digestive, and respiratory. Some of the more effective drugs such as DDT cannot be used for immediate protection because they kill slowly. Others have a rapid "knockdown" effect but may fail to kill and so allow the insect to revive. Many commercial preparations for use in and around buildings combine these two types to good advantage.

DDT (dichlorodiphenyl trichloroethane) is a mixture of two isomers, the structural formulas of which are shown in Figure 15. It is a white crystalline powder, nearly insoluble in water, moderately soluble in petroleum oils, and readily soluble in many organic solvents. This chemical is lethal to most arthropod vectors of disease and has been used extensively in combating mosquitoes, cockroaches, houseflies, bedbugs, and other pests. Topical application—as a 10 percent dusting powder or in combination with other insecticides as a liquid—is very effective against lice and fleas. It has no ovicidal and little, if any, scabicidal action. Al-p, p′—DDT

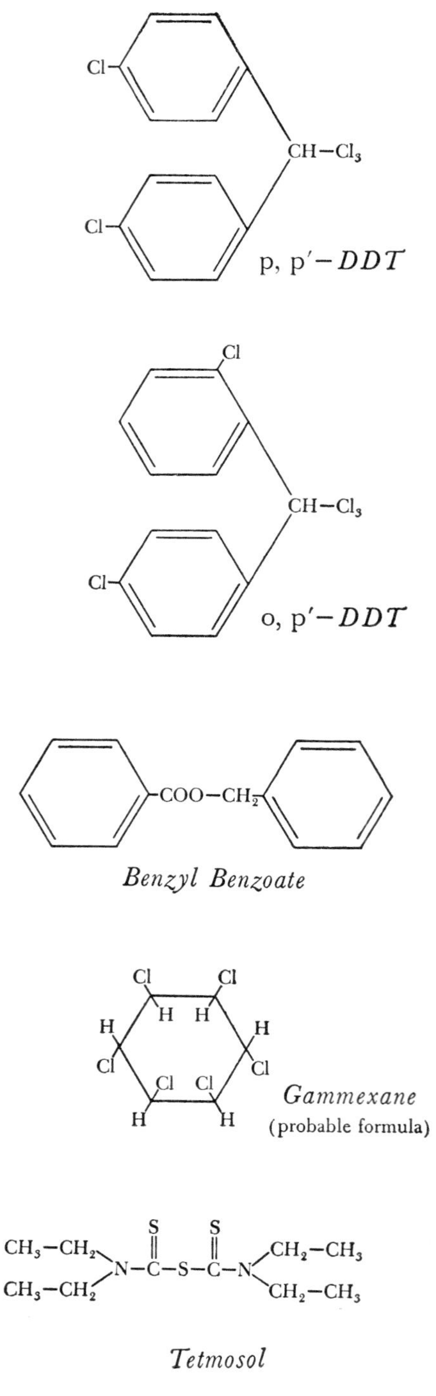

o, p′—DDT

Benzyl Benzoate

Gammexane
(probable formula)

Tetmosol

FIGURE 15—*Structural Formulas of Some*
Insecticides

though it does not attack the louse egg, it remains effective longer than the usual hatching period and consequently kills as the lice emerge. When ordinary woolen underwear is treated with solutions or emulsions containing 1.5 to 2 percent of DDT, the garments will control lice effectively, even after being laundered four or five times.

Solutions of DDT are absorbed through the skin and, if applied repeatedly or in high enough concentration, may be toxic. In animals, concentrations up to 5 percent are safe for topical application, provided drug accumulation from prolonged treatment is avoided. Three to five months' exposure to saturated atmospheres of 5 percent DDT in kerosene has not produced toxicity in man. When used as recommended for the control of human parasites, DDT is not harmful.

Symptoms of DDT poisoning in man are headache, nausea, vomiting, dizziness, apprehension, nervous instability, stiffness and pain in the jaws, aching and heaviness of the extremities, muscular weakness, tremor, and paresthesias. No specific antidote has been discovered. Sedatives and injections of calcium salts (p. 344) are indicated in severe cases for the relief of those symptoms which are caused by increased excitability of the central nervous system.

Benzyl Benzoate (for formula, see Figure 15) is a volatile oily liquid of pungent taste and characteristic odor prepared synthetically or obtained from the balsams of Peru and Tolu. It is very slightly soluble in water and glycerin but is miscible with various organic solvents. When administered by mouth, benzyl benzoate has a slight antispasmodic action, but it is rarely used for this purpose because of the existence of more active compounds.

Benzyl benzoate has long been used for the treatment of scabies and is generally considered to be the most effective single preparation available. One treatment with a 25 percent emulsion is successful in most cases. Burning and stinging usually follow topical application of this strength. Secondary chemical dermatitis is sometimes troublesome and may become severe if treatment is repeated under the misconception that the infection is still active. Benzyl benzoate also attacks lice and their embryonated ova, but with less efficiency than in the case of scabies. Impregnation of clothing with emulsions of benzyl benzoate is an effective method for preventing attack by itch mites (chiggers). In addition to its parasiticidal properties, the compound may be used as a solvent for DDT.

Systemic toxicity from repeated local application of benzyl benzoate does not develop in dogs, cattle, horses, sheep, or pigs, but cats are particularly susceptible and develop symptoms in two or three days. Aside from skin irritation, no toxic symptoms have been noted in man.

Liquid 'Topocide' (Benzyl Benzoate Compound, Topical, Lilly) is a special liquid preparation used for eradication of body lice, pubic lice, and the itch mite, *Sarcoptes scabiei*. It contains in each 100 cc.:

    benzyl benzoate........................12.5 Gm.
    Benzocaine............................. 2 Gm.
    DDT................................... 1 Gm.
    Water, Bentonite Magma, and polyoxyalkylene deriva-
    tives of sorbitan monooleate comprise the inert ingredients,
    which approximate 85 percent (w/w).

One application to the affected skin and hair usually is sufficient to eliminate either type of parasite.

Sulfur in the precipitated form, usually incorporated into an ointment, has long been used for treatment of scabies. When in contact with the skin in the presence of alkalies, it forms hydrogen sulfide and pentathionic acid, which are believed to attack the organisms. It also has some keratolytic action (see p. 482). Repeated application of a 2.5 to 10 percent ointment is necessary for treatment of scabies. This not infrequently causes chemical dermatitis. Mitigal (dimethyl-thianthrene) is an oily compound containing about 25 percent organic sulfur. More effective preparations are now available.

Larkspur Tincture, N.F., is parasiticidal and has been used particularly for treatment of pediculosis capitis. It has been largely replaced by more efficient preparations. Since it does not attack ova, treatment is complicated. Toxicity from skin absorption may occur.

Ethyl Aminobenzoate (Benzocaine) is an ovicide which is also detrimental to lice and to the parasite of scabies. In addition, it is a mild local anesthetic (for discussion of this action, see p. 446). These properties make it useful in combination with other parasiticides. Ethyl aminobenzoate is soluble in oil and in fat solvents. Because of its relative insolubility in water, it is practically nontoxic and almost free of local irritant action.

Gammexane (666) is the gamma isomer of benzene hexachloride (for structural formula, see Figure 15). Like DDT, it has residual toxicity for arthropods, including lice, fleas, flies, ticks, and bedbugs. It is relatively insoluble in water and is stable at high temperatures. Residual deposits are less persistent than those of DDT. A possible disadvantage of gammexane is that poisoning in animals occurs suddenly and is irreversible, whereas DDT produces well-defined premonitory signs of intoxication before lethal amounts have been absorbed. However, the amounts of gammexane required as an insecticide can be applied to the skin with little danger.

Mercuric Chloride (bichloride of mercury) is effective against head lice when applied to the hair and scalp twice daily for three or four days as a 1:500 to 1:1,000 solution in 50 percent alcohol. In more dilute solutions or as mild mercurial ointment, it may be used for body and crab lice. Treatment is prolonged and is more painful than with newer, rapidly acting, nonirritating parasiticides.

Tetmosol (tetraethylthiuram monosulfide; for structural formula, see Figure 15) is a scabicide prepared in a 25 percent alcoholic solution. This can be used full strength for adults but is quite painful. Generally it is diluted with distilled water, 1:4, just before use. The resulting emulsion is applied once or twice daily for three days.

Rotenone is the active principle of derris root. It has been used as a 1 or 2 percent suspension applied once or twice daily for two or three days. Burning is often severe, and dermatitis is not uncommon.

INSECT REPELLENTS

Insect repellents are substances for application to the skin or for impregnation of clothing to prevent or discourage mosquitoes, flies, mites, and other arthropods from attacking. They may be, but commonly are not, insecticidal. It is believed that the repellent action is due to odor which, though not necessarily so to man, is disagreeable to pests.

Volatile oils have long been used as insect repellents. Oil of citronella and oil of pennyroyal, either alone or in combination with other substances, are quite effective for intervals of an hour or two. A mixture of two parts oil of citronella, two parts Camphor Spirit, and one part oil of cedar has been a popular remedy. The smoke from smoldering pyrethrum powder may be used with fair success to dispel mosquitoes from dwellings.

Newer repellents developed during World War II are considerably more efficient and, when applied

to the skin, will protect for several hours. The duration of action depends mostly upon the amount of
perspiration and the type of attacking insect. The
repellents are applied evenly to all exposed surfaces. Untreated areas will not be protected. Im-
pregnating clothing by spraying or rinsing in dilute
solutions is very effective and under ideal circumstances will provide repellent action for several
weeks.

The individual compounds vary in degree of
activity and in the species of arthropod affected.
Dimethyl phthalate affects larval mites such as
chiggers, most *Anopheles* mosquitoes, and some species of the *Aëdes* genus. It is nontoxic to man.
Dibutyl phthalate and benzyl benzoate are of little
value against mosquitoes but will prevent skin infestation by mites. Among the most effective miti-
cides are diphenyl carbonate and *p*-cresyl benzoate.
Indalone (*n*-butyl mesityl oxide oxalate) is especially active against biting flies but is much less so
against malarial mosquitoes. It tends to cause
dermatitis in the presence of copious perspiration.

Rutgers 612 (2-ethylhexanediol-1,3) repels most
mosquitoes (including the salt-water varieties), chiggers, biting flies, fleas, and bedbugs. It is nontoxic
and nonirritating to man but will cause dermatitis
if diluted with alcohol. Other repellents include
2-phenylcyclohexanol, 2-cyclohexyl cyclohexanol,
and dimethyl carbate.

Mixtures are more effective than the single compounds. One known as 622 consists of six parts
dimethyl phthalate, two parts Indalone, and two
parts Rutgers 612. It is used for mosquitoes, sand
flies, chiggers, ticks, fleas, mites, and gnats and will
give protection for one to six hours. When applied
to clothing by sprays or other means, activity
is maintained for several days. Another combination, NMRI 448, is a mixture of seven parts
2-phenylcyclohexanol and three parts 2-cyclohexyl
cyclohexanol. NMRI 201 consists of 1,2,3,4-tetra ·
hydro-beta-naphthol (Tetralol) and 2-phenylcy-
clohexanol-3,7. The latter is said to protect for a
period of about seven hours on dry skin and for
about three hours on sweating skin.

BIOLOGICAL THERAPY

INTRODUCTION

Because of the very great number of possible variations in conception and processing of biological
products intended for any given use, it has not been
deemed practicable to describe all which are available to the physician. Discussion of individual preparations is therefore largely limited to Lilly products, since these embody the considered conclusions
of the Research Staff of Eli Lilly and Company.
The general principles set forth below apply, of
course, to all biological preparations.

Biological products and subjects for discussion include the following:

Antigens administered to stimulate active immunity against infection.
Antibody-containing serums to provide passive
immunity against infection.
Antigens administered for the production of
fever.
Antigens administered to reduce allergic hypersensitivity to the same antigens.
Antigens used for diagnostic tests.

Serum or plasma to supply needed substances
other than antibodies.
Storage of biologicals.

Infection involves two living entities, the infectious agent and the host. For infection to occur,
not only (1) must the infectious agent invade the
tissues of the host, but (2) the latter must suffer
injury thereby, and typically (3) it must react to
the invasion and injury in certain ways which may
be considered as attempts at defense.

Pathogenic organisms may injure the host's tissues by means of:

1. An extracellular toxin, or exotoxin, as in diphtheria and
   tetanus.
2. An intracellular toxin, or endotoxin, set free only upon
   the death of the invading organism, as in typhoid fever.
3. The ordinary proteins of the bacterial cell, as may be
   possible in bacterial allergy.
4. Mechanical obstruction of blood vessels, as in anthrax.
5. Actual destruction of cells, as in malaria.

The reaction of the host may be local or systemic
or both. Locally at the site of infection there may
be vasodilation, exudation of fluid, infiltration with
leukocytes, and even necrosis of tissue, with resulting redness and heat, swelling, pain and tenderness, and ulceration or abscess formation. The

systemic reaction may include malaise progressing to prostration, fever, tachycardia (or, with some infections, bradycardia), alteration of the leukocyte count, and production of antibodies. Many other local and systemic reactions are seen with particular infectious agents and under special circumstances.

The power of a host to resist or overcome infection is termed "immunity." The reciprocal of immunity is "susceptibility." Many factors influence immunity, their relative importance varying with the infectious agent. They may act through tissue cells, white blood and migratory extravascular cells, and circulating or fixed antibodies of various sorts. Immunity may be altered, at least temporarily, by many types of influences which include such things as weather changes, exposure to cold or dampness, severe hemorrhage, overwhelming infection, fatigue, severe hypothyroidism, and nutritional status.

Immunity to a given infectious agent may be:

I. Present throughout the lifetime of the individual. This natural immunity may be peculiar to the individual or common to the race or species.

II. Acquired at some time during the life of the individual.
   A. Passive immunity.
      1. Naturally acquired by the child *in utero* through passive transfer of antibodies from the mother.
      2. Artificially produced by parenteral administration of antibody-containing serums from animals or human beings.
   B. Active immunity.
      1. The result of having and recovering from an infection with the given or a related organism.
      2. The result of repeated exposure to doses of an organism which are too small to produce clinical infection.
      3. The result of unknown factors.
      4. The purposeful result of administration of suitable *antigens*.

An *antigen* is any substance which stimulates the production of antibodies, including specific antibody, or which reacts with specific antibody in some observable way. Similarly, an *antibody* is any substance which is produced by the body cells in response to stimulation by an antigen and which reacts specifically with it. A complete antigen is one that is capable not only of reacting with antibody but also of stimulating its production. A partial antigen, or *hapten*, is one which is capable of reacting with antibody but not of stimulating antibody formation. Some types of antibodies circulate in the blood and reach all parts of the body to which blood flows. Other (sessile) antibodies appear to be confined within the cells of certain tissues, conferring on them a "local immunity" or "tissue immunity" which may be very high.

ANTIGENS ADMINISTERED TO STIMULATE ACTIVE IMMUNITY AGAINST INFECTION

Measures employed to increase immunity to certain infections include the administration of antigens. The question has not been fully answered, but it seems likely that a particular antigen can give rise to only one type of antibody and that the reaction between an antigen and a particular type of antibody can result in only one kind of phenomenon. Thus, when, as frequently happens, the injection of a vaccine containing a given kind of bacterial cell results in production of a number of different antibodies, it is probable that the cell contained a corresponding number of antigens.

The presence of more than one antigen in a given bacterial cell is exemplified by the pneumococcus. Every pneumococcus, so far as has been determined, contains at least two different kinds of antigen. One of these kinds can be identified by the quellung, or capsule-swelling, reaction described by Neufeld. The other is the one that gives rise to the heterophile antibody discovered by Forssman. The antigen identified by the capsule-swelling reaction is not the same in all pneumococci. In fact, pneumococci are divided into a considerable number of types based on differences in the capsular antigen. If a horse is immunized with only one of these types of pneumococci, serum later obtained from that horse will be effective only in a pneumococcal infection due to that type.

The pneumococcus administered to that horse contains also the heterophile antigen; but since the horse is unable to respond to heterophile antigen by the production of heterophile antibody, none of this antibody is ever present in horse serum. Rabbits, cattle, and human beings respond to administration of the heterophile antigen. If a rabbit were immunized with one type of pneumococcus, the serum from this animal would contain at least two kinds of antibodies—the antibody specific for the capsular antigen of that type and the heterophile antibody. The heterophile antibody is specific for the heterophile antigen. Although the heterophile antigen is widely distributed among pathogenic bacteria and thus has a broad application, it is in no sense "nonspecific."

A number of factors have an important influence on the effectiveness of active immunization:

1. The antigenic value of the product used. Though the response in human patients is the ultimate test of antigenicity, a practical indication is given by the antibody titer in animals after a standard immunization procedure. In the case of tox-

oids, precipitation with aluminum potassium sulfate (alum) increases antigenicity, in part by slowing absorption and thus prolonging the antigenic stimulus.

2. Route of administration. In general, antigens are most effective when injected into the subcutaneous tissue. Intracutaneous injection of small doses of fluid antigens may be used in the presence of hypersensitivity and other special indications. The value of intracutaneous inoculation for producing basic immunity has been questioned, and its effectiveness for secondary stimulation is not fully evaluated. Intramuscular or intravenous injection of unmodified antigens is followed by more rapid absorption and destruction or excretion of the antigen, with a correspondingly briefer antigenic stimulus. However, alum-precipitated antigens are given intramuscularly by preference and never intravenously or intracutaneously.

Most antigens are destroyed by the digestive juices; however, in recent years, certain ones have been prepared in forms which are relatively resistant to digestion and which therefore may be absorbed to exert antigenic activity after oral administration. Obviously, a higher dosage must be employed than for parenteral injection.

3. Number of doses. If a sufficient interval is allowed between doses, every successive administration is followed by an increase in antibody production. Although a "one-shot" antigen remains as an ideal, experience has shown that for satisfactory clinical immunity against such diseases as diphtheria, tetanus, and pertussis, a minimum of two injections of alum-precipitated antigen or three doses of fluid antigen is required. When less than full doses are given, the number of injections must be greater.

4. Quantity administered. The quantity of antigen to be administered depends on the potency of the antigen, the route of administration, the number of doses, and the interval between them. A given amount of antigen is more effective if divided into two or three doses than if given all at once.

5. Interval between doses. The period between doses is of extreme importance. If the interval is insufficient, the response to the succeeding dose is both smaller and slower than if the interval has been adequate to allow the preceding dose to complete its action. The optimal interval varies for different antigens. In general, it is shorter for fluid preparations (one to three or four weeks) than for alum-precipitated types, which should be given at intervals of one to three months.

6. Reaction following injections. There have been many attempts to prepare antigens of high potency which would produce little or no reaction. However, it has been found that in the absence of local reaction, effective immunity develops less frequently. As an example, it has been shown that when tetanus toxoid which produces little local reaction is given mixed with sufficient typhoid vaccine to produce moderate local reaction, the resulting immunity to tetanus is much greater and develops more rapidly than when the two substances are injected at the same time but at different sites. The ideal would seem to be the production of some local reaction but not sufficient to cause more than minor discomfort to the patient.

7. Combination of antigens. The combination of antigens before injection has the advantage of reducing the number of injections. With certain antigens it has the additional advantage of producing a greater immunity to each antigen, apparently because of increased local reaction. There is evidence, however, that when too many antigens are introduced simultaneously, the antibody response to each is less than if they had been given separately. Tests indicate that diphtheria toxoid, tetanus toxoid, and pertussis vaccine, or any two of them, can be combined without loss of immunity response.

8. Individual variation in response. There is an unpredictable difference in the response of individuals regardless of other factors. When tests are not made or are not available to determine immunity response (p. 338) after administration of antigens, it may be advisable to give an extra dose of antigen beyond the minimum recommended.

9. Stimulating doses. Following active immunization and the resultant increase in antibody titer, there is a varying rate of decrease in demonstrable antibodies which is manifested clinically by increasing susceptibility to infection. In order to maintain effective protection, it is necessary to restimulate antibody production by administration of single "boosting" doses of antigen. With tetanus and diphtheria it appears that once basic immunity has been established, the ability to respond to additional injections of toxoid is kept for many years, perhaps indefinitely. This is not true in all types of immunization. The antibody response to additional antigen administration appears within a few days and nearly always exceeds that obtained from basic immunization, even though protective titers have fallen too low to be measured by present methods.

10. Passive immunity (including that which is inherited) blocks stimulation of the mechanism by which immunity is produced and thus prevents active immunization. This blocking occurs in infants born of mothers immune to diphtheria and has been demonstrated in nonimmune individuals treated simultaneously with tetanus antitoxin and tetanus toxoid. After the passive immunity is lost, active immunity can be induced without difficulty.

It has been pointed out above that a certain amount of local reaction is necessary to the production of active immunity. Individual biological responses are not always predictable after injection of an antigen, any more than they are after exposure to and invasion of an infecting organism. There are other factors concerned in the occurrence of reactions after administration of antigens: too large a dose for the patient's tolerance; too-short intervals between doses; improper placement of the inoculum in the tissues; trauma from the injection; use of a syringe that has not been freed of reacting substances from a previous injection; and incorrect sterilization of the needle and syringe.

Reactions may be systemic as well as local. They may be due to the inherent toxicity of the bacterial proteins. Such reactions are manifested by malaise and fever and are the rule after the administration of certain antigens such as typhoid vaccine. In other rare cases allergic reactions may occur. Bacterial allergy (and even anaphylaxis) exists and can be demonstrated with all the mechanism of true protein allergy. Bacterial allergy may have a role in arthritis, fibrositis, nephritis, and other conditions. Intravenous injection of bacterial antigens involves the risk of protein shock and should be made only with appropriate safeguards.

There are two distinct types of bacterial hypersensitiveness—one that elicits the ordinary type of response to protein allergy (p. 264), and one which calls forth special types such as the tuberculin (p. 339) and id (p. 268) reactions. Immediate reactions may be difficult to control because of their severity and rapidity of development. Once the reaction is recognized (angioneurotic edema, sneezing, rhinorrhea, bronchial asthma, shock), treatment should be instituted as for anaphylactic shock (p. 269).

There are other factors of unknown nature that influence reactions to vaccines and other types of medication. When large numbers of injections are given over a period of time, a definite variation in incidence or severity of reactions, or both, may be observed to be correlated with the time of day, the season of the year, or the recurrence of certain weather conditions.

Antigens used for development of active immunity include the following: (1) virus vaccines, (2) rickettsial vaccines, (3) toxoids, (4) bacterial vaccines (suspensions of dead but physically intact bacteria), (5) lysates, and (6) undenatured bacterial antigens.

VIRUS VACCINES

Smallpox Vaccine (Vaccine Virus)—The event which first foreshadowed the modern development of active immunization to infection was Jenner's use of the virus of vaccinia, or cowpox, to produce active immunity to smallpox. The practice has changed little since his day. Protection is relatively complete but does not last indefinitely, and revaccination is necessary. The first vaccination may be carried out early in life, any time after the umbilicus has healed. It is usually postponed until after the third month and is preferably carried out during the cooler months, when the vaccine is less susceptible to deterioration and there is less likelihood of secondary infection. Vaccination should be repeated at the time of entrance into school and again in early adult life. All persons exposed directly or indirectly to smallpox should be vaccinated or revaccinated immediately, unless they have had smallpox.

The present vaccine is essentially the same as the original Jenner vaccine, except that calf lymph is used instead of human lymph and bacterial contamination is successfully controlled by the use of glycerin and ripening. It is supplied in capillary tubes. Smallpox vaccine must be kept very cold (preferably below freezing). When not properly refrigerated, it loses its activity very rapidly (see Table 34, p. 340).

The preferred site of vaccination is the upper arm, where there is less risk of secondary infection. By the present methods of vaccination, the scars can be kept small and in an inconspicuous area. The skin at the site is cleansed with ether or acetone and allowed to dry. The capillary tube of vaccine is broken at both ends, and the vaccine is expressed onto the skin with the rubber bulb. A sterile needle is held parallel to the skin surface, and the pointed end is pressed against the skin (about ten times for primary immunization and twenty or thirty times for revaccination), firmly enough to break the cornified outer layer of the epidermis but not sufficiently to draw blood. The punctures should cover an area no larger than 1/8 inch in diameter. The drop of virus may be wiped off immediately. Dressings should not be used.

Proper aftercare of the vaccination is essential. Severe local lesions due to secondary infection are largely preventable by proper technic of vaccination and aftercare. Shields, pads, gauze, or other dressings are contraindicated, since they are considered to predispose to serious complications. A few layers of gauze fastened to the lining of the garment worn next to the site of inoculation may be used if necessary.

Among others, the following may be listed as causes of failure of vaccination:

1. Use of improperly stored vaccine.
2. Too-deep scarification, with bleeding.
3. Application to the skin site of denatured alcohol or antiseptics that destroy the virus before it can be absorbed.
4. Exposure of the area to sunlight within the first four hours after inoculation.

After vaccination with an active vaccine, one of three reactions may be expected to occur, and failure to obtain one of them is an indication for revaccination:

1. Vaccinia, or the typical "take," indicating lack of previous immunity. A small macule appears, usually on the third day, which gradually changes into a papule with red areola. Vesiculation begins about the fifth day and progresses to form by the seventh to ninth day a flat, yellow-gray, umbilicated, multilocular lesion, about 1/2 inch in diameter, with surrounding redness and swelling. Desiccation begins on the tenth or eleventh day and proceeds rapidly. The crust usually separates in the third week or later, leaving the characteristic scar. The lesion is usually tense, itching, and sore, with regional lymphadenopathy. The systemic symptoms of infection may occur, usually from the fifth or sixth to the eighth or ninth days.

2. Vaccinoid, or mild "take," indicating the presence of partial immunity usually resulting from previous vaccination. The course resembles that of vaccinia except that it is shorter and milder in every way.

3. An immune reaction indicative of a satisfactory immunity resulting from previous vaccination or an attack of smallpox. An itching papule of

variable size appears, reaching its maximum within forty-eight hours.

In primary vaccinations the site should be examined on the ninth and fourteenth days. In secondary vaccinations it should be inspected at the end of two days for an immune reaction and, if negative, again between four and seven days for vaccinoid.

Since immunity is developed in about eight days after successful vaccination and since smallpox has an incubation period of about fourteen days, it is possible to vaccinate contacts promptly after exposure. The duration of immunity after vaccination is variable but usually is five to seven years and may be much longer.

A number of complications may follow vaccination. In rare instances, the vesicle may become purulent and extend beyond its normal diameter. If this occurs, the vesicle should be opened, and a strong antiseptic solution should be applied. Moist dressings may be required for a few days. Accessory vesicles sometimes develop around the vaccination site, particularly when the skin has been cleansed too vigorously. Autoinoculations sometimes occur because of accidental transfer of virus from the site of vaccination. It is advisable to caution patients regarding this possibility, particularly as to contamination of the eyelids, on which lesions may be of serious consequence.

Generalized vaccinia is a rare but serious complication that occurs as crops of secondary lesions for four to six weeks after vaccination. It may be fatal to those who are debilitated or who have skin eruptions or eczema. Rather than vaccinate such persons, it may be advisable to isolate them during epidemics of smallpox, making sure that all contacts have been successfully vaccinated.

Skin eruptions may appear during or shortly after the height of reaction; they are self-limited and require no treatment. Tetanus and demyelination encephalitis are serious complications which are becoming increasingly rare. Available evidence indicates that vaccination during pregnancy does not lead to congenital malformation of the baby. Vaccination may occasionally produce false positive serologic tests for syphilis.

Rabies Vaccine is used in the preventive treatment of rabies (p. 30). According to corrected mortality statistics, when rabies vaccine is given promptly and in adequate amounts, protection is afforded in 99 to 99.5 percent of cases exposed to rabies. The prognosis in a given case depends much upon the location and severity of the bite. Bites above the

shoulders are apt to be followed by such a short incubation period (because of the short distance the virus travels to reach the brain) that it may not be possible to produce immunity in time to prevent the disease. In such cases, especially careful and thorough local treatment of the wound is urgently indicated, and the course of rabies vaccine should be started at once. Some recommend that three or four doses of vaccine be given at different sites each day. Severe bites on other parts of the body are likewise more dangerous than less extensive ones.

Vaccination against rabies should be undertaken when the situation fulfills one of the criteria listed below regarding the biting animal and one regarding the bitten individual:

A. Criteria regarding the biting animal
   1. When it is clinically rabid, even though examination of the brain fails to reveal Negri bodies.
   2. When Negri bodies are found, regardless of whether there were clinical manifestations.
   3. When it disappears after biting or cannot be identified.
   4. When it bites without provocation and is immediately killed.
B. Criteria regarding the bitten person
   1. There are visible wounds into or through the bare skin made by the teeth or claws of the animal.
   2. Wounds were inflicted through clothing which was torn by the teeth of the animal.
   3. Fresh, open wounds of any origin have been contaminated by the saliva of a rabid animal.

Vaccination against rabies is *not* indicated under the following circumstances:

   1. When exposure is limited to contact with saliva on the unbroken skin or mucous membrane or on pre-existing wounds more than twenty-four hours old.
   2. When the teeth of the animal merely bruise but do not break the skin.
   3. When exposure consists only in handling rabid or exposed animals or objects contaminated with saliva.
   4. When milk from a rabid animal has been ingested.
   5. When bites or scratches were inflicted at least seven days before the clinical onset of rabies in the attacking animal.

The vaccine is a suspension of a standardized powder obtained by desiccating in the frozen state the pulverized brains of rabbits which have been killed after becoming completely paralyzed following inoculation with fixed virus. The antigenicity of the vaccine is determined by the Habel mouse technic.

A complete treatment consists in one daily subcutaneous injection for a period of fourteen days. All doses are of the same strength (2,000 Harris units) and are the same for children as for adults. Before injection, the vaccine should be warmed by holding the vial in the hand for a few minutes. Injections are made into the subcutaneous tissue, preferably of the right and left lateral regions of the abdomen alternately. Care should be taken to avoid the inguinal regions. The arms are not suitable sites.

Local reaction to the injections is common and is manifested by redness, tenderness, induration, and sometimes itching. Occasionally systemic symptoms occur, with malaise, numbness, tingling sensations, insomnia, or even unusual drowsiness; these are possible symptoms of demyelination encephalitis and call for discontinuation of treatment. Encephalitis may be fatal.

Rarely, allergic reactions such as urticaria are seen. Very rarely, the serious complication of treatment paralysis may develop, carrying a mortality as high as 30 percent. Treatment need not disturb the patient's daily routine, but he should be advised against excesses of all kinds, fatigue, exposure to cold, emotional strain, and violent exercise.

The induced immunity rarely persists as long as a year and cannot be depended upon for more than three months. Re-exposure more than three months after immunization should be followed by a second course of vaccine injections.

Influenza Virus Vaccine (Types A and B)—Influenza virus vaccine has been developed in the past few years to produce active immunity to influenza due to Types A and B virus. Its use in the presence of epidemics has reduced the incidence of infection by approximately 70 percent. The duration of immunity is probably not longer than a few months.

For production of the vaccine, the viruses are grown in the allantoic fluid of incubated hen eggs. There are several methods for separating the virus from the egg proteins: cold hemagglutination, adsorption on calcium phosphate, and ultracentrifugation. The amount of virus is measured by cold hemagglutination and by mouse immunity tests.

One subcutaneous injection of 1 cc. of the vaccine has been the immunizing procedure used with success in the armed forces. For children one may give a total of 1 cc. in divided doses in the course of a week. The vial should be shaken well before the dose is withdrawn. For those who wish to maintain immunity throughout the winter, it is suggested that the injection be repeated at intervals of approximately three months.

About two-thirds of patients may be expected to have local reactions, with varying degrees of redness, tenderness, and induration. About 2 percent may be expected to have systemic reactions, with chilliness, generalized aching, headache, and occasionally fever. Because of the low protein content of the vaccine, the formalin which it contains is likely to produce immediate stinging on injection. This effect is of brief duration and has no other significance.

Allergic reactions are possible and may be due to the antigen itself or to the egg protein on which it is grown. Ratner advises that all persons be tested intradermally with undiluted vaccine, 0.02 cc., before each and every dose is administered. If the test dose is negative or doubtful, the vaccine can be given with impunity. If a moderate local reaction ensues, the vaccine can be administered, but with the added precaution of simultaneous subcutaneous injection of 2 or 3 minims (0.13 to 0.2 cc.) of Epinephrine Solution (1:1,000). If a large local reaction is obtained, the epinephrine should be given before the vaccine; and the latter should be given either in divided doses at one, two, or three-day intervals, or it may be given intradermally in 0.1-cc. doses, repeated several times. If a test dose induces a systemic reaction, the vaccine should be withheld unconditionally.

Mumps Vaccine is a suspension of killed mumps virus in isotonic sodium chloride solution, preserved with 'Merthiolate,' 1:10,000. The virus is grown in embryonated chicken eggs. After incubation for about seven days, the periembryonic fluid is removed aseptically and dialyzed for recovery of the raw virus. Inactivation is accomplished with ultraviolet radiation. The killed virus is concentrated and purified with alcohol. Tests for antigenicity, sterility, and safety are performed according to specifications of the National Institutes of Health of the United States Public Health Service.

Mumps vaccine is a recent development in immunology, and consequently indications for general use are not clear-cut. Adults who are susceptible to infection (as shown by lack of circulating complement-fixing antigen or a negative skin test [see p. 338]) may be immunized. Complement-fixation titers increase within one week; therefore, vaccination of nonimmune adults after exposure is a logical procedure. Epidemics of mumps are prone to occur in segregated populations, such as in the armed forces, schools, asylums, and orphanages and among medical students and nurses. These may be prevented by routine administration of the vaccine to all susceptible individuals; or, if already established, they may be aborted by immediate vaccination. Routine immunization before adolescence is not recommended on the basis that the artificially induced immunity may wane and permit infection to occur at an older age when there is greater danger from complications. It is not known whether induced immunity in infants and children may be maintained indefinitely by administration of boosting doses. Immunity to mumps is found in many individuals who never have had clinical manifestations of parotitis. It is possible that actively immunized children may develop subclinical infections and thereby acquire permanent protection. Until these points have been clarified, administration of mumps vaccine to infants and children should be limited to special circumstances in which the need for protection outweighs any possible disadvantages.

Individuals who are allergic to eggs may develop severe reactions and should not be immunized with the vaccine.

For active immunization against mumps, two injections of 1 cc. each are given subcutaneously five to ten days apart. The site of injection should not have been used previously for administration of other antigens. Previously immunized individuals with waning immunity or after exposure to infection may be given a single stimulating, or boosting, dose of 0.5 to 1 cc. subcutaneously. Local and systemic reactions are usually mild. Slight erythema with some tenderness and, rarely, induration may develop at the site of injection. Fever and malaise are uncommon.

Since the vaccine is prepared from the embryonic fluid of chicken eggs, it should not be administered in the presence of allergy to egg proteins. Studies show that egg vaccines are not dangerous for 99.5 percent of the general population, including allergic individuals not sensitive to egg.

RICKETTSIAL VACCINES

Rocky Mountain Spotted Fever Vaccine is administered to produce active immunity against Rocky Mountain spotted fever (p. 18). It is prepared by the yolk-sac method.

Adults are given either three injections of 1 cc. or two injections of 2 cc. subcutaneously or intramuscularly at intervals of one week. Children under ten years of age should receive 0.5 cc. at weekly intervals for three doses. A course of immunization gives full protection for one year against mild strains but not against many highly virulent strains. A boosting dose should be given annually, preferably before the start of the tick season.

Because of the possibility of egg allergy, Ratner advises the same precautions before each injection as with influenza virus vaccine (p. 323).

Immunization is contraindicated in the presence of debilitating disease or latent or active infections.

The vaccine is effective only in prophylaxis; it is of no value if given after the bite of an infected tick.

TOXOIDS

Toxoids are derivatives of exotoxins prepared by treating the toxins with formalin in such a way that all toxicity is lost but full antigenicity is maintained. Toxoids have largely replaced toxin-antitoxin mixtures because they contain no serum and consequently cannot sensitize patients to serum. Alum-precipitated toxoids are preferred by most investigators over fluid toxoids because of their greater antigenicity.

Diphtheria Toxoid, Fluid, is given for production of active immunity against diphtheria (p. 3). Diphtheria toxin is obtained in the usual way by growing a good toxin-producing strain of diphtheria bacillus (*Corynebacterium diphtheriae*) in special media. After incubation the culture is filtered, and the potent toxin filtrate is treated with formalin and incubated until all toxicity is lost. Detoxification must be so nearly complete that five human doses, when injected into guinea pigs weighing 300 Gm., will cause no signs of diphtheria-toxin poisoning, either locally or generally, within thirty days. After detoxification, the toxoid is purified by a process of fractionation with methanol at subfreezing temperatures which removes practically all of the inert, nonantigenic protein.

Toxoid is given by subcutaneous injection in three 0.5-cc. doses at intervals of three or four weeks. Three injections will engender in four months an antitoxin titer of 0.01 unit or more of antitoxin per cubic centimeter of blood serum in approximately 96 percent of Schick-positive cases, and this titer is maintained for at least two years.

Plain toxoid is well borne by children up to six years of age. Pronounced local and systemic reactions may occur in older children and adults. These reactions are mostly accounted for by hypersensitiveness to diphtheria-bacillus proteins of the toxoid preparation. This sensitization is acquired through contact with the diphtheria bacillus as the individual becomes older, or it may develop from previous injections of toxoid.

Diphtheria Toxoid, Alum Precipitated, also is used to produce active immunity against diphtheria. It has the advantage over fluid toxoid of much greater antigenicity, inducing a much higher and more lasting titer of antitoxin. It is prepared by treating fluid toxoid with alum. Since practically all of the inert, nonantigenic proteins have previously been removed by the purification process, only small amounts of alum are required to effect complete precipitation.

To produce immunity, two doses of 0.5 cc. are given subcutaneously, with an interval of a month or more between them. An interval of two or three months gives a somewhat more effective immunity. Alum-precipitated toxoid should be given intramuscularly or deposited deep in the subcutaneous tissue between the muscle fascia and overlying layer of subcutaneous fat.

As in the case of plain toxoid, the alum-precipitated toxoid contains diphtheria-bacillus proteins and may produce reactions in the older age groups. A nodule may appear at the site of injection and sometimes persists for several weeks. The most frequent local reaction consists in redness, induration, tenderness, and pain of varying grades of intensity. The systemic reaction is not severe in younger children, although there may be some restlessness, irritability, and slight coryza. Rarely, even in the young children, there may be more severe reactions.

An optimal age for beginning immunization with diphtheria toxoid cannot be designated on the basis of present evidence. Conservative groups recommend administration sometime after six months of age, preferably at eight or nine months. Public health authorities believe that immunization should be completed by the age of six months. Others suggest that injections be started early, between the first and third months of life.

If early immunization is practiced, it probably should be limited to those infants whose mothers are known to be Schick-positive. However, it has been reported that low titers of inherited diphtheria antitoxin, too small to influence the skin test, may interfere with production of active immunity. On the other hand, successful active immunization has been accomplished in the presence of passively acquired antitoxin. In view of the conflicting evidence, it seems particularly important that all individuals who are immunized early receive the benefit of a boosting, or stimulating, dose of toxoid sometime before two years of age.

When infants have been successfully immunized against diphtheria, a variable proportion will have very little protection at the age of four or five years. However, a single injection of toxoid rapidly renews immunity. Protective antibody levels are attained within a few days and continue to increase at an accelerated rate for a week or more to titers higher than those following primary immunization or recovery from the disease itself. A boosting dose

of diphtheria toxoid should be given to all previously immunized children before they enter school. Many recommend that an injection be given one year after basic immunization or by the age of two years. Revaccination should be performed in the presence of an epidemic; but, owing to the short incubation time of the disease, this procedure cannot be used to prevent diphtheria following exposure.

Routine administration of diphtheria toxoid to adults is neither a practical nor a safe procedure. Many have acquired sensitivity to proteins of the diphtheria bacillus and will develop serious allergic reactions when toxoid is given. If immunization is to be carried out, it should be reserved only for those who are susceptible as determined by the Schick test, and then not until a Moloney test for sensitivity is known to be negative. When the latter is positive, it may be possible to immunize by observing the proper precautions.

Tetanus Toxoid, Fluid, is given to produce active immunity against tetanus (p. 12). Tetanus toxoid is prepared by addition of 0.4 percent formalin to highly potent tetanus toxin and incubation for several weeks. When detoxification is complete, the toxoid is purified by a fractionation process which removes practically all of the inert, nonantigenic protein.

Persons engaged in civil and military pursuits in which the risk of tetanus is great should be immunized. Immunization should be advised for subjects who are naturally sensitive to animal serum proteins or for those who have acquired sensitization through previous administration of tetanus or other antitoxins and for whom the injection of tetanus antitoxin is more or less hazardous.

The actively immunized person is usually protected against tetanus which may arise from those accidents and wounds too minor to suggest prophylactic administration of antitoxin. In this group of injuries belong ordinary and electrical burns, effects of exposure to cold, excoriations under casts, and even pinpricks—to say nothing of the numerous slight injuries of childhood, such as cuts, bruises, and cement burns.

For basic immunity, three doses of 0.5 cc. each of fluid toxoid are administered subcutaneously at intervals of three or four weeks. An additional dose of 0.5 cc. one year later is recommended.

The duration of basic immunity produced by the usual two doses of alum-precipitated tetanus toxoid or by the three doses of the fluid type is not exactly known, but it is generally believed to remain effective for one or two years. Basic immunity may decline at a relatively rapid rate; but following renewal by a boosting dose of toxoid, the blood antitoxin increases within a few days to higher levels than those produced by the primary two or three doses of toxoid. In addition, these levels persist for longer periods of time. Thus, even if the antitoxin has declined to a very low level, it is possible to protect against exposure to tetanus infection by administering a single dose of toxoid. This procedure avoids the development of serum-protein sensitivity from the use of tetanus antitoxin and maintains immunity well beyond the incubation period of the disease.

The longest interval following basic immunization with tetanus toxoid at which boosting doses will be effective is not definitely known. There is evidence that once primary immunity is established, the immune mechanism is able to respond years later.

Tetanus Toxoid, Alum Precipitated, also is used for the production of active immunity against tetanus. It has the advantage over fluid toxoid of much greater antigenicity, inducing a higher and more lasting titer of antitoxin. Alum-precipitated tetanus toxoid is prepared by precipitating the purified fluid tetanus toxoid with alum, washing the precipitate, and resuspending it in isotonic sodium chloride solution. Because the toxoid is so highly purified, relatively small amounts of alum are required to produce complete precipitation. 'Merthiolate,' 1:10,000, is used as a preservative.

Two doses of 0.5 cc. of alum-precipitated tetanus toxoid are injected subcutaneously with an interval of one month or more between doses. An additional dose of 0.5 cc. one year later is recommended. In the event of injury and possible exposure to *Clostridium tetani*, a single subcutaneous injection of 0.5 cc. of either alum-precipitated or fluid toxoid is given as soon as possible. Stimulating doses may also be indicated before secondary operations on or manipulations of old wounds. If the injury should occur less than one month after initial or basic immunization or if there is any doubt as to the immune status, tetanus antitoxin must be used.

Active immunization with tetanus toxoid causes the production of circulating antitoxin, which reaches a maximum in three to five months. This is maintained for variable lengths of time and then gradually recedes. Once basic immunity has been established, an additional dose of tetanus toxoid will cause a very prompt rise in antitoxin, which usually reaches protective levels in three days and

continues to rise to levels considerably greater than can be produced by prophylactic doses of the antitoxin.

Local and systemic reactions may be observed after either the plain tetanus toxoid or the alum-precipitated product; but for the most part, they are moderate. Subjects are not hypersensitive to the tetanus-bacillus proteins (as they may be to the diphtheria-bacillus proteins) despite previous contact with the tetanus bacillus.

Diphtheria-Tetanus Toxoids Combined — Diphtheria-Tetanus Toxoids Combined, Fluid, is a solution of purified diphtheria and tetanus toxoids in isotonic sodium chloride solution, preserved with 'Merthiolate,' 1:10,000.

Diphtheria-Tetanus Toxoids Combined, Alum Precipitated, is a suspension of alum-precipitated, purified diphtheria and tetanus toxoids in isotonic sodium chloride solution, preserved with 'Merthiolate,' 1:10,000.

Each toxoid in both the fluid and alum-precipitated preparations is prepared and standardized as described under the individual toxoids. The purification process removes practically all of the inert proteins, thus reducing the incidence and severity of reactions, particularly those at the site of injection. Since the nonantigenic proteins are removed, very little alum is required to produce complete precipitation.

Diphtheria-Tetanus Toxoids Combined, Fluid, is given subcutaneously in three doses of 0.5 cc. each, at intervals of three to four weeks.

The injections of Diphtheria-Tetanus Toxoids Combined, Alum Precipitated, are made deep subcutaneously or intramuscularly in an area where no previous antigen injections have been made. The first dose is 0.5 cc., followed after an interval of one or more months with a second 0.5-cc. dose.

The boosting dose of either preparation is 0.25 to 0.5 cc.

When immunization is carried out in the preschool age, the reactions to the combined toxoids are no more frequent or severe than those following diphtheria alum-precipitated toxoid. Older children and adults may have developed sensitivity to proteins of the diphtheria bacillus and should not be immunized without preliminary testing, as described under Diphtheria Toxoid, Alum Precipitated, above.

BACTERIAL ANTIGENS

Bacterial antigens are employed to induce active immunity to the proteins of the bacteria themselves. Various preparations differ from each other as to (1) the organism, or even strain, represented, and (2) the method by which the organisms are killed.

The expression "bacterial vaccine" usually refers to a suspension in physiological salt solution of dead but physically intact bacteria. The organisms may have been killed by heat, by chemicals, or by physical means such as ultraviolet light. The potency of vaccines of this type is ordinarily expressed as the number of bacteria per cc., and the volume of the individual dose is regulated accordingly.

Bacteria can also be killed and their proteins liberated by the addition of bacteriophage. Bacterial antigens prepared in this way have been termed "lysates." Lysis by bacteriophage produces less denaturation of the bacterial proteins than does heat or chemicals. When lysates are applied topically to an infected area, the bacteriophage is believed to exert a specific effect which apparently does not occur after injection. However, most of the effect of lysates, even on topical application, is believed to depend on the production of active immunity to the bacterial proteins.

A third method of killing bacteria, and the one which appears to produce a minimum of denaturation of the bacterial proteins, is mechanical disruption by prolonged grinding in a ball mill. Such preparations are known as "undenatured bacterial antigens." They are prepared from washed bacterial cells and are therefore free of medium, bacterial metabolites, and protein split products. Ultrafiltration removes any intact and viable bacteria. The product is standardized on the basis of nitrogen content.

Pertussis Vaccine (Prophylactic) is given to induce active immunity to whooping cough (p.15). It is a fluid type of vaccine prepared from recently isolated strains of *H. pertussis* of demonstrated phase I characteristics and high antigenicity. The vaccine is an unwashed suspension of organisms, killed by formalin, in physiological salt solution and preserved with 'Merthiolate,' 1:10,000. The concentration is 50,000 million killed organisms per cc.

The vaccine is administered subcutaneously in three doses of 0.5 cc. each, at intervals of three or four weeks. No two injections should be made in the same skin area, and injections should not be made at the site of a previous vaccination. Great care must always be taken not to inject into a vein or skin capillary.

The total immunizing dose provided by the three injections is 75,000 million organisms, which is less

than that employed prior to 1950. This reduction was made possible by development of the mouse challenge test, which permits selection of strains with maximum antigenicity. Previously, it was necessary to give from 80,000 million to as high as 120,000 million organisms to compensate for "soft," or less antigenic, strains that could not be identified.

Those who have undergone primary immunization in the first year should receive a boosting dose of 0.25 to 0.5 cc. at about two years of age. All previously immunized children should be given a boosting dose at five or six before entrance into school. Similar doses are indicated during epidemics and particularly after known intimate exposure.

Local reactions are ordinarily moderate, with redness, tenderness, and induration of varied intensity. Occasionally, fever and restlessness will be observed during the first thirty-six hours after injection. Convulsions (with or without fever) develop rarely and are believed to represent an individual peculiarity, possibly due to previous sensitization to pertussis organisms. Should convulsions occur, subsequent injections are given with extreme caution or not at all. Children who have systemic reactions should be kept quieter than usual after the vaccine injections.

If unusually severe reactions occur, the subsequent scheduled doses should not be increased, but additional injections of divided doses should be made to bring the total volume to that intended. Older children tend to develop more severe reactions. The Pertussis Agglutination Test (p. 339) is available to determine the response to immunization.

Pertussis Vaccine (Prophylactic), Alum Precipitated, is administered to produce active immunity to whooping cough (p. 15). As is the case with the diphtheria and tetanus toxoids (pp. 324 and 326), the alum-precipitated pertussis vaccine induces a higher titer of antibodies than the ordinary vaccine. Each cc. represents 25,000 million killed *H pertussis*. The amount of alum contained in the maximum dose is less than 20 mg.

Basic immunity is established by the administration of three 0.5-cc. doses of alum-precipitated pertussis vaccine at intervals of one or more months. A stimulating dose of 0.5 cc. or less should be given a year after the completion of basic immunization. For children receiving primary vaccination early in life, a second stimulating dose (that is, fifth injection) of 0.5 cc. is advised before entrance into school at the age of five or six years. Since immunity is relative and may be overcome by large doses of infective organisms, a stimulating dose should be given as soon as possible after intimate exposure.

The injections are best given intramuscularly or deep in the subcutaneous tissues. Care should be taken to avoid depositing the vaccine immediately beneath the skin, in the upper part of the subcutaneous layer of fat, or in sites which have received previous inoculations.

Reactions are similar to those observed after alum-precipitated diphtheria toxoid in young children (see p. 324). There are indurated nodules at the site of injection; these persist for some time, gradually decreasing in size and disappearing. If the tissue irritation is severe at the site of injection, there will be a migration of leukocytes to the area, with resulting fluctuation. Occasionally, the area may become a sterile abscess. The factors concerned in reactions are the insoluble alum (which acts as a tissue irritant of varying degree, depending on individual tissue susceptibility) and pertussis-bacillus protein and endotoxins. There will be some local and general reaction from the first dose, and somewhat more may be expected after the second and third. Intramuscular injection largely eliminates the more severe local reactions.

'Perdipigen, Fluid,' (Pertussis-Diphtheria Immunizing, Lilly) is given to produce active immunity to both diphtheria and whooping cough. The combined antigen accomplishes this result with no more local reaction than would be expected from the administration of either antigen alone. The fluid diphtheria toxoid and pertussis vaccine are prepared and standardized separately and then combined, each cc. of the combination representing 50,000 million killed *H. pertussis*. The total immunizing dose of 1.5 cc. contains the same amount of diphtheria toxoid that is required when it is given separately.

Combined immunization against diphtheria and whooping cough can be given any time after six months of age, preferably about the eighth or ninth month. By this time active immunization can be produced more readily, since interference by the passive diphtheria immunity inherited from the mother has been largely eliminated. Some authorities recommend that injections be started at three months of age. 'Perdipigen, Fluid,' is given subcutaneously in three 0.5-cc. doses three or four weeks apart. Revaccination is recommended with a single dose of 0.25 to 0.5 cc. at about two years of age and again before entrance to school.

'Perdipigen, Alum Precipitated,' (Pertussis-Diphtheria Immunizing, Lilly) is also used to induce active immunity to both diphtheria and whooping cough. It bears the same relation to 'Perdipigen, Fluid,' that the alum-precipitated diphtheria toxoid and pertussis vaccine bear to the fluid toxoid and vaccine. Each cc. of 'Perdipigen, Alum Precipitated,' represents 25,000 million killed alum-precipitated pertussis organisms. The total dose of 1.5 cc. contains the same amount of alum-precipitated diphtheria toxoid that is required when it is given separately.

Three injections of 0.5 cc. of 'Perdipigen, Alum Precipitated,' are given at intervals of one month or more. Injections are best given intramuscularly or, if preferred, deep in the subcutaneous tissue. Boosting doses are given as recommended for the fluid combination.

The most frequent local reaction consists in inflammation, induration, and tenderness. Severe local reactions with liquefaction and sterile abscess formation occur rarely and can generally be prevented by intramuscular injection. General reactions may occur, with fever, malaise, and restlessness. Some increase in the severity of either or both types may be expected to follow the second and third doses. Older children and adults may have developed sensitivity to diphtheria toxoid and should not be immunized routinely unless the Schick test is positive and the Moloney test is negative.

Diphtheria-Tetanus Toxoids and Pertussis Vaccine Combined—Diphtheria-Tetanus Toxoids and Pertussis Vaccine Combined, Fluid, is a suspension of formalin-killed, phase I *H. pertussis* in a solution of purified diphtheria and tetanus toxoids, preserved with 'Merthiolate,' 1:10,000. The individual ingredients are prepared and standardized as described previously. Each cc. contains 50,000 million killed whooping cough organisms. The total immunizing dose of 1.5 cc. contains the same amount of each toxoid that is required when they are given separately. Practically all of the inert proteins are removed from the toxoids by the purification process. Diphtheria-Tetanus Toxoids and Pertussis Vaccine Combined, Alum Precipitated, is prepared in the same manner except that each ingredient is precipitated with alum. Each cc. contains 25,000 million killed pertussis organisms. The total immunizing dose of 1.5 cc. contains the same amount of each toxoid as is required when they are given separately. Since purification of the toxoids removes practically all of the inert protein, very little alum is required to produce complete precipitation. The alum content, therefore, is considerably less than the maximal limits of 20 mg. per dose.

Combined immunization against diphtheria, tetanus, and whooping cough should be performed between six and twelve months of age, preferably at eight or nine months. The site for administration should be chosen away from previous injections and in an area providing lax skin with abundant subcutaneous tissue. The usual aseptic precautions are necessary.

The alum-precipitated preparation is given in three doses of 0.5 cc. each, at intervals of one or more months. The injections are best made intramuscularly; or, if preferred, they may be given deep in the subcutaneous tissue. Revaccination with a single injection of 0.25 to 0.5 cc. one or two years after primary immunization and again at five or six years of age is desirable. If preferred, the individual antigens may be used. Active immunization with the fluid combination consists of three subcutaneous injections of 0.5 cc. each, given three or four weeks apart. A dose of 0.25 to 0.5 cc. is adequate for revaccination.

Whenever an immunized individual is exposed to tetanus, a stimulating dose of either fluid or alum-precipitated tetanus toxoid should be given as soon after injury as possible.

The Schick test (p. 338) may be applied six to twelve months after immunization. Fewer pseudopositive reactions will be obtained with the longer interval. The test may be omitted if a stimulating dose of diphtheria toxoid is substituted. The pertussis agglutination test (p. 339) should be performed three or four months after the last dose of vaccine. There is no practical test for measuring protection against tetanus.

As a rule, reactions to the combined antigen are not severe; but inasmuch as the response of an individual to biological therapy cannot always be predicted, varying degrees of reaction are to be expected. The most frequent local reaction is inflammation, induration, and tenderness beginning about twenty-four hours after injection and persisting for two or three days. General reactions are characterized by fever, malaise, and restlessness. Since allergic reactions to diphtheria toxoid may occur in older individuals, they should not be immunized unless the Schick test is positive and the Moloney test is negative.

Typhoid Vaccine is given to produce active immunity to typhoid fever (p. 14). The protection is not complete, but the incidence of the disease in vaccinated groups is approximately only one-fourth that in similar unvaccinated groups. The vaccine is prepared from a virulent smooth strain of *Eber-*

thella typhosa of complete antigenic composition; the bacteria are heat-killed. Each cc. contains 1,000 million organisms.

The vaccine is administered subcutaneously in the arm or other suitable site. Three injections of 0.5 cc. each are given at intervals of five to ten days. Children should be vaccinated in the second year of life. Intracutaneous administration is not recommended for basic, or primary, immunization but may be employed for revaccination.

In administering typhoid vaccine, it is extremely important not to inject the dose into the circulation. Such an accident would cause a severe nonspecific protein reaction with chills and fever. For this reason, intramuscular injection is avoided; and on subcutaneous injection, suction is applied to the plunger after the needle is inserted, to make certain that the tip of the needle is not in a blood vessel. The purposeful intravenous injection of typhoid vaccine for nonspecific effects is discussed on page 336.

The injection of typhoid vaccine produces one or several of a group of local and constitutional symptoms which usually are not severe. The local reaction at the site of injection consists in redness, induration, and edema associated with pain. The general reaction is characterized by malaise, headache, and fever. The severity of reaction when the vaccine is given subcutaneously tends to increase with successive revaccinations.

In areas where typhoid fever is found, revaccination of previously immunized individuals by means of a single stimulating dose of vaccine every two or three years should protect most of them against the disease. Intracutaneous administration of 0.1 cc. of a potent vaccine is the preferred method. A subcutaneous dose of 0.5 cc. will also produce satisfactory stimulation of immunity but may cause more severe reactions. In highly endemic areas or in the presence of an epidemic, more frequent revaccination is indicated.

Typhoid-Paratyphoid Vaccine, also known as triple typhoid vaccine or "T.A.B.," is given to induce active immunity not only to typhoid fever but also to paratyphoid infections. It contains in each cc. 1,000 million heat-killed typhoid bacilli and 250 million each of *Salmonella paratyphi* and *S. schottmuelleri* (paratyphoid bacilli A and B). 'Merthiolate' is used as a preservative. This vaccine is used in the same way as Typhoid Vaccine.

Staphylococcus 'U B A' (Undenatured Bacterial Antigen, Lilly) contains undenatured bacterial antigens of staphylococci of the *aureus* type, 0.025

mg. nitrogen per cc., and staphylococci of the *albus* type, 0.025 mg. nitrogen per cc. It is used for treatment of chronic or recurrent staphylococcus infections. No active immunity is produced.

For best results in chronic or recurrent infections, a series of injections is necessary. An initial dose of 0.1 cc. may be tried. If this causes a severe reaction, the next injection may be 0.01 cc. or even less. The dose is increased gradually at three-day intervals until clinical improvement is evident. Injections are then continued, perhaps for several weeks, at intervals of three to seven days, but without increase in dosage. Severe local or focal reaction is an indication for reduction in dosage and more gradual increase thereafter. In acute cases, injections may be given daily.

'Staphylo-Jel' (Lysed Staphylococcus Antigen Jelly, Lilly) is a solution of bacteriophage-lysed staphylococci (75 percent) and streptococci (25 percent) incorporated in a water-soluble jelly base. 'Staphylo-Jel' is applied locally in the treatment of epithelial surface staphylococcus infections.

Streptococcus Vaccine (Intravenous) is a suspension of killed streptococci of a strain used by Clawson and Wetherby in the treatment of arthritis. It has been used in both rheumatoid and osteoarthritis.

The initial intravenous dose in chronic cases is usually 100 million organisms. If the reaction is not too severe, an injection is given each week, and each dose is increased by 100 million until 800 million are being given. If clinical improvement has followed this course of eight injections, the intravenous dose of 800 million is repeated once a month for a time. If no improvement has been seen, larger doses—e.g., 1,200; 1,600; 2,000; and 2,400 million— are given at intervals of two weeks. In the absence of benefit from these larger doses, vaccine treatment is discontinued. If there is improvement only after the larger doses, such dosage is repeated at intervals of two to four weeks.

The initial dose should ordinarily be less than 100 million in acute phases of arthritis with persistent fever or for patients in whom the risk of a possibly severe reaction is undesirable. Slow injection has a tendency to reduce or avoid reaction. Some degree of reaction follows injection in about 50 percent of cases. The treatment is contraindicated in pregnancy and glomerulonephritis.

Streptococcus Vaccine (Arthritis Strains) is prepared according to the method of E. C. Rosenow

for treatment of arthritis. It is a suspension of killed green-producing streptococci having elective localizing power and other specific properties characteristic of streptococci found by Rosenow in foci of infection in cases of arthritis. In chronic arthritis it is usual to begin with 2 million organisms injected subcutaneously. If there is little or no local or focal reaction, the dose is increased by 2 million weekly. After a dose of 20 million is reached, the dose is increased by 10 percent each time. If after the first or any subsequent injection there is a decided local or, particularly, a focal reaction, the dose is reduced to the point where such a reaction does not occur. It is then increased more slowly. The persistence of induration at the site of injection is evidence of overdosage. The duration of treatment, size of dose, and interval between injections are determined by the patient's condition and response. If there is no response to the above schedule in eight weeks, the vaccine should be discontinued. In some instances, intravenous administration may be more effective than subcutaneous. Initial intravenous dosage is usually 200,000 organisms in 10 cc. of physiological salt solution, given very slowly and cautiously.

Streptococcus Vaccine (Fibrositis Strains) is prepared according to the method of E. C. Rosenow for treatment of fibrositis. It is a suspension of killed green-producing streptococci having elective localizing power and other specific properties characteristic of streptococci found by Rosenow in foci of infection in cases of fibrositis. It is used in the same way as Streptococcus Vaccine (Arthritis Strains).

Streptococcus 'U B A' contains undenatured antigens of streptococci—hemolytic and viridans strains, 0.02 mg. nitrogen per cc. each, and indifferent strains, 0.01 mg. nitrogen per cc. It is intended for treatment of streptococcus infections, and particularly those associated with chronic arthritis. It may be given subcutaneously or intradermally. Subcutaneously the first dose is usually 0.01 cc., and each succeeding dose is increased by 0.01 to 0.05 cc. until 1 cc. is reached. Three doses are given weekly over a period of six to eighteen weeks, after which the interval is gradually lengthened to several weeks. The initial intradermal dose is 0.1 cc. or less, and injections are given twice weekly, the dose being gradually increased to 0.5 cc. Intradermal and subcutaneous treatment may be given together. As with other vaccines given for chronic infections, any decided local or focal reaction requires reduction of dosage and a more grad-ual subsequent increase.

Streptococcus-Staphylococcus Vaccine is given to induce active immunity to streptococcus and staph-ylococcus infections. Each cc. contains killed or-ganisms as follows:

streptococci........................... 200 million
Staph. aureus..........................1,000 million
Staph. albus...........................1,000 million

The vaccine is given subcutaneously at intervals of three to seven days. A suggested dosage schedule is 0.125, 0.25, 0.5, 1, 1 cc., and so on. Severe reaction is an indication for reduction of dosage.

Staphylococcus-Streptococcus 'U B A' contains undenatured antigens of staphylococci and strepto-cocci, 0.025 mg. nitrogen each per cc. It is in-tended for treatment of chronic mixed staphylococ-cus and streptococcus infections, including those associated with arthritis. The dosage and method of administration of Staphylococcus 'U B A' (p. 329) are suitable for Staphylococcus-Streptococcus 'U B A.'

Respiratory 'U B A' contains undenatured bac-terial antigens of:

pneumococci..............0.015 mg. nitrogen per cc.
streptococci..............0.015 mg. nitrogen per cc.
H. influenzae..............0.01 mg. nitrogen per cc.
M. catarrhalis..............0.0025 mg. nitrogen per cc.
staphylococci..............0.0075 mg. nitrogen per cc.

The preparation is intended for parenteral or topical administration with a view to developing immunity to the bacteria represented in the for-mula. These bacteria are either primary or second-ary invaders in various infections of the respiratory tract. The antigen has been used with much success in chronic purulent sinusitis, both by topical and parenteral administration, and also as a prophy-laxis against certain bacterial infections which are most common during the winter months.

In the treatment of chronic purulent sinusitis, it has been administered subcutaneously, intracu-taneously, and topically. Although the dose must be individualized, a program that has met the needs of many patients has been as follows: initial dose, 0.1 cc. intradermally and 0.1 cc. subcutane-ously; the subcutaneous dose is increased by 0.1 cc. at each succeeding injection until the tenth dose, the interval being three to five days; beyond the tenth dose the treatment may be continued at weekly intervals with 0.1 cc. intradermally and 1 cc. subcutaneously. At each visit the nasal pas-

sages may be cleared of pus, crusts, or scabs and the turbinates shrunk with an appropriate vaso-constrictor (p. 362). The antigen (1 to 1.5 cc. diluted with an equal quantity of 1 percent ephedrine sul-fate or other vasoconstrictor in physiological salt solution) is then instilled topically into the sinuses by the Proetz displacement method (p. 377).

For prophylaxis of bacterial infections of the re-spiratory tract the following schedule may be fol-lowed, provided little or no reaction occurs: initial dose, 0.5 cc. subcutaneously; then four doses of 1 cc. at weekly intervals; then doses of 1 cc. at in-tervals of two to four weeks throughout the winter months. Such prophylactic injections may well be-gin in the early fall. If the initial or any subsequent dose causes moderate or severe reaction at the site of injection, in the form of nasal symptoms, or as systemic effects, the dose is reduced until no reaction follows and is then gradually increased to 1 cc. No dose should be increased if the interval since the preceding dose is more than seven days.

H. Influenzae-Pneumococcus Vaccine is prepared by the method of E. C. Rosenow. Each cc. contains the following killed organisms:

pneumococci.....................:........1,500 million
Streptococcus viridans.....................1,500 million
hemolytic streptococci...................1,000 million
Staph. aureus........................... 500 million
H. influenzae........................... 500 million

Its purpose is to develop active immunity to the bacteria represented in the formula. Since these organisms are frequent primary or secondary in-vaders in various infections of the respiratory tract, the immunity so obtained will tend to prevent or modify such infections.

The initial prophylactic dose in the average case is 0.5 cc. injected subcutaneously. If this should cause severe reaction, the next dose should be smaller. If no reaction occurs, the next dose may be 1 cc. five to seven days later. The third dose may be 1.5 cc. after a similar interval. The vaccine should then be repeated at intervals of three weeks throughout the winter season. The doses for chil-dren may be 0.1 cc., 0.2 cc., and 0.3 cc., or more according to age.

If at any time untoward reaction follows an in-jection, the next dose should be reduced. If the dose is excessive, symptoms resembling those of a common cold may result and remain a few hours. Overdosage may prevent the immunity response.

H. Influenzae Mixed Vaccine is given to induce active immunity to the organisms represented in the formula below. These organisms are frequent primary or secondary invaders in various infections of the respiratory tract. Active immunity to them tends to prevent or modify such infections.

The most concentrated mixture (No. 4) contains in each cc. killed organisms as follows:

H. influenzae	500 million
M. catarrhalis	100 million
streptococci	500 million
Bacillus Friedländer	250 million
Staph. aureus	500 million
Staph. albus	500 million
pneumococci	1,500 million

The vaccine is ordinarily administered subcutaneously. When injections are begun in the early fall, the interval between doses may be five to seven days. The initial dose is usually 0.1 cc. of Mixture No. 4, or a proportionately larger dose of one of the other mixtures. If no serious reactions occur, successive doses of Mixture No. 4 may be 0.25 cc., 0.5 cc., and 1 cc. Thereafter, to maintain immunity, 1 cc. is injected at intervals of two to four weeks. If it is desired to produce immunity as quickly as possible, the intervals between the first four doses may be as short as two days. Children tolerate the vaccine relatively well. Children of six years or older can usually receive the adult dose; younger children are ordinarily given half as much.

As with other vaccines, severe reaction is an indication for reduction of dosage. Symptoms suggestive of rhinitis a few hours after an injection may mean that the dose was somewhat excessive.

Catarrhalis Vaccine Combined offers another combination of antigens for induction of active immunity against organisms which are frequent primary or secondary invaders in infection of the respiratory tract. The most concentrated mixture (No. 4) contains in each cc. killed organisms as follows:

M. catarrhalis	200 million
Bacillus Friedländer	200 million
pneumococci	100 million
streptococci	100 million
Staph. aureus	400 million
Staph. albus	200 million

Dosage and administration are the same as for H. Influenzae Mixed Vaccine (see above).

'Ento-Lysate' (**Lysed Respiratory Antigen, Lilly**) is a solution of bacteriophage-lysed *M. catarrhalis*, pneumococci, staphylococci, and streptococci of various types. '**Ento-Jel**' (**Lysed Respiratory An-**

tigen Jelly, Lilly) is prepared by incorporating the lysate in a water-soluble jelly.

'Ento-Lysate' is administered locally or systemically to stimulate the production of immunity against the bacteria represented in the formula. Since these organisms are frequent primary or secondary invaders in various infections, the immunity so obtained would tend to prevent or modify such infections.

The preparation used and method of administration depend upon the requirements of the case. 'Ento-Jel' is suitable for local application to the nasal mucous membrane or to the conjunctiva. In rhinitis or sinusitis, 'Ento-Lysate' may be administered, 2 cc. in each nostril, by the Proetz displacement technic (p. 377). This treatment may be repeated three times a week.

For subcutaneous injection of 'Ento-Lysate' to provide systemic immunity in acute infections, the initial dose may be 0.1 cc. In succeeding visits, which may be at intervals of one to two days, the dose is gradually increased (provided no severe reactions occur) until 1 cc. or more is being given. For chronic cases, the interval may be three to five days. In prophylaxis of possible future infections, the subcutaneous doses may be respectively 0.25, 0.5, 0.75, and 1 cc. at intervals of three to seven days. To maintain the immunity, doses of 1 cc. may thereafter be injected at intervals of one to four weeks.

Local application of 'Ento-Lysate' or 'Ento-Jel' is usually nonirritating, but occasionally a patient is hypersensitive to the proteins in the preparation. If subcutaneous injection causes severe reaction, the next dose should be smaller.

Entoral is a dry powdered vaccine supplied in pulvules. Each pulvule contains killed:

pneumococci	40,000 million
streptococci	15,000 million
H. influenzae	2,500 million
M. catarrhalis	2,500 million

When administered orally, Entoral is capable of inciting the production of specific bacterial antibodies and heterophile antibody in sufficient amounts to increase materially the resistance of many individuals to the bacteria which most frequently are present in respiratory infections. When administered to appropriate experimental animals in adequate dosage, it incites sufficient immunity to protect them against inoculations of virulent pneumococci representing 1,000 minimal lethal doses. Each pulvule contains between 80 and 100 heterophile antigenic units. Because of the heterophile antibody, development of which is stimulated by the heterophile antigen, the resulting immunity protects not only against the bacteria represented in the formula but against other bacteria which are susceptible to this antibody.

Entoral is used as a prophylactic of bacterial respiratory infections which are most likely to occur during cold weather. It supplies no immunity against various virus infections of the respiratory tract, but it may modify them favorably by preventing secondary bacterial invasion. It can also prevent primary bacterial invasion by the organisms represented in the formula and by other heterophile-antibody-susceptible bacteria.

The usual dosage plan is one pulvule by mouth thirty minutes or more before breakfast. This is repeated daily for seven days as an initial immunizing dose and then is taken twice weekly for maintenance of the immunity. Preferably the immunizing series is begun early in the fall a week or two before the usual onset of cold weather and is discontinued at the season when cold weather ordinarily ceases. In the North Temperate Zone it may be started in September and discontinued in April, during which interval approximately sixty pulvules will have been used. Experience indicates that whereas the lower maintenance dosage of one pulvule a week may be sufficient for some, it is inadequate for many others. A few will need more than the recommended two pulvules weekly. Children under five are frequently given half the contents of a pulvule suspended in water at the same intervals. The antigens in Entoral are relatively resistant to gastric juice and bile. Entoral is absorbed if taken after meals, but not as completely as when taken on an empty, resting stomach.

Entoral may be employed as maintenance therapy following initial subcutaneous immunization by means of some heterophile-antigen-containing vaccine like Respiratory 'U B A.'

Entoral is nontoxic, but in occasional cases reactions occur. These are apparently due to hypersensitivity. They include nasal blocking or "stuffiness," gastro-intestinal discomfort, and, in rare instances, urticaria. The nasal blocking may cease to appear if the patient persists in the prescribed dose. It is better, however, to reduce the dose temporarily to half the contents of a pulvule. If the reaction continues or if other symptoms of hypersensitivity appear, it is desirable to change to an injectable respiratory vaccine and to hyposensitize the patient, beginning with a small dose of diluted vaccine and working up gradually as in administration of allergens (see Hay Fever, p. 265).

ANTIBODY-CONTAINING SERUMS TO PROVIDE PASSIVE IMMUNITY AGAINST INFECTION

Antibodies (p. 319) may be of several types, as determined by the phenomena that follow their interaction with antigens. If bacteria or other cells containing a given antigen are clumped together after the interaction, the antibody is termed an "agglutinin." If clouding with flocculent precipitation of antigen-containing particles occurs, the antibody is referred to as a "precipitin." If the cells or particles containing the antigen break down and go into solution, the antibody is called a "lysin." Similarly, neutralization of a toxin is performed by an "antitoxin"; and increased susceptibility to phagocytosis is induced by an "opsonin." Other antibodies have been described as "alexin-fixing," "bactericidal," or "virucidal." Clinically, antibodies are distinguished as being antibacterial or antitoxic.

Most circulating antibodies occur in the globulin of the blood serum. The antitoxins have been further localized to the pseudoglobulin fraction, whereas other antibodies are found in the euglobulins. Efforts at concentration and refinement of serums aim to isolate the fractions highest in antibody titer.

Sessile antibodies also occur which are attached to tissue cells. It has not been established whether these antibodies are or are not the same as the circulating antibodies.

Antibodies to be used therapeutically (see also Introduction, p. 318) are usually produced by active immunization of an animal, such as the horse or rabbit. The serum, after collection, is processed in such a way as to concentrate the antibody-containing fraction and eliminate or modify, insofar as possible, all other protein fractions. Against some infections, human convalescent or immune serum is used.

Since the advent of powerful antibacterial drugs such as the antibiotics and sulfonamides, many of the antibacterial serums are no longer used except when these drugs fail. The antitoxins continue to be widely employed in the immediate prophylaxis and treatment of gas gangrene, tetanus, and diphtheria. Proper use of diphtheria and tetanus toxoids to produce active immunity to these two diseases is preferred; but after a susceptible individual has been exposed, there is not sufficient time for active immunity to develop, and reliance must be placed on administration of serums conferring passive immunity.

The basic requirements of antiserums or antitoxins are (1) proper valency, (2) high potency, (3) maximal concentration and purification, (4) adequate dosage, and (5) administration by the proper route.

Absorption of antibody following subcutaneous injection is slower than after intramuscular or intravenous injection. Therefore antitoxin for prophylaxis is best given subcutaneously, whereas for therapy the other routes are preferred. The first therapeutic dose is often given intravenously for rapid effect. The duration of adequate passive immunity following a single dose is seven to thirty days or more, depending on the size of the dose. After previous injections of serum from the same animal, the antibody is eliminated more rapidly.

Since the antibodies given to provide passive immunity are themselves proteins derived from the serum of other than the human species, they may act as antigens in the human body, inducing allergy or hypersensitivity. As a rule, the manifestations of hypersensitivity to serum preparations are mild and without danger. However, cases are on record in which fatal anaphylactic shock (p. 269) has followed a single injection or even an intradermal skin test. Fatalities after second injections are very rare, although alarming symptoms may occur. Every care and caution should be exercised in the administration of serums, but the possibility of anaphylaxis is not to be compared with the danger incurred in withholding serum from cases in which it is indicated.

All patients who are to receive therapy of this type should be questioned about previous serum injections (including toxin-antitoxin) or ingestion of horseflesh. A history should also be obtained as to symptoms of asthma, hay fever, or hives, since patients having such symptoms are likely to be sensitive to many proteins, including horse serum. Horse asthmatics, especially, should never be given serum products.

Skin and ophthalmic tests have been employed in an effort to detect those patients who will have unfavorable reactions to serum therapy. Unfortunately, such tests are not infallible. Patients with positive tests may have no systemic reaction on administration of serum, and patients with negative tests may have serious reactions.

In spite of their fallibility, there is some correlation between the results of sensitivity tests and the incidence of reactions. If they are to be employed, the intradermal test is usually performed first. Normal horse serum or the antiserum to be injected is diluted 1:100 or 1:10 with physiological salt solution, and 0.1 cc. is injected intracutaneously. In cases in which hypersensitivity is suspected, it is better to use the weaker dilution. A positive reaction occurs in fifteen minutes and is indicated by the development of a wheal with a red flare and pseudopodia. A syringe of Epinephrine Injection, U.S.P., (1:1,000) should be available.

If the intradermal test is positive, it is customary to perform the eye test. A drop of undiluted serum, or a 1:10 or 1:100 dilution in some instances, is instilled into the conjunctiva. A positive reaction appears in from ten to twenty minutes as a diffuse reddening with a watery discharge and itching. When the reaction has developed, it should be controlled by instillation of epinephrine into the eye. The test is of no value in young children, for they may wash out the serum by crying.

If the skin test is positive and the eye test negative, administration of serum should be preceded by "desensitization." If both skin and eye tests are positive, serum should not be given unless circumstances make it mandatory. Even then, serum should not be given intravenously in the presence of a positive eye test. Although "desensitization" may reduce somewhat the frequency and severity of reactions following reinjection of serum, it cannot be counted on to have this effect in patients subject to allergy. Persons naturally sensitive to horse serum cannot be desensitized. However, the desensitization procedure has value in that development of reactions following the early small doses gives warning of extreme sensitivity while the administration of larger amounts can still be avoided and the symptoms can still be controlled by epinephrine.

In patients suspected, on the basis of allergic history or positive skin and eye tests, of being liable to untoward reactions, the following procedures may be employed. If the serum is to be given subcutaneously or intramuscularly:

1. Inject subcutaneously 0.3 cc. (5 minims) Epinephrine Injection (1:1,000) (see p. 424) and at the same time, but not in the same place, 0.05 cc. of a 1:20 dilution of the therapeutic antiserum in physiological salt solution.

2. Repeat serum injection at half-hour intervals, giving in order, 0.1, 0.2, 0.5, 1, 2, and 4 cc., and so on until the total volume is given.

3. Repeat epinephrine injection at hourly intervals until serum administration is completed, increasing the dose to 0.5 cc. or 1 cc. if signs of reaction occur. The dose of epinephrine should be modified for children according to age.

If the serum is to be given intravenously:

1. Proceed as above, giving epinephrine and serum subcutaneously.

2. After the 1-cc. injection of diluted serum, the subcutaneous administration is discontinued; one-half hour later, intravenous injection is begun with 0.1 cc. of serum diluted

to 1 cc. with physiological salt solution, to be followed at similar intervals by 0.2 cc. diluted to 1 cc., 0.5 cc. diluted to 1 cc., 1 cc. undiluted, 2 cc., 4 cc., and so on until the entire dose has been given (intravenous injections should be given very slowly).

3. Hourly subcutaneous administration of epinephrine is continued as in the preceding schedule.

4. If there is the least sign of a reaction (dyspnea, palpitation, itching or burning of skin), discontinue the injections immediately and give Epinephrine Injection at once in a dose of 0.3 to 0.5 cc. After the symptoms disappear, start injection again, but in a smaller dose and more slowly.

Coca states that when reinjection of therapeutic serum is urgently indicated, it is useless to apply the cutaneous test or the procedure of desensitization as a precautionary measure. The physician must be governed in such a situation wholly by the exigencies of the patient's condition.

Even in those not subject to allergy, there frequently occurs after a variable incubation period a train of symptoms classified together as serum sickness. This is discussed on page 268.

Diphtheria Antitoxin, Purified, Concentrated, is prepared from the serum of horses actively immunized against the toxin of *Corynebacterium diphtheriae*. It should be given as early as possible in all cases of diphtheria (p. 3) except to those individuals in whom serum products are absolutely contraindicated (p. 334). Doses and routes of injection are governed by the severity and duration of the disease. For early diphtheria, in which the membrane is limited to the tonsils, 10,000 to 20,000 units of antitoxin are considered sufficient. Nasopharyngeal involvement, with membrane formation, calls for at least 40,000 units. Severely toxic cases, especially if in the fifth or sixth day of disease, require doses of 50,000 or 60,000 to possibly 200,000 units. Opinion differs as to whether larger doses accomplish more than those of 60,000 units. Intramuscular injection is generally preferred, maximum absorption being attained in sixteen to eighteen hours. The intravenous route provides immediately available antitoxin and may be indicated in very toxic cases. If the response has not been satisfactory within twelve to twenty-four hours, additional quantities can be given—at a new site and preferably in a different extremity.

Prophylactic administration of diphtheria antitoxin to susceptible individuals who have been heavily exposed to diphtheria is indicated when it is impossible to perform daily examinations, including cultures of the nose and throat. When close observation after exposure is possible, the use of diphtheria antitoxin may be reserved for those who are Schick-positive and show virulent diphtheria

organisms by culture. Nose and throat cultures will usually show sufficient growth for identification within twenty-four to forty-eight hours, at which time a fairly accurate reading of the Schick test (p. 338) can also be made. The subcutaneous or intramuscular injection of 1,000 to 2,000 units will provide protection for approximately ten to twenty-one days.

Tetanus Antitoxin, Purified, Concentrated, is prepared from the serum of horses actively immunized against the toxin of *Clostridium tetani*. It should be given prophylactically as early as possible to all nonimmune patients who have been exposed to possible tetanus (p. 12) infection. Persistent surgical cleansing of the wound is also mandatory (p. 12). *Early* administration of the antitoxin is most important, and dosage should be adequate. Doses of 1,500 units have been recommended, but this amount is effective for only seven or, at the most, ten days. For routine prophylaxis, 5,000 units are now considered the optimal dose and can be expected to protect for approximately three weeks. When contamination is suspected in wounds of the head or neck or in compound fractures, 8,000 to 10,000 units should be given. Antitoxin should also be administered to all nonimmune persons at least twenty-four hours before manipulation of old wounds or operations which might activate foci of latent infection.

In contrast to the prophylactic use of tetanus antitoxin discussed above, the therapeutic use, in which the antitoxin is given only after clinical evidence of tetanus is present, has been subjected to question (see p. 12). In any case, its success depends on how much toxin has already been fixed in the nervous system at the time treatment is begun. Antitoxin has no influence on toxin which has already entered nerve cells. Since it cannot be determined beforehand whether a fraction of a lethal toxic dose or one or more lethal doses have been fixed, any patient showing symptoms of tetanus should probably receive tetanus antitoxin at once. The usual dosage is 30,000 to 60,000 units, regardless of body weight. Larger doses or repeated administrations probably do not improve the results. Intramuscular injection is preferred in the majority of cases. Suitable precautions should be observed (see preceding page).

When a wound is to undergo surgical treatment, dissemination of preformed toxin from the wound site can be prevented by infiltration of antitoxin into the surrounding area an hour beforehand. Intraspinal injection of antitoxin is no longer favored.

Gas-Gangrene Antitoxin (Combined) Concentrated is prepared from the serum of horses actively immunized against the toxins of *Clostridium perfringens* and *Cl. septicum* (vibrion septique). It may be used in the treatment of gas gangrene (p. 5) simultaneously with the sulfonamides and penicillin. In treatment, 20,000 to 100,000 units are given intravenously as early as possible, of course with suitable precautions (p. 334 to p. 335). Additional doses, as required, may be given at intervals of four to six hours. In prophylaxis, similar or smaller doses are given intramuscularly. The possibility of tetanus as an additional infection must always be considered.

Hyperimmune Human or Rabbit Serum for Whooping Cough is obtained from healthy persons or rabbits that have been actively immunized against *H. pertussis*. It is used in treatment of the disease or in prevention following exposure in those not previously immunized, but results vary considerably. If it is to be given, administration should be early and in adequate dosage. As with all passive immunity, the protection is temporary.

The usual dosage of unmodified human hyperimmune serum is as follows. For prophylaxis following exposure, two intramuscular or intravenous injections of 20 cc. are given; if the first can be made within forty-eight hours after exposure, the second is made five days later; if the first injection is given more than two days after exposure, the second should be given three days after the first. If paroxysms have already begun, the minimum course should be three 20-cc. injections spaced forty-eight hours apart; in case of relapse, an additional 20 cc. may be necessary. Seriously ill children, especially those with bronchopneumonia, should receive 50 to 100 cc. intravenously.

The dosage of hyperimmune rabbit serum should be that recommended by the manufacturer. Refined and concentrated human serum is several times more potent than the unmodified product and is used in doses as recommended by the manufacturer.

Immune Globulin (Human Immune Globulin, U.S.P.) is obtained from human placentas and provides a source of passive immunity to *measles*. Immune globulin therapy is indicated to *prevent* the disease in physically debilitated individuals and young infants or to stop epidemics in institutions. Doses of 2 to 10 cc. are injected intramuscularly as soon as possible after exposure and before the fourth day of incubation. The duration of immunity due to convalescent serum is usually about three weeks.

Infants whose mothers have had the disease usually inherit passive immunity for about six months.

Placental globulin may be given to *modify* measles in normal susceptible individuals following exposure. The injection is made on the sixth or seventh day after exposure or on the second day after the rash has appeared on the individual from whom the infection was acquired. The usual dose is 2 to 5 cc.

The gamma globulin fraction of human plasma may be used similarly in doses of 0.02 to 0.025 cc. per lb. of body weight for modification, and 0.1 cc. or more per lb. for prevention.

When modification is successful, the incubation period is sometimes prolonged and the prodromal period almost suppressed. Koplik's spots do not develop. The eruption is mild and often fleeting and is not accompanied by constitutional symptoms or complications. Permanent immunity is almost always produced.

ANTIGENS ADMINISTERED FOR THE PRODUCTION OF FEVER

Intravenous administration of a bacterial vaccine is likely to be followed by a febrile reaction. Such an episode tends to mobilize the various defenses of the body and produce "nonspecific" immunity which may be useful in combating certain infections or inflammations, particularly chorea (p. 48) and ocular inflammations (p. 241). The vasodilation which accompanies the reaction may also be useful in certain forms of arterial disease (especially thromboangiitis obliterans, p. 76) and in trigeminal neuralgia (p. 163).

Though many kinds of foreign protein have been used to produce fever, preparations of typhoid vaccine are commonly employed because of their effectiveness, ready availability, and satisfactory standardization. Typhoid-Paratyphoid Vaccine (p. 329) may be employed, but Typhoid H Antigen is generally preferred.

Typhoid H Antigen is obtained from the flagella of motile typhoid bacilli. The febrile reaction following intravenous injection of Typhoid Vaccine (which contains the so-called O antigen from the bodies of the bacilli) usually begins one to two hours after the injection and is preceded by a chill. When a similar injection of Typhoid H Antigen is given, the febrile reaction begins in four to eight hours and is not preceded by chill in most cases. Because of this latter quality, Typhoid H Antigen is preferred for inducing nonspecific febrile reactions.

Typhoid H Antigen is given intravenously. The average initial dose for young or middle-aged men with no evidence of cardiac disease, anemia, or other debilitating conditions is 25,000,000 to 40,000,000 organisms; for females, 15,000,000 to 30,000,000. Care must be taken to avoid unduly severe reactions, and it is better to start with too small rather than too large a dose. In subsequent injections the dose of antigen is increased each time as much as is thought necessary to obtain the desired febrile reaction. The usual increases vary from 20,000,000 to 50,000,000, depending upon the reaction obtained after the previous injection. In treatment of ocular inflammations, a lesser degree of response is usually desired than in peripheral arterial disease.

After administration of the antigen, the temperature is taken at hourly intervals unless it exceeds 40°C. (104°F.), when it is taken every thirty minutes. Blankets and hot-water bottles are applied to the patient after the temperature begins to rise. To promote the patient's comfort, a hypodermic injection of codeine sulfate (1/4 to 1/2 grain) is usually given a half hour after the vaccine. It may be repeated at three-hour intervals.

Temperatures of 41°C. (106°F.) are considered excessive. After such a reaction, no increase in dosage is made at the next injection. Immediate treatment consists in placing an icecap on the patient's head and giving acetylsalicylic acid, 5 grains, by mouth. If the temperature reaches 41.7°C. (107°F.), all covering should be removed, and the patient should be given a tepid sponge bath or, if he is unduly distressed, a tub bath with the water at 38°C. (100.4°F.). Cold water can be added slowly. Rectal administration of acetylsalicylic acid, 10 grains, may be helpful.

For most indications, fever treatment is given every second, third, or fourth day, depending on the patient and the condition being treated. In chorea it is given daily unless the temperature is still above 100°F. on the morning following a treatment, in which case that day is skipped. Five to ten treatments usually constitute a course. The patient's cardiovascular system should be carefully watched for evidence of overstrain or failure. Daily urinalysis should be performed. The appearance of protein or blood is an indication to stop the treatments.

Fever therapy is contraindicated for elderly, asthenic, cachectic, arteriosclerotic, or anemic patients, and for those with cardiac disease or with obvious subacute or latent infections other than what is being treated.

ANTIGENS ADMINISTERED TO REDUCE ALLERGIC HYPERSENSITIVITY TO THE SAME ANTIGEN

It is chiefly in the treatment of clinical allergy (p. 264)—asthma, hay fever, urticaria, and the like—that antigens are administered to reduce allergic hypersensitivity to the same antigens. These antigens are administered in the form of extracts of pollen, house dust, epidermal substances (hair, feathers, dander), food, and other substances which people may inhale, ingest, or otherwise encounter.

The earliest extracts for treatment of allergy were made using physiological salt solution or glycerin. They are still widely used. They have, however, the disadvantage of rapid absorption and hence brief antigenic activity. Precipitated antigens have been prepared which are only slowly dissolved and absorbed after injection, allowing a more prolonged antigenic effect. These have the additional advantage of accurate standardization which facilitates treatment, especially in highly sensitive patients. Although most antigens are given hypodermically, certain ones are absorbed from the gastro-intestinal tract and may therefore be given by mouth.

'Panoral' is a sterilized, stable, whole-pollen preparation for oral administration. Spring Type 'Panoral' contains the pollen of timothy, June grass, orchard grass, and redtop. Fall Type 'Panoral' contains equal parts of pollen from giant and short ragweed.

Experiments with the blood and urine of patients orally treated with pollen have shown that (1) an appreciable amount of pollen is absorbed through the gastro-intestinal tract, and (2) reagin and allergen coexist in the circulating blood at the height of treatment.

As with other hyposensitizing agents, the treatment is preferably begun eight weeks or more before the season is due to start (preseasonal). Treatment begun after the season has started (coseasonal) is not as satisfactory. Giving treatment throughout the year (perennial) may be necessary in difficult cases. Literature suggesting dosage schedules is available to physicians upon request.

Reactions sometimes occur, taking the form of hay-fever symptoms, gastro-intestinal distress (colic or diarrhea), headache, dizziness, exhaustion, urticaria, or other dermatitis.

Oral pollen therapy is not advised in patients

suffering from gastro-intestinal disturbances, such as peptic ulcer, colitis, or chronic indigestion.

Trichophyton 'U F A' (see p. 339)

Tuberculin (see p. 339)

ANTIGENS USED FOR DIAGNOSTIC TESTS

Antigens may be useful in a number of ways for determining the state of immunity. They may be injected into the patient to detect the presence of neutralizing antibodies, as in the Schick test. They may be injected to ascertain the existence of sensitivity which has been induced by infection with the organism from which the given antigen was obtained, as in the case of Tuberculin. They may be mixed with the patient's blood in vitro to determine the adequacy of the patient's antibody response to active immunization, as in the Pertussis Agglutination Test.

The antigens described below have been in use for some time and are generally accepted. New ones for other conditions are developed from time to time, and physicians are invited to inquire of the Lilly Research Laboratories, Indianapolis, Indiana, concerning any in which they are interested.

Mumps Skin-Test Antigen—Recovery from mumps, whether the classical parotitis or the more obscure systemic type of infection, produces a lasting immunity. This immunity causes specific skin hypersensitivity to the virus which may be detected by intradermal injection of mumps skin-test antigen.

The test may be employed at any age for determining susceptibility to mumps. It is particularly useful during and after adolescence to identify those who should be protected against the disease and its complications which so frequently develop in this age group. Because of the relatively long incubation period of mumps, there is time to apply the test after exposure and to vaccinate individuals requiring protection. As a matter of fact, the test itself produces some increase in immunity. However, active immunization with mumps vaccine or repeated tests do not affect the skin reaction.

The antigen is prepared in the same manner as Mumps Vaccine (p. 323) except it is more dilute. The vaccine should not be used for skin testing. The test is performed by injecting 0.1 cc. of skin-test antigen intracutaneously. A control test is not necessary. The reaction should be examined in twenty-four to thirty-six hours. An area of erythema 1.5 cm. or more in diameter, with or without indura-

tion, indicates immunity. Conversely, a negative reaction indicates susceptibility to infection. Pseudopositive reactions may develop in the presence of hypersensitivity to egg protein.

The Schick Test is performed to ascertain susceptibility to diphtheria (p. 3). It may be applied two months to one year after active immunization against diphtheria to determine the establishment of immunity. It is also used as a screening test in persons six years of age or older who have not previously been immunized. Because older children and adults tend to exhibit unpleasant reactions after immunizing procedures, it is advisable to immunize only known susceptibles in these groups. Children under six are immunized without previous testing, because of the high percentage who are susceptible and the low incidence of reactions.

For the test, 0.1 cc. of the Schick Test Solution (containing diphtheria toxin) is injected intradermally on the flexor surface of the forearm. Because of the frequency of pseudoreactions due to sensitivity to diphtheria-bacillus protein, it is advisable to make an intradermal injection of 0.1 cc. of Schick Control Solution in the other arm. The Control Solution is made from the same lot of toxin as the Test Solution, but it has been heated sufficiently to destroy the toxin while leaving uninjured the substances responsible for pseudoreactions.

A positive reaction will occur only at the site of injection of the Test Solution. It means *susceptibility* to diphtheria. Absence of reaction indicates immunity. A positive reaction is best read on the fourth or fifth day (if no control has been used, reading on the seventh day may help eliminate errors due to pseudoreactions). It is characterized by redness and infiltration which appear in twenty-four to thirty-six hours and persist four or five days. The reaction gradually disappears, leaving a persistent desquamating area of brownish pigmentation.

A pseudoreaction will occur at the sites of injection of both the Test Solution and the Control Solution. It appears earlier than the true positive reaction and usually disappears in forty-eight hours, leaving no pigmentation. It is occasionally seen in persons who have natural antitoxin.

The positive-combined reaction is one in which the positive reaction and a pseudoreaction overlap. Doubtful reading should be interpreted as positive. Children with positive or positive-combined reactions are susceptible to diphtheria. Sometimes a negative Schick test will be accompanied by a positive control; such individuals are immune.

Tuberculin is used chiefly for diagnosis of tuberculous infection (p. 12), principally in the form of the Mantoux or intradermal test. Occasionally it is used therapeutically; initial doses are extremely small and are increased gradually as in a series of hyposensitizing doses in allergy. Proper therapeutic use requires considerable skill and experience.

Old Tuberculin is prepared by boiling, filtering, and concentrating a bouillon culture of tubercle bacilli. Former preparations varied in potency, but it is now possible to standardize the antigenicity of tuberculin in such a way as to assure equal potency of all manufactured lots.

One cc. of standard Tuberculin, Old, Human, Concentrated, is sometimes referred to as 1,000 milligrams O.T. One cc. of a 1:10 dilution (0.1 cc. O.T. + 0.9 cc. saline) would then contain 100 mg. Similarly, a 1:100 dilution would contain 10 mg. per cc., and so on. Such dilutions should be prepared fresh every two weeks.

The Mantoux test may be performed by injecting intracutaneously 0.1 cc. of a 1:1,000 dilution of Old Tuberculin. The injection is usually made in the flexor surface of the forearm. A positive reaction consists in infiltration and hyperemia about the site; it appears in a few hours, reaches its maximum in about forty-eight hours, and ordinarily disappears in six to ten days.

If the test is negative but there is still reason to suspect tuberculosis, it may be in order to repeat the test using 1:100 O.T. Many physicians hesitate to use the 1:1,000 dilution until after they have obtained a negative test with a 1:10,000. Otherwise this larger dose might be followed by necrosis and scar formation. Very occasionally, when caution is highly desirable, the initial dose is with 1:100,000. If this is negative, it is followed by 1:10,000, and if still negative, by 1:1,000.

A positive reaction means only that the patient has had contact with the tubercle bacillus; it is not an indication of clinical activity. It is of great significance before the age of two, but after that its importance diminishes. About 90 percent of adults have positive reactions. On the other hand, a negative reaction is very significant in ruling out tuberculosis. It must be recalled, however, that the test may become negative in very advanced progressive tuberculosis and in the presence of certain other diseases, such as measles.

The Pertussis Agglutination Test is performed after active immunization to whooping cough (p. 15) to determine the antigenic response. This test is not of value in measuring immunity many months

or years after immunization, nor is it sufficiently sensitive to demonstrate immunity following recovery from the disease.

The test should be performed three to four months after conclusion of the first immunizing course or about two weeks after a stimulating dose of vaccine. The antigen is a standardized, colored, homogeneous suspension of killed pertussis bacilli. A drop of antigen is placed on a white porcelain spot plate, a piece of hard-surfaced white cardboard, a piece of heavy letter paper, or a comparator card,* and to it is added a somewhat smaller drop of the patient's blood, either fresh or citrated. The combined drop is spread with a toothpick, match, or other suitable mixing rod to form a circle about one-half inch in diameter which is then gently rocked back and forth for one minute. Too-long agitation will cause the clumped antigen to form a blue ring at the margin of the drop. Sodium citrate contained in the pertussis antigen will prevent coagulation.

The entire test can be conducted and read in two or three minutes, since only a minute's agitation is required for the incubation period.

A positive result is observed as a granulation or clumping of the blue antigen on the reddish background of blood (see Color Section, Plate 44). A negative reaction is indicated by a diffuse reddish-blue color. Pronounced granulation signifies a satisfactory response to immunization. A negative or weakly positive test is an indication for an additional dose of pertussis vaccine. This additional dose should be followed in two weeks by another agglutination test.

Trichophyton 'U F A' may be used as a skin test for diagnosis of fungus infection (p. 229) or therapeutically to reduce hypersensitivity to *Trichophyton interdigitale*. The antigen is prepared from mass cultures of *T. interdigitale* by the method used in preparing undenatured bacterial antigens (p. 329).

For the skin test, 0.1 cc. of Trichophyton 'U F A' may be diluted with 0.4 cc. of sterile physiological salt solution. An intradermal injection of 0.1 cc. of this dilution is then made, usually into the flexor surface of the forearm. As a control, one may also inject intracutaneously 0.1 cc. of sterile physiological salt solution, either in the same arm at a distance of about two inches or in the other arm. The sites should be examined twenty-four to forty-eight hours later. If the saline injection has given no reaction and the injection of 'U F A' has caused a

*Supplied with Test Kit.

340   Drugs—Actions and Uses □

moderate or considerable wheal or papule surrounded by a zone of erythema, the test is considered positive. In highly sensitive patients a vesicular or eczematous reaction develops. In some
instances the reaction may not appear for five to
seven days. Occasionally an immediate reaction in
twenty to thirty minutes may develop.

A negative test is presumptive evidence of the
absence of infection with *T. interdigitale* or related
organisms (there is considerable cross immunity to
the various fungi that produce superficial skin infection). A positive test does not, however, establish the mycotic nature of an existing eruption,
since it may be related to a previous infection.

Hyposensitization is sometimes helpful in patients with a positive skin test who have an exaggerated reaction at the site of infection (not due to
secondary bacterial infection) or who develop id
reactions (p. 268). Hyposensitization is begun with
an intracutaneous injection of 0.1 cc. of a 1:100,000
dilution of Trichophyton 'U F A.' If reactions do
not occur, subsequent doses may be 0.2 and 0.3
cc. of 1:100,000, followed by 0.05, 0.1, 0.2, and
0.3 cc. of 1:10,000 and later of 1:1,000, 1:100, etc.,
until improvement in the id reaction is observed.
The dose that is followed by improvement is then
repeated as long as improvement continues. Any
decided reaction to the injections is an indication
for reduction of the dose.

SERUM OR PLASMA TO SUPPLY NEEDED SUBSTANCES OTHER THAN ANTIBODIES

At present, the only generally accepted use of
serum or plasma to supply substances other than
antibodies is the intravenous administration of citrated human plasma to furnish plasma protein in
treating shock (p. 90). The plasma is supplied in
dry form and is reconstituted by solution in sterile
distilled water. Because of the use of pooled blood
and the absence of erythrocytes, typing is unnecessary and reactions are infrequent. The danger of
homologous serum jaundice (p. 140) can apparently
be eliminated or greatly reduced by ultraviolet irradiation of the plasma.

A pint of reconstituted plasma contains approximately as much protein as a quart of whole blood.
In severe shock, several pints of plasma may be
necessary. Whole blood is apparently somewhat
more effective than plasma, and the use of the
latter is largely restricted to situations in which
whole blood is not quickly obtainable.

STORAGE OF BIOLOGICALS

Because their active principles are protein in nature, biological preparations deteriorate when exposed to light and much more rapidly when subjected to heat. Care must therefore be exercised in
their storage. *All biological products are best stored
under refrigeration.*

Most susceptible to inactivation is smallpox vaccine, which must be kept very cold, preferably
below freezing, during the interval between manufacture and use. The effect of temperature is shown
in Table 34.

TABLE 34—*The Effect of Temperature on the
Potency of Smallpox Vaccine*

Temperature	Duration of Exposure	Effect on Vaccine
140°F.	5 min.	Inactive
132°F.	5 min.	Much weakened
98°F.*	3 to 4 days	Inactive
70°F.	1 to 3 weeks	Weakened
50°F.	3 to 6 months	Still alive but very weak
10°F.†	4 years	Still alive

*The temperature of a coat pocket.
†Freezing of itself does not harm smallpox vaccine.

Serums and antitoxins retain their potency for
years when properly refrigerated. Undue heat may
coagulate them as it does egg white. Unconcentrated
serums may develop a precipitate during storage
which does not as a rule interfere with their use.
Freezing should be avoided, since it may cause
breakage of the container, contamination from un-
seating the rubber stopper, or the appearance of a
precipitate in the product.

Bacterial antigens deteriorate slowly at 45°F.
They can be frozen once or twice without significant damage. Toxoids are rather stable, but they
should not be subjected to high temperatures for
prolonged periods. Recommended temperatures
are listed in Table 35.

TABLE 35—*Recommended Temperatures for
Storage of Biologicals*

	Optimum	Highest Permissible
Smallpox vaccine...	Below 32°F.	32°F.
Serums and antitoxins........	35°F.	50°F.
Bacterial antigens...	35° to 45°F.	50°F.
Toxoids...........	35° to 45°F.	50°F.

Federal law requires that packages of biological products be marked with the date prior to which the contents can be expected, beyond reasonable doubt, to yield their specific results. This time limit presupposes protection from light and heat; and if such protection is not given, the value of the time limit is destroyed as an index of potency of the product.

The following are the usual limits between release of the product and expiration date:

Smallpox vaccine........................ 3 months
Rabies vaccine........................... 6 months
Schick test.............................12 months
Bacterial antigens.......................18 months
Diphtheria toxoid, tetanus toxoid, and the
   combined diphtheria-tetanus toxoids....... 2 years
Antitoxins.............................. 3 years
Tuberculin............................. 5 years

Expiration dates are not to be interpreted as dates on which the potency of the product suddenly falls from the labeled value to zero. There is a gradual and continuous loss of potency of all biological material with time; therefore, the product is supplied with a sufficient excess of potency before release so that under proper storage conditions it will on the expiration date have beyond reasonable doubt a potency at least equal to that stated on the label. Slightly outdated material can be expected to have slightly less than the stated potency, and the loss will naturally be slower in those products having the longer limits between release and expiration. When an emergency exists and a fresh preparation cannot be obtained at once, the physician can use outdated material with reasonable assurance of efficacy if proper allowance is made for loss of potency.

WATER, SALTS, AND OSMOTIC AGENTS

WATER

Water is the medium in which life exists. Practically all, if not all, metabolic processes take place in solution. Because a certain amount of water is being constantly and inevitably lost to the body, frequent replenishments are necessary to prevent serious disorders of body function. Water balance and its disturbances are discussed beginning on page 49.

Water as such is not given parenterally because of its hypotonicity. Instead, it is given as dextrose solution (see p. 349). The dextrose is promptly removed by the liver and other tissues. A 5 percent dextrose solution is isotonic with the extracellular fluids and is the strength employed when the primary need is for water rather than for carbohydrate. Dextrose solutions are best given by intravenous drip.

IONS

Sodium is the principal basic ion of the extracellular fluids (p. 50). Its normal level in the plasma is about 142 milliequivalents per liter (327 mg. per 100 cc.). The tissue-cell membranes are normally impermeable to it. Aside from its osmotic action and its basic properties, it is pharmacologically inert. It has two important functions in the body: If there is an adequate supply of body water, the volume of extracellular fluid is largely determined by the total body content of sodium, and the degree of intracellular hydration is mainly dependent on the concentration of sodium in the extracellular fluid (see Disturbances of Fluid and Electrolyte Balance, p. 49). It is thus apparent that sodium intake and excretion are always important in any condition affecting fluid balance.

Sodium is contained in most foods and some drinking waters. Diets low in the element will be found on page 585. Sodium is also present in all body secretions (sweat, milk, digestive juices). It is excreted principally through the kidneys, which thereby exert a major influence over the volume and osmotic properties of the extracellular fluids. The amount excreted depends primarily on the extent of reabsorption from the glomerular filtrate by the epithelial cells of the proximal tubules. In turn, this reabsorption is governed by the supply of sodium factor secreted by the adrenal cortex (p. 460). There is an apparent reciprocal relationship in the renal excretion of sodium and potassium.

SODIUM EXCESS may be relative or absolute or both, depending on the availability of water and the state of renal function. It is encountered when sodium excretion fails to keep pace with sodium intake for one of the following reasons: (1) The intake exceeds the normal excretory capacity of the kidneys; (2) renal excretory capacity is limited by a deficiency of water (the kidneys can concentrate sodium chloride only to about 1.8 percent); or (3) renal function has been disturbed by crush syndrome, cardiac failure, or other disorder.

Sodium excess in the presence of adequate water gives rise to edema (see p. 53). The combination of acute relative or absolute sodium excess and water deficiency gives rise to a different type of manifestation, the exact clinical picture of which depends on other factors as yet poorly understood. Hoarseness and a sensation of "heavy eyelids" are the most common symptoms. Others include lethargy, somnolence, thirst, anorexia, nausea, and vomiting. There may also be irritability or depression, disorientation, muscle in-co-ordination, edema, and, at the same time, oliguria or anuria with nitrogen retention.

This acute syndrome of sodium excess is readily brought on postoperatively and after injury (see Crush Syndrome, p. 222) by the exclusive use of isotonic sodium chloride solution to supply the need for water (see Water, above). It may also be induced by drinking sea water to satisfy thirst. Other names for the same syndrome are "salt block" and "acute salt intolerance."

Sodium excess can be prevented by limiting sodium intake to body needs and excretory capacity. The needs of the patient who has been injured or operated on are discussed on page 58. Once sodium is present in excess, the patient should be given water (by mouth if possible, by intravenous infusion of 5 percent dextrose solution if necessary) in sufficient quantity to reduce the electrolyte concentration of the body fluids to normal and to permit the kidneys to excrete the excess salt.

SODIUM DEFICIENCY results from excessive loss of sodium salts, as in extreme sweating, acidosis, terminal glomerulonephritis, vomiting, diarrhea, or drainage of gastro-intestinal secretions or from wounds or burns. It is part of the picture of electrolyte deficiency (see Dehydration, p. 56). It is an important factor in heat prostration (p. 273). Its various aspects are discussed under those subjects. The abdominal or other muscle cramps which some people experience during hot weather are due to sodium deficiency with relative water excess and may be prevented by increasing salt intake.

When sodium is administered, it is usually as the chloride. In acidosis, it is given as the bicarbonate or lactate. For preparations containing sodium, see page 348 *et seq.*

Potassium is the principal basic ion of the body cells. It is present in muscle to the extent of about 112 milliequivalents per liter (mEq/L.) of muscle

water, and in the plasma to only about 5 mEq/L. (about 20 mg. per 100 cc.). Potassium is necessary to cell function, and complete deprivation causes eventual death. Nevertheless, the exact mechanism of its action is not understood. It plays an important part in the transmission of impulses along nerves and is also concerned in some way with the release of acetylcholine at synapses and nerve endings (see p. 416). Potassium has a vagus-like effect on the heart and, in addition, has what seems to be an independent action on both impulse conduction and muscle contractility. It has great influence on the function of skeletal muscle, some of which may be due to its action on nerves and nerve endings. Potassium therapy seems to be specific for familial periodic paralysis. It has a moderate effect in myasthenia gravis. It antagonizes the action of curare (p. 447). It intensifies the symptoms of myotonia congenita.

Potassium is rapidly absorbed after ingestion of most of its salts. Much of it is removed by the liver and gradually liberated into the blood. Potassium is excreted chiefly by the kidneys, and under ordinary circumstances an excess of ingested potassium is excreted more rapidly than is a comparable excess of sodium. There is an apparent reciprocal relationship in the renal excretion of sodium and potassium. The presence of an excess of one leads to increased excretion of the other. There is consequently potassium retention in adrenal cortical insufficiency (p. 183), but the mechanism is not understood.

POTASSIUM INTOXICATION—Abnormally high plasma levels of potassium lead to the syndrome of potassium intoxication. There is considerable individual variation, but, in general, levels of 7.5 mEq/L. (30 mg. per 100 cc.) produce paresthesias of the hands and feet. At about the same level the T waves of the electrocardiogram are elevated. At about 9 to 9.5 mEq/L. (35 to 37 mg. per 100 cc.) the P waves disappear. As the level increases, the ST segment is depressed. The QRS complex spreads (from slowing of intraventricular conduction) and becomes a biphasic curve, and the heart slows. Cardiac arrest and death may occur when the level of 10 or 11 mEq/L. (39 to 43 mg. per 100 cc.) is exceeded.

In some patients, elevation of plasma potassium is associated with flaccid paralysis of the skeletal muscles, generally of ascending type. It usually develops in the course of a few minutes, in contrast to organic paralyses. Paradoxically, it may resemble clinically the paralysis induced by too *low* a level of serum potassium (see following page).

Elevations of plasma potassium may occur in severe renal insufficiency, in untreated adrenal cortical insufficiency, in crush syndrome (p. 222), and following intravenous injection of solutions containing higher concentrations of potassium than does plasma. Oral administration of single doses of potassium salts containing 80 to 100 mg. of potassium per Kg. of body weight may be toxic in normal individuals. Subdivision of dosage eliminates the danger if renal function is normal.

Therapeutic administration of potassium salts to patients having a blood urea or nonprotein nitrogen level of 100 or more mg. per 100 cc. should be preceded by an oral test dose of 5 Gm. of potassium bicarbonate, with electrocardiograms and determinations of serum potassium before and 90 and 180 minutes after ingestion of the drug. Urine specimens should be collected over the two ninety-minute periods and total potassium excretion determined. The normal rise in serum potassium is not more than 1.25 mEq/L. (5 mg. per 100 cc.), and the normal excretion is 50 or more percent. Patients with normal tolerance can be given potassium salts with safety. Some uremic individuals have an intracellular deficit of potassium, and they may have a normal rise in serum potassium coupled with a low urinary excretion.

The treatment of potassium intoxication is intravenous administration of isotonic or hypertonic (3 percent) sodium chloride solution. Doses of 12 to 15 Gm. may have to be given in this manner before improvement is noted; 15 to 25 Gm. of sodium chloride should be given daily until clinical manifestations have disappeared and the serum potassium level has returned to normal.

POTASSIUM DEFICIENCY—Deficiency of potassium may be intracellular, extracellular, or both. It may result from:

Abnormally low intake of potassium as compared with sodium, as in low-potassium diets or when body fluids are being maintained by parenteral administration of solutions containing only sodium, chloride, and dextrose.
High excretion of potassium, as in hyperadrenalism or after overdoses of desoxycorticosterone (p. 460).
Alkalosis, when severe or persistent.
Extreme electrolyte loss even when accompanied by acidosis, as in severe diarrhea in infants, diabetic acidosis, and some cases of renal failure.
Trauma to muscles (Crush Syndrome, p. 222), in which the muscle cells lose their ability to retain potassium.
Injury due to cold.

In fact, a certain degree of potassium deficiency is to be expected in alkalosis, diabetic acidosis, and severe diarrhea in infants; and potassium salts should usually be included in therapy.

When one or more of the factors listed above are

in operation, potassium ions ordinarily pass out of the cells and are replaced by sodium ions. This transfer of sodium from the extracellular fluids may seriously increase any extracellular sodium deficit already present. When electrolyte deficiency is multiple and severe, as in infants with diarrhea, the adjustment may not take place.

Extracellular potassium deficiency is, of course, associated with abnormally low levels of serum potassium. The latter cause lowering of the T waves in the electrocardiogram, and they may induce a rapidly developing skeletal motor paralysis which is clinically indistinguishable from that of abnormally high serum potassium.

However, normal or high levels of serum potassium may be associated with intracellular potassium deficiency, particularly in infants with diarrhea and patients in severe diabetic acidosis. Thus, neither serum potassium levels nor clinical signs are sure diagnostic aids in potassium deficiency, and a tentative diagnosis must be made largely by recognition of the conditions likely to be associated with this disturbance.

It is generally agreed that potassium should be administered by mouth if possible, in the form of potassium salts or foods rich in potassium (broth, meat extracts, meat itself, and most cereals, vegetables, and fruits). There is some difference of opinion regarding parenteral administration. Darrow recommends for infantile diarrhea a solution containing:

sodium chloride.........................0.44 percent
potassium chloride......................0.27 percent
sodium bicarbonate.....................0.40 percent
(A similar quantity of sodium ions is supplied by substituting for the sodium bicarbonate 30 cc. of one-sixth-molar sodium lactate solution per 100 cc. of final solution.)

This yields the following ions:

sodium..............................123 mEq/L.
potassium............................ 36 mEq/L.
chloride.............................111 mEq/L.
bicarbonate.......................... 48 mEq/L.

Darrow gives 40 to 80 cc. of this solution per Kg. of body weight (20 to 40 cc. per lb.) per twenty-four hours, preferably by hypodermoclysis. The total dose should be given in not less than four hours and preferably over eight or more. The patient should receive dextrose intravenously at the same time because there is evidence that the uptake of dextrose by muscle cells facilitates the uptake of potassium ions. The solution is given only after dehydration has been treated with intravenous sodium chloride and dextrose solutions (20 to 40 cc. per Kg.), complemented by blood transfusions in all patients likely to be suffering from shock. The above solution, diluted with two or three parts of 5 or 10 percent dextrose solution, can be given by mouth in the same total quantities when there is no likelihood of vomiting.

For alkalosis, Darrow suggests a solution containing 0.29 percent sodium chloride and 0.37 percent potassium chloride, which yields 50 mEq/L. each of sodium and potassium and 100 mEq/L. of chloride. However, such a solution has apparently not had extensive use.

It is again emphasized that potassium salts must be given with great caution by hypodermoclysis and with even greater caution by vein. Administration should be slow, the patient should be watched carefully, and it is best to have a urine flow previously established. The most serious dangers of hyperpotassemia are heart block and erythema with subsequent desquamation.

PREPARATIONS OF POTASSIUM—Most of the salts of potassium which are employed therapeutically are given for the effect of the acid portion of the molecule. Examples are the bromide, iodide, permanganate, and penicillin salts of potassium. When the effect of potassium is desired, potassium chloride is usually chosen. Exceptions are the use of the more powerful potassium nitrate as a diuretic and the administration of potassium gluconate in allergic disorders.

Tablets and concentrated solutions of potassium chloride and nitrate are likely to produce gastric irritation when taken by mouth. These drugs are therefore usually given either in dilute solution or as 'Enseals.' One gram of potassium chloride may be taken in a wineglassful of milk, fruit juice, or tomato juice, or in more dilute solution for children. For extremely large quantities, the patient may make up the following each day, to be taken at mealtime in three equally divided doses:

    milk, 1 quart
    cream, 1/2 cup
    egg, 1
    sugar, 2 tablespoonfuls
    potassium chloride, 30 Gm.

Potassium gluconate seldom produces gastric irritation, but it has two disadvantages: In contrast to the chloride and nitrate, which are neutral, it has a net alkaline reaction which favors sodium retention; and the high molecular weight of gluconic acid makes it necessary to give three times as much potassium gluconate as chloride to obtain the same amount of potassium.

THERAPEUTIC USES—The pharmacologic effect of potassium may be useful in a number of conditions. In the rare disease, familial periodic paraly-

sis, attacks can be prevented by oral administration each evening of 5 Gm. of potassium chloride. The same dose, perhaps repeated after three hours, relieves attacks. Potassium should be administered intravenously only in an extreme emergency, and then very slowly as not more than 50 cc. of a 2 percent solution.

In myasthenia gravis, symptomatic improvement may result from single oral doses of 12 Gm. of potassium chloride or doses of 4 to 6 Gm. repeated six times daily. Potassium works well in combination with neostigmine (p. 251).

The ectopic beats caused by digitalis can be abolished, often for considerable periods, by a single oral dose of 5 or 10 Gm. of potassium chloride.

Potassium salts have been employed in conditions marked by local or general sodium retention and edema. In all of these, administration of potassium should be accompanied by restriction of sodium intake to 1 or 2 Gm. daily (see p. 53). The use of potassium salts as diuretics against generalized edema is discussed on page 352. In Ménière's disease (p. 244), a significant proportion of patients find their symptoms reduced in intensity by ingestion of 6 to 10 Gm. of potassium chloride daily in divided dosage. Potassium chloride has been helpful in a few cases of allergy (asthma and chronic urticaria), especially in children. The total daily adult dose is 2 to 6 Gm. or more, and it must be combined with a low-sodium diet (p. 585).

Calcium* ions are necessary for normal body function; they lessen the irritability of all tissues (of particular importance is their effect on neuromuscular excitability and cardiac rhythmicity), they diminish the permeability of cell membranes, and they are essential in the clotting of blood (p. 373).

Calcium does not occur in the blood cells but only in the plasma. One portion is in combination with the plasma proteins (largely the albumin fraction); it is nondiffusible and physiologically inactive. Its amount varies with the plasma protein level, the normal range being 4.5 to 6 mg. of calcium per 100 cc. of serum. The remainder is diffusible and contains the ionized calcium which alone possesses physiological activity. The normal level of the diffusible portion is 4.5 to 5.5 mg. per 100 cc. of serum. Unfortunately, the percentage of diffusible calcium which is ionized, or even ionizable, cannot as yet be accurately estimated. Thus, the blood level of physiologically active calcium cannot be determined directly, and one is

---
* For the physiology and therapeutic use of calcium in other than ionic form, see page 505.

forced to guess at it from measurements of total serum calcium, which is normally 9 to 11.5 mg. per 100 cc. The guessing is made more accurate if one knows the plasma protein level, for one can then estimate and discount the level of protein-bound calcium. If, in addition, the inorganic phosphate level is known, the approximation becomes closer because of the known inverse relationship between serum phosphate and ionizable calcium. It is therefore important that the physician always order determinations of plasma protein and serum inorganic phosphate in addition to serum calcium.

The concentration of ionized calcium in the blood is influenced by the following factors:

1. The amount of calcium absorbed from the alimentary tract (see p. 506).

2. The pH of the blood. The percentage of ionizable calcium which is actually ionized at any particular time varies with the hydrogen-ion concentration.

3. Serum phosphate level (p. 347). There is a roughly reciprocal relationship between the blood levels of ionizable calcium and of inorganic phosphate.

4. The intake of vitamin D (including the vitamin D formed by ultraviolet irradiation of the skin) (p. 494).

5. The supply of parathyroid hormone (see p. 195).

Hypercalcemia reduces neuromuscular excitability, giving rise to weakness, loss of appetite (and consequent loss of weight), constipation, muscle and joint pains, and abdominal pain. The effects on the heart are more serious; as calcium level rises progressively, there are extreme slowing, flattening, and then inversion of T and P waves in the electrocardiogram and sinus arrest. In animals, other disturbances have been noted.

As might be inferred from the above listing, hypercalcemia is observed clinically in hyperparathyroidism (p. 197), in massive overdosage of vitamin D (p. 495), and sometimes in chronic acidosis or hypoxia such as may develop in advanced nephritis with uremia, chronic pulmonary emphysema, pneumoconiosis, and the like. It also occurs, for unknown reasons, in erythremia (p. 101), multiple myeloma (p. 105), and extensive metastatic neoplasms of the skeleton.

Treatment of hypercalcemia should be directed primarily at the underlying cause. In emergency, to reduce the immediate effects, one can increase the pH and the level of phosphate in the plasma by intravenous administration of sodium lactate (p. 349) and sodium phosphate, Na_2HPO_4 (p. 347).

The principal symptoms associated with hypocalcemia result from increased neuromuscular excitability. The clinical picture is called "tetany" and is described under Hypoparathyroidism (p. 195). In addition to hypoparathyroidism, hypocalcemia is observed in vitamin D deficiency (rickets, osteomalacia, p. 496) and deficient calcium intake or absorption (p. 495). Alkalosis may produce tetany without change in serum calcium level by reducing the ionization of calcium. In nephrosis there may be a fall in serum calcium level due to the low serum protein; it does not affect the physiologically active calcium. In chronic glomerulonephritis, hypocalcemia may be secondary to phosphate retention.

Treatment is directed at the principal causative factor (see listing above; for tetany due to alkalosis, see p. 61). In the emergency treatment of hypocalcemia, it is sometimes advisable to administer calcium salts intravenously, since this is the most rapid method of elevating the level of blood calcium. Dosage and precautions are discussed below.

For rapid ionic effects, calcium is injected either intravenously or intramuscularly. Calcium chloride has been used, but it has the disadvantage of being extremely irritating; consequently, it can be given only by the intravenous route and with the utmost precautions against extravasation. Calcium is generally injected as a salt of one of the sugar acids. Because of the variation in molecular weights, different quantities are required to obtain a given amount of calcium ion. The listing below gives some of the more important salts, the concentrations usually employed, and the quantities which yield 0.1 Gm. of calcium ion:

> 7.4 cc. of 5 percent calcium chloride
> 3.7 cc. of 10 percent calcium chloride
> 5.6 cc. of Ampoules Calcium Glucoheptonate, Lilly
> 5.6 cc. of 'Gluco-Calcium' (Calcium Salts of Sugar Acids, Lilly)
> 11.1 cc. of 10 percent calcium gluconate
> 15.4 cc. of 5 percent calcium lactate
> 7.7 cc. of 10 percent calcium levulinate

Although the calcium salts of the sugar acids are all relatively nonirritating in adults, calcium glucoheptonate seems to be the best tolerated. When the volume to be injected exceeds 3 cc., however, the intravenous route is preferred. In contrast, the muscle of infants and young children is relatively intolerant of all calcium salts, and intramuscular injection is contraindicated with the exception that, in emergency when technical difficulties make intravenous injection impossible, calcium glucoheptonate may be given intramuscularly to very young patients.

Intravenous injection should always be slow,

with the patient lying down. The maximum rate recommended for an adult is 36 mg. of calcium ion per minute; this quantity is contained in:

    2.65 cc. of 5 percent calcium chloride
    1.33 cc. of 10 percent calcium chloride
    2   cc. of Ampoules Calcium Glucoheptonate, Lilly
    2   cc. of 'Gluco-Calcium'
    4   cc. of 10 percent calcium gluconate
    5.5 cc. of 5 percent calcium lactate
    2.75 cc. of 10 percent calcium levulinate

Even with slow injection, many patients will vomit and there may be a slight, transient increase in systolic and diastolic arterial pressures. Faster injection causes a wave of peripheral vasodilation that is felt subjectively as warmth. More rapid injection may lead to circulatory collapse and death or to manifestations of hypercalcemia (discussed above). Other indications of too-rapid injection include tingling sensations, a calcium taste, or a sense of oppression. Great caution should be exercised in parenteral administration of calcium to patients under the influence of digitalis or a related drug (see p. 356).

In hypocalcemia the parenteral route for calcium is justified only in the presence of tetany with laryngeal spasm, and administration should then be intravenous. The usual doses are listed below, and the *minimum time* for injection of the entire dose is *eight minutes*:

    20 cc. of 5 percent calcium chloride
    10 cc. of 10 percent calcium chloride
    15 cc. of Ampoules Calcium Glucoheptonate, Lilly
    15 cc. of 'Gluco-Calcium'
    30 cc. of 10 percent calcium gluconate
    40 cc. of 5 percent calcium lactate
    20 cc. of 10 percent calcium levulinate

The amount of calcium ion in each dose is 0.27 Gm.

When the need is less urgent, the blood calcium level should be raised by administration of parathyroid extract (p. 475) or vitamin D (p. 494), supplemented by calcium salts by mouth (p. 506).

Calcium is a requisite for uterine motility, which varies according to the level of available calcium ion. In an occasional obstetrical case, the parturient uterus will be unresponsive to oxytocic agents without apparent reason. Determinations of serum calcium have not been reported for such patients; but it has been demonstrated that in most, if not all, of them the uterus responds dramatically to the intravenous injection of calcium. In cases of postpartum hemorrhage due to uterine atony, intravenous calcium has been a lifesaving procedure when the uterus has not responded to oxytocics. It is recommended that ampoules be kept in the delivery room for emergency use. The dosage for

hypocalcemia (see above) is appropriate, and the same precautions must be observed.

Calcium intravenously is an antidote to the systemic effects of overdosage of magnesium (see below). It also relieves the pain from muscle spasm following spider bites.

Intravenous calcium has been successful in relieving intestinal, ureteral, and biliary colic (including lead colic) and the abdominal pain, diarrhea, and tenesmus of intestinal tuberculosis. However, it should probably be employed only if the more common symptomatic agents are ineffective (see Morphine, p. 399, Papaverine, p. 363, Nitrites, p. 364, and Antidiarrheics, p. 387).

Magnesium is an ion vital to life. It is essential to proper functioning of the neuromuscular system, is necessary to activity of phosphatases, and plays an important part in the energy transfer during muscular contraction. In high concentration it is depressant to the central nervous system, an effect which is directly antagonized by calcium.

Like potassium, magnesium is an intracellular ion. It is present in cell fluid to the extent of about 44 milliequivalents per liter (about 54 mg. per 100 cc.), whereas the normal plasma level is about 1.6 to 2.5 mEq/L. (2 to 3 mg. per 100 cc. of serum). Approximately 80 percent of the plasma magnesium is ionized and diffusible.

Abnormally low levels of plasma magnesium may occur during hypoparathyroidism, chronic glomerulonephritis, epilepsy, or without known cause. As the plasma level drops below 1 mEq/L., muscular twitchings develop. Lower levels may induce generalized convulsions. In patients with glomerulonephritis, 15 Gm. of magnesium sulfate by mouth are followed in a few hours by rise in the plasma level and subsidence of twitchings or convulsions. For more rapid effects, magnesium can be given by injection (see below).

Abnormally high levels of serum magnesium may follow parenteral injections of magnesium salts or even oral administration in patients with severely impaired renal function, or they may occur spontaneously in renal failure. Drowsiness is observed at levels of 6.5 to 8.5 mEq/L. (8 to 10 mg. per 100 cc.), and coma occurs sometimes at levels of 8.5 mEq and regularly at 14 mEq (17 mg.). Intravenous calcium is an immediate antidote for the central-nervous-system effects of magnesium (for dosage and precautions, see p. 346), but in renal failure the possibility of concomitant hypercalcemia must be kept in mind. High levels of serum magnesium also depress intracardiac conduction, with increase in P-R interval, widening of the QRS complex, and occasional S-A or A-V block. First there is tachycardia and, later, bradycardia. These effects are not influenced by calcium therapy.

Magnesium is given parenterally as the sulfate ($MgSO_4 \cdot 7H_2O$, of which magnesium represents about 10 percent). The dose varies with need and with rate of administration. One may give, for example, 2 cc. of 50 percent solution (containing 0.1 Gm. magnesium) intramuscularly, 20 cc. of 10 percent solution (0.2 Gm. magnesium) intramuscularly, or 500 cc. of 2 percent solution (1 Gm. magnesium) intravenously over a thirty to sixty-minute period. The adequacy of the dose is judged by the clinical effect, and it may be repeated as the condition warrants.

Certain precautions should be observed. The knee jerks should be tested before each dose; if they are absent, no more magnesium should be given until they return. Administration beyond the point of suppression of knee jerks may cause temporary failure of the respiratory center, necessitating artificial respiration or intravenous administration of calcium. Ampoules of injectable calcium should be available whenever magnesium is administered parenterally.

Magnesium should be given very cautiously in the presence of serious impairment of renal function. Magnesium is excreted almost entirely by the kidneys, and impaired excretion leads to rapid rise in blood level.

Magnesium is administered parenterally in treatment of convulsive states. It has been used extensively in eclampsia, but other methods threaten to supersede it (p. 213). It may prove helpful in the immediate control of convulsions or generalized muscular twitchings from any cause, but particularly in epilepsy, glomerulonephritis, and hypoparathyroidism. Because of the possible occurrence of a low plasma magnesium level in these three conditions, it may be advisable to draw blood for a magnesium determination before administering treatment. Magnesium may be given in conjunction with barbiturates or narcotics, making possible —in fact, necessitating—reduction in dosage of the latter.

Magnesium has also been advocated as a myometrial relaxant in uterine tetany, especially that from oxytocic agents, and in dysmenorrhea.

Chloride is the chief acidic ion of the extracellular fluid. It is essential because of its unique property of neutralizing basic ions and supplying osmotic effect without pharmacologic action. It has been

aptly termed "osmotic stuffing." This same capacity makes the chloride salts advantageous forms for administering basic therapeutic agents.

The normal level of plasma chloride is 103 mEq/L. (about 365 mg. chloride ion per 100 cc., or about 600 mg. expressed as sodium chloride). A relative deficiency of chloride ions accompanies alkalosis (see Dehydration, p. 56, and Alkalosis, p. 61). In acidosis (p. 59), chloride is displaced by other fixed acids which are less readily excreted by the kidneys.

Chloride may be administered as the neutral sodium chloride (for dosage, see pp. 58 and 348) or the acid-producing ammonium chloride (p. 352), depending on the acid-base balance. When special basic ions, such as potassium, are required, they are usually given as chlorides.

Chloride is given therapeutically to prevent or treat deficiency. It is also used in treating bromide and iodide intoxication.

Phosphate—Phosphorus (see also p. 505) is an essential element occurring in bone and the nucleoproteins and playing an important role in the metabolism of fat and carbohydrate, the formation of thrombin, and blood coagulation. Phosphates, largely in organic combination, are the principal acidic ions of the intracellular fluids. They also act as buffers because of the differing tendencies of the hydrogen ions to dissociate. At normal pH (7.4), about 80 percent of inorganic phosphate occurs as the disodium salt, Na_2HPO_4 (dibasic sodium phosphate or, with seven molecules of water of crystallization, Sodium Phosphate, U.S.P.), and the remainder as the monosodium salt, NaH_2PO_4 (sodium acid phosphate or, with one molecule of water of crystallization, Sodium Biphosphate, U.S.P.).

In the extracellular fluids, inorganic phosphate occurs in low concentration that of the plasma being normally about 1.6 to 2.4 mEq/L. (about 3 to 4.5 mg. per 100 cc. of serum) in adults and 2.1 to 3.2 mEq/L. (4 to 6 mg. per 100 cc. of serum) in children. There is a reciprocal relationship between the levels of inorganic phosphate and calcium ions (p. 345). After ingestion and during utilization of carbohydrate, there is normally a fall in plasma phosphate.

The phosphate ion itself has little or no pharmacologic effect. Hypophosphatemia occurs in hypercalcemia (p. 345) from any cause—including hyperparathyroidism, rickets and osteomalacia (hypovitaminosis D), and sprue—and temporarily during increased carbohydrate utilization. Hyperphosphatemia is observed in hypocalcemia (see p. 345 and also Hypoparathyroidism, p. 195), hypervitaminosis D (p. 495), in some cases of renal failure, and during the healing of fractures.

The phosphate ion as such has no therapeutic indication. Phosphate occurs abundantly in the average diet, and a primary deficiency has not been recognized. However, phosphate is bound by aluminum hydroxide (p. 382); and when the latter is administered, the patient should be assured a high phosphate intake to prevent deficiency.

ELECTROLYTE SOLUTIONS

Electrolyte solutions are administered for restoration or maintenance of the body stores of ionized salts (see Disturbances of Fluid and Electrolyte Balance, p. 49). The principal ions are sodium, potassium, chloride, and either bicarbonate or lactate (the latter two are equivalent inasmuch as lactate is burned in the body to form carbonic acid and water). The ionic content of various solutions is given in Table 36. Since none of them provides a significant quantity of potassium, this ion must be supplied separately (see p. 343).

Provided they are isotonic, electrolyte solutions can be administered by hypodermoclysis. However, it is usually more satisfactory to give them by intravenous drip, the rate depending on the state of the circulation.

Blood or **Blood Plasma** is obviously the most complete replacement therapy because it contains not only all the necessary ions but also the protein needed to maintain blood volume. It is indicated when electrolyte deficiency is severe enough to cause shock (see pp. 56 and 90). It is administered intravenously as often as necessary to prevent or relieve shock. Individual doses range from 10 to 30 cc. per Kg. (5 to 14 cc. per lb.) of usual body weight.

Isotonic Sodium Chloride Solution, U.S.P., containing 0.9 percent sodium chloride, is the simplest solution in common use. It does not closely approximate the composition of plasma (see Table 36) or interstitial fluid (see p. 50), for it contains relatively too much chloride. It is indicated chiefly, then, in alkalosis (p. 61) (in which there is a relative deficiency of chloride) and in mild electrolyte deficiency in the presence of adequate renal function (under which circumstances the excess of chloride can be selectively excreted).

Ringer's Solution, U.S.P., contains:

```
sodium chloride......................0.86   percent
potassium chloride...................0.03   percent
calcium chloride (CaCl₂ · 2H₂O).........0.033 percent
```

It is intended to provide an isotonic solution which, though still relatively simple, more closely approximates the composition of plasma and interstitial fluid than does Isotonic Sodium Chloride Solution. It fulfills these intentions to a certain degree (see table); but it does not contain a therapeutically significant quantity of potassium and, like sodium chloride solution, it is relatively high in chloride ion. It has the same indications as Isotonic Sodium Chloride Solution.

Lactated Ringer's Solution, U.S.P., has the following composition:

```
sodium lactate.......................0.31 percent
sodium chloride......................0.60 percent
potassium chloride...................0.03 percent
calcium chloride (CaCl₂ · 2H₂O)..........0.02 percent
```

It comes the closest of any of the common solutions to the actual ionic make-up of interstitial fluid. It

TABLE 36 — *Ionic Content of Electrolyte Solutions*

Preparation	Ions Supplied, in mEq/L.				
	Na+	K+	Ca++	Cl⁻	HCO₃⁻*
Blood plasma..	142	5	5	103	27
Isotonic Sodium Chloride Solution, U.S.P.............	154	0	0	154	0
Ringer's Solution, U.S.P............................	147	4	4	155	0
Lactated Ringer's Solution, U.S.P...................	130	4	3	109	28
Sodium Lactate Solution, 1/6 Molar.................	167	0	0	0	167
Mixture of 1 part 1/6-Molar Sodium Lactate and 3 parts Isotonic Sodium Chloride Solution................	157	0	0	115	42
Mixture of equal parts 1/6-Molar Sodium Lactate and Isotonic Sodium Chloride Solution................	161	0	0	77	84

* Or lactate, which is burned to form carbonic acid and water.

is therefore appropriate as replacement of electrolyte loss when disturbance of acid-base balance is not severe. It is especially indicated in the presence of impaired renal function, when the kidneys are not well able to excrete or reabsorb ions selectively.

Lactated Ringer's Solution is usually supplied in concentrated form. *This concentrated solution must be suitably diluted with sterile distilled water before use.*

Sodium Lactate Solution, One-Sixth Molar, containing 1.87 percent $CH_3 \cdot CH(OH) \cdot COO \cdot Na$, is an approximately isotonic preparation which supplies only the sodium ion. The lactate is oxidized in the body. It is useful in the treatment of acidosis (p. 59), in which the primary ionic deficit is of sodium. It may also be administered to alkalinize the urine, as during sulfonamide therapy (p. 295).

Mixtures of one-sixth-molar sodium lactate solution and Isotonic Sodium Chloride Solution may be employed. One part of the lactate solution combined with three parts of the chloride solution yields a product which corresponds fairly well to interstitial fluid (see Table 36) and may thus be used in the same way as Lactated Ringer's Solution. A mixture of equal parts of the lactate and chloride solutions provides a fluid suitable for treatment of acidosis which, in contrast to sodium lactate alone, supplies a certain amount of chloride along with the sodium.

Sodium lactate is usually supplied as a one-molar solution *which must be diluted with five volumes of sterile distilled water before use.*

DEXTROSE SOLUTIONS

Dextrose solutions are the most satisfactory source of either carbohydrate or water when these substances must be supplied parenterally. Unless there is some disturbance of carbohydrate metabolism such as untreated diabetes mellitus, the dextrose is rapidly removed by the liver and tissues. A 5 percent solution of dextrose is isotonic with plasma and extracellular fluid, and a liter of such a solution provides 50 Gm. of carbohydrate or 200 calories. The purely nutritional phases of dextrose are discussed beginning on page 253. It may be pointed out here that carbohydrate (100 Gm. or more a day) may itself decrease the rate of dehydration, probably by three actions: production of water of oxidation (60 cc. per 100 Gm.); reduction of catabolism of protein and consequent diminution in obligatory urine volume; and avoidance of ketosis and resultant electrolyte and water loss in urine.

When dextrose solution is given primarily for its water content, the 5 percent solution is used. This is suitable for intravenous administration; it should be given by hypodermoclysis only when mixed with at least an equal volume of isotonic electrolyte solution. A 10 or even a 15 percent solution may be given intravenously (never by hypodermoclysis) when the amount of carbohydrate to be given would carry with it an undesirably large amount of water if administered as a 5 percent solution. The more concentrated solutions tend to be irritating and may induce phlebothrombosis. They should not be given too rapidly (see p. 285); and intravenous administration should never be stopped abruptly, particularly after prolonged clysis, because of the danger of compensatory hypoglycemia. Rather, the rate should be gradually diminished over a period of an hour or two.

Dextrose solution provides an excellent medium for parenteral administration of water before, during, and after operation. It is of no value in treating shock or as replacement of electrolyte losses.

Extremely concentrated dextrose solutions have been given intravenously as osmotic agents; they are discussed on page 353.

DIURETICS

Diuresis is the result of diminished reabsorption of glomerular filtrate. The reabsorptive capacity of the tubules (p. 218) is so great that only in extreme renal failure is urine volume influenced by the rate of glomerular filtration.

Diuretics are employed in the treatment of edema. They are most effective in cardiac edema, the mechanism of which seems to involve the kidneys (p. 54). They are less useful in nephritic edema and are rarely helpful in edema which is entirely extrarenal in origin.

Water is the simplest diuretic. Extra water ingested by a normal person is usually eliminated within four hours, most of it within two hours. Diuresis does not begin, however, until thirty to sixty minutes after water is ingested. In the interval, water is absorbed from the intestine and, presumably because it dilutes the blood and lowers osmotic pressure, escapes rapidly into the tissue spaces, carrying salt with it.

One assumes that these changes in the blood inhibit the output of posterior pituitary hormone, thus diminishing distal tubular reabsorption and increasing urine volume. As equilibrium is restored, pituitary hormone output rises to its previous level. Confirmatory evidence for this explanation is found in the observation that the onset of such a water diuresis can be delayed in dog or man by the injection of posterior pituitary hormone. It can also be delayed in an identical manner by emotional stress in dogs having completely denervated kidneys, presumably through an effect on the posterior pituitary.

In edematous patients, water may induce diuresis provided sodium intake is kept very low. Without an adequate supply of water, diuresis is impossible.

Digitalis—In cardiac decompensation with obvious or latent edema, the administration of digitalis is often followed within a few days by profuse diuresis. However, digitalis is not a diuretic in itself. Rather, its diuretic effect is brought about by improvement in circulation when this has been impaired (p. 63).

Salts—Various salts are of value in the treatment of edema, particularly as adjuvants to digitalis, the xanthines, and the mercurial diuretics. Their usefulness is due partly to their ability to alter the ionic and acid-base balance of the blood and tissue fluids and partly to their ability to diminish reabsorption of water in the renal tubules.

An excess of alkali or of sodium, or a high sodium-potassium ratio in the mineral intake, favors retention of fluid in the tissue spaces. Acids, which promote excretion of sodium, aid in combating edema. However, only the fixed acids—those which are not oxidized in the body—behave in this fashion.

To be effective, all the diuretic salts must be taken in quantities of 90 to 180 grains (6 to 12 Gm.) a day, and administration should be intermittent. They are usually given for periods of three to five days, with rest periods following. Since the maximum effect is ordinarily obtained on the second or third day after initiation of therapy, administration should be started one or two days before other diuretics such as the xanthines or mercurials are given.

All the diuretic salts are somewhat irritating to the stomach, particularly in the large doses necessary for therapeutic effect. They are therefore commonly administered as 'Enseals' (p. 282).

Renal insufficiency with elevated blood urea is an absolute contraindication to the administration of the diuretic salts, since they accumulate in the body when not excreted in the urine.

Because of the importance of acid-base balance in the genesis and continuance of edema, diuretic salts are usually classified in two groups: the acid-producing salts and the neutral salts.

THE ACID-PRODUCING SALTS—*Ammonium chloride* is perhaps the most widely used of the acidifying salts. The ammonia contained in the compound is transformed into urea in the liver, leaving hydrochloric acid in the blood. The chloride radical tends to produce a shift toward acidity and is particularly helpful when the chloride of the plasma is abnormally low. The shift carries with it the danger of severe acidosis, which must be kept in mind when large amounts of ammonium chloride are being given. Such an acidosis is capable of producing renal insufficiency. The chloride in itself is nontoxic.

According to Keith, *ammonium nitrate* in daily doses of 180 grains (12 Gm.) is the most efficient of the acid-producing salts, and it has a minimum tendency to produce nausea. It does not cause so great a shift in acid-base balance as ammonium chloride; consequently, the danger of producing acidosis and renal insufficiency is lessened considerably. Ammonium nitrate may produce methemoglobinemia, but this is transient if administration of the salt is promptly discontinued. In rare instances, nitrite intoxication has been observed in patients with constipation.

Calcium chloride has been used as an acidifying diuretic. Acid is produced because most of the calcium remains in the intestine, allowing the chloride radical to enter the blood stream without neutralization. Mainly because of the irritant properties of this salt, it has been superseded, for the most part, by ammonium chloride and ammonium nitrate.

NEUTRAL SALTS—Keith and Binger have concluded that *potassium nitrate* is the most potent diuretic of all the salts, whether neutral or acid-producing. Potassium salts should be withheld from patients with anuria or extreme oliguria, or when the blood urea is over 100 mg. per 100 cc. The potential dangers of nitrates are set forth in the paragraph on ammonium nitrate above.

Potassium chloride, though somewhat less potent as a diuretic than the nitrate, is perhaps better suited for long-continued administration since it may be used in part as a substitute for table salt.

Small initial doses of potassium salts are advised, with 185 grains (12.5 Gm.) as a daily maximum dose. Other potassium salts seem to be less effective than the chloride and nitrate. For other uses of potassium salts, see page 344.

The Xanthines are potent diuretics. Although surpassed in power by the mercurials, they are relatively nontoxic and are less irritating to tissues.

The chemical and pharmacologic properties of the xanthines and their clinical use as antispasmodics, vasodilators, and cardiac stimulants are discussed on page 358. Their diuretic effect seems to depend on a depression of renal tubular reabsorption. The theophylline compounds are generally recognized as the most powerful.

As diuretics, the xanthines are used most frequently as adjuncts to digitalis in treating the edema of cardiac failure (p. 54). They induce less effective diuresis in edema from other causes. The usual total daily dose is 1 to 2 Gm. When taken by mouth, the total daily quantity may be given in two doses, one at seven and the other at ten o'clock in the morning, so that diuresis will occur during the day and the patient's sleep will not be disturbed. If given in the form of 'Enseals' 'Monotheamin,' the daily dose can be administered in the late evening, and diuresis will begin the following morning.

As diuretics, the xanthines are best given intermittently. Administration may be continued for from one to four days, depending on tolerance and results; thereafter a rest period of several days is usually advisable. The xanthines can advantageously be combined with the diuretic salts.

An augmentation of diuresis has been observed when the xanthines are administered concomitantly with the mercurial diuretics. The xanthine diuretics include the following:

theophylline and its derivatives
aminophylline
'Monotheamin'
theobromine and its salts
caffeine and its salts

The Mercurial Diuretics are the most potent diuretics known. They produce a powerful depression of renal tubular reabsorption, which is, however, apparently limited to the distal convoluted tubule. Although most effective in the edema of cardiac failure, they may occasionally be useful in other conditions, including hepatic cirrhosis and nephrosis, provided the liver and kidneys have some degree of function remaining.

The earlier organic mercurial diuretics were frequently toxic. These properties have been reduced in the newer preparations; and, recently, combinations of organic mercurial compounds with theophylline have shown still further decrease in irritant properties and considerable increase in diuretic potency.

The mercurial diuretics are contraindicated in acute nephritis and in ulcerative colitis and should not be given to patients with an idiosyncrasy to mercury. Renal or hepatic insufficiency is also a contraindication; but when elevation of blood urea is due only to circulatory failure, the compounds may be used. The sodium intake in patients receiving mercurial diuretics should not be restricted too greatly, and care should be taken that diuresis is not too drastic, lest dehydration and electrolyte deficiency supervene (p. 56). When these preparations are used repeatedly over prolonged periods, the urine should be examined at regular intervals for protein, casts, and blood.

Relatively inactive by mouth, the mercurial diuretics are usually given by injection. Those containing theophylline may be given intramuscularly, and this route is preferred because of its freedom from systemic reactions. In rare instances, death has followed intravenous injection. The diuresis from mercurials is frequently enhanced by preliminary administration of the acid-producing salts.

Hypertonic Solutions, when given intravenously, tend to produce diuresis by temporarily altering the osmotic pressure of the blood and glomerular filtrate. Solutions of the sugars and sugar alcohols are usually employed for this purpose, since they produce no disturbance of ionic equilibrium. They are discussed on page 352.

Urea has been reported to be an effective diuretic in cases of heart failure and of nephrosis. The mechanism is osmotic. A natural waste product of protein metabolism, urea produces no symptoms of toxicity until the blood level approaches 150 mg. per 100 cc., when anorexia, nausea, lassitude, and weakness may be noted.

To be effective as a diuretic, urea must be taken in quantities of 20 to 100 Gm. daily in divided doses. Because of its somewhat disagreeable taste, urea is usually administered in fruit juice or syrup of acacia and is best taken after meals to minimize gastric disturbance. It is well suited for long administration in chronic conditions.

ANTIDIURETICS

The only antidiuretic substance of practical importance is the principle of the posterior pituitary gland (p. 473). It acts by increasing reabsorption in the distal tubule of the kidney. Because the pituitary principle cannot increase the reabsorptive *capacity* of the distal tubule, and because the distal tubule is responsible for only a part of the reabsorptive process, it can compensate to only a limited extent for failure of reabsorption higher in the tubule. Though effective against water diuresis, the pituitary principle has little effect on osmotic diuresis (salts, sugars, urea) or tubule-inhibitory diuresis (xanthines and mercury).

The **Posterior Pituitary** principle constitutes specific therapy in diabetes insipidus (p. 194). Posterior Pituitary, U.S.P., which is a powder, can be insufflated into the nose three or four times daily in amounts averaging 40 mg. In the occasional patient who suffers nasal irritation from the powder, pituitary extract (solution) may be injected subcutaneously twice daily in doses of 5 to 10 U.S.P. Units. Suspensions in oil are available which lessen the frequency of injection. Pituitary preparations are ineffective by mouth.

ACIDIFIERS AND ALKALIZERS *

Except in treating acidosis (p. 59), alkalosis (p. 61), and some cases of gastric anacidity (p. 384), acidifiers and alkalizers are used almost entirely to modify the reaction of the urine. Such modification may be useful in treating urinary tract infection (p. 224), during sulfonamide administration (p. 295), and in persons susceptible to renal calculus (p. 223). The action on the urine follows from the function of the kidneys in maintaining a constant pH in the plasma; any excess of basic or acidic ions is excreted in the urine. Thus, except when renal function is seriously impaired, the reaction of the urine can be altered at will by administering actual or potential acids or alkalies.

Ammonium Chloride and **Ammonium Nitrate** are effective in acidifying the urine (for their **diuretic** action, see p. 350). The dosage cannot be fixed in advance but must be adjusted in accordance with the pH actually obtained in the urine (for determination of urinary pH, see p. 521). **Sodium Biphosphate** (sodium acid phosphate), $NaH_2PO_4 \cdot H_2O$, acts in the body as a monobasic acid. It has no advantage over other acidifiers, but it has traditionally been given with methenamine (p. 310). The usual dose is 15 to 40 grains (1 to 2.5 Gm.) four to six times daily.

Sodium Bicarbonate (p. 383) is perhaps the most widely used alkalizing agent. For the prevention of crystalluria during sulfonamide therapy (p. 295), an average daily dosage of 15 or 16 Gm. has been recommended to be given in six subdivided doses.

---

* For gastric antacids, see page 382.

In all cases, dosage should be governed by the pH of the urine (p. 521). When large amounts of sodium bicarbonate are taken by mouth, the resultant neutralization of gastric acidity may interfere with digestion and give rise to symptoms. To prevent gastric disturbance, **Sodium Citrate** (p. 376) or a solution of **Sodium Lactate** (p. 349) may be given dissolved in fruit juice. The effect of 1 Gm. of sodium bicarbonate is reproduced by 1.17 Gm. of sodium citrate or 1.33 Gm. of sodium lactate. **Potassium Bicarbonate** and **Potassium Citrate** are sometimes used in place of the sodium salts. They have no advantage in most cases but may be preferred during cardiac failure because of the tendency of the sodium ion to produce edema. However, the potassium ion may be toxic in the presence of adrenal insufficiency or severe renal failure (p. 223).

OSMOTIC AGENTS

All solutes exert osmotic effects. The term "osmotic agent" is used here to designate substances which increase the effective osmotic pressure of the blood plasma and thus tend to maintain or increase plasma volume. (The general subject of body water and its distribution is discussed beginning on page 49.) Blood and its derivatives are useful in treating hemorrhage and shock. Hypertonic solutions have a limited place in reducing the volume of interstitial fluid in the brain and thus reducing intracranial pressure in the presence of trauma, tumor, or abscess of the brain or in anticipation of operation on the brain. Most osmotic agents have a diuretic action also, by virtue of the increase in plasma volume.

Blood and Its Derivatives—The most satisfactory agent for inducing a prolonged increase in plasma osmotic pressure is plasma protein itself, and especially the albumin fraction. Following hemorrhage and in the initial treatment of shock or severe burns, whole blood is the agent of choice. The miminum dose should be 500 cc., and more is often advantageous (up to 1,500 cc. in shock and burns, and 3,000 cc. after hemorrhage). When it is unnecessary or undesirable to increase further the number of red blood cells or when whole blood is not available, plasma may be given as a supplement to whole blood or as a substitute. Since whole blood is about 55 percent plasma (v/v), 55 cc. of plasma provide the same quantity of protein as 100 cc. of whole blood. For details of dosage and management, see under the condition to be treated (Acute Blood Loss, p. 94; Shock, p. 90; Burns, p. 270).

If it is advisable to give plasma protein with a minimum of fluid, reconstituted plasma can be employed in twice the normal strength or a concentrated solution of plasma albumin may be used.

The Sugars—When it is desired to reduce the volume of the brain, hypertonic solutions of the sugars or sugar alcohols are generally employed. They can be given in sufficient quantity to produce sharp rises in plasma osmotic pressure, and they have the advantage over inorganic salts of causing no disturbance of ionic equilibrium.

Dextrose has been used as an osmotic agent, but it has disadvantages. The effect is brief because the sugar diffuses rapidly into the tissues, especially the liver. When given in effective quantities (75 to 100 Gm.), it is likely to disturb carbohydrate metabolism. After an initial reduction of intracranial pressure, there is a secondary rise because of the osmotic effect of the dextrose which has diffused into the cerebral tissues and fluids.

Sucrose and sorbitol, however, do not pass from the blood vessels into the tissues, are not utilized, and are excreted almost quantitatively in the urine. The effect is therefore more prolonged and without secondary rebound, and there is no interference with carbohydrate metabolism. Because the molecule of sorbitol is smaller than that of sucrose, the osmotic effect per gram is greater. With solutions of equal tonicity, sucrose is apparently more effective than sorbitol or dextrose. The usual intravenous dose of sucrose is 100 to 200 cc. of 50 percent solution; that of sorbitol, 50 cc. of 50 percent solution. At least ten minutes, and preferably thirty to forty minutes, should be taken for the injection.

Sucrose and dextrose have been shown to produce temporary hydropic degeneration of the renal tubular epithelium unaccompanied by detectable alteration in kidney function. Even though no clinically demonstrable harm has resulted, injections should probably not be repeated more frequently than at intervals of several weeks.

DRUGS AFFECTING PRINCIPALLY THE CARDIOVASCULAR SYSTEM

CIRCULATORY STIMULANTS

The Digitalis Group

A large number of glycosides* of plant origin, and some from animal sources, have actions on the heart of a type which may be useful in the treatment of cardiac failure. Only a few, however, have established a place in therapeutics, and of these the most widely used are obtained from digitalis.

Plants of the genus *Digitalis* (foxglove) yield a number of cardioactive glycosides. The best known are digitoxin, which is present in both *D. purpurea* and *D. lanata*, and digoxin, which occurs only in *D. lanata*. Their formulas are shown in Figure 16.

Digitoxose is a rare sugar. The aglycone* is composed of a cyclopentenophenanthrene steroid plus an unsaturated lactone. The digitalis principles are therefore members of the steroid family, which includes cholesterol, the bile acids, vitamin D, and the sex and adrenal hormones. The digitalis action,

---

* The term "glycoside" is applied to a substance containing one or more carbohydrate groups in combination with some other type of organic chemical group. The "other group" is known as the aglycone.

however, requires the presence of the lactone group, which is not present in these other compounds.

Pharmacologically, the cardiac glycosides appear to be more closely related to the adreno-cortical hormones than to other naturally occurring steroids, and it has been suggested that their beneficial effect in cardiac failure may be due in part to a cortin-like action upon the myocardium. It seems probable that the digitalis glycosides act in three ways (a single glycoside is capable of producing all of the effects of whole digitalis leaf):

1. Direct action on the cardiac muscle, by which contractility is stimulated at the same time that conductivity is depressed. Thus, contraction is made more efficient, but the tendency toward conduction block is increased. The conduction block is beneficial in auricular fibrillation, where it assists in slowing the ventricular rate by lessening the number of the auricular impulses reaching the ventricles. With toxic doses of digitalis, however, this same influence may produce partial or complete heart block and other undesirable effects.

2. The point is disputed, but there is some evidence that the digitalis glycosides diminish venous tone and consequently venous pressure. The normal

heart responds to lowered venous pressure by re-duced output; but in some cases of heart failure with low initial output, lowering venous pressure results in increased output. This action may be of great importance in "low-output failure" (p. 65).

3. Stimulation of the vagus nerve, tending to slow the auricular rate and to produce other func-tional changes, most of which are opposite to but very much less intense than the direct effect of digitalis on the heart muscle.

There are no absolute contraindications to the administration of digitalis. In general, it can be said that the drug should be used for the treatment of actual or threatened congestive heart failure with low cardiac output, for the control of ventric-ular rate in auricular fibrillation, and in some cases as preparation for the administration of quin-idine (p. 360). It is not helpful and should not be given in peripheral vascular collapse or other changes in hemodynamics such as may accom-pany shock, anemia, or severe infection.

Digitalis should be given very cautiously in the presence of hypercalcemia because of the additive effect of the latter (see p. 356). In the absence of heart failure, the effect of digitalis on conduction makes the drug dangerous in the presence of mul-tiple ventricular extrasystoles, ventricular tachy-cardia, angina pectoris, coronary occlusion (recent or old), hypersensitivity of the carotid sinus, Adams-Stokes syndrome, or partial heart block. It should be given cautiously and in low dosage to patients whose heart muscle has been severely damaged by arteriosclerosis or senescence.

The clinical effectiveness of the cardiac glyco-sides depends, among other factors, on their con-centration in the body. A definite percentage of this concentration—a percentage which varies from one person to another—is excreted each day, so that the absolute amount excreted depends partly on the volume of tissue and body fluid in which the drug is distributed and partly on the level of glycoside in the tissues and body fluids.

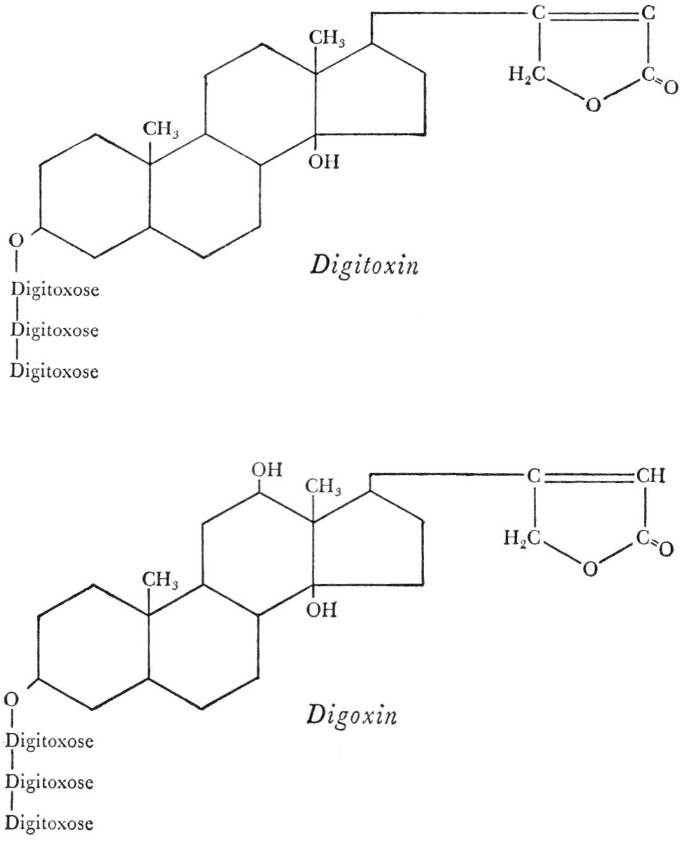

FIGURE 16 — *Structural Formulas of Digitalis Glycosides*

Initially, one can establish a therapeutic concentration slowly or rapidly, depending on the physician's preference and the patient's condition. If it is established rapidly, by administering relatively large initial doses, it is maintained by continuing smaller (maintenance) doses which are just sufficient to balance excretion. Since the rate of excretion cannot be predicted, the maintenance dose for each patient must be determined by trial on an individual basis. If the maintenance dose is too large, a toxic concentration will eventually be reached. If the maintenance dose is too small, the therapeutic effect will slowly be lost.

If the therapeutic concentration is to be established gradually by prolonged administration of relatively small doses, there will be an early period of increasing concentration of glycoside in the body. As the body concentration increases, the absolute excretion increases to the point where it balances the dose administered, and the body concentration thereafter remains constant as long as the given dose is continued. If the dosage has been too large for that individual, a toxic level will be reached; if the dosage has been too small, the level remains below the optimal therapeutic.

With digitoxin, 0.2 mg. daily, about three weeks are required for the establishment of equilibrium; similarly, when the drug is discontinued, about three weeks must elapse before all digitalis effect is lost. It is therefore apparent that, with either slow or rapid administration, the patient must be followed closely for at least three weeks before the suitability of a given maintenance dose can be determined. Because of its digitoxin content, whole leaf has a similar period of action. Digoxin is excreted more rapidly, and equilibrium is reached and lost more quickly.

The management of dosage is also influenced by the patient's cardiac rhythm. In the presence of auricular fibrillation and a rapid ventricular rate, the effect of therapy is usually striking, adequate dosage being followed by a great reduction in pulse rate, improvement in subjective and objective signs of heart failure, and frequently profuse diuresis. The concentration of drug in the patient is built up to the point where the ventricular rate drops to 80 or somewhat below, after which the dosage is adjusted to that which will just maintain such a rate. In the presence of hyperthyroidism, larger dosage is required, and it may not be possible to reduce the ventricular rate below 100 or 120 with safe doses of digitalis until the metabolic rate has been reduced.

Patients with cardiac failure, but with either regular rhythm or auricular fibrillation associated with slow ventricular rate in the untreated state, less frequently experience a dramatic improvement and diuresis. In patients with regular hearts, the pulse rate is not helpful in gauging dosage; and loss of appetite, slight nausea, prolonged A-V conduction time as shown in the electrocardiogram, or coupled beats are the only sure evidence that the maximal therapeutic effect has been passed. When these manifestations occur, the drug is omitted until they disappear, and then a maintenance dosage is begun which is smaller than that producing intoxication. There is no advantage in maintaining dosage at toxic or barely subtoxic levels, and it is best to reduce the dose to a maintenance level as soon as a satisfactory improvement occurs in the signs and symptoms of decompensation.

Anorexia, nausea, and vomiting are the most widely recognized indications of digitalis overdosage. The same symptoms may, however, be produced by cardiac failure itself or by the hepatic congestion which may go with it. A distinction can usually be made because the anorexia and nausea produced by digitalis are ordinarily accompanied by a sense of dizziness and fullness in the head which are lacking with the other two causes. Overdoses of digitalis reverse the gradient of gastro-intestinal motility through an effect on the central nervous system. The glycosides themselves are irritating to the alimentary tract only in doses much larger than the therapeutic. It is rare for the inert ingredients of the digitalis leaf to cause symptoms.

There are many signs and symptoms of digitalis overdosage, and they do not appear in any regular order. Frequent early indications are headache and nervous irritability. Greenish-yellow vision and flickering sensations are common. In fact, so many kinds of visual disturbances have been reported that one is justified in suspecting any unexplained visual symptom of being an early indication of digitalis overdosage. Abdominal pain, paresthesias, tingling of the extremities, and neuralgia (particularly of the mandibular branch of the trigeminal nerve, simulating toothache) have been described.

Other manifestations include restlessness, inability to think clearly, mental confusion, drowsiness, disorientation regarding time and place, hallucinations, delirium, occasional acute psychopathic outbreaks, and, rarely, convulsions. These features frequently are evident only at night and often are attributed to cerebral anoxia arising solely from the cardiac condition. A false interpretation sometimes leads to continued overdosage of digitalis and results in even more serious manifestations of poisoning.

Heart block of various degrees, auricular fibrillation, auricular standstill, and even ventricular fibrillation may occur. These may appear as early, and sometimes as the sole, manifestations of overdosage. Ventricular fibrillation, if of more than very brief duration, is invariably fatal.

Frequently a warning of impending heart block will be given by the regular recurrence of extrasystoles (the so-called "pulsus bigeminus," or coupled rhythm). The sudden appearance of this phenomenon in a patient receiving digitalis calls for withdrawal of the drug until the previously existing rhythm has been resumed. However, the presence of occasional extrasystoles in a patient who has received no digitalis is not a contraindication to use of the drug, and the appearance of irregularly recurring extrasystoles during digitalis administration does not necessarily have the same significance as pulsus bigeminus.

Overdosage of digitalis leads to alteration in the T waves of the electrocardiogram beyond those seen with therapeutic amounts; and in animals, overdosage may lead to coronary vasoconstriction and the development of degenerative lesions in the myocardium.

From all of the above considerations, it is evident that proper dosage is a matter of the patient's safety as well as his comfort.

Rapid diuresis should be avoided in edematous cardiacs who have been under the full influence of digitalis for a few days. In such patients there has been an opportunity for digitalis storage in the edema fluid, and rapid reabsorption of the edema may produce "spontaneous redigitalization" and digitalis intoxication. Of course, such a precaution is not necessary in patients not fully under the influence of digitalis.

Great caution should be exercised in administering calcium intravenously to patients under the influence of digitalis, for elevation of the serum calcium increases the effectiveness of the drug and deaths have been reported from intoxication induced in this way. Calcium salts by mouth are safe because they do not significantly elevate blood calcium.

PREPARATIONS OF DIGITALIS AND RELATED DRUGS

Until the recent isolation of the more important glycosides, dried leaves and extracts of them were the only preparations of digitalis available. Of necessity, standardization was biological. The glycosides, now available in pure form, can be expected in time to replace the older preparations.

Digitoxin, U.S.P., is the principal glycoside present in the official species, *Digitalis purpurea*. Its chemical formula is shown on page 354. It is a white, crystalline substance which is insoluble in water, very slightly soluble in ether, and soluble in alcohol.

Clinical studies have indicated that digitoxin has approximately 1,000 times the potency of Digitalis, U.S.P. (the leaf preparation). Thus, 0.1 mg. of digitoxin is, in general, equivalent to 0.1 Gm. of Digitalis, U.S.P., or to 1 U.S.P. Digitalis Unit. In corresponding doses, digitoxin and standard leaf digitalis produce their therapeutic effects in the same length of time (earliest effects on oral administration, two to four hours; maximum, six to twenty-four hours), and these effects have approximately the same duration (one to three weeks, depending on dosage level).

Digitoxin has the following desirable properties. It is a stable chemical compound. It is completely absorbed from the gastro-intestinal tract but can, if necessary, be given intravenously in the same dosage. However, it acts rapidly enough after oral administration so that intravenous injection is rarely necessary unless the patient can take nothing at all by mouth. The relatively prolonged action, like that of whole-leaf digitalis, makes for easy maintenance.

Unless the situation is very urgent, it is usual to give 0.6 mg. of digitoxin by mouth, to be followed by 0.4 mg. every six, twelve, or twenty-four hours until a full effect is obtained, usually within two or three days. By this method, the total quantity needed will seldom be more than 1.8 mg. before the dosage can be reduced to a maintenance level. If it is important that the effect begin in less than two hours, the first dose can be given by vein; this route reduces the latent period to about half an hour.

Larger initial doses have been used by some, and there is considerable experience with 1.2 mg. given by mouth at one time. Within six to ten hours after such an initial dose, (1) many, if not most, patients will exhibit considerable therapeutic effect, (2) about 2 percent can be expected to have minor toxic manifestations, and (3) an occasional patient may be severely intoxicated. This last possibility is a strong argument against routine use of the method. Before such a large single dose is given, it is especially important to ascertain that the patient has had no digitalis preparation during the previous three weeks. The full doses of digitoxin should not be given by vein.

When the patient's susceptibility to digitalis has been enhanced by coronary artery disease, severe "chronic myocarditis," or impairment of the intra-cardiac conduction mechanism, it is best to obtain the digitalis effect by slow cumulation. The start-ing daily dose of digitoxin should be 0.2 or 0.4 mg. When the desired effect has been obtained, the dosage is reduced to the maintenance level. If more than four weeks are required, it is evident that the patient's excretion rate is unusually high, and the dose must be increased.

As explained on page 355, the maintenance dos-age must be individualized by trial. Usually it will fall within the limits of 0.1 to 0.3 mg. daily.

Digoxin, U.S.P., is obtained from *Digitalis lanata.* Its chemical formula is shown on page 354. In appearance and physical properties it is much like digitoxin, from which it differs chemically only in having a hydroxyl group on carbon atom 12 of the steroid ring structure.

Digoxin is more rapidly but less completely ab-sorbed from the gastro-intestinal tract than is digi-toxin. It is likewise more rapidly eliminated, about half being gone in twenty-four hours and five-sixths in forty-eight.

With digoxin, it is usual to give 1, 1.5, or 2 mg. by mouth initially, to be followed by 0.5 or 1 mg. every six hours until the therapeutic effect is ob-tained. The average dose given in this way is 3.75 mg. The oral maintenance dose is 0.25 to 1.25 mg. daily. For intravenous administration the initial dose is 1 mg., followed by 0.5 mg. every six hours as necessary.

Even though the somewhat more rapid action of digoxin makes it preferable to digitoxin in those relatively few emergencies in which the time dif-ferential may be important, ouabain (see below) is still the drug of choice when speed is the primary consideration. It is true that the relatively short duration of action of digoxin hastens the recovery from overdoses, but under reasonably careful super-vision, serious toxicity need seldom be encountered with digitoxin or whole-leaf preparations. More importantly, the brief action of digoxin makes more difficult the maintenance of a full therapeutic ef-fect over the long periods usually necessary in heart disease.

Lanatoside C, U.S.P., is closely related to digoxin, from which it differs by inclusion of a dextrose molecule and an acetyl group. However, its absorp-tion from the gastro-intestinal tract is irregular and quite incomplete; consequently the oral dose is several times larger than for digoxin and is more variable in different individuals (the average initial dose is 7.5 to 10 mg. in the first two or three days, followed by maintenance doses of 0.5 to 3 mg. daily).

As between digoxin and lanatoside C, the ad-vantage would appear to lie with digoxin for oral administration, whereas lanatoside C would seem to be preferable for intravenous injection because of its greater solubility and lesser tendency to pro-duce local irritation. The intravenous dose of lana-toside C is 1.2 to 1.6 mg., followed by 0.4 mg. every four to eight hours until the full effect is obtained.

Digitalis, U.S.P., represents the dried leaves of *Digitalis purpurea.* It is the classical preparation. The natural content of glycosides is variable, and bio-assay has been employed to effect greater uni-formity of the prepared medication. For many years the frog was the assay animal, and ouabain was the standard with which digitalis preparations were compared. This method was, however, con-sidered unsatisfactory; consequently, in U.S.P. XI (1936) an actual lot of digitalis was chosen as the reference preparation and a new standard was set up which included the U.S.P. Digitalis Unit (equal to the International Unit and contained in 0.1 Gm. of U.S.P. Digitalis). Digitalis, U.S.P. XI, was more potent than Digitalis, U.S.P. X, probably by 25 to 30 percent, although the point was controversial.

In U.S.P. XII (1942) a new reference standard was chosen, and the cat was substituted for the frog as the assay animal. No further change has been made. Though Digitalis, U.S.P. XII, XIII, and XIV, is weaker than Digitalis, U.S.P. XI, there is controversy over the amount of difference. Probably the present potency is much like that of U.S.P. X, although the change in assay animal and the inherent variability in bio-assay make a de-finitive answer impossible.

Digitalis, U.S.P., is administered by mouth. For rapid digitalization, 6 U.S.P. Units (0.6 Gm.) may be given, followed by 2 or 3 U.S.P. Units every eight to twelve hours until a therapeutic effect is obtained or evidence of overdosage appears, usu-ally after a total of 16 or 18 U.S.P. Units. The average maintenance dose is 1 or 2 U.S.P. Units. The same precautions should be employed as with digitoxin.

Digitalis Tincture, U.S.P., is preferred by some to the powdered leaf. It is so standardized that 1 cc. contains 1 U.S.P. Digitalis Unit.

Ouabain, U.S.P., is a glycoside obtained from the seeds of *Strophanthus gratus.* It is the most rapid act-ing of the cardiac glycosides and is given intravenously when a digitalis action must be obtained in the shortest possible time. Its effects can be noted in three or four minutes following intravenous injection. They reach a maximum in one-half to two hours and last a total of twenty-four to seventy-two hours. For a patient who has not received a digitalis-type preparation for three weeks, the usual intravenous dose is 0.3 to 0.5 mg., followed by 0.1 mg. every half to one hour until an effect is obtained or a total of 1 mg. has been given.

Ouabain has, however, two disadvantages. It is quite irritating when injected outside a vein, and its action is so brief as to create a problem in maintenance. It has been suggested that at the time of the first intravenous dose of ouabain, the patient take by mouth 0.6 mg. of digitoxin or 6 U.S.P. Units of digitalis (more or less, depending on the patient's weight), maintenance doses being started the following day. When urgency is less than extreme, digitoxin would seem to be preferable to ouabain from the beginning. Ouabain is not administered by mouth because of variable absorption.

Strophanthin, N.F., is a glycoside or mixture of glycosides obtained from *Strophanthus kombé.* Its action and dosage are the same as those of ouabain, over which it has no advantage.

The Xanthine Group

Caffeine, theobromine, theophylline, and their salts and derivatives are often termed collectively "the xanthines." Related chemically and pharmacologically, these compounds have been found useful as cardiac stimulants, diuretics, coronary dilators in angina pectoris and coronary artery disease, and in the symptomatic treatment of asthma. The xanthines are found naturally in coffee, tea, cocoa (chocolate), kola, and certain other plants used for beverage and condiment purposes.

The formula of xanthine is shown in Figure 17. Caffeine is 1:3:7-trimethylxanthine; theobromine is 3:7-dimethylxanthine; and theophylline is 1:3-dimethylxanthine. The intensity of the various actions is shown in Table 37.

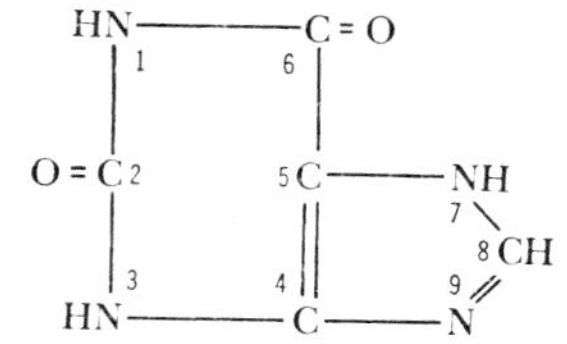

FIGURE 17—*Structural Formula of Xanthine*

TABLE 37 — *Comparative Potency of Xanthine Derivatives, 1 Indicating Highest Potency*

Drug	Cardiac Stimulation	Coronary Dilation	Diuresis	Bronchodilation	C.N.S. Stimulation
Theophylline .	1	1	1	1	2
Caffeine	3	3	3	–	1
Theobromine .	2	2	2	–	3

The xanthines have a number of actions on the cardiovascular system, some of which are mutually antagonistic. They stimulate the myocardium directly, increasing cardiac output independently of other factors. They also tend directly to increase heart rate; but in addition they stimulate the vagus center, which tends to slow the heart, so that the net effect on heart rate cannot always be predicted. There is a direct vasodilator effect and also a stimulant effect on the vasomotor center which gives rise to vasoconstrictor impulses. In therapeutic doses, the vasodilator effect predominates. Coronary blood flow is apparently increased because of coronary vasodilation plus increased cardiac output. Pulmonary arterial pressure falls. On the other hand, systemic blood pressure usually rises slightly, the effect of increased cardiac output predominating over other conflicting factors. However, if a xanthine is injected rapidly by vein, there is a sharp, but usually transitory, fall in systemic arterial pressure.

These drugs also cause relaxation of other types of smooth muscle. In the case of theophylline, this action has been valuable for relaxing bronchospasm in allergic asthma. In asthma of cardiac origin, the relief is thought to be due principally to lowering of pulmonary arterial pressure.

The xanthines are potent diuretics which increase the renal excretion of sodium (see Body Water, p. 49, and Edema, p. 53). The mechanism by which sodium excretion is augmented is unknown.

Caffeine and theophylline stimulate the central nervous system; the former, particularly, induces keener appreciation of sensory stimuli, more rapid flow of thought, quicker reaction time, and relief of sleepiness and fatigue. They also have a mild stimulant effect on the medullary centers controlling respiration and vasomotor and vagus tone, and they may increase basal metabolic rate to some extent.

There seem to be few or no contraindications to xanthine therapy. After prolonged use, these drugs may become less effective, particularly in their diuretic and vasodilator actions. Habituation to caffeine is the rule, with headache as the most common withdrawal symptom.

The xanthines are well absorbed after either oral or parenteral administration, but after ingestion they tend to produce gastric discomfort, nausea, and even vomiting. A portion of these drugs is excreted in the urine, but most is broken down to urea, and not to uric acid as might be expected from the chemical structure. They are therefore not contraindicated in gout.

THEOPHYLLINE

Because of its potency, theophylline is the xanthine most used for cardiac stimulant, coronary vasodilator, diuretic, and bronchodilator effects. In congestive heart failure (p. 63), it is valuable as a supplement to digitalis; in addition to increasing cardiac output, it often gives relief from paroxysmal nocturnal dyspnea and from Cheyne-Stokes respiration, and it may induce or increase diuresis in those cases which have not responded well to digitalis or the combination of digitalis and a mercurial diuretic. In coronary disease (p. 67), its administration over long periods has been recommended. It is useful by the intravenous or rectal route for relief of either cardiac or allergic asthma (particularly in those patients who no longer respond to epinephrine); and one theophylline preparation, 'Monotheamin,' is effective by mouth for prevention of asthma.

Aminophylline, U.S.P., (theophylline ethylenediamine, $[C_7H_8N_4O_2]_2 \cdot [NH_2 \cdot CH_2 \cdot CH_2 \cdot NH_2] \cdot 2H_2O$) contains 75 to 82 percent anhydrous theophylline. It is probably the most widely used preparation of theophylline. It can be given by mouth, by rectum, or parenterally. The oral route is usually satisfactory for cardiac and diuretic effects that are not urgent. The oral or rectal dose is 0.1 to 0.4 Gm. three or four times daily, usually beginning with the smaller dose. Adequate dosage varies among individuals. The drug should be given with meals to minimize gastro-intestinal side-effects. When patients are apprehensive, excitable, or restless, aminophylline may advantageously be combined with a barbiturate. For diuretic effects the drug is usually administered for three or four consecutive days. During the following three or four days the patient is allowed a rest period or is given a theobromine preparation.

Rectal administration is said to give rapid and powerful effects, especially in asthma. The usual dose is 0.25 to 0.5 Gm. If this route does not give satisfactory results, the drug may be given intravenously in the same dosage; it is dissolved in 10 to 20 cc. of water (2.5 percent solution) or in 50 cc. of 5 percent dextrose solution. Extravasation is painful. *Intravenous administration must always be very slow.* Deaths have been reported following rapid intravenous injection. The dose may be repeated as needed.

Intramuscular injection is seldom employed; the drug often causes local pain, and when oral administration is ineffective or too slow, the rectal or intravenous route is generally advisable.

'Monotheamin' (Theamin, Lilly) is similar to aminophylline except that it contains monoethanolamine, $NH_2 \cdot CH_2 \cdot CH_2OH$, instead of ethylenediamine. In dosage and action it is similar to aminophylline. The following advantages are claimed for 'Monotheamin': Instead of being a variable mixture which decomposes readily, it is a definite chemical compound of fixed properties (74.68 percent theophylline) and satisfactory stability; it is more soluble than aminophylline; and it is effective in preventing asthmatic attacks in many individuals when given by mouth. It is commonly prescribed as 'Enseals' to avoid all possibility of gastro-intestinal irritation.

Theophylline and Sodium Acetate, N.F., (55 to 65 percent theophylline) may be administered by mouth, but not parenterally. It is less soluble than the amine-containing derivatives, and it is believed by many to be more irritating to the gastro-intestinal tract.

Theophylline, U.S.P., is only slightly soluble (1:120) in water. Apparently it is infrequently prescribed.

THEOBROMINE

Theobromine has therapeutic properties similar to those of theophylline; it is less potent, but its action is more enduring. It is often given in courses of three or four days alternating with theophylline. Since it has almost no capacity to stimulate the central nervous system, it is advantageous in those few instances when that property of theophylline is troublesome.

Theobromine and its salts are given only by mouth. Like theophylline derivatives, they tend to irritate the gastro-intestinal tract, but possibly to a lesser degree. The dosage is 0.3 to 1 Gm. three or four times a day with meals. Available preparations include the following:

Theobromine and Sodium Acetate, U.S.P., containing 55 to 65 percent theobromine.
Theobromine and Sodium Salicylate, N.F., containing not less than 46.5 percent theobromine.
Theocalcin (calcium theobromine and calcium salicylate), containing not less than 44 percent calcium theobromine.

CAFFEINE

The therapeutic use of caffeine is now largely limited to stimulation of the central nervous system. It is valuable in cases of poisoning by central depressants, and particularly by morphine. It is also used extensively, generally in combination with analgesics and hypnotics, in treating headache, including migraine.

Caffeine is usually given as Caffeine and Sodium Benzoate, U.S.P., containing 47 to 50 percent caffeine. This substance can be given by mouth or by intramuscular injection. The usual dose is 0.5 Gm. Citrated Caffeine, N.F., (48 to 52 percent caffeine) may be given by mouth, usually in doses of 0.3 Gm. In emergency, caffeine may be administered as an enema of strong coffee (an average cup contains 0.1 to 0.15 Gm. caffeine base).

CIRCULATORY DEPRESSANTS

Depression of the heart as a whole is seldom desirable. However, it is sometimes of great value to be able to depress selectively certain phases of cardiac function. Two drugs are at present useful in this field. Quinidine slows conduction in the heart and lengthens the refractory period (albeit with some degree of depression of contractility as well); and methacholine mimics the cardio-inhibitory effects of vagus stimulation.

QUINIDINE

Quinidine is an optical isomer of quinine (for structural formula, see Figure 10, p. 302). It occurs in small quantities with quinine in cinchona bark. It is administered as the sulfate, which is a white crystalline powder soluble in water to about 1 percent. Like quinine, it is intensely bitter.

Quinidine has the same general pharmacologic and therapeutic properties as quinine except for the action on the heart. Both quinine and quinidine depress myocardial contractility and lengthen the refractory period following contraction. However, quinidine is ten to twenty times as potent with respect to lengthening the refractory period, and

cardiac effects can be obtained largely without the systemic effects of quinine administration. A further advantage of quinidine as a cardiac drug is that, in proportion to its therapeutically desirable action on refractory period, it has less of the therapeutically undesirable depressive effect on contractility than does quinine. The actions of quinidine and their electrocardiographic manifestations are summarized in Table 38.

Quinidine sulfate is rapidly absorbed from the gastro-intestinal tract and rapidly excreted. After a single dose, it appears in the urine in a few minutes and the maximum blood concentration is reached within an hour. The drug should therefore be given at frequent intervals. About one-third of administered quinidine is excreted in the urine; the remainder is destroyed in the body, probably by the liver.

Although quinidine is employed infrequently, its unique properties make it extremely important when the need arises. If satisfactory results are to be obtained and the patient is to be safeguarded from unnecessary risk, the drug must be handled skillfully. The following paragraphs outline its clinical use.

Except in emergency, quinidine sulfate is administered by mouth. An initial dose of 0.2 Gm. (3 grains) is usually given as a test for idiosyncrasy. If no untoward symptoms follow, larger doses are employed at regular intervals until either the desired effect is obtained or minor side-effects appear.

TABLE 38—*Effects of Quinidine on the Heart*

Action of Drug	Clinical Effect	Change in ECG
To Lengthen Refractory Period		
1. Of S-A node	Slowing of heart rate if regular	Greater interval between P waves
2. Of auricular muscle	Slowing of circus movement in auricular fibrillation or flutter	Longer cycles in F waves in flutter
3. Of A-V node	a. Slowing of ventricular rate in auricular fibrillation	Greater interval between QRS complexes
	b. After very large doses, various degrees of block	Lengthening of P-R interval
To Slow Conduction		
1. In auricle	Usually none	Lengthening of P-R interval
2. In ventricle	Usually none	Widening of QRS complex, deviation of the ST segment, and inversion and widening of T waves

In *auricular fibrillation*, quinidine may be useful as an aid in restoring and maintaining normal rhythm. In general, restoration of normal rhythm is considered advisable only when there is little or no organic heart disease and the arrhythmia is of short duration (for further discussion, see Auricular Fibrillation, p. 71). If the ventricular rate is rapid, it is first controlled by digitalis. If the rate is slow, some cardiologists administer digitalis as a precaution, whereas others do not.

The initial dose of quinidine sulfate is 0.1 Gm. (1 1/2 grains), which is repeated for a total of three doses the first day. If no side-effects are noted, the dosage is gradually increased until by the tenth day the patient is taking 0.6 Gm., or 9 grains, three or four times daily. If normal rhythm has not returned after three days at this dosage, the drug is discontinued and no further trial is made, for it is considered that normal rhythm would be unduly difficult to maintain should it be established by even larger doses. If normal rhythm is restored by the above regimen, the dose of the drug is gradually reduced to 0.1 or 0.2 Gm. three times daily. It may be necessary to continue administration indefinitely to prevent recurrence of the arrhythmia. Quinidine may also be given prophylactically to patients subject to recurrent paroxysmal auricular fibrillation.

In *ventricular tachycardia* (see p. 71), massive doses of quinidine may be required. If the disorder is causing a rapid failure of the circulation, the physician should give quinidine sulfate or lactate intravenously at once, employing, if necessary, an impromptu 1 percent solution (the exact concentration is not too important) sterilized by boiling. A visible-recording electrocardiograph should be attached to the patient, and both the patient and his electrocardiogram should be watched by competent observers while the solution is administered very slowly with frequent pauses. The injection is stopped at once when any one of the following occurs:

1. Sinus rhythm is restored.
2. Side-effects of more than trivial nature arise.
3. The duration of the QRS complex is prolonged in excess of 25 percent beyond that observed prior to the injection.
4. The P waves disappear.

Except in emergency, the quinidine should be given by mouth. After a test dose of 0.2 Gm., increasing doses up to 0.6 Gm. are given at two-hour intervals. The heart is examined before each dose; when the rate has been reduced to 120 per minute (without restoration of normal rhythm), an elec-trocardiogram should be obtained. In some instances, larger doses may be required, but the amount should not be increased beyond that which either prolongs the original duration of the QRS complex by 25 percent or almost abolishes the P waves. In many instances it may be advisable to continue the drug for a time in lower dosage to prevent recurrence.

Quinidine may be of value in those cases of *auricular flutter* which do not respond to digitalis (see p. 71). The technic of administration is the same as in auricular fibrillation.

In *paroxysmal auricular tachycardia*, quinidine may prove effective when other measures have failed (see p. 70). Because of its potential hazards, however, it is reserved for desperate cases.

Quinidine may also be indicated when it is of serious importance to stop *extrasystoles* (p. 69), as (1) when they are extremely disturbing to the patient; (2) when, in the presence of rheumatic valvular disease, they may appear to be forerunners of auricular fibrillation; or (3) when, after acute coronary occlusion (p. 69), they may herald ventricular tachycardia.

There is considerable variation in the response to and tolerance for quinidine. Overdoses may themselves produce disorder of cardiac rhythm, including extrasystoles, tachycardias, auricular or ventricular fibrillation, heart block, and cardiac arrest. Cardiac arrest and ventricular fibrillation may cause sudden death. These undesirable effects are more likely to occur in patients with severe myocardial disease than in those with functional arrhythmia in the presence of a relatively normal heart muscle.

Idiosyncrasy is not uncommon and is manifested by dizziness, nausea and vomiting, shock, cyanosis, cold sweat, and respiratory distress, including in some instances temporary cessation of respiration. It should be tested for by a small initial dose in every patient. Very rarely, quinidine may produce cinchonism, with disturbances of hearing and vision, gastro-intestinal symptoms, skin rashes, localized edema, headache, fever, apprehension, excitement, confusion, coma, and even death.

There are no absolute contraindications to quinidine therapy except idiosyncrasy or a history of severe cinchonism. In general, however, the drug should not be given to patients with congestive heart failure, severe mitral stenosis, auricular fibrillation of long standing or in a badly damaged heart, intraventricular conduction defects, or a previous history of embolic phenomena from thrombi originating from within the heart.

METHACHOLINE

Methacholine (acetyl-beta-methylcholine, Mecholyl) is a cholinergic drug which mimics the effect of vagus stimulation (see Table 44, p. 417, for details). Its properties and general uses are discussed on page 417. The cardio-inhibitory action of the drug may be valuable in stopping attacks of *paroxysmal auricular tachycardia* which do not respond to physical measures. Administration is a hospital procedure. For details of indications, contraindications, administration, and dosage, see pages 70 and 417.

SYSTEMIC VASOCONSTRICTORS

The over-all control of vasomotor tone is exercised by the vasomotor center, which is located in the medulla oblongata along the floor of the fourth ventricle. From this center, vasoconstrictor impulses travel in the sympathetic (adrenergic) portion of the autonomic nervous system (p. 416) to the smooth muscle of the arterioles and, presumably, of the venules. These vessels are normally in a state of tone; systemic arterial diastolic pressure varies directly with the three factors vasomotor tone, heart rate, and cardiac output.

The most important systemic vasoconstrictor drugs are the sympathomimetic amines (for general discussion, see p. 422). Posterior pituitary hormone (p. 473) has a powerful vasoconstrictor effect, but it is seldom used clinically for this purpose because of its strong action on the coronary vessels.

Occasionally the patient's response to vasopressor drugs will be misjudged, particularly during anesthesia, and an undesirable or dangerous acute hypertension may develop. It may be overcome by intravenous administration of sodium nitrite (p. 364).

Ephedrine is probably the drug most widely used for systemic vasoconstrictor effect—that is, for control of neurogenic hypotension such as may be seen during high spinal or caudal anesthesia or in postural hypotension. The general properties and uses of ephedrine are discussed beginning on page 426.

Depending on the urgency of the situation, ephedrine may be administered (as the sulfate or hydrochloride) by mouth (25 to 50 mg.), hypodermically (25 or 50 mg. as initial dose, 25 mg. subsequently), or intravenously (5, 10, or even 25 mg. if injected very slowly and if smaller doses prove ineffective). The usual period between administration and onset of effect varies with the route and the state of the circulation: After oral doses it is thirty to sixty minutes; after hypodermic administration, ten to twenty minutes if the circulation is efficient; and after intravenous injection, about three minutes.

Administration can be repeated as needed. In general, no more than 100 mg. should be given over any eight-hour period; excessive doses may lead to diminished response. For contraindications and side-effects, see page 428.

'Clopane Hydrochloride' (Cyclopentamine Hydrochloride, Lilly) has properties similar to those of ephedrine hydrochloride or sulfate and is employed as a systemic vasoconstrictor in the same dosage. 'Clopane Hydrochloride' has the advantage, however, of almost complete freedom from side-effects (as distinguished from excessive therapeutic effects due to overdosage). The general properties of the drug are discussed on page 430.

Neo-Synephrine, administered as the hydrochloride, has an extremely powerful vasopressor action. Therapeutic doses seldom produce side-effects. Dosage, administration, and precautions are set forth on page 429.

Epinephrine is, next to arterenol, probably the most potent vasopressor drug known. However, it is seldom employed therapeutically for its action on blood pressure because (1) the effect of a single injection lasts only a few minutes; (2) there is a brief period of hypotension following the pressor effect; and (3), for sustained action, the drug must be given intravenously in a dosage that usually causes unpleasant symptoms.

Oenethyl, 2-methylaminoheptane, has also been suggested as a vasopressor drug during anesthesia. It has little effect on blood pressure in unanesthetized individuals. In those under anesthesia, the effect on systolic pressure is usually greater than that on diastolic pressure. The full effect of a given dose of Oenethyl appears to follow slowly after the initial effect. As a result, the correct dosage may be difficult to estimate. Repeated doses tend to produce diminished response. For dosage and further discussion, see page 431.

SYSTEMIC VASODILATORS

Systemic vasodilation is produced by relaxation of vasomotor tone or blocking of the vasomotor impulses at some level (see Systemic Vasoconstrictors, above). Temporary regional vasodilation may be achieved by sympathectomy or regional anesthesia (p. 440). Some degree of vasomotor tone generally returns months after sympathectomy. A number of agents have been discovered which are capable of blocking adrenergic nerve endings; their clinical usefulness is limited (see p. 431). Ethyl alcohol relaxes vasomotor tone, apparently by depressing the vasomotor center. This action is not employed clinically. Those vasodilator drugs which are used therapeutically relax the arteriolar smooth muscle directly. Some of them also relax smooth muscle in other organs and are thus antispasmodic (see p. 434).

Clinically, systemic vasodilators are used to abate vasomotor spasm. They have a place in the treatment of peripheral, coronary, and pulmonary arterial embolism or occlusion, angina pectoris, coronary disease, and certain forms of peripheral vascular disease. They are not of value in hypertension.

PAPAVERINE

Papaverine is a derivative of benzyl isoquinoline (see Figure 18) which occurs naturally in the opium poppy along with morphine. In spite of its continued inclusion under narcotic laws, papaverine differs significantly from morphine in chemical structure (compare Figure 18 with Figure 26, p. 399), and the two drugs are quite unlike in pharmacologic and therapeutic properties. Most importantly, no case of tolerance, habituation, or addiction to papaverine has ever been reported.

Papaverine is administered as the hydrochloride. This salt is a white crystalline substance of slightly bitter taste. It is soluble to about 2.5 percent in water. It also dissolves in alcohol and in chloroform but is practically insoluble in ether. Almost all of the drug used in medicine is now made synthetically. Impromptu solutions are subject to deterioration, but properly prepared ampoules are stable indefinitely if protected from light and from excessive heat.

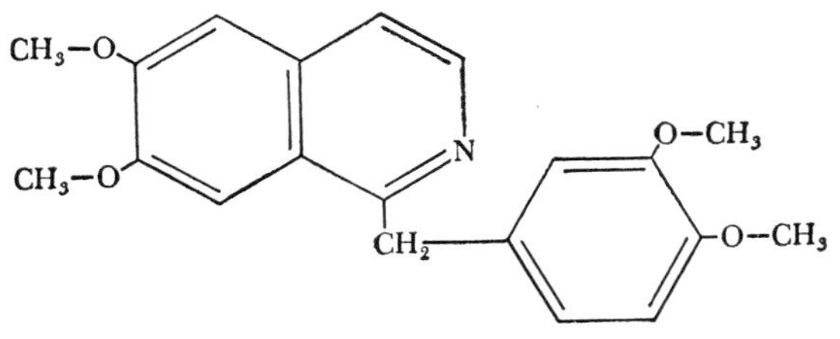

FIGURE 18—*Structural Formula of Papaverine*

The chief therapeutic property of papaverine is to relax the tonus of smooth muscle of all kinds, including the coronary arteries, without interference with normal contractions. The action is apparently direct on the muscle cells themselves. In addition, papaverine diminishes the irritability of the cardiac auricles and ventricles to extrinsic stimuli and prolongs the refractory period. The drug has a feeble analgesic effect on the central nervous system. In large doses there may be a sedative effect as well; but since it lacks the subjectively pleasant aspect of morphine narcosis, patients do not wish to continue use of the drug on account of this feature. Papaverine apparently makes the respiratory center more sensitive to stimulation by carbon dioxide. It has also a slight local-anesthetic action which is unimportant therapeutically. The drug is well absorbed from the gastro-intestinal tract. It is probably completely destroyed in the body, since neither it nor any immediate decomposition products have been recovered from the organs or excreta following hypodermic administration.

Papaverine is useful both as an antispasmodic and as a vasodilator. The former action is discussed on page 434. The vasodilator effect is particularly useful in:

Acute embolism or occlusion of the peripheral (p. 77), coronary (p. 67), or pulmonary (p. 119) arteries

Ergotism (p. 478)

It may also be of value in some cases of:

Angina pectoris (p. 66)

Cardiac extrasystoles (p. 69)

Thromboangiitis obliterans (p. 76)

Periarteritis nodosa (p. 77)

Raynaud's disease (p. 86)

In contrast to the antispasmodic effect on the smooth muscle of hollow viscera, the vasodilator effect of papaverine is not influenced by morphine, and the two drugs may be given together, without conflict, for their actions on the cardiovascular system.

When effects are needed quickly or when they have not followed oral administration, papaverine hydrochloride should be given intravenously. The dose may vary from 0.032 to 0.13 Gm. (1/2 to 2 grains). When the situation is urgent, a relatively large dose is recommended. To avoid the occasional occurrence of uncomfortable or alarming side-effects, papaverine hydrochloride must be given slowly over a timed period of one or two minutes. The injection may be repeated as often as needed.

For maintenance therapy and when rapid or

especially powerful effects are unnecessary, papaverine hydrochloride is given by mouth. The dosage varies with the patient and with the disease and must be determined by trial; the ordinary limits are 0.1 to 0.3 Gm. (1 1/2 to 5 grains) three, four, or five times daily. When oral therapy is contraindicated, the drug may be given intramuscularly in somewhat smaller dosage.

The toxicity of papaverine is low, and it has few contraindications. In complete A-V heart block (p. 72), the intravenous route should not be employed; and in other conditions in which the myocardium is depressed, intravenous administration should be very cautious lest it produce ectopic rhythms of ventricular origin—either premature beats or paroxysmal tachycardia. Side-effects sometimes observed include sweating, flushing of the face, and mild constipation. After rapid intravenous injection there may be transient rise in arterial pressure (averaging 12 mm. Hg), pulse rate, and respiratory rate. When large doses are continued over a long period of time, the sedative action may become prominent or even disturbing. In some conditions, such as acute coronary occlusion, this effect may be desirable. It may be emphasized that addiction to papaverine has never been reported.

NITRITES

The nitrite ion, $[NO_2]^-$, relaxes smooth muscle by direct action without impairing ability to contract on normal stimulation. Nitrite acts most strongly on the capillaries and venules and to a somewhat less extent on arterioles and arteries. The result is a decrease in arterial pressure; the systolic falls more than diastolic, and pulse pressure is therefore diminished. One would expect to find an increase in blood flow; but such a tendency is apparently balanced by a diminished filling of the heart in diastole (due to pooling of blood in the venules), for cardiac output is seldom altered significantly. There is a rise in pulse rate secondary to the fall in arterial pressure. Nitrites have no direct effect on the myocardium.

The response to nitrite varies in different vascular beds. The coronary vessels are apparently the most responsive; for, in spite of the fall in arterial pressure, there is a prolonged and relatively great increase in coronary blood flow which is the basis for the use of nitrites in angina pectoris. The skin of the face and neck, and occasionally the upper trunk, flushes readily to quick-acting nitrites but not to slow-acting ones. The meningeal vessels are easily responsive, thus accounting for the pulsating

headache which may be induced by nitrites. The visceral bed is moderately responsive, but the arterioles are often constricted, apparently as a reflex response to the fall in blood pressure. The pulmonary vessels are little affected.

Nitrite also relaxes the smooth muscle of the gastro-intestinal, biliary, urinary, and bronchial tracts. It often provides dramatic relief of colic (pain due to spasm) in these viscera. It may therefore be of value for symptomatic relief in biliary colic, lead colic, "green-apple colic" and its analogues, and ureteral colic. It is not used in asthma.

The soluble nitrites (and those nitrates having a nitrite action) are well absorbed from the gastrointestinal tract, and some are absorbable from the oral mucosa, skin, and lungs. About two-thirds of the drug is destroyed in the body, and the remainder is excreted in the urine as nitrite or nitrate.

For nitrite effect, either nitrites or certain organic nitrates can be given.

Sodium Nitrite, $NaNO_2$, is effective by either the oral or intravenous route. For oral administration, it is prescribed in solid form because ordinary solutions deteriorate within a few days. The drug is little employed, however, in angina pectoris because (1) it produces gastric irritation, especially in large doses; and (2) its duration of action is not great. The dose is 30 to 60 mg. It may be expected to take effect in ten to twenty minutes and remain effective for one to two hours.

Sodium nitrite by the intravenous route is of great value in combating acute hypertension due to overdosage of vasopressor drugs during anesthesia. A dose of 50 to 60 mg. (3/4 to 1 grain) is given slowly and may be repeated at intervals of three to five minutes until the desired reduction in pressure is achieved. One or two doses are usually sufficient. The effect lasts twenty to thirty minutes, by which time the acute action of the vasopressor drug has generally subsided.

Amyl Nitrite, $CH_3 \cdot CH(CH_3) \cdot CH_2 \cdot CH_2 \cdot NO_2$, is a clear, yellowish, volatile, flammable liquid with a peculiar pungent odor. It is usually supplied in fragile glass containers which are enclosed in a woven absorbent covering. For administration, the container is crushed, preferably in a handkerchief, and the vapor is inhaled deeply. Single doses larger than 0.2 cc. are seldom required.

Amyl nitrite is used for relief of attacks of angina pectoris. It acts within one to two minutes, but the duration is brief—often only a few minutes. It has now largely been displaced by nitroglycerin.

Nitroglycerin (glyceryl trinitrate, glonoin) is a volatile, explosive, yellowish liquid having the formula $C_3H_5(NO_3)_3$. For medicinal use, it is incorporated into tablets (ranging in strength from 0.16 to 1.3 mg. [1/400 to 1/50 grain]). These are not explosive, but the active agent escapes from them easily by evaporation. Such tablets should therefore be kept cool (a vest pocket is demonstrably worse than a coat pocket) and in a small bottle which is opened as infrequently as possible and is at all other times kept tightly stoppered with an impermeable closure.

Although chemically a nitrate, nitroglycerin has a nitrite action in the body. A tablet placed under the tongue takes effect within one or two minutes. The sublingual route is so satisfactory that others are seldom employed. It is recommended that hypodermic tablets be used for sublingual administration because of their rapid disintegration.

In some individuals, less than 0.1 mg. (1/650 grain) is sufficient for a discernible effect. In others, 0.4 or 0.6 mg. (1/150 or 1/100 grain) may be necessary. Until a patient's requirement is known, the smallest possible dose should be given initially; if it has had no therapeutic action or serious side-effect after five to seven minutes, a larger dose is given, and this sequence can be continued until one or the other type of effect is obtained.

Nitroglycerin is employed principally for the immediate relief of attacks of angina pectoris. The effect usually lasts thirty to forty-five minutes. It may also be extremely effective for relief of visceral smooth-muscle spasm, especially intestinal, biliary, or ureteral colic.

Erythrityl Tetranitrate (erythrol tetranitrate), $C_4H_6(NO_3)_4$, is an explosive solid which is insoluble in water. It is available as tablets to which sufficient lactose has been added to make the mixture nonexplosive. Like nitroglycerin, erythrityl tetranitrate has a nitrite effect in the body. Its action is too slow for satisfactory relief of angina pectoris, once an attack has developed. However, taken by mouth, it is of value for prevention of attacks. Its action begins in about fifteen minutes and persists for three or four hours. It is recommended before exercise and, in those patients subject to nocturnal attacks, at bedtime. The usual dose is 30 to 60 mg.

Mannitol Hexanitrate, $C_6H_8(NO_3)_6$, is an insoluble substance which in pure form is even more explosive than nitroglycerin. Diluted with at least nine parts of carbohydrate, it is safe for use. It has a nitrite action of even longer duration than

erythrityl tetranitrate and is used for the same purpose. The action usually begins in fifteen to thirty minutes and lasts four to six hours; the average dosage range is 15 to 60 mg.

The nitrites may have certain undesirable effects. Headache due to meningeal vasodilation is common; it is usually transient, but with the longer-acting drugs (especially erythrityl tetranitrate) it may be annoyingly persistent. Circulatory collapse has been reported from therapeutic doses; lesser grades of circulatory inadequacy (failure of venous return) may give rise to nausea and vomiting, weakness, restlessness, pallor, sweating, or syncope. Such manifestations are treated by placing the patient supine with head low and moving the extremities to facilitate venous return. Epinephrine and other vasoconstrictors are contraindicated.

The intraocular pressure may rise; accordingly, nitrites should be used cautiously, if at all, in the presence of actual or incipient glaucoma. Intracranial pressure is also increased.

Large doses of nitrites cause methemoglobinemia. This condition is usually undesirable (especially in the presence of anemia), but in cyanide poisoning it may be lifesaving because it offers a rapid means of separating cyanide from hemoglobin. For the technic of treating cyanide poisoning, see page 557.

Continued use of any one member of the nitrite group leads to tolerance which begins in a few days and is fully developed in two to three weeks. On discontinuation, susceptibility is again established after a week or two. Sometimes cross tolerance extends to other nitrites. Nitrites should, therefore, be given in the smallest effective dosage and should not be continued longer than two weeks without a rest period.

XANTHINES

The xanthines induce vasodilation of the coronary arteries and, to an even greater extent, of the pulmonary arterioles. They have been given over long periods to prevent or minimize attacks of angina pectoris and to combat reflex vasospasm in diseased coronary arteries in the absence of angina. By the intravenous route, they are effective therapy for cardiac asthma.

Of the xanthine group of drugs, theophylline has the greatest vasodilator action. It is usually given as aminophylline or 'Monotheamin'—0.25 to 0.5 Gm. intravenously, or 0.1 to 0.4 Gm. by mouth three or four times daily. For a general discussion and for further details regarding dosage, administration, and precautions, see under Circulatory Stimulants, page 358.

NICOTINIC ACID

When given in large doses, nicotinic acid (and its sodium, ammonium, and monoethanolamine salts, but not nicotinamide) acts as a vasodilator, causing flushing, burning, and itching of the skin along with increased cutaneous and intracranial blood flow and elevated skin temperature. The effect involves mainly the head and upper part of the body, and there is no significant change in pulse rate or blood pressure. Sometimes there is dizziness, pulsating headache, nausea, and vomiting. The more general properties and uses of nicotinic acid are discussed beginning on page 487.

The vasodilator action of nicotinic acid is of value in the treatment of Ménière's disease (p. 244), migraine (p. 161), and some cases of trigeminal neuralgia. Therapy is usually continued over a period of months or years. The regimen of Atkinson provides an initial intramuscular dose of 25 to 35 mg. to determine the response of the patient. The following six or eight injections are given at daily intervals by the intravenous route, starting with 20 to 30 mg. (on the basis of response to the intramuscular dose) and increasing the dose each time by 5 mg. to a limit of 50 mg. if that much can be tolerated. The patients are then taught to administer to themselves 25 to 50 mg. intramuscularly at intervals of one or two days as may be indicated by experience and the severity of the symptoms of the disease. During this period, 50 to 100 mg. are taken by mouth daily in divided doses. As the response allows, the patient gradually discontinues injections and continues maintenance therapy by mouth.

Nicotinic acid produces most intense vasodilation when given by the intravenous route; the onset begins in a few seconds. After oral administration the onset is delayed for twenty to thirty minutes, and the action persists for several hours. Intramuscular injection produces effects which are intermediate in both duration and intensity.

HISTAMINE

Histamine (beta-imidazolylethylamine; for structural formula, see Figure 19) is a basic substance which may be obtained by decarboxylation of the amino acid histidine (Figure 6, p. 258). Histamine occurs in all body tissues, but normally in bound and inactive form. Its physiological function is un-

known. However, either it or closely related compounds (the so-called "H-substances") are believed to be the mediators of many types of allergic reactions (see p. 264).

Histamine affects almost all tissues. It is a very powerful capillary dilator, acting directly on the contractile mechanism. Large doses increase capillary permeability, with loss of plasma protein and local edema. Intradermal injection of histamine gives rise to the triple response of Sir Thomas Lewis (local dilation of small vessels, local edema [urticaria] from increased capillary permeability, and reflex arteriolar dilation of the surrounding skin), which is also seen after local injury and in clinical urticaria (p. 267).

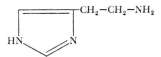

FIGURE 19—*Structural Formula of Histamine*

There are great species differences in the reaction of the arterioles to histamine. In man, there is arteriolar relaxation, which is especially noteworthy in the meninges, brain, and skin. Cerebral, ocular, and cutaneous blood flow are increased, and there is a rise in intraocular and spinal-fluid pressure, as with the nitrites. Similarly, the pulsating headache caused by histamine is due to meningeal vasodilation.

The extreme capillary and arteriolar relaxation induced by histamine leads to a pronounced fall in blood pressure. With large doses of the drug, acute circulatory failure (p. 63) may ensue. With smaller doses, compensatory mechanisms may prevent more than a slight change in the general circulation.

Histamine stimulates many of the glands of external secretion, including the salivary and intestinal. The greatest effect, however, is on those of the stomach, for which histamine provides a maximal secretory stimulus. They respond with a copious flow of gastric juice of high acidity. Because of this property, histamine is employed as a test for the secretory capacity of the stomach (see p. 127).

Histamine also causes contraction of the smooth muscle of the uterus and the bronchi. It has little or no direct action on the heart. The drug in all its actions is specifically antagonized by epinephrine.

Histamine is inactive when taken by mouth, probably because of destruction by the enzyme histaminase, which is present in the intestinal mucosa. When given parenterally, it is rapidly absorbed and rapidly destroyed. Intravenous doses of 0.1 mg. in normal individuals are followed within half a minute by intense flushing of the head and upper trunk, fall in blood pressure, increase in pulse rate (compensatory), and rise in spinal-fluid pressure. After an additional half minute, the blood pressure and spinal-fluid pressure are returning to normal and headache is beginning. The flush subsides in three or four minutes, and the headache in seven or eight. During continuous intravenous infusion of histamine, headache is rare.

Histamine is usually administered as the acid phosphate (2 molecules of phosphoric acid to 1 of histamine), which is stable and water-soluble. Since the molecular weight of histamine acid phosphate is 307.15 and that of histamine itself is 111.15, 2.75 mg. of the salt are required to obtain 1 mg. of the active principle.

When histamine is used as a test of gastric secretion, it is administered subcutaneously. The usual dose is 0.1 mg. of the base per 10 Kg. of body weight; some investigators limit the total dose to 0.5 mg. A solution containing 1 mg. of histamine base (2.75 mg. of the acid phosphate) per cc. is generally employed; the dose of such a solution is then 0.1 cc. per 10 Kg.

Histamine may be administered therapeutically in Ménière's disease (p. 244) and in histaminic cephalalgia (p. 145). The favorable results have been attributed by some to a hyposensitizing action on the assumption that the conditions are due, at least in part, to hypersensitivity to histamine. The drug is usually given subcutaneously in very small initial dosage which is gradually increased. Concentrations of histamine base of 1:10,000 (0.1 mg. per cc.) to as low as 1:100,000 have been used. In migraine, it has also been given by intravenous drip over a period of hours. For details of dosage and administration, see under the various diseases.

Initial doses of histamine should be conservative because of the variability of responsiveness. Flushing and early headache are to be expected as side-effects. Excessive dosage may induce a metallic taste, vomiting, diarrhea, bronchoconstriction (asthma), undue fall in blood pressure, or even shock. Epinephrine (p. 422) is an antidote. Histamine should not be given to patients with arteriosclerosis, advanced cardiovascular or peripheral vascular disease, or peptic ulcer or to patients subject to asthma.

SCLEROSING SOLUTIONS

Sclerosing solutions are preparations which, when injected into veins, serous spaces, or tissues, cause obliterative scarring of the injected area. Such solutions are used for the treatment of varicose veins, hernia, hydrocele, and hemorrhoids.

Sclerosing solutions should be of low toxicity to permit repeated injections and to avoid the production of pain and cramps in the injected area. The solutions used in the treatment of varicose veins and hemorrhoids should produce a firm, nonfriable, adherent clot, and not just a thrombosis. They should not cause a sloughing if extravasation occurs; they should not result in allergic reactions; and they should possess bactericidal properties. The solutions used for the treatment of hernia and hydrocele should have these same properties, except that in these conditions the formation of a blood clot is not the objective.

The following sclerosing solutions are listed in the order of increasing sclerosing and clot-forming power. The dosages mentioned are for the treatment of varicose veins.

Invert Sugar is used in solutions containing 7.5

Gm. in 10 cc. of sterile distilled water. Two to 20 cc. of the solution are injected. Rarely are there cramps with this sclerosing agent, and there is a minimal tendency toward sloughing if the solution is inadvertently injected around the vein or if it leaks out of the vein. Invert sugar has the disadvantage of forming a rather soft clot which may recanalize.

Sodium Chloride—Five to 20 cc. of a 20 percent solution are considered sufficient for one treatment. Cramps are likely to follow the injection, and sloughing may be rather extensive if the solution is placed in the perivascular space.

Sodium Psylliate (Sylnasol) is the sodium soap of the fatty acids of psyllium seed oil. It is used in 5 and 10 percent solutions in dosages of 2 to 5 cc. Because the drug is irritating, the solutions are prepared with 2 percent benzyl alcohol (p. 447), which has local anesthetic properties. There is a little tendency toward sloughing if the material is accidentally injected perivenously. Renal colic has been reported as an untoward reaction.

Sodium Ricinoleate is the sodium soap of the fatty acids of castor oil. It is used in 0.5 to 5 percent solutions in amounts of 2 to 5 cc.

Sodium Morrhuate is the sodium soap of the fatty acids of cod liver oil. It is considered by many to be the best sclerosing agent available. A 5 percent solution is used in dosages of 2 to 10 cc. It does not cause cramping; it is nontoxic, produces a firm thrombus, and is least likely to cause sloughing. An occasional patient may be encountered who shows signs of sensitivity, as evidenced by a dermatitis or mild systemic shock.

Monoethanolamine Oleate, 5 percent solution, is used in doses of 2 to 5 cc. This is a solution of an ester of a fatty acid, and its advantages and untoward reactions are the same as for sodium morrhuate.

Quinine Hydrochloride and Urethane is used in 2-cc. doses of a solution containing 0.266 Gm. of quinine hydrochloride and 0.133 Gm. of urethane. This solution forms a firm thrombus; however, idiosyncrasy is frequently observed, and sloughing is common if the solution is injected perivenously. Reactions become more frequent with repeated injections or with injection of more than 2 cc. at a dose.

Sodium Salicylate, 30 to 40 percent solution, is used in dosages of 1 to 3 cc. A strong clot is formed; however, there may be intense cramping pain in the extremity and much soreness along the course of the vein. Patients often refuse the second injection because of the intense discomfort.

For the treatment of hernia, hemorrhoids, and hydrocele, the advantages and disadvantages of various sclerosing solutions are the same as indicated for the treatment of varicose veins. Sodium morrhuate, and quinine hydrochloride and urethane, are the two solutions of choice for the treatment of these three conditions. Dosages vary with the condition treated and its extent.

DRUGS ACTING ON THE BLOOD OR BLOOD-FORMING ORGANS

HEMATINICS

Hematinics are substances which under proper conditions are effective in increasing the hemoglobin and red cell content of the blood. They are indicated in the presence of anemia (see p. 94). The hematinics are of varied nature and include iron, copper, manganese, liver, vitamin B_{12}, and folic acid.

IRON

Iron occurs in the nucleus of all body cells. Its clinical importance, however, stems from its presence in hemoglobin. Iron is an essential constituent of the hemoglobin molecule. Unless it is supplied in adequate quantities, the maturation of red blood cells is retarded, the number released from the bone marrow into the circulation is reduced, and those red cells which are released have a subnormal hemoglobin content.

Reserve iron is normally present in the spleen and bone marrow. In the presence of an adequate reserve, an iron intake of 12 to 15 mg. daily is sufficient for an adult. When iron reserves are depleted, a larger intake is necessary for normal blood formation.

Inorganic iron is absorbed throughout the gastrointestinal tract. However, most absorption takes place in the upper part of the small intestine. It is believed that iron is absorbed only in the ferrous state. Absorption is apparently reduced by the absence of free acid in the gastric juice and is influenced also by the state of the iron reserves; when these are low, more iron is absorbed. Iron is excreted only in minute amounts. The iron content of the body (about 4 Gm. in an adult) is controlled by regulation of absorption rather than by excretion. The principal sources of iron in the diet are liver, lean beef, egg yolk, whole-grain cereals, molasses, and certain vegetables and fruits. The normal diet contains adequate quantities. Contrary to previous belief, spinach is a poor source of iron because the element is present in a form that is not well absorbed.

Iron is indicated as a therapeutic agent (1) whenever there is a deficiency of iron (from blood loss or because of poor absorption) and (2) whenever the demand is unusually great (as in prematurity, periods of rapid growth, pregnancy, and lactation). Even though iron injected parenterally is effectively utilized, this route is considered inadvisable in most cases because (1) oral medication can also be made effective and (2) a therapeutic dose of the preparations now available for injection is often followed by severe reactions (believed to be due to precipitation of the preparation in the blood stream or at the site of injection).

For oral administration, inorganic salts of iron appear to be the most desirable; ferrous salts are preferred to ferric compounds because (1) they are more readily absorbed, (2) they are effective in smaller doses, and (3) they produce less gastrointestinal irritation. Iron is available in many forms; the following are the most important:

Ferrous Sulfate, U.S.P., $FeSO_4 \cdot 7H_2O$, containing 20 percent iron; sometimes preferred in enteric coating. The usual dose is 5 grains three times daily after meals.

Saccharated Ferrous Carbonate, N.F., containing 7.2 percent iron. The usual dose is 5 grains three times daily after meals.

Ferrous Carbonate Pills, N.F., (Blaud's pills) each pill containing 29 mg. of iron. The usual dose is 3 to 5 pills three times daily after meals.

Ferrous Gluconate, N.F., $Fe(C_6H_{11}O_7)_2 \cdot 2H_2O$, containing 11.5 percent iron; considered to be one of the least irritating of the salts of iron. The usual dose is 5 grains three times daily after meals.

Ferric Ammonium Citrate, U.S.P., (iron and ammonium citrates) containing about 17.5 percent iron; considered to be less irritating than other ferric salts. The usual dose is 22 1/2 to 30 grains (1.5 to 2 Gm.) three times daily after meals.

Reduced Iron, N.F. The usual dose is 10 to 15 grains three times daily before meals.

Although there is variation from one compound to another and among different individuals, all inorganic iron compounds are capable of causing gastrointestinal irritation (gastric discomfort, constipation, or diarrhea) if taken by mouth in large amounts. In patients known to have an irritable gastro-intestinal tract, the dosage of iron should be slowly raised to the therapeutic level.

Iron is contraindicated in hemochromatosis, in which there is already excessive storage and possibly increased absorption of the element.

COPPER

It has been demonstrated that small amounts of copper are required to supplement iron in the cure of certain nutritional anemias of experimental animals. The element is believed to act as a catalyst in some stages of hemoglobin synthesis. However, it seems doubtful that added copper is necessary in the treatment of iron deficiency in human be-

ings. An abnormally high blood level of copper is a characteristic finding in such anemias, and most diets contain sufficient copper for a normal supply. In addition, the iron preparations available for therapeutic use contain enough copper as an impurity to supply the needs for hemoglobin synthesis.

MANGANESE

In certain experimental anemias, the element manganese has a supplementing effect that is similar to but less pronounced than that of copper. It is likewise present in most iron preparations, and there is no apparent need for larger quantities in human therapy.

LIVER

The liver is the storage depot for the maturation factor which is necessary for development of red blood cells beyond the megaloblast stage. Deficiency of this factor is the immediate cause of the macrocytic anemias which may be present in pernicious anemia (p. 96). A similar deficiency may occur in the macrocytic anemias of sprue (p. 133), pregnancy and the puerperium, infancy, and nutritional deficiency. Liver or extracts of liver are indicated as a source of the maturation factor in pernicious anemia, and either liver extract or folic acid (p. 371) is indicated in the other macrocytic anemias listed or in any macrocytic anemia in which there is megaloblastic hyperplasia of the bone marrow. In subacute combined degeneration of the spinal cord, which is usually associated with pernicious anemia, liver or liver extract in adequate quantities stops the progress of the lesions.

Daily administration of whole liver over long periods of time and in the quantities usually needed is impractical in most patients. Liver extracts are available for oral use that are highly effective in uncomplicated pernicious anemia. Incubation of the liver extract with stomach tissue greatly increases its potency. However, many patients with pernicious anemia or some other macrocytic anemia are unable to ingest sufficient liver extract to maintain the blood at normal levels or to prevent neurological lesions.

Liver extracts are from thirty to one hundred times more effective when given parenterally than when taken by mouth. The injection of highly purified liver extracts has been found to be the most readily administered, economical, and efficient type of therapy for Addisonian pernicious anemia. Such highly purified extracts are also extremely effective in preventing advancement of the neurological lesions of pernicious anemia; in some instances, the lesions actually regress.

Less purified liver extracts contain (in addition to the maturation factor) various members of the vitamin B complex (including trace amounts of folic acid) and possibly other as yet unidentified factors. These so-called crude liver extracts may be preferred (orally or by injection) for the treatment of the nutritional macrocytic anemias (sprue, macrocytic anemia of pregnancy, and so on); in such anemias, the highly purified liver extracts are sometimes ineffective.

Liver extracts have also been recommended in treatment of x-ray sickness, as a stimulant to leukocytosis, in the treatment of various liver diseases, and as a source of the unidentified fractions of the vitamin B complex.

Liver extracts are standardized for maturation factor by administration to patients with proved pernicious anemia. The U.S.P. has established two units for antianemia potency, one for oral and one for parenteral preparations. They are not interchangeable. If a manufacturer wishes to state the potency of his liver extract in terms of U.S.P. Units, he must submit protocols of trials of each lot of the extract to the U.S.P. Anti-anemia Preparations Advisory Board. On the basis of such protocols, the Board assigns a potency to each lot in terms of U.S.P. Units. One U.S.P. Unit (Oral or Injectable) is "that amount of an otherwise acceptable product which produces, when administered daily, clinical and hematopoietic responses in Addisonian pernicious anemia that are considered by the Board to be satisfactory." The responses are judged by the rise in reticulocyte (young red blood cell) count and the subsequent increase in red cell and hemoglobin level.

In the average uncomplicated case of pernicious anemia in relapse, the initial dosage of parenteral liver extract should be 10 to 20 U.S.P. Units (Injectable) intramuscularly each day for three days. In complicated cases, the injections may be repeated for seven days. The response to treatment is usually definite and in many instances dramatic. Within two or three days, the patient usually becomes more alert and the appetite improves. The first response in the blood is seen in two to ten days, depending on the dosage of liver extract, and consists in a rise in the number of reticulocytes (compare Plates 33 and 35). The maximum reticulocyte count is reached in seven to twelve days, and its height depends on the initial red blood cell count. The total red cell count begins to increase,

and under adequate therapy it reaches normal in six to eight weeks. The gastro-intestinal symptoms usually disappear in one to two weeks, and glossitis subsides. Dyspnea and weakness disappear gradually as the red count increases. For a time, edema may actually increase. Symptoms of nervous-system lesions are slower in responding. Those of brief duration may eventually disappear entirely, whereas any of long standing may change very slowly or not at all.

After the initial few days of most intensive treatment, doses of 10 to 20 units should be given every seven to ten days for a period of at least several weeks. After the blood has returned to normal, the dosage may be reduced in uncomplicated cases, but it should amount to 1 or 1 1/2 units for each elapsed day. Since the maturation factor is stored in the liver, very frequent injection is unnecessary, but the intervals should not be longer than two weeks. Patients with neurological lesions should continue to receive 2 to 3 units per elapsed day for a year or, if the lesions are still improving at the end of this period, until they are stationary.

Oral therapy is most satisfactory for maintenance in the majority of uncomplicated cases. The daily requirement is usually 1 or 2 U.S.P. Units (Oral), and it is best given in subdivided doses three times daily before meals.

The maintenance requirement varies from one individual to another and from time to time in the same individual. In general, the requirement is increased by old age, neurological involvement, infections, the presence of malignancy, chronic blood loss, and degenerative complications (such as arteriosclerosis). Criteria for adequate dosage are (1) maintenance of red blood cell count, red cell size, and hemoglobin content of the blood at normal levels, (2) disappearance of gastro-intestinal symptoms, and (3) cessation of progress in neurological lesions.

A complete physical examination and a complete blood count should be performed every three months. If the blood is not normal, if there are gastro-intestinal symptoms attributable to the disease, or if there is evidence of an advancing neurological lesion, the dosage of liver extract should be increased in those patients who are on parenteral therapy; those who are taking oral medication should be transferred at once to parenteral therapy. The presence of infection usually increases the requirement 50 to 100 percent.

The management of other macrocytic anemias (including the dosage of liver extract) follows the same principles as in pernicious anemia.

Parenteral liver extract sometimes proves irritating. Local reactions can be minimized by the use of intramuscular rather than subcutaneous injections. Rarely, patients may become allergic to liver extracts. The allergy is usually to the proteins of liver tissue rather than to the species of animal from which the liver was obtained. Sensitization is most commonly manifested when injections are resumed after a rest period. Epinephrine (p. 422) usually controls such allergic reactions. Desensitization is difficult but may be attempted (see Allergy, p. 265). Most such patients should be changed over to crystalline vitamin B_{12} (see below).

VITAMIN B_{12}

Vitamin B_{12} is a red crystalline compound containing cobalt, phosphorus, and nitrogen. Its exact structure is not yet known. It was first isolated from commercial purified liver extracts but is now usually prepared from culture broths of grisein-producing strains of *Streptomyces griseus* (other strains of this fungus produce streptomycin). Vitamin B_{12} is closely related to or possibly identical with a previously unidentified chick-growth factor ("animal protein factor") which is present in fish meal, liver, cow manure, and other crude protein-containing materials and is necessary for the hatching of hen eggs and for optimal growth of chicks.

Vitamin B_{12} appears to be either the maturation factor for red blood cells (see under Pernicious Anemia, p. 96) or else its precursor, the extrinsic factor. When administered parenterally, it is highly effective in the treatment of pernicious anemia; it produces a satisfactory clinical and hematological response and prevents the progress of neurological lesions. Orally, vitamin B_{12} is very much less effective, although its potency is greatly enhanced by incubation with normal gastric juice. Patients sensitive to liver extracts can take vitamin B_{12} without reaction. There are no known contraindications to the substance.

The dosage requirements vary in the same way as do those of liver extract. In general, it may be considered that 1 microgram of vitamin B_{12} injected parenterally is the equivalent of 1 U.S.P. Unit (Injectable). The criteria for adequacy of dosage are the same as for liver extract (see above). Vitamin B_{12} may be administered subcutaneously or intramuscularly. The effective oral dose has not been established, but it appears to be prohibitively high.

Patients having macrocytic anemias of nutritional origin (sprue, pregnancy) may in some instances fail to respond to vitamin B_{12}, even though they respond to either liver extract or folic acid.

FOLIC ACID

Folic acid (pteroylglutamic acid) belongs to the group of compounds called "pterins," which were first recognized in the wings of butterflies. Its structural formula is shown in Figure 20. Folic acid is one of the more recently isolated members of the vitamin B complex. It is an indispensable constituent of all tissues, particularly those in a state of rapid growth. However, its exact function is unknown. It is contained in foods of both animal and vegetable origin, and, in addition, it is synthesized and released by the intestinal flora. These sources provide an adequate supply for normal needs. The minimal daily requirement is not known.

Certain related compounds such as aminopterin act as antagonists to folic acid (presumably by blocking enzyme systems). It is believed that some of the effects of these antagonists, such as stomatitis, hemorrhagic manifestations, and bloody diarrhea, are manifestations of folic acid deficiency.

Folic acid is best known for its influence on the bone marrow. It appears to be necessary for the transformation of megaloblasts into red blood cells. However, it is not the maturation factor present in liver extract, nor is it the extrinsic factor. Administration of folic acid in pernicious anemia is generally followed by a definite hematological response. Sometimes, however, response is incomplete, or a relapse will occur later in spite of continued therapy. Frequently, the gastro-intestinal symptoms are not relieved, or the neurological lesions progress greatly during treatment. Folic

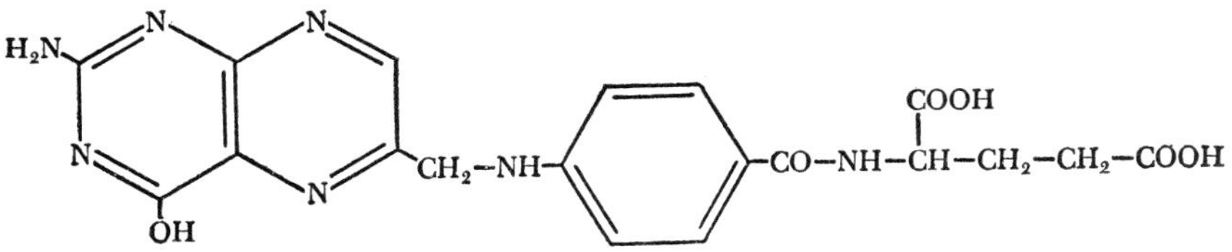

FIGURE 20—*Structural Formula of Folic Acid*

acid is not, therefore, recommended as the sole therapeutic agent in pernicious anemia.

On the other hand, folic acid produces a satisfactory remission in sprue, tropical macrocytic anemia, "refractory megaloblastic anemia," the macrocytic anemia of pregnancy and the puerperium, and the megaloblastic anemia of infancy. These anemias seldom respond to vitamin B_{12} or to *purified* liver extract.

Folic acid is not effective in treatment of aplastic anemia, iron-deficiency anemia, leukemia, the leukopenia of influenza, and general reductions in bone-marrow activity of unknown origin. It has been reported to precipitate exacerbations of chronic myelogenous leukemia.

Administration may be intravenous, intramuscular, oral, or rectal. Oral and parenteral effectiveness are similar, but daily oral therapy is apparently more efficacious than periodic injection. Initial oral dosage of folic acid is 10 to 40 mg. daily; the maintenance dose is 5 to 10 mg. daily. The drug is relatively nontoxic.

DRUGS USED TO INCREASE THE WHITE CELL COUNT

A number of drugs have been used to increase the white blood cell count. It is doubtful whether any of them will increase the low white count associated with certain infections (such as influenza or typhoid fever), but the administration of a few drugs to patients having agranulocytosis (p. 102) has been followed by an increase in the number of granulocytes in some patients.

Nucleic Acid Derivatives—*Pentnucleotide* is a solution of the sodium salts of four pentose nucleotides derived from the nucleic acids of yeast. In animals it stimulates the precursors of the leukocytes in the bone marrow, especially if they have been depressed. In many cases of agranulocytosis, its administration has been followed in three to five days by a return of the granulocytes. However, the relationship has not been established with certainty as one of cause and effect, for similar recoveries have occurred spontaneously.

For seriously ill patients, the recommended dose is 20 cc. twice daily by intramuscular injection. After four days the individual dose is reduced to 10 cc. Treatment is continued until there is a definite increase in granulocytes, but not for longer than ten days. The intravenous route is not recommended because of untoward reactions. In some instances, intramuscular injection may be followed by transient symptoms of chill, fever, precordial distress, or a feeling of tension followed by lethargy.

Liver Extracts are highly effective in increasing the white blood cell count of patients suffering a relapse of pernicious anemia and have been recommended in other leukopenias and in agranulocytosis.

Pyridoxine (vitamin B_6), one of the components of vitamin B complex, has been recommended in the treatment of agranulocytosis. The daily intravenous injection of from 125 to 200 mg. of pyridoxine hydrochloride has been followed by prompt clinical improvement in a few patients. The possible mechanism of action, if any, is not known, and, as with Pentnucleotide, the results may be a matter of coincidence.

DRUGS USED TO REDUCE THE WHITE CELL COUNT

Reduction in the number of circulating white blood cells is desirable only in leukemia. Even here, it constitutes symptomatic treatment rather than cure (see p. 103).

Urethane, $NH_2 \cdot COO \cdot CH_2 \cdot CH_3$, is the ethyl ester of carbamic acid. For many years it has been extensively employed as a hypnotic in laboratory animals (it is relatively ineffective in man). It is also combined with quinine hydrochloride as a sclerosing agent in varicose veins (p. 368). Its current clinical interest follows from the observation that it acts as a selective metabolic inhibitor for white blood cells. Leukemic cells are much more susceptible than are normal white cells. The most susceptible are early myeloid cells. Urethane has shown clinical usefulness in chronic leukemia and multiple myeloma.

In chronic leukemia (either lymphatic or myeloid), the drug produces a more mature type of blood picture and leads to a decrease in size of the lymph nodes and spleen. The remission is not permanent, however, and it is less complete than that which follows x-ray therapy. The drug may be of value as a supplement to x-ray or after x-ray has become ineffective. It is not beneficial in acute leukemia.

The usual initial dosage of urethane in leukemia is 1 Gm. three times daily by mouth. After the white count begins to decline, the dose is reduced to 0.5 to 2 Gm. daily, depending on the response. Dosage should be kept as small as is consistent with a satisfactory fall in white count. In a few instances, as much as 6 Gm. must be given daily before an effect is noted. When the white count has been reduced to about 20,000 per cu. mm., the drug should be discontinued. Therapy is resumed if the count rises significantly or there is clinical relapse. Attempts to reduce the white count to a normal level or to return the spleen to normal size may end in fatal agranulocytosis.

Favorable clinical responses to urethane have also been observed in multiple myeloma. The usual dosage is 1 Gm. three times daily. Sometimes three months or more of therapy are required before improvement begins.

Because of the frequency of gastro-intestinal irritation (anorexia, nausea, vomiting, diarrhea), urethane is best given in enteric coating. Some investigators have preferred daily intravenous injection of a concentrated solution. Within the usual dosage range, serious toxic effects are rare. However, there is a possibility that large doses of the drug may be toxic to the liver. Drowsiness is occasionally encountered from therapeutic doses.

DRUGS USED TO ALTER BLOOD COAGULATION

Coagulation, or clotting, of blood is still not fully understood. The uncertainties have to do particularly (1) with the possibility that what appear to be primary substances may, in fact, be derived from still more fundamental compounds, and (2) with the role of substances which are essential to the process but which are needed in such small quantities as to escape detection. According to present concepts, four primary substances are required:

1. Prothrombin, a water-soluble glycoprotein which is formed in the liver. Its normal concentration in the blood is about 20 mg. per 100 cc.
2. Fibrinogen, a labile protein which is presumably formed in the liver. Its normal concentration in the blood is about 0.4 Gm. per 100 cc.
3. Calcium ions.
4. Thromboplastin (thrombokinase). There is difference of opinion regarding the nature of thromboplastin. Some consider it identical with the phospholipid cephalin. Others believe it to be a lipoprotein from which cephalin is released by hydrolysis. Whatever its exact structure, thromboplastin occurs in all body cells. It is especially abundant in brain, lung, thymus, and testicular tissue and in the blood platelets.

The process of blood coagulation can be shown in its simplest terms thus:

1. Prothrombin + thromboplastin + calcium ions ⟶ thrombin.
2. Thrombin + fibrinogen ⟶ fibrin.

The nature of the reaction between prothrombin and thromboplastin is in dispute. Since trypsin and snake venoms act in the absence of calcium to change prothrombin to thrombin, it has been argued that thromboplastin and calcium combine to form an enzyme. On the other hand, thromboplastin is quantitatively consumed in the process, which suggests that the reaction is chemical. Regardless of its method of formation, thrombin is apparently an enzyme. It acts on fibrinogen to produce fibrin, which separates from the blood as a netlike gel that holds the formed elements of the blood in its interstices. Intact platelets in the interior of the mass collect at the intersections of the strands of fibrin and form large knotlike bodies; at the same time, the strands become bent, twisted, and shortened, thus bringing about retraction of the clot (syneresis). The clot, or thrombus, is red if it contains red blood cells. If it does not, the color is that of plasma (white thrombus).

Since the plasma normally contains prothrombin, fibrinogen, and calcium ions, it is plain that clotting occurs when, and only when, thromboplastin is supplied either from injured tissue cells or from damaged or disintegrated platelets. Drugs that influence blood coagulation do so by acting on one or more of these primary factors.

VITAMIN K

The term "vitamin K" refers to a group of substances, derivatives of naphthoquinone, which have the common property of being essential for the production of prothrombin by the liver. Vitamin K and its therapeutic use are discussed on page 499.

PROTAMINE

Protamine is a complex protein-like substance which occurs in combination with nucleic acid in the sperm of salmon and other fish. With Insulin it forms an insoluble compound which is useful because of its slow absorption after subcutaneous injection (see p. 451). In adequate quantities, protamine also acts as an anticoagulant. It is an antithromboplastin. However, protamine and heparin (see below) have a stronger attraction for each other than for the elements of the blood. Thus, they neutralize each other as anticoagulants.

Protamine is therefore of value as a therapeutic agent to counteract overdoses of heparin. If hemorrhage has followed administration of heparin, protamine sulfate is useful as emergency treatment. The 1 percent solution of protamine sulfate (as supplied) is diluted with a sufficient volume of an electrolyte solution (p. 348) to facilitate slow administration; it is then injected slowly by vein over a period of one to three minutes. The total dose should be the same, mg. for mg., as the quantity of heparin which had been administered in the previous three or four hours. The amount of protamine sulfate given at one time, however, should not exceed 50 mg.

During abnormal bleeding in certain cases of leukemia and other blood diseases and after irradiation, protamine sulfate may be effective in checking the hemorrhagic tendency. The best response has been in patients whose blood showed the following characteristics:

1. An increased amount of circulating heparin-like substance.
2. Prolonged clotting time of whole blood.
3. Usually, but not invariably, a low platelet count.
4. Normal or near-normal prothrombin time.
5. No evidence of true hereditary hemophilia.
6. Adequate fibrinogen.
7. No evidence of increased fibrinolysin.

In the spontaneous hemorrhagic diseases, protamine therapy is best accompanied by transfusions of fresh whole blood. The suggested daily dosage of protamine sulfate is 5 to 8 mg. per Kg. (2.3 to 3.6 mg. per lb.) of body weight. For the average adult, this amounts to about 300 mg. per day. It is given in divided doses five to six hours apart. The protamine sulfate solution is diluted to 300 or 500 cc. with electrolyte solution and is administered slowly by vein over a period of thirty to forty minutes. If bleeding has stopped, the total daily dose is reduced by 50 percent after three days. If it has not been affected by this time, further administration of protamine is not likely to be of benefit.

The toxicity of protamine sulfate is extremely low. Very rarely, sensitivity may be encountered.

HEPARIN

Heparin is a complex mucopolysaccharide resembling chondroitinsulfuric acid. It has a negative electric charge—in fact, the strongest electric charge of any organic compound found in the animal body. This high negative charge is associated with a very powerful anticoagulant action. Heparin prevents the action of thromboplastin on prothrombin to produce thrombin (antithromboplastin activity), and it also inactivates thrombin itself. Substances with strong positive charges, such as protamine (see above), prevent the anticoagulant action of heparin.

Heparin occurs in many organs, but especially in the liver and lungs. It appears to be the granular substance observed in the mast cells of Ehrlich,

which occur mainly in connective tissue in the walls of blood vessels and the vicinity of capillaries.

Heparin Sodium, U.S.P., is assayed for anticoagulant effect on sheep plasma. It must contain not less than 100 U.S.P. Heparin Units per mg. The U.S.P. Heparin Unit is equal to the Provisional International Heparin Unit.

The clinical effect of heparin is to prolong the clotting time of the blood. It has proved of value for prevention or retardation of intravascular thrombosis in: phlebothrombosis; embolism or occlusion of peripheral, pulmonary, or coronary arteries; arteriosclerosis obliterans; thromboangiitis obliterans; erythremia; and the like.

The immediate aim of heparin therapy is to increase the clotting time of the blood to a more or less arbitrary level so that dangerous clotting may be prevented. The simplest technic is to administer 50 to 150 mg. of sodium heparin slowly by vein through a very fine needle four times daily. Until the desired prolongation has been obtained, clotting time should be determined before each injection. After maintenance dosage has been established, tests can be somewhat less frequent. A more troublesome but possibly more physiological method is constant intravenous drip of a solution containing 0.1 mg. per cc. (obtained by diluting the more concentrated solution with electrolyte solution [p. 348]). The rate is regulated to administer 10 to 20 mg. (100 to 200 cc.) per hour until a therapeutic effect is obtained (as indicated by frequent tests of clotting time), and the speed of injection is then adjusted to maintain the effect. Sodium heparin is also available in media containing gelatin or vasoconstrictors or both, from which it is slowly absorbed. Effects lasting about a day can usually be obtained from intramuscular injection of 300 to 400 mg. of such a preparation. Maintenance dosage is somewhat smaller.

The amount of heparin necessary to produce a given prolongation of clotting time will vary greatly in different patients and, occasionally, from day to day in the same patient. *Dosage must be controlled by frequent determinations of coagulation time.* Most investigators recommend maintaining coagulation time at fifteen minutes as determined by the capillary tube method or three times the normal value (twenty to forty-five minutes) as measured by the Lee-White technic (p. 529). The period of heparin therapy is determined by the specific condition which is under treatment.

If the clotting time is prolonged to a dangerous point, the drug should be discontinued at once; because of the brief action of heparin, the clotting time will be reduced within a few hours. If immediate counteraction is desired, protamine sulfate should be used (see above).

No specific toxic action of heparin has been demonstrated, and the only untoward effects seem to be those incidental to hemorrhage following overdosage or too-early administration after hemorrhage or trauma. Since heparin does not affect clots already formed, difficulty is not likely to be encountered if postoperative administration is withheld until oozing from the operative site is completely stopped. Heparin should not be given to patients with a pre-existing tendency toward bleeding, such as occurs in hemophilia, purpura, or jaundice.

DICUMAROL

Dicumarol (bishydroxycoumarin) is a substance originally isolated from spoiled sweet clover. It is the factor in improperly cured hay or silage prepared from common sweet clover which produces hemorrhagic disease in cattle. The chemical formula of Dicumarol is shown in Figure 21.

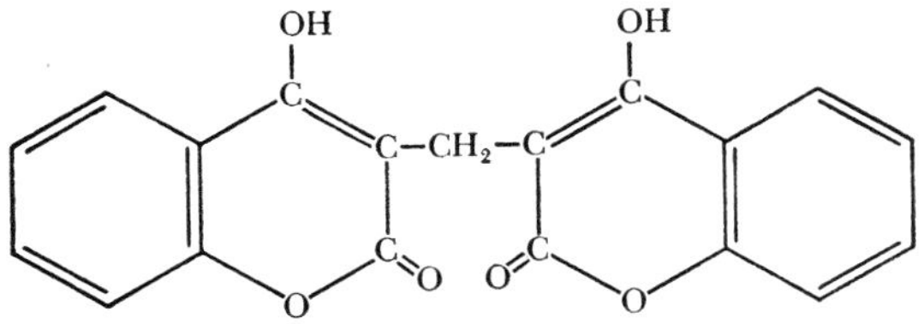

FIGURE 21 — *Structural Formula of Dicumarol*

The drug acts by preventing formation of prothrombin in the liver. The concentration of prothrombin in the blood is thus reduced, and the prothrombin time is increased (see p. 373). Dicumarol is employed clinically as an anticoagulant for the same purposes as heparin (see above). However, as shown in Table 39, its mode of action and its administration are quite different.

Dicumarol is an extremely potent drug which tends to have a prolonged and cumulative action. Overdosage may result in severe hemorrhage. Since patients vary in their response to the drug, *dosage can be controlled only by determining the prothrombin time each day.* Clotting-time or bleeding-time determinations are of no value in measuring the effects of Dicumarol. Dicumarol should be administered only to hospitalized patients and only when there are facilities for (1) daily prothrombin-time determinations and (2) immediate transfusion of fresh blood of a compatible type, should it be needed.

TABLE 39 — *Comparison of Heparin and Dicumarol*

	Heparin	Dicumarol
Source	Mast cells of Ehrlich	Spoiled sweet clover
Mode of Action	Blocks action of prothrombin	Blocks formation of prothrombin
Onset of Action	Immediate	Delayed 24 to 72 hours
Duration of Action	Transitory	Prolonged
Method of Administration	Parenteral	Oral
Toxicity	Only that incidental to hemorrhage	Only that incidental to hemorrhage
Dosage	Controlled by clotting time	Controlled by prothrombin time
Counteraction	Protamine sulfate	Vitamin K; transfusions

Dicumarol is contraindicated in patients (1) who are bleeding from any cause (except possibly menstruation), have purpura of any type, or are obviously malnourished; (2) who have ulcerating or granulomatous lesions; or (3) who have subacute bacterial endocarditis. It is probably contraindicated during pregnancy. Fever intensifies the action of the drug, as do salicylates and their derivatives. In patients undergoing continuous tube drainage of the stomach or small intestine, Dicumarol therapy is inadvisable because of the difficulty of obtaining absorption by either the oral or the rectal route. Such patients should be given heparin. Postoperative use of Dicumarol should be very cautious, particularly after operative procedures on the brain or spinal cord.

Dicumarol is administered by mouth. Because its effect does not begin for twenty-four to seventy-two hours, a schedule such as the following is suggested:

Day 1. Determine prothrombin time, preferably by the Quick technic (p. 529). If it is normal, give a dose of 200 to 300 mg. Dicumarol (patients of average size and good condition should receive 300 mg.). If prothrombin time is prolonged, a smaller dose should be given.

Day 2. Determine prothrombin time and translate into percentage of prothrombin activity according to the prothrombin activity curve determined by the hospital clinical laboratory for that particular lot of thromboplastin reagent. If the prothrombin activity is greater than 25 percent, 100 to 200 mg. of Dicumarol are given.

Day 3 and subsequently. Determine prothrombin activity as above, and do not administer Dicumarol until the result of the test is known. Give no Dicumarol on any day when the prothrombin activity is less than 25 percent. If the prothrombin activity is 25 percent or more, 50 to 200 mg. are given, according to the patient's previous response.

It is desirable to keep the prothrombin time between 15 and 30 percent of normal. Hemorrhagic complications rarely occur unless the prothrombin time falls below 10 percent. Nevertheless, all patients receiving the drug should be watched carefully for any evidence of hemorrhage. At the first indication of bleeding, transfusions of fresh whole blood should be given and repeated, if necessary, until the bleeding is controlled. Preliminary reports indicate that vitamin K_1 (p. 499) or vitamin K_1 oxide may be an effective antidote to Dicumarol when administered as an emulsion intravenously in doses of 0.5 to 3 Gm. Other vitamin K preparations appear to have no value. After the return of prothrombin time to the desired therapeutic range, Dicumarol therapy is resumed.

Treatment is usually continued for fourteen to twenty-eight days after the last episode of thromboembolic activity. It has been suggested that anticoagulant therapy should be maintained about forty days in patients with coronary thrombosis, about five days in patients with phlebothrombosis below the knee, and about ten days in patients with phlebothrombosis extending above the knee. Patients having recurring thrombotic phenomena have been maintained on Dicumarol therapy for indefinite periods of time. After a period of study, the maintenance dose of the drug is determined with sufficient accuracy to allow them to return to their usual activities. Prothrombin time may be checked weekly.

CITRATE

The salts of citric acid (for formula, see Figure 22) are effective anticoagulants in vitro because the citrate ion combines with calcium to form the nonionizable calcium citrate. Coagulation of blood requires calcium ions (see p. 344). The effect of the citrate is overcome by the addition of ionizable salts of calcium. In vivo, the citrates do not act as anticoagulants, because they cannot be given in sufficient quantity to combine with all the calcium present in and available to the blood. Actually, very large doses of citrates increase rather than decrease the coagulability of the blood, probably through a compensatory mechanism. Sodium and potassium citrates have been administered systemically as alkalizing agents (see p. 352).

Sodium citrate is useful as an anticoagulant in collecting blood for transfusion or for laboratory tests. A concentration of 0.25 percent is adequate. A more concentrated solution is placed in the receiving vessel, and the blood is drawn into it. A 2.5 percent solution is effective when diluted to ten times its volume with blood, whereas a 5 percent solution may be diluted to twenty times.

$$\begin{array}{c} CH_2-COOH \\ | \\ HOC-COOH \\ | \\ CH_2-COOH \end{array}$$

FIGURE 22—*Structural Formula of Citric Acid*

DRUGS AFFECTING PRINCIPALLY THE RESPIRATORY SYSTEM

NASAL VASOCONSTRICTORS

Nasal vasoconstrictors are drugs which, on topical application to the nasal mucosa, produce local vasoconstriction with shrinkage. They have been used to improve drainage of the paranasal sinuses in sinusitis and for symptomatic relief of nasal congestion in sinusitis, rhinitis, the common cold, and nasal allergy. However, their use is declining, partly because better results can often be obtained by systemic administration of adrenergic and vasopressor drugs, and partly because of abuse. In allergy, their local application may prove irritating.

When used with due regard for the physiology of the nose, vasoconstrictors do no harm. However, it is easy to abuse them by too-frequent application of excessively strong concentrations. Like other tissues, the nasal mucosa requires a certain amount of blood flow to supply it with oxygen and food materials and to carry away the end products of metabolism. Excessive concentrations of nasal vasoconstrictors cause too great a reduction in mucosal blood supply, with resultant tissue hypoxia and accumulation of waste products. Such a situation is especially undesirable in the presence of infection. When an excessive vasoconstrictor effect wears off, it is followed by a period of excessive vasodilation and congestion (secondary hyperemia). The patient may be even more uncomfortable than before the vasoconstrictor was applied, and he is tempted to renew the application. A vicious cycle of tissue hypoxia and compensatory hyperemia is thus set up which may result in serious damage to the mucosa.

The drugs used as nasal vasoconstrictors are adrenergic (p. 422), and some of them have a vasopressor action when given systemically in adequate dosage. Some may be applied to the nasal mucosa as vapors, whereas others are used as solutions in water or oil.

In general, the volatile agents in inhaler form are least irritating and reach all parts of the mucosa most readily except in the presence of complete blockage, when they are totally ineffective. For administration, the inhaler is inserted into one nostril and the patient inhales slowly while the other nostril is occluded. Two or three such inhalations on each side are usually sufficient. When blocking is severe but not complete, inhalation may be repeated at five-minute intervals until all parts of the nose are open or it is evident that they will not open. Vasoconstrictor vapors may also be introduced into the paranasal sinuses by the technic of Proetz (see below).

Aqueous solutions of the salts of vasoconstrictor drugs exert a more powerful action than do vapors, and they may be effective on repeated application when the nose is completely blocked. However, they are slightly more irritant than vapor and, as ordinarily administered, do not reach all parts of the incompletely blocked nose as adequately. They may be applied by patient or physician as drops or spray for their effect on the nasal mucosa, on cotton pledgets by the physician, or by the Proetz displacement technic for introduction into the sinuses.

For nasal effect, the spray is generally more satisfactory than drops. The nozzle should first be directed at a right angle to the general plane of the face and then progressively upward until parallel with the profile of the nose. Finally, the tip should be turned upward and inserted well into the nostril to cover the very upper surface of the mucosa.

The instillation of drops with the head merely tilted backward is totally ineffective, for the medication passes only along the floor of the nose and into the nasopharynx, from which it is usually swallowed. A number of technics are satisfactory. In one, the patient lies across a bed or table with the head over the edge exactly upside down. Two or three drops are then instilled into each nostril. While the patient breathes through his mouth, the head is slowly rotated from side to side. After

twenty to thirty seconds, the patient sits up and leans forward with the face parallel to the floor. He remains in this position for a minute or two to allow the medication to pass over the turbinates and to permit drainage of any excess.

Another satisfactory posture is the lateral head-low position. The patient lies on one side with the lower shoulder supported by a pillow in such a way that the head is inclined downward at an angle of about 45 degrees. The patient breathes through his mouth. Twenty to thirty seconds after the medication is instilled into the lower nostril, the head is rotated to a face-downward position to allow drainage of excess. The patient is then turned, and the application is repeated on the other side.

Oil solutions are now little used because they have two serious disadvantages; the oil tends (1) to impede ciliary activity and (2) to pass down the nasopharynx and enter the trachea and bronchi, from which it is taken up by leukocytes and deposited in the tracheobronchial lymph glands with resultant lymphatic blockage. This latter complication occurs particularly in children. In infants and in enfeebled adults with weak cough reflexes, oils (especially mineral oils) are contraindicated for nasal application because they may produce lipoid pneumonia.

For introduction of vasoconstrictors, anti-infective agents, or other drugs into the paranasal sinuses, the displacement technic of Proetz is valuable. The nose is cleaned, and the mucosa is shrunk by a vasoconstrictor. The patient is placed on his back with head hyperextended until the ear and chin are in vertical alignment. An aqueous solution of the desired agent, warmed to body temperature, is instilled into the nares along the septum. The physician occludes one naris with his finger and applies two to five pounds of negative pressure repeatedly to the other naris while the patient maintains the posterior nares closed by a raised palate. The correct position of the palate is that assumed during enunciation of the letter "K." This "K" position is maintained throughout the procedure, and the patient breathes through his mouth.

No more than 2 cc. should be instilled into each nostril at one time. This fluid should disappear from the nasal cavity after eight to twelve alternations in pressure. An additional instillation is usually made to bring the total volume administered to 8 cc.

The volatile vasoconstrictors can be introduced into the sinuses by a slightly modified technic. The cotton cylinder containing the drug should be placed in a container, one end of which has (or can be connected with) an olive tip for application to a naris; a hole of no greater diameter than 1/64 inch is bored in the other end. The nose is prepared as for introduction of a fluid. However, since gravity is not required for entry of the vapor, the patient may remain sitting. Instead of closing the opposite naris, the physician inserts the perforated olive tip of the container into it. The negative pressure draws the vasoconstrictor into the nose at the same time that it reduces the pressure. The alternations of pressure are made by removing the suction tip. Volatile agents may be introduced into the sinuses by the displacement technic during acute sinusitis because they cannot spread infection as fluids might.

Ephedrine was the first of the nasal vasoconstrictors and is still the most widely used. Its general properties are discussed on page 426. It is available in many forms for nasal application, including the following:

Ephedrine sulfate or hydrochloride solution, 3 percent, with sufficient sodium chloride to make an isotonic solution. Such a solution is generally diluted with an equal volume of isotonic salt solution before use, in order to yield a 1.5 percent strength.
Ephedrine sulfate solution, 1 percent, with antiseptics (such as 'Merthiolate,' 1:5,000).
Ephedrine gluconate solution (equivalent to 1 percent ephedrine alkaloid), aromatized, made isotonic with dextrose. Such preparations are available with or without antiseptics (see 'I-sedrin Plain' and 'I-sedrin Compound,' p. 603).
Ephedrine jelly, 1 percent, with or without antiseptics.
Ephedrine inhalant, aromatized, with or without antiseptics, and containing 1 percent ephedrine base in a light oil.

The vasoconstrictor action of ephedrine begins within a minute or two after local application and lasts two to four hours. With 1 or 1.5 percent solutions there is no secondary hyperemia. Insomnia and other manifestations of central-nervous-system stimulation are uncommon following topical application of ephedrine. They are combated by the barbiturates (p. 392).

'Clopane Hydrochloride' (Cyclopentamine Hydrochloride, Lilly) is a more potent nasal vasoconstrictor than ephedrine hydrochloride or sulfate and has the additional advantage of a much lower incidence of side-effects. It is applied as a 0.5 percent solution in the same way as ephedrine salts. It does not induce secondary hyperemia. As a rule, three hours should elapse between administrations. For the general properties of 'Clopane Hydrochloride,' see page 430.

'Tuamine' (Tuaminoheptane, Lilly) is a powerful nasal vasoconstrictor without side-effects. It is volatile and is employed in inhaler form. Administra-

tion is seldom required more frequently than at hourly intervals.

'Tuamine Sulfate' (Tuaminoheptane Sulfate, Lilly) is a solid which is soluble in water. A 1 percent solution has a more potent and enduring nasal vasoconstrictor action than a 2 percent solution of an ephedrine salt. Release is gradual and is not followed by secondary engorgement. A 2 percent solution is available, but it should be reserved for use in the physician's office; it is too powerful for use by the patient. For Proetz displacement therapy, a 0.2 solution is adequate. The structural formula of 'Tuamine' is shown in Figure 34, page 423.

'Forthane' (Methylhexamine, Lilly) is an isomer of 'Tuamine.' Like 'Tuamine,' it is volatile and is about four times as potent as a nasal vasoconstrictor. The effect lasts a half hour or more. No side-effects have been reported. For structural formula, see Figure 34, page 423.

Benzedrex (see Figure 34, p. 423, for structural formula) also is a volatile substance available in inhaler form as a nasal vasoconstrictor. It is free of side-effects.

Neo-Synephrine Hydrochloride is employed as a nasal vasoconstrictor in 0.25 or 0.5 percent solution or emulsion or in jelly (0.5 percent). It has a relatively prolonged action without secondary hyperemia. Side-effects are rare. In resistant cases, a 1 percent solution may be used. For a general discussion of the drug, see page 429.

Propadrine Hydrochloride is applied as a 1 percent solution or 0.66 percent jelly for nasal vasoconstriction. The effect is said to be more prolonged than that of ephedrine, and central-nervous-system stimulation is said to be less common. For general discussion, see page 430.

Vonedrine (see also p. 430) is a volatile vasoconstrictor which may be used in inhaler form. The levulinate is applied as a 0.5 percent solution. The onset of effect is somewhat slower than that of ephedrine salts, but the action is somewhat more prolonged. There is no secondary hyperemia and little tendency to stimulation of the central nervous system.

Privine Hydrochloride has an extremely powerful and prolonged nasal vasoconstrictor action; a 0.05 percent solution or jelly may be effective for six to eight hours. These properties make it easily abused, with resulting secondary hyperemia. Consistent abuse may lead to serious mucosal damage. Only 2 or 3 drops (in children, 1 or 2 drops) should be instilled into each nostril, and administration should not be repeated until the effect has definitely worn off. For a general discussion, see page 431.

Methamphetamine Hydrochloride (desoxyephedrine hydrochloride) is best known as a stimulant to the central nervous system, but it also has nasal vasoconstrictor properties. For reasons of compatibility, it is the vasoconstrictor agent which is combined with sodium sulfathiazole in 'Thizodrin' (Sodium Sulfathiazole and Desoxyephedrine, Lilly). 'Thizodrin' may be employed when vasoconstriction is desired in addition to the effects of sulfathiazole locally on the nasal mucosa. For further discussion of desoxyephedrine, see Methamphetamine, page 428; of sulfathiazole, page 293. The exact composition of 'Thizodrin' appears on page 604.

DRUGS AFFECTING COUGH AND EXPECTORATION

Cough and expectoration are useful insofar as they aid in clearing the bronchial tract of secretion and discharge. However, they represent only a part of the system for removal of bronchial secretions. These secretions are normally transported upward by a number of mechanisms. In the bronchioles they are moved by cough—partly by the force of the sudden air current and partly by the reflex tussive squeeze in which the lumina are actually closed somewhat in the manner of upward peristalsis. In the bronchi there is continuous upward transport by the cilia (which do not extend into the bronchioles). During all of this period, reabsorption of the secretion is taking place; its rate is influenced by many factors. The matter which escapes reabsorption in its upward passage is finally coughed up and either expectorated or swallowed.

Obstruction of the respiratory passages is determined much more by the viscosity of the bronchial secretion than by its volume; within limits, the more fluid the secretion, the easier it is to bring up. The amount expectorated is also affected not only by the volume secreted but by the volume which is reabsorbed. Volume and viscosity are unrelated properties, and it is possible to influence them independently. Inhaled gases and systemically administered drugs have important effects on both character and quantity of secretion and on the cough reflex. The most important are discussed below.

A number of types of cough may be distinguished. The *useful cough* brings up secretion and aids in clearing the respiratory tract. A *useless cough* is one which is not stimulated by the presence of an accumulation of secretion but rather by mechanical irritation, as from pressure on the trachea or bronchi. Potentially useful coughs may be *tight* or *unproductive*, a situation which is alleviated by measures which liquefy the sputum. An *insufficient cough* may be observed in very weak patients. An extremely *loose cough* may indicate that the secretion is too liquid to be raised easily, in which case antiexpectorants are indicated.

EXPECTORANTS

An expectorant will be considered in this discussion as a drug which reduces the viscosity of bronchial secretion, thus facilitating upward passage and expectoration.

Steam or a very moist atmosphere is a simple yet extremely effective agent for lessening the viscosity of bronchial secretions. Steam may be inhaled for half-hourly periods under a sheet or towel draped over the head, or the room may be saturated with steam from a boiling kettle or with moisture from a mechanical vaporizer. Benzoin Tincture is commonly added to the water which is boiled to provide steam for inhalation. It probably does no more than add a pleasant odor.

Carbon Dioxide also lessens the viscosity of bronchial secretions but in addition causes hyperemia in those portions which are diseased. Apparently the hyperemia increases reabsorption, for both volume and viscosity of the sputum are diminished at the same time. A combination of 5 percent carbon dioxide and steam is even more effective. Patients vary in their tolerance for carbon dioxide; some, especially those with pulmonary emphysema, may be able to take a 10 percent concentration, whereas others may find 2 to 3 percent intolerable. A 5 percent concentration produces a satisfactory liquefaction of sputum. It may be inhaled constantly or for periods of a few minutes at frequent intervals.

Drugs are in general less effective than either steam or carbon dioxide. However, the combination of steam, carbon dioxide, and drugs is more effective than any combination of a lesser number of agents.

AMMONIUM CHLORIDE reduces both the viscosity and the pH of bronchial secretions. It is commonly given in doses of 0.3 to 0.5 Gm. (5 to 7.5 grains) every one or two hours. The taste is best disguised in a syrup, such as Wild Cherry, Citric Acid, Orange, Tolu Balsam, or Acacia, or in Terpin Hydrate Elixir. A full glass of water is taken with each dose. Enteric-coated tablets are not recommended as expectorants.

IODIDES, either sodium or potassium, also reduce viscosity and lower *p*H of bronchial secretions. They are especially used in the treatment of asthma and chronic bronchitis. They are considered too irritating to be given in the presence of acute inflammation. They are contraindicated in all forms of tuberculosis. Dosage of either salt is 0.06 to 0.3 Gm. (1 to 5 grains) every three to four hours. For children, Hydriodic Acid Syrup may be diluted to four parts with a fruit syrup, 1 dram of the mixture being given every three to four hours.

IPECAC is a nauseant expectorant which reduces the viscosity of the bronchial secretion without influencing *p*H. It is usually prescribed as Ipecac Syrup. The dosage for adults is 8 to 15 minims (0.5 to 1 cc.) every four hours. Children are usually given 5 minims for the first year of age and an additional minim for each additional year up to the adult dose.

ANTIEXPECTORANTS

Oxygen is probably the most potent agent for increasing the viscosity of bronchial secretion. This tendency is not diminished by passage of the oxygen through a water bottle. However, when oxygen is administered with steam *and* 5 percent carbon dioxide, the viscosity of sputum is lowered. Oxygen alone causes drying of secretions and makes them cling to the bronchial mucous membranes in the form of crusts, which may produce obstruction.

Codeine is used to depress the cough reflex by central action in those patients in whom coughing is in excess of that needed to keep the respiratory passages reasonably clear. Codeine is usually prescribed as the sulfate or the more soluble phosphate. Only small doses are required to dull the cough reflex—5 to 10 mg. (1/12 to 1/6 grain). Large doses of codeine (over 60 mg., or 1 grain) may actually increase the cough reflex and should therefore be avoided in cough. However, after twenty-four hours of administration, even small doses of codeine increase the viscosity of sputum progressively as the drug is continued. Even when codeine is combined with an efficient expectorant, the influence of the codeine is predominant. *Codeine should not be*

used when fluidity of the sputum is a therapeutic objective.

A general discussion of codeine will be found on page 403.

Methadon Hydrochloride ('Dolophine Hydrochloride') depresses the cough reflex by central action in a manner similar to that of codeine. However, the effect of a single dose of methadon is of longer duration. The quantities required (0.75 to 1 mg. every four to eight hours, usually as a syrup) are not sufficient for analgesic effects or side reactions. It is not known whether continued administration of methadon increases the viscosity of sputum as does codeine. For a general discussion of methadon, see page 403.

Dihydrocodeinone (Hycodan, Dicodid) bears the same chemical relationship to codeine that dihydromorphinone bears to morphine (see Figure 26, p. 399). It acts on cough in the same way as codeine, but the effect lasts longer, and the side-effect of constipation is said to be less frequent. However, the drug is reported to induce addiction about as easily as morphine.

Dihydrocodeinone may be presumed to have the same effect as codeine on the viscosity of sputum during continued administration. The usual adult dosage of the hydrochloride or bitartrate is 5 to 15 mg. every six to eight hours, preferably immediately after meals. Children under two years of age should receive one-fourth the adult dose; children over two, one-half.

Atropine has been found to act as a powerful antiexpectorant; it decreases the production of sputum and greatly increases the viscosity of the unexpectorated material.

Irritants—In chronic bronchitis, mild irritants have been used in an effort to stimulate repair. Such are creosote and guaiacol. They apparently act as antiexpectorants, and their therapeutic value is questionable. They should not be given in acute bronchitis. Clinical doses may cause gastro-intestinal irritation. Large doses may be toxic, resulting in cardiovascular collapse.

Creosote carbonate, calcium creosotate, or guaiacol carbonate is given in doses of 5 to 15 grains (0.3 to 1 Gm.) orally with milk every four hours.

Terpin hydrate has been given to diminish an abundant, and especially a liquid, sputum in chronic cough. To be effective, it should be given in doses of 5 grains (0.3 Gm.) three times a day. Such a dosage is not difficult in capsules, but it is rather impractical with Terpin Hydrate Elixir, N.F., which contains only 1 grain per dram.

RESPIRATORY STIMULANTS

Respiration is controlled by the respiratory center, which is located on the floor of the fourth ventricle in the medulla oblongata. The respiratory center responds to both sensory and chemical stimuli of various sorts.

The basic control of respiration is chemical, and the normal stimulation depends on oxygen want of the center itself and decrease in pH of the blood (accumulation of carbon dioxide). These two chemical stimuli acting singly have different effects. Acidity alone induces the Kussmaul type of respiration, which is characteristic of severe acidosis. Oxygen want acting alone induces Cheyne-Stokes respiration. Many other chemical substances stimulate respiration, some of them as part of a general stimulant effect on the central nervous system.

Many sensory influences act on respiration. The normal, automatic breathing is conditioned by many reflexes originating in the mucosa of the respiratory passages, the diaphragm and intercostal muscles, the carotid body, and possibly other structures. Respiration is also greatly affected by stimuli from the cerebral cortex and by strong emotion of any kind, but particularly by pain.

Therapeutic respiratory stimulation is of value mainly to counteract respiratory depression induced by certain drugs. Depression of the respiratory center in the course of disease is usually the result of fatigue following prolonged respiratory stimulation due to hypoxia or acidosis. In a situation of this kind, administration of a respiratory stimulant is useless and often harmful; the proper treatment is early recognition and treatment of the hypoxia or acidosis. Thus in diabetic coma, respiration is stimulated by the presence of the acetone bodies and hypoxia. Central-nervous-system stimulants are of little or no value; but if, in addition to specific measures, oxygen is administered, the speed of recovery may be enhanced. Likewise, in asphyxia neonatorum, the infant's respiratory center has already been strongly stimulated by oxygen want and carbon-dioxide accumulation; the treatment is clearance of the air passages and administration of oxygen rather than injection of respiratory-stimulant drugs.

Picrotoxin is one of the most powerful known stimulants of the central nervous system, including the respiratory center. It is employed therapeutically in treatment of overdosage of certain central-nervous-system depressants, particularly the barbiturates. For details of use, see page 395.

Metrazol is a powerful central-nervous-system stimulant which has somewhat more action on the lower centers (including the respiratory center) and spinal cord than has picrotoxin. It is apparently less valuable than picrotoxin in treating overdoses of central depressants. It is used principally as a convulsant in the treatment of schizophrenia. For further discussion of the drug, see page 389.

Nikethamide (Coramine) is the diethylamide of nicotinic acid, $C_5H_4N \cdot CO \cdot N(CH_2 \cdot CH_3)_2$. In doses of 0.25 to 0.75 Gm. (1 to 3 cc. of a 25 percent solution), it is a respiratory stimulant which has been used to treat overdosage of morphine, tribromoethanol (Avertin), and inhalation anesthetics. Against barbiturate intoxication it is less effective than picrotoxin or Metrazol. Its effects on the cardiovascular system are controversial. It may be given orally, subcutaneously, or intravenously. Very large doses are convulsive.

Caffeine (for general properties, see p. 360) has a powerful stimulant action on the central nervous system which includes the respiratory center. Stimulation is most readily obtained when respiration is acutely depressed by some drug antagonist such as chloral hydrate or morphine. However, in chronic poisoning as in uremia, the drug produces little benefit. Caffeine and Sodium Benzoate, U.S.P., is employed in doses of 0.13 to 0.25 Gm. (2 to 4 grains) subcutaneously (or, in emergency, intravenously) for respiratory stimulation—particularly in morphine poisoning and Cheyne-Stokes respiration. Doses of more than 0.5 Gm. may produce undesirable psychic stimulation.

Lobeline is a pyridine derivative which is related chemically and pharmacologically to nicotine. It has in the past been used as a respiratory stimulant, especially for resuscitation of the newborn, but the action is uncertain and brief, and the drug may be toxic.

Ammonia, NH_3, is an irritant gas; when inhaled in dilute form, it stimulates both the respiratory and vasomotor centers reflexly from the sensory endings of the trigeminal nerve in the nasal mucosa. In the form of a few whiffs of Aromatic Ammonia Spirit, U.S.P., it is employed in syncope (fainting) of nervous or emotional origin.

DRUGS GIVEN FOR THEIR ACTION
ON THE ALIMENTARY TRACT

Mouthwashes

Proper mouth care is even more important during illness than it is in health. Especial attention is necessary in very weak or unconscious patients, those with fever, and those taking either nothing by mouth or liquid diets requiring no mastication. When practical, the toothbrush should be used after every meal. It is especially important to cleanse the mouth after a milk drink.

When the mucous membrane is very dry or cracked, one of the following should be applied frequently:

Light liquid petrolatum

A mixture of light liquid petrolatum, 3 parts, and glycerin, 1 part

Rose Water Ointment, U.S.P. (cold cream)

Foul or infected mouths may be cleansed with potassium permanganate solution, a tablet or a few crystals being dissolved in water and diluted to a rose or port wine color.

In febrile but conscious patients, one may use a solution of sodium bicarbonate and sodium chloride, 1 teaspoonful of each in a pint of warm water, or the more pleasant Alkaline Aromatic Solution, N.F., which contains:

potassium bicarbonate	20	Gm.
sodium borate	20	Gm.
thymol	0.5	Gm.
eucalyptol	1	cc.
methyl salicylate	0.5	cc.
Amaranth Solution	14	cc.
alcohol	50	cc.
glycerin	100	cc.
distilled water, to make	1,000	cc.

It may be used undiluted or with up to 4 volumes of water.

When a mild bacteriostatic effect is desired, sodium peroxide or sodium perborate may be used, either as a powder with a toothbrush or in strong or saturated solution. The perborate should not be swallowed.

Antacids and Adsorbents

Gastric antacids are drugs which reduce the acidity of the contents of the stomach. Adsorbents are colloidal substances having the power to bind or hold other substances which may include mineral acids, bacteria, toxins, and also digestive enzymes.

Gastric antacids comprise two kinds of substances: adsorbents, which bind hydrochloric acid physically; and actual or potential alkalies, which combine with acid chemically.

The adsorbents are useful in diarrhea (p. 132) and food poisoning (p. 271). Antacids are employed in hyperchlorhydria and peptic ulcer (p. 128); although they may be of great benefit in tiding a patient over an acute exacerbation of peptic ulcer, many clinicians believe that their continuous use in large doses is not only futile but may actually be harmful.

The ideal antacid has the following properties: (1) It is an effective neutralizing agent; (2) it does not cause systemic alkalosis; (3) it does not lead to "rebound" stimulation of acid secretion; (4) it does not interfere with digestive processes; (5) it does not cause diarrhea or constipation; (6) it does not release carbon dioxide on contact with acid; (7) it does not irritate the stomach. Some of the more commonly used adsorbents and antacids are discussed below and are compared in Table 40.

Kaolin is a hydrated aluminum silicate which is an effective adsorbent for bacteria and many toxic substances. It has protective as well as adsorbent properties. It is useful in diarrhea, particularly that of infectious origin, and in food poisoning. Because it has relatively little adsorbent power for acids, it is not used as an antacid. Alone, kaolin tends to settle out of suspension and form a dense, inactive mass. For this reason it is usually prescribed with aluminum hydroxide, acacia, pectin, or some other suspending agent. The dose may be from 5 to 30 Gm. every few hours.

Aluminum Hydroxide, $Al(OH)_3$, in colloidal form is widely employed in the treatment of peptic ulcer and acute diarrhea. As shown in Table 40, it fulfills in rather high degree the more important criteria for a satisfactory antacid. Its slight astringent action is an advantage in diarrhea but tends to produce constipation in peptic ulcer. A more serious disadvantage is its binding of phosphate, which may lead to deficient absorption of the latter ion unless the intake is high.

Colloidal aluminum hydroxide is available in solid or liquid form. It is most commonly administered as an aqueous suspension, such as Aluminum Hydroxide Gel, U.S.P. Most suspensions contain approximately 4 percent, expressed as aluminum oxide; and 1 cc. is usually capable of neutralizing 10 to 15 cc. of N/10 hydrochloric acid.

Aluminum Hydroxide Gel can be given in doses of 10 to 20 cc. every few hours. During acute exacerbations of peptic ulcer, it may be given by the constant-drip method, 5 or 6 drops per minute being delivered through a stomach tube day and night for ten days. Dried Aluminum Hydroxide Gel, U.S.P., may be given in solid form in doses of 0.6 to 2 Gm. every few hours. The dried form is not as efficacious as the gel.

Aluminum Phosphate, $AlPO_4$, is somewhat similar to aluminum hydroxide in properties and mode of action. It has the advantage of not interfering with phosphate absorption and the disadvantage of being only 50 percent as effective. Aluminum Phosphate Gel, U.S.P., contains approximately 4 percent of the active agent. The usual dose is 15 to 30 cc. of suspension every two hours during acute exacerbations of peptic ulcer. Like Aluminum Hydroxide Gel, it may be given by the continuous-drip technic, but at the rate of 10 to 12 drops an hour.

Magnesium Trisilicate, $Mg_2Si_3O_8 \cdot nH_2O$, is a very effective adsorbent in both peptic ulcer and diarrhea (see Table 40). One Gm. neutralizes approximately 155 cc. of N/10 hydrochloric acid within four hours. Although the greatest effectiveness is obtained during the first hour after ingestion, it continues to be effective for many hours thereafter. The drug is almost insoluble, but large doses may cause diarrhea because of the formation of magnesium chloride. Magnesium trisilicate may be prescribed as powder, tablets, capsules, or suspension. The usual dose is 0.5 to 2 Gm. every few

hours. Sometimes it is given in combination with aluminum hydroxide.

Calcium Carbonate, $CaCO_3$, is an effective antacid. It is practically insoluble. It reacts with hydrochloric acid to produce calcium chloride. Its principal disadvantage is that it tends to be constipating, and it lacks the demulcent properties of the antacids discussed above. One Gm. neutralizes about 210 cc. of N/10 hydrochloric acid. The average adult dose is 0.6 to 2 Gm.

Magnesium Oxide, MgO, is insoluble but reacts with hydrochloric acid to form the soluble magnesium chloride, small amounts of which may be absorbed. In cases of extreme impairment of renal function, it may produce the symptoms of magnesium poisoning (p. 346). It tends to be laxative, and because of this property it has been used alternately with or in conjunction with calcium carbonate. One Gm. of magnesium oxide neutralizes approximately 500 cc. of N/10 hydrochloric acid. The average adult dose is 0.6 to 2 Gm.

Magnesium Hydroxide, $Mg(OH)_2$, is very similar to magnesium oxide except that it is usually dispensed as an aqueous suspension (Magnesia Magma, U.S.P., milk of magnesia) containing between 7 and 8.5 percent of the drug. One teaspoonful of Magnesia Magma is equivalent to approximately 0.35 Gm. magnesium oxide. The average dose as an antacid is 1 Gm.

Sodium Bicarbonate, $NaHCO_3$, is an effective antacid, but its many disadvantages make it undesirable. Perhaps its most serious defect is the production of systemic alkalosis through its ready solubility and rapid systemic absorption. It acts

TABLE 40—*Comparison of Antacids*

	Aluminum Hydroxide	Aluminum Phosphate	Magnesium Trisilicate	Calcium Carbonate	Magnesium Oxide	Magnesium Hydroxide	Sodium Bicarbonate
Acid-binding power	++	+	++	++	++	++	+++
Adsorbent action	Yes	Yes	Yes	No	No	No	No
Demulcent effect	Yes	Yes	Yes	No	No	No	No
Systemic alkalosis	No	No	No	No	No	No	Yes
"Rebound" secretion	No	No	No	No	No	No	Yes
Digestive interference	No	No	No	No	No	No	Yes
May cause { Diarrhea	No	No	Yes	No	Yes	Yes	No
Constipation	Yes	No	No	Yes	No	No	No
Releases CO_2	No	No	No	Yes	No	No	Yes
Gastric irritation	No	No	No	No	No	No	No

quickly but briefly. Its additional disadvantages are indicated in Table 40. One Gm. of sodium bicarbonate neutralizes 120 cc. of N/10 hydrochloric acid. The dose is 0.6 to 2 Gm.

Digestants

Digestants are drugs which are administered as aids to digestion in the alimentary tract. True digestants are specific substances capable of replacing those normally found in the alimentary tract which are necessary for the digestion of foodstuffs. They should be prescribed only in the presence of actual deficiency.

Hydrochloric Acid—Anacidity (the absence of free hydrochloric acid from the stomach) may be associated with symptoms of indigestion and diarrhea, although in most individuals with the condition no symptoms can be attributed to it. If symptoms are present, they may disappear on administration of the acid.

Diluted Hydrochloric Acid, U.S.P., (10 percent HCl) may be given in doses of 4 to 10 cc. The dose is well diluted with water and sipped with meals through a straw placed far back in the mouth to avoid contact of the acid with the teeth.

Glutamic acid hydrochloride is the hydrochloride of an amino acid. It releases hydrochloric acid on contact with water. This preparation can therefore be used as a substitute for hydrochloric acid, with the advantage of avoiding hazard to the teeth.

Pepsin, N.F., is a substance containing a proteolytic enzyme secreted in the stomach which initiates hydrolysis of proteins. This action normally is an important factor in digestion; however, it is not indispensable, since the enzymes of the intestine attack native proteins. Some peptic activity is always present when the pH of gastric contents is below 7, but there is none when the pH is above 7. In most patients the administration of hydrochloric acid alone will relieve the symptoms attributed to anacidity, but occasionally pepsin is prescribed with the acid. The usual dose of pepsin is 0.5 to 1 Gm. after meals.

Pancreatin, U.S.P., contains the pancreatic enzymes, amylase, trypsin, and lipase, obtained from fresh hog pancreas. It has been administered in digestive disorders, but there is some doubt as to its effectiveness. A large proportion of the activity is probably destroyed in the stomach unless it is administered in enteric-coated tablets, and one cannot be certain that the release from an enteric coating will be uniformly high enough in the intestine to provide effective digestion. The usual dose is 0.3 to 1 Gm. after meals.

Bile and Bile Salts—Of the constituents of bile, only the bile salts are essential for normal digestion. They facilitate the digestion of fats and the absorption of fatty acids, carotene, vitamin A, the vitamins D, and vitamin K. For further discussion, see under Cholagogues and Choleretics, page 387.

Laxatives and Cathartics

Interest in the eliminative functions arises in the child at an early age and persists in conscious or subconscious channels throughout life. It is therefore not surprising that drugs affecting intestinal elimination should be among the oldest known. Drugs promoting defecation have been termed "laxatives" or "cathartics." The former term carries the connotation of a loosening and is the antonym for constipative. The term "cathartic" carries the connotation of cleansing and implies a stronger action than does laxative.

Laxatives are probably the drugs most frequently taken by the American public, yet they have little real usefulness. They aggravate rather than relieve constipation (see p. 130). Their occasional use is probably without harm, but their frequent or habitual use is contraindicated and may produce serious gastro-intestinal disturbances.

Strong laxatives may have value in treating certain food and drug poisonings (pp. 271 and 551); they are used routinely after anthelmintics (p. 311); and they are sometimes given before x-ray examination of the gastro-intestinal tract. Castor oil may be helpful in connection with induction of labor (p. 214).

Laxatives and cathartics can be classified according to their mode of action into three main groups:

1. Irritant drugs, which increase peristalsis by irritating the mucosa or by stimulating the intestinal muscle directly.

2. Substances which increase the bulk of the intestinal contents.
   Saline cathartics, which attract water to provide bulk, and which are also irritating because of their hypertonicity.
   Hydrophilic colloids and indigestible fiber.

3. Emollient laxatives.

Only those most commonly used will be discussed.

Cascara Sagrada, the "sacred bark," obtained from *Rhamnus purshiana*, is extensively used as a laxative. It contains emodin derivatives and, in spite of its usually mild action, is technically classed with the group of irritant cathartics. A therapeutic dose usually leads to a single soft evacuation, without discomfort or griping, six to twenty-four (generally about eight) hours after ingestion. It is therefore ordinarily taken at bedtime. The emodin cathartics act only on the large intestine. Some of the active principle is absorbed and may be excreted in the milk in sufficient quantity to affect a nursing baby.

Official preparations include the following:

Aromatic Cascara Sagrada Fluidextract, U.S.P., the most commonly used preparation, which is made palatable by treatment with magnesia to remove bitter principles. The usual dose is 4 cc.
Cascara Sagrada Fluidextract, U.S.P., which is effective but bitter. The usual dose is 2 cc.
Cascara Sagrada Extract Tablets, U.S.P., which are less reliable than the liquid extracts. The usual dose is 0.3 Gm. (5 grains).

Senna, the leaves of *Cassia acutifolia* or *C. angustifolia*, like cascara sagrada, contains emodin derivatives, but it is more active. Griping, which is commonly produced by official preparations, is thought to be due to resins rather than to the cathartic agent. Official preparations include Senna Fluidextract, N.F., (dose, 2 cc.) and Senna Syrup, N.F. (dose, 8 cc.).

Castor Oil, U.S.P., obtained from the seed of *Ricinus communis*, is the triglyceride of the unsaturated hydroxy fatty acid, ricinoleic acid. Castor oil itself is a bland emollient. However, when it is digested in the intestine, the ricinoleic acid which is liberated is highly irritant and stimulating to the small intestine, and the intestinal contents are rapidly propelled into and through the colon. The fluid nature of the stool is due to lack of fluid absorption from the bowel rather than to fluid diffusion into it.

A therapeutic dose of castor oil, namely 15 to 30 cc. in an adult, usually produces one or two semifluid stools within two to six hours. Because any excess of oil is excreted with the stool, castor oil is a relatively safe cathartic. The objectionable taste is partly disguised in Aromatic Castor Oil, N.F., and in various proprietary preparations.

Phenolphthalein, U.S.P., is a relatively nontoxic laxative which apparently acts by direct stimulation of the smooth muscle of the intestine, particularly the colon. It is insoluble in water and hence passes through the stomach without change. It dissolves in the alkaline intestinal contents. About 15 percent is absorbed and excreted in conjugated form in the urine. After large doses, enough free phenolphthalein may be excreted so that an alkaline urine may be colored red, as may alkaline intestinal contents or the return from a soapsuds enema after ordinary doses. The color should not be mistaken for blood.

Rarely, hypersusceptible individuals may undergo excessive purgation, with colic and even collapse. Again rarely, others may develop a skin rash (Color Section, Plate 20) which may persist for long periods and flare up whenever the drug is taken.

The effective dose of phenolphthalein averages 0.2 Gm. (3 grains), and it is generally followed in four to eight hours by a soft movement. Children and the aged may require larger doses. Because of the availability of phenolphthalein in the form of laxative candy and gum, extreme overdosage in children is sometimes encountered. If the patient is seen within two hours after the overdose was taken, a therapeutic dose of castor oil is given. This sweeps out the insoluble and more slowly acting phenolphthalein. The patient is kept quiet but not in bed. If diarrhea develops beyond that expected from the castor oil, give Activated Charcoal, U.S.P., every hour in teaspoonful doses suspended in half a glass of milk, water, or a carbonated beverage such as ginger ale or Coca-Cola. If more than two hours have elapsed since the overdose, the castor oil is not given, but the Activated Charcoal is administered regardless of whether or not diarrhea occurs. The charcoal is capable of adsorbing the phenolphthalein and preventing its laxative action. An excess of charcoal is harmless.

The Saline Cathartics are salts which contain ions that are only slowly absorbed from the gastrointestinal tract. When large amounts of such salts are taken, the resulting hypertonic solution leads to diffusion of fluid into the lumen from the intestinal mucosa. The relatively large volume of fluid (and possibly the hypertonicity of the fluid) stimulates peristalsis, and a liquid evacuation results.

Magnesium Sulfate, $MgSO_4 \cdot 7H_2O$, is a commonly used and efficient saline cathartic. Twenty to 40 percent of the magnesium is absorbed and may be toxic in the presence of extremely impaired renal function (see p. 346). The drug is very bitter, but the taste is partly masked by acids. The usual dose is 15 Gm., taken in a small quantity of water or, preferably, diluted lemon juice.

Magnesium Citrate Solution, U.S.P., contains about 1.75 percent magnesium citrate, with added flavoring and sufficient potassium bicarbonate and citric acid to make it effervescent. It is in effect a more palatable substitute for magnesium sulfate. The average dose is 200 cc.

Magnesia Magma, U.S.P., (milk of magnesia) is used as a laxative as well as an antacid (p. 383). It is very mild in action. The laxative dose is 15 to 30 cc.

Sodium Sulfate, $Na_2SO_4 \cdot 10H_2O$, (Glauber's salt) is an effective saline cathartic and has the advantage over magnesium salts of being nontoxic after absorption. The taste, however, is extremely objectionable. The usual dose is 15 Gm.

Sodium Phosphate, $Na_2HPO_4 \cdot 7H_2O$, (disodium acid phosphate) is effective but is milder in action than sodium or magnesium sulfate. The taste is not unpleasant. It is nontoxic on absorption. The usual dose is 4 to 8 Gm. It may also be given as Effervescent Sodium Phosphate, U.S.P., containing added sodium bicarbonate, tartaric acid, and citric acid; the dose is 10 Gm. taken dissolved in half a glass of water.

The Hydrophilic Colloids act mechanically by increasing the bulk of the intestinal contents and thus stimulating peristalsis. They are of value in certain cases of chronic constipation in which the stools are small and desiccated.

Methylcellulose, a synthetic substance made by treating cellulose with methyl chloride, is a relatively inert hydrophilic colloid which has recently been introduced as a bulk laxative. It is apparently nontoxic and nonantigenic. The average dose is 1.5 to 4.5 Gm. with one or two glasses of water two or three times a day.

Agar, U.S.P., is a hydrophilic colloidal substance obtained from certain marine algae. It contains much indigestible hemicellulose. It may be obtained shredded or as a powder, and it is taken in doses of 10 to 40 Gm. daily as a cereal, as a jelly (after solution in hot water and subsequent cooling), or incorporated in food.

Plantago Seed, N.F., (psyllium seed) obtained from *Plantago psyllium*, *P. indica*, or *P. ovata*, contains hydrophilic colloidal material. The seeds are taken (without chewing) mixed with fruit juice, or

the gelatinous mass which results from putting them into hot water can be mixed with food. The usual dose is 4 to 15 Gm. one to three times daily. Generous quantities of fluid should be taken with and after plantago seed to avoid the possibility of their swelling in the esophagus and producing obstruction.

Grinding of plantago seed releases a pigment which is deposited in the renal tubule cells in experimental animals. Although such pigment is not known to be harmful, grinding or chewing of plantago seed is not recommended.

Bran, obtained in the milling of wheat, contains about 20 percent of cellulose and has been used to add bulk to the intestinal contents. Several tablespoonfuls may be taken daily as breakfast food or incorporated in muffins or cookies. An excess may, however, be irritating and may aggravate rather than ameliorate spastic constipation.

Liquid Petrolatum (mineral oil) is the principal emollient laxative. It is indigestible. The very small quantities that are absorbed lodge in the mesenteric lymph nodes and the liver. Liquid petrolatum lubricates the feces and prevents their excessive desiccation. It has been advocated for keeping the feces soft after hemorrhoidectomy, in cardiovascular disease, or after abdominal operations, i.e., when straining at stool must be avoided.

The advisability of its clinical use, however, has been gravely questioned. When it mixes with food, liquid petrolatum tends to coat the particles and impede their contact with the digestive enzymes. It speeds passage of the food through the small intestine. This combination of actions may result in defective digestion and absorption of food and in excessive fermentation by bacteria. The symptoms of indigestion (p. 127) may result. In addition, liquid petrolatum may impede absorption of carotene, vitamin A, vitamin D, calcium, phosphates, and vitamin K. It has been thought by some to retard healing of rectal and anorectal lesions and incisions.

If liquid petrolatum is used, it is best taken once a day at bedtime, at least three hours after food. If administration is to be prolonged, special attention must be given to high intake of those substances with the absorption of which it may interfere.

Three official forms are available:

Liquid Petrolatum, U.S.P. (heavy white mineral oil)
Light Liquid Petrolatum, N.F. (light mineral oil)
Liquid Petrolatum Emulsion, U.S.P., containing 50 percent oil in a syrup with acacia

The usual dose is 15 to 45 cc. of oil.

Antidiarrheics

Antidiarrheics are drugs given to control excessive looseness of the bowels. Such drugs are, however, purely symptomatic, and their administration should accompany a search for and treatment of the underlying cause. In the presence of diarrhea it is necessary to maintain fluid and electrolyte balance (p. 56) by administering fluid and electrolytes—parenterally if need be.

Opium and its derivatives have been used as antidiarrheics for many centuries. The action on the bowel is purely local and is due to morphine. The secretion of the stomach, pancreas, and small intestine and of bile is diminished, and the tone of the gastro-intestinal smooth muscle, including the sphincters, is increased. Peristalsis is thus greatly lessened or abolished. For use of the opium alkaloids in diarrhea, see page 402.

Adsorbents may be useful in diarrhea by binding toxins and bacteria. Some of them are slightly astringent. Those most commonly employed include magnesium trisilicate, aluminum hydroxide, aluminum phosphate, and kaolin. Detailed discussion begins on page 382. Because of its content of pectin, scraped raw apple has been employed in diarrhea in infants, the dose being 1 to 2 tablespoonfuls at frequent intervals.

Astringents, such as tannic acid, have also been employed against diarrhea. They are probably less desirable than the adsorbents. Tannic acid is generally given in the form of acetyltannic acid, which is relatively insoluble in acid and consequently does not begin to act until it reaches the intestine. The dose for children is 0.2 to 1 Gm. every few hours. In various forms of dysentery and in chronic ulcerative colitis, a 2 percent solution of tannic acid given as an enema may afford some degree of symptomatic relief.

Chemically Inert Powders may help control diarrhea by coating the wall of the intestine and acting as protectives. They are probably inferior to the adsorbents. Among them are the following:

Bismuth Subcarbonate, U.S.P.; average dose, 2 to 5 Gm. every few hours.
Bismuth Magma, N.F., an aqueous suspension of bismuth subcarbonate and bismuth hydroxide yielding about 5.5 percent Bi_2O_3; average dose, 15 to 60 cc. (1 to 4 tablespoonfuls) every few hours.
Bismuth Subgallate, N.F., which also exerts a slight astringent action; average dose, 2 to 5 Gm. every few hours.
Bismuth Subnitrate, N.F., which is now little used because of the possibility of its producing nitrite poisoning (p. 365).

Emetics

An emetic is a drug which produces vomiting. It may act reflexly from irritant action on the gastrointestinal tract or directly from stimulation of the vomiting center in the medulla. Emetics have a very limited therapeutic use and have been replaced to a great extent by the stomach tube. They are occasionally used to treat patients with acute food and drug poisoning, to control unruly alcoholic patients, and to stop paroxysms of auricular tachycardia.

The hypodermic injection of apomorphine hydrochloride in 5 to 10-mg. doses usually produces vomiting in 10 to 15 minutes by its central action. The drug has a strong central-depressant action, however, and the dose should never be repeated. Apomorphine may cause dangerous depression or death in patients who are in shock from corrosive poisons, narcotized from overdoses of sedatives, or too inebriated to stand unaided.

Copper sulfate, 0.25 to 0.5 Gm., zinc sulfate, 1 to 2 Gm., or mustard, 1 teaspoonful, taken in a glass of warm water may produce vomiting by local irritant action. The stomach tube is more effective, however.

Ipecac acts both locally and centrally; but because vomiting is not produced for thirty to sixty minutes, it is of no value in an emergency, and the stomach tube is more satisfactory. It is usually given as Ipecac Syrup, U.S.P., in doses of 1 tablespoonful for adults and 1/4 to 1 teaspoonful for infants.

Cholagogues and Choleretics

Cholagogues are agents that promote emptying of the gall bladder, whereas choleretics primarily increase the flow of bile. The most effective stimulus for the discharge of bile from the gall bladder is fatty food, particularly egg yolk, cream, or olive oil. Magnesium sulfate when placed in the duodenum also causes evacuation of the gall bladder and relaxation of the sphincter of Oddi.

The natural and most powerful choleretics are the bile salts. These are stable substances, the sodium salts of the bile acids. The bile acids occur in the bile in conjugated or unconjugated form. The latter consist of the steroids, cholic and desoxycholic acid. The structural formula of cholic acid is shown in Figure 23.

Desoxycholic acid lacks the oxygen atom at position 7. The conjugated bile acids are formed by the chemical combination of cholic acid with taurine ($NH_2 \cdot CH_2 \cdot CH_2 \cdot SO_2 \cdot OH$) or with glycine (gly-

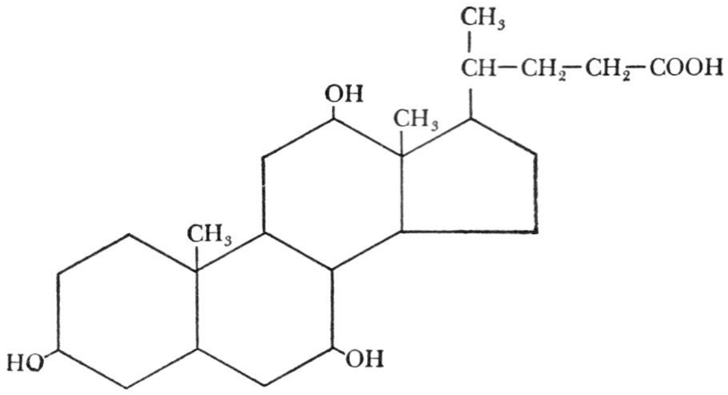

FIGURE 23 — *Structural Formula of Cholic Acid*

cocoll; $NH_2 \cdot CH_2 \cdot COOH$). Chemical treatment outside the body may oxidize the bile acids, the hydroxy groups being replaced by keto groups.

The bile salts have the following physiological functions:

1. They aid in the emulsification and absorption of fats and increase the effectiveness of pancreatic lipase.

2. After aiding in digestion, 80 to 90 percent of the bile acids are absorbed into the portal circulation and carried to the liver, where they promote secretion of bile by the liver.

3. They aid in the absorption of iron and calcium and are necessary to the absorption of carotene and vitamins A, D, E, and K.

4. They aid in the maintenance of normal intestinal motility.

5. They retard excessive growth in the intestine of the colon bacillus and putrefactive organisms.

6. They prevent precipitation of cholesterol and fatty acids in the gall bladder.

The unoxidized conjugated bile salts are the best choleretics, their administration being followed by an increased flow of bile containing an increased concentration of normal bile salts.

Bile salt therapy may be of value in the following types of cases:

1. In the immediate postoperative period following cholecystectomy, as replacement therapy during the interval when most of the bile is being drained to the outside.

2. After the continuity of the biliary tract has been restored following cholecystectomy, to approximate the action of gall-bladder bile and thus facilitate return to a reasonably normal diet.

3. Indigestion of the "gall bladder" type (see p. 143).

4. Biliary dyskinesia, or motor disturbance of the biliary tract in the absence of organic biliary disease or following cholecystectomy.

5. Indigestion accompanying cirrhosis or other liver disease in which production of bile acids is impaired.

6. Constipation, particularly if associated with hepatic insufficiency.

7. In conjunction with vitamin K therapy for hypoprothrombinemia (p. 501).

8. In pancreatic disease characterized by steatorrhea (p. 144).

Caution should be exercised in giving bile salts to patients with a stone in the cystic or common duct. Bile salts are contraindicated in the presence of extreme biliary obstruction.

Many forms of bile preparations are available, including Ox Bile Extract, U.S.P. The most effective are those consisting of unoxidized conjugated bile salts. In one of the most satisfactory of these (p. 608), iron takes the place of sodium as basic ion. The iron bile salts are insoluble in acid and thus pass through the stomach without disturbing its function. In the alkaline medium of the intestine, however, they dissolve readily at the optimum point for emulsification and absorption of food.

The average daily dose of bile salts is 0.3 to 2 Gm. (5 to 30 grains), taken in divided doses during meals. It is generally advised that the dosage regimen be initiated with 5 grains daily for three to five days, with subsequent gradual increase until the patient experiences loose stools or abdominal cramps. The dosage is then reduced to the highest that causes no undesired effects. For a few patients this optimum dosage will be as small as 2 1/2 grains daily.

In conjunction with vitamin K therapy for hypoprothrombinemia, the daily dosage of bile salts should not be greater than 25 grains.

DRUGS HAVING PRINCIPAL EFFECT
ON THE CENTRAL NERVOUS SYSTEM

CENTRAL-NERVOUS-SYSTEM STIMULANTS

Drugs may stimulate different parts of the central nervous system, separately or together. However, most drugs having such an effect act on other parts of the body as well, and the actions of many of them on the central nervous system must be considered as side-effects. Such drugs include atropine, the local anesthetics, some of the adrenergic drugs (p. 422), salicylates, and phenol.

The proper use of central-nervous-system stimulants is limited almost entirely to emergencies. The most important have to do with the respiratory center. A general discussion of respiratory stimulation begins on page 381. Stimulation of the vasomotor center may sometimes be desirable. Although no drug has a selective action on this center, it usually responds with the respiratory center to drugs which stimulate the latter. In addition, it is possible by the use of systemic vasoconstrictor drugs to induce peripheral vasoconstriction independently of the vasomotor center. Stimulation of the central nervous system in general may be advisable following overdoses of depressant drugs.

Picrotoxin is a neutral principle with the empirical formula $C_{30}H_{34}O_{13}$. It occurs in cocculus indicus, which is the seed of the East Indian vine *Anamirta cocculus*. Picrotoxin is one of the most powerful known stimulants of the central nervous system. It is particularly effective for the respiratory center. The drug is employed clinically in treating overdosage of the barbiturates, for which it is probably the most effective antidote. This use is discussed on page 395. Overdoses produce convulsions.

Metrazol (pentylenetetrazol, pentamethylenetetrazole) is also a powerful stimulant to the central nervous system. Its chemical structure is shown in Figure 24. It acts primarily on the higher centers but also on the respiratory, vasomotor, and vagus centers and on the spinal cord. As a treatment for overdoses of central-nervous-system depressants, it seems to be less valuable than picrotoxin, although it is extremely useful as an index of the severity of such poisoning (see p. 396).

Its principal use has been for shock therapy in schizophrenia, but it appears to be less satisfactory than Insulin for this purpose; the severity of Metrazol convulsions leads to a high incidence of fractures. As an antidote to central depression, the usual dose is 0.1 to 0.3 Gm. subcutaneously, intramuscularly, or intravenously as a 10 percent solution. To produce convulsions (shock therapy), 0.3 to 0.7 Gm. is injected intravenously. Aside from the production of convulsions, the drug is relatively nontoxic.

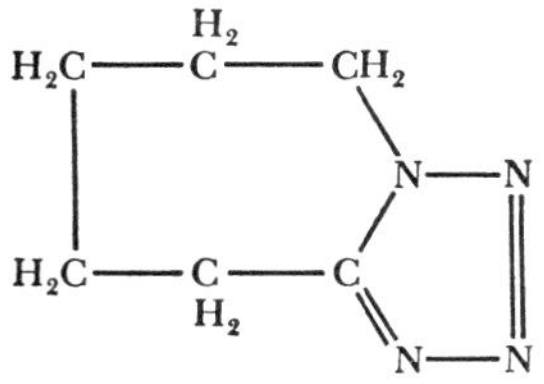

FIGURE 24 — *Structural Formula of Metrazol*

Caffeine is a member of the xanthine group of drugs. It is a central stimulant which is especially valuable in Cheyne-Stokes respiration and in morphine poisoning. It is discussed on page 360.

Strychnine is the principal alkaloid in nux vomica, the seed of an Asiatic tree. It increases the reflex excitability of the spinal cord and, in larger doses, sensitizes the cerebral cortex in such a way as to make the senses more acute. In still larger doses it produces convulsions. In former years, strychnine was much used as a "tonic." Actually, strychnine has no value as a tonic, and it is inferior to other drugs in the treatment of central depression. Strychnine poisoning should be treated as outlined on page 561.

d-Methamphetamine* stimulates the higher cerebral centers, decreasing the sense of fatigue, counteracting sleepiness, and, in most persons, increasing the urge to work. It is employed as a temporary measure in mild depressions, in acute alcoholic intoxication, and to counteract excessive effects of central depressants. It is also useful in postencephalitic paralysis agitans. Additional discussion, including dosage, begins on page 428.

d-Amphetamine (Dexedrine) has similar properties to d-methamphetamine. It is discussed on page 429.

---

* d-Methamphetamine hydrochloride is marketed by Eli Lilly and Company as 'Amphedroxyn Hydrochloride.'

SEDATIVES AND HYPNOTICS

Sedatives and hypnotics depress activity of the central nervous system and produce changes in the sensory, motor, intellectual, autonomic, and psychic reactions. Sedative drugs are used to allay mental excitement and produce mental calm. In general, they tend to cause lassitude and reduced mental activity. Hypnotic drugs are used to produce sleep.

The degree of central-nervous-system depression varies with the choice of drug, dose, route of administration, and mental state of the patient. These compounds have little or no analgesic properties and therefore may fail to produce sedation or sleep in the presence of pain or unduly severe extraneous stimuli. Under such circumstances they may produce delirium, confusional states, and restlessness. When combined with analgesic drugs, they render the analgesia more effective; but in the absence of pain, the combination does not potentiate sedative or hypnotic action. If the patient is cooperative and not unduly stimulated, sedation or hypnosis can be obtained with relatively small, nontoxic doses. Much larger doses are required in psychoses and extreme mental states and for the control of excitement and unrest in infants and children; and bizarre effects may be produced, particularly during the period of recovery from the subanesthetic stupor.

Drugs of many different kinds have sedative or hypnotic effects. The mechanism of this action is unknown. Only those preparations having special clinical usefulness are discussed here.

THE BARBITURATES

The parent molecule of the barbiturates is barbituric acid (malonyl urea; see Figure 25), which is formed as the result of condensing malonic acid, $HOOC \cdot CH_2 \cdot COOH$, and urea, $NH_2 \cdot CO \cdot NH_2$. Urea and barbituric acid themselves are devoid of sedative activity, but substitution of the hydrogen atoms of the malonic acid portion of the molecule with various organic radicals produces a number of useful compounds, as illustrated in Figure 25. As a general rule, the duration of action decreases as the side chains become longer or more complex; but as the number of carbon atoms increases beyond five or six, the sedative effect decreases and convulsive properties may appear. The same change in action tends to follow substitution at the nitrogen atoms. Substitution of sulfur for oxygen at the urea carbon atom yields rapidly acting compounds such as Pentothal Sodium. The barbiturates are weakly acidic and are sparingly soluble in water. They readily form soluble salts of alkaline reaction that are unstable in solution.

The barbiturates are central-nervous-system depressants which can be made to provide almost any degree of depression from light sedation through deep hypnosis. They appear to act on the thalamic portion of the diencephalon. Phenobarbital is known to depress cortical activity, which accounts for its effectiveness in epilepsy (see p. 170).

Oral administration of hypnotic doses of the barbiturates is usually followed by slight slowing of respiration, probably as a result of the attendant hypnosis. Larger doses depress the respiratory center directly, and death from massive overdosage is due as a rule to respiratory failure. The margin between the amount of barbiturate which will cause respiratory failure and that responsible for cardiac arrest is sufficiently wide to permit the successful application of artificial respiration in combating the effects of overdosage. Respiratory depression is more likely to occur during intravenous administration, for the degree of depression is dependent not only upon the total dose but upon the rate of injection as well. Slow administration is essential.

The sedative and hypnotic doses of the barbiturates used clinically cause no significant change in circulation. Because of a vagus-inhibiting effect, the heart rate may be slightly quickened. Large doses of the barbiturates given orally or by rapid intravenous injection cause a fall in blood pressure due to vasodilation, but generally there is a rather prompt return to normal. In anesthetic doses, cardiovascular reflexes are diminished and the carotid sinus is depressed; but there is no direct toxicity to the myocardium, nor is the rhythm or conduction of the heart affected.

The blood constituents are not altered by barbiturate medication in moderate doses, and there is no appreciable change in blood-sugar concentration unless depression of such depth is produced that acidosis results.

The basal metabolic rate is reduced by large doses of barbiturates, but quantities sufficient for light hypnosis cause no significant depression below the resting level. Sedative and hypnotic doses lower the body temperature slightly. Kidney function is not seriously affected by barbiturate medication, provided (1) there is not a prolonged period of deep depression and (2) hepatic function is unimpaired.

Distribution of barbiturates in body tissues and fluids has not been completely determined. There is no greater concentration in the brain than in other tissues, and analysis of spinal fluid has revealed insignificant amounts even after administration of large doses. Following intravenous injection, the drug remains in the blood in appreciable quantities for only a few minutes.

Barbiturates are transported through the placenta to the fetus and may thus cause depression

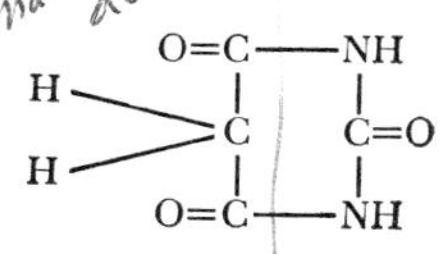

Barbituric Acid

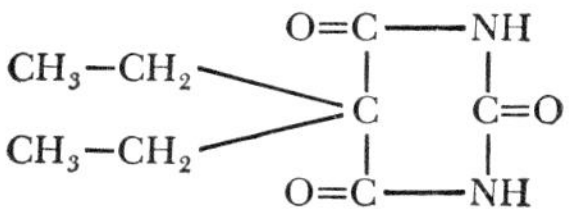

Barbital
(Veronal)

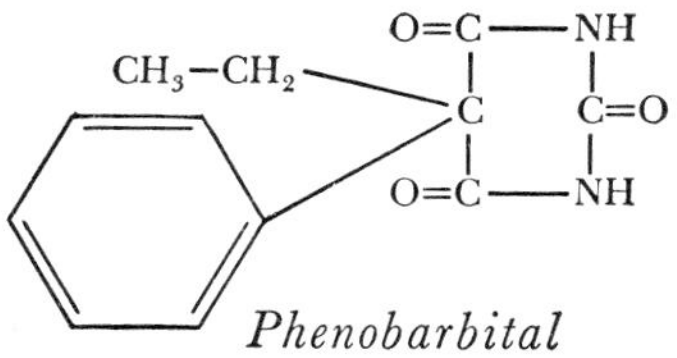

Phenobarbital
(Luminal)

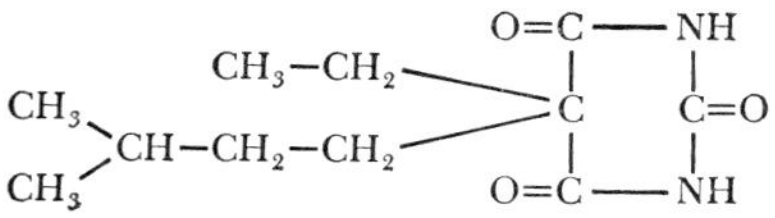

'Amytal'
(Amobarbital)

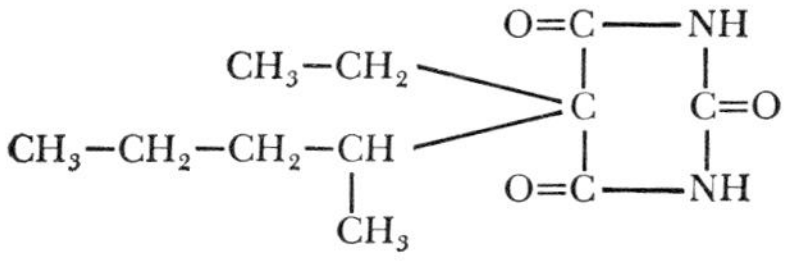

Pentobarbital
(Nembutal)

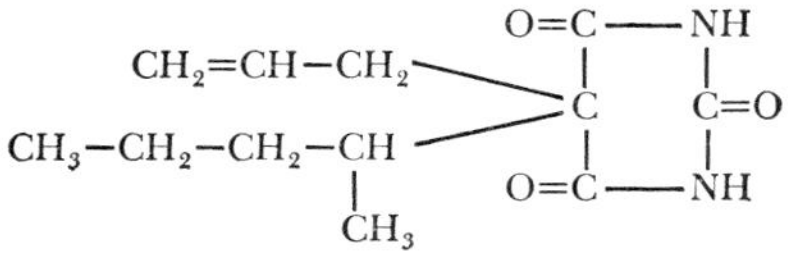

'Seconal'
(Secobarbital)

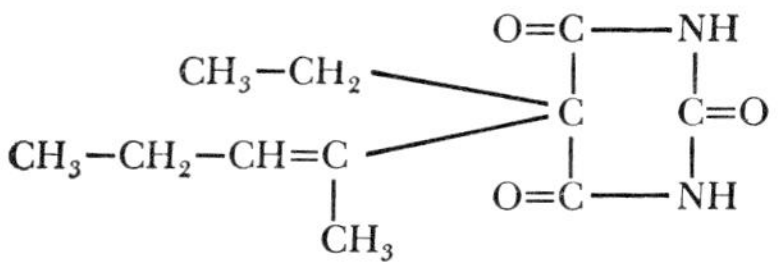

Vinbarbital
(Delvinal)

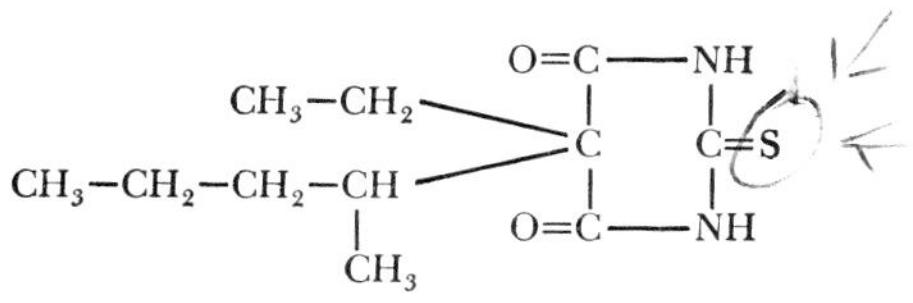

Pentothal
(Thiopental)

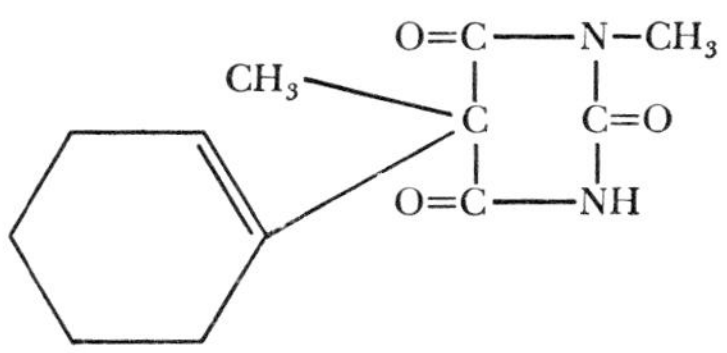

Evipal

FIGURE 25—*Structural Formulas of the Barbiturates*

of the newborn when excessive doses are used in obstetrics. The barbiturates may appear in breast milk but not in sufficient amounts to harm a nursing infant.

The body eliminates barbiturates in two ways— by excretion through the kidneys and by destruction in the liver. The longer-acting compounds barbital and phenobarbital depend to a greater extent upon the kidneys for elimination, which probably accounts in part for their prolonged effect. As much as 85 percent of the total amount of barbital administered has been recovered in the urine, and the drug may be excreted for a period of several days. Damage to renal tissue appreciably extends the period of action of barbital and phenobarbital. The shorter-acting drugs are broken down in the body, probably in the liver, and are not recovered in the urine when the dosage is within the sedative range. These drugs do not depend upon an intact renal system for excretion, but their effect is prolonged when there is extensive liver damage.

Clinical Use—The barbiturates may be given orally, rectally, intramuscularly, or intravenously. The oral route is the one most commonly used, and the desired depth of sedative or hypnotic effect is obtained through proper selection of drug and dose. Rectal administration may be indicated in infants or in patients who do not tolerate drugs orally. In extreme emergencies, when very prompt action is required, barbiturates may be given intravenously as sodium salts. (Of course, the ultrashort-acting barbiturates administered for surgical anesthesia must of necessity be given intravenously.) However, the intravenous route is not without danger, and special caution must be observed in preparing solutions and in making injections (see p. 394). In lesser emergencies or when intravenous administration is not practical, the drugs can be given intramuscularly. Because of the alkalinity of the salts, they are not suited for subcutaneous injection.

A large number of barbiturates are available for clinical use. Closely related compounds give essentially the same therapeutic effects; small variations in pharmacologic action have no clinical significance. The sodium salts act somewhat more rapidly than the free acids, and slightly larger doses are generally required to produce the same effect. Therefore, selection of a barbiturate for a given clinical indication depends primarily on its duration of action and the physician's experience with the drug. Selection of the free barbiturate or the sodium salt (when both forms are available) depends on how quickly the onset is desired. Four groups of compounds are recognized; they, their principal members, and their average dosage are presented in Table 41.

Infants and children are said to tolerate relatively larger doses than adults, but this probably is explained by differences in mental reactions. Most adults readily accept sedation or hypnosis and co-operate by mental adjustment. Under stress, young patients rarely have the ability to acquire mental composure, and consequently they maintain resistance to the disturbing situation. In children, therefore, the barbiturates often must be used as chemical brakes in doses approaching the upper limits of tolerance. This requires considerable caution, since, on the basis of weight, toxicity is probably the same in infants and adults. Average doses have been suggested on the basis of age, but these should be modified according to the condition and the response of the patient. Table 42 may be used as a guide for oral or rectal administration of long, moderate, and short-acting barbiturates.

SEDATIVE ACTION—Sedation may be useful in many disorders, including hypertension, undesirable effects from cerebral stimulants (ephedrine, xanthine diuretics, etc.), hyperthyroidism, paralysis agitans, dysmenorrhea, chorea, allergic

TABLE 41—*Principal Barbiturates, Their Duration of Action, and Their Average Adult Hypnotic Dose**

Long-Acting	Moderate-Acting	Short-Acting	Ultrashort-Acting (for Anesthesia)
Barbital, 0.3 to 0.5 Gm.	'Amytal' and 'Amytal Sodium,' 0.1 to 0.3 Gm.	'Seconal' and 'Seconal Sodium,' 0.1 to 0.2 Gm.	Pentothal Sodium
Phenobarbital and phenobarbital sodium, 0.1 to 0.2 Gm.	Pentobarbital sodium, 0.1 to 0.2 Gm.	Vinbarbital Sodium (Delvinal Sodium), 0.1 to 0.2 Gm.	Evipal Soluble

* The sedative dose is usually one-fourth to one-third the hypnotic dose and may be repeated three or four times daily.

TABLE 42—*Average Dosage of Barbiturates*
on the Basis of Age

1 to 3 months................0.015 to 0.03 Gm.
(1/4 to 1/2 grain)
3 to 6 months................0.03 to 0.05 Gm.
(1/2 to 3/4 grain)
6 to 36 months................0.05 to 0.065 Gm.
(3/4 to 1 grain)
3 to 8 years.................0.05 to 0.10 Gm.
(3/4 to 1 1/2 grains)
8 to 15 years.................0.065 to 0.12 Gm.
(1 to 2 grains)

disorders, nausea or vomiting of functional origin, motion sickness, labyrinthitis, heart failure, reactions to immunizations, spasmodic croup, emotional crises, and nervous tension. It may also allay nervousness and apprehension related to infectious and other diseases or to diagnostic and therapeutic procedures, particularly with pediatric patients and in connection with surgical procedures.

Usually the longer-acting barbiturates are prescribed when continuous or prolonged sedation is indicated; but in the presence of impaired kidney function (as in hypertension), the moderately long-acting drugs are preferred because they are destroyed in the body and do not depend upon the kidneys for elimination. They have a sufficiently long duration of action for use in prolonged sedation and may be prescribed three or four times daily without danger of cumulative effect.

HYPNOTIC ACTION—The ability of the barbiturates to induce sleep is employed to relieve insomnia caused by mental unrest, excitement, fear, worry, apprehension, or extreme fatigue. Sleeplessness caused by physical discomfort does not respond well to these compounds. Usually a rapid onset of hypnotic effect with a short duration of action is desirable; for, once started, sleep will in most cases continue normally. 'Seconal Sodium' is ideal for this purpose; in adequate dosage it usually brings sleep within fifteen to twenty minutes, and its effect is dissipated within a few hours. The patient wakens refreshed and free of the aftereffects which sometimes are apparent following use of longer-acting barbiturates. Rarely is more than 0.1 Gm. (1 1/2 grains) of 'Seconal Sodium' needed, and often 0.05 Gm. (3/4 grain) is sufficient.

For those patients who sleep well during the first part of the night but who have insomnia during the early morning hours, 'Enseals' 'Seconal Sodium' may be prescribed. Because of their coating, these tablets release the barbiturate in the intestine after a period of four to seven hours, and a dose taken at bedtime becomes effective several hours later.

When prompt but more prolonged hypnotic effect is required, Tuinal may be prescribed. This product, which combines equal parts of 'Seconal Sodium' and 'Amytal Sodium,' may be given in doses of 0.1 Gm. (1 1/2 grains) for simple insomnia. For more profound hypnosis of longer duration, 0.2 Gm. (3 grains) may be administered.

The type of insomnia encountered or the physical disorder which may be associated with it may make necessary the administration of a longer-acting barbiturate. In the order of increasing duration of action, 'Seconal Sodium' is followed by pentobarbital sodium, 'Amytal Sodium,' 'Amytal,' barbital, and phenobarbital.

It should be noted that use of a barbiturate night after night usually is not good practice. It is more logical for the physician to investigate the cause of insomnia and prescribe measures for its correction rather than to countenance continued use of hypnotic drugs.

ANTICONVULSANT ACTION—The barbiturates are effective in controlling convulsions. The sodium salts of the moderate or short-acting preparations are employed intramuscularly or intravenously in convulsions due to fever, eclampsia, cerebral hemorrhage, tetanus, rabies, local anesthetic agents, and overdoses of certain drugs such as picrotoxin and strychnine, and in convulsions occurring during general anesthesia.

'Amytal Sodium,' for example, is particularly effective in the spasms of tetanus (p. 12). The initial dose may be 0.5 Gm. (7 1/2 grains) parenterally. Control may then be maintained by doses of 0.3 to 0.8 Gm. (5 to 12 grains) by mouth or rectum every four hours. The dosage of pentobarbital sodium or phenobarbital sodium is similar, in case one of them is preferred. The respirations and degree of muscular relaxation should be noted carefully because, when convulsions cease, deep coma with respiratory failure may supervene if too much barbiturate has been given.

'Seconal Sodium' may be preferred for some cases of tetanus (particularly in children) and for convulsions from other causes, because of its rapid onset and short duration of action. Doses for oral or rectal administration are calculated on the basis of 0.2 to 0.25 Gm. (3 to 4 grains) every three to four hours for a five-year-old child.

Phenobarbital is also of value in convulsions due to transient causes. It is the drug of choice in the symptomatic treatment of epilepsy; its use in this condition is discussed on page 170.

PREMEDICATION FOR ANESTHESIA—Hypnotic doses of the short or moderately long-acting barbiturates are employed extensively as premedication for local, regional, and inhalation anesthesia. They allay apprehension and fear, facilitate smooth induction of inhalation anesthesia, and reduce the amount of anesthetic required. When morphine and atropine are used preoperatively with a barbiturate, their dosage should be reduced because of synergistic action and possible respiratory depression.

As ANESTHETIC AGENTS—Most barbiturates are not satisfactory anesthetic agents, but the ultrashort-acting compounds such as Pentothal Sodium and Evipal Soluble (the sodium salt) are widely used. They are not well suited to prolonged operations and should in general be limited to procedures requiring twenty minutes or less. Since they are given intravenously, their action is prompt and not without untoward side-effects. Therefore, they should be administered by an adequately trained anesthetist. This form of anesthesia is contraindicated in patients with impaired liver function, shock, hypotension, pulmonary disease, or debilitation.

IN OBSTETRICS—The barbiturates have been employed extensively to produce amnesia in obstetric patients. The initial dose is administered when labor is definitely established, with regular pains and beginning dilation of the cervix. The patient is encouraged to take fluids and to relax and sleep between contractions. Average doses are shown in Table 43. Very large doses are inadvisable; quantities sufficient to produce complete analgesia or amnesia carry a risk of respiratory and vascular depression in the mother. The larger doses also seem to contribute to increased restlessness. Supplemental medication during the first and second stages of labor may include morphine, scopolamine, paraldehyde, or rectal oil-ether in doses adjusted downward to allow for synergism.

The barbiturates pass through the placenta to enter the fetal circulation and may exert a depressant effect upon the infant. Occasionally there is difficulty in resuscitating the child following birth, but this does not occur if the doses are carefully adjusted to the mother's requirements and are kept within the low range. Barbiturates, like opiates and other drugs which may affect fetal respiration adversely, should be withheld if delivery is anticipated within two hours from the time the medication is to be administered. Suspected immaturity of the fetus is an indication for extreme caution in the use of any hypnotic or analgesic drug; consideration should be given to local or regional anesthesia for management of the labor.

IN PSYCHIATRY—Production of narcosis and controlled hypnosis has become an accepted procedure for certain psychiatric patients. 'Amytal Sodium' has been selected as the drug of choice and usually is given by slow intravenous injection. Depending upon the effect desired, doses vary from 0.2 to 0.6 Gm. (3 to 9 grains).

PARENTERAL ADMINISTRATION—When prompt action is essential, the barbiturates can be given parenterally. Intramuscular injection is safer than intravenous but does not take effect as rapidly. 'Amytal Sodium' is ordinarily administered as a 10 percent solution; pentobarbital sodium, 'Seconal Sodium,' and phenobarbital sodium, as 5 percent. For intramuscular injection, not more than 5 cc. should be deposited at any one site.

Intravenous injection should be slow; with the solutions mentioned above, the rate should not exceed 1 cc. per minute. Rapid injection carries two serious dangers: (1) the risk of immediate collapse (speed shock; see p. 285), and (2) the possibility of serious overdosage. The *full* effect of intravenously administered phenobarbital and pentobarbital may be somewhat delayed; unless the injection is made very slowly, the eventual degree of depression may be underestimated. Regardless of

TABLE 43—*Average Doses of Barbiturates in Obstetrics*

	'Seconal Sodium'	'Amytal Sodium'	Pentobarbital Sodium
Initial dose when labor is definitely established	0.2 to 0.3 Gm. (3 to 4 1/2 grs.)	0.2 to 0.4 Gm. (3 to 6 grs.)	0.1 to 0.2 Gm. (1 1/2 to 3 grs.)
Subsequent doses at 1 to 3-hour intervals	0.1 to 0.2 Gm. (1 1/2 to 3 grs.)	0.2 to 0.4 Gm. (3 to 6 grs.)	0.1 to 0.2 Gm. (1 1/2 to 3 grs.)
Total dose	0.8 Gm. (12 grs.)	1 Gm. (15 1/2 grs.)	0.5 Gm. (7 1/2 grs.)

any previous decision regarding dosage, the desired therapeutic effect should be constantly watched for during injection; and if it begins to develop sooner than anticipated, administration should be stopped immediately.

Doses for parenteral administration vary with the condition of the patient and the effect desired. Maximum single doses are 1 Gm. (15 grains) of 'Amytal Sodium' and 0.5 Gm. (7 1/2 grains) of pentobarbital sodium or 'Seconal Sodium.' Average doses are much smaller.

Solutions of 'Seconal Sodium,' 'Amytal Sodium,' pentobarbital sodium, and phenobarbital sodium for parenteral administration should be prepared only from the sealed ampoules of sterile anhydrous drug. They should be prepared with sterile distilled water, which is introduced slowly into the ampoule by means of a sterile syringe and needle. The ampoule is then rotated to facilitate solution; several minutes may be required. Shaking should be avoided. If solutions are not absolutely clear after being prepared for five minutes, they should be discarded. Since these solutions are affected by exposure to air, no more than thirty minutes should elapse from the time an ampoule is opened until it is used.

Contraindications and Side-Effects—The barbiturates should be prescribed with caution in patients with advanced cardiovascular-renal disease or impaired liver function. When kidney damage is present, the shorter-acting drugs which are destroyed in the liver are preferred. In the presence of extensive liver damage, even these should be used cautiously.

Unusual reactions are likely to be encountered in hyperthyroidism, diabetes mellitus, severe anemia, and cardiac failure; the barbiturates may be valuable drugs in these conditions, but they should be employed carefully. Debilitated patients and those of advanced age may respond more profoundly than younger individuals, and therefore smaller doses are indicated. Patients with pulmonary infections should not be given amounts sufficient to impair the cough reflex. Prolonged use of large doses of a barbiturate is inadvisable during pregnancy; such chronic administration may harm the fetus because of its greater susceptibility to these drugs.

The effect of barbiturates is potentiated by morphine and its analogues, and the depression produced is considerably prolonged. Alcohol also is synergistic.

Toxic reactions to barbiturates may occur in the course of clinical use as a result of overdosage or because of individual susceptibility to the drug, but death from the doses used for sedation and hypnosis is practically unknown. Hypersensitivity may be manifested in a number of ways. Ordinary doses in susceptible individuals may produce temporary mental disturbances characterized by excitement, delirium, and even hallucinations. Skin eruptions due to phenobarbital have not been unusual, and hyperpyrexia has been noted following barbiturate medication.

Habituation to the barbiturates parallels alcoholism and narcotic addiction in certain respects. The patient who has developed dependence on a barbiturate usually employs the drug as an escape mechanism (see p. 147). For this reason, it is frequently almost impossible to correct the condition without psychiatric treatment. There is no specific regimen to follow when an attempt is made to overcome habituation. A desire to co-operate must be manifested by the patient. Abrupt withdrawal has been practiced and appears to provide satisfactory results in some cases. However, when large quantities of barbiturates have been ingested for a long time, abrupt withdrawal may be followed by convulsive seizures or psychotic manifestations or both. Under such circumstances, the drug may be withdrawn gradually or some other sedative may be substituted and later withdrawn. In ordinary cases, small quantities of the bromides and belladonna may be helpful during the trying period of the first few days. Adequate rest and freedom from worry should be encouraged.

Barbiturate Poisoning—Severe acute barbiturate poisoning usually when five to ten times the full oral, hypnotic dose is taken; and when fifteen times the usual dose is absorbed, fatality is likely to result. Death has resulted from the combined effects of a barbiturate and alcohol when each was present in a concentration which was high but ordinarily would not have been fatal.

The common symptoms of acute barbiturate poisoning are drowsiness, mental confusion, and headache, with the depression progressing to profound sleep or coma. Mild excitement, along with ataxia and slurring speech similar to that seen with alcoholic intoxication, may precede depression. The pulse is weak and rapid, and respiration is depressed to such an extent that anoxia becomes evident. The blood pressure and temperature fall, although the latter may rise again above normal levels. The skin becomes moist and cyanotic, and the pupils first contract and then dilate as anoxia supervenes. The reflexes become sluggish and the urine scanty.

In the management of severe barbiturate intoxication, close supervision of the patient is essential. If there is respiratory embarrassment, an adequate airway is provided and oxygen is administered. Repeated tracheal suction may be needed to clear obstructing mucus. If there is evidence of circulatory collapse (p. 63), oxygen therapy is supplemented by, first, transfusion of plasma or whole blood and, later, electrolyte and dextrose solutions. In some patients, artificial respiration (with a tight-fitting face mask and oxygen rebreather bag) may be necessary for a time. In most patients gastric lavage is desirable, even if the drug was taken some hours before. Catharsis may be beneficial, and for this purpose 2 to 3 oz. of a saline cathartic such as sodium phosphate may be left in the stomach after the last washing. The patient's position should be changed frequently and body temperature maintained.

In mild cases, adequate stimulation may be provided by hypodermic administration of 25 to 50 mg. (3/8 to 3/4 grain) of ephedrine sulfate and 0.5 Gm. (7 1/2 grains) of caffeine and sodium benzoate. Intoxication may be considered to be severe if unconsciousness prior to hospitalization was prolonged, if coma is associated with loss of reflexes, or if respiratory depression is evident. In such cases, more powerful stimulation is required.

Probably the most effective agent for severe barbiturate poisoning is picrotoxin (p. 389). It is, however, a potentially dangerous drug which must be used with due care. The diagnosis of barbiturate poisoning should be definitely established before administration of picrotoxin, for the drug may prove disastrous if the patient is not suffering from such intoxication. Furthermore, it should be employed only in severe cases.

For patients in coma, administration may begin with intravenous injection at the rate of 3 mg. per minute, which may be continued until the corneal reflex returns or signs of stimulation occur (such as increased respiratory activity, muscular twitching, or oscillation of the eyeballs). This state is then maintained by repetition of similar or smaller doses as the patient again becomes more depressed; a common requirement is 3 to 6 mg. every hour or two, but doses may have to be repeated every fifteen minutes. If the patient is receiving intravenous fluids, the injections may be made into the rubber tubing. Otherwise, maintenance doses may well be given intramuscularly.

Active reflexes and involuntary movements should be demonstrable at all times. There is great individual variation in the amount of picrotoxin needed, and as much as 1 or 2 Gm. has been employed in extreme cases. Overdosage of picrotoxin is to be carefully avoided. It is manifested by convulsions.

Metrazol (p. 389) is also effective as a central stimulant, but its brief action has appeared to make it best applicable as an index to the depth of coma in barbiturate poisoning. A dose of 100 mg. is given intravenously. If there is no reaction within a few minutes, 200 mg. are administered. Doses of 300 and, finally, 400 mg. are then injected if there is still no response. Such test doses are repeated periodically and serve as indices to the condition of the patient and the dosage of picrotoxin.

When the patient begins to respond with preconvulsive twitchings to progressively smaller doses of picrotoxin, cortical stimulation with methamphetamine (p. 428) or d-amphetamine (Dexedrine) (p. 429) may be undertaken. Doses of 10 to 30 mg. are given by slow intravenous injection at intervals of thirty to sixty minutes until some degree of consciousness returns. If injection is too rapid, laryngospasm may develop. Blood pressure usually increases after each dose, as does the quality of respiration. Overdoses may produce temporary hypertension.

Stimulatory treatment is tapered off gradually. With severe poisoning by long-acting barbiturates (such as phenobarbital), it may have to be continued for five to seven days. Patients must be observed for several days for the possibility of relapse. Ample fluids and diuretic agents such as the xanthines (p. 358) may aid excretion of the drug. Despite frequent changes of position, most patients with severe intoxication develop pneumonia. They may therefore be given antibiotics prophylactically.

After recovery, patients who have voluntarily taken overdoses of barbiturates should be placed under the care of a psychiatrist.

CHRONIC INTOXICATION with the barbiturates may occur, particularly with the long-acting drugs. It develops gradually when barbiturates have been taken over a long period in doses sufficient to produce a cumulative toxic effect. The symptoms may present striking incongruities and, unless the physician is suspicious of drug intoxication, are easily confused with other syndromes, such as paresis, encephalitis, multiple sclerosis, brain tumor, and acute psychosis. Drowsiness, loss of mental acuity, failing memory, incoherent speech, mental depression, confusion, and disorientation may be present.

In more severe cases there are neurological findings also: vertigo, ataxia, nystagmus, diplopia, strabismus, paresis of the limbs, and numbness and tingling. Deep reflexes may be increased, decreased, or absent entirely. Gastro-intestinal disturbances may occur, such as anorexia, obstipation, foul breath, and coated tongue. There may be an erythematous, pruritic rash, particularly with phenobarbital intoxication. This may involve the tongue and produce an appearance somewhat like that in measles or scarlet fever. Fever may be present. Examination of the urine may show protein and casts. Sometimes there is loss of weight and secondary anemia.

Treatment of chronic intoxication involves, first, withdrawal of the drug; then, provision of adequate nutrition and other supportive measures; and finally, if possible, treatment of the condition for which the drug was originally taken. Improvement may require three weeks to a month.

THE BROMIDES

The bromide ion produces depression of the central nervous system. It is administered as the sodium, potassium, or ammonium salt, each of which is a water-soluble, saline-tasting, crystalline powder. Bromine-containing organic compounds which do not release the element in ionic form do not have sedative properties.

Bromides were formerly much used as sedatives and hypnotics. Because of their slow onset of action and potential toxicity, they have largely been replaced by the barbiturates. They have anticonvulsant activity and sometimes can be used to advantage in epilepsy when other anticonvulsive drugs have failed to give proper control.

In therapeutic doses, bromides cause mental calmness, sedation, drowsiness, and sleep. The sleep is neither as deep nor as refreshing as that produced by the barbiturates, chloral hydrate, or paraldehyde and often is followed by a so-called hangover. Larger doses impair mental function and cause motor in-co-ordination, lethargy, disorientation, delirium, stupor, and coma.

The soluble bromide salts are readily absorbed from the gastro-intestinal tract in a manner similar to chlorides. High concentrations in the stomach produce gastritis and, occasionally, vomiting, which can be avoided by administering the drugs after meals or with large amounts of water.

Bromide is excreted in the urine in the same manner as chloride—in fact, the kidneys do not distinguish between them. If there is a relative deficiency of chloride in the body, bromide will be retained as well. If there is a relative excess of chloride so that excretion is high, bromide will be excreted also. Under ordinary circumstances, 1 Gm. of sodium bromide may require two to three weeks for complete excretion.

Exact dose recommendations for bromides cannot be given. Moderate sedation in adults can usually be obtained with 3 to 5 Gm. of sodium bromide daily. This amount may be toxic in the presence of dehydration, impaired renal function, or an inadequate diet with low chloride intake. For epilepsy, the dose is the smallest amount that will control the individual case; it should not be sufficient to increase the blood bromide level above 125 mg. per 100 cc. Adults usually require an average of 1 to 3 Gm. three times daily.

There is some variation in the bromine content of the several inorganic salts, but this is not of clinical significance. However, the basic ion may be of some importance when large doses are given. In epilepsy, for example, in which the hydrating effect of sodium is undesirable, potassium bromide or a mixture of sodium, potassium, and ammonium bromides may be employed. Ammonium bromide has an acidifying and dehydrating effect similar to that of ammonium chloride (see p. 350).

Bromism, or poisoning from prolonged use of bromides, continues to occur even though more efficient and less dangerous sedatives and hypnotics are available. The symptoms, which develop slowly and insidiously, are influenced individually by constitutional and personality factors. They may include any or all of the following: impaired mental processes, loss of memory, drowsiness, dermatitis or bromide rash, disturbed consciousness, disorientation, and emotional disturbances; and, in severe cases, delirium, delusions, vivid auditory and visual hallucinations, violent mania, lethargy, and coma. Neurological manifestations include tremors of the hands, lips, and tongue, speech defects, weakness, sluggishness of movement, motor in-co-ordination, faulty gait, ataxia, altered deep or superficial reflexes, and a positive Babinski sign.

Bromism may be confused with chronic alcoholism, encephalitis, and similar entities. The blood level of bromide provides an index to the presence and severity of intoxication. One to 1.5 mg. bromide per 100 cc. serum are normally present. Levels above 100 mg. per 100 cc. are likely to be associated with toxic symptoms. Psychosis may appear at a level of 150 to 250 mg. However, the presence or absence of symptoms depends also on other factors, such as the state of general health and nutrition, hydration, chloride intake, and state of renal function.

The treatment of bromide poisoning is begun by removing all possible sources of the drug. A daily dose of 4 to 10 Gm. of sodium chloride is given by mouth to hasten excretion of the bromide ion. Fluid intake is maintained at not less than 4,000 cc. per day. Constipation is relieved if present. Skin lesions usually clear spontaneously but may be treated with antipruritic lotions for symptomatic relief. Such procedures as cold, wet-sheet baths and continuous tub baths may be given to allay insomnia and excitement. Sedatives are usually contraindicated; but when required to control extreme excitement, morphine or, preferably, paraldehyde may be used. Recovery usually is complete in three or four weeks.

CHLORAL HYDRATE

Chloral hydrate, $CCl_3 \cdot CH(OH)_2$, is a chlorinated derivative of ethyl alcohol employed principally as a sedative and soporific. The drug has little effect upon blood pressure, respiration, or the heart. It is absorbed readily from the gastro-intestinal tract and eliminated by the urine.

The principal uses of chloral hydrate are similar to those of the barbiturates and paraldehyde, although the barbiturates are used more frequently. Chloral hydrate as a sedative will produce an effect in ten or fifteen minutes, and sleep occurs within an hour. The sleep resulting from this drug is quiet, deep, and unaccompanied by dreams and lasts five to eight hours. The patient may be readily aroused and suffers no aftereffects. The drug is also useful for persons undergoing morphine or alcohol withdrawal and in delirium tremens. Chloral hydrate is contraindicated in persons suffering renal or hepatic impairment, severe cardiac disease, or gastritis. It is not suitable for general anesthesia because of the high dose required. As with all hypnotics, its powers as an analgesic are weak. The drug has an unpleasant taste and a tendency to produce gastric irritation.

The usual hypnotic dose is 0.5 to 1 Gm., although as much as 2 Gm. may be given if necessary. It is administered by mouth or, in oil solution, by rectum. It should not be given in an alcoholic vehicle because of a possible increase in toxicity. It is too irritating for parenteral administration. The lethal dose is approximately 10 Gm., although death has occurred from smaller doses.

Steady use of chloral hydrate is hazardous, since the drug operates within a narrow margin of safety.

Individuals may develop tolerance which may be suddenly broken by liver damage or at the time of an overdose, and death may result. Acute chloral intoxication may manifest itself by stupor, extreme vasodilation, low blood pressure, fall in body temperature, slow respiration, and cyanosis. There may also be gastric irritation, vomiting, pin-point pupils, and a skin rash. Acute poisoning may be treated by gastric lavage, warmth, circulatory and respiratory stimulants, and artificial respiration when needed. In chronic poisoning, the most certain procedures are withdrawal of the drug and measures to build up the patient's health, besides correcting the cause of the habituation.

PARALDEHYDE

Paraldehyde is a polymer of acetaldehyde with an action on the central nervous system similar to that of chloral hydrate. It is absorbed rapidly from the gastro-intestinal tract and from intramuscular sites of injection. It is thought to be destroyed to the extent of about 80 percent in the liver, the remainder being excreted mostly by the lungs. The drug should not be used in the presence of liver disease or gastroenteritis. It is difficult to dispense in palatable form.

Although paraldehyde produces hypnosis more promptly than any other sedative, it is little used in ambulatory cases because of the offensive odor it imparts to the breath. Under suitable conditions, however, it is a desirable hypnotic which produces sleep in ten to fifteen minutes without aftereffects. These properties make it useful when rapid sedation is required, as in delirium tremens and strychnine or cocaine convulsions.

The usual dose is 3 to 8 cc., which may be increased to 10 or 15 cc. if necessary. In delirium tremens, the dose is 15 to 30 cc. It is generally given by mouth and is perhaps least unpalatable when taken chilled on cracked ice. It may also be administered rectally, dissolved in one or two ounces of oil. In extreme cases it may be injected intravenously, although this route carries with it the possibility of circulatory collapse or pulmonary edema. Intravenous dosage is 4 to 5 cc. It should be given very slowly, and medication should be stopped as soon as the desired degree of depression is reached.

ANALGESICS AND ANTIPYRETICS

The analgesic and antipyretic drugs include a small, heterogeneous group of compounds which are used principally for the symptomatic relief of pain and fever. The salicylates, acetanilid, aceto-phenetidin, antipyrine, aminopyrine, and cincho-phen affect both pain and fever. When they were first used in medicine, their antipyretic action was considered the most important, but today they are employed chiefly to produce analgesia. The opium alkaloids and the synthetic morphine substitutes have no antipyretic action but are outstanding analgesics. Colchicine is included for its pain-relieving properties in acute gout, but since it is of no value in other types of pain, it cannot be classed as a true analgesic.

Quinine is only weakly antipyretic except against the fever of malaria, which it controls directly by destruction of the parasites. It also has analgesic properties quite similar to those of the salicylates and, therefore, is used in many coryza remedies. Alcohol produces analgesia, euphoria, and hypnosis. Its effect on the pain threshold is more prompt and slightly greater than that of aspirin. Caffeine alone does not relieve pain, but frequently it is combined with the weaker analgesic drugs for the control of headache. Its mode of action is not clear but may be associated with cerebral vascular changes. Barbiturates potentiate the action of analgesics but do not themselves reduce pain. Analgesics do not potentiate the hypnotic action of barbiturates. Other drugs such as the anesthetics and antispasmodics relieve pain but are not classed as analgesics because of differences in modes of action.

Opium Alkaloids and Synthetic Morphine Substitutes

Opium is obtained from the milky exudate (latex) of the unripe seed capsules of the Oriental poppy, *Papaver somniferum*. It contains many alkaloids, of which morphine, codeine, and papaverine are clinically important. Papaverine is quite different chemically, pharmacologically, and therapeutically from morphine and codeine; it is discussed on page 363.

Morphine is the most important of the opium alkaloids. A large number of derivatives have been prepared from it; those of greatest interest are dihydromorphinone (Dilaudid), methyldihydro-morphinone (metopon), diacetylmorphine (heroin), and apomorphine (for which, see p. 387). Pantopon is a purified mixture of opium alkaloids containing about 50 percent morphine; its properties closely resemble those of morphine. Two compounds have been synthesized which are chemically unrelated to morphine and lack many of its

disadvantages but are nevertheless potent analgesics; they are methadon and Demerol (isonipecaine).

MORPHINE

Morphine is the principal member of the phenanthrene group of opium alkaloids. It constitutes about 10 percent of opium. Its structural formula is shown in Figure 26. The outstanding therapeutic property of morphine is its ability to relieve pain. This is believed to be accomplished by a selective action on pain centers in the optic thalami. Con-

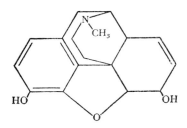

Morphine

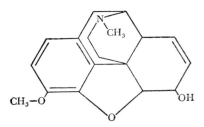

Codeine

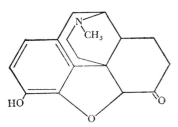

Dihydromorphinone (Dilaudid)

FIGURE 26—*Structural Formulas of Morphine and Certain Derivatives*

tinuous dull pain is relieved more readily than sharp intermittent pain, and larger doses are required to control existing pain than that beginning after medication has taken effect. For some reason, the pain of tabetic crises is peculiarly resistant. In the presence of severe pain, analgesia is obtained before the pain threshold has reached its maximum. This is due to alteration in the pattern of reaction; although the individual continues to be aware of the pain, he is not disturbed and tolerates it without anxiety or fear. In addition to these direct effects on pain threshold and reaction pattern, the opiate promotes sleep, which in itself raises the threshold as much as 50 percent.

Administration of morphine in moderate doses (up to 15 mg. in an adult) produces euphoria, muscular relaxation, freedom from anxiety, rapid flow of uncontrolled thought and imagination, inability to concentrate, lethargy, dimness of vision, apathy, and eventually sleep. Respiration is depressed, the pupils are somewhat constricted, hunger is abolished, and vomiting may occur. With full therapeutic doses (15 to 20 mg.), the psychological effects give way shortly to deep dreamless sleep; respirations are definitely slowed, and the pupils are considerably constricted. Recovery from large doses is characterized by mental depression, constipation, nausea, and vomiting.

The depression of respiration is due to direct action on the respiratory center and is proportional to the dose. In morphine poisoning, the cause of death is respiratory arrest. The cough reflex is depressed by small doses and is abolished by large ones. Morphine stimulates the reflex centers of the spinal cord and consequently is contraindicated in strychnine poisoning, tetanus, status epilepticus, and similar convulsive states.

The smooth-muscle tone in the gastro-intestinal tract is increased. Thus, gastric emptying is delayed because of decreased peristalsis and contraction of the pyloric sphincter. Similarly, in the small bowel, propulsive peristalsis is diminished and muscular tone is increased; emptying of the large bowel is delayed and there is increased absorption of water, with resultant constipation. The muscular tone and amplitude of contractions of the ureters are increased. Ordinarily this would aggravate the pain of renal colic, but such an effect is overridden by the strong central analgesic action. Large doses of morphine may cause urinary retention due to increase in tone of the bladder sphincter and dulling of bladder sensation. Moderate doses increase considerably the pressure in the biliary tract and may cause epigastric distress or even biliary colic;

but, as in renal colic, the pain is brought under control by central analgesic action.

Therapeutic doses of morphine tend to have a slight bronchoconstrictor and vasodilator action. However, they do not cause significant changes in blood pressure, cardiac action, or body temperature. Although uterine muscle is not affected directly, large doses may interrupt or retard labor because of the parturient's failure to reinforce the uterine contractions by voluntary effort.

Morphine is well absorbed from the gastro-intestinal tract and subcutaneous tissue. It is not absorbed by intact skin but will pass through abraded skin and all mucous membranes. It is not stored appreciably, since withdrawal symptoms appear in addicts within a few hours after the drug is stopped. It readily passes the placental barrier and will cause addiction in infants born of mothers receiving the drug regularly. Morphine is eliminated principally by the kidneys but does appear in all excreta. A large portion is destroyed in the body, probably by the liver.

Indications and Use—Relief of severe pain is the most important therapeutic indication for morphine. As stated previously, the drug is more effective when given before the onset of pain, and dull continuous pain is more readily controlled than is sharp intermittent pain, but sufficiently large doses will relieve almost all types. However, very large doses should be given with the utmost caution for pain that may be relieved suddenly, as by passage of a small ureteral or biliary stone. Under such circumstances, removal of the cause of pain may be followed by the symptoms of acute morphine poisoning (see p. 402).

Morphine is particularly effective for the relief of pain due to smooth-muscle spasm, as in renal or biliary colic. However, papaverine (p. 363) appears to offer a more physiological approach to relief of smooth-muscle spasm. If papaverine is to be used, morphine should be withheld, since it opposes and overrides the relaxing effect of the papaverine. Atropine will overcome morphine-induced ureteral spasm, but it has no effect on biliary spasm. It must be given in large doses to counteract the increased gastro-intestinal muscle tone induced by morphine.

Acute vascular occlusion is an outstanding indication for morphine, regardless of whether the occlusion is coronary, pulmonary, or peripheral. Here, papaverine and morphine are synergistic rather than antagonistic. Morphine is also employed routinely as preanesthetic medication but should

ters, and it appears to have no direct action on the pregnant uterus. In contrast to codeine and to methadon, Demerol is of no value against cough.

Demerol is a mild sedative in ordinary therapeutic doses. Occasionally euphoria is produced. As with morphine, addiction and tolerance occur. The drug does not usually cause significant respiratory depression except in the aged and in the presence of expanding intracranial lesions. Dizziness, particularly in ambulant patients, is the most frequent untoward side-effect; profuse sweating is also common, but nausea and vomiting are noted only occasionally. The drug is readily absorbed and, for the most part, is inactivated in the liver, a small portion being excreted in the urine.

Demerol is used to relieve severe pain, to decrease gastro-intestinal hypermotility, for preanesthetic and postoperative medication, and to produce analgesia during labor. It may be administered orally, but results are less satisfactory than with the intramuscular route. Intravenous injection has been used. Doses of the hydrochloride range from 25 to 150 mg. (3/8 to 2 1/2 grains). For preanesthetic and obstetrical analgesia, doses of 100 to 150 mg. are usually employed.

Drugs Having Both Analgesic and Antipyretic Effects

The drugs having both analgesic and antipyretic effects are less potent against pain than are morphine and its substitutes, but they have the advantage of being non-narcotic. They act in the same manner, namely, by raising the pain threshold through depression of pain centers in the thalamus.

The chief application of compounds in this group is for control of pain associated with arthralgias, neuralgias, myalgias, cephalalgias, and similar conditions. They are of little or no value in the presence of severe pain, particularly if it is of visceral or traumatic origin. Therapeutic doses do not dull consciousness or the special senses, nor do they reduce motor activity.

All analgesics have a maximum effect, or ceiling, beyond which little or no additional increase in the pain threshold is obtained, even though doses are increased considerably. However, the duration of action is prolonged by larger doses. Combinations of analgesic drugs do not increase the maximum effect, the ultimate threshold being that of the most active component. However, a combination of submaximal doses of different analgesics may produce a maximum effect while minimizing the side-effects of each constituent drug.

Ordinary doses of salicylates and related compounds have little effect on normal body temperatures. In the presence of fever, however, these drugs act directly on the heat-regulating centers of the hypothalamic nuclei. Through an unknown mechanism, blood volume is increased at the expense of the extravascular fluids, and there is peripheral vasodilation, increased cutaneous blood flow, and usually sweating. These actions combine to increase the rate of dissipation of body heat. Since heat production is not altered, body temperature falls.

Antipyretics do not act on the etiology of disease but are used (1) to obtain symptomatic relief when fever is the chief cause of distress and (2) to protect against dangerously high temperatures. They do not influence the duration of illness or prevent complications. Their routine use in ordinary, mild fevers is no longer recommended. They may make the diagnosis of unidentified fevers more difficult by distorting the normal pattern of the temperature curve. In the event that the usual therapeutic doses fail to produce the desired effect, large doses should not be employed, since they add little and may be toxic.

SALICYLATES

Salicylates were among the first drugs to be synthesized. Since then, their use has steadily increased. At one time it was believed that compounds derived from natural sources were superior in therapeutic action to the same compounds of synthetic origin. This has now been completely disproved, not only for salicylates but for other compounds as well.

The parent compound is salicylic acid (ortho-hydroxybenzoic acid), the formula of which appears in Figure 28. The hydroxyl group must be in the ortho position; the meta and para-hydroxybenzoic acids are without analgesic properties. Salicylic acid is too irritating for internal use; but by altering either the COOH or the OH group, various compounds suitable for oral administration can be synthesized. Substitution in the COOH radical gives esters of salicylic acid, such as methyl salicylate (oil of wintergreen), whereas retaining the carboxyl group and substituting at OH gives salicylate esters of organic acids, as represented by acetylsalicylic acid (aspirin). Formulas are shown in Figure 28. In addition, simple salts of salicylic acid, such as sodium salicylate, may be prepared.

Salicylic acid and its salts and esters are readily absorbed from the intact skin. The rate varies somewhat, depending upon the length of the carbon side chain. On oral administration, absorption

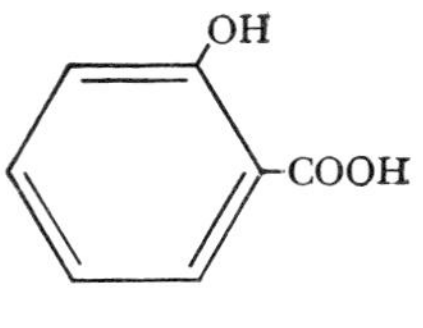

Salicylic Acid

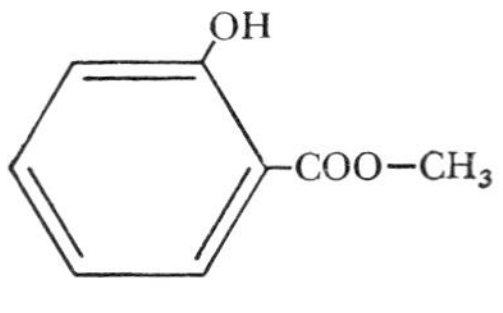

Methyl Salicylate

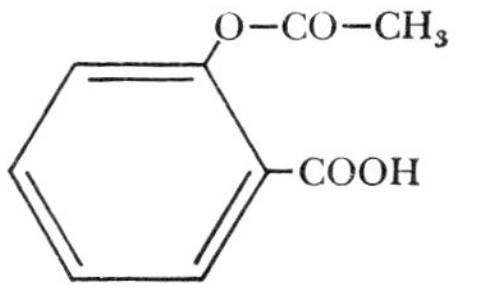

Acetylsalicylic Acid
(Aspirin)

FIGURE 28—*Structural Formulas of Salicylic Acid*
and Certain Derivatives

is influenced by the emptying time of the stomach. The upper intestinal tract absorbs salicylates much faster than the lower, but the difference is not great enough to preclude rectal administration. As a matter of fact, the compounds are among the most rapidly absorbed drugs, regardless of the route of administration.

After ingestion, peak blood levels occur in from one and one-half to four hours, depending on the compound used. Sodium salicylate is absorbed about twice as fast as aspirin. Blood levels are proportional to the dose given. A large part is bound to plasma proteins. There is no selective distribution in the body; salicylate is found in all tissues and fluids but in no higher concentration in pathological fluids (such as joint effusions) than in blood.

Excretion is mainly by way of the urine, although some appears in sweat and saliva. Elimination begins in a few hours and is complete within twenty-four to forty-eight hours. When salicylates are administered, the nonglucose reducing substances in the urine are increased, and false positive tests for sugar may be observed. Excretion is most rapid in alkaline urine (at pH 7.7 the rate is approxi-

mately ten times that at pH 6.0). This explains the apparent increase in tolerance to salicylates when they are given with sodium bicarbonate. Development of gastric disturbance soon after oral administration is due to local irritation; nausea and vomiting of later onset are of central origin. Alkalies relieve both types, the first by local action and the second by increasing renal excretion and thus reducing the blood level. Combined therapy with salicylate and alkali (usually sodium bicarbonate) may reduce plasma levels as much as 33 percent in adults and 50 percent in children. On the other hand, administration of para-aminobenzoic acid decreases urinary excretion and causes plasma levels to rise two to five times.

Salicylates have both analgesic and antipyretic effects (for general discussion, see p. 405). In addition, they increase the urinary excretion of uric acid. Blood prothrombin is reduced by large doses, but whether sufficiently to produce hemorrhage is debated. There is evidence that prothrombin levels return to normal spontaneously even though salicylates are continued; but, on the other hand, cases of severe hemorrhage with low blood prothrombin have been reported. As a precaution, it has been recommended that 1 mg. of menadione (p. 499) be given for each gram of salicylate. If liver function is impaired, much larger doses of vitamin K are required.

Oral administration of sodium salicylate or aspirin sometimes causes immediate vomiting, supposedly due to irritation of the gastric mucosa. However, attempts to demonstrate such irritation in animals and man by direct examination have failed. Abnormally high blood sedimentation rates are sharply reduced by salicylates, and, if the medication is stopped before the underlying condition is removed, a secondary rise will occur. This effect is most evident in initial attacks of rheumatic fever and may not occur in later ones.

The respiratory rate is increased by large doses of salicylates, mainly through direct stimulation of the respiratory center. Occasionally, the hyperpnea is of the Kussmaul type and may be difficult to distinguish from that of diabetic acidosis. Severe dyspnea may develop when plasma levels are 35 mg. percent or above. The increase in respiration produces alkalosis, with decrease in plasma carbon-dioxide level and excretion of an alkaline urine. If continued, the increased bicarbonate excretion may result in secondary acidosis which may proceed to ketosis. Salicylates do not cause primary acidosis.

Free salicylic acid is quite irritating to skin and mucous membranes and is used therapeutically as a keratolytic (see p. 482). Methyl salicylate also is irritating and is used externally in liniments as a counterirritant. Phenyl salicylate (salol) has been used for coating enteric tablets; however, it is not well suited to this purpose. It has also been incorporated into ointments for protection of the skin against ultraviolet rays.

Aspirin (acetylsalicylic acid, 'A.S.A.') is used principally as an antipyretic and for relief of the pain and discomfort of headache, arthralgia, neuralgia, coryza, and acute rheumatic fever. The dosage varies between 0.3 and 1 Gm. (5 and 15 grains), although, as discussed previously, large doses merely prolong the action without adding appreciably to the degree of analgesia. Large doses, 10 to 16 Gm. daily, are used for rheumatic fever (p. 46). Aspirin is unstable in solution and hence cannot be given in liquid form.

Sodium salicylate is comparable in action and dosage to aspirin. In contrast to aspirin, it is quite soluble and may be given intravenously. Although this route is sometimes used, it does not seem to improve results. Since it is not without danger, it cannot be recommended. Sodium salicylate is sometimes injected into local varicosities for its sclerosing effect (see p. 368).

The salicylates occasionally produce mild toxic symptoms of salicylism when given in large doses. The syndrome consists in headache, dizziness, tinnitus, impaired hearing, dimness of vision, mental confusion, sweating, thirst, nausea, vomiting, diarrhea, and increased respiratory and pulse rates. At times there may develop restlessness, incoherent speech, excitement, mania, hallucinations, and delirium. Such reactions may occur after administration of 12 Gm. or more in a period of twelve to twenty-four hours. Recovery usually is prompt if salicylates are withdrawn. Large toxic doses may also cause dyspnea and acidosis, as described previously.

As poisoning progresses, the patient becomes stuporous, lapses into coma, and dies from cardiovascular collapse and respiratory failure. The fatal dose is variable. Death has resulted from oral ingestion of 20 to 40 Gm., and recovery has followed taking as much as 80 Gm. There is no specific antidote for salicylate poisoning.

Idiosyncrasy to salicylates, and particularly to aspirin, usually manifests itself as skin rashes (see p. 227) and anaphylactic-like reactions. The rash may be erythematous, scarlatiniform, pruritic, eczematoid, or desquamative; frequently it is urticarial. In highly sensitive individuals, asthma and angioneurotic edema may develop. It is important to know that most cases of salicylate sensitivity occur in patients with asthma or other forms of allergy.

ACETANILID AND ACETOPHENETIDIN

Acetanilid and acetophenetidin (phenacetin) are effective analgesics and antipyretics; but, because of frequent untoward side-effects, they have largely been replaced by the salicylates. They are chemically related to phenol (hydroxybenzene) and aniline (aminobenzene), as will be seen from their structural formulas (Figure 29). Aniline, itself, is antipyretic but is much too toxic for clinical use. It is believed that the pharmacologic action of these compounds is brought about by conversion in the body to para-aminophenol, which also is toxic when administered in quantity. Alteration of the hydroxyl and amino radicals of para-aminophenol reduces toxicity without significantly impairing activity. A large number of compounds have been prepared, of which acetanilid and acetophenetidin are the important survivors.

The modes of action of acetanilid and acetophenetidin are the same as those of the salicylates (see p. 405). The two drugs are rapidly absorbed from the intestinal tract and are conjugated in the body with glucuronic acid and sulfuric acid, in which form they are promptly excreted in the urine. Their presence may give the urine a dark amber or wine color which, on prolonged exposure to air, may change to dark brown or black. They give a positive indophenol test.

Both compounds are given orally, the average single adult doses being 0.2 Gm. of acetanilid and 0.3 Gm. of acetophenetidin. Neither should be prescribed in combination with antipyrine because liquefaction results. When given with other analgesic drugs, the action is somewhat smoother and more efficient. Such mixtures are less toxic, since the dose of each component is then reduced to one half or less.

Acetanilid is more toxic than acetophenetidin, but neither possesses a high degree of toxicity. Poisoning, either acute or chronic, usually results from medicinal misuse. There is considerable individual variation in susceptibility; although uncommon, fatalities have been reported. Recovery has occurred after ingestion of as much as 8 Gm. of acetanilid, but smaller amounts may be fatal.

Acute poisoning is characterized by formation of methemoglobin and sulfhemoglobin, which cause the skin, mucous membranes, and fingernails to develop a bluish cyanotic color. Spectroscopic examination may detect the altered blood pigment, but the test is not always positive. Symptoms commonly encountered are dyspnea, vertigo, weakness, and anginal pain. Severe cases exhibit vascular collapse, with prostration, rapid shallow respirations, weak pulse, and subnormal temperature. As anoxia progresses, shock may ensue, and terminally there develop collapse, coma, and asphyxial convulsions. There is no specific treatment. Gastric lavage and catharsis are in order if the toxic dose was recently ingested. Artificial respiration, oxygen and carbon-dioxide inhalation, and blood transfusion may be necessary. Administration of alkalies may prevent further precipitation of hemoglobin and aid in the reconversion of methemoglobin. When methemoglobinemia is severe, methylene blue (methylthionine chloride) may be administered intravenously (1 to 2 mg. per Kg. of body weight).

Chronic poisoning from regular continuous ingestion is insidious in onset and may be difficult to diagnose unless a positive history of drug administration can be obtained. It is encountered much more frequently than acute poisoning. Self-administration of these drugs sometimes is continued for long periods without symptoms, when suddenly toxicity develops. The manifestations of chronic poisoning are the same as the early ones of the acute form. In addition, there may be anorexia, digestive disturbances, loss of weight, insomnia, and leukocytosis. Treatment consists in withdrawing the drug, correcting whatever condition may have instigated use of the drug, and administering iron salts for anemia. If the methemoglobinemia does not demand immediate relief, recovery can be accelerated by daily oral administration of 400 to 1,000 mg. of ascorbic acid given in divided doses for several days. When untreated, the bluish discoloration may require several weeks to disappear completely.

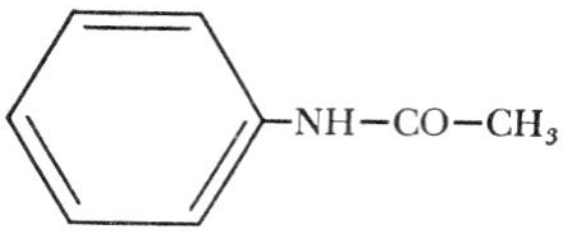

Acetanilid

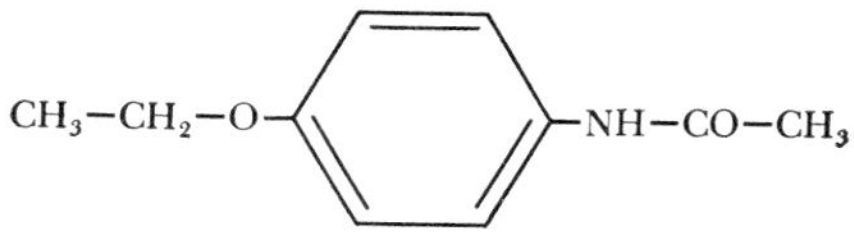

Acetophenetidin
(Phenacetin)

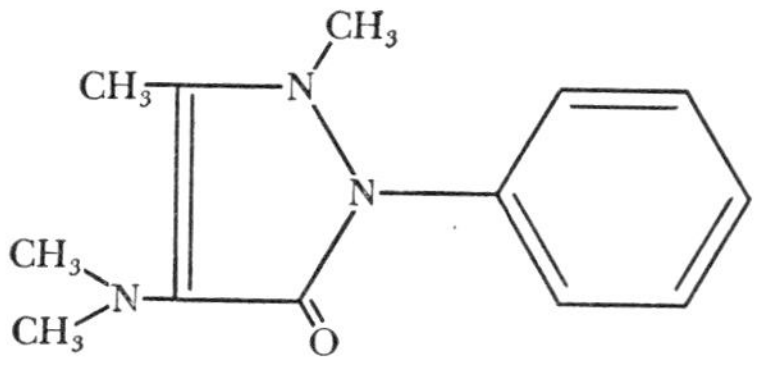

Aminopyrine
(Pyramidon)

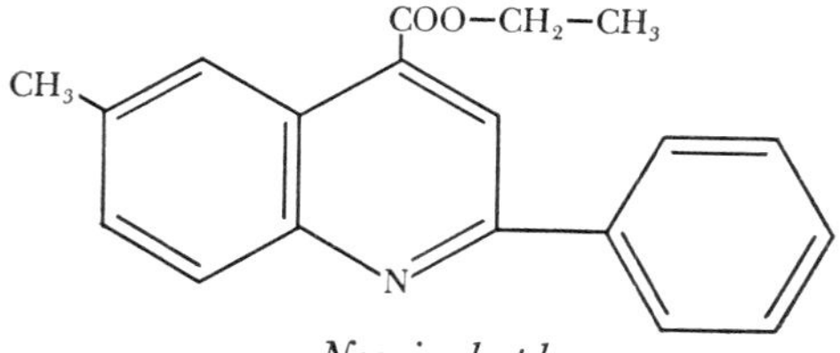

Neocinchophen

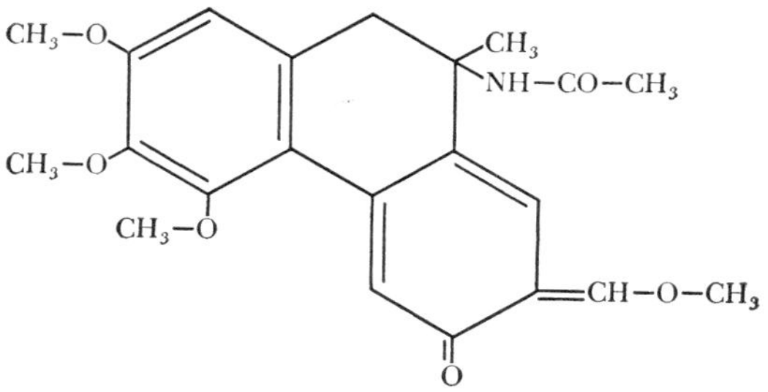

Colchicine

FIGURE 29—*Structural Formulas of Certain Analgesic Drugs*

AMINOPYRINE AND ANTIPYRINE

Aminopyrine (amidopyrine, Pyramidon) and antipyrine (phenazone) were among the early synthetic antipyretic compounds. Like the other antipyretics, they are now more commonly administered for their analgesic effect. In mode of action, they are similar to the salicylates and the aminophenol derivatives (see p. 405). The formula of aminopyrine is shown in Figure 29; antipyrine differs in lacking the dimethylamino group which appears in the lower left-hand corner.

Aminopyrine is considered to be the most active of the non-narcotic analgesics, but it is little used because of its tendency to produce the dangerous side-effect of agranulocytosis (p. 102). The drug is given by mouth in doses of 0.3 Gm. (5 grains) every four hours.

The action of antipyrine is more rapid in onset and of shorter duration than that of aminopyrine. The drug is given orally in doses of 0.3 to 0.6 Gm. about every four hours. Since analgesics are often combined in reduced doses, it should be remembered that liquefaction results if antipyrine is mixed with acetanilid or acetophenetidin.

Poisoning from antipyrine and aminopyrine is quite similar to that from acetanilid and acetophenetidin, except that methemoglobinemia seldom occurs. Allowing for this difference, treatment is the same. Dermatitis medicamentosa is more common with antipyrine, whereas sensitivity to aminopyrine is more often manifested by herpetic lesions about the lips and angioneurotic edema. Agranulocytosis has not been observed with antipyrine.

CINCHOPHEN AND NEOCINCHOPHEN

Cinchophen and neocinchophen are synthetic compounds derived from quinoline carboxylic acid. The formula of neocinchophen is shown in Figure 29; cinchophen differs from it in lacking (1) the ethyl group attached to the carboxylic acid group and (2) the methyl group in the upper left-hand corner. Both compounds have analgesic and antipyretic properties but were introduced into medicine primarily for the treatment of gout (p. 248). They increase the urinary excretion of urates and uric acid in a manner similar to the salicylates but to a considerably greater degree. It is believed that this effect is due to direct alteration of the renal threshold for these substances.

The two drugs are adequately absorbed from the intestinal tract and probably undergo decomposition in the tissues, since only small amounts are excreted in the urine. Both compounds produce minor untoward side-effects consisting in drug rashes, urticaria, gastro-intestinal disturbances, and even anaphylactic-like reactions. Their chief drawback is the severe and often fatal toxic hepatitis that occurs in unpredictable fashion. Neocinchophen is said to be less toxic, but this has not been definitely established. Many authorities believe that neither drug is indispensable, and that responsibility for their use rests entirely with the physician. The use of either is unwarranted if relief can be obtained with salicylates or colchicine.

In chronic gout, cinchophen is given in doses of 0.5 to 1.5 Gm. (7 1/2 to 25 grains) three or four times daily, suspended in large quantities of water. Some recommend limiting use of the drug to three consecutive days per week. The dose of neocinchophen is 0.3 to 0.5 Gm. (5 to 7 1/2 grains) four to six times daily. With either drug, the urine should be alkalinized to prevent precipitation of uric acid in the urinary tract. Acute gout is treated with 0.5 Gm. of cinchophen or 0.3 Gm. of neocinchophen every two or three hours for five or six doses.

COLCHICINE

Colchicine is an alkaloid derived from the seeds and corm of the autumn crocus. It has the formula shown in Figure 29. Colchicine and extracts containing it (colchicum) have long been used em·pirically for the treatment of gout (p. 248). It has no other therapeutic uses. The mechanism of its action is not known. The drug has no effect on uric acid metabolism or on other types of pain.

Colchicine is of little or no value in chronic gout, but it quickly reduces the pain, swelling, and redness of acute attacks, provided therapy is started early. It is best given in the form of tablets because the wine and tincture give irregular results. The dose is 1 mg. repeated every two or three hours. As a rule, symptoms are controlled after four to eight doses.

Side-effects from the use of colchicine are due to overdosage and, regardless of the amount given, appear after a latent period of several hours. They consist in burning sensations in the throat, abdominal pain, nausea, vomiting, and diarrhea which becomes profuse, watery, and bloody. As fluid, electrolyte, and blood plasma are lost and vascular damage takes place, shock may result. There are usually also hematuria and oliguria, due to kidney damage. All of these processes combine to reduce the patient's strength and to increase muscular depression; the pulse becomes rapid and weak, and as paralysis of the nervous system ensues, death may occur from respiratory failure. The fatal single dose of colchicine has been estimated at 8 mg. Treatment of overdoses is symptomatic.

GENERAL ANESTHETICS

Anesthesia may be defined as the blocking of sensation in general or of pain in particular. Block of pain alone is technically referred to as analgesia. Anesthesia may be the result of psychic forces, as in hysterical anesthesia. For clinical purposes it is usually produced by means of drugs. When the block occurs in the brain, the term "general anesthesia" is used. When the block is peripheral to the brain, the term "regional anesthesia" is applied.

Agents producing general anesthesia have been introduced into the body by all conceivable routes. The most common routes are, however, the pulmonary (by inhalation), intravenous, and rectal.

INHALATION ANESTHETICS

Inhalation anesthesia is one of the oldest forms of general anesthesia, and it is still the most common procedure for surgery. The agents employed are gases or volatile liquids.

Ordinarily, inhalation anesthesia is administered by one of four methods:

1. The open method, such as the use of a wire face mask covered with gauze for volatile anesthetic agents or the use of an open-end delivery tube for insufflation of gases under pressure. The method is simple and has a wide margin of safety.

2. The semiopen method, which is similar to the open method except for an increased amount of dead space under the mask to permit accumulation of carbon dioxide. The method is used chiefly during induction of anesthesia when it is desirable to stimulate respiration with the accumulated carbon dioxide.

3. The closed method, with the use of an anesthetic machine, oxygen and other gases under pressure, face mask with delivery tubes for the gases, anesthesia bag, and a soda-lime canister for the absorption of carbon dioxide. In this setup, there is no escape of the patient's expired air to the outside. This method possesses the advantages of economy of agent, greater safety against fire or explosions, faster induction, more-even maintenance of anesthesia, greater controllability of respiration and its aberrations, less heat and fluid loss through respiration, and quicker emergence from anesthesia. It requires much greater skill on the part of the anesthetist than do the open methods.

4. The semiclosed method, which is essentially similar to method 3, except that a graduated escape valve is placed in the circuit. With the soda-lime canister shut off and the escape valve partially open, carbon dioxide accumulates in the anesthesia system and, along with some increased resistance to respiration, serves to augment thoracic excursions.

The administration of inhalation anesthesia may be divided into four periods: induction, mainte-

nance, emergence, and recovery. It is possible to produce successively four stages of anesthesia:

1. Analgesia, with dulling of pain and some dulling of consciousness but seldom unconsciousness.

2. Excitement or delirium, with loss of consciousness and loss of cortical control of subcortical motor activity.

3. Surgical anesthesia, with loss of consciousness and of all skeletal motor activity of central origin, a variable degree of skeletal muscular relaxation, and, ideally, a minimal interference with the functions of the circulatory and respiratory systems. The stage is subdivided into four planes on the basis of disappearance of various reflexes and degree of respiratory depression.

4. Respiratory or bulbar paralysis, with cessation of function of medullary centers and death of the patient.

Inhalation anesthesia is greatly facilitated by premedication designed to allay apprehension and fear, dull pain, and depress or abolish undesirable reflex activities. The opiates (p. 399) are the drugs of choice for eliminating pain or apprehension. Many anesthetists precede them with a barbiturate (p. 390) to diminish central-nervous-system irritability still further. The belladonna drugs, and particularly atropine (p. 420), are commonly employed to control undesirable reflex activity (such as excessive mucus secretion), which, during anesthesia, involves mostly the cholinergic (parasympathetic) system. Dosage of these drugs depends on age; true weight; the presence of fear, pain, fever, toxemia, cachexia, or acidosis; the status of the central nervous, circulatory, and respiratory systems; the surgery contemplated; and the choice of anesthetic agent and technic.

Inhalation anesthesia has the following advantages:

1. A wide margin of applicability and effectiveness.
2. Rapid control of depth of anesthesia and of depression of the central nervous system.
3. Nondependence on tissue for destruction of the agent.

Perhaps the chief disadvantage of inhalation anesthesia is the postanesthetic incidence of, first, pulmonary complications (such as atelectasis, bronchitis, and pneumonia) and, second, nausea, vomiting, and abdominal distention. The pulmonary complications can apparently be largely eliminated by a combination of (1) skillful administration of anesthesia, (2) bronchoscopic aspiration of mucus from the bronchial tree under direct vision at the beginning of the recovery period, and (3) periodic turning of the patient from side to side and deep-breathing exercises during the first few postoperative or postpartum days.

Successful anesthesia which is satisfactory to the surgeon and safe for the patient depends primarily on the knowledge and skill of the anesthetist.

Ether (diethyl ether), $CH_3 \cdot CH_2 \cdot O \cdot CH_2 \cdot CH_3$, is the oldest anesthetic agent in common use and is generally regarded as having the largest factor of immediate safety. It is a clear, colorless, volatile liquid which boils at 34.6°C. (94.3°F.) and is soluble in water to the extent of about 8 percent (w/v). The vapor is pungent, irritating, and, when mixed with air, extremely inflammable and explosive. It decomposes readily, and the U.S.P. warns that it is not to be used for anesthesia if it has been removed from the original container longer than twenty-four hours.

Ether exerts an effect on most tissues of the body and on all major systems. It is a central-nervous-system depressant, yet at the same time it has some stimulating effect on the sympathetic system. Ether is a total anesthetic agent, one that can fatally depress the central nervous system without hypoxia. In this action, there is a progressive depression of the nervous system in the following order: cerebrum, cerebellum, midbrain, spinal cord and medulla. The effect of ether on the respiratory system consists in an increased rate and minute volume, and excessive mucus secretion. These reactions are reflex or peripheral in origin. Cessation of respiration follows medullary paralysis, as seen in overdoses of ether. The cardiovascular system shows some sympathomimetic effects. The blood pressure, pulse rate, and cardiac output are slightly increased. Ether apparently exerts no specific action on the myocardium or automatic tissues of the heart. The gastro-intestinal tract generally exhibits an initial stimulation seen in salivation, nausea, and vomiting. This is followed by a pronounced depression of both the secretory and motor activity of the alimentary tract. Liver and kidney functions are depressed as revealed by common laboratory tests. These organs show not only functional but also morphologic changes following ether anesthesia. Although such effects are significant, particularly in organs already diseased, they are generally temporary in nature. The spleen contracts during ether anesthesia. Peripheral arterioles dilate, facilitating diaphoresis and a decrease in body temperature. Skeletal muscles relax as the result of spinal-cord depression.

Ether exerts the following effects on the blood: moderate hyperglycemia; increase in nonprotein nitrogen, urea, ammonia, and white and red blood cells; and a decrease in carbon-dioxide combining power, phosphates, and lipids.

The following changes may be noted in the urine after ether anesthesia: mild glycosuria, albuminuria, phosphaturia, and occasionally ketonuria.

The continued popular use of ether for over one hundred years is undoubtedly due to an appreciation of its many advantages. It is a cheap, readily available, and transportable agent which is stable (when properly packaged) and practically free of impurities. It can be used by the open-drop or closed system of anesthesia with a wide margin of safety in providing adequate muscular relaxation. Like all other anesthetic agents, ether anesthesia has its limitations and contraindications. Some contraindications, absolute or relative, may be listed as follows:

1. Acute infectious diseases of the respiratory tract.
2. Pulmonary tuberculosis.
3. Acute hepatic disease.
4. Acute nephritis.
5. Diabetes insipidus.
6. Malignant hypertension.
7. Peripheral vascular collapse or shock.
8. Dehydration with or without acidosis.
9. Use of cautery, flame, fluoroscopy, x-ray apparatus.
10. Greatly increased intracranial pressure.
11. Prematurity (in obstetrics).

Ether is also given rectally as an analgesic agent in obstetrics. A mixture of ether, 75 cc. (2 1/2 fl.oz.), and olive or mineral oil, 45 cc. (1 1/2 fl.oz.), is instilled high into the rectum between pains. Sometimes paraldehyde, 8 cc. (2 dr.), is added. The procedure is simple, but there is danger of narcotization of the baby, the patient is predisposed to uterine atony and hemorrhage, and many women dislike the aftereffects of ether.

Vinethene (vinyl ether, Vinesthene, divinyl oxide), $CH_2 : CH \cdot O \cdot CH : CH_2$, is an unsaturated aliphatic ether of vinyl alcohol. It is a clear, colorless fluid with a garliclike, slightly irritant odor. It is very volatile, with a boiling point of 28.3°C. (83°F.). It is inflammable and explosive and is decomposed by heat, sunlight, or air. Hence, Vinethene is supplied in amber, tightly sealed bottles with 4 percent absolute alcohol and 0.01 percent aromatic amine as a stabilizer.

Pharmacologically, Vinethene is a total anesthetic agent and acts not unlike diethyl ether. Its effects on the central nervous system differ from ether in that in man it is prone to stimulate the production of tremors or convulsions. Moreover, concentrations adequate for surgical anesthesia damage the liver and, to a lesser extent, the kidneys. For this reason its use is limited to open-drop administration for short (40 minutes) minor procedures or as an inducing agent for ether. In safe concentrations it does not produce deep relaxation. **It has the same contraindications as has ether.**

Ethyl Chloride, $CH_3 \cdot CH_2 \cdot Cl$, is a clear, colorless, nonirritating liquid which boils at 12.5°C. (54.5°F.). It is inflammable and is readily decomposed by light, heat, moisture, and acids. It acts much like chloroform. It is a total anesthetic agent and, in excess, produces death by respiratory and circulatory paralysis. The central nervous system is progressively depressed from the cortex to the medulla. Respirations are gradually depressed to complete apnea when high concentrations are given. The myocardium may be irritated under ethyl chloride anesthesia to produce serious, if not fatal, arrhythmia. The blood pressure is decreased by means of depression of the vasomotor center and of the myocardium. The secretory and motor activity of the gastro-intestinal tract is decreased. Muscular relaxation is generally moderate with safe doses. Ethyl chloride also decreases liver and kidney functions.

The use of ethyl chloride has been restricted to short minor procedures or to induction for ether anesthesia. It occasionally is employed as a topical agent, the vaporization of the liquid producing low or freezing temperatures of the skin. Its margin of safety, which is greater than that of chloroform, is definitely less than in the case of diethyl ether or Vinethene. It has many contraindications as an inhalant agent and should not be used in the following conditions:

1. Heart disease.
2. Malignant hypertension.
3. Peripheral vascular collapse or shock.
4. Hepatic disease.
5. Nephritis.
6. Diabetes mellitus.
7. Dehydration, with or without acidosis.
8. Use of cautery, flame, fluoroscopy, x-ray apparatus.
9. Prolonged procedures or those requiring great muscular relaxation.

Chloroform (trichloromethane), $CHCl_3$, is a clear, volatile liquid with a sweet, nonirritating odor. It boils at 61°C. (142°F.) and is noninflammable. A powerful total anesthetic, it acts rapidly, is easy to administer, and is pleasant to the patient. However, chloroform tends to cause cardiac arrhythmias, and high concentrations damage the liver and kidneys. It is now little used in the United States.

Nitrous Oxide, N_2O, is one of the oldest anesthetic agents still in common use. It is a clear, colorless, sweet-tasting gas which is nonirritating to the respiratory tract. It has a boiling point of −89°C. It is fairly stable under pressure and is noninflammable, but it will support combustion. Nitrous oxide is very soluble in tissues, accounting in large

measure for the quick induction of and emergence from anesthesia.

Nitrous oxide has narcotic properties but by itself is not a total anesthetic agent, and it is not lethal at one atmosphere of pressure when the partial pressure of oxygen is within normal limits. It is given mixed with oxygen, and the common practice today is not to exceed an 80:20 mixture. At this concentration and with the customary premedication given to the patient, the central nervous system can be depressed to third-stage, first-plane anesthesia. Respirations are quiet, of normal minute volume, and not accompanied by stimulation of mucus secretion. Both the blood pressure and pulse rate remain unchanged. The motor and secretory activity of the gastro-intestinal tract similarly remains within normal limits. The functions of the liver and kidney are not significantly altered. Skeletal muscles are only slightly and inadequately relaxed. Injurious and often irreversible effects to the central nervous system with evidence of hypoxial damage are noted when nitrous oxide is administered to the exclusion of adequate amounts of oxygen.

Nitrous-oxide-oxygen anesthesia in varying concentrations up to 80:20 percent is now commonly employed for induction to ether anesthesia, for short minor procedures requiring little or no muscular relaxation, or for light narcosis in conjunction with Pentothal Sodium, curare, or spinal anesthesia. Its intermittent use for obstetrical analgesia is still popular in many hospitals of the country. Age presents no limitation. Fundamentally, the use of nitrous-oxide-oxygen anesthesia may be contraindicated when there is actual or potential oxygen want or when extreme muscular relaxation is desired. The availability of safer agents and technics justifies this contention.

Ethylene, $CH_2 : CH_2$, is an unsaturated hydrocarbon gas which boils at −103°C. It is a relatively new anesthetic agent but one which has been well established. It is colorless and nonirritating but has a characteristic unpleasant odor. Ethylene is explosive in air or oxygen mixtures used in anesthesia. It is rapidly diffusible in the body. Like other inhalant agents, it is not destroyed in the body but eliminated almost entirely through the pulmonary route.

Pharmacologically, ethylene is more potent than nitrous oxide, and, in deep anesthesia, its action is augmented by a variable degree of hypoxia. Depression of the central nervous system to first-plane, third-stage anesthesia can be obtained safely without hypoxia in a premedicated patient. In the absence of hypoxia, the respiratory minute volume remains the same or is slightly decreased, and the blood pressure and pulse rate are essentially unaffected. There is no effect on the myocardium per se. Similarly, hepatic and renal functions are not affected. The motility of the gastro-intestinal tract is only slightly decreased. The skeletal muscles are relaxed by ethylene-oxygen mixture but generally to a degree not ideal for upper abdominal surgery.

Ethylene is an accepted anesthetic agent and is particularly popular in Midwestern hospitals. Its disagreeable odor, explosiveness, and lack of potency in providing great muscular relaxation for upper abdominal surgery are its main disadvantages. However, it has proved very useful for short minor surgery, as an inducing agent to ether anesthesia, for surgical procedures not requiring profound muscular relaxation, and as a supplement to the use of Pentothal Sodium, curare, and spinal anesthesia. In potency, it is greater than nitrous oxide and less than ether or cyclopropane. Like nitrous-oxide-oxygen mixtures, ethylene should not be administered to the exclusion of oxygen for narcosis; and, like cyclopropane, it should not be employed when cautery, x-ray apparatus, diathermy, or the like is used in the operating room.

Cyclopropane (trimethylene) is a pleasant, colorless, sweet-smelling gas which is nonirritating to the mucous membranes of the body. Its structural formula is shown in Figure 30. It boils at −34°C., is water and fat-soluble, and is explosive in air or oxygen at concentrations used for anesthesia. It is stable and contains perhaps insignificant amounts of impurities such as propylene, propane, and cyclohexane.

FIGURE 30 — *Structural Formula of Cyclopropane*

Pharmacologically, cyclopropane is a total anesthetic agent and can be lethal even in high oxygen concentrations. The central nervous system can be gradually narcotized from slight analgesia to medullary paralysis. Respirations are progressively depressed and generally disappear before circulatory failure is noted. Apnea from direct respiratory-center depression may be seen in light cyclopropane anesthesia in patients who are heavily premedicated. The blood pressure remains essentially the same, although it may be depressed during deep cyclopropane anesthesia. The heart rate is generally decreased, with an early and temporary increase in cardiac output. The cardiac mechanism may be irritated by cyclopropane, particularly when it is under the influence of hypoxia or increased epinephrine secretion or both. Arrhythmias may be noted, ranging from benign, occasional premature ventricular systoles to heart block, ventricular tachycardia, and ventricular fibrillation. Such arrhythmias have been prevented by the use of ether anesthesia, quinidine sulfate, intravenous administration of procaine hydrochloride solution, or sympatholytic agents. In light cyclopropane anesthesia, the movements and secretions of the gastro-intestinal tract may be increased; in deeper planes (third stage, second plane), both are depressed. The spleen becomes enlarged during cyclopropane anesthesia. There is no effect on the function of the liver or kidneys. Skeletal muscles are relaxed, although not to the degree seen in ether or spinal anesthesia. No clinically significant blood or urine changes are noted.

Cyclopropane is now commonly employed for practically all major and minor types of surgery per se or as an inducing agent to ether anesthesia, as a supplement to spinal or other forms of regional anesthesia, or in conjunction with curare preparations administered intravenously. Age is no contraindication. Because of its explosiveness, it is often administered in air or helium mixtures and always with other safeguards such as the Horton intercoupler. Surgical anesthesia may be produced with 20 to 25 percent concentrations in oxygen. Hence, cyanosis should never be experienced with cyclopropane anesthesia. Because of its potency and the absence of respiratory stimulation, induction is rapid and maintenance quiet. Its use should not be attempted by the novice without supervision. Like all other anesthetic agents, it should not be administered indiscriminately. It should not be employed in cases with acute cardiac arrhythmias, in those in whom epinephrine is to be used, or when the use of cautery, x-ray apparatus, or other source of spark or flame is contemplated during surgery. It has proved to be an excellent anesthetic agent in trained hands for poor-risk patients or for those in circulatory collapse who do not show the contraindications mentioned.

ANTICONVULSANTS

Anticonvulsants are drugs given to prevent or stop convulsive and equivalent seizures. A discussion of convulsions and their causes will be found under

Convulsions in Childhood, page 146, and Epilepsy, page 170. For the immediate control of convulsions, a general anesthesia with chloroform or ether is preferred. For prevention of convulsions and for immediate control when a general anesthetic is contraindicated or not available, one of the preparations discussed below may be suitable.

THE BARBITURATES*

The barbiturates are the drugs of choice in convulsions due to a transient cause, such as fever, and in the grand-mal type of epilepsy. Their action is associated with slowing of the abnormally rapid brain waves. In petit mal and psychomotor attacks, in which the brain waves are abnormally slow, the barbiturates may sometimes accentuate attacks and may therefore be unsatisfactory.

Phenobarbital is the most satisfactory barbiturate in epilepsy. For treatment of status epilepticus and other types of severe persistent convulsions, the sodium salt may be given intramuscularly or even (cautiously!) intravenously in doses of 0.13 to 0.5 Gm. (2 to 8 grains); or doses of 2 to 3 mg. per lb. of body weight may be given every fifteen or twenty minutes until the convulsions stop (usually after the second or third injection).

The average daily dose in epilepsy may be as small as 30 mg. (1/2 grain) in a child or as much as 0.6 Gm. (10 grains) in an adult. The average for an adult is 0.05 to 0.13 Gm. (3/4 to 2 grains). Initial dosage should be small, and it should be slowly increased (usually at intervals of seven to ten days) until the lowest dose is found which gives satisfactory control. If attacks occur only at night, all or the major part of the dose may be taken at bedtime; if attacks are diurnal, the principal dose is taken on arising; otherwise the dose may be subdivided equally. In some cases, phenobarbital can be effectively combined with one of the hydantoin derivatives or with the ketogenic diet.

If excessive hypnosis occurs, it may be counteracted by cerebral stimulants (p. 389) or by gradual reduction of the phenobarbital and addition of other anticonvulsant drugs. Status epilepticus frequently results if phenobarbital is stopped suddenly.

Once established, therapy with phenobarbital should be maintained until the patient has been free of attacks for one or two years. A trial without therapy may be in order at the end of such a period.

* A comprehensive discussion of the barbiturates will be found on page 390. Here the presentation is limited to their use in convulsive states.

If the drug is discontinued for any reason, it should be withdrawn gradually to avoid the possibility of severe seizures or status epilepticus.

Drowsiness or tipsiness is a sign of overdosage. Allergy in the form of skin eruption is occasionally seen (p. 227). Petit mal and psychomotor seizures may be aggravated.

Other Barbiturates having a shorter action may be used in recurrent convulsions from such causes as eclampsia and strychnine poisoning but are of no value in epilepsy.

THE HYDANTOINATES

The hydantoinates are analogous to the barbiturates, being derivatives of glycolyl urea as compared with malonyl urea. Their basic structure is shown in Figure 31. The hydantoinates diminish the frequency of the spike waves in the electroencephalogram which are characteristic of convulsive seizures. At the same time they do not depress other phases of cerebral function and have less sedative effect than the barbiturates.

'Thiantoin Sodium' (Phethenylate Sodium, Lilly), sodium 5-phenyl-5-thienyl hydantoinate, is probably the most useful of the hydantoinates. It differs from others in this group in being capable of controlling not only grand mal but also psychomotor seizures and petit mal. In addition, its relatively low toxicity allows administration of larger doses with less danger of undesirable reactions, thus facilitating control of severe, resistant cases.

As with all anticonvulsant drugs, the dosage should be the smallest that is effective. For the majority of patients, 0.13 Gm. (2 grains) two to four times daily, before or after meals, is adequate. In resistant cases, as much as three times this dosage may be required. When the drug cannot be administered by mouth, the pulvules may be punctured at each end and given rectally.

Toxic effects are less common than with other hydantoinates. Gum hypertrophy is an uncommon complication that is usually mild when it does occur. Average doses do not cause sedation. Gastrointestinal symptoms are uncommon and can usually be overcome by varying the time of administration with relation to meals. Patients requiring large doses may develop vertigo, ataxia, or disequilibrium. In such cases the drug should be stopped at once. Skin rash is uncommon. When it occurs, therapy should be discontinued until the rash has disappeared. The drug may then be tried again, begin-

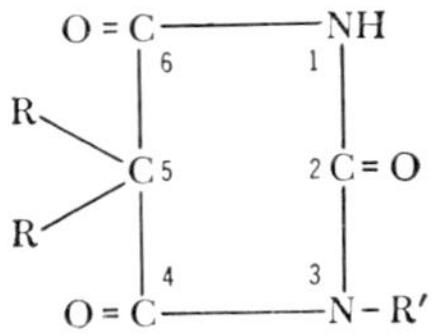

Barbiturates

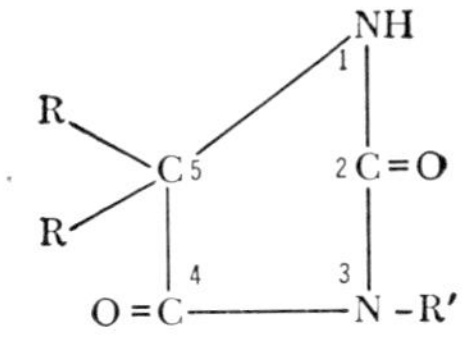

Hydantoinates

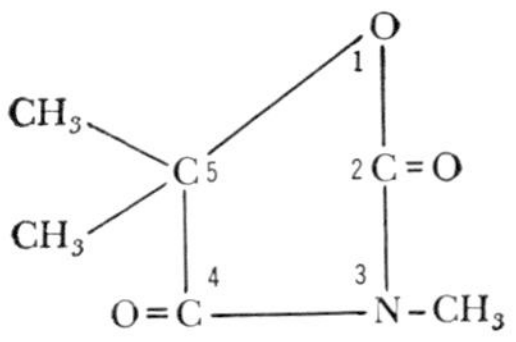

Tridione

FIGURE 31—*Basic Structure of the Anticonvulsant Drugs. The symbols "R" stand for hydrocarbon radicals, and "R'" stands for either hydrogen or a hydrocarbon radical.*

ning with very small doses and increasing gradually to the desired amount.

The transition from phenobarbital or other drugs to 'Thiantoin Sodium' should be made gradually, with some overlapping of dosage.

Diphenylhydantoin Sodium (Dilantin Sodium), sodium 5,5-diphenyl hydantoinate, is the oldest of this group of compounds. It is most valuable in grand mal.

Diphenylhydantoin sodium is administered by mouth. The usual initial dosage in both adults and children is 0.1 Gm. two or three times daily, and this is gradually increased until satisfactory control is obtained. Several days are required at a given dosage before its full effectiveness is manifest. Most adults can tolerate 0.3 to 0.4 Gm. daily without toxic effects.

Toxic effects from the drug are rather common. They may involve the gums, skin, gastro-intestinal tract, or central nervous system. Diphenylhydantoin sodium sometimes causes gastric distress, which can usually be prevented by administration with half a glass of water during or just after meals. If distress persists, 1 cc. of Diluted Hydrochloric Acid may be added to the water. Early manifestations of toxicity are giddiness, ataxia, nervousness, tremor, nystagmus, head nodding, blurring of vision, pain in the eyes, and slurring of speech. They are usually promptly relieved by reduction of dosage.

Hyperplasia of the gums is common in children and young adults. Occasionally the gums bleed or are painful on pressure. These effects are seldom serious and need not interfere with therapy. They are infrequently encountered when oral hygiene is good. Skin eruptions, usually of scarlatiniform type, are occasionally seen; they are usually mild and disappear promptly without alteration of dosage.

Mesantoin, 3-methyl-5,5-phenylethyl hydantoin, is similar therapeutically to diphenylhydantoin sodium. It is less potent, but it has the advantage of rarely causing gum hypertrophy. It is, therefore, used as an alternative to diphenylhydantoin sodium in patients who develop hypertrophy of the gums from the latter drug. Substitution of Mesantoin should take place gradually over a period of three to four weeks, the dosage of the new drug being gradually increased as that of diphenylhydantoin sodium is diminished.

Mesantoin is effective in grand mal and to a less extent in psychomotor epilepsy. It has little or no effect on petit mal seizures, and at times these become more frequent. As with other anticonvulsive drugs, the dosage is adjusted to the smallest which is effective. Children usually require 0.1 to 0.4 Gm. daily, and adults usually need 0.2 to 0.6 Gm. Soporific effects are not uncommon and may require counteraction with central-nervous-system stimulants (p. 389). Skin rashes are encountered more frequently than with other hydantoin anticonvulsants. Agranulocytosis (p. 102) may occur and in some instances has been fatal. Fever and lymphadenopathy are also seen.

TRIDIONE

Tridione (trimethadione) is 3,5,5-trimethyloxazolidine-2,4-dione. Its structural formula is shown in Figure 31. It is similar in basic structure to the hydantoinates, but it has an oxygen atom in place of one of the nitrogens of the latter.

Experience with Tridione has varied considerably. It seems to be of value only in petit mal. It is not uncommon for patients who have petit mal or psychomotor seizures in addition to grand mal to find that it is only the grand mal which is controlled by phenobarbital or a hydantoinate or a combination of the two. Under these circumstances, the addition of Tridione often affords complete control. In other situations in which medication has been unsuccessful, a combination of the three drugs may give good results. The usual dose of Tridione is 0.3 Gm. three or more times daily.

A distinct limitation to the usefulness of Tridione has been the occurrence of severe, and even fatal, aplastic anemia or agranulocytosis. Patients re-

ceiving the drug should, therefore, have blood counts at least once a month, including hemoglobin determination, red and white cell counts, differential count, and platelet count. The drug should be discontinued if any of these is substantially below normal. Tridione should not be given to patients known to be susceptible to blood dyscrasias.

The more common side-effects of the drug are visual and include blurring of vision, sensitivity to light, impairment of acuity, and deficient color discrimination. Other side-effects include drowsiness, vertigo, irritability, and skin eruptions. All of these disappear when the drug is discontinued.

DRUGS HAVING PRINCIPAL EFFECT ON THE PERIPHERAL NERVOUS SYSTEM AND EFFECTOR ORGANS

Recent investigations into neuromuscular chemistry and physiology have resulted in considerable revision of fundamental concepts in these fields. It has been conceived that the transmission of impulses from nerve endings to effector organs (muscle and gland), and at synapses in autonomic ganglia, is mediated by chemical substances. Postganglionic sympathetic (thoracolumbar) autonomic fibers act on effector organs by liberation of a mixture of epinephrine (Adrenalin) and a closely related substance (see p. 425). For this reason these nerves have been termed "adrenergic."

The other chemical mediator is acetylcholine, which is liberated in connection with the transfer of impulses as follows:

1. Between certain postganglionic autonomic fibers and effector organs.
   a. All such parasympathetic (craniosacral) fibers and the effector organs which they supply.
   b. Certain fibers arising from nerve cells in the sympathetic (thoracolumbar) ganglia, and effector organs consisting of sweat glands and certain blood vessels.
2. Between preganglionic nerve fibers and:
   a. All ganglionic nerve cells (postganglionic fibers) in both sympathetic and parasympathetic autonomic ganglia.
   b. The epinephrine-secreting cells of the adrenal medulla.
3. Between somatic motor fibers and the cells of skeletal muscle.

All of the nerves listed above are termed "cholinergic." Stimulation limited to Class 1 above is termed "muscarinic action," because the cholinergic action of muscarine (p. 418) is limited (for practical purposes) to this class. Similarly, stimula-

tion limited to Classes 2 and 3 is called "nicotinic action." Atropine (p. 420) blocks cholinergic effects on effector organs of Class 1, nicotine in large doses blocks Class 2 responses, and curare (p. 447) blocks Class 3 actions.

The normal responses of various effector organs to cholinergic and adrenergic stimuli are listed in Table 44.

DRUGS STIMULATING STRUCTURES INNERVATED BY CHOLINERGIC NERVES

The stimulation achieved by the acetylcholine liberated by cholinergic nerves is normally brief because of the presence of an enzyme, cholinesterase, which splits acetylcholine into acetic acid and the pharmacologically weak choline. Cholinergic effects can therefore be achieved in two ways: either by applying a drug having an action like that of acetylcholine; or by applying a drug which inhibits cholinesterase and allows continued and cumulative effect of the naturally produced acetylcholine.

DIRECTLY CHOLINERGIC DRUGS

Most drugs of this type are esters or other derivatives of choline (see Figure 32, p. 418, for chemical formulas). Acetylcholine is, of course, the typical cholinergic substance, since it is the actual chemical mediator of cholinergic nerve impulses. It is of little clinical use, however: (1) because of its rapid destruction; and (2) because, when given systemically, it stimulates *all* autonomic ganglion cells in addition to cholinergic effector organs.

TABLE 44 — *Responses of Effector Organs to Autonomic Nerve Impulses*

	Cholinergic Impulses	Adrenergic Impulses
HEART		
Rate	Slowed	Accelerated
Output	Decreased	Increased
Conduction mechanism	A-V block, vagal arrest	Ventricular extrasystoles, tachycardia, fibrillation
BLOOD VESSELS		
Coronary	Constricted	Dilated
Cerebral	Dilated	Constricted
Pulmonary	Dilated	Constricted
Abdominal visceral	———	Constricted
Skeletal muscle	Dilated	Dilated, constricted
Skin and mucosal	Dilated	Constricted
LUNG		
Bronchial muscle	Constricted	Dilated
Bronchial glands	Secretion	Inhibited?
STOMACH AND INTESTINE		
Muscle tone and motility	Increased	Decreased
Sphincters	Usually relaxed	Usually contracted
Digestive glands	Secretion	Inhibition
GALL BLADDER AND DUCTS	Contracted	Relaxed?
URETER		
Muscle tone and motility	Increased	Decreased
URINARY BLADDER		
Detrusor muscle	Contracted	Relaxed
Trigone and sphincter	Relaxed	Contracted
UTERUS (Human)		
Pregnant		
Muscle of corpus	Relaxed?	Stimulated?
Circular muscle of cervix	Constricted?	Relaxed?
Nonpregnant	Variable	Stimulated?
EYE		
Iris	Miosis	Mydriasis
Ciliary muscle	Accommodated (near vision)	Relaxed (distant vision)
Smooth muscle of orbit	———	Constricted (exophthalmos)
SKIN		
Pilomotor muscles	———	Contracted
Sweat glands	Secretion (general)	Secretion (restricted)
SPLEEN (Capsule)	———	Constricted
ADRENAL MEDULLA	Secretion of epinephrine	———
LIVER		Glycogenolysis
SALIVARY GLANDS	Secretion (profuse, watery)	Secretion (scanty, thick)
LACRIMAL GLANDS	Secretion	———
GLANDS OF NOSE AND PHARYNX	Secretion	———
AUTONOMIC GANGLION CELLS	Stimulated	———
SKELETAL MUSCLE	Stimulated	———

Methacholine (acetyl-beta-methylcholine, Mecholyl), given as the chloride or bromide, has two advantages over acetylcholine: It is less rapidly inactivated; and it has little effect on autonomic ganglion cells (nicotinic action). It thus stimulates only cholinergic autonomic effector organs and, to a lesser extent, skeletal muscle. Its principal clinical uses, with dosages, are as follows:

Paroxysmal auricular tachycardia (p. 70), 15 to 50 mg. (varies with age and weight) hypodermically.

Raynaud's disease (p. 86), 20 to 100 mg. or more by mouth three times daily, or by iontophoresis of a 0.2 percent solution.

Vascular spasm, as in thrombophlebitis, 200 to 500 mg. by mouth, or by iontophoresis of a 0.2 percent solution.

Abdominal distention, 20 to 50 mg. Hypodermically (with caution!).

Megacolon, 100 to 200 mg. by mouth once or twice daily.

The effect of methacholine, like that of acetylcholine, is potentiated by physostigmine and similar drugs (see below) and inhibited by atropine. Methacholine should not be given intravenously. Large doses should never be used until the effect of small doses has been tried. Great care is necessary in combining it with physostigmine or Prostigmine. Because of the side-effects, patients receiving the drug by injection should be in bed and lying down, with a bedpan in place.

The effect of the subcutaneously injected drug can be enhanced by massage of the site. It can be limited by applying a tourniquet proximal to the site, or it can be immediately arrested by intravenous injection of atropine sulfate, 0.5 to 1 mg. (1/120 to 1/60 grain). A sterile solution of atropine sulfate should always be on hand when choline esters are injected. The drug is contraindicated in hyperthyroidism (danger of auricular fibrillation) and asthma (bronchoconstrictor effect).

Carbachol (carbaminoylcholine chloride, Doryl) is also a powerful cholinergic drug. It differs from methacholine (and resembles acetylcholine) in having a powerful effect on autonomic ganglia. It differs from both the other agents in being impervious to the action of cholinesterase. Its effect is therefore neither enhanced nor prolonged by physostigmine or Prostigmine.

Therapeutically, carbachol has been used to relieve spasm in vascular disease and to stimulate emptying of the urinary bladder during retention after surgical operations, parturition, or lesions of the spinal cord. The usual initial clinical dose is 0.25 mg. by hypodermic injection. To induce emptying of the bladder, this dose may need to be repeated once or twice at half-hour intervals.

The same contraindications and precautions should apply to carbachol as to methacholine. Care is especially necessary in patients who are very ill or in shock.

Muscarine is not employed clinically, but it is the active agent in poisoning by the mushroom

Amanita muscaria. Muscarine stimulates the effector organs innervated by postganglionic cholinergic fibers. It has little action on ganglionic nerve cells, the adrenal medulla, or skeletal muscle. The effects of muscarine can therefore be predicted from the column headed "Cholinergic Impulses" in Table 44. Its action is inhibited by atropine.

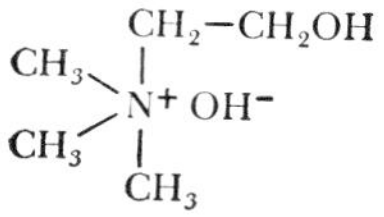

Choline

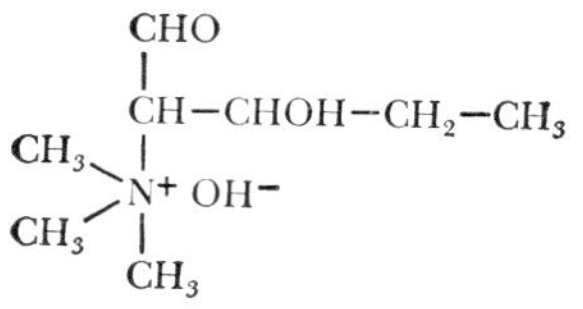

Muscarine

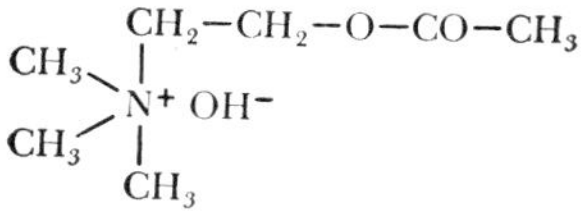

Acetylcholine

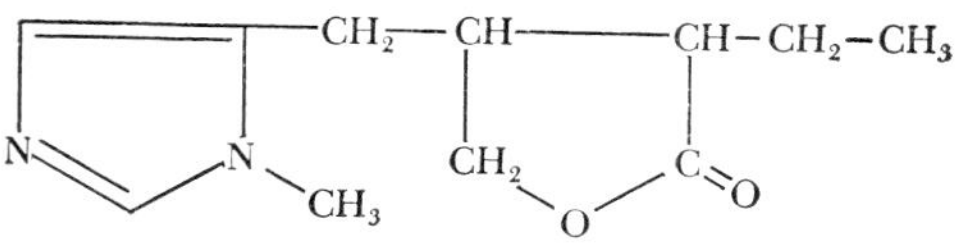

Pilocarpine

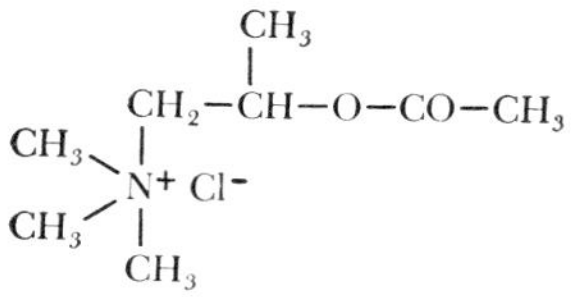

Methacholine Chloride
(*Acetyl-beta-methylcholine Chloride, Mecholyl*)

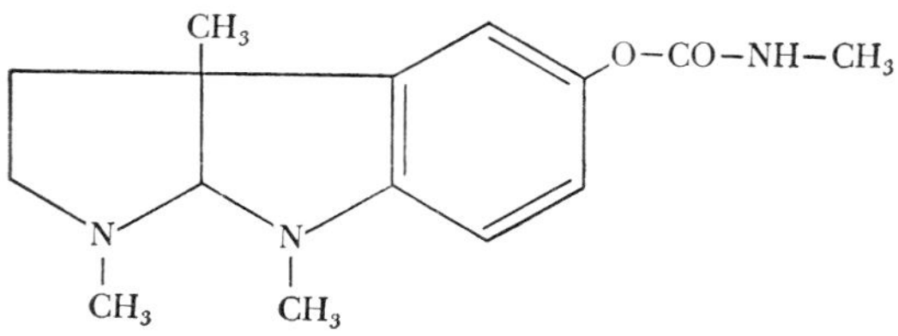

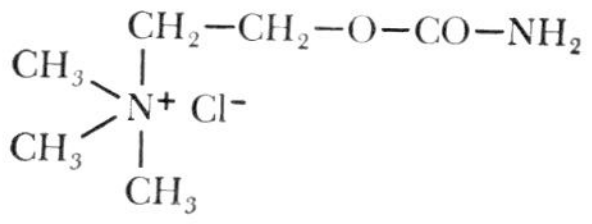

Carbachol
(*Carbaminoylcholine Chloride, Doryl*)

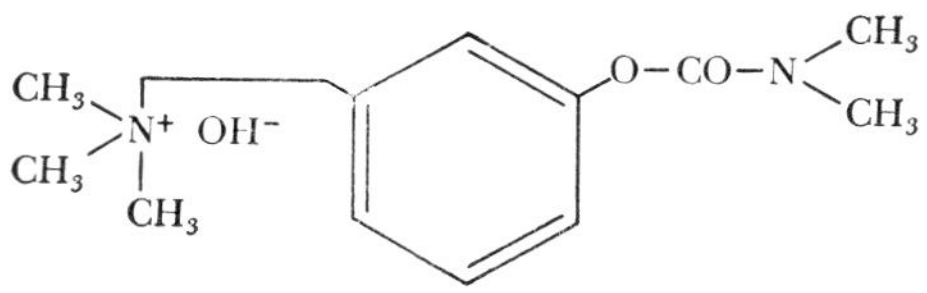

Physostigmine

Prostigmine

Figure 32 — *Structural Formulas of Cholinergic Substances*

Pilocarpine, like muscarine, stimulates the smooth muscle and gland cells innervated by postganglionic cholinergic fibers and has little effect on cells innervated by preganglionic and somatic motor fibers. Sweat and salivary glands and the iris are especially responsive to the drug, and its practical use is connected with these organs.

Pilocarpine (as the nitrate) is mainly given by local application, as drops or ointment (0.5 to 3 percent), to the eyes to produce miosis and increase drainage of intraocular fluid in glaucoma (p. 241) or to overcome the mydriasis of atropine (p. 420). In the past, pilocarpine was used as a diaphoretic (10 to 15 mg. [1/6 to 1/4 grain] hypodermically), but the side-effects may be distressing and sometimes dangerous.

The drug has a certain usefulness in counteracting the peripheral autonomic effects in atropine poisoning, but it does not influence the more serious features, namely, the central toxic actions. The effects of pilocarpine can be neutralized by suitable doses of atropine.

INHIBITORS OF CHOLINESTERASE

Certain phenyl esters of alkylcarbamic acids are potent and specific inhibitors of cholinesterase activity (see Figure 32). By preventing hydrolysis of acetylcholine and some of its derivatives, these compounds increase and prolong the effects of parasympathetic nerve stimulation and of certain administered choline derivatives. In this sense they are cholinergic drugs. Two of them are used in medicine: physostigmine (eserine) and Prostigmine.

Physostigmine is extracted from the Calabar bean, indigenous to West Africa. Perhaps its main therapeutic use is to produce miosis and improve drainage of intraocular fluid in glaucoma (p. 241). Water solutions in glass tend to deteriorate with formation of a pink or red-brown color. Discolored solutions should be discarded. Boric acid acts as a preservative. Solutions may be irritating. Local anesthetic drugs may be incorporated with them.

Physostigmine (1 to 2 mg. [1/60 to 1/30 grain] hypodermically) has been used to promote intestinal motility in abdominal distention (see Methacholine, p. 417). Sometimes larger doses are required, but these should be administered only in nontoxic cases and after simpler measures have failed. Physostigmine has been used in myasthenia gravis (p. 250), but the results are less satisfactory than those with Prostigmine.

Because the cholinesterase of ganglion cells of both sympathetic and parasympathetic ganglia is inhibited by physostigmine, the response to physostigmine is not always predictable when the drug is given systemically. In some instances or with some organs, the adrenergic response may exceed the cholinergic. Atropine inhibits the more dangerous features of physostigmine poisoning, namely, the effects on the respiratory tract and circulation.

Prostigmine (neostigmine) is a synthetic compound. In most of its effects it closely resembles physostigmine. However, for reasons as yet unknown, it has proved more effective in counteracting the weakness of myasthenia gravis (p. 250). These drugs doubtless act by preventing destruction of acetylcholine at the somatic motor-nerve endings. The effect in this disease is so specific that Prostigmine is useful as a diagnostic test in doubtful cases.

The initial hypodermic dose of Prostigmine in myasthenia gravis is usually 0.5 mg. (as the methylsulfate), which is increased if necessary. A response is seen after ten to thirty minutes and persists four to six hours. Injections are usually repeated three or four times daily.

Oral administration may also be effective. The dose is 15 to 30 mg. (as the bromide) three times daily. Each dose takes effect in one to two hours. With the large doses necessary for oral therapy, the muscarinic effects (p. 416) may become troublesome. To avoid them, the patient takes atropine sulfate, 0.3 mg. (1/200 grain), or Belladonna Tincture, 0.6 to 1.5 cc. (10 to 22 minims), three times daily. Many clinicians prefer to combine Prostigmine with ephedrine or some other adrenergic drug (p. 426) or with choline esters (p. 416) in the treatment of myasthenia gravis.

Prostigmine is also used for the relief of abdominal distention in the same way as physostigmine, or in bladder atony as carbachol (p. 417) is used. It has had limited use in atrophic rhinitis (p. 111), as a miotic (p. 436), and to relax spastic muscles associated with rheumatoid arthritis (p. 247).

DRUGS INHIBITING STRUCTURES INNERVATED BY POSTGANGLIONIC CHOLINERGIC NERVES

The most important drugs of this group are the alkaloids of the belladonna plants. Of greatest usefulness are atropine and scopolamine. The presence of an asymmetric carbon atom (shown in bold face in the structural formulas in Figure 33) results in stereoisomerism, the nomenclature of which is confusing. Atropine is racemic hyoscyamine and is the chief active ingredient of belladonna and stramonium. Scopolamine is levorotatory hyoscine and is found in extracts of hyoscyamus. Racemic hyoscine is called atroscine.

Atropine has two types of action: One is on the central nervous system; the other and more important is inhibition of smooth muscle and glands innervated by postganglionic cholinergic nerves. This latter action is strongest in blocking the muscarinic actions of cholinergic drugs (p. 416); it is less effective against cholinergic nerve stimulation, probably because in the latter case the acetylcholine is liberated within the effector cell and distal to the site of action of atropine. The exact mechanism of atropine block of cholinergic response is unknown, but it is not through prevention of the release of acetylcholine.

This parasympatholytic action of atropine has many clinical uses. In the eye, the drug prevents contraction of both the constrictor muscle of the iris and the ciliary body, resulting in mydriasis and loss of accommodation. The clinical use of atropine as a mydriatic and cycloplegic is discussed on page 436.

In the respiratory tract, atropine reduces mucosal secretion and dilates the bronchial tree. In common colds and hay fever, the drug may induce symptomatic relief from excessive nasal secretion (atropine sulfate, 0.2 to 0.3 mg. [1/300 to 1/200 grain]; Belladonna Tincture, U.S.P., 2 or 3 minims; or Belladonna Extract, U.S.P., 0.015 or 0.03 Gm. [1/4 or 1/2 grain], repeated as needed). Clinically, atropine has proved relatively ineffective in bronchial asthma (p. 265), contrary to theoretical expectation. In so-called "cardiac asthma" (p. 64), it is sometimes given in combination with morphine. Atropine is much used to prevent excessive bronchial secretion during general anesthesia (p. 410).

Atropine or belladonna is widely employed in gastro-intestinal disorders; suitable doses diminish spasm and excess motor activity without interfering seriously with digestive processes. They are especially valuable in functional and nervous indigestion, in which one of them can advantageously be combined with mild sedation (for instance, as a mixture of Belladonna Tincture and Phenobarbital Elixir, or as tablets containing phenobarbital and Belladonna Extract). They are also useful in mu-

cous or ulcerative colitis, dysenteries, lead colic, and spastic constipation. (See also Antispasmodics, p. 434.)

When liquid medication is desired for oral administration, Belladonna Tincture is usually employed. Its advantage of extreme flexibility in dosage is important in treating gastro-intestinal disturbances, in which dosage may vary greatly. It is best to start with 0.3 to 0.6 cc. (5 to 10 minims) three times daily before meals. Sometimes a dose

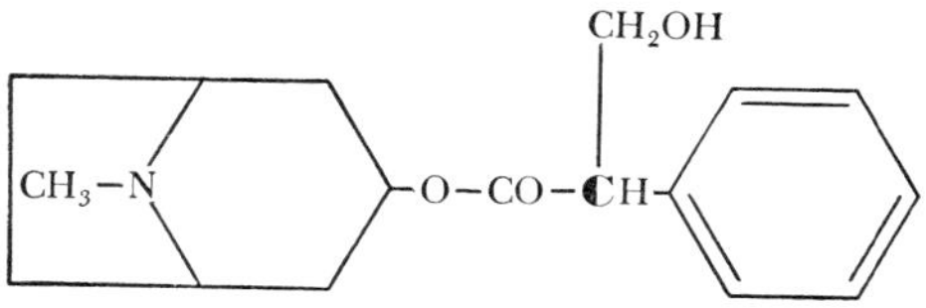

Atropine
(Conventional representation)

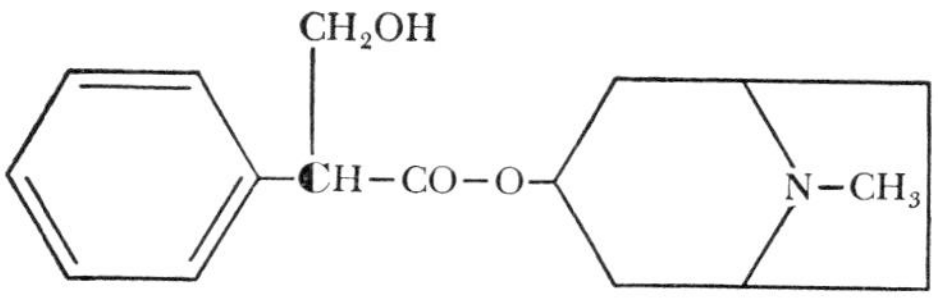

Atropine
(To show relationship to cocaine, p. 446)

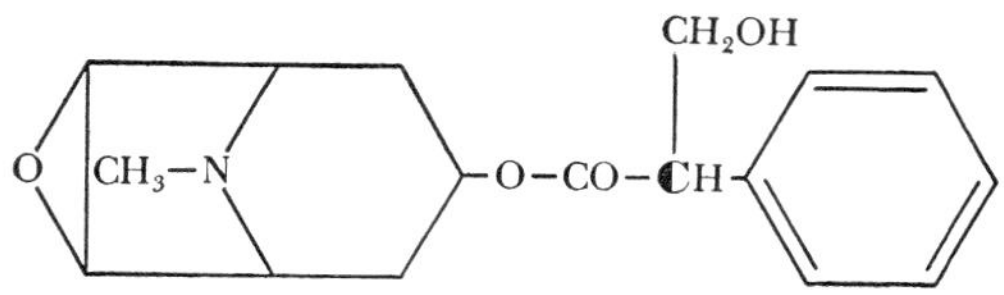

Scopolamine

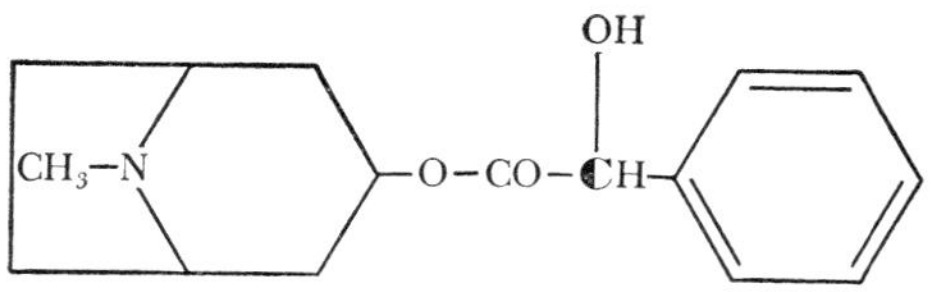

Homatropine

FIGURE 33 — *Structural Formulas of Anticholinergic (Cholinergic Inhibitory) Drugs* at bedtime is given as well. For solid medication, Tablets Belladonna Extract may be given. The usual single starting dose is 16 mg. (1/4 grain). The dose of either is adjusted upward or downward to the minimum necessary for symptomatic relief. Occasionally, relief cannot be obtained without undesirable side-effects.

Atropine is sometimes useful in ureteral colic (see Antispasmodics, p. 434). Its action in inhibiting excessive detrusor tone makes it helpful in enuresis in children (p. 225) and for lessening the urgency and frequency of urination in patients with spastic paraplegia.

Occasionally, atropine is of value in cardiovascular disease. In some cases it may abolish premature beats (p. 69). It is often helpful in preventing syncope when this is due to bradycardia or to complete systolic arrest from abnormally active carotid sinus reflexes.

With respect to the central nervous system, doses of 0.5 to 1 mg. (1/120 to 1/60 grain) of atropine are mildly stimulating. After larger doses there may be mental disturbances (see listing below). Still larger doses are depressing, and death in atropine poisoning is usually due to paralysis of the medullary centers. On certain central motor mechanisms the effect is depressive from the beginning, and atropine or one of the related drugs is useful as symptomatic treatment of paralysis agitans (p. 172). Stramonium Extract or Tincture is often the most effective preparation. The reason is unknown, since most of the action of stramonium is due to atropine.

Toxic effects from overdosage of atropine are not uncommon, especially in children, and patients taking the belladonna drugs over long periods or in large doses should be acquainted with them. Individual tolerance varies greatly, but on the average the following systemic doses are likely to produce the following effects:

0.5 mg. (1/120 grain)	Slight dryness of nose and mouth; slight slowing of heart.
1 mg. (1/60 grain)	Greater dryness of nose and mouth, with thirst; slowing, then acceleration, of heart; slight mydriasis.
2 mg. (1/30 grain)	Very dry mouth; rapid heart, with palpitation; mydriasis, slight blurring of near vision; inhibition of sweating.
5 mg. (1/12 grain)	Increase in above symptoms plus disturbance of speech; difficulty in swallowing; headache; hot, dry skin; restlessness, with fatigue.
10 mg. (1/6 grain) and over	Above symptoms to extreme degree, plus ataxia, excitement, disorientation, hallucinations, delirium, and coma.
65 mg. (1 grain)	May be fatal.

If one is in doubt as to the diagnosis of poisoning with one of the belladonna alkaloids, the hypodermic injection of 10 to 30 mg. of methacholine (p. 417) may be helpful. If the characteristic cholinergic effects do not follow (such as miosis, salivation, sweating, urination, peristalsis), belladonna poisoning is almost certainly present. Treatment is outlined on page 554.

The two isomers contained in atropine have quantitatively similar central actions, but the peripheral effects are due almost entirely to the levo isomer, hyoscyamine. Unfortunately, the latter substance when alone is unstable, changing in time to the racemic mixture, atropine.

Scopolamine, or levo hyoscine, is much more active than its dextro isomer. Its peripheral action differs quantitatively from that of atropine, being more pronounced on the iris, ciliary muscle, and salivary, bronchial, and sweat glands, and less intense and of briefer duration on the heart, intestine, and bronchial muscle. However, the dominance of its central effects has limited its clinical use to their production.

In contrast to atropine, scopolamine seems to be a primary central depressant. Doses of 0.5 mg. (1/120 grain) as the hydrobromide usually cause drowsiness and dreamless sleep. Sometimes, however, an opposite effect is obtained, namely, excitement, restlessness, hallucinations, and even delirium. Scopolamine is often used instead of atropine for administration with morphine prior to general anesthesia. It has a similar effect on bronchial secretion, with the advantage of a central sedative rather than a stimulant action. Scopolamine is also combined with morphine or a barbiturate for obstetrical analgesia. It may be useful as a sedative in various psychoses and maniacal states, in delirium tremens, and in the withdrawal treatment of narcotic or alcohol addiction.

Homatropine, a synthetic substance, has effects qualitatively similar to those of atropine but weaker and of shorter duration. It is used to produce mydriasis and cycloplegia in adults in whom the prolonged action of atropine may be dangerous. It is administered in 1 or 2 percent solution as the hydrobromide. (See p. 436 for discussion.)

Eucatropine (Euphthalmine), another synthetic preparation resembling atropine in qualitative effects, is employed as a mydriatic when cycloplegia is not desired. It is used in 5 or 10 percent solution as the hydrochloride. (See p. 436 for discussion.)

DRUGS STIMULATING STRUCTURES INNERVATED BY ADRENERGIC NERVES

A large number of chemical substances have been discovered which act qualitatively on effector organs in much the same way as does stimulation of postganglionic sympathetic nerve fibers. However, the details and intensity of action vary widely from one compound to another. The actual chemical mediators at the nerve endings of this portion of the autonomic system appear to be epinephrine (Adrenalin) and arterenol in varying ratio. Because the role of epinephrine was suspected first, the term "adrenergic" has been applied both to the sympathetic (thoracolumbar) system and to the drugs which stimulate it (for a listing of adrenergic effects, see Table 44, p. 417). These drugs are also referred to as "sympathomimetic" and, because of their chemical nature, as "sympathomimetic amines." The number of substances having some degree of adrenergic activity is so great that only those which have unusual properties or are widely used clinically will be discussed here.

EPINEPHRINE AND ITS IMMEDIATE DERIVATIVES

Epinephrine (Adrenalin, Suprarenin) is one of the substances secreted by the adrenal medulla (p. 187), and it is one of the chemical mediators at postganglionic sympathetic nerve endings. It was the first hormone to be isolated in crystalline form. Its chemical formula is shown in Figure 34. The presence of an asymmetric carbon atom (the second, or beta, from the amine group) makes possible optical isomerism. The epinephrine secreted by the adrenal medulla is levorotatory. The dextro isomer has the same qualitative action but only about one-twentieth the potency. Epinephrine, U.S.P., is the levorotatory form.

Epinephrine is relatively unstable, both in the body and outside, and its action is comparatively short, although not so brief as that of the parasym-

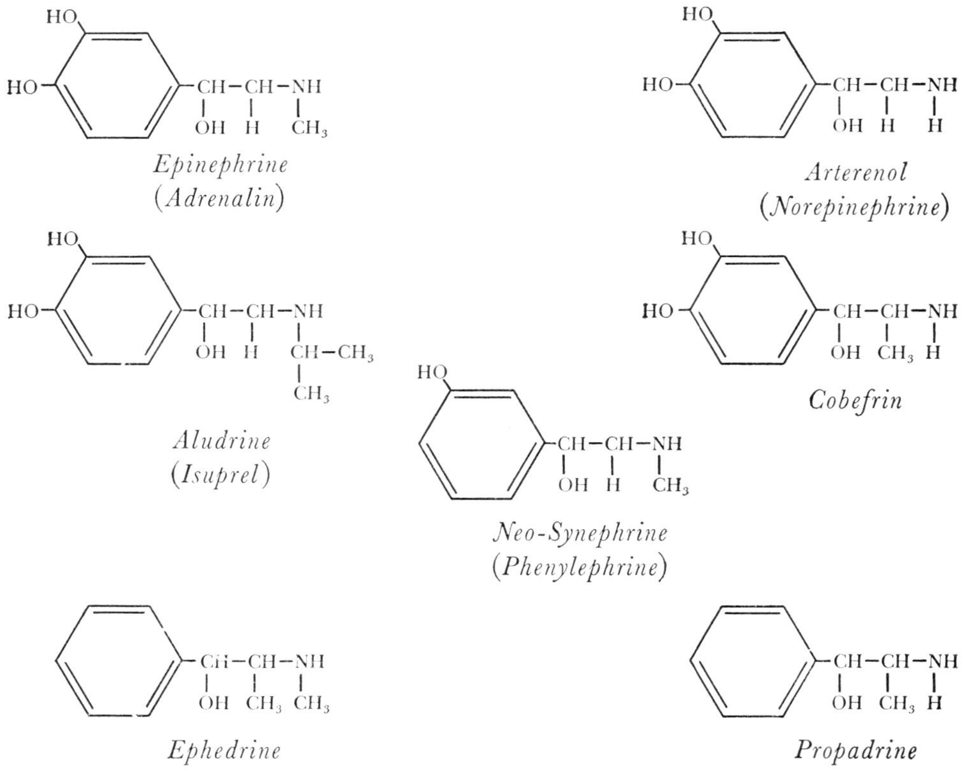

FIGURE 34 — Structural Formulas of Adrenergic Substances

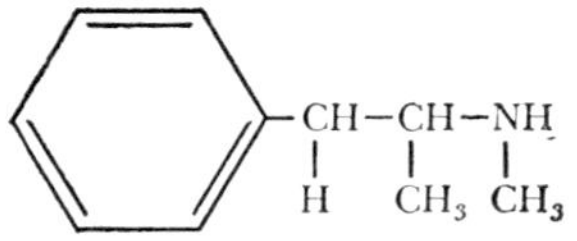

CH—CH—NH
| | |
H   CH₃ CH₃

Methamphetamine*
(*Desoxyephedrine*)

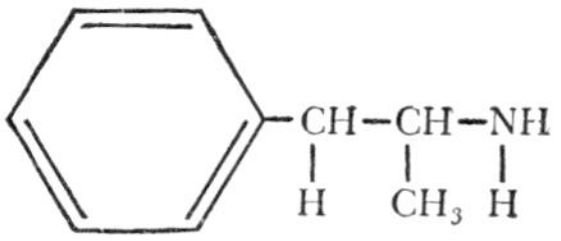

CH—CH—NH
| | |
H   CH₃   H

Amphetamine
(*Benzedrine*)

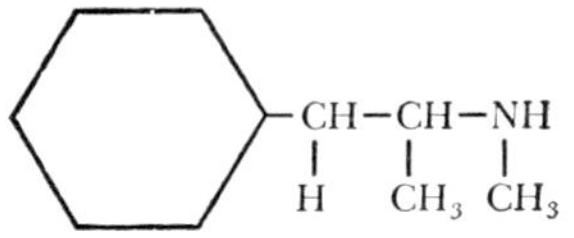

CH—CH—NH
| | |
H   CH₃ CH₃

Benzedrex

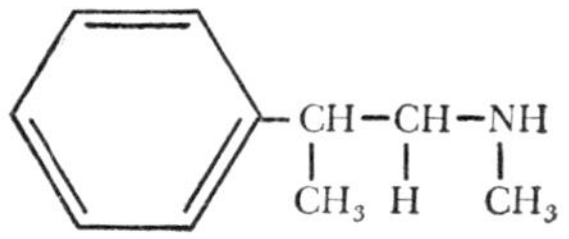

CH—CH—NH
| | |
CH₃ H   CH₃

Vonedrine

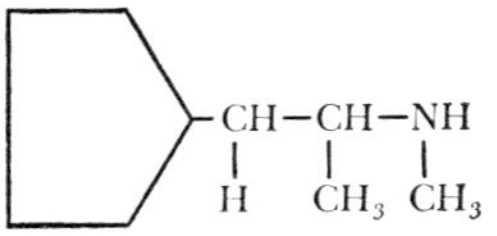

CH—CH—NH
| | |
H   CH₃ CH₃

Cyclopentamine †

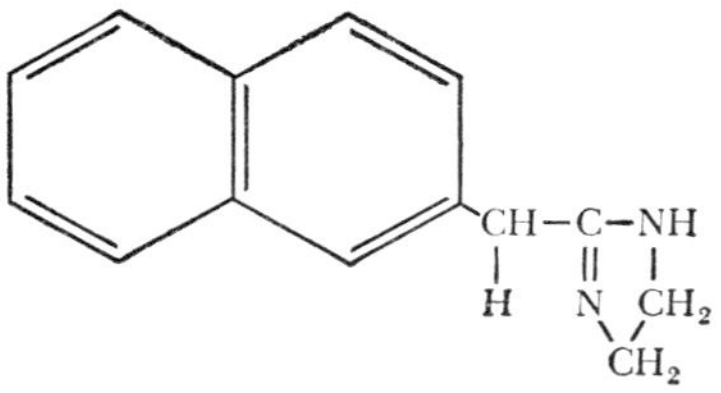

CH—C—NH
| ‖ |
H   N   CH₂
       \   /
       CH₂

Privine

$CH_3-CH_2-CH_2-CH_2-CH-CH-NH$
                         | | |
                        H   CH₃   H

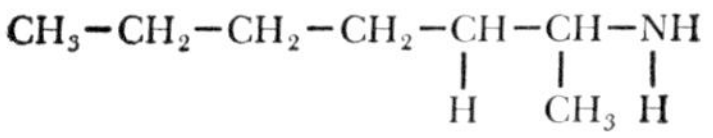

2-Aminoheptane
(*'Tuamine'*)

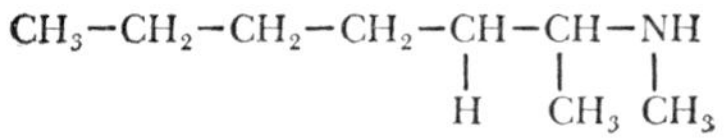

$CH_3-CH_2-CH_2-CH_2-CH-CH-NH$
                         | | |
                        H   CH₃ CH₃

2-Methylaminoheptane
(*Oenethyl*)

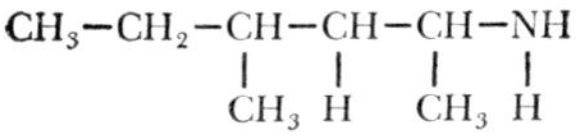

$CH_3-CH_2-CH-CH-CH-NH$
              | | | |
             CH₃ H   CH₃ H

2-Amino-4-methylhexane
(*'Forthane'*)

* Methamphetamine hydrochloride is marketed by Eli Lilly and Company as 'Amphedroxyn Hydrochloride.'
† Cyclopentamine hydrochloride is marketed by Eli Lilly and Company as 'Clopane Hydrochloride.'

FIGURE 34 (*Continued*) — *Structural Formulas of Adrenergic Substances*

pathetic mediator, acetylcholine. It is destroyed by oxidation rather than by a specific enzyme as is the case with acetylcholine. When administered therapeutically by the subcutaneous route, epinephrine induces local vasoconstriction which slows its absorption and prolongs its action. The drug is quickly destroyed in the gastro-intestinal tract and thus has no therapeutic effect when given orally.

Epinephrine appears to act directly on effector cells. A listing of these actions will be found in the column headed "Adrenergic Impulses" in Table 44 (p. 417). It will be noted that epinephrine stimulates some types of effector organs and inhibits others. The responsiveness of all these tissues is greatly enhanced by denervation, and consequently the action of the hormone is greater on regions of the body which are affected by sympathetic nerve block or sympathectomy.

The response of the individual patient to epinephrine cannot always be predicted because of the mutual antagonism of some of the individual effects listed in Table 44, factors related to disease, and compensatory and other reactions. Cardiac stroke volume is almost always increased, and systolic blood pressure is usually elevated 10 to 70 mm. Hg by doses of 0.5 mg. However, total blood flow may be either increased or decreased, depending on the relative extent of vasoconstriction in some areas as compared with vasodilation in others. Increased blood flow may lead to a fall rather than a rise in diastolic arterial pressure. Similarly, bradycardia may represent a compensatory reaction to increased cardiac output and systolic pressure, even though the direct action of epinephrine on the heart includes acceleration of rate.

Epinephrine is made available in the following forms:

Epinephrine Solution, U.S.P., containing epinephrine hydrochloride, 1:1,000 (1 mg. per cc.).
Epinephrine Injection, U.S.P., containing a sterile solution of the hydrochloride, 1:1,000.
Epinephrine Inhalation, U.S.P., containing the hydrochloride, 1:100, in distilled water.
Epinephrine in Oil, 1:500, a suspension for intramuscular injection for slow absorption and prolonged effect.

Epinephrine and its salts must be protected from light and alkali, which greatly accelerate the rate of destruction.

In Allergy—Epinephrine was for many years the most effective drug for symptomatic relief in asthma, urticaria, angioneurotic edema, serum sickness, and anaphylactic shock. Its place is now being challenged by the antihistaminic drugs (p. 509), certain xanthine derivatives (p. 358), and, in asthma, aludrine (p. 425).

In asthma of allergic origin, epinephrine usually induces prompt relief. It is most simply administered by inhalation of the 1:100 solution (Epinephrine Inhalation, U.S.P.) from a special nebulizer (see p. 266). Relief generally begins immediately and may persist for an hour or two. Two to four properly performed inhalations constitute a dose. The quantity of drug required is usually so small that side-effects are rare.

Very severe paroxysms may necessitate subcutaneous injection of the 1:1,000 solution (*the 1:100 inhalant must never be injected*). The usual initial dose is 0.2 to 0.3 cc. (3 to 5 minims). If no relief is obtained in five minutes, the site of injection is massaged. If another five-minute period passes without effect, the injection is repeated. Seldom are more than three such doses required. Children must receive proportionately smaller quantities. Excessive dosage is to be avoided, especially in children. For effects lasting four to twenty-four hours, 0.5 to 1.5 cc. of the 1:500 suspension in oil may be given

intramuscularly. The oil suspension should be employed only after a preliminary trial of an aqueous solution has elicited a satisfactory response. The effect of the oil preparation begins fifteen to twenty minutes after injection.

When epinephrine is used repeatedly over a period of days or weeks, tolerance is likely to develop. A rest period from the drug, during which aludrine or a xanthine is used, ordinarily restores responsiveness. Epinephrine should be used cautiously in chronic asthmatics who have pulmonary emphysema and may have some degree of myocardial degeneration.

In urticaria, angioneurotic edema, and serum sickness, epinephrine is usually inferior to the antihistaminic drugs. In urgent cases or those in which the antihistaminics are ineffective, epinephrine hydrochloride may be given subcutaneously as in asthma. When allergic swellings obstruct respiration, epinephrine should be administered at once, either by inhalation or subcutaneously.

Epinephrine is the drug of choice in treating anaphylactic shock. Doses should be comparatively large, and the intravenous route should be employed in emergency (for details, see p. 269).

As a Vasoconstrictor—Epinephrine hydrochloride is commonly added to solutions of local anesthetic agents. The resulting local vasoconstriction slows absorption of the anesthetic agent with the result that the duration of anesthesia is prolonged and the incidence of systemic toxicity is reduced. For infiltration, a final concentration of 1:200,000 epinephrine hydrochloride is adequate. For regional anesthesia, including nerve, epidural, and caudal block, the concentration should be 1:100,000. For small injections into vascular areas such as the gums, it may be 1:50,000. Moderate prolongation of spinal anesthesia may be achieved by adding 0.5 to 1 mg. (0.5 to 1 cc. of 1:1,000 solution) to 1 or 2 cc. of spinal anesthetic solution.

Epinephrine hydrochloride has been applied topically as a hemostatic agent in concentrations of 1:50,000 to 1:2,000. Capillary and arteriolar, but not venous, bleeding can be controlled by application of a spray or of cotton or gauze pledgets moistened with the solution. However, secondary hyperemia usually occurs after the vasoconstrictor effect has worn off, and for this reason preference is usually given to other methods of control. The same disadvantage militates against epinephrine as a nasal vasoconstrictor. It is sometimes used in the eye in concentrations no stronger than 1:4,000.

In spite of its potency, epinephrine is seldom used for systemic pressor effect (increase in blood pressure). The reason is threefold: The effect lasts only a few minutes; it is followed by a brief period of hypotension before the blood pressure returns to the original level; and, for consistent pressor effects, the drug must be given intravenously in a dosage that usually causes unpleasant symptoms (see below). Paradoxically, very small doses of epinephrine produce brief generalized vasodilation, slight fall in systolic arterial pressure, and somewhat greater fall in diastolic pressure.

As a Cardiac Stimulant—In cardiac arrest for other reasons than chronic myocardial failure, epinephrine may occasionally restore function, although it is probably inferior to direct cardiac massage. A dose of 0.5 cc. of 1:1,000 is injected into the heart muscle and ventricle. Sometimes the drug itself in such high direct doses induces ventricular fibrillation. If arrest is incomplete and some heart sounds are audible, 0.05 to 0.2 cc. may be given intravenously very slowly in 10 cc. of isotonic salt solution.

Intracardiac injection as above may sometimes restore cardiac function in Adams-Stokes syncope (p. 73). For prevention of attacks, 0.3 to 0.5 cc. of the 1:1,000 solution may be given every two hours, or 0.5 to 1 cc. of the oil suspension, 1:500, may be given at longer intervals; however, ephedrine is just as effective as a prophylactic and has the advantage of oral administration.

In "cardiac asthma," epinephrine is probably contraindicated. This condition is now better treated by the xanthine drugs (p. 358). Epinephrine has no value and may be harmful in heart failure or shock (for discussion, see p. 90).

In Hypoglycemia—In severe hypoglycemia, subcutaneous injection of 0.5 cc. of epinephrine hydrochloride solution, 1:1,000, may prove effective in raising the blood sugar, but only if the liver contains an adequate store of glycogen.

Side-Effects—Epinephrine has an extremely low systemic toxicity. Its side-effects are exaggerations of its physiological effects. With overdoses or in extremely susceptible individuals, there may be anxiety, tenseness, restlessness, headache (usually throbbing), nausea, respiratory difficulty, palpitation, tachycardia, cardiac arrhythmias, weakness, dangerous elevation of blood pressure, and even cerebral hemorrhage.

Hyperthyroid individuals are particularly susceptible to epinephrine, and in them it should be used very cautiously. It may likewise prove dangerous in the presence of arteriosclerosis and, particularly, cerebral arteriosclerosis. It is contraindicated in hypertension and in shock.

Initial doses should be small until the patient's response has been ascertained. Great care should be taken to avoid inadvertent injection into a vein. Among the cardiac arrhythmias which may be caused by epinephrine is ventricular fibrillation, which is fatal if continued for more than a few minutes. Ventricular fibrillation is relatively easily produced in patients under general anesthesia, and in them the drug should be used with great caution. The same is true of those with organic heart disease.

l-Arterenol, *l*-norepinephrine, is believed to be the precursor of epinephrine in the body and to be liberated, along with epinephrine, from the adrenal medulla and at postganglionic sympathetic nerve endings. Chemically, arterenol differs from epinephrine by the absence of a methyl group on the amino nitrogen (see Figure 34, p. 422). A number of tissues appear to be capable of methylating arterenol to produce epinephrine.

Pharmacologically, arterenol differs from epinephrine mainly in that, (1) as a pressor drug, it is about one-third more potent, has a greater duration of action, and has no period of secondary hypotension; (2) it is much less toxic; and (3) its action is not reversed by ergotoxine or ergotamine. This last difference suggests a different site of action of the two drugs, but it is of no clinical importance because the doses of the two ergot alkaloids required to reverse the action of epinephrine are toxic in man.

Both in the adrenal medulla and at postganglionic sympathetic nerve endings, the mixture of arterenol and epinephrine which is liberated is a variable one. As stimulation continues, the methylation of arterenol to epinephrine lags behind production of arterenol, and the liberated mixture contains a progressively higher fraction of the latter drug, with a corresponding increase in vasoconstrictor and pressor effects.

l-Arterenol is used clinically as a local vasoconstrictor in connection with local and regional anesthesia.

Aludrine (isopropylepinephrine, Aleudrin, Isuprel, Isonorin) differs from epinephrine in that it has an isopropyl group attached to the nitrogen in place of the methyl group (see Figure 34, p. 422). This change appears to diminish those actions of epinephrine which are fundamentally excitatory and to augment those which are inhibitory. Thus, aludrine has practically no vasoconstrictor action but in larger doses may cause vasodilation and fall in blood pressure. On the other hand, it is extremely effective in producing bronchodilation. The racemic form is used in medicine.

Therapeutically, aludrine is employed in the symptomatic treatment of asthma (p. 265). As a bronchodilator, it is several times as powerful as epinephrine and affords relief in many cases that have become resistant to epinephrine and the xanthines. The route of administration has great influence on both therapeutic action and undesired side-effects. The dose must be suited to each patient, for there is great variation in different individuals as to the amount required for therapeutic action and for appearance of side-effects.

Aludrine is administered as the hydrochloride or sulfate. It is most effective when inhaled as a nebulized mist of a preparation such as '*Aerolin*' (Cyclopentamine and Aludrine Compound, Lilly), in which it is combined with other agents. The active ingredients of 'Aerolin' are:

'Clopane Hydrochloride' (Cyclopentamine Hydrochloride, Lilly)	0.5	percent (w/v)
aludrine sulfate	0.25	percent (w/v)
atropine sulfate	0.1	percent (w/v)
procaine hydrochloride	0.2	percent (w/v)
propylene glycol	80	percent (v/v)
distilled water	q.s.	

When properly administered, 'Aerolin' is apparently the most effective known agent for the relief of asthmatic attacks. Its dosage and administration are discussed on page 266.

The next most effective route for administration of aludrine (as the hydrochloride; 'Aerolin' is suitable only for inhalation) is the sublingual. It works well in the early abortion of mild asthma but is less beneficial in cases of moderate severity and of little or no value in severe asthma. The usual adult sublingual dose is 10 mg. If relief is to be obtained from this dose, it will probably appear in five to ten minutes. If no relief and no important side-effects have been observed in fifteen minutes, the dose may be repeated. A third dose may be given after an additional quarter hour if there is still no relief and no serious side-effects. On later occasions, initial doses of 15 or 20 mg. may be feasible in patients not responding to smaller doses. Care must be taken to instruct the patient regarding the technic of sublingual administration (p. 283); swallowing of the drug is to be avoided. Mild and fleeting side-effects can be expected in about one-third of patients.

Subcutaneous injection of aludrine salts should be reserved for the more serious cases not responding to inhalation or sublingual administration. Because of the local vasodilator effect, absorption is very rapid, and both therapeutic effects and side reactions are intensified. Therapeutic effect is less

prolonged (two to three hours) than after the other two routes. The initial subcutaneous dose for adults should be 0.0625 mg. (0.25 cc. of the 1:4,000 solution). If this proves inadequate and the side-effects are not excessive, the next dose may be 0.5 cc. Eventually, the optimal dose for the individual is found. Dosage for children is in proportion to body weight. In the presence of a vicious asthmatic cycle, it may be necessary to repeat the subcutaneous dose every two hours. After six such doses, sublingual administration should be substituted if it is effective by that time.

Oral administration of aludrine is not recommended. The therapeutic effect is relatively slight, and the side-effects are relatively great.

The most frequent side-effect of aludrine is tachycardia, which may cause palpitation. Some rise in pulse rate can be expected, and there is an accompanying increase in cardiac work. In severe asthma with anoxia, dosage should be cautious until it is evident that the heart muscle is not being adversely affected by the stimulation induced by the drug. Ordinarily the acceleration of rate appears in one or two minutes and disappears in less than fifteen minutes.

With therapeutic doses the blood pressure may rise, fall, or remain the same. Sometimes there is a rise in systolic and a fall in diastolic pressure. A precipitate fall in both systolic and diastolic pressure has been reported. Other side-effects include, in order of decreasing frequency, nausea, headache, nervousness, tremor, dizziness, precordial ache, weakness, sweating, and related symptoms.

Aludrine should be used cautiously in the presence of myocardial degeneration, acute myocardial damage, limited cardiac reserve, and hyperthyroidism.

Ephedrine occurs in plants of the genus *Ephedra*, one of which is the Chinese herb ma huang. Its actions are basically like those of epinephrine, but it differs both chemically and pharmacologically in important respects. Its chemical structure lacks the two hydroxyl groups on the benzene ring, and there is a methyl group on the alpha carbon atom (next to the amine group; see Figure 34, p. 422). The presence of two asymmetric carbon atoms makes possible six forms (four isomers and two combinations of isomers): *l*, *d*, and *dl*-ephedrine and *l*, *d*, and *dl*-pseudoephedrine. Only *l*-ephedrine is official in the U.S.P., and it is the form discussed here. *dl*-Ephedrine (racephedrine) has about three-fourths the potency of *l*-ephedrine. Racephedrine Hydrochloride is official in the N.F.

Ephedrine appears to have a different mode of action from epinephrine as evidenced by the following laboratory observations and by the clinical observations in the succeeding paragraph: Ephedrine does not evoke increased responses from denervated effector organs or after large doses of cocaine; its action is not reversed by ergotoxine; and it has relatively little action on isolated tissues.

In further contrast to epinephrine, ephedrine is stable and is effective on oral administration. It is more rapidly absorbed than epinephrine after subcutaneous injection because of the lesser degree of local vasoconstriction. It has a longer duration of action but, if repeated too frequently, may induce a progressively diminished response (tachyphylaxis). The action of ephedrine on arterioles is less than that of epinephrine, but that on veins is greater; following a pressor effect of ephedrine, there is no secondary hypotension. Ephedrine has a pronounced stimulating effect on the central nervous system. Its mydriatic effect is useful clinically (see p. 436), and it is of some value in the treatment of myasthenia gravis (p. 250).

Ephedrine is most commonly administered as the hydrochloride or sulfate. Both are stable and freely soluble in water. The sulfate should not be added to solutions containing calcium (such as Ringer's Solution) because of the insolubility of calcium sulfate. For systemic administration, ephedrine salts are available in ampoules, hypodermic tablets, capsules, elixir, and syrup. In some of these and in enteric coating, sedative or other drugs are also present. For topical application as vasoconstrictors and decongestants, ephedrine salts are supplied as aqueous solutions and jellies with and without additional medication. An oil solution of ephedrine base has also been used as a nasal spray.

IN ALLERGY—Ephedrine is extremely useful in the symptomatic treatment of hay fever and asthma. It is of little value against acute urticaria, angioneurotic edema, serum sickness, or anaphylaxis but may have prophylactic value in chronic urticaria. In hay fever, the hydrochloride or sulfate is given by mouth in doses of 10 to 50 mg. (1/6 to 3/4 grain). It acts as a nasal and conjunctival vasoconstrictor to reduce congestion and edema and the discomfort which results from them. It has less effect on the watery nasal secretion. The action usually lasts three to seven hours. Ephedrine can with advantage be combined with antihistaminics (p. 509). Solutions or jellies of ephedrine salts may be applied to the nose, but in hay fever the drug is less effective by this route and the solution is usually irritating to the allergic mucous membrane.

In asthma, ephedrine salts may be given by mouth or hypodermically in doses of 25 to 50 mg. (3/8 to 3/4 grain). In treatment of attacks, ephedrine is much less powerful than epinephrine and is useful only in mild paroxysms; its onset of action is slower, but the duration of action (usually four hours) is longer than that of aqueous solutions of epinephrine hydrochloride. The principal value of ephedrine in asthma is for prevention of attacks, for which the oral route is adequately effective. It can often be combined advantageously with one of the xanthine drugs (p. 358). Dosage should be repeated three to six times daily.

Because of the common side-effects of nervousness, tremor, and wakefulness (which are, however, less intense than those from epinephrine), and because allergic patients frequently benefit by sedation, ephedrine is often given in combination with a barbiturate in allergic conditions.

DURING ANESTHESIA—In spinal and epidural (including caudal) anesthesia, there is commonly a reduction in arterial pressure due to a blocking of tonic vasomotor impulses to the abdominal viscera and legs. Ephedrine salts are valuable aids in preventing and correcting this hypotension.

Dosage and administration are discussed beginning on page 439.

IN HEART DISEASE—In complete heart block with syncopal seizures (Adams-Stokes syndrome), ephedrine salts taken by mouth may prevent the periods of asystole which lead to syncope. The minimal effective dosage (usually 15 to 30 mg. three times daily) should be employed, since administration must usually be continued indefinitely, and unnecessarily large doses may be harmful because of the usual presence of serious organic heart disease. The exact cause of the asystole should be determined, if possible, because ephedrine is contraindicated if the seizures are due to ventricular prefibrillation.

Like epinephrine, ephedrine is not of value and may be harmful in the treatment of heart failure or shock.

OTHER USES—The nasal congestion and discomfort which accompany the common cold, acute or chronic sinusitis, and other nasal infections can often be substantially relieved by ephedrine. The drug may be given systemically as 25 to 50 mg. of the sulfate or hydrochloride by mouth every four to six hours, or it may be applied topically to the nasal mucosa as an aqueous solution of an ephedrine salt, 1 to 3 percent, or an oil solution of ephedrine base, 1 percent. There is no secondary hyperemia following the use of ephedrine.

In postural hypotension with syncopal attacks (p. 85), ephedrine sulfate, 25 to 50 mg. every two to four hours by mouth, often prevents fainting. The first daily dose is taken an hour before arising.

Ephedrine is useful as a supplement to Prostigmine in myasthenia gravis (p. 250). Doses of 10 to 25 mg. two or three times daily should seldom be exceeded, for larger doses may aggravate rather than relieve the weakness. The mechanism of relief is not known, although it has been noted that under certain circumstances ephedrine can prevent the effects of skeletal muscular fatigue in animals.

The central nervous stimulation of ephedrine may be useful in combating overdoses of depressant drugs such as morphine and the barbiturates, although it is probably inferior to methamphetamine (see below) for this purpose. The dosage and frequency of administration must be governed by the patient's condition; the initial dose may be 50 mg. by hypodermic injection.

Ephedrine has value in certain types of cough, including that of whooping cough, probably because of its bronchodilator action. It is for this reason a common ingredient of cough syrups. In doses of 10 to 50 mg. three times daily, it is a valuable symptomatic measure in narcolepsy. Its use as a mydriatic is discussed on page 436, and in enuresis on page 225.

SIDE-EFFECTS—Ephedrine in therapeutic doses is likely to produce insomnia and nervousness. Less frequently it gives rise to tremor, palpitation, dizziness, warmth, sweating, and headache. These side-effects are in most patients completely controlled by ordinary doses of the barbiturates. Uncommonly, patients may complain of nausea, vomiting, anorexia, or precordial pain. Spasm of the vesical sphincter may lead to difficulty in urination. Cardiac arrhythmias are a rare complication. Contact dermatitis from topical application has been reported.

In general, the same precautions and contraindications apply to ephedrine as to epinephrine (p. 425), although perhaps not so stringently. However, ephedrine should be used cautiously in the presence of organic heart disease (compensated or decompensated), hypertension, hyperthyroidism, and angina pectoris and during therapy with digitalis.

Ephedrine does not produce addiction or chronic intoxication.

Methamphetamine (desoxyephedrine) is related chemically to both amphetamine (discussed below) and ephedrine (see Figure 34, p. 423). It is stable and is active on oral administration. An asymmetric carbon atom is responsible for optical isomerism. The dextrorotatory form is the most potent in its central effects.

Pharmacologically, d-methamphetamine differs greatly from ephedrine in that the central stimulant effects completely overshadow the adrenergic actions. d-Methamphetamine hydrochloride ('Amphedroxyn Hydrochloride,' Methedrine Hydrochloride, Pervitin Hydrochloride), when given in doses of 2.5 to 5 mg. by mouth, elevates the mood, increases the urge to work, and counteracts sleepiness and the feeling of fatigue in most persons, with only slight elevation of blood pressure and pulse. The euphoric effects begin ten to sixty minutes after administration and continue for six to twelve or, in some instances after large doses, as long as thirty-six hours. The drug does not improve intelligence, but it increases attention and speed in performance tests without affecting reaction time. The result apparently is achieved by facilitating the use of reserve energy. Total performance over a period of weeks does not seem to be improved, and the need for rest and sleep is not reduced.

Therapeutically, d-methamphetamine may be useful for temporary or emergency use as a cerebral stimulant and to impart a sense of decreased fatigue and sleepiness. It may be employed in postoperative depression, mild nervous depression, and to counteract overdoses of depressant drugs such as morphine and barbiturates (see pp. 399 and 390). The usual dose is 2.5 mg. once or twice daily. The first dose is taken on arising; if a second dose is taken, it should be at or before noon.

d-Methamphetamine, in doses of 2.5 or 5 mg., is effective in overcoming the symptoms of alcoholic intoxication. In narcolepsy, 2.5 to 7.5 mg. two or three times daily may afford symptomatic relief. Doses of 15 mg. reduce appetite in about 30 percent of patients. The drug may be useful in postencephalitic Parkinsonism, but it is contraindicated in that due to arteriosclerosis; the average dosage is 2.5 to 5 mg. daily.

In clinical use a total daily dose of 10 mg. should seldom be exceeded. Overdoses may produce insomnia, restlessness, weakness, dyspnea, tachycardia, cardiac arrhythmia, mydriasis, and nausea and vomiting. Allergy (urticaria) has been reported. The lethal human dose is apparently very high, for no fatalities have been reported.

The possibilities for abuse of methamphetamine are obvious. Just as in addiction to morphine or alcohol, such abuse generally indicates an inadequate personality seeking an escape mechanism.

Patients of this type should not be given an opportunity to acquaint themselves with the properties of methamphetamine. Continued use may lead to tolerance.

Methamphetamine is also contraindicated in patients with myocardial degeneration, coronary disease, hypertension, hyperthyroidism, or arteriosclerotic Parkinson's disease. It should be avoided in hyperexcitable, agitated, or elderly individuals and in those known to be unusually susceptible to the effects of adrenergic drugs.

When applied topically to the nasal mucosa, racemic methamphetamine has a vasoconstrictor action similar to that of ephedrine. Its hydrochloride is employed particularly in combination with sodium sulfathiazole, with which ephedrine salts are incompatible. The quantities of methamphetamine absorbed seldom exert systemic effects.

Amphetamine (Benzedrine) differs chemically from methamphetamine in the absence of a methyl group on the nitrogen atom (see Figure 34, p. 423). The asymmetric alpha carbon atom in the side chain makes possible optical isomerism. As with methamphetamine, the dextrorotatory isomer has the more powerful central effects.

Racemic amphetamine (Benzedrine), like ephedrine and epinephrine, is adrenergic (see Table 44, p. 417). It has, in addition, a strong stimulating effect on the central nervous system like that of methamphetamine. Amphetamine is very slowly destroyed in the body, and much of it is excreted in the urine. The volatility of amphetamine base led to its administration by inhalation as a nasal vasoconstrictor; but the side-effects of nervousness and insomnia were common, and there was great possibility for abuse of the central nervous effects. It is no longer available in inhaler form.

d-Amphetamine (Dexedrine), because of the greater ratio of central nervous to adrenergic effects, is to be preferred to racemic amphetamine when central effects are desired. *d*-Amphetamine is used for the same purposes as *d*-methamphetamine but is apparently less potent except in the matter of diminishing appetite. Average doses of *d*-amphetamine sulfate are as follows: for euphoric and central-nervous-system stimulant effects, 5 to 15 mg. daily, one-half the dose on arising, the other half before noon; in narcolepsy, 10 to 50 mg. daily, subdivided as required; for reduction of appetite, 15 to 20 mg. daily in three equal doses taken before breakfast, at 11 a.m., and at 4 p.m.; in postencephalitic Parkinsonism, 10 to 25 mg. daily, one-half on arising, the other half before noon.

d-Amphetamine is subject to the same precautions and contraindications as methamphetamine, and the side-effects are, in general, similar. Perhaps because it has been in clinical use longer than methamphetamine, a greater variety of side-effects has been reported with amphetamine, usually following overdosage. They include (in addition to those given under methamphetamine) talkativeness, irritability, tremors, confusion, delirium, hallucinations, panic states, and suicidal or homicidal tendencies. Fatigue and depression commonly follow the central stimulation. Deaths have occurred.

Neo-Synephrine (phenylephrine) differs from epinephrine in lacking that hydroxyl group which is in the para position on the benzene ring to the side chain (see Figure 34, p. 422). It is an adrenergic drug with important therapeutic differences from both epinephrine and ephedrine. It has an asymmetric carbon atom (in the beta position), and the levorotatory form, which is the most active, is used in medicine.

The predominant action of Neo-Synephrine is on the vascular system. It raises blood pressure, largely by peripheral vasoconstriction, but cardiac output may be increased also. In comparison with epinephrine, Neo-Synephrine and its salts are more stable, and their effects are more lasting. With therapeutic doses, the side-effects of anxiety, tremor, nervousness, and headache, so common with epinephrine, are seldom seen. The principal clinical uses are as a vasopressor during spinal anesthesia and as a topical nasal vasoconstrictor.

As a pressor drug, Neo-Synephrine Hydrochloride is usually given subcutaneously in doses of 1 to 10 mg.; the initial dose should not exceed 5 mg., and subsequent injections should be no more frequent than every ten or fifteen minutes. The effect of subcutaneous injection usually lasts one or two hours. In emergency, the drug may be given slowly and cautiously by vein in quantities of 0.5 to 3 mg. The pressor action of Neo-Synephrine is more positive than that of ephedrine; this makes Neo-Synephrine of great value in extreme emergency but necessitates caution in its use and great care to avoid overdosage. Oral doses of 10 to 25 mg. usually have pressor effects which may be useful in such conditions as orthostatic hypotension. In therapeutic doses, Neo-Synephrine does not lose its effectiveness on repeated administration and does not affect the central nervous system.

As a nasal vasoconstrictor for topical application, Neo-Synephrine Hydrochloride is employed as an aqueous solution of 0.25, 0.5, or, in resistant cases,

1 percent concentration or as a 0.5 percent jelly. It has a relatively prolonged action without secondary hyperemia.

Therapeutic doses of Neo-Synephrine very seldom produce side-effects. However, dosage must be carefully regulated to avoid undesirably high elevations of arterial pressure. The same other general contraindications and precautions apply to Neo-Synephrine as to epinephrine.

Cobefrin is closely related to epinephrine both chemically and pharmacologically. The methyl group which in epinephrine is attached to the nitrogen atom is in Cobefrin attached to the first (alpha) carbon atom of the side chain (see Figure 34, p. 422). Therapeutically, the two are similar, but Cobefrin is less potent. Its clinical use is limited to the production of local vasoconstriction in solutions of local anesthetic agents, particularly in the dental field. Cobefrin Hydrochloride is employed in concentrations of 1:80,000 to 1:10,000, which correspond to concentrations of epinephrine hydrochloride of 1:400,000 to 1:50,000.

Propadrine (phenylpropanolamine) occurs in small amounts with ephedrine in plants of the genus *Ephedra*. It differs chemically from ephedrine only in the absence of a methyl group on the nitrogen (see Figure 34, p. 422). As with ephedrine, the presence of two asymmetric carbon atoms (alpha and beta of the side chain) makes possible six optical isomers. The pseudopropadrines are relatively inactive; the *d*, *l*, and *dl*-propadrines are similar in potency and have an action much like that of ephedrine. The racemic (*dl*) form is available for clinical use.

Therapeutically, Propadrine Hydrochloride is employed by systemic administration in allergy and by topical application as a nasal vasoconstrictor (see p. 378) in the same manner as ephedrine. The oral dose is 3/8 to 3/4 grain every two to four hours as needed. The drug is applied to the nasal mucosa usually as a 1 percent solution or a 0.66 percent jelly. The effect is said to be more prolonged than that of ephedrine, and central-nervous-system stimulation appears to be less common. The general contraindications and precautions which apply to ephedrine apply also to Propadrine.

Vonedrine (phenylpropylmethylamine) is an adrenergic drug which differs chemically from ephedrine in two ways: It contains no hydroxyl group, and the methyl group attached to the first (alpha) carbon atom of the side chain in ephedrine is joined instead to the second (beta) carbon atom

in Vonedrine (see Figure 34, p. 423). The racemic preparation is used in medicine.

The base is volatile and is employed in inhaler form as a nasal vasoconstrictor. Shrinkage is produced without blanching; the effect is reasonably prolonged; and there is no secondary congestion or hyperemia. The levulinate salt is applied to the nose as a 0.5 percent solution. The onset of effect is slower than that of ephedrine salts but is somewhat more prolonged. There is less tendency toward central-nervous-system stimulation.

Benzedrex, 1-cyclohexyl-2-methylaminopropane, differs chemically from methamphetamine in that the ring is saturated and hence has an aliphatic rather than an aromatic character (see Figure 34, p. 423). This chemical change results in a great alteration of pharmacologic properties; Benzedrex is volatile and has relatively little effect on the central nervous system. It is used clinically in inhaler form as a nasal vasoconstrictor.

OTHER CYCLIC COMPOUNDS

Cyclopentamine, the hydrochloride of which is marketed by Eli Lilly and Company as 'Clopane Hydrochloride,' is related chemically to methamphetamine and Benzedrex; it has the same side chain, but the ring structure consists of only five carbon atoms and is saturated (see Figure 34, p. 423). As with Benzedrex, saturation of the ring brings a recession in the ability to stimulate the central nervous system.

'Clopane Hydrochloride' is employed therapeutically because of its powerful vasoconstrictor action. As a pressor agent during anesthesia, it is of about the same potency as ephedrine and is given subcutaneously in the same dosage—usually 25 mg. (for details of use, see p. 439). In emergency, 5 to 10 mg. may be given very slowly by vein.

Applied topically to the nasal mucosa, a 0.5 percent aqueous solution of 'Clopane Hydrochloride' has about the same potency as 1 or 2 percent 'Tuamine Sulfate' (see below) and a more powerful and enduring action than 3 percent ephedrine sulfate. There is no secondary engorgement after the effect wears off. For associated decongestant and anti-infective action, 'Clopane Hydrochloride' can be combined with penicillin. The 0.5 percent solution may also be applied to the eye to produce mydriasis without cycloplegia. The drug is one of the important constituents of 'Aerolin' (p. 426); the latter is a very potent bronchodilator which affords symptomatic relief in asthma.

As with any pressor drug, systemic administration of 'Clopane Hydrochloride' should be cautious, especially in the presence of vascular disease or hyperthyroidism. Side-effects, as distinct from excessive therapeutic effects due to overdosage, are apparently extremely rare.

Privine (naphazoline) follows in only a general way the chemical pattern of previously discussed adrenergic drugs (see Figure 34, p. 423); there is the double ring of naphthalene in place of the benzene or cyclopentyl single ring, and the side chain contains a second amino nitrogen and has been condensed into a ring. When applied topically to the nasal mucosa, Privine Hydrochloride has an extremely powerful and prolonged vasoconstrictor action. A 0.05 percent solution or jelly is usually effective for several (often six to eight) hours. The extreme potency of the drug necessitates great caution in its use. Only two or three drops (in children, one or two drops) should be instilled into each nostril, and administration should be repeated only after the effect has worn off. Excessive use may cause local anoxia from extreme reduction in local blood flow, with resultant secondary hyperemia and congestion or more serious tissue damage. If overdosage has taken place and the drug is reapplied to overcome the secondary engorgement, a vicious cycle may be set up. Stronger solutions than 0.05 percent should not be used except by the physician in his office.

When the drug is correctly used, side-effects are apparently very rare. Solutions should be kept out of contact with aluminum.

STRAIGHT-CHAIN COMPOUNDS

'Tuamine' (Tuaminoheptane, Lilly) is a straight-chain aliphatic compound (see Figure 34, p. 423) which has a powerful topical vasoconstrictor action without side-effects. The base is volatile and is employed in inhaler form as a nasal vasoconstrictor. Solution 'Tuamine Sulfate,' 1 or 2 percent, may be applied topically for the same purpose; the stronger solution should be reserved for use in the physician's office. The 1 percent solution has a more powerful and enduring action than 2 percent ephedrine sulfate; release is gradual and is not followed by secondary engorgement. For displacement therapy by the Proetz technic, a 0.2 percent solution is adequate.

No side-effects have been reported. Oral administration of relatively large doses has not raised the blood pressure of normal individuals.

'Forthane' (Methylhexamine, Lilly) is 2-amino-4-methylhexane and is an isomer of 'Tuamine' (see Figure 34, p. 423). It is volatile, like 'Tuamine,' but is about four times as potent. It, also, is employed in inhaler form as a nasal vasoconstrictor. One or two inhalations through each nostril are usually sufficient, and the effect lasts one-half hour or more. No side-effects have been reported.

Oenethyl, 2-methylaminoheptane, is the methyl derivative of 2-aminoheptane and bears the same chemical relation to it that epinephrine bears to arterenol (see Figure 34, p. 423). Oenethyl has been employed clinically as a pressor drug in connection with anesthesia. It has a longer duration of action than epinephrine and differs also in raising both systolic and diastolic pressures. The elevation is ordinarily greater in the systolic pressure, with the result that pulse pressure is increased.

The drug has little pressor effect on unanesthetized individuals. In those under anesthesia, intramuscular doses of 75 to 100 mg. begin to take effect usually in two to three minutes, but the action is not maximal for about ten minutes. When systolic pressure is below 60 mm. Hg, intramuscular doses are ineffective. Intravenous injection initiates a response in one to two minutes which does not become maximal for about five minutes. It has been recommended that doses of 5 to 10 mg. be injected intravenously fifteen to thirty seconds apart until a satisfactory response is obtained (usually after 25 mg.), at which time an intramuscular dose is given which is double the total quantity previously administered by the intravenous route. It has been observed, however, that the final blood pressure attained is usually higher than the preanesthetic level, a result which is not always desirable.

Oenethyl displays tachyphylaxis (diminished response on repeated doses), and administration by continuous drip has not been satisfactory. Therapeutic doses increase respiratory rate in most patients and may cause pupillary dilation lasting about thirty minutes. If the drug is given to patients already under inhalation anesthesia, extrasystoles may be observed. Side-effects include nausea, dizziness, and pallor—usually mild.

DRUGS INHIBITING STRUCTURES INNERVATED BY ADRENERGIC NERVES

For many years chemists and pharmacologists have sought agents which would inhibit the structures innervated by adrenergic nerves in a manner analogous to that in which atropine and related drugs inhibit the structures innervated by cholinergic nerves. Until recently, the nearest approach was the ergot alkaloids ergotamine and ergotoxine, which inhibit adrenergic responses in animals. However, the doses required are in the toxic range, and the drugs could not be used clinically for this purpose.

During the past ten years several new drugs have become available which are steps toward the goal. Some of them block one or more phases of the action of epinephrine, an effect which is termed "adrenolytic." Others are capable of blocking one or more phases of the excitatory type of response to sympathetic stimulation and therefore are termed "sympatholytic." The clinical use of all of them must still be considered as experimental.

Benodaine (benzodioxane, 933 F) is 2-(1-piperidylmethyl)-1,4-benzodioxane. It is a stable substance, the structural formula of which is shown in Figure 35. Benodaine has the ability to prevent the action of epinephrine, particularly on blood pressure. It is thus adrenolytic. Because of its similarity in structure to epinephrine (compare Figure 35 with Figure 34, p. 422), Benodaine is thought to act by occupying the receptors for epinephrine and thus blocking access of the latter to the effector organs.

Not all phases of the action of Benodaine are understood. It has been employed as a diagnostic agent for epinephrine-producing tumors (pheochromocytoma and paraganglioma) as a cause of hypertension. For this purpose a dose of 10 mg. of Benodaine Hydrochloride per square meter of body surface (for calculation, see nomogram, p. 569) is given. The patient must rest quietly in a supine posture until the pulse rate and blood pressure have become stabilized. The Benodaine in 0.2 per cent solution is then injected intravenously over a period of two minutes. The pulse and blood pressure are recorded every minute for fifteen minutes. If the patient's hypertension is due to epinephrine, a significant fall in blood pressure can be expected to take place from a few seconds to four minutes after the injection. The pressure usually returns to the preinjection level within fifteen minutes, and when it does, the readings can be discontinued. The interpretation of the test is not absolute: A fall in blood pressure following Benodaine has been recorded in a case of renal hypertension, and a rise in a case of hypertensive vascular disease.

Benodaine has been suggested as a blocking agent during operations for the removal of epinephrine-producing tumors, for the purpose of forestalling the dangerous effects of the large quantities of epinephrine which may be released during the inevitable manipulation of the tumor. Such use should probably be cautious until more experience is gained.

Side-effects are fairly common after the intravenous injection of Benodaine. They usually last no longer than two or three minutes, although occasionally they may persist for twenty to twenty-five minutes. They include tachycardia, palpitation, substernal pressure, precordial distress, flushing, cold and clammy extremities, nervousness, apprehension, dizziness, mild headache, hyperpnea, and sighing respirations. No permanent or serious side-effects have been reported.

Dibenamine, N,N-dibenzyl-beta-chloroethylamine (for structural formula, see Figure 35), has sympatholytic as well as adrenolytic properties. It not only blocks but also reverses the vasopressor response to all doses of epinephrine; it blocks the vasopressor and vasoconstrictor effects of Neo-Synephrine (p. 429); and it diminishes the vasopressor but not the vasoconstrictor response to ephedrine (p. 426). It blocks the anticurare action of epinephrine. On the other hand, Dibenamine does not influence the following effects of epinephrine: increase in heart rate and cardiac output, relaxation of the intestine and nonpregnant uterus (cat), hyperpnea, and rise in blood sugar. It would seem that Dibenamine must block some essential step in the excitatory process— a step which occurs between the site of action of certain sympathomimetic agents and the final contractile mechanism of the smooth muscle cell.

Even more than with Benodaine, the clinical use of Dibenamine is still experimental. It lowers blood pressure in certain types of hypertensive patients, but its local irritant properties make it an impractical agent for prolonged therapy. It has been used with excellent effect to protect against cardiac arrhythmias during anesthesia with cyclopropane. It has also been employed in the management of certain psychopathologic states—as an adjunct to diminish symptoms related to anxiety, fear, anger, and associated conditions and believed to be mediated through the sympathetic nervous system.

Dibenamine is effective by the oral, intramuscular, and intravenous routes, but it produces sufficient local irritation to make the intravenous route the only practical one. Even when given carefully by vein, it tends to produce venospasm and phlebothrombosis. The usual intravenous dose of the hydrochloride is 4 to 6 mg. per Kg. (1.8 to 2.7 mg.

per lb.) of body weight. It is administered in 500 or more cc. of isotonic salt solution over a period of thirty to sixty minutes. The maximum action is exerted during the first twenty-four hours. However, in some patients the response to sympathomimetic agents is altered for several days.

Side-effects to Dibenamine are common. They fall into three groups:

1. Local irritation.

2. Vasodilation—congestion of the nasal mucosa, tingling of the feet, sweating, and postural hypo-

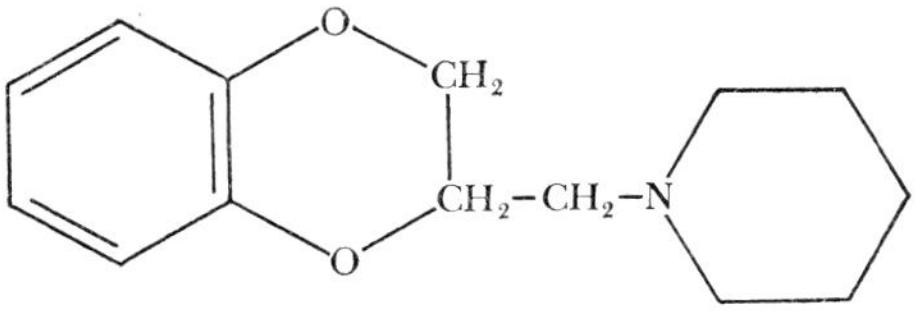

Benodaine

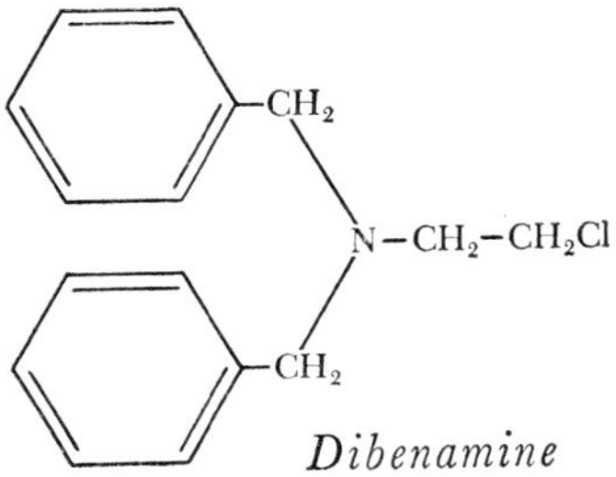

Dibenamine

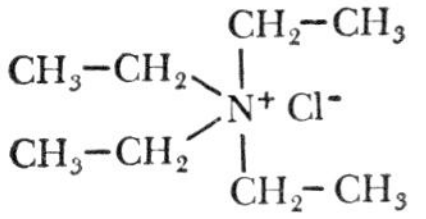

Tetraethylammonium Chloride
(Etamon Chloride)

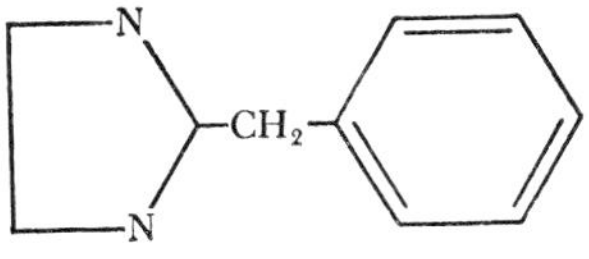

Priscoline

FIGURE 35—*Structural Formulas of Antiadrenergic Drugs*

tension with severe vertigo and faintness on standing. This last effect may persist for twenty-four hours.

3. General toxic effects, including nausea, palpitation, dizziness (as distinguished from vertigo), restlessness, irritability, psychotic episodes, drowsiness, and convulsions.

Tetraethylammonium (T.E.A.) compounds (for formula, see Figure 35) have the property of blocking the transmission of nerve impulses at autonomic ganglia. The effects are complex and are mutually antagonistic to those of both adrenergic and cholinergic substances, including the tetra*methyl*ammonium compounds.

Perhaps the most valuable clinical application of tetraethylammonium compounds at present is the production of sympathetic block of the extremities in such conditions as thrombophlebitis, causalgia, post-traumatic states, Raynaud's disease, acrocyanosis, and peripheral vascular disease. Tetraethylammonium is also useful in evaluating vasomotor tone but has not been of value as a test for selection of those hypertensive patients who may be expected to benefit from sympathectomy. It is not effective in the medical management of hypertension, even though it produces a temporary fall in arterial pressure. It has been used as a diagnostic agent for epinephrine-producing tumors in the same way as Benodaine (p. 432) and for reduction of gastro-intestinal tone and motility as a therapeutic measure and in connection with x-ray studies.

Tetraethylammonium bromide or chloride (the latter is also known as Etamon Chloride) is effective on intramuscular or intravenous injection but not by mouth. The usual intravenous dose is 4 to 6 mg. per Kg. (1.8 to 2.7 mg. per lb.) of body weight, given over a period of 90 to 120 seconds. If it is injected as an intravenous infusion at the rate of 8 to 12 mg. total per minute, much of its effect is retained without significant reduction in blood pressure. Relatively large doses can be given intramuscularly.

Some of the side-effects encountered with tetraethylammonium compounds are physiological actions to be expected of an agent which blocks autonomic ganglia: loss of accommodation, hypotension in the upright posture (producing vertigo and faintness) and in the supine as well, reduced gastro-intestinal motility, and inability to void. Others include sleepiness, excitability, tingling of the extremities, ventricular extrasystoles (with large doses), and purpura. Death has been reported following intravenous administration.

Priscoline (Priscol) is 2-benzylimidazoline (for structural formula, see Figure 35). It has several types of action which vary in different species of animals. Some of them depend on dosage. In small doses (15 mg.) the drug is adrenolytic (i.e., it blocks the action of adrenergic drugs) with respect to blood pressure. In larger doses it is sympatholytic as well (i.e., it blocks the effect of the sympathetic nervous system on blood pressure). It does not influence depressor or dilator actions. Priscoline also displays cholinergic effects: It stimulates the gastro-intestinal tract, including gastric secretion, and in this action is blocked by atropine. It also has some histamine-like effects in animals.

The drug has been used clinically for its vasodilator effect in peripheral vascular disease, Raynaud's disease, thrombophlebitis, post-traumatic states, causalgia, and other conditions marked by vasospasm. Relief has also been reported from pain and spasm in acute anterior poliomyelitis, from pain and vomiting in syphilitic gastric crisis, and from pain associated with tabes dorsalis.

Priscoline is effective orally or by any parenteral route. The usual dose is 25 mg. every three or four hours. If the response is not satisfactory and if no side-effects have occurred, the dose may be increased to 50 mg. Children over five can receive doses half this size; children under five, one-fifth. As the dosage is increased, side-effects occur usually in the following order:

1. Flushing of the face and upper trunk.
2. Warming of the extremities with a diminution in the temperature gradient from the trunk to the extremities.
3. Increase in heart rate (10 to 20 beats per minute).
4. Either slight rise or fall in blood pressure while patient is recumbent.
5. Increased pilomotor activity (goose flesh) with brief tingling or chilliness.
6. Diminution, loss, and finally reversal of response to epinephrine.
7. Increased peristalsis.
8. Postural hypotension.
9. Muscular twitching.
10. Diminution or loss of response to pressor reflexes.

In case of undue fall in blood pressure, posterior pituitary extract (p. 473) is usually effective as an antidote. Nausea, vomiting, abdominal pain, or diarrhea is ordinarily controlled by atropine.

Priscoline should be given cautiously, if at all, to patients with gastritis, peptic ulcer, or coronary arteriosclerosis.

ANTISPASMODICS

The term "antispasmodics" refers to drugs which relax spasm of smooth muscle, particularly that of hollow viscera; "spasmolytics" is a synonym. Drugs which relax the smooth muscle of blood vessels are spoken of as "vasodilators" (for discussion, see p. 362). Antispasmodics must also be differentiated from anticonvulsants (p. 413), which are drugs that prevent convulsions, or spasms of central origin, involving skeletal muscle.

The hollow viscera, the smooth muscle of which most often gives rise to clinical syndromes, are the bronchi, intestines, ureters, and bile ducts. In all of these, the muscle is stimulated by the cholinergic (parasympathetic) division of the autonomic nervous system and inhibited by the adrenergic (sympathetic). Accordingly, spasm of visceral smooth muscle can theoretically be relaxed by drugs which act in any of three different ways: (1) by inhibition of the cholinergic system; (2) by stimulation of the adrenergic system; or (3) by a direct relaxing effect on the muscle itself. Actually, the smooth muscle of the different viscera differs in its responsiveness to these modes of attack. Even though dysmenorrhea is believed to be due to spasm of the smooth muscle of the uterus, the responses of the myometrium are sufficiently individual to necessitate a separate discussion, which will be found beginning on page 205.

Belladonna Alkaloids, and especially atropine, act by inhibiting cholinergic responses. They affect all smooth muscle which responds to cholinergic impulses, but their clinical effectiveness is greatest in spastic conditions of the gastro-intestinal tract, including indigestion, spastic constipation, irritable colon, and lead colic. They are also useful in ureteral and biliary colic, in the urgency and frequency of urination which may accompany spastic paraplegia, and in the enuresis of children. The belladonna alkaloids are of little value in asthma. For dosage and administration, see page 420.

Adrenergic Drugs (epinephrine, ephedrine, and related compounds) are of practical value against spasm of the bronchi only (asthma). Aludrine is the most effective, followed in order by epinephrine and ephedrine. For discussion of the drugs themselves, see page 422; for their use in asthma, see page 265.

Papaverine relaxes smooth-muscle spasm by direct action. It is both an antispasmodic and a vasodilator. As an antispasmodic, it is effective on the intestine, ureters, and bile ducts, but it is relatively ineffective on the bronchi. However, when papaverine is employed in the treatment of visceral spasm, morphine should be omitted, since the lat-

ter, while dulling the perception of the pain, actually aggravates its cause and at the same time
overrides the relaxing effect of papaverine. For dosage and administration of papaverine, see page 363.

Nitrites are effective antispasmodics and vasodilators by direct action on the muscle. They often
bring immediate and dramatic relief from intestinal, biliary, or ureteral colic when administered
sublingually or by inhalation. They are not of
value in asthma. A discussion of nitrite preparations, dosage, and administration will be found on
page 364.

The Xanthine Compounds, such as aminophylline
and 'Monotheamin' (Theamin, Lilly), are antispasmodic in their action on the bronchial tree.

They are relatively ineffective against spasm of
other hollow viscera. For discussion of the compounds themselves, see page 358; for their use in
asthma, see page 265.

Synthetic Compounds—Many new chemical substances have been synthesized in an attempt to find
a compound which would combine the desirable
antispasmodic properties of atropine and papaverine without side-effects.

Several such preparations are now in clinical
use. Some of them are moderately effective against
gastro-intestinal spasm, as in peptic ulcer, indigestion, and spastic colon, but there is some difference
of opinion as to their advantage over atropine.
Chemical formulas are shown in Figure 36 (compare with Figure 33, p. 420, and Figure 57, p. 510).

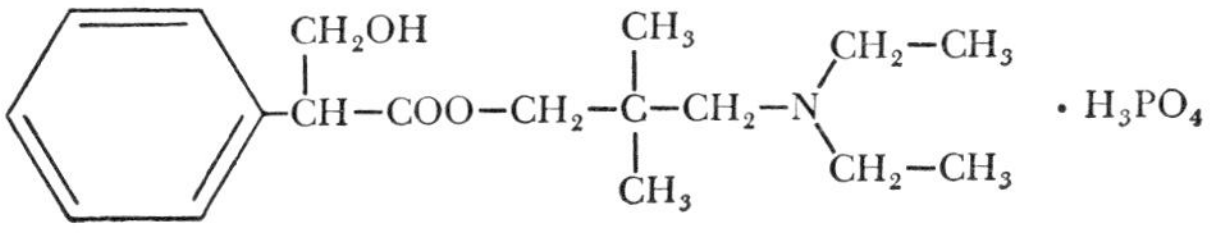

Syntropan

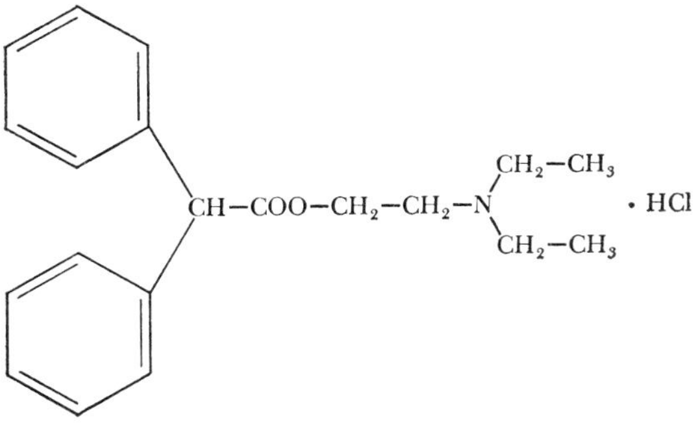

Trasentine

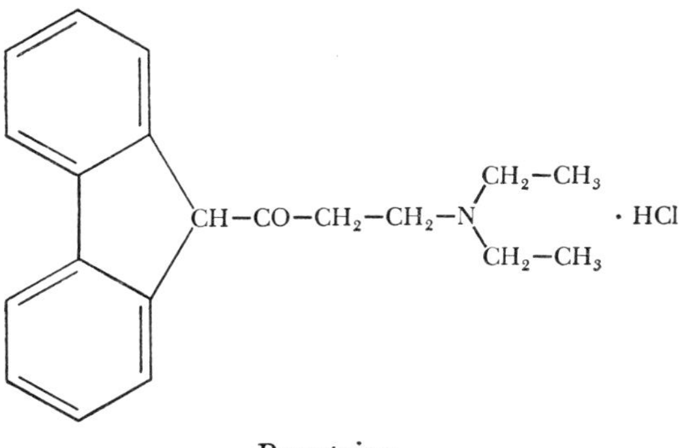

Pavatrine

FIGURE 36—*Structural Formulas of Synthethic Antispasmodics*

Syntropan is given either orally in doses of 50 mg. before meals and at bedtime or subcutaneously in 10-mg. doses as needed. The oral dose of Trasentine is 75 to 150 mg. before meals and at bedtime; the intramuscular dose, 50 mg. Pavatrine is given by mouth in doses of 125 to 250 mg. before meals and at bedtime.

MIOTICS

Miotics act on the eye to cause (1) constriction of the pupil (miosis) and (2) spasm of the muscle of the ciliary body (accommodation). Two mechanisms exist for such action:

1. Parasympathetic stimulation.
2. Sympathetic inhibition.

Morphine produces miosis by the second mechanism. Miosis for clinical purposes is usually achieved by the first mechanism.

Miosis is useful in the treatment of glaucoma (p. 241), after the application of mydriatics and cycloplegics, and, alternating with mydriasis, for the prevention and treatment of adhesions between the iris and the capsule of the lens in iritis and iridocyclitis (p. 241).

Physostigmine (p. 419) and pilocarpine (p. 419) are the drugs usually employed. The former is the more powerful. It is usually applied to the conjunctiva in a 0.2 percent solution as the salicylate. If a more intense effect is necessary, 0.5 to 1 percent solutions can be used. Pilocarpine, as the nitrate, is used in 1 percent concentration. Sometimes the two drugs are combined, to take advantage of their different modes of action. Patients who develop an idiosyncrasy to one of these preparations can be given a 3 percent solution of Prostigmine Bromide (p. 419) or a 0.75 percent solution of carbachol (p. 417). For prolonged effects, instillation is repeated two or three times daily; one or two drops is a sufficient amount.

MYDRIATICS
AND CYCLOPLEGICS

Mydriasis is dilation of the pupil of the eye. Cycloplegia is paralysis of accommodation. The two can be produced by either:

1. Parasympathetic inhibition, or
2. Sympathetic stimulation.

When either of these forces is increased, mydriasis first occurs progressively, and then cycloplegia. Thus, considerable mydriatic effect can be obtained without cycloplegia, but cycloplegia cannot be produced without mydriasis.

The two effects together are useful during active inflammation of the internal structures of the eye (iritis, iridocyclitis, keratitis); the local rest so obtained relieves pain and promotes healing, and the mydriasis helps prevent adhesions. For such a purpose a prolonged maximal effect is desired.

Cycloplegia is often required for refraction. Children are liable to spasm of the accommodation which can be abolished only by a strong cycloplegic effect. In adults, such spasm is both less frequent and easier to overcome.

Mydriasis alone is useful as an aid in ophthalmoscopic examination of the fundus, and alternate mydriasis and miosis are employed to break up adhesions between the iris and neighboring structures. Extreme or prolonged mydriasis tends to impair absorption of intraocular fluid and thus to increase intraocular pressure. In susceptible persons, injudicious mydriasis may precipitate an acute attack of glaucoma (p. 241) with ensuing blindness. Special care is necessary in those over forty years of age.

Atropine (p. 420) is the most powerful mydriatic and cycloplegic. It acts through inhibition of parasympathetic (cholinergic) response. When it is applied to the conjunctiva as the sulfate in 1 percent solution, mydriasis usually begins within fifteen minutes and persists for ten to fourteen days. Cycloplegia begins a few minutes later and is less persistent; in young children repeated instillations are necessary for complete cycloplegia, and the action lasts only two or three days. Because of the extreme effects, atropine is especially valuable in inflammations of the uveal tract. The same property makes it inadvisable as an aid to ophthalmoscopy, and for refraction in adults.

Atropine sulfate, usually in 1 percent strength, may be employed either in aqueous solution or ointment. One or two drops of solution are instilled into the conjunctival sac, and pressure is maintained below the inner canthus of the eye for five to ten minutes to prevent passage of the solution through the nasolacrimal duct into the nose, from which absorption may be sufficient to produce undesirable systemic effects, especially in children. Stronger solutions than 1 percent may be used (with caution!) if necessary, and instillation may be repeated at intervals of a few hours if extreme effects are desired or if inflammation speeds absorption. In susceptible persons atropine may be irritating, producing acute edema or chronic conjunctivitis. Because of the danger of glaucoma, intraocular pressure should always be tested before atropine is used as a mydriatic or cycloplegic.

When the action of atropine is no longer needed, mydriasis and photophobia may be overcome, at least partially, by instillation of a solution of physostigmine salicylate, 0.2 percent (p. 419), or pilocarpine nitrate, 1 percent (p. 419).

Homatropine Hydrobromide in 2 percent solution provides a briefer cycloplegia (twelve to twenty-four hours) which is adequate in adults. Discussion of this compound appears on page 421.

Mydriasis without cycloplegia can be obtained with:

Eucatropine Hydrochloride, 2 or 5 percent (p.421)
'Clopane Hydrochloride,' 0.5 percent (p. 430)
Neo-Synephrine Hydrochloride, 2.5 percent (p. 429)
Ephedrine Sulfate, 3 percent (p. 426)
Amphetamine Sulfate, 3 percent (p. 429)
Epinephrine Hydrochloride, 1 percent (p. 422)

The last five preparations act by sympathetic stimulation. Dilation of the pupil for ophthalmoscopic examination is usually obtained with one drop of the above solutions. A drop of 1 percent pilocarpine nitrate after the examination is a wise precaution.

LOCAL ANESTHETICS

The term "local anesthetic" is applied to drugs which abolish for the time being the conductivity of nerve fibers. The term is also used to designate infiltration anesthesia. A generic term for all the procedures by which peripheral nerves are blocked is "regional anesthesia" (compare with General Anesthesia, p. 410).

Regional anesthesia has a number of forms, based on the relative "peripherality" of the site of application of the anesthetic drug. Beginning with the most central, they include the following:

1. Spinal anesthesia (subdural, subarachnoid).
2. Epidural (peridural) anesthesia, of which caudal anesthesia is a special form.
3. Nerve block.
4. Paravertebral sympathetic block.
5. Field block.
6. Local infiltration.
7. Topical application.

In addition, the analgesic power of low temperatures has been employed to produce local anesthesia (crymoanesthesia).

In contrast to general anesthesia (see p. 410), regional anesthesia has the following characteristics:

1. No effect on consciousness. This is often desirable in poor-risk patients. Consciousness may be depressed, if necessary, by premedication or by supplementary general anesthesia.
2. Analgesia can be restricted to the site of operation.
3. Minimal interference in the functioning of the respiratory and cardiovascular systems and their compensatory mechanisms.
4. No significant alteration in the water and electrolyte balance or in heat regulation.
5. Simple, portable, relatively inexpensive equipment.
6. The agents are abundant, stable, nonexplosive, and easily transportable.
7. In properly selected cases and properly executed procedures, the margin of safety is wide.
8. There are fewer, and commonly less severe, postanesthetic complications than after inhalation anesthesia.
9. Less postoperative time and care are required of the attending personnel.

Limitations or contraindications to regional anesthesia include the following points:

1. Except in the continuous spinal and epidural technics, the limited duration of effect may impose a time restriction on the surgeon.
2. Time and technical ability are necessary to perform the various procedures.
3. Not all patients are suited by temperament and other considerations to regional anesthesia.
4. Anatomical limitations and contraindications to certain procedures.
5. Infection or trauma near anatomical landmarks or site of the procedure.
6. Idiosyncrasy to or toxicity from the drug employed.
7. The presence of multiple wounds in different parts of the body may necessitate too many block procedures and an excess of agent.
8. Occasionally there is inadequate relaxation and exposure of the operative field.
9. Some forms of regional anesthesia, such as local infiltration, may distort the anatomy of the surgical field.

For consistent success in regional anesthesia, certain principles must be followed:

1. The operator must have a thorough knowledge of:
   a. The indications, contraindications, and limitations pertaining to each regional procedure.
   b. The origin, anatomical path, and function of the nerves to be anesthetized.
   c. The anatomical landmarks for each block procedure.
   d. The pharmacology, optimum concentration, and maximum volume of the agent to be employed.
2. Patients must be selected with care. Unpleasant consequences may follow the use of regional anesthesia in patients who are:
   a. Fearful of the procedure to be used.
   b. Unduly apprehensive.
   c. Neurotic.
   d. Suffering from organic disease of the nervous system.
3. Patients should be adequately sedated with premedication and their confidence assured.
4. Prophylactic medication should be employed against toxicity from the anesthetic agent, and means of treatment should be at hand in case symptoms of toxicity or idiosyncrasy develop.
5. Proper needles, syringes, and other equipment should be available and surgically sterile. The area of the patient's body for the insertion of needles should be sterile as for surgical procedures.

6. Solutions of anesthetic agents should be freshly made or ampoules of prepared solutions should be freshly opened; they should be sterile and in the desired concentration and volume.

7. After the regional anesthetic procedure has been completed and the proper interval allowed for anesthesia to develop, patients should be checked for success or failure of the block before being draped for surgery. Signs of toxicity should be quickly noted and treated.

SPINAL ANESTHESIA

Spinal anesthesia results from the deposition of a suitable anesthetic agent in the subarachnoid space. The agent blocks the conduction of nerve impulses cephalad from the level of deposition and from a number of higher segments, depending on the degree of flow or diffusion of the agent. Spinal anesthesia produces complete sensory (afferent) and visceral efferent (including vasomotor) block and, unless the agent is extremely dilute, somatic motor (skeletal muscle) block.

In establishing spinal anesthesia, a single injection may be made, or a needle or catheter may be left in place so that repeated injections are possible. The latter technic is termed "continuous spinal anesthesia." The single-injection technic has the advantage of simplicity. However, the continuous technic is only slightly more difficult, and it has the following advantages:

1. Anesthesia can be prolonged indefinitely.
2. Anesthesia and motor block can be materially diminished or, in some instances, abolished in a matter of minutes by withdrawing the 5 to 10 cc. of spinal fluid which contain the anesthetic agent.
3. The level of anesthesia can be raised or lowered at will by injecting or withdrawing fluid.
4. Very low concentrations of agent can be used, thus minimizing the chance of toxicity.

Low or minimal spinal anesthesia by single injection affords adequate sensory block and relaxation for perineal operations and for vaginal delivery. The descriptive term "saddle block" has been applied to this procedure, even though analgesia must extend to the tenth thoracic segment to control uterine pain. Often the anesthetic agent is weighted by incorporation of dextrose into the vehicle. Following injection, such an agent can be kept low in the spinal canal by the force of gravity. Moderate prolongation of anesthesia may be achieved by addition of 0.5 to 1 mg. of epinephrine hydrochloride (p. 422) to 1 or 2 cc. of spinal anesthetic solution.

Spinal anesthesia is compatible with active pulmonary tuberculosis, bronchiectasis, asthma, and drug addiction; inhalation anesthesia is usually contraindicated in these conditions.

In addition to those for regional anesthesia in general, listed on page 437, spinal anesthesia has the following absolute contraindications:

1. Organic disease of the central nervous system, no matter how mild.
2. Disease of the vertebral column.
3. Chronic backache.
4. Unfavorable skin conditions at site of proposed lumbar puncture.
5. Secondary anemia with hemoglobin below 50 percent.
6. Primary anemia, even when controlled.
7. Septicemia.
8. Lack of experience on the part of the anesthetist.
9. Lack of personnel or equipment in the operating theater to care for the patient in an emergency.

Spinal anesthesia is usually contraindicated by:

10. Difficulty in performing lumbar puncture.
11. Severe debility.
12. Extreme hypotension, relative or absolute.
13. Emotional instability.
14. Fear of spinal anesthesia by the patient.
15. Adverse effects after previous spinal anesthesia.
16. Possibility of severe hemorrhage during operation.

Shock, whether from hemorrhage or other causes, must be brought under control before induction of spinal anesthesia.

The height of anesthesia obtained can be controlled by varying the site and speed of injection, the volume of solution injected, the specific gravity of the solution, and the position of the patient after injection. Other factors being constant, the level may also vary slightly with different agents.

Too high a level of anesthesia temporarily paralyzes the nerves controlling respiration. Respiration may cease abruptly, or involvement of only part of the respiratory muscles may produce a gradually cumulative anoxemia which ultimately results in sudden cardiovascular collapse. Patients should be watched carefully and treated promptly for early signs of hypoxia. Such patients should be given oxygen through a patent airway, by artificial means if necessary, until anesthesia recedes and the patient can resume adequate automatic breathing. If it is deemed advisable to hasten the return of the patient's own respiratory function, up to 20 cc. of spinal fluid can be removed from the lumbar region; the volume withdrawn depends on the desired amount of lowering of the level of motor block and anesthesia. In case of respiratory paralysis, no other treatment than the above is necessary or advisable. In case of cardiovascular collapse, oxygen may be supplemented by subcutaneous or cautious intravenous administration of adrenergic drugs such as epinephrine, Neo-Synephrine, ephedrine, or 'Clopane Hydrochloride.'

Unless the level of anesthesia is higher than the

third lumbar segment, spinal anesthesia has no discernible effect on the vasomotor system. As this level is exceeded, however, a progressively greater portion of the system is blocked from below upward. As the middle thoracic segments are reached, the vasomotor fibers to the abdominal viscera are involved, and pooling of blood in them and in the legs may be extensive enough to reduce the return of blood to the heart sufficiently to cause a fall in arterial pressure. Since an extreme or prolonged fall may be harmful, the blood pressure should be closely watched; as a rule, the systolic pressure should not be allowed to fall below 80 mm. Hg or half the preoperative level, whichever is higher.

Low blood pressure during spinal anesthesia may be combated by (1) raising the patient's legs 15° to 30°, thus returning pooled blood from these members; (2) administering oxygen; and (3) using pressor drugs (see p. 362). Except in patients with hypertension, 25 mg. of ephedrine sulfate or 'Clopane Hydrochloride' (p. 430) are usually injected intramuscularly immediately before lumbar puncture is done. In the presence of hypertension, the injection is delayed until there is evidence of beginning anesthesia. If the systolic pressure falls to 80 mm. Hg or half the preoperative level, whichever is higher, 25 mg. of ephedrine sulfate or 'Clopane Hydrochloride' may be given slowly by vein. If the pressure does not rise within two or three minutes, the injection may be repeated. However, if the excessive fall in blood pressure persists after the first intravenous injection, it is generally due not to the spinal anesthesia but to other conditions which cause shock, such as hemorrhage, traction on the mesentery, or some previously undiscovered pathologic condition of the cardiovascular system. For treatment of shock, see page 90.

In poor-risk and older patients, injection of a pressor drug before lumbar puncture is made, or injection of too large a dose, may be followed by an extreme and prolonged rise of blood pressure resulting in a cerebral accident. In such patients, it is better to await the onset of anesthesia and then administer small doses as they are needed. Frequent intravenous injection of 5 or 10 mg. of ephedrine sulfate or 'Clopane Hydrochloride' may enable the anesthetist to keep the pressure at the exact level desired.

Nausea may be a troublesome phenomenon during spinal anesthesia. It is thought to be due to sudden alterations in blood pressure. When it is due to fall in blood pressure, the measures discussed in the previous paragraphs should be employed. If the anesthesia has risen rapidly to a higher level than is needed, lowering of the level may afford relief in cases in which the continuous technic is being employed.

Spinal anesthesia itself causes few sequelae. Backache may be due to trauma by the needle or to lack of support in the lumbar region while the patient is on the operating table. Headache may follow lumbar puncture even in the absence of spinal anesthesia. Sometimes it can be controlled by hypodermic administration of 0.5 Gm. caffeine and sodium benzoate. If it is troublesome, it can be relieved by either intrathecal injection of 5 to 20 cc. of 5 percent dextrose in isotonic sodium chloride solution or epidural (caudal) injection of 30 to 100 cc. of isotonic sodium chloride solution. For intrathecal injection, a 22-gauge needle is used and care is taken to avoid unnecessary trauma to the dura.

As a persistent sequela, permanent disability due to injury of nerve tissue has occurred, paralysis of the legs or of the vesical or anal musculature being the most common. The most frequent cause seems to be employment of too concentrated a solution of local anesthetic agent. Other factors include preexisting organic disease of the nervous system and mechanical injury to nerve tissue by the lumbar puncture needle.

The agents most commonly used for spinal anesthesia are procaine (p. 442), 'Metycaine' (p. 443), Pontocaine (p. 445), and Nupercaine (p. 445).

EPIDURAL ANESTHESIA

Epidural (peridural) anesthesia is accomplished by depositing a local anesthetic agent beneath the ligamentum flavum in the epidural space, where it acts on nerve trunks as they emerge from the dura peripheral to the posterior root ganglia. The dura is not penetrated. The insertion of a catheter makes possible a "continuous" technic, whereby anesthesia can be prolonged indefinitely.

As in spinal anesthesia, epidural anesthesia produces sensory (afferent), visceral efferent (autonomic), and somatic efferent (skeletal muscle) block. In epidural anesthesia, however, there is more gradation between the different modalities of nerve function, both in intensity and in speed of onset of effect: Vasomotor block may take place minutes before there is noticeable blunting of pain; complete loss of pain may precede by a minute or two complete loss of touch; and this last may precede by half an hour or more complete loss of skeletal motor power, depending on the concentration of anesthetic agent (see also p. 441).

When compared with continuous spinal anesthesia, continuous epidural anesthesia has the following advantages:

1. Less danger of residual nerve damage.
2. Greater separation of the level of anesthesia and the level of skeletal motor block, so that a high level of anesthesia can be produced with less danger of respiratory paralysis (see p. 438).
3. Relatively less motor block, so that patients can still move voluntarily.
4. When, as during labor, the patient is to be left free to move in bed, the epidural technic carries less danger of displacement of the catheter or trauma to the patient.
5. Better tolerated by seriously ill and handicapped patients.
6. Applicable to some cases of disease of the central nervous system in which spinal anesthesia would be contraindicated.
7. Absence of postanesthetic headache.
8. Postoperative pain can be controlled by leaving the catheter in place and injecting additional quantities of agent as required, thus reducing the need for sedatives and narcotics.

Except as noted above, epidural anesthesia has the same advantages, disadvantages, limitations, and contraindications as regional anesthesia in general and spinal anesthesia in particular. When properly executed, the technic of lumbar epidural anesthesia may be easier than spinal anesthesia. In comparison with spinal, the principal disadvantage of epidural is the slower onset of effect (ten to thirty minutes as against about five minutes).

The epidural technics appear to be particularly advantageous in the field of obstetrics—for pain relief during labor and delivery and for cesarean section.

The agents most frequently used for epidural and caudal anesthesia are 'Metycaine' (p. 443), procaine (p. 442), and Pontocaine (p. 445). The duration of anesthesia can be considerably prolonged by the addition of sufficient epinephrine hydrochloride (p. 424) to produce a concentration in the anesthetic solution of 1:100,000.

Caudal Anesthesia is a form of epidural anesthesia in which the needle or catheter is inserted into the caudal epidural space through the sacral hiatus instead of into the lumbar epidural space between the spines of lumbar vertebrae. It has the same advantages and disadvantages as the lumbar technic with the following exceptions:

1. The caudal technic is generally considered to be more difficult.
2. The site of insertion of the caudal needle is more liable to contamination during labor and delivery.
3. A larger volume of agent must be injected caudally to produce a similar level of *abdominal* anesthesia.
4. A smaller volume of agent is required by caudal than by lumbar epidural injection to produce *sacral* (perineal) anesthesia.

NERVE BLOCK

"Nerve block" is the term applied to the deposition of a local anesthetic agent in the immediate vicinity of a nerve trunk. It is obvious that many varieties of block fall into this category. The more central the site of block, the more extensive will be the region anesthetized.

The various nerve blocks confine anesthesia to the site of distribution of the peripheral nerve which is blocked. This avoids extensive vasomotor effects and requires relatively little anesthetic agent. These features may be of considerable advantage in poor-risk cases. On the other hand, nerve block is the most difficult of the various regional blocks, requiring exact knowledge of the anatomy of nerves and landmarks and considerable skill for consistent success.

Sympathetic Ganglion Block (paravertebral sympathetic block) results when the local anesthetic agent is deposited at or near the thoracolumbar sympathetic ganglia which lie in a chain alongside the bodies of the vertebrae. It is used chiefly in treating vasospasm in such conditions as arterial embolism or occlusion of the legs, thrombophlebitis, peripheral arterial disease, and post-traumatic vasomotor disturbances.

As with other nerve blocks, technical skill and experience are necessary for success. The same end can be accomplished, with the additional feature of anesthesia, by high spinal or epidural anesthesia.

The agents commonly employed for nerve block are procaine (p. 442) and 'Metycaine' (p. 443). Addition of epinephrine hydrochloride as in epidural block (see above) provides a similar prolongation of anesthetic effect.

FIELD BLOCK

Field block is produced by injecting a local anesthetic agent into superficial and deep fascial layers along a line so as to block the many terminal nerve filaments and some smaller nerve trunks which pass across the line into the area of operation. Field block is used particularly for moderately large areas such as quadrants of the abdomen. It may provide muscular relaxation as well as analgesia. It has the advantage of being simpler technically than nerve block, and it anesthetizes a larger and deeper area than infiltration. However, unless it is skillfully done, anesthesia may be spotty.

The agents most frequently used for field block are procaine (p. 442) and 'Metycaine' (p. 443).

LOCAL INFILTRATION

Local infiltration is achieved by injecting a local anesthetic agent directly into the tissue which is to be anesthetized. It is suitable for superficial skin areas and is adequate for suturing lacerations or tendons, removing superficial foreign bodies, and the like. It does not provide muscular relaxation and is not suitable for prolonged operations or for very large or multiple areas. Solutions of local anesthetic agents should not be injected into areas which are infected or edematous.

The agent most frequently used for local infiltration is procaine (p. 442). Local anesthesia with any agent is prolonged and intensified by addition to the anesthetic solution of sufficient epinephrine hydrochloride (p. 424) to produce a final concentration of 1:200,000.

TOPICAL APPLICATION

Topical application of local anesthetics may be effective on mucous membranes and on damaged skin. Intact skin is impervious to them. On mucous membranes topical anesthesia affords relief in painful conditions, abolishes reflexes originating in the mucous membrane, and permits operations or otherwise painful procedures. However, anesthesia is limited to the surface, and pain arising in deeper structures is not affected. Areas that are very large, edematous, infected, or extremely vascular are poorly anesthetized. Topical anesthesia should be applied cautiously, if at all, to infected, traumatized, or vascular membranes; they may permit rapid absorption and toxic effects.

Certain topical anesthetics have a satisfactory effect on damaged skin and are useful in burns (including sunburn), abrasions, and certain other types of skin lesions.

The agents most frequently used for topical anesthesia are cocaine (p. 446), 'Surfacaine' (p. 446), Pontocaine (p. 445), and 'Metycaine' (p. 443).

CRYMOANESTHESIA

Crymoanesthesia is analgesia produced by lowering the temperature of the tissues. A temperature of 4° to 5°C. (about 40°F.) provides optimal analgesic effect without damage. The technic is used particularly with devitalized tissues and has the advantage of (1) greatly reducing metabolic requirements at a time when the local circulation is inadequate and (2) minimizing absorption of toxic products from the damaged area.

LOCAL ANESTHETIC AGENTS

A great many substances have local anesthetic properties, but comparatively few have been satisfactory for clinical use. The first to be employed in scientific medicine was cocaine. Its high toxicity led to experimentation which resulted in the synthesis of procaine. All local anesthetics follow in a general way the structure of these two substances.

Local anesthetic agents act by blocking the passage of impulses along nerves. The mechanism for all except Nupercaine is probably interference with an enzyme system which is concerned with restoration of potential following the passage of an impulse. If applied to a nerve in sufficient concentration, a local anesthetic agent causes irreversible changes (i.e., kills the nerve). In lesser concentrations, the changes are reversible. It is those concentrations producing reversible block which are employed clinically. With such concentrations the block is not absolute; extremely strong impulses are capable of breaking through.

Nerve fibers of different kinds vary in their susceptibility to local anesthetic agents, the small unmedullated fibers (unlocalized pain, vasomotor efferent) being the most susceptible and the large, heavily medullated fibers (skeletal muscle motor) being the least susceptible. As the concentration of agent is increased from zero, nerves serving different functions are affected in approximately the following order (different conditions may modify the relative positions somewhat):

Vasomotor efferent
Cold
Warmth (heat, burning)
Pain (unlocalized, diffuse)
Pain (localized)
Touch, deep pressure, joint sense, position sense
    (the last is often lost after skeletal motor)
Skeletal motor

It is thus possible (although for various reasons not always practicable) to administer a local anesthetic in such concentration that only vasomotor effects are obtained, or only vasomotor, temperature sensory, and pain sensory. When higher concentrations are administered, as in spinal or epidural anesthesia, not only do the different types of nerves go out of function in the above order, but those listed first may be affected one or more segments higher than those low on the list. This is particularly noticeable in epidural anesthesia (see p. 439). As anesthesia wears off, functions return in the opposite order from their disappearance. In a patient under continuous spinal anesthesia, for instance, the return of awareness of the legs is an indication for administration of a supplementary dose, since it warns that pain sensation will probably be restored very soon.

Regional anesthesia wears off because of absorption of the agent into the blood or lymph. Agents which are benzoates are destroyed in the blood by enzymes which split the benzoate esters. It was formerly thought that destruction took place entirely in the liver. It is possible to prolong certain forms of regional anesthesia by adding a vasoconstrictor which retards absorption. Such vasoconstrictors are discussed on page 362. Retardation of absorption has the additional advantage of reducing the danger of intoxication by the local anesthetic agent.

When the rate of absorption of local anesthetics exceeds the rate at which they are destroyed, the level in the blood may rise to the point at which systemic toxic effects begin to appear. Toxic reactions are characteristically biphasic (see Table 45); however, in mild overdoses only the first phase may occur, whereas in overwhelming doses the first phase may last only a few seconds and the second phase may dominate the picture. Different individuals vary greatly in their susceptibility and in the extent to which the various systems are involved.

After inadvertent intravenous injection, a reaction, if it occurs, will begin within a few seconds. Most commonly, toxic effects follow the use of overly great volumes or concentrations for topical application or local infiltration. Such reactions usually begin twenty to forty minutes after administration. Their onset may be rapid or insidious. Because of the rapidity with which the drugs are destroyed, late systemic toxic effects do not occur.

TABLE 45—*Systemic Toxic Effects of Local Anesthetic Agents*

System	First Phase	Second Phase
Central nervous	Numbness, nervousness, apprehension, restlessness, dizziness, tinnitus, disorientation, tremors, convulsions	Unconsciousness, coma, death
Autonomic nervous	Excitement, pallor, perspiration	Paralysis of both adrenergic and cholinergic parts
Cardiovascular	Rise in blood pressure, bradycardia	Fall in blood pressure to shock level, tachycardia
Respiratory	Hyperpnea, polypnea	Central respiratory depression
Gastrointestinal	Salivation, nausea, vomiting	

The following steps are recommended to prevent reactions:

1. Inquiry of the patient for history of proved idiosyncrasy to any one agent.
2. Premedication with a barbiturate (0.1 to 0.2 Gm. [1 1/2 to 3 grains] of 'Seconal Sodium' or pentobarbital sodium).
3. Use of clear, colorless solutions of agents (with expiration date if agent is unstable).
4. Use of the most dilute solution capable of producing the desired effect (a given quantity of drug is less toxic in dilute than in concentrated solution; thus, 100 cc. of 0.5 percent solution have a greater margin of safety than 50 cc. of 1 percent).
5. Employment of minimum volume necessary.
6. Addition of a local vasoconstrictor, such as epinephrine, which reduces the rate of absorption of the drug (see p. 424).
7. Aspiration of the needle, by drawing back of the plunger, in two planes before injection (except in spinal anesthesia).
8. Having always available a central-nervous-system depressant for immediate intravenous use (such as a solution of Pentothal Sodium, 2.5 percent).

If a reaction occurs, it should be treated at once by:

1. Immediate cessation of administration of local anesthetic agent.
2. Placing patient in supine posture.
3. Intravenous injection of a barbiturate (Pentothal Sodium, 'Seconal Sodium,' pentobarbital sodium, 'Amytal Sodium') in an amount sufficient to prevent or relieve muscular rigidity.
4. Maintenance of a patent airway and an adequate minute volume of respiration, preferably with pure oxygen and the closed CO_2-absorption system.
5. Treatment of shock if present (see p. 90).
6. Other symptomatic measures if indicated.

Rarely, patients will show true allergy to local anesthetic agents, with bronchospasm, urticaria, angioneurotic edema, or dermatitis. Such reactions usually respond to hypodermic injection of epinephrine hydrochloride, 0.2 to 0.3 cc. of 1:1,000, or to intravenous injection of an antihistaminic drug, such as 'Histadyl' (p. 509).

Procaine (Novocain), the oldest of the synthetic local anesthetic agents, is still one of the most popular. Chemically, it is the diethylaminoethyl ester of para-aminobenzoic acid (for structural formula, see Figure 37). Procaine itself is only slightly soluble in water and has an alkaline reaction. It is used in the form of the hydrochloride, which is extremely soluble and is somewhat acid. Solutions of procaine hydrochloride are decomposed rapidly by alkali and more slowly by light, air, and boiling. Solutions should preferably be fresh.

Procaine is used for all types of regional anesthesia except topical. It is clinically ineffective on mucous membranes. The usual range of concen-

TABLE 46—*Concentrations and Maximum Injections of Procaine Hydrochloride in Regional Anesthesia*

Type of Regional Anesthesia	Procaine Hydrochloride Concentration	Maximum Volume
Spinal	3 %	6 cc.
	5 %	3 cc.
Epidural	1 %	50–75 cc.
	2 %	20–50 cc.
Nerve block	1 %	100 cc.
	2 %	50 cc.
Sympathetic ganglion block	1 %	50 cc.
	2 %	40 cc.
Field block or local infiltration	0.5 %	150–200 cc.
	1 %	100 cc.

trations and maximum single injections for the various procedures is shown in Table 46. Submaximal injections can usually be repeated every twenty minutes, and maximal injections every forty.

The onset of action depends on the concentration, volume, and method employed. Its effect is noted in one to three minutes after local infiltration or spinal injection and ten to twenty minutes after epidural or sympathetic ganglion block. The duration of action depends on many factors. In most regional blocks it averages about forty minutes without epinephrine and sixty with. For spinal anesthesia, the usual maximum dose is 1 mg. per lb. of body weight or 150 mg. total, whichever is the smaller.

Procaine combines chemically with penicillin to form an insoluble compound which is administered to provide a deposit for slow absorption and prolonged effect of the penicillin (see p. 288).

Procaine is incompatible with the sulfonamide group of drugs because one of its breakdown products is para-aminobenzoic acid (see p. 294). Procaine should therefore not be used for anesthesia in patients receiving sulfonamides. The small amounts of procaine released from procaine penicillin are believed to be insufficient to interfere with concomitant sulfonamide action.

'Metycaine' (Piperocaine, Lilly) differs chemically from procaine principally in being a benzoate instead of an aminobenzoate and in having the nitrogen at the other end of the molecule incorporated into a six-membered ring (see Figure 37). Like procaine, 'Metycaine' itself is a base which is relatively insoluble in water. It is employed as the hydrochloride, which is extremely soluble in water and is somewhat acid (pH of solutions, about 3.8 to 4.2). Both the base and the hydrochloride are

stable and withstand exposure to light, air, and repeated autoclaving.

'Metycaine Hydrochloride' is used for all types of regional anesthesia and also for topical anesthesia. As compared with procaine hydrochloride, 'Metycaine Hydrochloride' takes effect in about two-thirds the time, endures about 50 percent longer, is about one-third more potent, and gives a more profound and certain anesthesia. Its toxicity in clinical use is no greater than that of procaine. The usual range of concentrations and maximum single injections for the various procedures is shown in Table 47. Submaximal injections can be repeated every twenty minutes, and maximal every forty.

For spinal anesthesia, 1.5 percent 'Metycaine Hydrochloride' in Ringer's Solution produces full sensory and autonomic block, satisfactory relaxation, and usually a satisfactory skeletal motor block. A high level can be maintained with less danger of respiratory paralysis than when more concentrated solutions are used. The 1.5 percent concentration is ideal for continuous spinal. Its only disadvantage for the single-injection technic is the slightly shorter duration of action than is obtained with higher concentrations. The minimum recommended volume for an initial injection is 1 cc. (15 mg.) in the cachectic and debilitated individual and 2 cc. (30 mg.) in the average patient. One cc. may be satisfactory as a supplementary injection in continuous spinal anesthesia or as an initial dose in individuals with short vertebral columns. The volume of a single injection should in general be no greater

TABLE 47—*Concentrations and Maximum Single Administrations of 'Metycaine Hydrochloride' in Regional Anesthesia*

Type of Regional Anesthesia	'Metycaine Hydrochloride' Concentration	Maximum Volume
Spinal	1.5 %	4 cc.
	5 %	3 cc.
Epidural	1 %	40 cc.
	1.5 %	40 cc.
	2 %	30 cc.
Nerve block	1 %	40 cc.
	2 %	25 cc.
Sympathetic ganglion block	1 %	40 cc.
	2 %	25 cc.
Field block	0.5 %	75 cc.
Local infiltration	0.25 %	125 cc.
	0.5 %	75 cc.
Topical anesthesia	2 %	10 cc.
	5 %	3 cc.
Instillation into hollow viscus	0.25 %	100 cc.

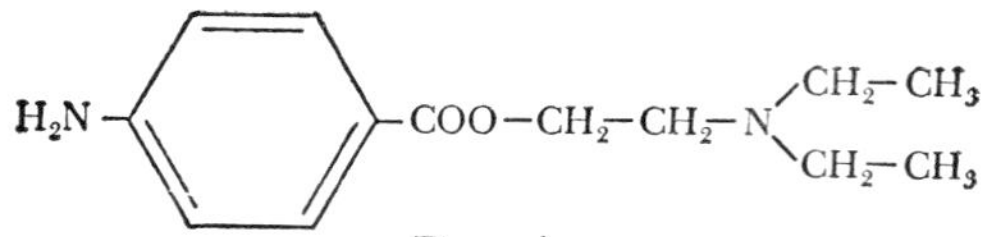

Procaine

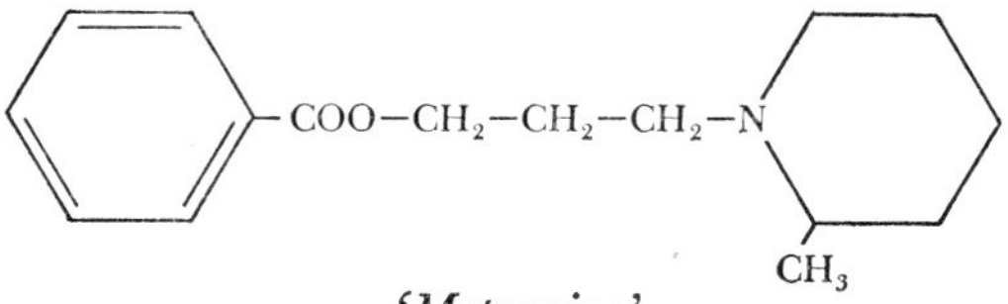

'Metycaine'

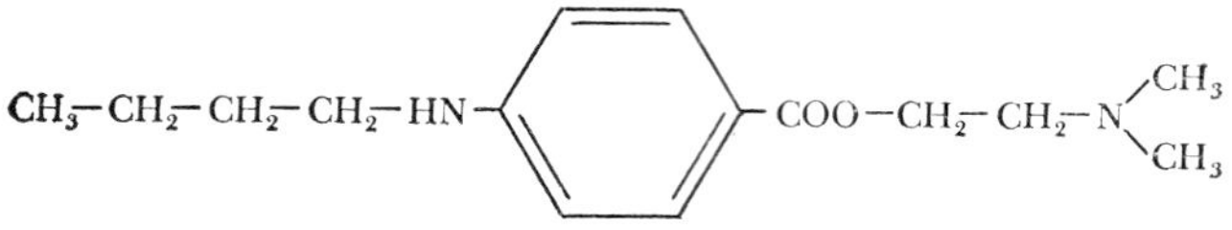

Pontocaine (Tetracaine)

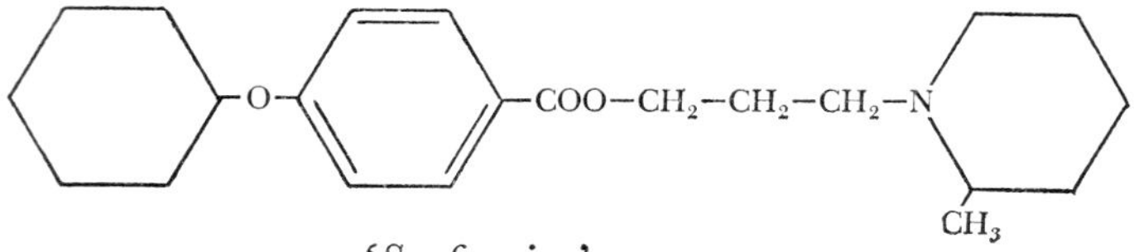

'Surfacaine'

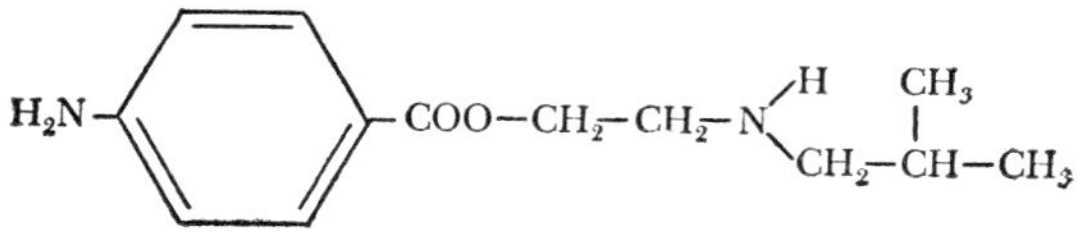

Monocaine

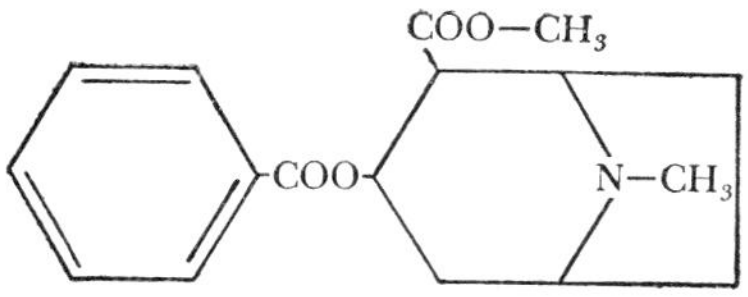

Cocaine

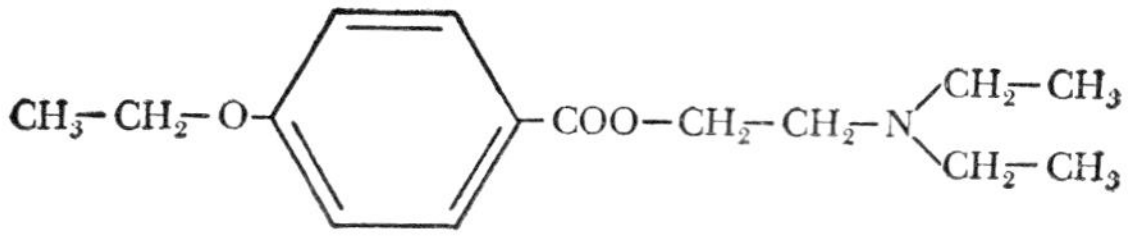

Intracaine

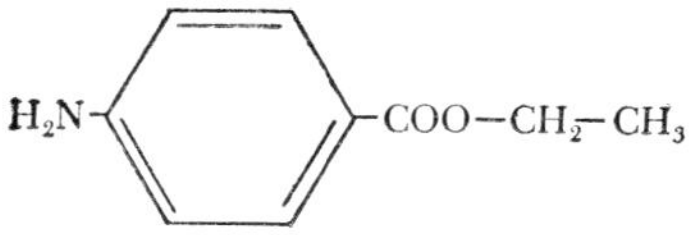

Ethyl Aminobenzoate (Benzocaine)

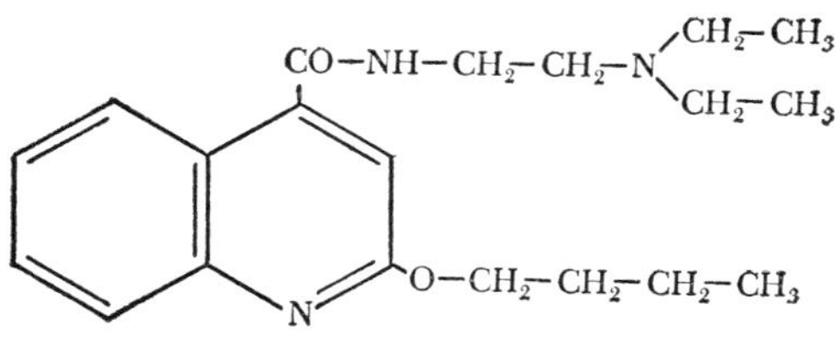

Nupercaine

FIGURE 37—*Structural Formulas of Some Local Anesthetics*

than 4 cc., with no further injection until pharmacologic effect is ascertained.

A 3, 4, or 5 percent solution produces full sensory, autonomic, and skeletal motor block. With the 5 percent solution, anesthesia can be expected to persist at least sixty minutes in all cases and as long as 100 minutes in about half the cases. Under no circumstances should more concentrated solutions than 5 percent be used for spinal anesthesia.

A 3 percent solution in 5 percent dextrose has proved popular for saddle block anesthesia in obstetrics. With 1 cc. (30 mg.), anesthesia usually lasts more than an hour, and the addition of 0.4 cc. of epinephrine hydrochloride, 1:1,000, increases the duration by about thirty minutes. For single-injection spinal anesthesia, the usual maximum dosage of 'Metycaine Hydrochloride' is 3/4 mg. per lb. of body weight or 150 mg. total, whichever is smaller.

Pontocaine (tetracaine) is rather similar to procaine chemically except for the normal butyl group attached to the amino group in the aminobenzoic acid portion of the molecule (see Figure 37). This substitution prevents interference with sulfonamide action, and Pontocaine is compatible with sulfonamides, in contrast to procaine. Pontocaine is stable and, like other local anesthetics, is used as the hydrochloride.

Therapeutically, Pontocaine is more like cocaine (p. 446) than like procaine. It is effective for topical anesthesia. It is much more potent than procaine and also more toxic. It is used principally for spinal and topical anesthesia and to a certain extent for epidural anesthesia. Table 48 shows the usual range of concentrations and maximum single administrations.

Pontocaine produces spinal anesthesia lasting usually one and one-half to two hours. The onset of anesthesia is rather slow, requiring seven to twelve minutes. The onset can be speeded by ad-

ministration in 5 to 10 percent dextrose solution or by addition of procaine. Even with small doses, the duration of action can be extended by administration in dextrose solution with addition of 40 to 50 mg. of ephedrine sulfate. The usual dosage for spinal anesthesia is 10 to 15 mg.

In epidural anesthesia, the action of Pontocaine lasts about twice as long as that of procaine. However, the onset may be delayed as much as forty minutes, and analgesia is often incomplete.

Pontocaine induces profound topical anesthesia of relatively long duration. However, its toxicity has limited its use to small areas, and consequently it is employed only in the eye, nose, and throat. For the nose and throat, a 1 or 2 percent solution is usually combined with an equal volume of epinephrine hydrochloride, 1:1,000. Barbiturate premedication is especially important before Pontocaine.

Nupercaine is a derivative of cinchoninic acid (3-carboxyquinoline). Its structural formula is shown in Figure 37. It is employed as the hydrochloride, which is freely soluble and which is stable in acid or neutral solution but is decomposed by even weak alkali. Nupercaine is an extremely potent and extremely toxic local anesthetic which is used for spinal and topical anesthesia. Its physical and pharmacologic properties are sufficiently different from those of most other local anesthetic agents to warrant special familiarity with them before the drug is used.

For spinal anesthesia, Nupercaine is usually given in 1:1,500 concentration (0.067 percent). Through choice of diluent, the solution can be made hypobaric (light) or hyperbaric (heavy), so that it will tend to rise or fall in the spinal canal after injection. The patient's position must be adjusted accordingly. Anesthesia usually lasts two and one-half to three hours. The total dose should seldom exceed 10 mg. of Nupercaine. Because of the slow onset of effect from Nupercaine (twenty to twenty-five minutes), it is often combined with short-acting agents. By the time the prompt anesthesia which they produce has worn off, the action of the Nupercaine is fully established.

Nupercaine, 1:400, in 5 or 10 percent dextrose has been extensively used in saddle block anesthesia in obstetrics. After 2.5 or 3.75 mg. in this medium, anesthesia usually lasts one and one-half to two hours, with an occasional instance of three hours.

Since Nupercaine causes a transient early vasodilation, it is combined with epinephrine for topical application. As in spinal anesthesia, the effect is prolonged, but the onset is slow. The concentra-

TABLE 48 — *Concentrations and Maximum Single Administrations of Pontocaine Hydrochloride in Regional Anesthesia*

Type of Regional Anesthesia	Pontocaine Hydrochloride Concentration	Maximum Volume
Spinal	0.3 %	4 cc.
	0.5 %	4 cc.
	1 %	2 cc.
Epidural	0.15 %	30 cc.
	0.2 %	25 cc.
Topical		
Eye	0.5 %	2 cc.
Nose and throat	1 %	4 cc.

TABLE 49—*Concentrations and Maximum Volumes of Nupercaine Hydrochloride in Topical Anesthesia*

Area of Application	Nupercaine Hydrochloride Concentration	Maximum Volume
Eye	1:1,000	3 drops
	1:3,000	9 drops
Nose and throat	1:50	5 cc.
Wounds and damaged skin	1:2,000	20 cc.
	1:4,000	30 cc.
Urethra and bladder	1:1,000	10 cc.

tions employed and maximum volumes are shown in Table 49.

'Surfacaine' (Cyclomethycaine, Lilly) is related to 'Metycaine' (see Figure 37 for structural formula). It is used as the sulfate, which is stable and is soluble in water to about 1 percent.

'Surfacaine' is a powerful topical anesthetic agent with relatively low toxicity. It is effective on damaged or diseased skin and on rectal, vaginal, urethral, and bladder mucous membranes. Clinically, it is only partially effective on other mucous membranes and is completely ineffective in the eye. When injected, it is too irritating to be useful for regional anesthesia. Its salts are employed as solution (0.25 percent), jelly (0.75 percent), cream (0.5 percent), ointment (1 percent), suppositories (10 mg.), and lotion (0.5 percent), alone and combined with other ingredients.

It is useful in burns and abrasions, where it provides sufficient anesthesia for scrubbing and débridement; sunburn; dermatitis venenata and other lesions involving the superficial layers of the skin; painful rectal conditions, for symptomatic relief; painful vaginal conditions, including relief of pain and discomfort after repairs; and instrumentation of the lower urinary tract.

Anesthesia persists as long as the agent is in contact with the surface and for fifteen to thirty minutes after removal of the drug. The incidence of reactions and of sensitivity seems to be very low, and 'Surfacaine' preparations can be applied freely to large raw surfaces without fear of toxicity.

Cocaine, the first local anesthetic to be employed in scientific medicine, is the only one now in use which is found in nature (the leaves of *Erythroxylon coca* and related plants). Its structural formula is shown in Figure 37. It is used as the hydrochloride, which is stable and freely soluble in water.

Cocaine is a very potent and very toxic local anesthetic agent. It is now employed almost altogether for topical anesthesia of the eye, nose, throat,

and urethra. The concentrations applied to the conjunctiva vary from 0.5 to 4 percent, depending on the depth and duration of anesthesia desired; in this field, cocaine has the advantage of producing local vasoconstriction and the disadvantage of causing mydriasis and drying of the cornea. In the nose, throat, and urethra, concentrations vary from 4 to 10 percent.

Premedication (p. 394) is especially important with cocaine. Doses for the average adult, administered at one sitting, should not exceed the following:

Concentration	Maximum Volume
0.5 percent	10-20 cc.
1 percent	5-10 cc.
4 percent	3- 5 cc.
10 percent	1- 2 cc.

Monocaine is an isomer of procaine (see Figure 37 for structural formula) which is employed as the formate. It is said to act more quickly and for a longer period than procaine, but with slower and less profound skeletal motor block. It is used in the same way as procaine. The usual dose for spinal anesthesia is 50 to 100 mg.; and for local infiltration, nerve block, and epidural anesthesia a 1 percent solution is effective for about an hour. Like procaine, monocaine is incompatible with sulfonamides.

Intracaine differs from procaine in having an ethoxy group in place of the amino group in the para-aminobenzoic acid portion of the molecule (see Figure 37). As the hydrochloride it has been used for nerve and epidural block in 1 or 1.5 percent concentration, for spinal anesthesia as 25 to 75 mg. of 2.5 percent solution, and as 5 to 20 cc. of 1.5 or 2 percent solution for topical application to the urinary tract (2 to 5 percent for bronchoscopy). It is apparently more potent than procaine, but there is difference of opinion as to how much.

Ethyl Aminobenzoate (Benzocaine) is a relatively simple compound (see Figure 37) which is only slightly soluble in water and possesses only moderate anesthetic power. These qualities, together with its lack of toxicity, give it some usefulness as an analgesic dusting powder in painful wounds or lesions of the skin or accessible mucous membranes. It can also be applied in jelly or suppositories. When a greater degree of relief is desired, a more potent agent such as 'Surfacaine' should be used. Ethyl aminobenzoate has the further disadvantage of inducing a relatively high incidence of sensitivity.

Benzyl Alcohol, $C_6H_5 \cdot CH_2OH$, has been used in oil solutions of local anesthetic bases which are intended for local injection for prolonged effect, as after hemorrhoidectomy. The theory was that the local anesthetic base, being insoluble in aqueous media, would be slowly absorbed and would thus give rise to anesthesia for many hours or perhaps for several days. It has been found, however, that local anesthetic bases are as rapidly absorbed from oil solutions as are the salts of these bases from aqueous solutions. It has been demonstrated that the prolonged effect actually obtained from oil preparations is due to their content of benzyl alcohol, the action of which is to destroy nerve fibers. A 5 percent oil solution of benzyl alcohol destroys a considerable number of the fibers in small nerves, whereas a 10 percent solution destroys them all. Sensation and motor function return as the nerves regenerate.

CURARE

Curare has long been known as a poison used on the arrows and darts of certain South American Indians. It was used sporadically in medicine as an antidote for convulsions. Within the past ten years, the development of a practical biological assay and, more recently, the isolation of active principles in pure form have led to its widespread adoption as a relaxant of skeletal muscle, particularly in connection with general anesthesia.

Curare relaxes skeletal muscle by blocking nerve impulses at the myoneural junction. As the dosage is increased, there is progressive paralysis, with the diaphragm and respiratory muscles the last to be affected. There is no action on smooth or cardiac muscle or on the circulation. The active principles are destroyed in the liver and excreted by the kidneys. Prostigmine (p. 419) is a physiological antagonist.

The earliest medicinal preparations of curare were incompletely purified and could be standardized only biologically. The accepted procedure is to determine the quantity of drug necessary to paralyze completely the muscles lifting the head in 50 percent of a group of rabbits. The control and test groups are alternated or "crossed over." Hence the procedure is known as the "Head-Drop Crossover Test," and the biological unit is termed the "Head-Drop Unit." With crystalline preparations the dosage can be more precisely stated in milligrams.

Two crystalline preparations are available: *d*-tubocurarine chloride and the more potent dimethyl-tubocurarine iodide.

'Metubine Iodide' (Dimethyl-tubocurarine Iodide, Lilly) is the dimethyl ether of *d*-tubocurarine iodide. Its structural formula is shown in Figure 38. It is a stable white crystalline solid. Aqueous solutions are slightly acid, having a pH of 4 to 5. This acidity leads to transient precipitation when solutions of 'Metubine Iodide' are mixed with those of barbiturates utilized for intravenous anesthesia.

The action of 'Metubine Iodide' is like that of *d*-tubocurarine chloride. The former drug is several times more potent yet has at the same time much less tendency to depress the respiratory muscles. It thus has a wider margin of safety.

'Metubine Iodide' may be used in conjunction with general anesthesia to produce satisfactory relaxation when minimal quantities of anesthetic agent are administered or when anesthetic agents are employed which of themselves in safe dosage do not produce relaxation. It is of value in modifying the convulsive seizures and diminishing the apprehension induced in shock therapy.

'Metubine Iodide' is supplied in a solution containing 0.5 or 1 mg. per cc. In clinical practice, the 1-mg. concentration induces a response comparable to that from a 3-mg.-per-cc. concentration of *d*-tubocurarine chloride (see below). 'Metubine Iodide' in the 0.5-mg. strength has special application in children and debilitated patients.

The drug is administered intravenously as a rapid injection. Fractional injections should be avoided. Average initial doses will vary with the anesthetic agent: 1.5 to 3 mg. with ether, 4 to 6 mg. with nitrous oxide, 2 to 4 mg. with cyclopropane, and 4 to 6 mg. with Pentothal Sodium. For amelioration of convulsions during shock therapy, 3 mg. is an average dose. Satisfactory relaxation cannot be obtained with initial doses below 1 mg.

Relaxation following the initial dose may be expected to persist for twenty-five to ninety minutes (average, sixty). Supplemental injections of 0.5 to 1 mg. may be given as required.

Curare drugs in general are contraindicated in patients with pulmonary disease, respiratory depression, or respiratory embarrassment. They are also contraindicated in myasthenia gravis except in extremely small dosage as a diagnostic aid (they greatly accentuate the myasthenia). They should be administered only by those who are familiar with their effects.

Overdosage is to be carefully avoided. In case of respiratory embarrassment, prompt artificial respiration, with an airway and employing pure oxygen, is indicated. Prostigmine Methylsulfate (p. 419) should be kept on hand for immediate use

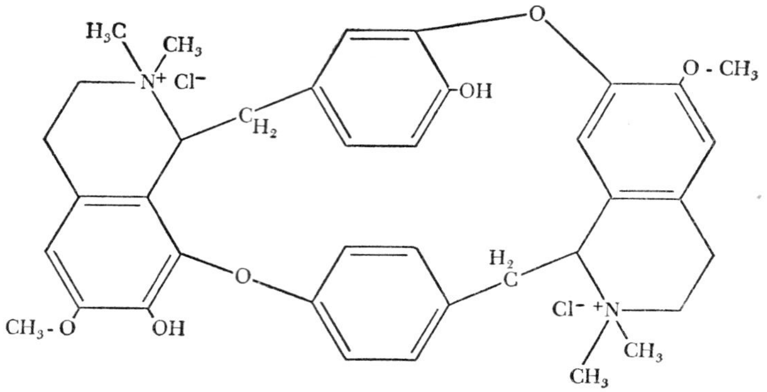

d-*Tubocurarine Chloride*

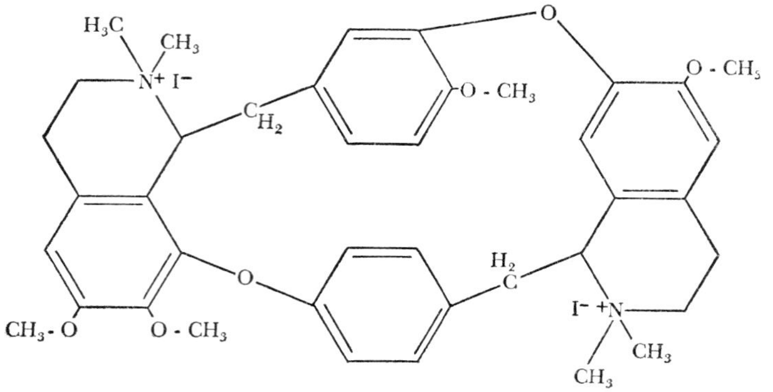

Dimethyl-tubocurarine Iodide

FIGURE 38 — *Structural Formulas of Curare Principles. Note that the nitrogen is everywhere pentavalent, forming "onium" compounds. The separation and ionic indications of the nitrogen and halogen atoms indicate the high degree of dissociation in solution, which is in contrast to the behavior of halogens attached to nitrogen in trivalent (amide) organic combination.*

as an antidote, the dose being 1 to 2 cc. of 1:2,000 solution intravenously. It is of value in mild overdosage, but it should not be given in the event of severe overdosage because both prostigmine and excessive doses of curare drugs tend to lower blood pressure and produce shock. There is no antidote for severe overdosage.

d-Tubocurarine Chloride was the first active curare principle to be isolated in pure form. Its structural formula is given in Figure 38. It, also, is a stable white crystalline compound. The stability of its solutions depends on their reaction; preparations having lower *p*H are more stable, even though they

cause a greater degree of temporary precipitation with barbiturates.

d-Tubocurarine chloride has the same indications as 'Metubine Iodide.' The former drug has a greater tendency to produce respiratory paralysis, however, and thus has a lower margin of safety. Its duration of action, averaging twenty to twenty-five minutes, is about 40 percent of that of 'Metubine Iodide.'

d-Tubocurarine chloride is supplied in a solution containing 3 mg. per cc. This quantity equals 20 Head-Drop Units. In contrast to 'Metubine Iodide,' *d*-tubocurarine chloride is administered intramuscularly or intravenously as a slow, sustained injection over a period of one to one and one-half minutes. As a precaution, the initial dose should be reduced to 20 units below the calculated amount. The speed of intravenous injection influences the result. Rapid administration enhances the effectiveness of a given dose; but if that dose is excessive, a dangerous situation may be produced.

During general anesthesia, in a patient of average weight, 40 to 60 units (2 to 3 cc.) may be given at the time the skin is incised. If further relaxation is needed, 20 to 30 units (1 to 1.5 cc.) may be given three to five minutes later. Supplemental doses of 20 units may be administered as required for long operations. As a general rule, dosage may be calculated on the basis of 1/2 unit per lb. of body weight.

In conjunction with shock therapy, the general rule of 1/2 unit per lb. may be followed, the patient receiving 20 units less than the calculated dose. The drug should be given intravenously and slowly. For diagnosis of myasthenia gravis, 1/15 to 1/5 the above dose is administered intravenously.

Contraindications and precautions for *d*-tubocurarine chloride are the same as for 'Metubine Iodide' (see above).

ENDOCRINE PREPARATIONS

INSULIN

Insulin is the antidiabetic principle of the pancreas. When pure, it is amorphous, but it crystallizes in the presence of small quantities of zinc or certain other metals. Insulin in the form of zinc-Insulin crystals behaves as a typical protein, having its optimum pH from 5.8 to 6.3. Insulin has been obtained in crystalline form from the islet tissue of practically all edible animals and from certain fishes (the only practical commercial sources have been beef and pork pancreas). Insulin from all these sources possesses the same physiological activity and has the same sulfur content, namely 3.2 percent.

The biological action of Insulin appears to be associated with the following groups: (1) dithio groups present as combined cystine; (2) certain amino groups which may be cystine; and (3) certain phenolic groups which may be tyrosine. The presence of tyrosine hydroxyl groups is regarded as being very important. The physiological properties of the molecule seem to be intimately associated with the manner in which the components are linked.

The most obvious physiological effect of Insulin is a fall in the level of sugar in the blood. In appropriate doses and under suitable conditions, Insulin enables the diabetic to utilize carbohydrates and fats in a comparatively satisfactory manner. The concentration of sugar in the blood is confined within normal limits; the urine becomes free of sugar and ketone bodies; and diabetic acidosis and coma are prevented. The effect of a dose ordinarily lasts for five or six hours or more. The antidiabetic effect of Insulin is essentially the same whether the solution is made from crystalline or noncrystalline preparations. Except in hypersensitive patients, experience has shown that Insulin of amorphous origin may be used interchangeably with Insulin made from zinc-Insulin crystals.

Although the exact mode or point of action is unknown, recent evidence indicates that it is concerned in the enzymatic phosphorylation of dextrose, which is facilitated by the hexokinase reaction. When administered to the diabetic animal fed with carbohydrates, Insulin brings about the restoration of carbohydrate metabolism and causes the deposition of glycogen in the liver. It affects the metabolism of fats indirectly by reducing the demand for oxidation of fat; the production of ketone bodies then diminishes to the point at which they can all be oxidized in the body, and consequently they disappear from the urine (see p. 59). The amount of dextrose that one unit of Insulin enables the body to utilize will vary greatly in different individuals and under various circumstances (such as the presence of infection or acidosis), but it is usually from 1 to 4 Gm.

Like other proteins, Insulin is destroyed in the gastro-intestinal tract and is not satisfactorily absorbed from the buccal mucosa. It is therefore given hypodermically. Insulin is apparently destroyed in the body. It does not appear in the urine in significant amounts.

Insulin is specific in the treatment of diabetic coma and acidosis. It is indicated in all cases of diabetes mellitus that demonstrate an inability to maintain normal weight and strength without hyperglycemia and glycosuria. Insulin is of particular value in the management of complications and in the treatment of diabetes in children, and it makes possible freedom from glycosuria and good mental and physical vigor in patients having severe diabetes.

Insulin has also been used successfully in the treatment of nondiabetic malnutrition, in which it stimulates the appetite and leads to a gain in weight. In schizophrenia, it has been used as a means of producing profound therapeutic hypoglycemic shock. The latter technic should be attempted only when a fully equipped ward is available under supervision of one who is qualified and thoroughly familiar with this method of treatment.

Hypoglycemia—The administration of an excessive dose of Insulin causes hypoglycemia (deficiency of sugar in the blood). This condition may also occur following increased work or exercise; when food is not being absorbed in the usual manner (as in illness with vomiting, diarrhea, delayed digestion, or the postponement or omission of a meal); when Insulin is given too long before a meal; when the patient's requirement of Insulin declines; or when large doses of Insulin are given at insufficient or irregular intervals. To avoid hypoglycemia and consequent reactions if a regular meal cannot be obtained, the amount of carbohydrate prescribed for this meal should be taken in the form of orange juice, syrup, candy, or bread and milk, without resorting to any change in the dose of Insulin. If it becomes necessary to omit a meal *on account of nausea or vomiting*, the physician should be notified and the urine should be tested every three or four hours. In any such instance, if sugar is being excreted at the stipulated time for the administration of Insulin, the prescribed dose should be injected; but if the urine is sugar-free at that time, the injection of Insulin may be postponed until sugar is again present. When the prescribed course of diet can again be followed, Insulin therapy should likewise be resumed.

The early symptoms of hypoglycemia may consist merely in a feeling of fatigue unwarranted by the activities of the patient. Hence *it is of utmost importance for the patient to understand clearly that the presence of vague symptoms of fatigue, headache, drowsiness, lassitude, tremulousness, or nausea demands immediate attention.* More severe symptoms of hypoglycemic reactions, such as weakness, sweating, tremor, or nervousness, may also develop, but these are more easily recognized. The occurrence of any of the above-mentioned symptoms calls for prompt and, if necessary, repeated administration of some form of carbohydrate. Candy or sugar is convenient

for this purpose and should always be carried by the patient. If the patient becomes delirious or mentally confused or suffers from loss of memory or delusions, diluted syrup or orange juice with sugar should be given by mouth. In severe hypoglycemic reactions, it may be desirable for the physician to inject intravenously from 15 to 20 Gm. of dextrose (d-glucose) in sterile solution.

UNMODIFIED INSULIN

Insulin may be employed as such or in modified forms. Unmodified Insulin is prepared from both amorphous and crystalline forms. The action of amorphous Insulin and Insulin made from zinc-Insulin crystals is identical. Both preparations are supplied as clear aqueous solutions containing either 40 or 80 U.S.P. Insulin Units per cc., and amorphous Insulin is available in a concentration of 100 units as well. All Insulin preparations bear a date of expiration on the outside of each package and should be placed in use prior to this date. Storage should be in a refrigerator, above freezing and below 59°F. Freezing should be avoided.

Unmodified Insulin is best employed in diabetes (see p. 174) under one of the following conditions:

1. In previously untreated diabetes until control is established and the patient's requirement of Insulin, if any, is known.
2. In emergencies and complications, when the need for Insulin may fluctuate rapidly.
3. As a supplement to longer-acting preparations when a quick and brief but powerful action is needed.
4. In very young children who are incapable of intelligently interpreting symptoms of hypoglycemia.

Unmodified Insulin is generally best administered fifteen to thirty minutes before a meal and is always given parenterally, usually by deep subcutaneous injection. The time, number, and amount of individual daily doses, as well as the distribution of food among the several meals of the day, must be determined for each patient in the light of blood-sugar and urinary-sugar findings during a period of close observation by the physician. The patient should remain under supervision because of the possibility of (1) changes in Insulin requirement and (2) complications.

Mild diabetics who excrete sugar chiefly in the morning may frequently be controlled with a single dose of Insulin given before breakfast. The dose upon beginning treatment may be 5 units, which is increased by 3 to 5 units every day or two until the urine becomes sugar-free. If glycosuria persists after the dose reaches 20 units or if sugar remains in the third and fourth fractional specimens during the day, a second dose will usually be required before the evening meal.

Severe cases having glycosuria in all urine specimens require at least two doses daily. Five to 10 units may be given before breakfast and dinner, and these amounts may be increased daily or every two days by 3 to 5 units until the urine is rendered sugar-free or doses have been increased to 20 to 30 units. Should glycosuria still persist, a dose at noon may be instituted, and sometimes a dose at night is necessary in order to prevent high blood-sugar levels and glycosuria during the early morning hours. The relatively short action of Insulin has been a disadvantage in severe cases, inasmuch as several doses daily may be required.

The doses required in the treatment of diabetic coma may be large. Diabetic acidosis and coma and their treatment are discussed beginning on page 59.

In nondiabetic malnutrition, the initial dose is usually 5 to 10 units one-half hour before meals. It is increased gradually until the stimulation of appetite is sufficient to insure the ingestion of adequate dietary intake; extra feedings are often provided, and sugar should be at hand in event of untoward hypoglycemia.

The doses used in schizophrenia likewise are variable and must be determined on the basis of the individual patient's response. Obviously, it is essential to have suitable dextrose solutions available for interruption of the profound hypoglycemia that is artificially induced.

MODIFIED INSULIN PREPARATIONS

Modified Insulin preparations were developed to meet two needs: control of blood-sugar level in the fasting state (which is often not possible even with multiple daily injections of unmodified Insulin), and reduction in number of daily injections. Modification is through combination with certain protein-like substances which are themselves protein precipitants: the protamines, histones, kyrines, and globins. Careful study indicated that protamine was likely to be the most useful clinically, and Protamine Zinc Insulin (the first modified Insulin to be made available) and NPH Insulin still have the widest application. Their great contribution to the control of diabetes is their peculiar attribute of controlling the nocturnal blood-sugar level.

By varying the ratio of protamine to Insulin, either in manufacture or afterward, preparations can be made which provide almost any desirable period of activity between the rapid action of In-

sulin and the slow, prolonged effect of Protamine Zinc Insulin itself. Such mixtures can be prepared as clear solutions or suspensions, according to whether they are acid or buffered toward neutrality. Similarly, various ranges of intermediate time-activity can be provided to fit the needs of the individual case by making suitable admixtures of Insulin and Protamine Zinc Insulin in the syringe just prior to injection. In this way, an almost infinite number of different degrees of rapidity in onset of effect and total duration of action can be provided (see Admixtures of Insulin and Protamine Zinc Insulin, p. 454). NPH Insulin (p. 453) closely duplicates the action of a mixture designed to fit the needs of the majority of patients.

Histone Zinc Insulin is available in South America; Globin Insulin with Zinc, both in the United States and abroad. They have shorter periods of action than has Protamine Zinc Insulin.

Protamine Zinc Insulin is in the form of a suspension of minute particles. When this preparation is brought into uniform suspension, each cc. contains either 40 or 80 units of Insulin, together with approximately 1.25 mg. of protamine and approximately 0.2 mg. of zinc per 100 units of the Insulin. The strength of the preparation is clearly stated on the labels of each package and vial. Doses are prescribed in terms of *units*. The *volume* of any prescribed dose will depend upon the strength of the preparation which is to be used.

In Protamine Zinc Insulin, the active material is the finely divided, insoluble, milky-white precipitate and not the clear supernatant fluid. To insure that a constant proportion of this precipitate is present in each dose injected, the vial should be rotated and inverted from end to end several times immediately before the withdrawal of each dose for injection. Failure to observe this precaution will lead to decided irregularity in the effects of individual doses. Vigorous shaking, with consequent frothing of the material, should be avoided as much as possible consistent with insuring a uniform suspension.

The fundamental difference between the effect of unmodified Insulin and the effect of Protamine Zinc Insulin is that the latter exhibits a prolonged blood-sugar-lowering action which lasts more than twenty-four hours. Fall of blood-sugar levels under the influence of Protamine Zinc Insulin may occasionally be so slow and gradual that hypoglycemia is produced without apparent symptoms or discomfort to the patient. A blood-sugar level which is probably low may be signified by symptoms such as weakness, nervousness, or sweating or simply by the occurrence of fatigue, drowsiness, headache, nausea, or tingling sensations in the extremities. If disregarded and not promptly and adequately treated, hypoglycemia may lead to stupor, unconsciousness, and possibly grave consequences. Because of its possible asymptomatic nature, hypoglycemia from Protamine Zinc Insulin is more serious than hypoglycemia from unmodified Insulin. It should receive even more careful attention from physician and patient (see p. 450).

Unmodified (soluble) Insulin is capable of balancing sudden influxes of exogenous carbohydrate (as with meals). It is not well suited to maintaining normal blood sugar during overnight fasting. In contrast, Protamine Zinc Insulin is well adapted to maintaining the blood-sugar level during fasting, whereas it is less effective in balancing exogenous carbohydrate. The postabsorptive (fasting) blood-sugar level in Insulin-treated cases of severity is characteristically elevated, but it falls during the daytime when Insulin is being injected prior to meals. With the use of Protamine Zinc Insulin in severe diabetes, however, the fasting blood-sugar level is low, and it ascends in the daytime because active Insulin is being released too slowly to compensate for the sudden influx of carbohydrate following meals.

Although its action becomes maximal in sixteen to twenty hours, the effect of a single dose of Protamine Zinc Insulin actually lasts much longer than twenty-four hours. Consequently, when doses are being given regularly each morning, the latter part of the effect of the dose given the first morning is superimposed on the first effects of the dose given on the second morning. This overlapping effect is one of the most important characteristics of Protamine Zinc Insulin. By protecting against nocturnal hyperglycemia, it literally "saves the day" for the diabetic.

The most satisfactory time for injection of Protamine Zinc Insulin, either accompanied or unaccompanied by treatment with unmodified Insulin, is usually before breakfast in the morning. Each case requires individual management. In many instances a period of careful observation under laboratory control, with frequent blood-sugar estimations and urine examinations, will be required before a proper readjustment of the blood-sugar level can be satisfactorily accomplished. The injection should be deeply subcutaneous, not intramuscular, and never intravenous.

NEW CASES OF UNCOMPLICATED DIABETES—Use of Protamine Zinc Insulin in previously untreated cases is usually a simple matter. One may begin with a dose of 10 units and increase this by 5 or 10 units each day or two until the total reaches 30 to 40 units, unless before that time it is evident that the urine specimens passed on arising in the morning or one-half hour thereafter (fasting) are becoming sugar-free. If glycosuria is persistent after meals (postprandial), the patient may take a separate injection of rapidly acting Insulin before breakfast at the same time as the injection of Protamine Zinc Insulin, beginning with 5 units as the dose of this separate injection and increasing this amount by 5 units each day until postprandial glycosuria is abolished. In making the subsequent changes in dosage which are necessary every day or two during the early period of readjustment, tests of two specimens of urine are especially important: the specimen at 11 a.m., which reflects the dosage of unmodified Insulin; and the specimen obtained upon arising in the morning, which reflects the dosage of Protamine Zinc Insulin. Increases or decreases of the doses, as indicated by the character of these two tests, may be made in amounts of 5 to 10 or more units. When the urine test before breakfast becomes sugar-free, further increases in the dose of Protamine Zinc Insulin will obviously result in hypoglycemia during the early morning hours.

CASES PREVIOUSLY TREATED WITH INSULIN—In long-standing cases of diabetes previously treated with Insulin, the substitution of Protamine Zinc Insulin for unmodified Insulin may best be made by replacing the entire requirement of Insulin by one daily injection of Protamine Zinc Insulin containing about three-fourths of the total number of units previously required. Then, if glycosuria persists in the late forenoon or early afternoon, readjustment of food intake or exercise is indicated, or a supplementary dose of unmodified Insulin may be given. Here again, the dose of Protamine Zinc Insulin is regulated by the amount of sugar in the urine specimen obtained upon arising in the morning (fasting) or the second specimen one-half hour later, whereas the dose of unmodified Insulin is adjusted according to the amount of sugar in the late morning or early afternoon specimens (postprandial). Aglycosuria upon arising in the morning precludes further additions to the dose of Protamine Zinc Insulin; otherwise, reactions will occur during the early morning hours.

During the first few days of substitution, it is important to keep in mind that in this initial period doses of unmodified Insulin may be needed until the more deliberate, prolonged action of Protamine

Zinc Insulin has become established. In such in-stances, the injections of both Protamine Zinc In-sulin and rapidly acting Insulin may be given at the same time but in different sites. If sugar appears in the late forenoon or early afternoon, more un-modified Insulin is needed; if the urine is sugar-free when the patient rises in the morning, the dose of Protamine Zinc Insulin may need diminution. If sugar appears late in the day or is evident when the patient arises in the morning, the dose of Protamine Zinc Insulin should be increased at three-day in-tervals until the urine becomes sugar-free. Too-rapid increase of the dose may result in attacks of hypoglycemia which may be profound and pro-longed. To prevent the occurrence of reactions in patients who are sugar-free, it is advisable to de-termine their blood-sugar levels at regular intervals and to reduce their doses of Protamine Zinc Insulin by from 3 to 5 units every few days as long as the urine remains sugar-free or until the optimum dos-age has been finally established. From several days to a few weeks may be required for satisfactory readjustment.

There has been general agreement that diabetes of moderate severity, requiring, for example, from 20 to 40 units of unmodified Insulin divided between two doses daily, can usually be controlled by giving a daily dose of from 20 to 40 units of Protamine Zinc Insulin in a single injection before breakfast.

NPH Insulin was developed to provide the effec-tiveness of mixtures of Insulin and Protamine Zinc Insulin given as a single daily dose. Extemporaneous mixtures are relatively inconvenient to prepare and carry the risk of error. NPH Insulin has similar time action to an extemporaneous mixture prepared from two parts of Insulin and one part of Protamine Zinc Insulin (2:1). At the same time, it is as stable and convenient to use as Protamine Zinc Insulin.

NPH Insulin is intermediate in action between the rapid, brief effect of Insulin and the delayed but prolonged effect of Protamine Zinc Insulin. However, the prolongation of activity of NPH In-sulin (about twenty-eight hours) is sufficient to as-sure an overlap of effect, thus maintaining a normal blood sugar after overnight fasting in the majority of cases. On the other hand, its action is sufficiently rapid in onset to provide adequate control of the after-breakfast rise in blood sugar which formerly might have required supplemental doses of un-modified Insulin.

NPH Insulin is supplied in the form of a suspen-sion of minute crystalline particles. Such crystals are a distinct entity. They are stable under proper conditions but change rapidly in the presence of serum. Each cc. contains either 40 or 80 units of Insulin and an amount of protamine sulfate suffi-cient to combine chemically with the Insulin pres-ent to form Protamine Zinc Insulin crystals.

The method of readjustment of the patient to NPH Insulin is the same as that discussed below under the heading "Admixtures of Insulin and Protamine Zinc Insulin in a Single Injection" (p. 454), the total dose of NPH being equal to the sum of the Insulin and Protamine Zinc Insulin units required. In uncomplicated cases, treatment may be started with a dose of 10 to 20 units; the dosage is revised upward or downward as necessary. The single injection is always given in the morning before breakfast. In severe cases of diabetes, it may be advantageous to supplement the dose of NPH Insulin with a separate dose of Insulin or to add Insulin to NPH Insulin in the same syringe. The necessity for supplemental doses is determined by the extent of daytime glycosuria. If unmodified In-sulin is mixed with NPH Insulin, the rules per-taining to Insulin-Protamine Zinc Insulin mixtures do not apply. The crystalline structure of NPH Insulin does not readily absorb the added Insulin; consequently, ratios of the two products are of less importance. The effect of the added Insulin is more nearly that of a similar dose of Insulin given by separate injection.

Globin Insulin with Zinc is a clear (acidified) preparation of Insulin modified by the addition of globin (from the hemoglobin of beef blood) and zinc chloride. It is marketed in concentrations of either 40 or 80 units per cc.

The pharmacology of Globin Insulin with Zinc is the same as that of Insulin with exception of the slower rate of onset and longer duration of effect. The greatest intensity of action occurs from about eight to twelve hours after injection, and the effect has practically disappeared at the end of twenty-four hours. Thus, it may not act long enough to maintain normal blood-sugar levels after the over-night fast when given once daily in severe cases; and the maximum effect may occur in late after-noon, a time when the actual Insulin requirement is usually low. The relatively high incidence of late-afternoon hypoglycemic reactions has led to the rec-ommendation that a midafternoon feeding or lunch be provided and that the breakfast consist of only 20 percent of the total food for the day, in order to compensate for the relatively weak effect in the morn-ing and strong effect in late afternoon, respectively.

The initial dose, which is usually given before

breakfast, may be approximately two-thirds of the total daily dose of unmodified Insulin. This dose is increased slowly as necessitated by glycosuria and hyperglycemia. If the patient has been previously taking Protamine Zinc Insulin, the first dose should be only about one-half the total dose of all Insulin formerly given. On subsequent days, dosage may be increased to two-thirds the total requirement, and then to the full amount as needed.

Admixtures of Insulin and Protamine Zinc Insulin in a Single Injection—The majority of diabetic patients can be satisfactorily controlled by unmodified Insulin if enough doses are given, or by a single dose of Protamine Zinc Insulin and (in cases of exceptional severity) one or more supplementary doses of rapidly acting Insulin. Various expedients of dietary rearrangement have been advocated in stabilizing patients of the latter group, such as (1) unequal apportionment of meals, (2) variation of the usual intervals between mealtimes, or (3) the provision of small lunches between meals and at bedtime. The purpose of these has been to adapt the inflow of exogenous carbohydrate more nearly to the rate at which active Insulin is released from the subcutaneous depot of insoluble modified Insulin. Recently, it has become apparent that injections of mixtures of Insulin and Protamine Zinc Insulin permit more highly individualized readjustment of each case, since the patient may employ a modification which is "tailor-made" to meet varying requirements of onset and duration of Insulin effect.

Extensive clinical studies have shown that suitable mixtures of Insulin and Protamine Zinc Insulin can be prepared which provide any desirable intermediate action between that of Insulin and that of Protamine Zinc Insulin with respect to promptness, intensity, and duration of effect. The most generally useful mixtures appear to be those made from approximately two parts of Insulin to one part of Protamine Zinc Insulin (referred to as a two-to-one mixture). A preparation having essentially the same effect as such a mixture is available in the form of NPH Insulin (see p. 453). Other mixtures must of necessity be made extemporaneously.

Because of the wide variability of dietary management in different clinics as well as variations in individual patients, it is probable that no single fixed proportion will be found suitable for the treatment of all cases. For practical purposes, mixtures made of equal parts of Insulin and Protamine Zinc Insulin do not show effects significantly different in action from those obtained when Pro-

tamine Zinc Insulin alone is used; also, the combinations containing more than three parts of Insulin to one part of Protamine Zinc Insulin result in too short a time activity and too great an intensity of effect during the daytime.

The method of readjustment of the hospitalized patient to a single-injection admixture is outlined in Table 50. In the uncomplicated case or in the outpatient department, treatment may be started directly by prescribing 9 to 21 units of a 2:1 mixture; this dose is then revised upward or downward, depending upon the response. In most hospitalized cases, however, there is an early period of several days after admission during which a complication is present, with consequent fluctuation in Insulin requirement necessitating daily or even hourly revision in Insulin dosage. It is only after conditions become reasonably well stabilized that any regimen should be undertaken which depends on a tolerably even balance between Insulin requirements and metabolic load.

The single injection is always given before breakfast each morning. The size of the dose of Protamine Zinc Insulin is determined by the conditions (blood sugar and glycosuria) in the fasting state, and the amount of Insulin is regulated by the same conditions during the daytime (feeding) hours. Glycosuria and hyperglycemia following meals call for more Insulin, whether it is being given separately or as one component of a mixture. If both the fasting and postprandial blood-sugar levels are too low, a reduced dosage is indicated, whereas, if both periods are poorly controlled, the total amount of the 2:1 mixture is increased. If only the fasting levels are too high, a greater proportion of Protamine Zinc Insulin is needed in the mixture; and if only the postprandial levels are high, a greater proportion of Insulin is indicated. Most cases require between two and three times as much Insulin as Protamine Zinc Insulin in making a mixture. In exceptional cases some further readjustments may be necessary, particularly during infections, when the usual course is to supplement the single injection of mixture with doses of unmodified Insulin given separately.

The admixture of Insulin and Protamine Zinc Insulin is a technic that is easy to perform but difficult to explain. *Patients must be actually shown how to make their mixtures.* The new feature to be learned is how to draw an air bubble into the syringe and roll it through to mix the doses. The dose of Insulin is always drawn into the syringe first; then the Protamine Zinc Insulin is added to make the total (so that the patient does not have to calculate).

TABLE 50—*Method of Readjustment of the Hospitalized Patient to a Single-Injection Admixture of Insulins*

METHOD

Recent Cases and Those Not Previously Treated	Patients Already Taking Insulin
I. A. First day— ⑩* units Protamine Zinc Insulin B. Increase daily by ⑤ to ⑩ units until urine is nearly sugar-free on arising, or until blood sugar (fasting) approaches normal levels.	I. A. Replace total daily dosage with three-fourths as much Protamine Zinc Insulin. B. Increase dose until urine is sugar-free on arising.

II. If glycosuria and hyperglycemia persist after ← II. meals, add supplementary doses of Insulin according to the Benedict test, e.g.:

Yellow	Orange	Red
5 units	10 units	15 units

III. Replace multiple injections with single-dose admixture:

   A. Replace total with 2:① mixture.

   B. If daytime glycosuria and hyperglycemia persist, increase Insulin content, e.g., 2 1/2:① ; 3:① .

   C. If postabsorptive (fasting) glycosuria and hyperglycemia occur, increase amount of Protamine Zinc Insulin in mixture, e.g., 3:② .

The criteria for adjustment of admixture are identical with those governing separate doses.

———

* Protamine Zinc Insulin is denoted by a circle. Ratio of mixture, e.g., 2:① , refers to proportions of Insulin and Protamine Zinc Insulin in terms of relative numbers of units. Mixtures are always made from preparations having the same concentration.

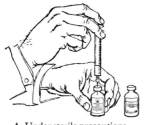

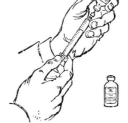

FIGURE 39—*Technic of Preparing Admixtures of Insulin and Protamine Zinc Insulin for Injection*

A. Under sterile precautions, inject volume of air equal to dose into top of vial of Protamine Zinc Insulin. Withdraw needle.

B. Inject air and withdraw proper dose of Insulin from vial in usual manner.

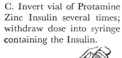
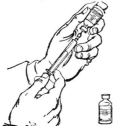

C. Invert vial of Protamine Zinc Insulin several times; withdraw dose into syringe containing the Insulin.

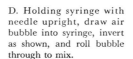
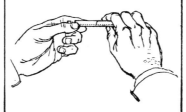

D. Holding syringe with needle upright, draw air bubble into syringe, invert as shown, and roll bubble through to mix.

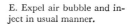
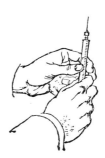

E. Expel air bubble and inject in usual manner.

Since all the daily doses are combined into one injection, the 80-unit-per-cc. concentrations are usually preferred in order to lessen the volume. Preparations of the same manufacturer should be used in order to keep conditions as constant as possible. In this connection, however, one need not be concerned about the effects that may be produced by an error of a unit or two in either direction, since it is obvious that one is working within a fairly broad zone of activity and the quick effect is not identical with the effect of unmodified Insulin. Because of the large doses sometimes given, a 2-cc.-capacity syringe calibrated for 80 and 160 units has been developed. The technic is demonstrated in Figure 39.

As an example, suppose that the dose is to be 30 units of Insulin and 15 units of Protamine Zinc Insulin (2:1 mixture). The total is 45 units. This mixture might be made from either U-40 or U-80 Insulin and from Protamine Zinc Insulin containing either 40 or 80 units per cc. Use only one concentration or the other. Do not attempt to mix different concentrations. The bulk of large doses should be reduced to 1 cc. or less whenever possible by using the 80-unit-per-cc. products. First, withdraw the clear Insulin up to the 30-unit mark in the manner described (Figure 39, p. 455); then draw into the syringe enough Protamine Zinc Insulin (15 units) to complete the dose, up to the 45-unit mark. Always withdraw the clear Insulin first. It will not matter if a drop of it enters the vial of Protamine Zinc Insulin, whereas if a small amount of Protamine Zinc Insulin gets into the vial of Insulin, it will cause the clear Insulin to become cloudy. Carefully follow each step of the method outlined. A little practice with two used Insulin vials which have been filled with water will increase proficiency and accuracy in this technic.

THYROID

Thyroid, U.S.P., (thyroid substance, desiccated thyroid) is "the cleaned, dried, and powdered thyroid gland previously deprived of connective tissue and fat. It is obtained from domesticated animals that are used for food by man." In contrast to the gonads, the thyroid stores relatively large quantities of its hormone in the form of thyroglobulin. The amino acid constituent of this protein which is essential for thyroid activity is thyroxin, the structural formula of which is shown in Figure 40. One other iodine-containing amino acid occurs in thyroglobulin—diiodotyrosine (see Figure 40)— and when thyroxin is present, diiodotyrosine has

FIGURE 40—*Structural Formulas of Thyroxin and Diiodotyrosine*

thyroid activity. The hormonal activity of thyroglobulin (for details, see p. 178) has been found to parallel its iodine content more closely than its thyroxin content or any other component or attribute. For this reason the organic iodine content of thyroid is the official index of potency.

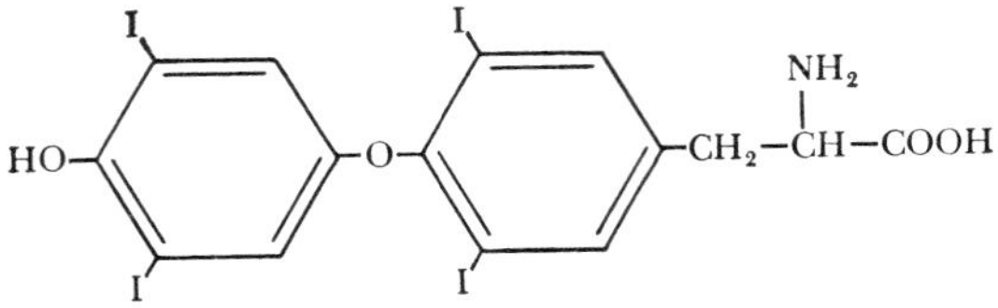

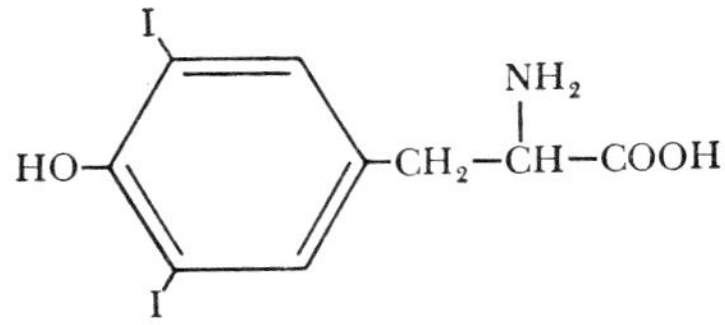

After desiccation, the thyroid glands of most food animals contain 0.3 to 0.35 percent organic iodine. The U.S.P. standard is 0.17 to 0.23 percent or, ideally, 0.2 percent. Therefore, desiccated thyroid is diluted with starch, lactose, or other inert material to the official iodine content. There is no advantage in using thyroid preparations which depart from the U.S.P. strength, and there is the chance of misunderstanding and consequent harm to the patient through improper dosage. For these reasons, only U.S.P. preparations should be specified.

The thyroid hormone is slow-acting; the full effect of a single dose is not manifest for about a week, and after this the action gradually diminishes. Parenteral administration does not hasten the activity. Thyroid is therefore given by mouth. It is nonirritating to the gastro-intestinal tract. Like other proteins, it appears to require digestion before it can be absorbed, and absorption seems to be complete. Evidently it is absorbed before it is fully broken down into amino acids, for thyroxin itself is irregularly and incompletely absorbed.

The slow action of thyroid makes daily dosage cumulative (there seems to be no advantage in subdividing the daily dose). It is not possible to gauge accurately the effect of a given dosage until it has been taken for ten to fourteen days. More frequent alteration of dosage makes for confusion. Because many of the actions of thyroid are trophic on such structures as the skin, nails, and hair, several weeks or months must elapse before the full effects of therapy can be observed.

Thyroid is specific and complete replacement therapy in myxedema (p. 178) and hypothyroidism (p. 180). It may also be useful in nephrosis (p. 220) and in menstrual disorders in the absence of definite hypothyroidism. It is of no value in the treatment of obesity.

Paradoxically, the dosage of thyroid varies inversely with the severity of hypothyroidism. In patients with myxedema (see p. 179), initial dosage should be 1/10 grain daily. If there is little or no response after two weeks, the dose may be increased to 1/4 grain, after another two weeks to 1/2 grain, and, if necessary, to 1 grain after an additional fortnight. Increases in dosage should be cautious and should be made only when it is certain that the previous dosage is proving inadequate. Underdosage is preferable to overdosage. Most patients require 1 to 1 1/2 grains daily.

Infant cretins may be started on 1/16 to 1/8 grain of thyroid daily. In most, the dose should be 1/4 to 1/2 grain by the sixth month and 1 grain or more by the third or fourth year. The maximum dosage is usually required during puberty, when it may be as much as 12 grains. Later it can usually be reduced. The dosage when myxedema develops during childhood is usually about the same as in cretins of similar age. In infancy and childhood it is best to err on the side of overdosage of thyroid, in contrast to the handling of myxedema in adults.

In mild or moderately severe hypothyroidism without myxedema, it is usually safe to start with a daily dose of 1 grain of thyroid, and the maintenance dose may be from 1 grain up; 2 to 3 grains are a common requirement, and as much as 6 grains is quite unusual.

Individuals with normal thyroid function can usually take 12 to 15 grains of thyroid daily before noting manifestations of overdosage. The normal thyroid-pituitary axis is capable of compensatory inhibition when thyroid is administered.

A useful objective indication of thyroid effect is the basal pulse rate. This is the pulse rate on first awakening in the morning. Most patients can easily be trained to place a watch or clock with a second hand at the bedside and to take their own pulses before even sitting up in bed on awakening. Of course, awakening must be spontaneous; an alarm clock may accelerate the pulse. A written record of the patient's observations is kept and brought to the office at each visit. A basal pulse rate of 72 or more before treatment makes hypothyroidism doubtful. As thyroid medication takes effect, the basal pulse rate increases. A consistent basal pulse rate higher than 80 suggests that no useful purpose is likely to be served by increasing dosage and, further, that dosage should probably be reduced.

The first response to thyroid in a mildly hypothyroid patient may be a slight rise in basal pulse rate or loss of a few pounds in body weight (actually due to loss of excess body water). The dosage level producing either or both of these effects may well be continued for a second ten-day period to ascertain more fully what it will accomplish. If symptoms are not satisfactorily ameliorated by the end of this second period, the dose is increased. It is likewise increased at the end of the first period if there has been no response. The maintenance dose is the smallest one which keeps the patient free of symptoms and signs of hypothyroidism.

The evidences of thyroid overdosage are the same as those of hyperthyroidism (p. 180). Palpitation, tachycardia, sweating, intolerance to heat, nervousness, tremor, fatigue, and dyspnea on exertion are common. On discontinuation of thyroid, they ordinarily disappear in a few days. When a maintenance dose of thyroid is discontinued in a patient with myxedema, it requires about three weeks for the basal metabolic rate to complete its decline.

A therapeutic trial of thyroid is the last court of appeal when the diagnosis of hypothyroidism is uncertain. It should not be undertaken casually. Two to three months of careful observation may be required, and this fact should be understood beforehand by the patient. A record of basal pulse rate is indispensable. If there is a question of anxiety or psychoneurosis, the patient may be given a placebo for two or three weeks to make clear any psychotherapeutic effect and to allow time for observing the range of basal pulse rate. The shift to thyroid medication is made as unostentatiously as possible. Dosage is increased at intervals of ten to fourteen days until one of three things happens: (1) The patient shows clinical improvement; (2) the basal pulse rate becomes consistently higher than 80; or (3) evidences of overdosage appear.

If the patient shows improvement in those signs and symptoms which can reasonably be attributed to hypothyroidism, and if the improvement has a sufficiently delayed onset as to make a psychotherapeutic factor unlikely (psychotherapeutic effects occurring in this situation are likely to be prompt; thyroid effects are much slower), then the diagnosis of hypothyroidism is considered to be confirmed, and a suitable maintenance dose is established. If the patient has a consistently high basal pulse rate or shows evidence of overdosage, the dosage is reduced to a level that will not cause these manifestations. If such a level is maintained for three or four weeks without clinical improvement, it can be concluded that the patient was not suffering from hypothyroidism, and the trial can be discontinued.

Thyroxin (see p. 456) may be useful under extraordinary circumstances when thyroid therapy is essential and the patient can take nothing by mouth. It may be given subcutaneously, intramuscularly, or intravenously. Dosage must be regulated in the same way as for thyroid. Cretins usually require 0.2 to 0.4 mg. daily or on alternate days. Myxedema usually responds to 1.5 to 2 mg. per day. The irregular and incomplete absorption of thyroxin from the gastro-intestinal tract makes it less useful than thyroid by mouth.

Iodinated Proteins—When suitably treated with iodine, casein and other proteins develop thyroid hormone activity. They have been used in veterinary medicine.

ANTITHYROID DRUGS

The term "antithyroid drugs" has been applied to a group of organic substances which tend to prevent the formation of thyroid hormone in the thyroid gland. All of these compounds contain nitrogen and sulfur, but their chemical structures are varied. A mild antithyroid action is possessed by thiocyanates (p. 512) and sulfonamides (p. 293). The drugs which are currently in clinical use for their antithyroid effect are the thiouracils: 2-thiouracil itself (for formula, see Figure 41), and the substituted derivatives 6-n-propylthiouracil and 6-methylthiouracil.

The antithyroid drugs prevent the formation of thyroglobulin, apparently by blocking an enzyme system essential to the iodination of tyrosine preparatory to formation of thyroxin (for the chemistry of thyroglobulin, see p. 456). These drugs have no influence on (1) release of preformed hormone from the thyroid gland or (2) utilization of released or administered thyroid hormone. There may, therefore, be a delay of weeks or months in the induction of remission when antithyroid drugs are given to hyperthyroid patients who have large

goiters or who have previously been treated with iodine, for in both of these situations there is likely to be a large store of preformed thyroglobulin in the thyroid gland.

The antithyroid drugs are employed clinically in the treatment of primary hyperthyroidism (p.180). In the average acute case not previously treated with iodine, adequate dosage of an antithyroid drug will be followed within a week by rapid improvement in signs and symptoms and a fall in basal metabolic rate. After the first two weeks, improvement continues at a slower rate, four to six weeks usually being required for complete disappearance of manifestations. Large glands (as in toxic nodular goiter), pretreatment with iodine, and the presence of other endocrine disturbances may delay the onset of improvement or slow its rate. Response is slow and incomplete also when dosage is inadequate.

Antithyroid drugs may be employed (1) to prepare patients for thyroidectomy or (2) as medical treatment in lieu of thyroidectomy. They are defi-

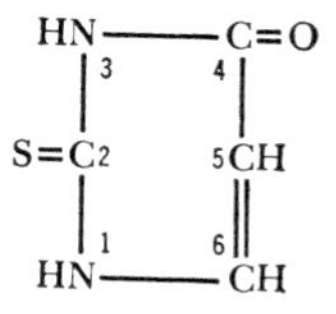

Thiouracil

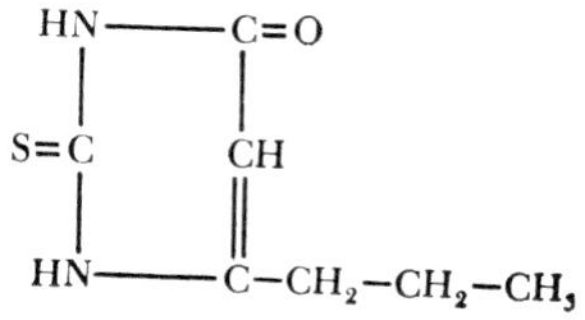

Propylthiouracil

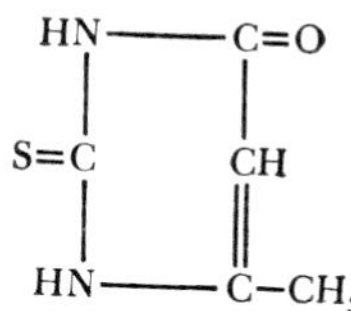

Methylthiouracil

FIGURE 41—*Structural Formulas of Antithyroid Drugs*

nitely indicated as preoperative therapy in all but the mildest cases, in which iodine alone suffices. In more severe cases, they have the advantage over iodine of providing complete control of the hyperthyroidism for an indefinite period, thus enabling the surgeon to operate on a patient who is at that time free of manifestations of the disease. The operative mortality and incidence of postoperative complications will be minimal under these circumstances.

As a preoperative measure, the antithyroid drugs are given until all manifestations of hyperthyroidism have disappeared and the patient has recuperated from them to as great an extent as is deemed possible (see p. 180). Thyroidectomy is then undertaken one week after discontinuation of the drug. During the last two or three weeks before operation, iodine should also be given in doses of 10 mg. daily (see p. 507). If the patient has been receiving iodine prior to beginning the antithyroid drug, it should be continued throughout the preparatory period. It is recommended that the period of preparation for operation never be less than five weeks. In severe and complicated cases, it may be several months. The antithyroid drugs are not given postoperatively.

In those patients who cannot or will not be operated on or who have suffered a recurrence of hyperthyroidism following thyroidectomy, the antithyroid drugs may be employed as medical treatment. As the patient becomes clinically well, the dosage should be reduced to a maintenance level to avoid the possibility of inducing hypothyroidism or myxedema. At this time, but not earlier, it is recommended that concomitant administration of iodine be begun, 10 to 30 mg. daily (see p. 507). Treatment should be continued without rest periods for twelve to eighteen months. At the end of such a period, the drug may be gradually discontinued. However, the patient should remain under observation for an additional year because of the possibility of recurrence. If the disease is to recur, it usually does so within five months. Factors favoring persistent remission are female sex, small goiter, and mild hyperthyroidism. As more experience is gained and greater skill is acquired in the employment of antithyroid drugs, the recurrence rate after their use is being reduced to approximately that following surgery.

Side-effects, apparently of allergic nature, may follow the administration of antithyroid drugs. The incidence varies with the particular drug. Such idiosyncrasy appears to be the only absolute contraindication to their use. Some patients may become allergic to only one drug, whereas others become allergic to all. Very large dosage and rest periods during therapy predispose to the development of allergy. Since the drugs may appear in the milk in significant quantities, women receiving them in the postpartum period should not nurse their babies. Antithyroid drugs are capable of passing the placental barrier, but there seems to be only a very small hazard to the fetus if the dosage is kept low and if iodine is given concomitantly.

The most serious side-effect of antithyroid drugs is agranulocytosis (severe granulocytopenia; p. 102). It may be fatal. All patients receiving these drugs should be instructed to report at once the occurrence of sore throats, fever, malaise, or any evidence of infection or illness. The physician himself should be alert to the early signs, since the prognosis seems to depend in considerable part on promptness of recognition and vigor of treatment. Because of the frequent spontaneous occurrence of leukopenia in hyperthyroidism, it is advisable to have a white blood and differential count before the institution of antithyroid therapy. Probably similar counts should be taken every week or ten days during the first two or three months of therapy, at least, and more frequently on the occurrence of any indication of illness, particularly of upper respiratory or throat infection. The treatment of agranulocytosis is discussed on page 102.

Temporary slight leukopenia is commonly seen in the first two or three weeks of therapy. It need cause no alarm unless the total white count drops to 4,500 or the percentage of granulocytes to 45.

Another serious side-effect requiring immediate and permanent discontinuation of that particular drug is drug fever. A third is a severe skin reaction, such as exfoliative dermatitis. Less-serious side-effects include skin rashes, nausea and vomiting, itching of the skin without eruption, headache, arthralgia, numbness of the skin, and drowsiness.

The antithyroid drugs are rapidly and effectively absorbed from the gastro-intestinal tract and are consequently administered by mouth. They are excreted promptly in the urine. For continued effect, therefore, they are given in subdivided doses— at six-hour intervals for initial therapy and at eight or twelve-hour intervals during maintenance.

Propylthiouracil (see Figure 41, p. 458, for formula) is at present the antithyroid drug of choice because of its low incidence of side-effects. Initial dosage of 200 to 300 mg. per day is recommended. A few patients may require as much as 400 mg. No patient with true hyperthyroidism will fail to respond if a suitable dose is given over a sufficient length of time. The maintenance dose may vary from 50 to 300 mg. daily. It must be established by trial.

The incidence of agranulocytosis due to propyl-thiouracil is apparently very low—of the order of 0.1 percent. Moderate leukopenia is seen in an additional 0.7 percent, and drug fever in about 0.3 percent. Skin rash (most frequently urticaria) is the commonest side-effect, being observed in 0.8 percent. The over-all incidence of side reactions is 2.7 percent. In many cases, the less-serious side-effects disappear spontaneously after a few days without alteration of therapy. In some, temporary discontinuation is advisable. In very few has permanent discontinuation been necessary. The administration of antihistaminic drugs (p. 509) is often of great benefit.

Thiouracil (for formula, see Figure 41, p. 458) was the first antithyroid drug to be used clinically. Its relatively high incidence of side-effects makes it much less desirable than propylthiouracil. The average initial dose was 0.4 to 0.6 Gm. daily, and the maintenance dose was 0.1 to 0.2 Gm. The over-all incidence of side-effects to thiouracil was 13 percent. The individual incidence was as follows: agranulocytosis, 2.5 percent; moderate leukopenia, 4.4 percent; drug fever, 2.7 percent; and skin rash, 3.3 percent.

Methylthiouracil (Muracil; see Figure 41, p. 458, for formula) has had more extensive use in Europe than in the United States. Initial dosage averages 300 mg. daily, and maintenance dosage is usually 100 to 200 mg. The over-all incidence of side-effects as represented in the published reports is about 12 percent. The individual incidences are agranulocytosis, about 0.3 percent; moderate leukopenia, 1.4 percent; drug fever, 4.4 to 5.5 percent; and skin rash, 3.5 to 4.2 percent.

ADRENOCORTICAL HORMONES

The adrenal cortices produce a large number of hormones. Some have principally estrogenic, androgenic, or progestational activity. Others may be considered as primary adrenocortical (corticoid) hormones. These specific adrenocortical hormones, which are essential to life, have a variety of actions; in addition, each different compound appears to have a different ratio of potencies in the various types of action. In general, the adrenocortical hormones can be classified according to whether their

activity is primarily on carbohydrate metabolism (gluco-corticoid) or on mineral metabolism (mineralo-corticoid). The life-maintaining action of the corticoids is probably due to a combination of these two effects, but it may well involve other actions not yet understood. Important androgenic and anabolic substances (N hormones) are also secreted by the adrenal cortex.

It should be emphasized that the steroids thus far isolated from the adrenal cortex account for only a small percentage of the total potency of adrenal extracts. Most of the activity resides in the amorphous fraction, the chemical nature of which is unknown.

MINERALO-CORTICOIDS

The steroids which have as their predominant action an influence on sodium and potassium metabolism are characterized by the absence of an oxygen atom at the eleventh carbon atom. The best known of this group are 11-desoxycorticosterone (desoxycorticosterone) and 11-desoxy-17-hydroxycorticosterone (Reichstein's Compound S), which are shown in Figure 42.

Desoxycorticosterone is the most powerful of this group. It is made synthetically and occurs in the adrenal cortex only in minute quantities if at all. Its actions may differ somewhat from those of other mineralo-corticoids. However, it is the only mineralo-corticoid now generally available.

The mineralo-corticoids cause retention of sodium and elimination of potassium. Most of this effect is exerted through the kidneys, in which these steroids act specifically on the cells of the proximal convoluted tubules to stimulate reabsorption of sodium; chloride and water are reabsorbed secondarily, and there is an increase in volume of the plasma and interstitial fluid. The renal excretion of potassium is increased, but the mechanism is not understood. In addition, the mineralo-corticoids influence capillary permeability and tissue affinity for electrolytes and water. These actions are associated with a decreased concentration of sodium and chloride in the sweat. Both the mineralo-corticoids and the gluco-corticoids exert slight androgenic and progestational effects.

Desoxycorticosterone acetate (DCA, Doca, Cortate, Percorten) is employed clinically in the treatment of Addison's disease (see p. 183). It is usually injected intramuscularly in oil solution. The average dose is 2 to 3 mg. daily, but in every case the dosage must be individualized to meet the needs

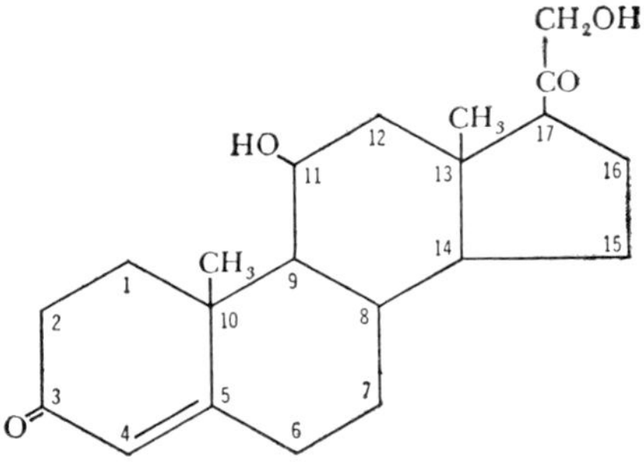

Corticosterone

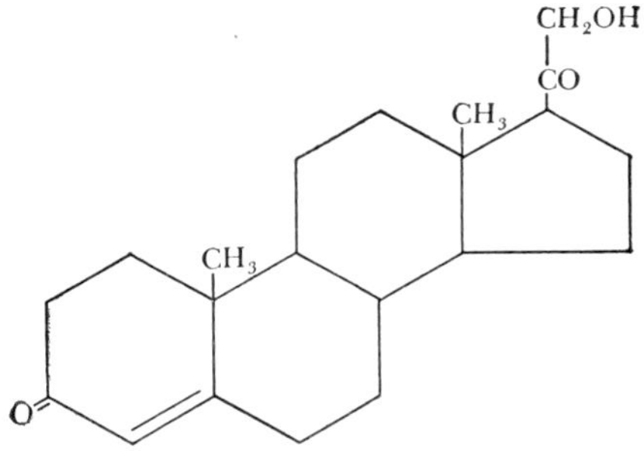

Desoxycorticosterone

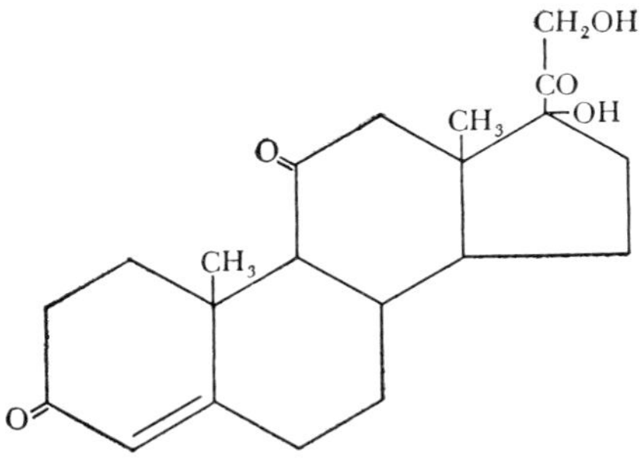

Cortisone
(Kendall's Compound E)

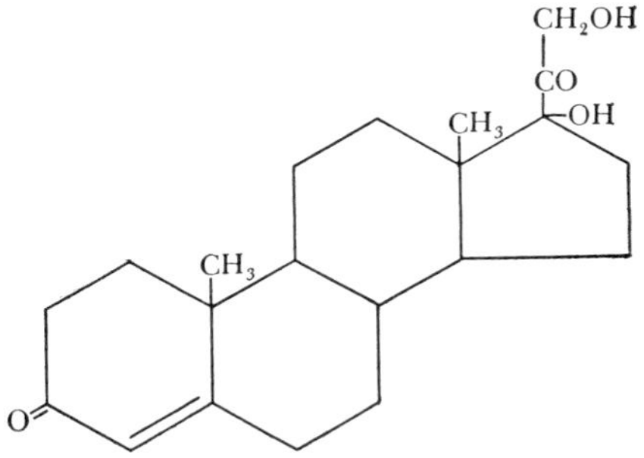

11-Desoxy-17-hydroxycorticosterone
(Reichstein's Compound S)

FIGURE 42—Structural Formulas of Some Adrenocortical Hormones

of the patient at the time. After the drug has been given for a considerable period and the requirement has been thoroughly established, pellets may be implanted in those patients whose requirements show little fluctuation. Pellet implantation has the advantage of eliminating constant injections, for one implantation is effective for months. However, it is a somewhat exacting procedure, and patients must be watched closely for danger signals of overdosage or hypoglycemia. Desoxycorticosterone acetate is also available dissolved in a mixture of propylene glycol and ethyl alcohol for sublingual or buccal administration. This route avoids the needle, but the dosage is rather uncertain.

Patients receiving desoxycorticosterone should have a definite intake of sodium, which may be in the form of the chloride, bicarbonate, or citrate (see p. 341). The usual intake is 3 to 5 Gm. in addition to that needed to season the food. Increasing the dose of sodium salts diminishes the requirement of hormone, and vice versa. Patients receiving hormonal therapy should also take up to

2 Gm. of potassium daily in the diet to prevent potassium deficiency. Since desoxycorticosterone has no effect on carbohydrate metabolism, it is especially important that Addisonian patients receiving it have a high carbohydrate intake. There should be frequent feedings, including one at bedtime.

As therapy in Addison's disease, desoxycorticosterone has two disadvantages. One is its lack of effect on carbohydrate metabolism; dangerous or even fatal hypoglycemia and asthenia may occur in patients otherwise well controlled. The other is the fact that overdoses are toxic. Overretention of sodium causes edema and increased plasma volume and may lead to hypertension, proteinuria, cardiac dilatation, heart failure, and angina pectoris. Hypopotassemia may cause replacement of tissue potassium with sodium; the result is muscular weakness or paralysis (see p. 342). Prolonged overdosage may induce degenerative changes in the arteries, including nephrosclerosis (p. 221). These manifestations are rare if patients are carefully followed on minimal effective dosage.

Administration of desoxycorticosterone to patients with functioning adrenals may lead to compensatory atrophy of the adrenals and diminution of output of gluco-corticoids as well as mineralocorticoids.

GLUCO-CORTICOIDS

Only those steroids having an oxygen atom attached to the eleventh carbon atom have gluco-corticoid activity. Several such compounds exist. Perhaps the two best known are corticosterone and cortisone, which are shown in Figure 42 (p. 461). Being more readily available, cortisone is discussed as typical of the group. It should be emphasized, however, that the different compounds vary in their relative potency for different effects.

Cortisone (Kendall's Compound E) has the following direct and indirect effects on carbohydrate metabolism:

1. Increase in conversion of exogenous carbohydrate to glycogen.
2. Increase in conversion of endogenous protein to carbohydrate (gluconeogenesis). This conversion of amino-acid radicals to dextrose is antianabolic, but it is not catabolic.
3. Increased mobilization and utilization of fat, thereby sparing carbohydrate.
4. Diminished oxidation of available carbohydrate.
5. Increase in blood-sugar level, probably as the result of Effects 1, 2, 3, and 4.

Cortisone has an action on sodium and potassium metabolism which is quantitatively about 3 per cent of that of desoxycorticosterone. The mechanism of action of the two is different, however; and when they are given together in certain relative dosages, they may tend to neutralize each other in electrolyte effect.

Cortisone (and other gluco-corticoids having a hydroxyl group attached to the seventeenth carbon atom) also causes lysis of lymphoid tissue, with diminution in size of the lymph nodes and thymus. It produces (1) a lymphocytopenia, (2) a sharp drop in eosinophil count, and (3) a neutrophilic leukocytosis which is usually sufficient to cause a slight increase in the total white blood cell count. The steroid also increases the renal excretion of uric acid. These effects of the gluco-corticoids have been employed as a test of the reserve power of the adrenals to respond to adrenocorticotrophic hormone (see p. 473).

The gluco-corticoids play an important part in meeting certain types of stress, such as infection, trauma (including burns), solar and roentgen irradiation, intoxications of various sorts, extremes of temperature, excessive exertion, strong emotion, malnutrition, and the effects of some drugs. The response to stress has been termed "the alarm reaction" by Selye. When the stress is acute, the immediate response has two phases. The first is shock (see also p. 90), marked by decrease in muscle tone and body temperature, tachycardia, hemoconcentration, anuria, edema, decrease in blood chlorides, acidosis, a transitory rise and then fall in blood sugar, formation of gastric and intestinal ulcers, and leukopenia followed by leukocytosis. This phase may last from a few minutes to a day.

Unless the patient dies, the shock phase is followed by the countershock phase, the most characteristic feature of which appears to be an increased secretion of gluco-corticoids by the adrenal cortex. The stress, acting either through neural pathways or humorally by means of toxic products, stimulates certain regions of the hypothalamus to secrete a hormone (of unknown nature) which acts on the anterior pituitary in such a way as to cause an outpouring of adrenocorticotrophic hormone (ACTH). Epinephrine (in doses of 0.3 mg. for an adult) has the same effect, but it is not the usual stimulus during stress. The ACTH acts on the adrenals to cause (1) enlargement of the cortex with signs of increased activity in the cells, and (2) release of hormones in which the gluco-corticoids appear to predominate. These gluco-corticoids have their usual effects, which include acute involution of the thymus and other lymphoid organs and a reversal of most features of the shock phase; there is increase in blood volume and dilution of blood constituents, increase in blood levels of chloride and sugar, tendency toward alkalosis, and often a rise in body temperature.

If the stress continues, the countershock phase of the alarm reaction passes into the stage of resistance, in which the lesions produced by the stressing stimulus regress, and resistance to the stimulus reaches a peak. The role of the adrenal cortex in the production of specific antibodies is controversial; in fact, much of the mechanism by which the gluco-corticoids increase resistance to stress is still wholly unknown. If the stress is too extreme or continues for too long a period, the power of response wears out; and the organism enters the stage of exhaustion, with reappearance of many of the manifestations of the shock phase.

The ability of the 11,17-oxycorticoids to counteract the effects of damaging agents is strikingly shown in the results of administration of cortisone and of ACTH in rheumatoid arthritis, rheumatic fever, gout, lupus erythematosus, and other diseases. In rheumatoid arthritis, for instance, the daily injection of 100 mg. or more of cortisone acetate is followed within a few days by reduction of stiffness, diminution in articular tenderness and pain on motion, reduction of swelling, and great improvement in articular and muscular function; improved appetite and weight gain; increase in feeling of well-being sometimes amounting to euphoria; great reduction (sometimes to normal) in blood sedimentation rate; improvement in anemia; and return toward normal in plasma protein level and distribution. However, the effects seldom outlast the period of administration.

The response of these diseases to the 11,17-oxycorticoids is nonspecific and is not due to any action on the causative agent. This is demonstrated both by the temporary nature of the remissions and by the observation that the arthritis produced in animals by intra-articular injection of mustard or formaldehyde (and which mimics the lesions of rheumatoid arthritis in man) is completely prevented by administration of cortisone. Until more is known about these effects, their mechanism, and the side-effects, the administration of cortisone must be considered an experimental procedure.

Large doses of cortisone (of the order of 100 mg. daily) are capable of reproducing the clinical picture of Cushing's syndrome (p. 186). If the drug is stopped promptly, the manifestations cease. Similar doses have also induced psychoses of various types, some of which have persisted after withdrawal of medication. Diabetes mellitus has also been precipitated in susceptible individuals.

Cortisone is new as a therapeutic agent, and a number of years of careful study will be required before its usefulness and limitations are fully known. In addition to its dramatic effects in diseases not directly related to the adrenal glands, it should theoretically be an ideal preparation in Addison's disease. Even here, its value and manner of use are in dispute as of this writing.

ADRENAL EXTRACTS

Since the adrenals store little preformed hormone, the glands themselves are not rich sources of their secretions. However, some concentrated extracts do have activity. The most potent is a lipoid extract of pork glands (Lipo-Adrenal Cortex) which is standardized on both dogs and rats. Each cc. exerts the same amount (10 rat units) of survival-growth effect as 10 cc. of aqueous extract of beef glands and as much effect on muscle work in dogs as 2 mg. of cortisone. Daily intramuscular doses

of 1 or 2 cc. may suffice to maintain patients with Addison's disease (p. 183).

As just indicated, aqueous extracts of beef adrenals have only 10 percent of the activity of lipoid extracts of pork glands. They have the further disadvantage that their action lasts only a few hours. On the other hand, aqueous extracts may be useful for intravenous administration in the early treatment of Addisonian crisis (see p. 185).

Largely because the liver removes the steroids from the portal blood, adrenal preparations are unsatisfactory for oral administration.

ESTROGENS

The term "estrogen" means "a substance which produces estrus (sexual heat in female animals)." Estrus does not occur in women, but the principal actions of estrogens in them are outlined in Table 51.

Many different types of chemical substances have estrogenic activity. As a group, they are oil-soluble and water-insoluble. The estrogens produced by

TABLE 51 — *Principal Actions of Estrogens*

I. Systemic
  A. Influence deposition of subcutaneous fat to give feminine body contours
  B. Tend to induce retention of sodium and water
  C. Increase callus formation at fracture sites
  D. Increase calcification of bone
  E. May under certain circumstances accelerate closure of epiphyses
  F. Lower basal body temperature (see p. 203)

II. On endocrine glands
  A. Ovaries: necessary for ovulation
  B. Adrenal cortices: stimulate directly or indirectly
  C. Anterior pituitary: small doses stimulate release of luteinizing hormone, and large doses inhibit release of all gonadotrophins

III. On reproductive tract and secondary sexual characteristics
  A. Myometrium: stimulate development of adult size and architecture; sensitize to all types of stimuli
  B. Endometrium: stimulate formation of proliferative (follicular) phase; withdrawal (in absence of progesterone) followed in four to nine days (average, seven) by endometrial bleeding without loss of tissue
  C. Vaginal epithelium: stimulate proliferation and cornification
  D. Breasts: stimulate growth of duct system; cause development of fat and connective tissue typical of female breast
  E. Pubic hair: cause typical female escutcheon

the ovaries of various species are steroids and are thus related to progesterone, the adrenal and testicular hormones, cholesterol, the bile acids, the vitamins D, and digitalis glycosides. A major distinguishing feature of the steroid estrogens is their lack of a methyl group attached to the tenth carbon atom (Figure 43).

Estrone and estradiol are the estrogens produced by the human ovaries, and they may apparently be produced by testes and adrenal cortices as well. They can be converted, one to the other, in the ovaries and in other tissues. In the presence of progesterone, estrone is converted into the very

weak estrogen estriol, which is excreted in the urine as the glucuronate. Estradiol and estrone may also appear in the urine as glucuronates (in the human species; in the horse they are excreted as sulfates).

The major part, if not all, of the inactivation and conjugation of estrogens takes place in the liver. In the normal individual, only 2 to 6 percent of injected estrogen can be recovered in the urine in either active or inactive form; the remainder is evidently destroyed in the liver. When more estrogen is presented to the liver than it can metabolize promptly, the excess is secreted into the bile. In the

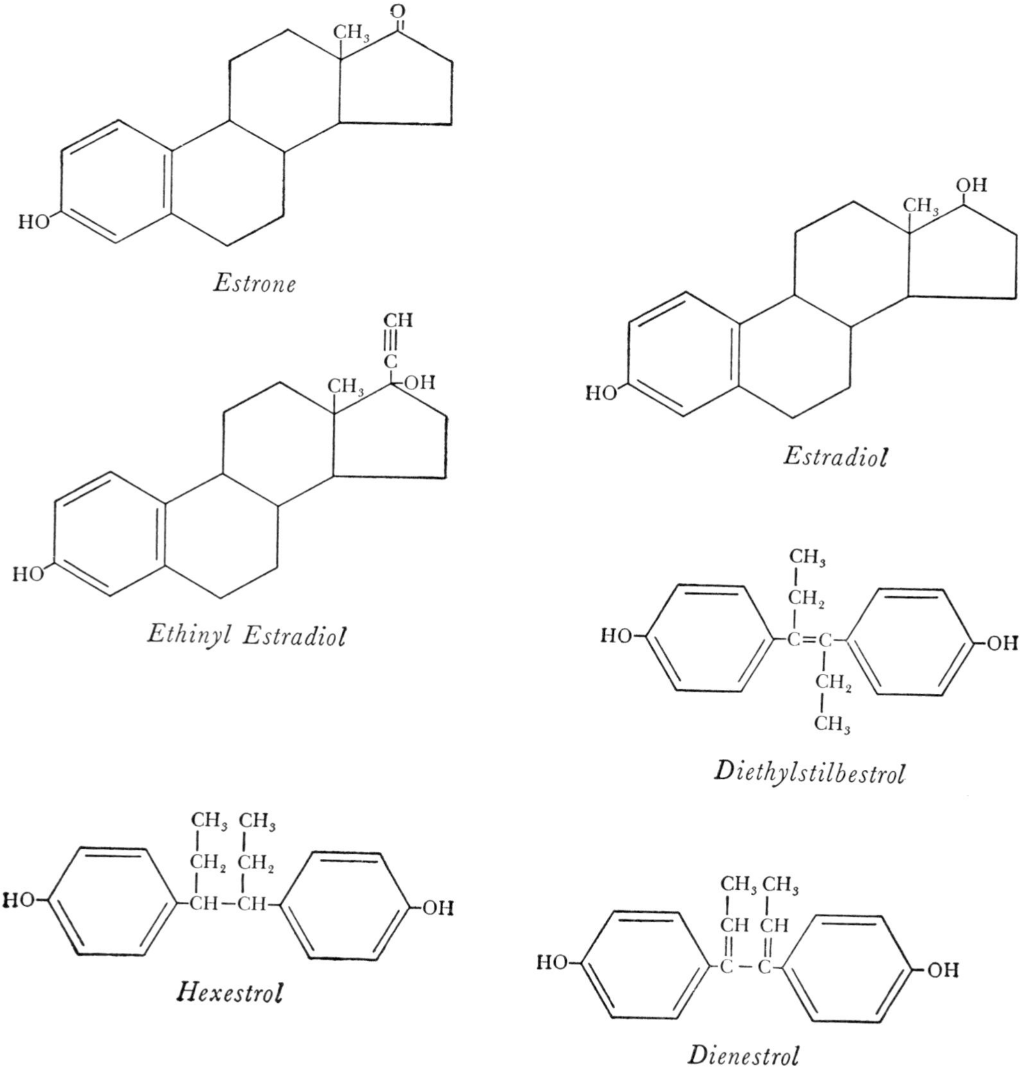

Estrone

Ethinyl Estradiol

Hexestrol

Estradiol

Diethylstilbestrol

Dienestrol

FIGURE 43 — *Structural Formulas of Estrogens*

bile, the estrogen passes into the intestine, only to be reabsorbed into the portal circulation. This enterohepatic circulation of estrogen serves to protect the body from the "excess" estrogen until the liver can destroy it.

These functions of the liver are impaired by extreme undernutrition or advanced liver disease; as a result, excessive estrogen effects (such as breast development in men and the appearance of spider angiomata in both men and women) occur in patients with cirrhosis and other severe hepatic diseases. The cycle of ovarian production of estrogen is discussed on page 202.

Estrogens have many clinical uses. Their oldest and most traditional use is in treatment of menopausal symptoms (for discussion, see p. 206). They are specific for senile vaginitis (p. 199). They are capable of inducing sexual development in women with prepuberal hypogonadism or ovarian agenesis (p. 188). They have proved useful in painful engorgement of the breasts postpartum (p. 216), functional uterine bleeding (p. 203), threatened or habitual abortion (p. 211), and for temporary control of carcinoma of the prostate in men (p. 217) and inoperable carcinoma of the breast in postmenopausal women (p. 201). They have also been effective in preventing toxemia of pregnancy (p. 212) and in preventing or alleviating mumps orchitis (p. 27).

A number of side-effects have been noted in connection with estrogen therapy. Most common is the occurrence of nausea, which may be severe enough to lead to vomiting. The incidence of nausea appears to differ significantly among various types of patients. Pregnant and postpartum women are the least susceptible, requiring single doses as large as 500 mg. of diethylstilbestrol, for instance, to produce nausea. Men, children, and nonpregnant women form an intermediate group in whom moderate doses seldom cause symptoms. Menopausal women and women subject to the nausea of pregnancy are most susceptible, a certain percentage being disturbed by dosages commonly prescribed for menopausal symptoms. Nausea and vomiting appear to be nonspecific responses which may be evoked by any estrogen if given in a sufficiently large dose in a form which is rapidly absorbed.

Other side-effects may be considered as exaggerated estrogenic effects. These include the production of uterine bleeding during continuous therapy (as distinguished from the withdrawal bleeding which occurs following discontinuation of physiological doses), the production of a hypertrophic endometrium (including the so-called "Swiss cheese" condition seen in endometrial biopsies), painful breasts, and vaginal soreness. The uterine bleeding and endometrial hypertrophy result from prolonged constant administration and can be prevented by cyclic therapy as described under treatment of menopausal symptoms (p. 207).

Comparatively rare side-effects include abdominal distress or pain, anorexia, diarrhea, lassitude, paresthesia, vertigo, headache, anxiety, insomnia, thirst, scotomata, and even psychotic episodes. Cutaneous rashes, purpura, and other apparently allergic reactions have been observed, some of which seem to be due to the estrogen and some to the oil vehicle. The actual toxicity of all the estrogens appears to be low.

When estrogens are administered over prolonged periods in cancer of the prostate, the following side-effects have been noted:

1. Loss of sexual power and some degree of genital atrophy.
2. Breast changes:
   a. Gross: enlargement of the breasts and pigmentation and increased sensitiveness of the nipples and areolae.
   b. Microscopic: proliferation and budding of the duct epithelium, increase in connective-tissue stroma, edema of the stroma, increased vascularity, and (after prolonged treatment) deposition of fat.
3. Dependent edema.
4. Metaplasia of the urethral epithelium.
5. Increase in density of the bones.

Many of the estrogens are potent agents, and none should be administered without a positive indication. The breasts and pelvic organs should be examined before treatment is begun and at intervals during therapy. The patient should be advised of the importance of remaining under supervision during estrogenic therapy. Estrogens should be avoided in *pre*menopausal women who have cancerous or precancerous lesions of the breast or cervix or who have a family history of high incidence of breast or genital malignancy. However, estrogens have caused regression of breast cancer in *post*menopausal women (see p. 201). Present evidence suggests strongly that, in the average woman, sensible estrogenic therapy carries no appreciable risk of initiating cancer.

The two practical sources of estrogens are chemical synthesis and the urine of pregnant mares. The latter contains estrone and estradiol as well as equilin, equilenin, and hippulin, which are peculiar to the horse. Estrone and estradiol can now be made synthetically from certain plant steroids. A number of estrogens that are partly or completely of synthetic origin are available for clinical use; they include ethinyl estradiol, diethylstilbestrol, hexestrol, dienestrol, and others.

The dosage of chemically pure estrogens can and should be stated in terms of weight. In 1932, when it was thought that estrone was the only natural estrogen, a conference held under the auspices of the Health Organisation of the League of Nations adopted an International Unit, which was defined as the specific estrus-producing activity contained in 0.1 microgram (0.0001 mg.) of a chosen standard preparation of estrone. Regulations were adopted covering the application of the International Standard to bio-assay. Later, estradiol was discovered, and it was found that no satisfactory comparison was possible between estrone and either estradiol or estradiol benzoate. Therefore, a second conference adopted an International Benzoate Unit, which was defined as the specific estrus-producing activity contained in 0.1 microgram of a chosen standard preparation of estradiol benzoate, and which was specifically stated to be in no way equivalent to the estrone standard. It was further agreed: "That in the opinion of this Conference it is desirable that, as rapidly and as far as possible, the production of preparations of the oestrus-producing hormones should be limited to pure preparations of the different forms of the hormone and its chemically defined derivatives or of mixtures thereof, so that the activity may be indicated in exact weights, and indications in biological units may be abandoned."

In the ensuing years it has been amply demonstrated that comparisons of estrogens by bio-assay on one species cannot be transferred to other species (including the human) and that the potency of mixtures of estrogens cannot be determined by bio-assay of any type. This means that the International Unit is valid only when used to assay preparations of pure estrone and that the International Benzoate Unit is valid only for preparations of pure estradiol benzoate. Along the same lines, it has been found that the attempt to compare the potency of different estrogens in human beings has led to such discordant results as to make the question appear unanswerable.

Even though exact measurement seems impossible, different estrogens do undoubtedly differ in potency and in duration of action. Part of such differences may be due to different rates of inactivation in the liver. It is possible that there are also relative differences in specific types of activity; e.g., two estrogens may have the same potency in stimulating vaginal cornification but different potencies in producing estrogen-withdrawal bleeding in the endometrium. The evidence indicates, however, that all estrogens have the same *qualitative* proper-

ties, which is to say that what one estrogen can do, any estrogen can do when administered in appropriate dosage. The facts that there are many different estrogens in clinical use and that some of them are especially popular for particular purposes are apparently due to such factors as potency, cost, and custom.

Estrone (theelin; see Figure 43, p. 464, for formula) was the first estrogen to be obtained in pure form. In that form it is available for injection or in vaginal suppositories. The original injectable preparation was a solution in oil, 0.1 to 1 mg. per cc. More recently it has been made available also as an aqueous suspension, 1 to 5 mg. per cc., which has the advantage of dispensing with the oil vehicle and providing a deposit of crystals for more prolonged absorption. Estrone as such is employed largely for treatment of menopausal symptoms and senile vaginitis, partly because of custom.

Within the past few years, estrone has been marketed in conjugated form for oral administration. Preparations contain the sodium sulfate salt-ester of estrone and smaller quantities of similarly conjugated forms of estradiol, equilin, equilenin, hippulin, and possibly other estrogens occurring in the urine of pregnant mares. In contrast to estrone itself, the conjugated forms are water-soluble. They are marketed under such names as 'Konogen,' Premarin, Conestron, and Amnestrogen. Because of their slightly varying composition, they are assayed biologically. Labeling in terms of milligrams of sodium estrone sulfate is a matter of convenience and means that the quantity of material contained in the tablet produced a vaginal response in the assay animal equal to that from the stated amount of pure sodium estrone sulfate.

Average dosage of estrone and conjugated estrone is summarized in Table 52.

Estradiol (alpha-estradiol; see Figure 43, p. 464, for formula) is available in a number of forms. For injection, it is employed as the benzoate (Progynon-B, Ovocylin Benzoate, Dimenformon Benzoate) or the dipropionate (Progynon-DP, Ovocylin Dipropionate, Dimenformon Dipropionate). These esters are more slowly absorbed than unesterified forms, the dipropionate more slowly than the benzoate. Suppositories are available for vaginal therapy, as is an ointment. Average established doses are found in Table 52. Estradiol preparations may be used for the other conditions listed therein; however, the dosage in them is either not established or is the subject of disagreement. Estradiol itself

☐ *Estrogens*

may be given by mouth (Tablets Progynon-DH, Ovocylin, Dimenformon), but the liver removes such a high percentage that relatively large doses are required.

Ethinyl Estradiol (Estinyl, Eticylol, Lynoral) is an estrogen of high potency made synthetically from estradiol (for formula, see Figure 43, p. 464). The ethinyl group protects the compound from attack in the liver, and it is therefore highly potent on oral administration. Average doses are found in Table 52.

Diethylstilbestrol (stilbestrol) was the first estrogen of totally synthetic origin to find clinical use.

Its chemical structure (see Figure 43, p. 464) is not related to that of the natural estrogens, yet it mimics their actions faithfully. Diethylstilbestrol is attacked by the liver relatively slowly. This fact and its high potency make it extremely effective on oral administration. It may be employed whenever estrogenic therapy is indicated; average dosage is shown in Table 52.

Hexestrol, Dienestrol, and Benzestrol (the formulas of hexestrol and dienestrol are shown in Figure 43, p. 464) are closely related to diethylstilbestrol in chemical structure. Hexestrol and Benzestrol are less potent than diethylstilbestrol. In some actions dienestrol is less potent as well, but with regard to

TABLE 52 — *Average Customary Doses of Estrogens**

Estrogen	Route of Adminis-tration	Meno-pausal Symptoms	Senile Vaginitis	Painful Engorge-ment of Breasts	Functional Uterine Bleeding	Cancer of Prostate Initial Phase	Cancer of Prostate Mainte-nance	Cancer of Breast	For Sexual Develop-ment
Diethylstilbestrol	O	0.1-1 mg./d.	0.1-1 mg./d.	15-60 mg. over 2-4 d.	5 mg. q. 4-6 hr.	3 mg./d.	1 mg./d.	15 mg./d.	0.5-5 mg./d.
	IM	0.25-1 mg. q. 2-7 d.	0.25-1 mg. q. 2-7 d.	10-40 mg. over 2-4 d.	5 mg. q. 8-12 hr.	5 mg. q. 3-4 d.	2-4 mg. q. 3-4 d.		
	V	0.5 mg./d.	0.5 mg./d.						
Estrone	IM	0.2-1 mg. q. 2-7 d.	0.2-1 mg. q. 2-7 d.						
	V		0.2 mg./d.						
Estrone (conjugated)	O	1.25-3.75 mg./d.	1.25-3.75 mg./d.						
Estradiol	V		0.04-0.4 mg./d.					30 mg./d.	
Estradiol benzoate	IM	0.17-1 mg. q. 2-7 d.	0.17-1 mg. q. 2-7 d.	13.3 mg. over 4 d.		1.7 mg. q. 1 or 2 d.			1-1.7 mg. q. 2 d.
Estradiol dipropionate	IM	0.1-5 mg. q. 5-28 d.	0.1-5 mg. q. 5-28 d.					5 mg. q. 3 d.	
Ethinyl estradiol	O	0.02-0.15 mg./d.	0.02-0.15 mg./d.	4.5-7.5 mg. over 3 d.		0.25-0.5 mg./d.	0.05-0.1 mg./d.	3 mg./d.	
Hexestrol	O	0.2-3 mg./d.	0.2-3 mg./d.	30-90 mg. over 2-4 d.					
	IM	1 mg. q. 2 d.	1 mg. q. 2 d.	30 mg. or more over 2-4 d.					
Dienestrol	O	0.1-1.5 mg./d.	0.1-1.5 mg./d.	1.5 mg. daily for 3 d., then 0.5 mg. daily for 7 d.				15 mg./d.	
Benzestrol	O	2-3 mg./d.	2-3 mg./d.	60 mg. over 4 d.					
	IM	2.5-5 mg. q. 4-7 d.	2.5-5 mg. q. 4-7 d.						

*The doses given in the table do not necessarily represent the comparative potencies of the various preparations; dosage is to a certain extent affected by custom independently of drug potency.

KEY: O=oral; IM=intramuscular; V=vaginal; d.=day or days.

others there is disagreement. Like diethylstilbestrol, they are resistant to hepatic destruction and are therefore appropriate for oral administration. Average doses appear in Table 52.

Mixed Natural Estrogens—Mixtures of natural estrogens are available for oral or parenteral administration. These are extracted from the urine of pregnant mares. They contain mostly estrone, but significant quantities of estradiol, equilin, equilenin, and hippulin are also present. Inevitably, the proportions of the different estrogens vary from one lot to another. The inadequacy of bio-assay as a measure of therapeutic potency of estrogens (see p. 466) places these preparations at a great disadvantage.

PROGESTERONE

Progesterone is a steroid normally produced by the corpus luteum of the ovary. In chemical structure (Figure 44) it is more closely related to the adrenal hormones (Figure 42, p. 461) than to its companion ovarian hormones, the estrogens (Figure 43, p. 464). As a matter of fact, progesterone has been found in adrenal glands.

Progesterone is secreted by the corpus luteum and probably also by the ovarian follicle just before maturation (for further discussion, see p. 202). It may be considered to be a hormone of pregnancy—actual or potential. Perhaps its principal site of action is the endometrium. In the absence of estrogen, progesterone has no effect on the endometrium; but following development of the proliferative phase of this mucous membrane in response to estrogen, progesterone causes the changes characteristic of the secretory, or progestational, phase. In this state, the epithelium becomes high and

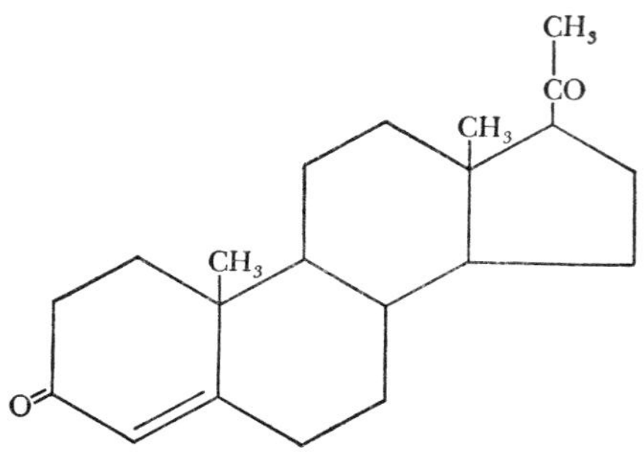

contains much glycogen, the glands become branched and dilated, and the stroma becomes more vascular. Nidation of a fertilized ovum will take place on the endometrium only when it is in the progestational phase. Once established, pregnancy continues only in the presence of progesterone. Withdrawal of the hormone leads to abortion.

Sudden withdrawal of progesterone in pregnant or nonpregnant women is followed in about forty-eight hours by uterine bleeding. In contrast to estrogen-withdrawal bleeding, that due to progesterone withdrawal is accompanied by sloughing of the mucous membrane. Normal menstruation is due to progesterone withdrawal (see p. 202).

Progesterone has a number of other important effects. It supplements the action of estrogen on the breasts, causing development of the lobules, or secreting elements. However, it does not initiate lactation. The hormone alters the contractility of the myometrium, lessening the frequency of contractions and increasing their amplitude. The vaginal mucosa becomes soft and the epithelium mucoid in type, resembling the condition present when amounts of estrogen act which are too small to produce cornification. Progesterone does not affect the basal metabolism, but it elevates the basal body temperature; this latter action is the basis for determination of ovulation by means of body temperature (see p. 203). Progesterone also tends to cause retention of sodium and water in the body.

Like other steroids, progesterone is fat-soluble and water-insoluble. It is well absorbed from the intestinal tract, but such a high percentage is removed by the liver following absorption into the portal venous system that oral administration is impractical. The hormone is converted in the body (apparently mostly by the liver) into the physiologically inactive substance pregnanediol. It is excreted as sodium pregnanediol glucuronate.

Progesterone has been employed in treatment of threatened or habitual abortion, dysmenorrhea, functional uterine bleeding, amenorrhea, endometrial hyperplasia, and puerperal afterpains. In threatened abortion, the dosage should be at least 10 mg. daily until symptoms have subsided. Recommended doses in prevention of habitual abortion have ranged from 1 to 5 mg. or more daily. Recent reports suggest that estrogen alone is more effective against habitual abortion and that estrogen alone or a combination of estrogen and progesterone is more effective against threatened abortion than is progesterone alone (see p. 211).

In pathological endometrial hyperplasia, prolonged therapy appears to be advisable: in the first

Progesterone

FIGURE 44 — *Structural Formula of Progesterone*

month, 5 mg. daily for ten days, beginning on the twelfth day before the expected onset of the next menstrual period; in the second month, the same dosage for eight days, beginning on the tenth day before the expected period; in the third month, for six days; and in the fourth month, for four days. Puerperal afterpains are usually controlled by a single dose of 1 mg. Dosage of progesterone for the other conditions named will be found under the condition: dysmenorrhea, page 205; functional uterine bleeding, page 204; and amenorrhea, page 205.

Progesterone is generally administered by intramuscular injection. It is rapidly absorbed and metabolized. For continuous effect it must be given daily. Recently, experiments have been conducted with sublingual administration.

Pregneninolone (anhydrohydroxyprogesterone, Pranone, Lutocylol, Progestoral) is a progesterone derivative in which the methyl ketone group and hydrogen at the seventeenth carbon atom (Figure 44) are replaced by a hydroxyl group and an ethinyl group (CH:C·), such as are present in ethinyl estradiol (Figure 43, p. 464). Pregneninolone is only slowly attacked by the liver and is therefore suitable for oral administration. It appears to mimic fairly closely the actions of progesterone.

When the drug is swallowed, the usual daily doses are as follows: habitual abortion, 5 to 10 mg.; threatened abortion, 10 to 15 mg.; functional uterine bleeding, 10 mg.; dysmenorrhea, 10 mg. If the drug is administered sublingually, the dose may be reduced by about half.

ANDROGENS

Androgens are substances which cause the development and maintenance of the male secondary sexual characteristics. They are analogous to estrogens (p. 463); but the analogy is incomplete, for the androgens have properties for which no counterparts are shown by estrogens. The androgens are steroids; the two which are employed therapeutically, testosterone and methyltestosterone, are shown in Figure 45. Other androgens, having somewhat different properties, are secreted by the adrenal glands (p. 183). Under certain unusual circumstances, ovarian tissue is capable of secreting androgens.

Testosterone is the principal and possibly the only androgen produced by the testes. It is secreted by the Leydig cells under the stimulus of luteinizing hormone from the anterior pituitary. Testosterone is the agent that mediates the development of the male accessory sex organs (penis, prostate), pubic hair, and beard and lowering of the voice, characteristic of puberty in men. It increases basal metabolic rate (10 to 45 percent) without affecting body temperature (compare with estrogen, p. 463, and progesterone, p. 468). It may lead to a slight decrease in carbohydrate tolerance; and it exerts a mild sodium-retaining action, which is, however, sometimes sufficient to cause water retention and edema.

Androgens exert several actions on the skin. In their absence, the skin is soft and young-looking. The face lacks deep furrows but carries numerous very fine wrinkles. The skin has a characteristic sallow color owing to the absence of pigment. The volume of blood in the skin is altered, as is capillary excitability. Androgen stimulates sebaceous secretion and is a prime but not the sole factor in the occurrence of acne vulgaris. The testicular hormone induces increased coarseness of body hair in general, in addition to stimulating growth of the beard and determining masculine distribution of pubic hair. It is a factor, along with adrenocortical hormones, in the growth of axillary hair. It induces increased bushiness of the eyebrows and development of hair between the eyebrows. It is a prerequisite for the common types of baldness observed in men, including the recession of hairline at the temples, which may begin in the middle twenties.

The most striking and important systemic effect of androgens is on protein metabolism. These steroids cause retention of nitrogen, potassium, and phosphate and increase in the mass of skeletal muscle, protein stores, and body weight. It seems probable that the heavier body musculature of men as compared with that of women is due in large part to a greater supply of testosterone and related substances.

The phosphate retention caused by androgens is often accompanied by calcium retention and increased maturation of bone structure. If the epiphyses are not closed, increase in height (growth in length of limb bones) occurs. Paradoxically, the prepuberal hypogonadal boy (who lacks androgen) is tall, with abnormally long limb bones, and androgens have been credited with slowing growth and with accelerating closure of epiphyses, thus permanently stopping growth. It seems probable that testicular hormone merely speeds up certain processes of bone development which would proceed more slowly to the same end without it.

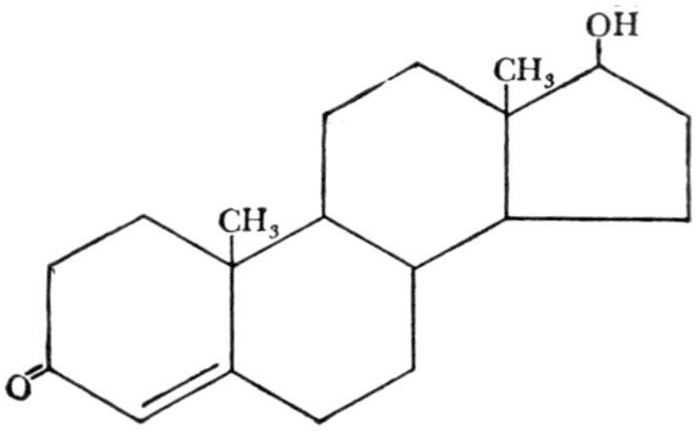

Testosterone

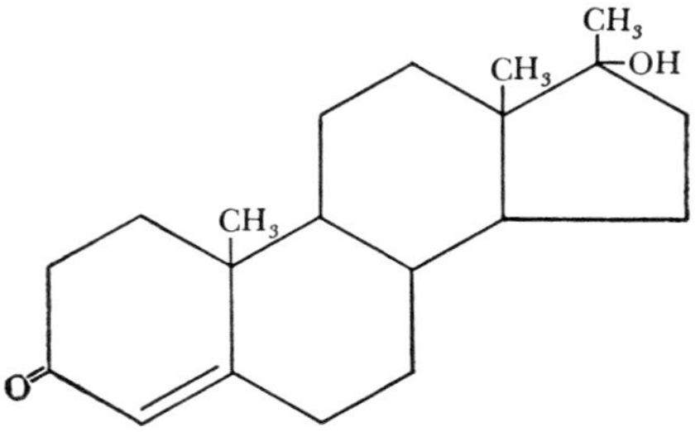

Methyltestosterone

FIGURE 45 — *Structural Formulas of Androgens*

When present in sufficient concentration in the blood, androgens tend to inhibit further release of gonadotrophin from the anterior pituitary. The administration of androgen may therefore impair or stop testicular function (both spermatogenesis and endogenous hormone production) in men and ovarian function in women.

Methyltestosterone has most of the properties of testosterone. There are apparently two principal differences. One is that whereas testosterone decreases the excretion of creatine, methyltestosterone increases it. The mechanism and significance of this observation are unknown. The other recognized difference is that methyltestosterone is relatively slowly destroyed in the liver; it is therefore suited for oral administration. Testosterone is rapidly inactivated by the liver and is therefore poorly suited for ingestion.

Administration and Dosage—Testosterone itself may be administered intramuscularly as an aqueous suspension or sublingually as tablets. More commonly, testosterone is administered as an oil solution of the propionate ester by intramuscular injection. Tablets of testosterone propionate are available for buccal or sublingual administration; however, methyltestosterone appears to be more

effective. Methyltestosterone tablets may be swallowed or may be allowed to dissolve under the tongue or between cheek and lower jaw; the latter route, permitting direct absorption into the blood stream, increases the efficacy by 30 to 50 percent. Because of the wide variation in individual requirements, the dosage of testosterone preparations must be established for each patient on the basis of trial. The doses suggested below are averages and do not necessarily apply to a given case.

In *adult testicular failure* (*primary postpuberal hypogonadism*), an average initial dosage of testosterone propionate by injection is 25 mg. three times weekly. The initial requirement of methyltestosterone by sublingual or buccal administration is 5 to 30 mg. daily. When methyltestosterone tablets are swallowed, the necessary daily dose is 15 to 100 mg. or more. After a satisfactory response has been obtained, dosage should be reduced, and the minimum necessary for maintenance should be determined by trial.

In *primary hypogonadism beginning before puberty*, a more complex problem is presented. The aim should be to initiate therapy and graduate dosage in such a way as to mimic natural puberty. Treatment may well be started at the age of 9 1/2 to 11 1/2 years for the purpose of advancing constitutional development. A daily dosage of 5 mg. methyltestosterone orally (swallowed) or buccally is adequate in the majority of cases. Parenteral medication is rarely necessary. Stimulation of growth, weight gain in the underweight, increased and more sustained physical energy, activity instead of sluggishness, and interest instead of disinterest in boyish activities are indications of constitutional improvement. As these become manifest, dosage may be increased to 10 mg. on alternate days and be kept at 5 mg. on the remaining days. Still further constitutional advance should occur following the increase in dosage, and growth of pubic hair and sexual development should gradually appear.

If sexual development is prematurely rapid, dosage is decreased. If very early or active penile response occurs on the 5-mg. daily dosage, the quantity must be reduced or given less frequently. Sometimes constitutional responses lag behind the penile response; when this occurs, it is considered best to be satisfied with slower general improvement in order to avoid precocious sexual development.

In general, underdosage is preferred to overdosage. Puberty is normally a gradual evolution requiring continued physical and psychological adjustment. For best eventual results, the process should not be hurried. Slight underdosage has the additional dual advantage of preventing complications like acne and of allowing maximum activity of the patient's own developmental forces.

As the age appropriate to full sexual development and function is reached, dosage may be increased to 10 or 15 mg. methyltestosterone daily, or more if necessary. When testicular deficiency is permanent, therapy must be continued indefinitely.

Androgens may also be useful in some cases of the following conditions; details of dosage and use are found under the several diseases: Addison's disease (p. 183), Cushing's syndrome (p. 186), carcinoma of the female breast (p. 201), functional uterine bleeding (p. 203), painful engorgement of the breasts postpartum (p. 216), and menopausal symptoms (p. 207).

Testosterone preparations should be administered only for a definite indication. Their potency and effects are such that indiscriminate use may be harmful.

Overdosage is to be avoided, particularly in women. Total quantities of 500 mg. or more of testosterone propionate per month (or equivalent quantities of methyltestosterone) are likely to produce masculinizing effects in women, such as enlargement of the clitoris, deepening of the voice, baldness, growth of beard, coarsening of body hair, and acne vulgaris. The first three of these changes, once accomplished, may show little or no regression when treatment is discontinued. *It is strongly advised that women receive no more than 75 mg. of testosterone propionate or its equivalent per week, or 300 mg. per month, except when necessary in the treatment of serious conditions such as mammary cancer.* Especial caution is desirable when the patient already has an unusually coarse growth of facial hair or other submasculine characteristics.

Since testosterone tends to inhibit gonadotrophin secretion by the anterior pituitary and since neither ovaries nor testes function in the absence of gonadotrophin, large doses of testosterone over long periods should be avoided when continued ovarian or testicular function is desired. Testosterone is particularly effective in suppressing spermatogenesis.

The ability of testosterone to cause closure of the epiphyses and thus permanently stop growth in height suggests caution in administration to adolescents. Adequate indications should be observed, and physiological doses should not be exceeded.

Testosterone is a powerful metabolic stimulant. Increased metabolism requires increased work by the cardiovascular system and places an increased strain on it. Testosterone therapy is therefore contraindicated in the presence of cardiovascular dis-

ease with the possible exception of uncomplicated angina pectoris. For the same reasons, androgenic therapy should be used very cautiously in older individuals.

The sodium-retaining action of testosterone leads to an increase in the volume of extracellular fluid and will result in edema if the increase is sufficiently great. Such fluid retention may be a factor in the heart failure which may occur as a complication of testosterone therapy.

The large doses required in breast cancer may induce hypercalcemia (p. 345), sometimes of dangerous degree. This complication should be watched for. If it appears to threaten the patient's life, it may be treated by intravenous infusion of 2.5 percent sodium citrate solution.

Testosterone and other androgens do not increase sexual potency in normal men. Unless impotence is due to testicular deficiency, androgen therapy is ineffective and may be harmful. Androgens have a stimulating effect on the growth of active prostatic cancer. Testosterone is therefore contraindicated in the presence of prostatic cancer, and it is advisable to examine for this condition any man past forty in whom androgenic therapy is contemplated. In addition, it has been demonstrated that a high percentage of men fifty years of age or older have foci of latent cancer in their prostates. Caution is therefore suggested in the use of testosterone in older men until more information is available as to the possible role of androgen in activating latent prostatic cancer.

ANTERIOR PITUITARY EXTRACTS AND RELATED PRINCIPLES

The hormones of the anterior pituitary gland (p. 191) are protein in nature. Some of them have been isolated in reasonably pure form. Although their normal functions are fairly well established, the clinical usefulness of extracts containing them is not yet clearly defined. Part of the difficulty appears to lie in the fact that the extracts are made from the anterior pituitaries of species other than the human. The hormones therefore act as foreign proteins and tend to induce allergy to themselves and immunity to their effects.

GROWTH FACTOR

The growth factor (somatotrophic factor, STH) of the anterior pituitary is one of the hormones influencing body growth (body growth is also influenced by androgens and thyroid hormone). Lack of it is a contributing cause of pituitary dwarfism; and an excess of it produces pituitary gigantism (p. 193) or acromegaly (p. 193), depending on whether the onset is before or after the epiphyses have closed.

The growth factor has been obtained in rather pure form but only in small quantities. Its exact composition is not known. Anterior pituitary extracts are available which are concentrated for growth factor but also contain small quantities of other pituitary factors. They have appeared to produce or initiate satisfactory growth in some cases of pituitary dwarfism. However, success is not universal. Some patients may develop immunity or allergy to them, or both. The dosage depends on the extract employed.

GONADOTROPHINS

The gonadotrophic hormones, or gonadotrophins, stimulate both ovaries and testes. Three of them are produced by the anterior pituitary; others are formed in the chorion and, later, the placenta during pregnancy. Their relation to the menstrual cycle is discussed on page 202.

Follicle-Stimulating Hormone (FSH, thylakentrin) from the anterior pituitary stimulates follicle growth in the ovaries without causing ovulation; in the testes it causes both development of the germinal epithelium and spermatogenesis. Pituitary extracts concentrated for follicle-stimulating hormone are available, but their clinical usefulness has not been established.

Luteinizing Hormone (LH) from the anterior pituitary acts in conjunction with FSH to stimulate further ovarian follicular development, which progresses to maturation and ovulation. As the follicle becomes sufficiently developed, estrogen is secreted. Continued action of LH on the postovulatory follicle causes formation of a corpus luteum. LH stimulates the interstitial cells (of Leydig) in the testes to secrete androgen and has for this reason also been termed "interstitial-cell-stimulating hormone (ICSH)."

Pituitary luteinizing hormone has been obtained in pure form. However, preparations available for clinical use contain follicle-stimulating hormone in addition. The indications for and therapeutic effects of such preparations are not agreed upon; there is some question as to whether they have actually induced ovulation in either normal women or those suffering from pituitary or ovarian dysfunction.

Luteotrophic Hormone (LTH) is the third pituitary gonadotrophin. It maintains the corpus luteum and stimulates it to secrete progesterone. It has no known effect on testes. There is evidence that LTH is identical with the lactogenic hormone, prolactin. If the mammary gland has been properly prepared by exposure to estrogen and progesterone, prolactin initiates lactation.

Pituitary extracts concentrated for their lactogenic effects are available; however, they have not proved especially helpful in stimulating deficient human lactation postpartum, perhaps because failure of lactation may be due to other factors than an inadequate supply of prolactin. Such preparations have not found general use for their luteotrophic properties. In addition, allergic reactions are not uncommon.

Chorionic Gonadotrophin is a protein which is secreted by the chorion and, later, the placenta during pregnancy. It is a luteinizing hormone the biological function of which is to maintain the corpus luteum of pregnancy and stimulate it to secrete estrogen and progesterone (see p. 207). It is excreted in the maternal urine in the human species, and its presence is the basis of a number of tests for pregnancy (see p. 207). The concentration in blood and urine increases rapidly in the first seven or eight weeks of pregnancy and then declines to relatively low levels, which are maintained until a few days after parturition.

The chorionic gonadotrophins of different mammalian species differ chemically, but all are glycoproteins. Human chorionic gonadotrophin, obtained from placentas and the urine of pregnancy, is available in highly purified form. An International Unit has been set up which is defined as the gonadotrophic activity of 0.1 mg. of an arbitrarily adopted standard preparation (from human sources) which is kept at the National Institute of Health in London.

Aside from its role in pregnancy, the most striking action of human chorionic gonadotrophin is its ability to stimulate secretion of androgen by the testes and thus to bring about descent of these organs when they are undescended. Chorionic gonadotrophin is employed clinically for this purpose when there is no mechanical bar to descent. The usual dosage is 150 to 750 I.U. two or three times weekly. If descent does not occur in six to eight weeks, therapy should be discontinued as unsuccessful. Overdosage, with excessive androgen production, may induce precocious puberty.

Chorionic gonadotrophin may also be employed as a diagnostic and therapeutic measure in male hypogonadotrophic hypogonadism (for details, see pp. 190 and 191). It has been used to check functional uterine bleeding in premenopausal women (p. 204). Chorionic gonadotrophin almost never induces either immunity or allergy.

Pregnant Mare Serum (PMS, equine gonadotrophin) contains equine chorionic gonadotrophin which, in contrast to the human type, has both luteinizing and follicle-stimulating properties. It is not excreted in the urine to any extent. An International Unit has been established which is defined as the gonadotrophic activity of 0.25 mg. of an arbitrarily adopted standard preparation housed at the National Institute of Health in London.

Theoretically, pregnant mare serum might appear to be indicated in hypogonadotrophic hypogonadism in either men or women (see pp. 191 and 189). Its practical usefulness is still in doubt. In men, average dosage is 500 I.U. intramuscularly on alternate days in courses of four weeks with a similar rest period. In women, dosage begins at 500 I.U. daily in the early part of the ovarian cycle and builds up to 2,000 I.U. on the fourteenth day, after which injections are discontinued.

Pregnant mare serum is contraindicated in patients sensitive to horse serum. Immunity to the clinical effects is likely to develop; for this reason, rest periods of four to six weeks should be allowed between courses.

THYROTROPHIN

Thyrotrophin (TTH, TSH) is an anterior pituitary hormone which stimulates the thyroid gland in such a way as to cause (1) hypertrophy and hyperplasia of the secretory epithelium and (2) increased uptake of iodine and amino acids, with formation and deposit of thyroglobulin in the colloid of the thyroid follicles (p. 178). Active thyrotrophin is also believed to induce absorption of water by the external ocular muscles and the tissues of the orbit, thus influencing the prominence of the eyes.

The activity of the thyroid gland is normally determined by the secretion of thyrotrophin. Circulating thyroid hormone tends to inhibit further output of thyrotrophin, thus providing a dynamic balance in thyroid and pituitary thyrotrophic function. Deficiency of thyrotrophin leads to hypothyroidism (p. 180), and excess induces hyperthyroidism (p. 180). Exophthalmos in hyperthyroidism is believed to be due, at least in part, to an excess of circulating active thyrotrophin. Excessive secretion of thyrotrophin is frequently a part of hyperpituitarism (p. 193).

The thyrotrophin of animals is available in fairly pure form. It has the drawback of tending to induce immunity when given over a continuous period of more than about four weeks. In addition, like other pituitary preparations, it must be given by injection. In almost all instances, thyroid substance by mouth is to be preferred for treatment of hypothyroidism (see p. 456).

ADRENOCORTICOTROPHIN

The adrenocorticotrophic hormone (adrenocorticotrophin, ACTH) is the anterior pituitary factor which stimulates hyperplasia and secretory activity in the adrenal cortices. Details of adrenal cortical function appear on page 183; the adrenocortical hormones are discussed on page 460. Deficiency of adrenocorticotrophin produces Addison's disease; excess produces Cushing's syndrome or the adrenogenital syndrome.

ACTH is now available in pure form. The supply is limited, however, since it is derived from animal pituitary glands. The preparation is effective in treating Addison's disease of pituitary origin. As with other anterior pituitary hormones of animal origin, prolonged administration tends to induce immunity and allergy. Current interest has been keenest in the experimental use of ACTH in rheumatoid arthritis, rheumatic fever, gout, lupus erythematosus, and other diseases which, in the main, appear to be either allergic or related to the so-called collagen diseases. In these conditions, ACTH acts by stimulating the adrenal cortices to produce the characteristic adrenal steroids (see p. 460). As far as can be determined in short-term studies, the effects of ACTH in these diseases are the same as the effects of cortisone (p. 462). The effective dose of ACTH averages 25 mg. daily by intramuscular injection. The precautions and side-effects are the same as those of cortisone, with the additional possibility of allergy to ACTH.

POSTERIOR PITUITARY EXTRACTS

Posterior pituitary extracts contain three types of activity: vasopressor, antidiuretic, and oxytocic. Two principles can be distinguished—vasopressin, which has vasopressor, antidiuretic, and, in human beings, oxytocic activity; and oxytocin, which has only oxytocic properties. These two principles are polypeptides with molecular weights of about 2,000. However, there is some disagreement as to whether they represent original posterior pituitary secretions or whether they are breakdown products of a single original posterior pituitary hormone.

The response of the human uterus to posterior pituitary extracts is extremely variable, depending on the type of extract, the condition of the uterus (i.e., the phase of the menstrual cycle or the stage of pregnancy), and other factors not as yet understood. The relationships are complicated and unclear. In general, large doses of posterior pituitary extract may cause uterine tetany lasting up to ten minutes. This is followed by a series of clonic contractions which gradually diminish in strength and frequency. Smaller doses produce only the clonic contractions.

Since the active principle has not been isolated, posterior pituitary extracts must of necessity be assayed biologically. The test is made on uterine muscle of virgin guinea pigs, and 1 U.S.P. Posterior Pituitary Unit is represented by the contractile effect of 0.5 mg. of the U.S.P. Posterior Pituitary Reference Standard powder. Unfortunately, the response of the guinea-pig myometrium does not necessarily parallel that of the human myometrium; for vasopressor extracts, which have been treated in such a way as to reduce by 90 percent their oxytocic activity in the guinea pig, at the same time retaining pressor and antidiuretic activity, may under certain circumstances actually have an enhanced oxytocic activity on the human uterus.

Vasopressor activity is due to contraction of the smooth muscle of the arterioles by direct stimulation. The coronary vessels appear to be particularly susceptible, and therapeutic doses may reduce coronary blood flow as much as 90 percent. Unfortunately, the vasopressor action of posterior pituitary extract is of little clinical use for the following reasons: (1) The blood pressure sometimes fails to rise or actually falls, apparently because of compensatory mechanisms; (2) severe myocardial anoxia may result from the predominance of coronary vasoconstriction; and (3) the principle may stimulate intense peristalsis in the intestine, which may have inconvenient if not harmful consequences. Extracts may be assayed for vasopressor activity on dogs by the method of Hamilton and Rowe. One pressor unit (unofficial) is the pressor activity exerted by 0.5 mg. of U.S.P. Posterior Pituitary Reference Standard.

Antidiuretic activity, which is to date inseparable from vasopressor action, is exerted on the distal convoluted tubules of the nephrons in the kidneys. Under the stimulus of posterior pituitary hormone, the distal tubules absorb water and salt. The hormone is thus the final determinant of urine volume. Its absence leads to diabetes insipidus.

Posterior pituitary extracts are available in the following forms:

Posterior Pituitary, U.S.P., which is "the cleaned, dried, and powdered posterior lobe obtained from the pituitary body of domesticated animals which are used for food by man." It must be assayed for oxytocic activity and must have a potency of not less than 1 U.S.P. Posterior Pituitary Unit per mg. (Note that this is only half the potency of the U.S.P. Posterior Pituitary Reference Standard.)

Posterior Pituitary Injection, U.S.P., containing 10 U.S.P. Units (oxytocic) per cc. (and presumably 10 pressor units per cc.). This preparation is known unofficially as "obstetrical pituitary."

The unofficial "surgical pituitary," or Posterior Pituitary Extract for Surgical Use, containing 20 U.S.P. Units (oxytocic) per cc. and presumably 20 pressor units per cc.

Pitocin (oxytocin), an especially treated extract containing 10 U.S.P. Units (oxytocic) per cc. and less than 0.5 pressor unit per cc.

Pitressin (vasopressin), an especially treated extract containing 20 pressor units per cc. and less than 1 U.S.P. Unit (oxytocic) per cc. (as determined on the guinea-pig uterus; but note that oxytocic activity may be high for the human uterus, as described above).

Pitressin Tannate, a suspension in oil of the water-insoluble tannate of Pitressin, containing 5 pressor units per cc.

Posterior pituitary extracts are ineffective by mouth because the active principle, being protein, is destroyed in the gastro-intestinal tract. They are, however, fully effective when applied to the nasal mucosa; the powdered extract may be snuffed or blown into the nose, or aqueous extracts may be applied on cotton pledgets which are inserted between the nasal septum and turbinates. The aqueous extracts may also be injected subcutaneously, intramuscularly, or intravenously. Stimulation of peristalsis is uncommon following intranasal administration, as are side-effects of any kind. Intravenous injection carries an especially great risk of adverse reactions.

The oxytocic property of posterior pituitary extracts has led to their use for prevention or relief of postpartum and postabortal uterine atony. As compared with ergonovine (p. 476 and Table 53, p. 477), however, posterior pituitary has the disadvantage of being less potent, less enduring, less reliable, and less safe. Posterior pituitary may, nevertheless, prove useful in carefully selected cases for the induction of labor or to combat uterine atony during labor, purposes for which ergot preparations are contraindicated.

As a routine for the prevention of postpartum hemorrhage (p. 215), posterior pituitary extract is given in doses of 5 to 10 U.S.P. Units subcutaneously or intramuscularly. A clinical effect seldom lasts more than thirty minutes. For induction of labor or stimulation of uterine contractions before delivery, dosage should be cautious because of the unpredictability of the response. Initial doses should never be larger than 1 unit; many recommend only 1/2 unit. Intranasal administration has the advantage that absorption can be discontinued at any time. Overstimulation with production of uterine tetany may asphyxiate the child or cause uterine rupture.

The antidiuretic property of posterior pituitary extract makes it specific therapy for diabetes insipidus (see p. 194).

Its ability to stimulate intestinal smooth muscle leads to its occasional use in treating abdominal distention or intestinal paresis. The usual hypodermic dose is 5 to 10 pressor units (or U.S.P. Units in the case of unfractionated extracts). Before administering the drug, the physician must make certain that there is no mechanical obstruction in the intestine.

Posterior pituitary extract or its pressor fraction may be useful in the treatment of herpes zoster (see p. 21).

Systemic reactions to posterior pituitary are not uncommon. Many cases of "obstetrical shock" are actually "pituitary shock." The onset of such a reaction may come a few seconds after intravenous injection or thirty to sixty minutes after subcutaneous administration. The patient may complain of anxiety, dyspnea, or sometimes precordial pain, or she may have no complaints. Circulatory collapse or shock (p. 90) develops. The skin in whole or in part assumes either a dusky-purple or a bright-red color. Subcutaneous edema may develop. The patient may recover or die. If she recovers, a rash may appear after a few days. Such reactions are considered to be allergic. Treatment is as for shock (p. 91). An intravenous antihistaminic drug would seem worth a trial.

PARATHYROID EXTRACT

The parathyroid hormone serves the biological purpose of controlling the level of calcium ions in the blood. It has the solubility and general properties of a proteose (a substance intermediate between a protein and a peptone) and is the active principle of parathyroid extract. The probable mechanism of its action is discussed on page 195. Parathyroid extract is standardized for its ability to raise the serum calcium of normal dogs. One

U.S.P. Parathyroid Unit is "one one-hundredth of the amount required to raise the calcium content of 100 cc. of the blood serum of normal dogs 1 mg. within 16 to 18 hours after administration." Parathyroid extracts should be kept under refrigeration.

Parathyroid extract may be given subcutaneously, intramuscularly, or intravenously. The intramuscular route is generally preferred because (1) moderate inflammatory reactions sometimes occur following subcutaneous administration, and (2) systemic reactions occasionally follow intravenous injection. If intravenous administration is considered necessary, a preliminary skin test should be made; if the test is positive, desensitization should be undertaken as with serums (p. 334). Even if the skin test is negative, intravenous injection should be slow, and a solution of epinephrine should be available in case of reaction.

When injected intramuscularly, the parathyroid hormone acts after a latent period of about four hours and continues to be effective for about twenty hours. Intravenous injection shortens these times somewhat, and subcutaneous injection probably lengthens them. Since calcium salts injected intravenously raise the serum calcium level at once, they can be given by this route in emergency during the latent period before injected parathyroid extract becomes effective.

Parathyroid extract is employed principally in the early treatment of hypoparathyroidism (see p. 195) to tide the patient over a period of acute depression of parathyroid function such as may occur following thyroidectomy or removal of an actively secreting parathyroid adenoma. The dosage varies with the degree of hypocalcemia.

In tetany, an initial dose of 100 to 150 U.S.P. Parathyroid Units is usually adequate, although as much as 300 units may be necessary if the serum calcium is extremely low. Maintenance dosage for the average adult averages 20 to 40 units every twelve hours.

In infantile tetany with hypocalcemia, dosage should be cautious. An initial injection of 5 units may be given; if it is not effective, 10 units may be administered. A dose of 20 units should rarely be exceeded.

Parathyroid extract has appeared to be effective in some cases of thrombocytopenic purpura when other measures have failed. The mechanism of action is unknown and may be nonspecific. Doses of 10 to 20 units may be employed initially, which may be increased to a maximum of 100 units if necessary. As in other uses of parathyroid extract, intravenous calcium increases the effectiveness.

The hormone has also been advocated in fractures occurring in patients with a low level of serum calcium. The indications for and regimen of treatment are rather specific and detailed; they will be found in an article by Nelson, C. F., and Nelson, R. C.: Medical Management of Fractures, *J.A.M.A.*, *116:*184, 1941.

The dosage of parathyroid extract should always be controlled by determinations of serum calcium (see p. 344 for interpretation). The preparation should not be given in the presence of hyper-calcemia, and it should be used cautiously in patients with renal or cardiac disease. Overdoses produce hypercalcemia, which may be dangerous (for details, see p. 345). Because the parathyroid hormone causes withdrawal of calcium from the bones if no other supply is available, calcium salts should be given by mouth during parathyroid therapy (see p. 505).

Parathyroid extracts are not suitable for long-continued administration; they may be antigenic for some patients and induce immunity or allergy or both.

DRUGS AFFECTING UTERINE MOTILITY

The human myometrium is responsive to many nervous, physical, and chemical influences, the mechanism of which in many instances remains obscure. Although the uterine muscle has a rich autonomic nerve supply, the type of response to nerve stimulation and to autonomic drugs appears to vary with the level of estrogen and progesterone and perhaps other substances.

Drugs Stimulating the Myometrium

The patterns of uterine motility which are termed normal require the presence of estrogen and calcium. When stimulating drugs are added, they may initiate or intensify these patterns, or they may produce mass contraction of the entire organ. Tension on the myometrium, as during distention of the uterine cavity, lowers the threshold of response to stimulation.

Estrogen (p. 463) is necessary for normal myometrial contractility. Under its influence, the uterine muscle undergoes rhythmic contractions which, in the organ *in situ*, arise in the uterine tubes and course from one or the other of the cornua over the corpus and down to the cervix. The intensity of response varies with the level of estrogen. During a long period without estrogen, responsiveness to estrogen falls off greatly but returns over a period of time as estrogen is again supplied. Clinical use of the action of estrogens on the myometrium is made in connection with the induction of labor at term (p. 213).

Calcium is also necessary for uterine contraction, and responsiveness to oxytocics after parturition can usually be increased by intravenous injection of a calcium salt (p. 344). Such treatment may have great value in overcoming uterine atony immediately postpartum.

Quinine has long been thought to stimulate uterine contraction, but recent evidence indicates that such action is unreliable, and the use of quinine as an oxytocic seems inadvisable because of the possibility that it may induce deafness in the child.

OXYTOCICS

Oxytocics are literally substances which speed parturition. The term is now applied principally to drugs administered to promote uterine contraction *after* delivery. Those used clinically include certain ergot alkaloids and posterior pituitary extract.

Ergot is a fungus (*Claviceps purpurea*) which grows on rye and certain other grains. It contains a great many pharmacologically active substances as well as a number of alkaloids peculiar to itself. These alkaloids occur in pairs which are optical isomers: the levo forms are active, with oxytocic properties; the dextro forms are inactive. Of the levo forms, ergonovine, ergotoxine, and ergotamine have found clinical use.

Ergonovine, the maleate of which is marketed by Eli Lilly and Company as 'Ergotrate Maleate,' is the hydroxyisopropylamide of lysergic acid (see Figure 46). It is the simplest of the active ergot alkaloids and the only one which is water-soluble. In therapeutic doses (0.2 to 0.4 mg.), its only action is to induce tonic uterine contraction on which are superimposed clonic contractions. As myometrial tone returns to normal over a period of hours, the clonic contractions tend to increase in ampli-

tude. After very much smaller doses, only clonic
contractions may occur. Various properties of ergonovine are listed in Table 53.

Very large doses of ergonovine produce certain
sympathomimetic effects in animals, but blood pressure is not affected. Vasoconstriction may be sufficiently great to cause gangrene, but ergonovine is
very much less potent in this respect than ergotoxine and ergotamine, and there is no practical
danger of gangrene in connection with human use.
The acute toxicity of ergonovine for animals is
about one-fourth that of the other two alkaloids.

Therapeutically, ergonovine is used principally
for the prevention of the postpartum or postabortal
hemorrhage which results from uterine atony. It
is given as the maleate. It is generally administered

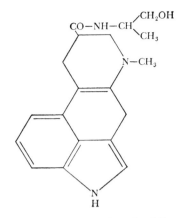

FIGURE 46 — *Structural Formula of Ergonovine*

TABLE 53 — *Comparison of Oxytocics*

	Ergonovine ('Ergotrate Maleate')	Ergotamine Ergotoxine	Posterior Pituitary
Onset of effect by different routes of administration			
Intravenous	15-60 seconds	5-45 minutes	15-60 seconds
Intramuscular	3-7 minutes	15-45 minutes	3-7 minutes
Oral	6-15 minutes	So slow as to be useless against postpartum hemorrhage	Ineffective
Duration of effect after absorption	3-8 hours	2-8 hours	30-60 minutes
Relative effectiveness, weight for weight	+++	+	Not comparable
Average dose	0.2 mg.	0.5 mg.	1-8 I.U.
Incidence of undesirable side-effects	Almost 0	++	++
Variation in action	Rare	Common	Very common
Mode of action	Stimulates muscle directly and through sympathetic nerve endings	Direct muscle stimulation	Direct muscle stimulation
Type of contraction from average dose	Tonic, later clonic	Tonic, later clonic	Clonic
Effect on blood pressure	None	May increase	Increases
Effect on pulse rate	None	None in absence of toxic effects	Increases
Effect on coronary blood flow	None	Possible decrease	Great decrease
Effect on urinary output	None	None	Diminution
Method of assay	By weight	By weight	Biological, on uterine muscle

either intravenously or intramuscularly following delivery of the placenta. Earlier administration—immediately after birth of the child or even after delivery of the anterior shoulder—reduces blood loss during the third stage but should be undertaken only by a trained obstetrical team in a hospital. If the patient has received spinal or caudal anesthesia, administration of ergonovine should be delayed until after delivery of the placenta, and the drug should be given by mouth or intramuscularly rather than intravenously.

Ergonovine maleate is usually given by mouth for the first three or four days postpartum (0.2 to 0.4 mg. two or three times daily) to prevent late hemorrhage and reduce the opportunity for puerperal infection. If the patient is to be at home or out of bed before the tenth day, ergonovine may be given until at least the fourteenth day. In the late puerperium, after abortion, or under other circumstances in which uterine contractility is less than it is immediately postpartum, larger doses may be required. When the administration of ergonovine at the end of parturition is not followed by uterine contraction, an intravenous injection of a calcium salt is recommended to restore uterine responsiveness. However, suitable precautions must be taken with regard to choice of patient and rate of injection (p. 345).

Ergonovine has also been used in the symptomatic treatment of migraine. It is less effective than ergotamine or ergotoxine by injection but is more effective by mouth than they are. The usual dosage is 0.2 mg. by injection, followed by 0.4 mg. by mouth at hourly intervals until the headache is relieved or until 2 mg. have been taken. Idiosyncrasy occurs but is rare.

Ergotoxine and **Ergotamine** are complex derivatives of lysergic acid, each containing a chain of amino acids joined by polypeptide linkage. Ergotamine appears to be a single substance, but ergotoxine has been shown to be a mixture of three closely related compounds, ergocristine, ergocryptine, and ergocornine. All five of these substances are pharmacologically and therapeutically indistinguishable. Although larger doses are required, they cause the same type of uterine contraction as ergonovine and have about the same duration of action. However, the onset of effect after injection is slower than with ergonovine; and on oral administration, in contrast to ergonovine, they are so poorly and irregularly absorbed as to be unreliable for oxytocic effect by this route (see Table 53, p. 477, for their comparative properties).

Their principal use is for the symptomatic treatment of migraine (p. 161), which they relieve apparently because of their vasoconstrictor action on the meningeal arteries. Ergotamine tartrate is commonly employed in doses of 0.25 to 0.5 mg. by subcutaneous or intramuscular injection. It may be repeated if necessary, but no more than 1 mg. should be given in a day, and no more than one course in a week. It can advantageously be combined with caffeine, 100 mg. of the latter to each 1 mg. of the ergot derivative.

These same vasoconstrictor properties of ergotamine and ergotoxine create a hazard of gangrene of the fingers or toes. The gangrene of ergotism is apparently due to these compounds, and gangrene has followed unsupervised or excessive dosage for therapeutic purposes. Ergotoxine and ergotamine are contraindicated in peripheral vascular disease, severe arteriosclerosis, and any other condition in which vasoconstriction would be harmful. Papaverine and other vasodilator drugs (p. 362) and sympathetic nerve block are probably the best antidotes.

Side-effects are common with ergotamine and ergotoxine, particularly after oral administration. They include nausea and vomiting, abdominal cramps, headache, weakness of the legs, muscle pains in the extremities, numbness and tingling of the fingers and toes, and precordial distress. Allergic phenomena occur, but they are rare.

Because of a lower incidence of side-effects, a synthetic derivative, dihydroergotamine, has been recommended in place of ergotamine for migraine. Dihydroergotamine has no action on the uterus.

Ergotamine and ergotoxine in relatively high concentrations inhibit the structures innervated by adrenergic (sympathetic) nerves. The doses required, however, would be toxic in man.

Methyl-Ergonovine (Methergine), the amide of lysergic acid and 1-hydroxy-2-aminobutane, has recently been introduced as an oxytocic agent. Pharmacologically, it is similar to ergonovine, and early clinical reports have not brought forth evidence of any therapeutic advantage over ergonovine.

Posterior Pituitary Extracts have oxytocic, pressor, and antidiuretic properties. These are discussed on page 473.

Drugs Inhibiting the Myometrium

There are few clinical indications for inhibition of uterine contraction, and there are no drugs which have such an action selectively. Uterine motility is impaired by most sedative and general anesthetic agents such as barbiturates, morphine (large doses), hyoscine (large doses), chloroform, and ether. Nitrous oxide is without effect. Ether appears to be the most effective in safe dosage, and a deep ether anesthesia is perhaps the most powerful means of relaxing constriction rings during labor or a postpartum uterus strongly contracted from ergonovine. During the period of relaxation, however, there may be danger of serious hemorrhage.

Epinephrine has been claimed to inhibit uterine motility, and doses of 0.3 mg. have been recommended for the relaxation of constriction rings during labor. Others maintain that any period of relaxation is brief and is merely compensatory for increased activity before or after. Perhaps other factors influence the response of the myometrium to epinephrine.

The **magnesium** ion (p. 346) has also been reported to relax uterine spasm when given intravenously in doses of 0.1 or 0.2 Gm. (as 2 cc. of 50 percent or 10 cc. of 20 percent magnesium sulfate).

DRUGS ACTING LOCALLY ON SKIN AND MUCOUS MEMBRANES*

Demulcents

Demulcents are bland substances, usually gummy or mucilaginous, which retain water and adhere to surfaces, affording mechanical protection and excluding air. On skin, which has an oily surface, the final result of prolonged contact with demulcents is a drying effect.

Starch, U.S.P., (cornstarch) made into a smooth paste with cold water, poured into boiling water with constant stirring, and then diluted with warm water to the desired consistency, is an extremely soothing application to irritated skin. A starch bath may be prepared by making a paste of 1/2 lb. of starch and 1/2 lb. of baking soda, adding a quart of boiling water slowly (because of effervescence) with vigorous stirring, and pouring into a half-filled bathtub of lukewarm water.

Glycerin, $CH_2OH \cdot CHOH \cdot CH_2OH$, is a valuable demulcent. It may be added to starch paste in amounts up to 20 percent to retard or prevent drying. In high concentrations, glycerin may be irritant because it is so intensely hygroscopic.

Jelly—When lubrication is desired, as for passage of instruments, a jelly may be used, containing acacia (10 to 15 percent), tragacanth (1 to 2.5 percent), or carboxymethylcellulose (2 percent). These and glycyrrhiza are also used to prepare suspensions of medication for oral administration.

Emollients

Emollients are bland oily preparations which are applied, usually in the form of ointments, to the skin to protect or soften the epidermis and prevent evaporation of moisture. The emollients may also be used as vehicles for certain drugs having local or systemic effects.

Commonly used emollients include the following:

Vegetable Oils—Cottonseed Oil, Olive Oil, Corn Oil, Expressed Almond Oil, Peanut Oil, and Theobroma Oil (cocoa butter), all U.S.P.

Animal Fats—Benzoinated Lard, N.F.; Wool Fat, U.S.P.; and Hydrous Wool Fat, U.S.P. (containing 25 to 30 percent water).

Waxes—White Wax and Yellow Wax, U.S.P., used to harden ointments.

Hydrocarbons—Petrolatum (petroleum jelly), White Petrolatum, Liquid Petrolatum (heavy white mineral oil), all U.S.P., and Light Liquid Petrolatum (light white mineral oil), N.F.

Mixtures of Emollients

Hydrophilic Petrolatum, U.S.P., containing:

cholesterol	3 percent
stearyl alcohol	3 percent
White Wax	8 percent
White Petrolatum	86 percent

Hydrophilic Petrolatum will hold up to three times its weight of water as a water-in-oil emulsion (see p. 481). It is useful as a vehicle for watery liquids or when it is undesirable to have moisture accumulate underneath the ointment. Sorboint (Lilly's absorbent ointment base) is very similar to Hydrophilic Petrolatum except for the addition of sufficient benzoin to provide an aroma.

* Except alimentary tract, for which see page 382.

Hydrophilic Ointment, U.S.P., containing:

methylparaben	0.025	percent
propylparaben	0.015	percent
sodium lauryl sulfate	1	percent
glycerin	12	percent
stearyl alcohol	25	percent
White Petrolatum	25	percent
water	37	percent

Hydrophilic Ointment serves a purpose similar to that of Hydrophilic Petrolatum. However, it includes water in its original composition. Methylparaben (methyl parahydroxybenzoate) and propylparaben (propyl parahydroxybenzoate) are included as preservatives. Sodium lauryl sulfate is a detergent, wetting agent, and emulsifier (p. 481).

Rose Water Ointment, U.S.P., ("cold cream") containing:

Spermaceti	12.5	percent
White Wax	12	percent
Expressed Almond Oil	56	percent
sodium borate	0.5	percent
Rose Water	5	percent
distilled water	14	percent
Rose Oil	0.02	percent

Cold cream is a useful emollient. It is a traditional application before and after exposure to sun and wind. U.S.P. XIV also includes Petrolatum Rose Water Ointment, in which Liquid Petrolatum is substituted for Expressed Almond Oil, gram for gram.

White Ointment, U.S.P., containing:

White Wax	5 percent
White Petrolatum	95 percent

The proportions of the ingredients may be varied to maintain a suitable consistency under different climatic conditions.

Yellow Ointment, U.S.P., is the same as White Ointment except for the substitution of Yellow Wax for White Wax and Petrolatum for White Petrolatum.

Carbowax Preparations—Carbowax is the name given to a series of compounds of high molecular weight which are polymers of ethylene glycol, $CH_2OH \cdot CH_2OH$. They are characterized structurally by a large number of ether linkages, and they are chemically quite inert and relatively nontoxic.

Carbowax 4000 (Polyethylene Glycol 4000, U.S.P.) has a molecular weight of about 3,600. It resembles hard paraffin in physical properties, but it is soluble in a wide variety of fluids: water, alcohol, acetone, and aromatic hydrocarbons. By combining Carbowax 4000 with varying proportions of propylene glycol or Carbowax 400 (Polyethylene Glycol 400, U.S.P.), a cream of any desired consistency can be obtained. Though such a cream contains no water, it is miscible with water in all proportions and washes off with water, leaving no residue. An official preparation is Polyethylene Glycol Ointment, U.S.P., containing equal parts by weight of Polyethylene Glycol 4000 and Polyethylene Glycol 400. For a softer ointment, not more than 20 percent of the Polyethylene Glycol 4000 may be replaced by an equal weight of Polyethylene Glycol 400.

Protectives

Protectives are insoluble and chemically inert substances which afford mechanical protection to the skin. Some of them absorb moisture; when these are applied in a finely divided state, the large surface they afford for evaporation gives them a drying as well as a protective effect.

The most complete mechanical protection is afforded by an application of **Flexible Collodion, U.S.P.**, which contains 2 percent camphor and 3 percent castor oil in collodion. The solvent is a mixture of 3 parts ether and 1 part alcohol. However, evaporation of insensible perspiration is retarded, and the skin may become macerated.

More commonly used as protectives are the finely powdered substances:

Talc, U.S.P., which is a native hydrous magnesium silicate.

Bentonite, U.S.P., which is a native colloidal hydrated aluminum silicate.

Zinc Oxide, U.S.P.

Calamine, U.S.P., which is a zinc oxide with a small amount of ferric oxide.

Zinc Stearate, U.S.P.

Prepared Chalk, N.F., which is a native form of calcium carbonate freed from most of its impurities by elutriation.

Precipitated Calcium Carbonate, U.S.P.

Starch, U.S.P. (powdered).

Lycopodium, consisting of the spores of a certain species of club moss.

Protectives are often included in pastes or emollient ointments (see above), such as:

Zinc Oxide Ointment, U.S.P., containing 20 percent.

Calamine Ointment, N.F., containing 17 percent.

Zinc Oxide Paste, U.S.P., (Lassar's Plain Zinc Paste) containing:

zinc oxide	25 percent
starch	25 percent
White Petrolatum	50 percent

Zinc Oxide Hard Paste, N.F., (Unna's Hard Zinc Paste) containing:

    zinc oxide...........................25 percent
    Purified Siliceous Earth, U.S.P.
      (infusorial earth)....................5 percent
    benzoinated lard ....70 percent

Zinc Oxide Soft Paste, N.F., (Unna's Soft Zinc Paste) containing:

    zinc oxide (in very fine powder)...........25 percent
    Precipitated Calcium Carbonate...........25 percent
    oleic acid..............................2.5 percent
    Linseed Oil............................25 percent
    Calcium Hydroxide Solution.............22.5 percent

Protectives are also incorporated into lotions which leave a powdery film on drying:

Calamine Lotion, U.S.P., containing:

    calamine................................80 Gm.
    zinc oxide..............................80 Gm.
    Polyethylene Glycol 400.................80 cc.
    Polyethylene Glycol 400 Monostearate........20 Gm.
    Water.................................900 cc.

Phenolated Calamine Lotion, N.F., containing 1 percent phenol.

Emulsifiers and Detergents

Emulsions are composed of two immiscible liquids, one of which is present as discontinuous droplets (the dispersed or internal phase) in a continuous medium of the other (the continuous or external phase). Emulsions are usually made up of oily and watery liquids and may exist as oil-in-water emulsions, in which water is the continuous phase, or water-in-oil emulsions, in which oil is the continuous phase. The type of emulsions does not depend primarily on which substance is present in greater quantity, but rather on the type of emulsifying agent.

The following emulsifying agents tend to produce oil-in-water emulsions:

    Sodium, potassium, and ammonium soaps (salts of fatty acids)
    Sulfated oils, such as sodium lauryl sulfate (see below)
    Mixtures of triethanolamine and fatty acids
    Gums, such as acacia and tragacanth
    Polyethers and polyalcohols (see Carbowax, p. 480)

The following emulsifying agents tend to produce water-in-oil emulsions:

    Calcium, zinc, and aluminum soaps
    Sterols (such as cholesterol) and sterol esters (such as wool fat)
    Fatty amides, secondary amides, and alkyloamides

Because the skin is an oily membrane, it is more easily wetted by water-in-oil emulsions, such as the hydrophilic ointments (p. 479). It has not been determined which type of emulsion is more favorable to absorption of medication.

Substances which are good oil-in-water emulsifying agents are usually good detergents as well, since the process of cleansing apparently involves emulsification or suspension of the foreign matter which is to be removed.

The most commonly used cleansing agents are the sodium, potassium, and ammonium soaps. They are for most purposes the most pleasant and satisfactory, and least harmful, detergents. Soaps are also antiseptic, not only indirectly by their detergent action but also by direct germicidal effect.

In certain conditions, such as abnormally dry skin or dermatitis, when it may be advisable to avoid soaps, vegetable oils or hydrocarbons may be used (see p. 227). One of the other detergents which is commonly employed is sodium lauryl sulfate, consisting chiefly of $CH_3 \cdot (CH_2)_{10} \cdot CH_2 \cdot O \cdot SO_3 \cdot Na$ with a small proportion of other sodium alkyl sulfates.

Astringents

Astringents have a nonpenetrating precipitant action on proteins. They act locally and superficially to produce a thin protective film of coagulated tissue.

Tannic Acid is a powerful astringent. It has been used particularly as a 5 percent solution in jelly for application to burns. The protective coating retards transudation of fluid and ingress of bacteria.

Tannic acid also forms insoluble complexes with heavy metals, glycosides, and alkaloids and is therefore useful as an antidote in poisoning with such substances.

Preparations of tannic acid include the following:

    Tannic Acid, N.F.
    Tannic Acid Glycerite, N.F., containing 20 percent
    Tannic Acid Ointment, N.F., containing 20 percent
    'Amertan,' containing 5 percent tannic acid in a water-soluble jelly base

Aluminum Salts are particularly useful as astringents in inflammations of mucous membranes and in many forms of acute dermatitis (p. 226).

Aluminum Acetate Solution, U.S.P., (Burow's Solution) contains about 5.3 percent aluminum acetate. It is usually diluted with 30 parts of water and applied as compresses.

Zinc Salts are especially useful as mild astringents and bacteriostatic agents on mucous membranes and skin. Zinc sulfate and zinc acetate are used particularly on the conjunctiva, as 0.1 to 1 percent solutions or as 0.5 percent ophthalmic ointment. Zinc oxide has a very slight astringent action in addition to its protective effect (see above).

Copper Salts are also astringent and mildly antiseptic, particularly against fungi. The sulfate is the salt usually employed, the strength varying from 0.1 to 3 percent.

Potassium Permanganate (p. 306) has a slight astringent action in addition to its antiseptic effect, and **magnesium sulfate** in concentrated solution is mildly astringent because of its hypertonicity.

Peeling or Softening Agents

In certain chronic infections and other disorders of the skin, it is desirable to soften the epidermis or cause the superficial layers to peel off or both. Sulfur and salicylic acid (orthohydroxybenzoic acid) are useful agents for this purpose.

Sulfur may be applied as:

White Lotion, N.F., containing 4 percent zinc sulfate and 4 percent Sulfurated Potash, N.F., in water.

Sulfurated Lime Solution, N.F., (Vleminckx's Solution) containing slaked lime and a total of 25 percent sulfur in water. For local application in acne vulgaris, it is diluted 1:15.

Sulfur Ointment, U.S.P., containing 10 percent (often a lower strength is desirable).

A solution in a mildly alkaline, penetrating vehicle. A preparation of this type, known as Intraderm Sulfur, contains:

```
sulfur (as sulfides and polysulfides).......0.75 percent
triethanolamine.......................10      percent
sodium mixed alkyl benzene sulfonates....11   percent
antipyrine............................11      percent
propylene glycol and water to make.....100    percent
```

It is used particularly in acne vulgaris.

Salicylic Acid is usually applied in 2 to 10 percent strength; official preparations include the following:

Benzoic and Salicylic Acid Ointment, N.F., (Whitfield's ointment) containing 12 percent benzoic acid and 6 percent salicylic acid.

Salicylic Collodion, N.F., containing 10 percent salicylic acid in Flexible Collodion, U.S.P.

Zinc Oxide Paste with Salicylic Acid, N.F., (Lassar's Zinc Paste with Salicylic Acid) containing 2 percent salicylic acid in Zinc Oxide Paste, U.S.P. (p. 480).

Irritants

Irritants were formerly used as "counterirritants," i.e., to produce by reflex means a vasodilation in internal organs. Counterirritation is less extensively used than formerly, and the principal use of irritant substances is now for local stimulation of the skin in certain skin diseases.

Coal Tar, obtained from the destructive distillation of bituminous coal, consists mostly of cresols and guaiacols. It is employed mainly in 1 to 5 percent concentration for local application in cases of psoriasis and other types of chronic dermatitis. Very prolonged use is inadvisable (see p. 277).

Coal Tar Ointment, U.S.P., contains 5 percent Coal Tar, U.S.P., in Zinc Oxide Paste, U.S.P. (see p. 480).

For psoriasis, many dermatologists prefer the formula of C. J. White:

```
Coal Tar...............................5 percent
zinc oxide.............................5 percent
starch................................45 percent
Petrolatum............................45 percent
```

It is made by first mixing the coal tar and zinc oxide thoroughly and allowing to stand for a day. Then the starch and petrolatum are thoroughly mixed, and the two pastes are worked together. A good preparation should be almost black in color and should smell of coal gas and tar.

Hair should be clipped short before coal tar ointment is applied. Treated areas may be lightly covered; tight bandaging is often followed by pustulation. One application should never be allowed to remain on the skin longer than twelve hours. At the end of this period the skin is cleansed with warm mineral oil. The ointment will stain clothing unless, at the time the latter is removed, the spots are impregnated from both sides with lard and then, after an interval of at least one hour, washed with soap and warm water.

Ichthammol, N.F., is prepared from the tar produced by the destructive distillation of certain bituminous schists. The tar is sulfonated and the product neutralized with ammonia. It is used in the same way as coal tar. Ichthammol Ointment, N.F., has a strength of 10 percent.

Peruvian Balsam, U.S.P., is used for mild stimulation of superficial wounds and chronic inflammations of the skin. It was at one time employed to treat scabies. It may be applied full strength or with any degree of dilution in an oily vehicle.

The exact physiological function of vitamin C is unknown. It is believed to take part in cellular respiration and to be essential in several oxidase enzyme systems. It is required for the production and maintenance of the collagen of all fibrous tissue, and thus the supply of it directly influences wound healing and the formation of dentine, cartilage, and the matrix of bone. Capillary fragility appears to depend primarily on the integrity of the intercellular cement substance. Under normal conditions, this is continually being replaced, possibly by the endothelial cells lining the capillaries. In the absence of vitamin C, synthesis of the intercellular material is inhibited and capillary hemorrhage occurs.

Vitamin C is essential for metabolism of the aromatic amino acids phenylalanine and tyrosine. Premature infants require relatively large amounts of protein; and, if vitamin C is withheld, abnormal metabolic products from incomplete breakdown of these two amino acids promptly appear in the urine. The vitamin is also involved in hemoglobin formation and in the maturation of erythrocytes.

Vitamin C Deficiency—Serious vitamin C deficiency causes the disease scurvy.

INFANTILE SCURVY is common in artificially fed infants but is exceedingly rare when breast milk is available. It usually develops during the second half-year of life and is infrequent after two years of age. The disease occurs more frequently than is generally recognized. The onset is insidious, with symptoms of vague digestive disturbances, anorexia, failure to gain weight, and increasing irritability. The infant cries on being handled, particularly when being elevated by the ankles for a change of diaper. Voluntary movement is painful. He lies quietly on his back and obviously avoids moving the legs and sometimes the arms. The legs are often maintained in the characteristic "pithed frog" position, with the thighs partially flexed and rotated externally and the legs semiflexed at the knees.

Hemorrhages may occur anywhere but are most frequent beneath the periosteum of long bones, in the gums (if teeth have erupted), and in the skin and mucous membranes. Subperiosteal hemorrhage is most common at the lower end of the femur and upper end of the humerus; less frequently it occurs about the wrists or ankles. The extravasation of blood strips the periosteum down to its attachment at the end of the bone. Consequently, when swelling is present, it never extends beyond the end of the bone and does not involve the joint. The gums become swollen and dark red

around the erupted teeth; they bleed easily when touched. Hemorrhage into the skin is not common in infants but may occur from slight trauma. Petechiae are sometimes scattered over the skin and mucous membranes. The costochondral junctions enlarge to give the "scorbutic rosary," which is sharp-feeling in contrast to the fusiform, rounded enlargement of rickets. Fever and secondary infection are common. Hypochromic anemia may be present.

When fully developed, the condition is readily recognized, but diagnosis may depend upon laboratory procedures. X-ray examination of the ends of long bones shows the typical "white lines" of scurvy with an adjacent zone of rarefaction on the shaft side. There may be separation of epiphyses and at times fractures through rarefied portions. Small spurs develop at the lateral margins of the shaft. The cortex is thin, and the shaft is less radiopaque. Subperiosteal hemorrhages may be evident. Plasma ascorbic acid is usually absent, and urinary excretion is almost nil.

ADULT SCURVY is uncommon but is encountered in the indigent, the insane, the alcoholic, and individuals taking sharply restricted diets for several months. It begins with weakness, loss of weight, and vague aches and pains in muscles and joints. There is increased susceptibility to infection; the latter may suddenly precipitate the classic picture. Hemorrhage develops at points of trauma and stress. Muscles are involved more commonly than in infants and become painfully indurated. Large areas of ecchymosis occur. Hemorrhagic gingivitis and petechial hemorrhages about the hair follicles are usually present. Since the adult bone is fully developed, there are no changes about the epiphyses, but subperiosteal bleeding may be found. Blood and urine analyses do not differ materially from those in infants.

TREATMENT—Ascorbic acid is specific and will relieve the pain of scurvy within one or two days. Infants and children are given from 50 to 100 mg. four times daily by mouth. If parenteral administration is necessary, intramuscular injection is preferred. Adults should be given 1,000 mg. of ascorbic acid daily in divided doses. Many cases of scurvy are complicated by other nutritional deficiencies which require dietary adjustment and administration of specific supplements.

Other Therapeutic Applications—As with the B complex vitamins, vitamin C deficiency may be produced by conditioning factors (Table 54, p. 484), and administration of the vitamin will speed recovery. Surgical patients, particularly those with gastro-intestinal disease, have particularly low vitamin reserves. Severe infections, wasting diseases, and burns also severely deplete the vitamin. Idiopathic methemoglobinemia may be relieved by oral administration of 150 mg. ascorbic acid two or three times daily; however, its action is not sufficiently prompt to be relied on as the sole therapy in acute cases.

VITAMIN A

Vitamin A exists in at least two forms: vitamin A_1, which is found in all animals and salt-water fish; and vitamin A_2, which occurs mostly in fresh-water fish. The latter probably is of no importance to mammals. Their chemical structures differ slightly, but they have the same qualitative and quantitative biological action. Vitamin A is an unsaturated alcohol which is soluble in oils and fat solvents and is fairly stable to heat but is very susceptible to oxidation (for structural formula of vitamin A_1, see Figure 52). In animals, it is stored as an ester, which is the form supplied in preparations obtained from fish liver oils for medicinal use. The synthetic vitamin in the form of the acetate and palmitate is also available and does not differ in biological activity from the natural form.

The U.S.P. Unit of vitamin A is the same as the International Unit and is equal to 0.344 microgram of vitamin A acetate. There are two official assay methods. The preferred one is spectrophotometric; a biological method may be employed on substances not suitable for spectrophotometry.

Plants do not contain vitamin A but synthesize provitamins, which are easily converted by animals into vitamin A. These provitamins belong to the class of carotenoids and are the most important natural sources of the vitamin for man and animals. Beta carotene is the most prevalent; its molecule contains two vitamin A_1 molecules joined at the ends of the side chains by removal of the hydroxyl groups. Other members of the group (such as alpha carotene, gamma carotene, and cryptoxanthin) are nutritionally important but, because of their asym-

metric structure, can yield but one molecule of vitamin A. Actually, however, the absorption and utilization of carotenes by the body is not efficient, and on a molecular basis their biological activity is only one-half to one-fourth that of vitamin A. They require the presence of fat and bile salts for intestinal absorption. Absorption is prevented by mineral oil and greatly inhibited by chronic diarrhea, pancreatic insufficiency, and sprue. The liver normally holds a large reserve of carotene which is gradually converted to vitamin A, supposedly by the enzyme carotenase. Carotene is not excreted in the urine or feces but does appear in breast milk; colostrum contains large amounts. Carotenemia develops when blood carotene levels exceed 250 micrograms per 100 cc. This is a harmless condition which may be confused with jaundice because of the yellow color imparted to the skin. It is readily differentiated, however, because the mucous membranes and sclera are not involved.

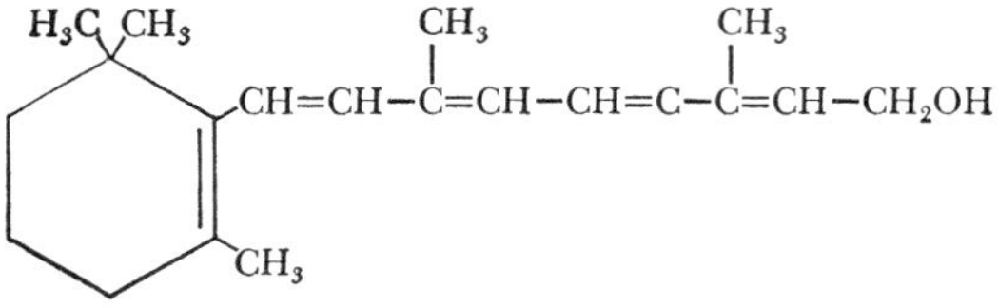

Vitamin A itself is readily absorbed from the upper intestine; fats and bile salts are not essential, although they enhance the process. Absorption of oil solutions is greatly impaired by pancreatic insufficiency; but if these are homogenized to give oil droplets 10 microns in diameter or less or if the vitamin is dissolved in propylene glycol, absorption will take place without fat digestion. Vitamin A ester is converted to the alcoholic form during passage through the intestinal wall but is promptly reconverted to the ester for transport by the blood and lymph. Plasma normally contains about 75 International Units per 100 cc. Faulty absorption is found in sprue, fibrocystic disease of the pancreas, vitamin B complex deficiency, colitis, infections (either enteral or systemic), and giardiasis. Mineral oil interferes with absorption, but not to so great an extent as in the case of carotene. There is disagreement regarding absorption and utilization of vitamin A when it is given parenterally in oil solution; when given in a fat solvent, it is readily utilized.

Large amounts of vitamin A are stored, 90 to 95 percent of it in the liver. Newborn infants have small reserves, regardless of dietary intake of the mother during pregnancy, and stores are not increased appreciably by milk feedings. Administration of vitamin A supplements brings prompt increase, however. The mechanism for mobilization of the liver stores has not been identified, but the stimulus is believed to originate in the central nervous system. Like the carotenes, vitamin A is excreted in milk but does not appear in the urine except in pathological conditions, and then only

FIGURE 52—*Structural Formula of Vitamin A_1*

when protein is present. The requirements are proportional to body weight, which suggests that the fundamental function of the vitamin is concerned with maintenance of structure rather than with metabolic activity. For optimal daily allowances, see Table 22 (p. 252).

Toxic manifestations have been recorded following administration of very large doses of vitamin A to animals. A few human cases of apparent vitamin A toxicity have been reported. Doses were considerably larger than those used for treatment of deficiency and in most instances had been continued for months or years. The manifestations include anorexia, irritability, and failure to gain weight. There is enlargement of the liver and sometimes the spleen; skeletal development is accelerated in children, with clubbing of the fingers, periosteal swellings, and bone tenderness. The hair becomes coarse and scanty. Hypoplastic anemia and leukopenia have been described. Serum levels of vitamin A are greatly increased. Apparent recovery follows soon after the vitamin is withheld.

Vitamin A Deficiency—When blood levels decrease below 60 units per 100 cc., early signs of deficiency develop. *Nyctalopia*, or faulty vision in dim light, is one of the earliest manifestations. The vitamin is the precursor of visual purple contained in the rod cells of the retina. Under the influence of light, visual purple breaks down into two constituents, which later recombine under the influence of vitamin A. Lack of the vitamin prevents the latter reaction and leads to photophobia and poor dark adaptation; patients adjust to dim light with great difficulty and may become blinded temporarily after sudden exposure to bright, glaring lights. Several types of ocular instruments for diagnosis of nyctalopia are available. The response to vitamin A administration is prompt provided that utilization is not impaired. Doses of 1,000 to 5,000 units may be sufficient, although amounts up to 25,000 units daily have been recommended.

More prolonged deficiency causes *xerophthalmia* with keratinization of the epithelial cells of the conjunctivae and tear ducts. The conjunctivae become dry and granular. Subjectively there are burning and itching, asthenopia, and photophobia. Small triangular white patches covered by white foamlike spots (known as Bitot's spots) appear just lateral to the cornea on the equator of the eye. Keratomalacia is uncommon in this country and is a late manifestation due to corneal involvement; it results in vascularization, secondary infection, and ulceration. Recovery may be complete, or

perforation of the cornea and destruction of the eye may take place. Permanent scarring of the cornea is common if ulcers have been present. Large daily doses of vitamin A, 25,000 to 100,000 units, are recommended for treatment.

Atrophy and keratinization of epithelium develop elsewhere, usually beginning in the respiratory mucosa and successively involving the mouth, tongue, salivary glands, renal pelves, ureters, bladder, and the skin. These changes predispose to secondary infection, and death from pneumonia is not uncommon in infants. Keratosis of the vaginal mucosa is frequent and often is a major factor in the etiology of senile vaginitis. The pathological changes in epithelium are the same, regardless of location. The normal cells become undermined with stratified epithelium which has failed to differentiate, but the basal cells remain intact. If the deficiency is relieved, complete regeneration is possible.

The skin changes which occur give rise to a characteristic appearance known as phrynoderma. There is excessive dryness, the hair becomes dull and brittle, and the skin is rough and scaly. The keratinized cells plug the pilosebaceous follicles, giving rise to small papules, each of which, if removed, leaves a small pit.

Specific treatment with vitamin A results in slow regeneration of involved epithelium and complete recovery. The process usually extends over several months, in contrast to the rapid response obtained in nyctalopia. Doses of 20,000 to 100,000 units daily are employed.

Other Therapeutic Applications of Vitamin A have been reported for conditions not necessarily associated with deficiency. The seborrheic acne of adolescence may be controlled with daily doses of 100,000 units continued for several months. Improvement begins two or three months after treatment is started and is first evidenced by a decrease in oiliness of the skin and reduction in size and number of the comedones. The pustules gradually decrease in number and severity. If treatment is stopped, relapse is likely to occur, but the condition will respond again to therapy.

Urinary calculi are prevalent in countries where severe vitamin A deficiency is common, and it is believed that the epithelial lesions in the urinary tract may furnish nuclei of desquamated cells for stone formation. The vitamin will not dissolve stones, but it may be of value in preventing recurrence. For this purpose, daily doses of 10,000 to 50,000 units have been recommended.

Vitamin A has been used in a variety of dermatoses characterized by keratinization, scaling, and excessive dryness of the skin. Results have not been uniformly good.

VITAMIN D

There are at least ten different compounds having vitamin D activity; two of these (D_2 and D_3) are important clinically. All have the same general chemical structure, being derived from cyclopentenophenanthrene, as are the sex hormones, the adrenocortical hormones, and the cardiac aglycones. Vitamin D is synthesized in nature and commercially by activation of certain sterols known as provitamins. This ordinarily is accomplished by ultraviolet irradiation or, for some pharmaceutical preparations, by exposure to an electronic stream.

Vitamin D_2 (calciferol; for formula, see Figure 53) is derived from the provitamin ergosterol, which is commonly found in plants. The ultraviolet activation process is not a single photochemical reaction but proceeds in steps in which intermediate products are formed; namely, lumisterol, tachysterol, calciferol, and toxisterol. None except calciferol have antirachitic activity. The older methods produced large amounts of these intermediate compounds; although modern methods have reduced them to a minimum, it is impossible to

eliminate their production entirely. The term "viosterol" is used to denote an unpurified irradiated ergosterol. There are several other methods for preparing vitamin D_2 synthetically, the two of most practical importance being the Whittier and Milas technics. In both methods, vaporized ergosterol under reduced pressure is subjected to bombardment by electrons. Vitamin D_2 is produced directly, without the intermediate products which accompany the irradiation process.

Vitamin D_3 has been called the "animal vitamin" because it is most abundant in animal tissues, in contrast to vitamin D_2, which is commonly found in plants. D_3 can by synthesized by the irradiation of 7-dehydrocholesterol. Its chemical formula is identical with that of D_2 except for the side chain (see Figure 53). Fish liver oils usually contain approximately half of the vitamin D in the form of D_3; the remainder is made up of several as yet unidentified components, of which one has many characteristics resembling vitamin D_2. Biological assays of these two vitamins show identical potencies in rats and human beings, but in chicks D_2 is considerably weaker insofar as its antirachitic effect is concerned.

In the pure state, vitamin D occurs as white, odorless crystals which are soluble in fats and in organic solvents. It is susceptible to heat, light,

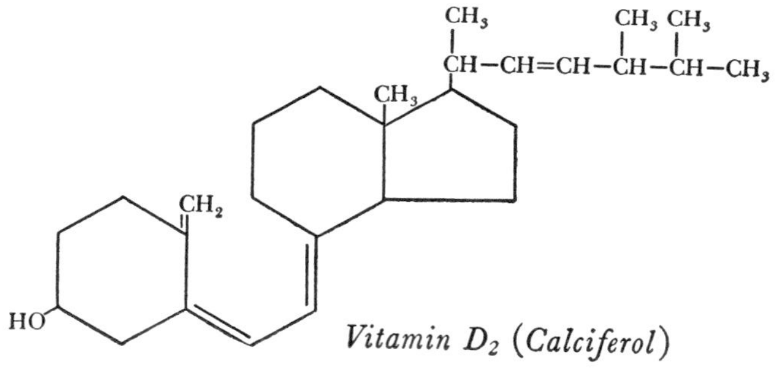

Vitamin D₂ (Calciferol)

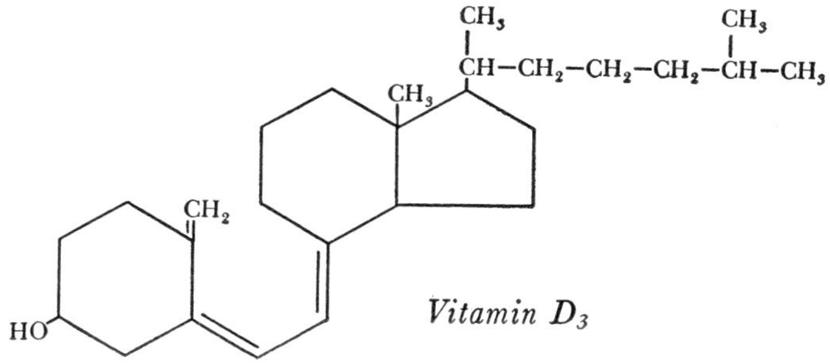

Vitamin D₃

FIGURE 53—*Structural Formulas of the Principal Vitamins D*

and oxidation. Oil solutions remain stable for many years when not exposed to air.

Vitamin D is not widely distributed in nature, and man cannot obtain sufficient quantities from the ordinary diet. The principal sources are (1) synthetic preparations and fish liver oils, (2) foods (such as milk and yeast) which have been fortified by ultraviolet irradiation, and (3) formation of vitamin D in the skin as the result of exposure to sunshine or ultraviolet rays.

Vitamin D is readily absorbed from the intestinal tract, particularly if bile salts are present. It penetrates the intact skin and can be utilized when given parenterally. On the basis of absorption studies of vitamin A, it is believed that intestinal absorption is retarded when fat digestion is impaired but that administration of homogenized material with fat globules less than 10 microns in diameter or of solutions of the vitamin in fat solvents (such as propylene glycol) permits absorption directly without digestion.

Little is known of the metabolism of vitamin D. The liver is the chief storage organ, and smaller amounts are found in the skin, brain, lungs, spleen, and bone. Liver disease interferes with storage and may lead to vitamin deficiency. The body conserves supplies efficiently; a single dose of 600,000 units will protect infants against rickets for several months. Vitamin D is excreted in milk in proportion to the amount received in the diet, but little is known about other routes of excretion.

The principal function of vitamin D is to maintain adequate supplies of calcium and phosphorus for growth and maintenance of bone. This is accomplished primarily by promoting intestinal absorption of these minerals. In addition, it probably acts locally in bone by assisting in the conversion of organic calcium and phosphorus to inorganic forms. In vitamin D deficiency, large amounts of unabsorbed calcium and phosphorus are excreted in the feces. Blood levels of phosphorus decrease because of lowering of the renal threshold, but serum calcium levels are better maintained because of decreased urinary excretion and increased mobilization from bone. Excessively large doses of vitamin D cause pronounced mobilization of calcium and phosphorus from bone, which increases blood levels and urinary excretion.

The International Unit for vitamin D is the antirachitic activity of 0.025 microgram of vitamin D_3. The U.S.P. Unit has the same potency. The U.S.P. assay method employs rats. The requirements for vitamin D have been established by the National Research Council at 400 International Units daily for infants, children, adolescents, and pregnant or lactating women. It formerly was believed that older children received sufficient amounts from natural sources, but this has been disproved and daily supplements are now recommended. It is possible to supply the requirements of infants by exposure to sunshine, but in most areas of the United States atmospheric conditions are too variable to rely upon this source. Not all authorities are in agreement regarding the adequacy of 400 units daily for young infants; some infants who are unusually susceptible to rickets will develop the disease on this dose, and consequently it has been suggested that, for routine prophylaxis, 800 to 1,000 units be used daily during the first year of life.

Toxicity—Regardless of the type of preparation used, vitamin D is potentially toxic when given regularly in large doses. Since individual susceptibility varies, no single toxic dose can be defined. Symptoms have developed in adults taking as little as 25,000 units daily; and, on the other hand, doses of 500,000 units have been tolerated for many months.

Early symptoms of hypervitaminosis D consist in anorexia, nausea, vomiting, abdominal cramps, frequent stools, pallor, lassitude, and frequent urination. Less common but more significant symptoms are vertigo, muscular weakness, paresthesia, headache, joint and muscle pain, tenderness of the teeth and gums, neuralgia of the mandibular branch of the trigeminal nerve, and impaired memory. Metastatic deposits of calcium may form in any organ or soft tissue and sometimes involve vital structures. Serum calcium may increase sufficiently to produce symptoms and signs of hypercalcemia (see p. 345). Kidney function is impaired, and, if vitamin administration is continued, renal failure may develop. Albuminuria and low specific gravity are seen early; scanty urine containing white and red blood cells and casts indicates more serious damage. Death may occur from uremia (p. 223).

Vitamin D in massive dosage should not be administered to old people with evidence of arteriosclerosis (particularly of the aorta) or to individuals who have renal stones. It should be used with caution in any patient with kidney disease, a sensitive colon, or disproportionate available supplies of calcium and phosphorus.

The prognosis of overdosage depends upon the amount of kidney damage and is good unless irreversible changes have taken place. Treatment consists in withholding the vitamin and employing measures to combat any existing uremia.

Vitamin D Deficiency in children predisposes to *rickets*. Premature infants are especially susceptible. Similar deficiency in adults may cause *osteomalacia* (hunger osteopathy, war osteopathy), which differs somewhat from rickets in its clinical manifestations but has the same basic rachitic process.

Although vitamin D is specific in the prevention and treatment of rickets, it is not the sole etiological factor. Depletion of calcium and phosphorus reserves is also important, and this is most likely to occur during periods of rapid bone growth. It is doubtful whether heredity is involved, but there probably is some unidentified constitutional factor, aside from prematurity and accelerated growth, which increases the susceptibility of certain infants. Dietary factors may be important, for the amounts and proportions of calcium and phosphorus must be correct: An excess of phosphorus may cause calcium deficiency by formation in the intestine of insoluble calcium phosphate, which is excreted in the feces; foods with an alkaline ash tend to decrease absorption of these metals; certain cereals, particularly oatmeal, contain phytic acid, which acts similarly; and excessive fat favors formation of calcium soaps which reduce the amount of available calcium. Rickets is sometimes precipitated by acute or chronic infections. Variations in renal function which increase urinary excretion of calcium and phosphorus may be important (so-called renal rickets is not included here since its pathogenesis is distinct). Dark-skinned races are more susceptible than Caucasians because of less absorption of the sun's ultraviolet rays.

The clinical manifestations of rickets depend primarily upon the failure of calcium phosphate to be deposited in the cartilage of growing bone. This accounts for the characteristic mushroom deformities and epiphyseal dislocations at the ends of long bones. Even in normal individuals, the calcium salts in previously formed bone are constantly being broken down and replaced. In rickets, the rate of removal is frequently accelerated and, since new salts cannot be laid down, the bones lose their normal rigidity. In addition to the presence of enlargement and dislocations at the epiphyses, various deformities are produced by the stress of gravity; and pathological fractures may occur, their nature depending upon age, rate of growth, postural habits, and severity of the disease.

It is no longer believed that early rickets is necessarily accompanied by restlessness, irritability, gastro-intestinal disturbances, and head sweating. One of the earliest signs is craniotabes, which appears in the second or third month and disappears by the eighth month even though the disease continues. Areas of softening develop in the occipital and parietal bones adjacent to the lambdoid sutures. Usually these are asymmetrical and about 3 cm. in diameter, but they may vary in size from 1 cm. to inclusion of the entire back of the skull. Careful pressure and release will reveal a parchmentlike sensation when the indented bone snaps back into position. Another early sign is enlargement of the costochondral junctions to give the "rachitic rosary," which is a fusiform type of deformity in contrast to the raised, sharp-feeling one found in scurvy. The epiphyseal enlargement at the ends of long bones can best be detected at the ends of the ulna and radius or the tibia and fibula.

The anterior fontanel fails to close and sometimes actually enlarges; but it usually disappears by the age of two and one-half years even though the disease continues. Thickening of the skull at the frontal and parietal eminences gives rise to the characteristic bossing. Flattening of the occipital region is common. In severe rickets, the pull of the diaphragm causes a depression (Harrison's groove) to form along the line of attachment at the lower part of the thorax. Prolonged rickets causes narrowing of the pelvic outlet. Bowlegs, knock-knees, and flat feet are common findings. Deformities of the spine develop from the effects of abnormal posture but not from structural changes.

Along with the skeletal lesions there develop weakness and relaxation of the muscles, which result in enlargement of the abdomen (potbelly) and delayed postural development. Growth may be considerably inhibited.

Diagnosis can be made by x-ray examination, but by the time the characteristic changes at the ends of long bones are demonstrable, the disease is well advanced. Blood analysis for calcium and phosphorus is helpful. Usually the calcium is in the normal range of 9.5 to 11 mg. per 100 cc. of serum, although at times it may be as low as 5 mg. When calcium is reduced below 8 mg., tetany frequently develops (see p. 195). In normal infants, the serum inorganic phosphate is about 5 mg. per 100 cc., but in rickets it is reduced and may be as low as 1 mg. In premature infants, rickets may develop without alteration of calcium or phosphorus concentrations. The alkaline phosphatase concentration of the blood normally is 5 to 15 Bodansky units, but in rickets it is increased to 20 to 60 units or more. This change is not specific, for it occurs in other conditions, including malignant tumors of bone and hyperparathyroidism.

Treatment—Rickets can be arrested with ordinary prophylactic doses of vitamin D (400 International Units daily), but the response will be delayed for two or three weeks. For treatment, daily doses of 5,000 units are more appropriate and should be continued for five or six weeks. Some cases are more resistant and require as much as 20,000 units or more. The response to treatment is best determined by x-ray examination; adequate treatment will produce a faint line of preliminary calcification across the epiphyseal cartilage in three weeks (sometimes as soon as eight days).

Other Therapeutic Uses—On the basis of pharmacologic effect, massive doses of vitamin D have been employed in the treatment of several diseases. Calciferol (vitamin D$_2$) or dihydrotachysterol (see below) provides the most satisfactory maintenance therapy for hypoparathyroidism (see p.196). Lupus vulgaris (tuberculosis of the skin) appears to respond to daily doses of 400,000 units, but patients must remain under close observation because of the frequent occurrence of mild toxic manifestations (see p. 345). The good results at one time reported in such conditions as rheumatoid arthritis, sarcoidosis, pemphigus, and scleroderma have not been confirmed. Treatment of them with vitamin D cannot be recommended.

DIHYDROTACHYSTEROL

Dihydrotachysterol (A.T. 10, Hytakerol) is an activated sterol obtained by reduction of tachysterol, which is one of the products that may be obtained by irradiation of ergosterol. Dihydrotachysterol has no appreciable antirachitic effect, but it has an action qualitatively like that of the parathyroid hormone (p. 195). It is used for maintenance therapy in hypoparathyroidism (p.196).

Dihydrotachysterol is administered by mouth. It acts on the serum calcium after a latent period which amounts to several days but is somewhat shorter than that for calciferol. In hypoparathyroidism, initial dosage may vary from 2.5 to 12.5 mg. daily. Maintenance dosage is typically 1.25 to 5.5 mg. once or twice a week. Because of the harmful effects of hypercalcemia, dosage should be controlled by tests of the excretion or serum level of calcium (see Treatment of Hypoparathyroidism, p. 196).

VITAMIN E

Vitamin E as it occurs in nature is a complex of at least four tocopherols—alpha, beta, gamma, and delta. As will be noted from the structural formulas (Figure 54, p. 498), all are homologues of alpha-tocopherol, and the beta and gamma compounds are isomers. They differ from each other only in the number and position of the methyl groups which are attached to the chroman nucleus. The tocopherols are soluble in oils and fat solvents and are insoluble in water. They are quite stable to alkali and to ordinary cooking processes but are oxidized in the presence of air, iron salts, and ultraviolet radiation and deteriorate rapidly when exposed to rancid fats. All are effective antioxidants, the gamma isomer being more active than the beta, which in turn is more effective than the alpha form.

Vitamin E is synthesized by plants and is widely distributed in them. Wheat germ oil, peanut oil, corn oil, and cottonseed oil are particularly good sources, and the green parts of plants contain moderate quantities. Animals are unable to form the tocopherols, and consequently animal tissues are poor sources. Fish liver oils and olive oil contain little of it.

The tocopherols are readily absorbed from the small intestine if fat digestion is normal, but the mechanism is not known. There is conflicting evidence in regard to utilization following intramuscular injection of oily solutions, but it appears that absorption from muscle does occur if the vitamin is dissolved in a fat solvent such as propylene glycol.

The total content of the normal human adult body has been estimated to be about 3.5 Gm.; its distribution is shown in Table 55. Little is known about the metabolism or function of vitamin E. It is not excreted in urine and probably is broken down in the body by oxidation. Normal serum tocopherol levels vary from 0.5 to 1.5 mg. per 100 cc. Low values are found in diseases which impair fat digestion, such as idiopathic steatorrhea, fibrocystic disease of the pancreas, biliary obstruction, nutritional macrocytic anemia, and diarrhea associated with achlorhydria, pellagra, and carcinoma of the stomach. High levels occur in diseases as-

TABLE 55 — *Tocopherol Content of Human Tissue*

Tissue	Tocopherol Content, mg. per 100 Gm.
Pancreas	5.5
Testis	2.8
Liver	2.5
Spleen	1.9
Lung	1.2
Heart	1.1
Skeletal muscle	1.0
Kidney	0.8

sociated with hypercholesteremia, such as diabetes mellitus, xanthomatosis, and glomerulosclerosis. Levels tend to rise during pregnancy. Patients with cardiovascular disease fall within the normal and high ranges. The clinical significance of these findings is not apparent.

If vitamin E deficiency occurs in man, it has not been recognized. Human requirements are completely unknown. It has been shown that an intake of 30 mg. of tocopherol per day increases blood levels to 1.2 mg. per 100 cc., beyond which no rise can be obtained even with large doses. On this basis, it has been suggested that the daily requirement for an adult lies somewhere between 15 and 30 mg. Deficiencies can be produced in animals; in different species, muscle dystrophy or sterility may be produced. Because of these observations, the vitamin has been used clinically for treatment of several neuromuscular disorders, including amyotrophic lateral sclerosis, progressive muscular dystrophy and atrophy, pseudohypertrophic muscular dystrophy, disseminated sclerosis, and certain myotonias. Some subjective improvement has been obtained, but there is no conclusive evidence that

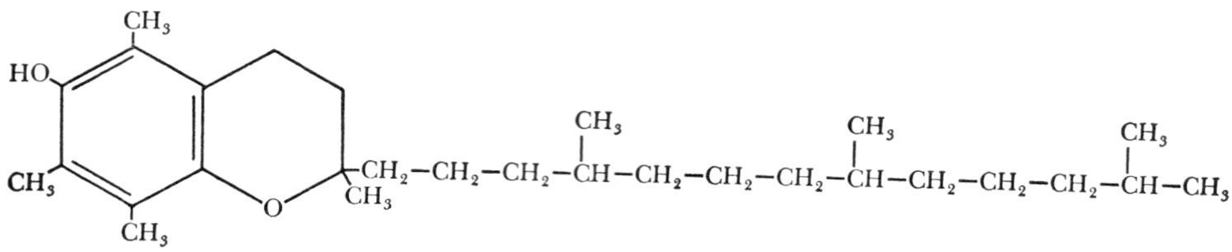

Alpha-Tocopherol

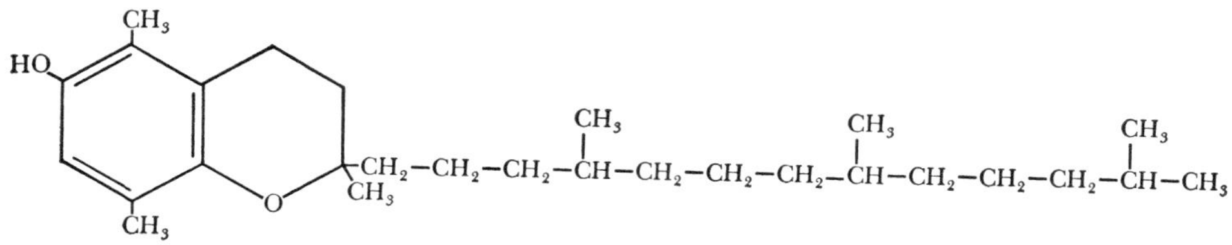

Beta-Tocopherol

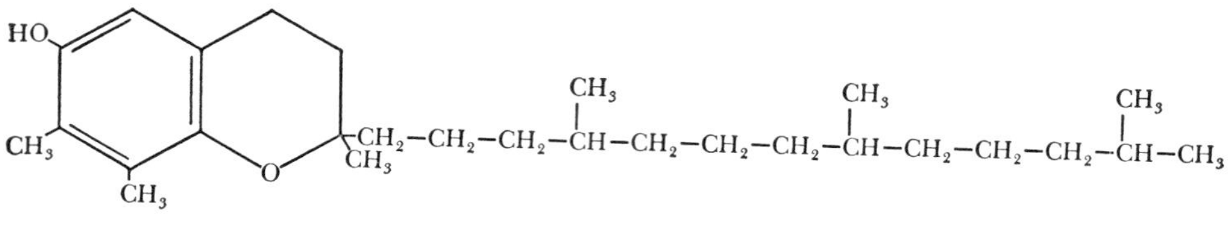

Gamma-Tocopherol

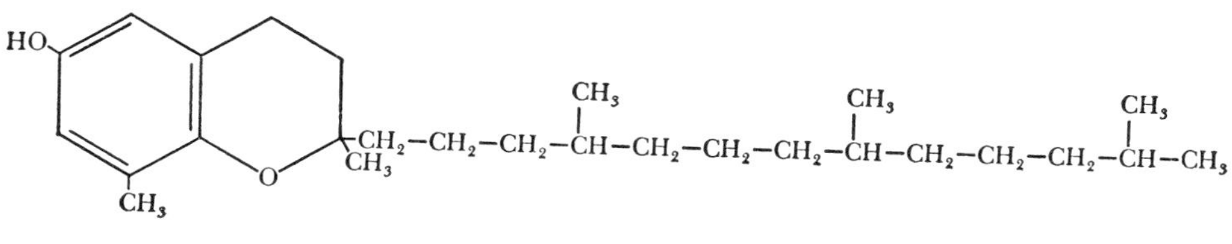

Delta-Tocopherol

FIGURE 54—*Structural Formulas of the Tocopherols (Vitamin E)*

the underlying pathology of these diseases is influenced. It is doubtful whether vitamin E is of value in treatment of male or female sterility. Threatened and habitual abortion have been treated with equivocal results.

Symptomatic relief of menopausal symptoms has been obtained with vitamin E. It is recommended particularly in cases suspected of having malignancy, when estrogens may be contraindicated. All types of vitamin E preparations have been used, but doses vary considerably and must be adjusted according to response. Although relief may be obtained with as little as 10 mg. once daily by mouth, 100 mg. three times daily are sometimes required.

The tocopherols have been used with some success in a group of diseases characterized by fibrosis. Primary fibrositis or so-called muscular rheumatism (p. 250) has responded to daily oral doses of 100 to 300 mg. of mixed natural tocopherols or similar amounts of synthetic alpha-tocopherol. Dupuytren's contracture has also been relieved, provided that treatment is instituted before permanent scarring or calcification has developed. Peyronie's disease, which is often associated with primary fibrositis, responds to vitamin E therapy. Treatment of fibrositis secondary to hypertrophic arthritis has not been successful. Urethral strictures of varied etiology have improved on daily doses of 300 mg.; resistant cases may require considerably more, in some instances as much as 1,200 mg. Such high doses have not caused toxic reactions.

There is considerable controversy as to the relative therapeutic activity of the individual tocopherols. It has been claimed that alpha-tocopherol (either the synthetic racemic acetate or the dextrorotatory ester from natural sources) is the only therapeutically active compound. In view of the failure of many competent investigators to confirm this claim, its validity seems at least doubtful. When clinical improvement has occurred following vitamin E therapy in the conditions named above, response has been obtained from all types of preparations, without regard to their content of alpha-tocopherol.

Two assay methods are most commonly employed. Spectrophotometric assay determines accurately the total quantity of tocopherols present but does not distinguish between the different members of the group. The bio-assay usually employed is the rat antisterility test, which measures the biological activity of all the tocopherols present with respect to antisterility effect (it should be recalled that similar activity has not been dem-onstrated with certainty for vitamin E in man). For the bio-assay, an International Unit has been established; it is the quantity of material which will enable 50 percent of vitamin-E-deficient pregnant rats to bear living litters. One mg. of racemic alpha-tocopherol acetate has about 1 International Unit of activity. The beta compound is about 40 percent as potent; and the gamma compound, about 8 percent. Little is known of the activity of delta-tocopherol.

VITAMIN K

Vitamin K activity is exhibited by a large number of naturally occurring and synthetic compounds which are derived from or related to menadione (2-methyl-1,4-naphthoquinone; for structural formula, see Figure 55, p. 500). The natural forms of vitamin K are of value from the nutritional standpoint but are no longer important therapeutically.

Menadione is a lemon-yellow, heat-stable crystalline powder that is soluble in oil and fat solvents but insoluble in water. It is susceptible to light and alkali. This compound is one of the most potent forms of vitamin K and is given by mouth and by intramuscular injection. It cannot be injected intravenously because of its insolubility in water.

Certain other quinones are water-soluble and can be given by all routes. They have identical qualitative actions and, if given in proper dosage, will produce identical effects. Their structural formulas are shown in Figure 55, and their relative doses are indicated in Table 56.

TABLE 56 — *Relative Doses of Substances Having Vitamin K Activity*

Substance	Dosage Equal to 1 mg. Menadione
Tetrasodium 2-methyl-1,4-naphtho-hydroquinone diphosphoric acid ester ('Kappadione,' Synkayvite) .	2 mg.
2-Methyl-1,4-naphthoquinone sodium bisulfite (Hykinone)	1.6 mg.
2-Methyl-4-amino-1-naphthol hydrochloride (Synkamin)	3 mg.

Menadione is absorbed from the intestinal tract if fat digestion is normal; although bile salts are not absolutely essential, their presence greatly facilitates absorption. The water-soluble compounds are absorbed directly. Little is known about the metabolism of vitamin K. Only small amounts are stored, and deficiency may develop within one week if the vitamin is withheld or cannot be ab-

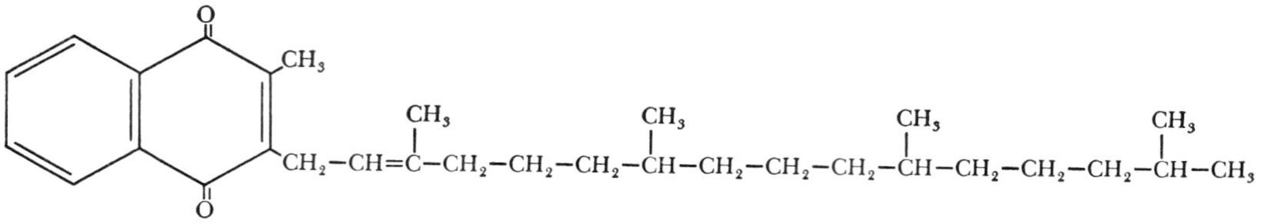

Vitamin K₁

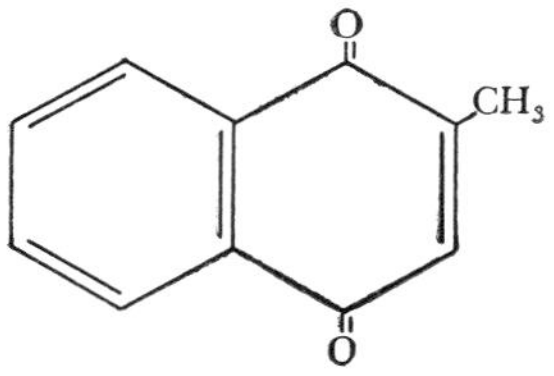

Menadione

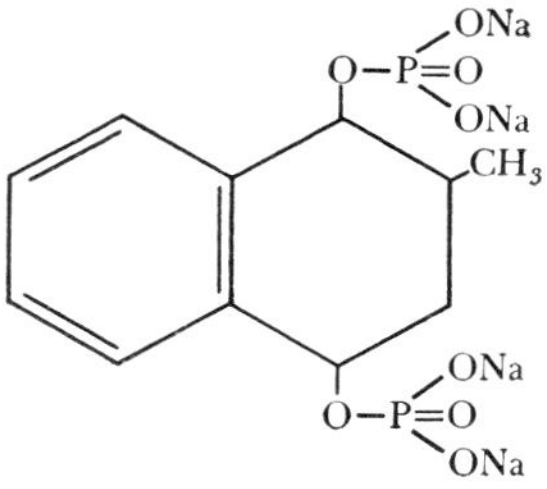

Tetrasodium 2-Methyl-1,4-naphthohydroquinone Diphosphoric Acid Ester ('Kappadione,' Synkayvite)

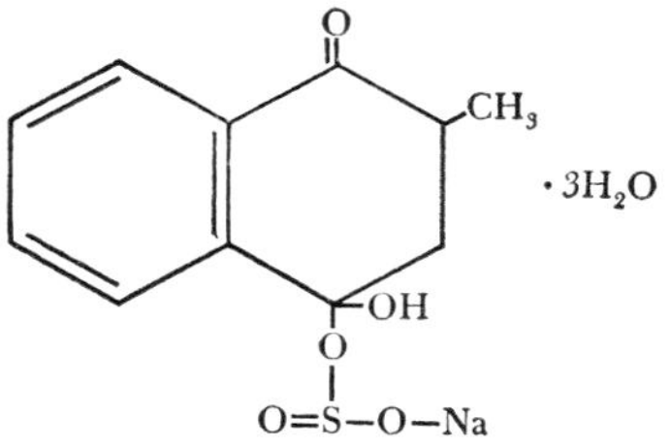

2-Methyl-1,4-naphthoquinone Sodium Bisulfite (Hykinone)

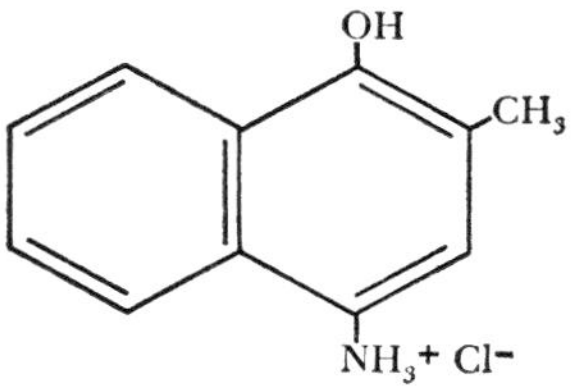

2-Methyl-4-amino-1-naphthol Hydrochloride (Synkamin)

FIGURE 55—*Structural Formulas of Some Substances Having Vitamin K Activity*

sorbed. Vitamin K appears in the feces, but this portion is believed to originate from the intestinal bacteria rather than from excretion.

Vitamin K appears to have but one function in the body. It is essential for the formation of prothrombin (see p. 107), but the mechanism of this action is not known. Vitamin K does not make up part of the prothrombin molecule; probably it stimulates synthesis by the liver. When the vitamin is not available to the liver or when synthesis is prevented by liver disease, blood prothrombin levels decrease and spontaneous hemorrhage appears.

Green plants are the richest sources of vitamin K. The daily requirement is not known; but when intestinal and liver function are normal, it is probably only a fraction of a milligram. However, in the presence of diarrhea, pancreatic steatorrhea, or impaired liver function, requirements are considerably increased.

Vitamin K is practically nontoxic. Doses ten times those recommended sometimes cause temporary hypotension. There is no reason to believe that large doses or continued therapy predispose to the occurrence of venous thrombosis.

Deficiency of Vitamin K as a primary disturbance is, for practical purposes, seen only in the newborn. It is discussed on page 108. As a secondary disorder, deficiency of vitamin K and prothrombin may be caused by a number of conditions. Operative procedures often are complicated by hemorrhage on this basis. When the possibility is suspected, vitamin K should be given preoperatively and continued postoperatively for several days. Parenteral administration is particularly advantageous, since oral medication may not be tolerated and absorption frequently is impaired.

Vitamin K is indicated in the presence of external biliary fistulas, impaired liver function, and biliary obstruction. Hypoprothrombinemia commonly complicates severe infections, particularly peritonitis which follows perforative appendicitis, ruptured peptic ulcer, or subdiaphragmatic or pelvic abscess; it frequently develops after severe burns and massive hemorrhage.

Hemorrhage is a common complication of jaundice and of sprue, pancreatic steatorrhea, ulcerative colitis, and other chronic diseases of the intestinal tract. Here, the water-soluble preparations are preferred because absorption is more certain. Vitamin K therapy is usually required in cirrhosis of the liver, toxic and infectious hepatitis, acute yellow atrophy, and neoplasms of this organ. When liver function is seriously impaired, the vitamin is not readily utilized, and blood transfusions may be required to control bleeding. Hemorrhagic manifestations in the course of acute and chronic infections may be due to diminished prothrombin, and further reduction may be caused by drugs; it has been shown that sulfonamides, salicylates, and barbiturates produce this effect in some cases.

Adult doses vary from 1 to 5 mg. of menadione daily or the equivalent in water-soluble preparations (Table 56). Biliary disease is an indication for simultaneous administration of bile salts when oil-soluble compounds are used orally. Infants are treated as described under hemorrhagic disease of the newborn (p.108).

Dicumarol and related drugs (p. 375) cause depression of prothrombin. The mechanism has not been identified, but it is not the same as that of vitamin K deficiency. Large doses of the several vitamin-K-active compounds have been employed with some success as antidotes to excessive Dicumarol action; but results are unpredictable, and accumulating evidence indicates that this application of vitamin K is not effective. However, in preliminary reports, vitamin K₁ (see Figure 55) or vitamin K₁ oxide, when given in an emulsion intravenously in doses of 0.5 to 3 Gm., is said to be an efficient antidote for Dicumarol.

VITAMIN P

Vitamin P is a term applied to several crude concentrates from plant sources and to a group of flavone glycosides which are believed necessary for maintenance of (1) normal capillary structure and (2), more specifically, capillary permeability. Of current interest are hesperidin, hesperidin methyl chalcone, and rutin (for structural formulas, see Figure 56). Eriodictyol, which is closely related chemically (see Figure 56), has only slight activity.

The flavones are naturally occurring yellow plant pigments. Hesperidin is a white, odorless, tasteless, crystalline powder which is almost insoluble in water, benzene, chloroform, and ether but which dissolves in alcohol and alkalies. Rutin occurs as light-yellow needles with similar solubilities except that it will dissolve in boiling water. Hesperidin methyl chalcone is a deep-yellow crystalline powder which is readily soluble in water, quite soluble in alcohol and acetone, and slightly soluble in ether. All are relatively stable. Hesperidin is extracted from the rinds of citrus fruits, rutin is obtained from young flowering buckwheat, and hesperidin methyl chalcone is prepared by methylation of hesperidin chalcone obtained from rinds of citrus fruits.

Although vitamin P is found in many fruits which also contain ascorbic acid, there is no constant relationship between the respective amounts of vitamin activity. For example, grapes are a potent source of vitamin P, but they have very little vitamin C. Generally speaking, fruits and green leaves are good sources of vitamin P, whereas roots and seeds have very little. Good sources are grapes, lemons, oranges, rose hips, blue plums, and black currants. Moderately good sources are grapefruit, apricots, cherries, blackberries, and blueberries. Little or no activity is found in tomatoes, lettuce, cabbage, cauliflower, turnips, parsnips, and potatoes.

The exact role of these and related compounds in nutrition has not been defined. Increase in capillary permeability has been observed in animals and man when they are removed from the diet, but results are inconstant and often cannot be duplicated. Methods for quantitative assay have been described, but they are not specific. Consequently, little is known about absorption, utilization, and excretion. When given orally or intravenously, they are relatively nontoxic, although rapid intravenous injection of hesperidin methyl chalcone reduces blood pressure sharply.

Vitamin P Deficiency—Although deficiency in man has been described, it has not been substantiated by independent investigators. The principal lesion is reported to consist of petechial hemorrhages in the skin and mucous membranes. The defect is described as distinct from the capillary lesion of scurvy, in which there is actual rupture of the vessel wall, giving rise to an oozing, more massive hemorrhage. When the petechial hemorrhages ap-

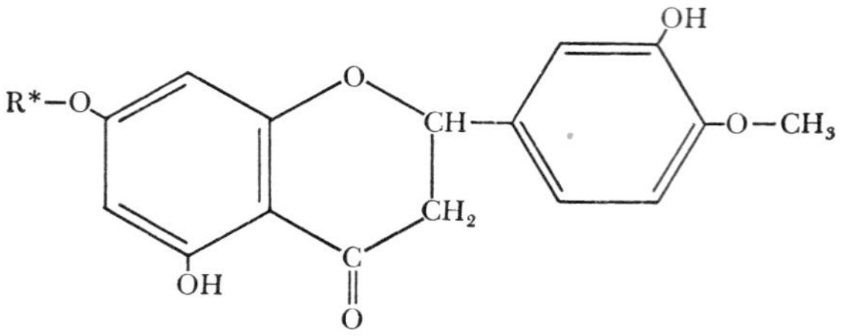

Hesperidin

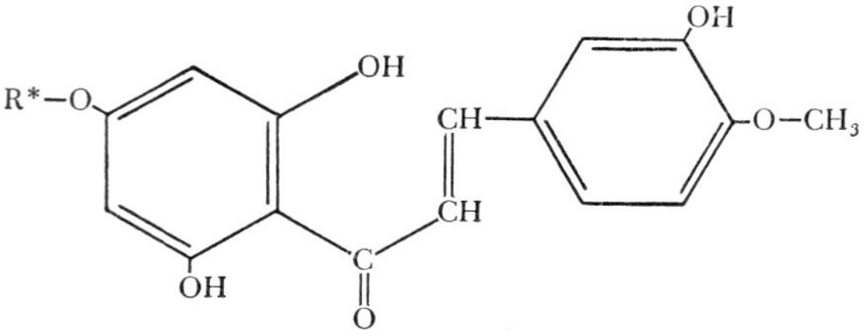

Hesperidin Chalcone

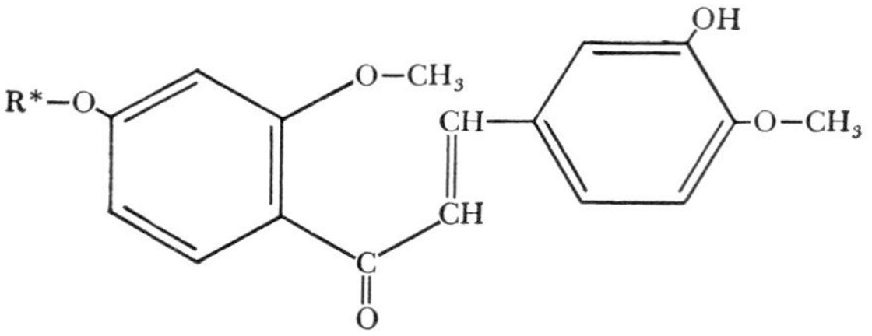

Hesperidin Methyl Chalcone

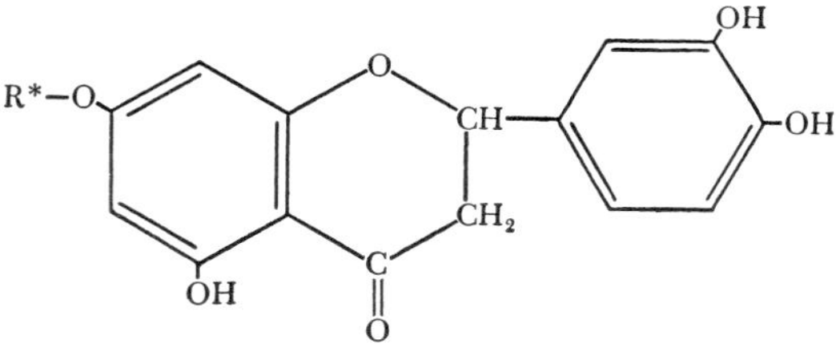

Eriodictyol

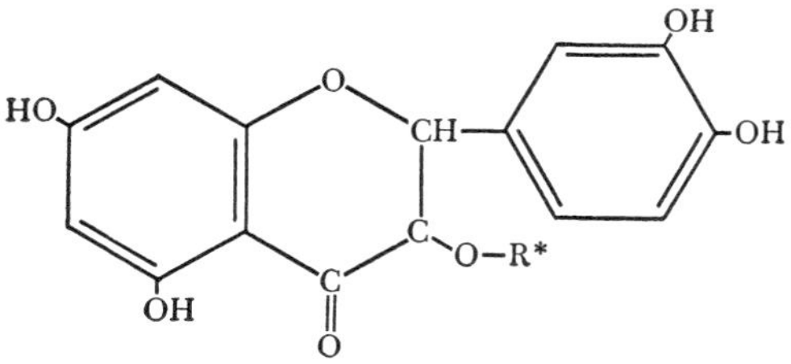

Rutin

*R = a sugar

FIGURE 56 — *Structural Formulas of Compounds with Vitamin P Activity*

peared spontaneously, there was noted lassitude, weakness, and pain in the shoulders, arms, and legs. Administration of vitamin P gave prompt relief within forty-eight hours. In severe deficiency, the petechiae appeared in areas of the skin subjected to external pressure from tight clothes or to the internal strain of increased intravenous pressure, as in the legs from an erect posture. They were characteristically small and were often perifollicular.

There are several methods for measuring capillary resistance or permeability, including Scarborough's modification of Hecht's negative pressure method, Wright and Lilienfeld's modification of Göthlin's technic for the Rumpel-Leede test, and Griffith and Lindauer's modification of the Göthlin test. All leave much to be desired, since at best they provide but crude approximations of capillary resistance. The negative and positive pressure technics do not give comparable results in the same individuals.

Evidence of increased capillary permeability may be encountered in a number of conditions, includ-

ing scurvy, multiple vitamin deficiencies, purpura, hypertension, and diabetes mellitus, as well as in many infectious and toxic states. Treatment with vitamin-P-active substances is not always successful and may even give inconstant results among patients with the same disease. Hereditary telangiectasia is not associated with recognized capillary defect, but, strangely enough, the massive hemorrhages peculiar to this condition have been controlled quite effectively with daily doses of 50 to 500 mg. Any of the three compounds described above may be used. If treatment is stopped, hemorrhages recur.

OTHER VITAMINS AND FACTORS

Other factors and supposed vitamins have been found or suspected at various times. Some of these are listed in Table 57, together with some of their reported properties.

TABLE 57—*Less Well Known Vitamins and Nutritional Factors*

Name	Synonym	Action	Remarks
Vitamin B_3	Williams-Waterman factor	Growth and weight maintenance in pigeons	May be pantothenic acid (filtrate factor II)
Vitamin B_4	Reader factor	Prevents specific type of paralysis in rats and chicks	Arginine? Glycine?
Vitamin B_5	Peters factor	Weight maintenance in pigeons	May be vitamin B_6 (filtrate factor I) or nicotinic acid
Vitamin B_7	Vitamin I	Absence accounts for gastrointestinal disturbances in pigeons	
Vitamin B_8	Adenylic acid	May increase effect of nicotinic acid in pellagra	Clinical studies being conducted
Vitamin B_{13}		A growth factor	No human application known to date
Vitamin B_{14}		Alleviates anemia and leukopenia in rats	No clinical studies
Vitamin B_c		Anemia in chicks and slow growth in young animals	Folic acid. Exhibits antianemia properties
Vitamin B_p	Antiperosis factor	In perotic chicks (hock disease or slipped tendon)	Probably not the only perosis-preventing substance
Vitamin B_T		Possible antianemia effect	May be related to Wills' factor
Vitamin B_x	Pantothenic acid		See Filtrate factor II
Factor W	Elvehjem factor, biotin	Growth of rats, chicks, and dogs	See Biotin *(Continued on next page)*

TABLE 57 (*Continued*)—*Less Well Known Vitamins and Nutritional Factors*

Name	Synonym	Action	Remarks
Biotin	Vitamin H (György), coenzyme R, anti-egg-white-injury factor, protective factor X (Boas), factor W (Elvehjem), factor S	Prevents "egg-white injury" and "spectacled eyes" in rats; growth factor for yeast and certain micro-organisms; antidermatitis factor for chicks	Avidin is toxic factor in egg white
Anti-gizzard-erosion factor		Gizzard erosion preventive in chicks	May be vitamin B_3
Factor U	Stokstad-Manning factor	Growth promotion in chicks	
Anti-spectacled-eye factor		Prevents incrustations about eyes in chicks. Also see Biotin and Inositol	Probably same as pantothenic acid. See Filtrate factor II
p-Aminobenzoic acid	Anti-gray-hair factor, chromotrichia factor, anticanitic factor, Bx factor	Chromotrichia factor for rat; growth factor for chick and certain bacteria	Clinical studies being conducted
Inositol	Antialopecia factor, inosite, bios I	Prevents loss of hair in rats and mice and "spectacled eyes" in rats. Promotes growth	Essential in fat metabolism. Considered a lipotropic agent
Vitamin H			See Biotin
Avidin		A protein capable of binding biotin	See Biotin
Filtrate factor I	Vitamin B_6		See Vitamin B_6
Filtrate factor II	Pantothenic acid		See Vitamin B_3 and Anti-gizzard-erosion factor
Vitamin I	Vitamin B_7		See Vitamin B_7
Vitamin J	Von Euler's factor, vitamin C_2	Antipneumonia factor in guinea pigs	No clinical studies
Vitamins or factors L_1 and L_2	Lactation vitamins	Believed necessary for lactation in rats	L_1 present in liver, L_2 present in yeast. Do not replace each other
Vitamin or factor M	Day's factor	Monkey pellagra and nutritional cytopenia factor	Probably a member of the vitamin B complex
Factor T	Platelet factor	Absence causes thrombocytosis in rats and man	
Grass-juice factor		Growth of rats and guinea pigs. May develop respiratory trouble in absence	Present in fresh grass and its juice; thus the name
Choline		With Mn is a perosis-preventing substance. Has lipotropic action	Essential in fat metabolism. A vitagen
P-P factor	Niacin, niacin amide		Nicotinic acid, nicotinamide
Aneurin			Is vitamin B_1 (thiamin)
Adermin			Is vitamin B_6 (pyridoxine)
Adenylic acid	Adenine nucleotide		See Vitamin B_8
Factor S			See Biotin
Mouse factor		Eye inflammation, blindness, and dermatitis in absence	Rats do not develop on same deficiency diet
Antistiffness factor	Wulzen factor	Deficient animals develop calcium deposits in muscle	Fat-soluble; heat labile; found in raw cream

MINERALS

Minerals make up a very small part of the body weight (calcium, the most abundant, accounts for only about 2 percent). Nevertheless, minerals are required for many vital physiological mechanisms, in which their roles are for the most part not clearly identified. Some help to make up a suitable medium for protoplasmic activity (see Body Water, p. 49); these also have important osmotic functions, and some of them are required for the maintenance of acid-base balance. Others make up part of specialized compounds; e.g., iron in hemoglobin and iodine in the thyroid hormone. Still others are important constituents of enzyme systems. A number are integral parts of bones and teeth. Except for these last, most of the minerals of the body are in solution.

The animal body requires seven principal mineral elements: calcium, magnesium, sodium, potassium, phosphorus, sulfur, and chlorine. At least six of the so-called trace minerals are also necessary: iron, copper, iodine, manganese, cobalt, and zinc. It is not known whether fluorine, aluminum, and boron are required by man. In an ordinary adequate diet, the different types of food supply about the following fractions of the mineral intake: milk, 40 percent; meat and eggs, 25 percent; cereals, 15 percent; vegetables, 15 percent; and fruits and nuts, 5 percent. The sodium and chloride are obtained from salt.

The daily requirements for calcium and iron are given in Table 22 (p. 252). For adults, the phosphorus allowance is about one and one-half times that of calcium. When the calcium requirement is relatively high (as in childhood, during the latter part of pregnancy, and during lactation), the phosphorus intake need be little greater than that of calcium. In actual practice, a diet that is adequate in calcium and protein is also adequate in phosphorus.

Adults require 1 to 2 mg. of copper daily and children about 0.05 mg. per Kg. of body weight. A diet adequate in other respects ordinarily contains this amount. The requirement for iodine is small and is discussed on page 507. Little is known of the importance of other minerals to man. If they are required, the amounts supplied by natural foods are apparently more than enough.

The inorganic elements are absorbed chiefly in the small intestine, although water and diffusible monovalent ions also can pass through the mucosa of the stomach and large intestine. Before absorption, the solutions of mineral salts are made isotonic or nearly so by the gastro-intestinal secretions. The polyvalent ions are absorbed somewhat more slowly than the monovalent. Magnesium sulfate, which has two divalent ions, is relatively poorly absorbed and so acts as a cathartic (p. 385). After absorption, the minerals are transported to the tissues by the blood and lymph.

The skeleton is the main depot for calcium, magnesium, sodium, phosphate, and the trace minerals. Muscle stores magnesium, potassium, and sodium. The liver is able to store bismuth, cadmium, chromium, cobalt, copper, gold, iron, manganese, nickel, silver, thallium, antimony, arsenic, molybdenum, selenium, and vanadium. Tin and arsenic are found in the skin. The thyroid contains most of the iodine.

The normal adult is in a state of mineral equilibrium, with intake and excretion balanced. However, growth necessitates a positive balance. Mineral retention is high during the last two months of fetal life; this need is reflected in the high incidence of mineral deficiency in premature infants, who are prone to develop anemia and rickets. During lactation, the output of calcium and phosphorus is increased considerably. Diarrhea increases intestinal excretion of potassium, sodium, and chloride, whereas dehydration raises urinary excretion.

Certain minerals are discussed in more detail as follows:

Sodium, p. 341
Potassium, p. 342
Magnesium, p. 346
Chloride, p. 347
Phosphate, p. 347
Iron, p. 368

Calcium and iodine are discussed below.

CALCIUM

Calcium, the most abundant mineral in the body, makes up about 2 percent of the body weight. It is important not only for its ionic effects (see p. 344) but also because calcium phosphate and carbonate are the principal constituents of bone. During lactation, calcium is required for milk formation. Requirements of calcium are given in Table 22 (p. 252).

Calcium occurs in food in both organic and inorganic form, but it is probably absorbed only as inorganic salts. Milk is the best dietary source (content: about 0.12 percent). Significant amounts of calcium are also obtained from those vegetables (e.g., carrots, kale, and mustard greens, but not spinach or beet greens) which do not contain oxalic acid. Hard water may supply considerable amounts.

Absorption takes place mainly in the upper part of the small intestine and is favored by an acid medium. Many other complicated factors influence calcium absorption; included in them are the following phases of the diet: the amount of carbohydrate, fat, and protein and the ratio of calcium to phosphate. Spinach, rhubarb, and other foods containing oxalic acid reduce calcium absorption because of the formation of insoluble calcium oxalate. Calcium also forms an insoluble salt with phytic acid (inositol-hexaphosphoric acid), which occurs in cereals. Calcium is excreted partly in the urine and partly through the small intestine, the route depending to a certain extent on the acid-base balance (alkalosis favors the intestine).

Calcium metabolism is greatly influenced by the supply of parathyroid hormone (see pp. 195 and 475) and vitamin D (see p. 494). The former has no influence on absorption of calcium; the latter probably does, although there is some disagreement.

For ionic effects, calcium must generally be given parenterally; indications, available preparations, dosage, and details of administration are discussed on page 344. Calcium is given by mouth in the presence of relative or absolute deficiency. Supplementary calcium may be indicated in late pregnancy, during lactation, and in the presence of hyperthyroidism (p. 180) or hypoparathyroidism (p. 195). The following salts are available:

Dicalcium phosphate (dicalcium orthophosphate; Dibasic Calcium Phosphate, U.S.P.), $CaHPO_4 \cdot 2H_2O$. One gram of calcium is supplied by 4.3 Gm. of the salt, which also contains 0.77 Gm. of phosphorus (2.4 Gm. of phosphate ion). Dicalcium phosphate is indicated particularly in pregnancy and other conditions in which supplements of both calcium and phosphorus are needed. It is not a suitable preparation when a low phosphorus intake is desired, as in hypoparathyroidism.

Calcium gluconate, $(CH_2OH \cdot [CHOH]_4 \cdot COO)_2Ca \cdot H_2O$. One gram of calcium is contained in 11.2 Gm. of the salt. It is possibly the most palatable of the calcium salts but has the lowest calcium content.

Calcium lactate, $(CH_3 \cdot CHOH \cdot COO)_2Ca \cdot 5H_2O$. One gram of calcium is found in 7.7 Gm. of the salt. It is relatively palatable.

Calcium chloride, $CaCl_2 \cdot 2H_2O$. One gram of calcium is supplied by 3.7 Gm. of the salt. It is the most efficient but the least palatable preparation and often produces gastro-intestinal symptoms. It is sometimes given as a 25 percent solution in syrup or elixir of glycyrrhiza.

For most indications, the oral dose of calcium itself is 2 to 4 Gm. Usually the total daily quantity does not have to be exact. The patient may measure it

out in teaspoonfuls of powdered salt, dissolve it in warm water, and take one-third of it two hours after each meal. To promote absorption, it is sometimes helpful to administer at the same time 1 or 2 cc. of Diluted Hydrochloric Acid, U.S.P. (p. 384).

IODINE

Iodine is of physiological importance because it is an essential constituent of the thyroid hormone (p. 456). It is not found in nature in the free form; but its salts are distributed widely, although sparsely and irregularly.

The metabolism and the effects of ingested iodine depend on the form and amount in which it is taken and on the state of the organism. Elemental iodine (as in Lugol's solution) is converted into inorganic iodide in the gastro-intestinal tract, and its systemic effect is therefore the same as that of a corresponding quantity of inorganic iodide. Sodium iodide is very rapidly and completely absorbed. Iodide ion is almost as rapidly absorbed when potassium iodide is ingested, but the potassium apparently remains in the gastro-intestinal tract; the rise in blood potassium is very small, whereas the rise in blood sodium after ingestion of potassium iodide is almost as great as after sodium iodide.

Iodine in loose organic combination is probably reduced to inorganic iodide in the gastro-intestinal tract. Iodine which is tightly bound to organic compounds, as in iodophthalein and iodopyracet (Diodrast), is unavailable to the organism. Thyroglobulin is digested in the gastro-intestinal tract like any other protein, and it seems probable that if any is absorbed undigested, the percentage must be extremely small. It is not known whether the digestive enzymes break thyroglobulin down to amino acids or merely to polypeptides or proteoses. Polypeptides containing thyroxin are well absorbed.

After absorption, iodide is distributed uniformly throughout the extracellular fluid in the same way as are chloride and thiocyanate. It appears very quickly in the milk and saliva. It is rapidly excreted in the urine and sweat but not in the feces. The follicle cells of the thyroid seem to be the only tissue in the body having a specific affinity for iodide, and this ion appears to have no part in the normal body economy except to act as a source of iodine for the manufacture of thyroid hormone. In contrast to the blood level of organic iodine (thyroid hormone), that of inorganic iodide would seem to be no more than a reflection of recent iodide intake and saturation of the organism.

Apparently it is only the iodide ion (i.e., inorganic iodine) that is taken up by the thyroid gland. The capacity of the gland for iodine has a definite limit, but on a low iodine intake the thyroid can concentrate the element to more than 10,000 times the blood level. Three factors apparently influence the rate of uptake of iodine by the thyroid. The first of these is the character of the local thyroid tissue; for instance, adenomata have a slower uptake and a lower iodine content than the surrounding normal tissue. The second is the blood level of inorganic iodide, which is a reflection of iodine intake; a high blood level tends to keep the colloid "saturated," so that the iodine content is relatively high and only a small part of a fresh increment of iodine is taken up. The third factor is the circulating level of thyrotrophin from the anterior pituitary gland; although iodine can be taken up and converted to diiodotyrosine and thyroxin in the absence of thyrotrophin, the process is speeded and made more complete by the latter, especially the conversion to thyroxin.

Although the need for iodine varies with caloric turnover, rate of growth, and the presence of pregnancy and is, besides, difficult to determine accurately, the minimal daily requirement has been judged to be 15 to 40 micrograms; the optimal for an average adult man, no more than 200 micrograms. Deficiency of iodine leads to thyroid hyperplasia and to simple goiter (see p. 178).

Iodine needs are ordinarily met by the small quantities contained in vegetables and drinking water. However, in some inland areas (in the United States, notably the north central and northwestern parts) the soil does not contain enough iodine to supply it to water and to growing plants. In these areas, the so-called goiter belts, deficiency is common. The simplest means of remedying the situation is the use, in cooking and at the table, of iodized salt containing 0.01 percent potassium iodide plus a stabilizer. Because of the efficiency of iodine conservation in the body, it is possible as an alternative to administer single prophylactic doses (50 mg. or more) twice yearly.

Iodine has a definite, although limited, ameliorating effect on hyperthyroidism, usually causing a fall of about 15 percent in the basal metabolic rate and a corresponding symptomatic improvement. The minimum dosage necessary to produce this effect is generally about 6 mg. of iodine per day, or roughly one hundred times the minimum daily physiological requirement. The response usually begins within a few days and levels off after a week. There appears to be no advantage in greatly exceeding 10 mg. daily. On the other hand, the preliminary administration of much smaller doses, such as 1 mg. daily, may in some cases interfere with subsequent response to adequate doses.

The advent of the antithyroid drugs (p. 458) has rendered obsolete the use of iodine as the sole preoperative medication preparatory to thyroidectomy, except in very mild cases. However, once hyperthyroidism has been brought under control by means of an antithyroid drug, iodine is valuable supplementary therapy; it causes involution of the gland and generally makes possible reduction in dosage of the antithyroid drug. For this purpose, a daily dosage of 10 mg. of iodine is adequate. As a preoperative measure, iodine is of value because the involution which it causes reduces the vascularity of the gland and makes the latter easier to handle at operation.

Iodine has also been used as a fibrolytic agent, as an "alterative," as an expectorant, and as an antiseptic. In syphilis and in other granulomatous diseases, such as leprosy, sporotrichosis, blastomycosis, and actinomycosis, the iodide ion in large doses appears to have a fibrolytic and healing action. Although recognizing that it is a nonspecific remedy, most syphilologists recommend it as an adjunct to bismuth and mercury in syphilis for its effect as a resolver of granulomatous processes, a stimulator of resistance in prolonged small-dose administration, and an aid in "loosening up" entrenched processes. Obviously such treatment is highly empirical, and there is no satisfactory explanation of its mechanism; iodide does not kill the organism or influence resistance in a measurable way. Its importance in connection with penicillin therapy is less certain, and as more-powerful specific treatment becomes available, the need for iodides can be expected to diminish.

In contrast to other granulomatous diseases, tuberculosis is adversely affected by iodides; their administration is often followed by exacerbation and spread of the disease process. Iodides are therefore considered to be strongly contraindicated in the presence of tuberculous infection.

The concept of general "alterative" medication has lost greatly in popularity as detailed knowledge of physiology and pharmacology has increased and the standards for clinical evaluation have become more critical. A generation ago, iodides were given almost routinely in arteriosclerosis and during convalescence from apoplexy. They are now little used in these conditions; if they have any action, it has not been objectively demonstrated and its possible mechanism is unknown.

Iodides have long been given as expectorants in asthma, chronic bronchitis, and the later stages of acute bronchitis. This use is described on page 380.

Free elemental iodine is an effective germicide, fungicide, amebicide, and virucide. This property is discussed on page 306.

All available evidence indicates that it is the iodide ion which is responsible for all the systemic actions of iodine. The simple salts, sodium or potassium iodide, administered by mouth, meet all the needs for systemic iodine therapy under ordinary circumstances. The sodium salt is prescribed only in solution because it is hygroscopic. It is less irritating to the gastro-intestinal tract than is the potassium salt. Potassium iodide may be given as tablets, but preferably in enteric coating. The saturated solutions have the great disadvantage of variability because of the extreme change of solubility of the salts with temperature. It is preferable to employ 100 percent solutions (w/v). For easier calculation of small dosage, one can employ a 21.23 percent solution of potassium iodide or a 19.17 percent solution of sodium iodide, the strength of each of which is such that one minim provides 10 mg. of iodine. The taste is well disguised by mixing each dose with rich milk a few hours before ingestion. Hydriodic Acid Syrup, U.S.P., may be more acceptable to children. Table 58 gives the iodine content of convenient quantities of commonly used preparations.

A traditional dosage form is Lugol's solution (compound iodine solution; Strong Iodine Solu-

TABLE 58 — *Iodine Content of Commonly Used Preparations*

Preparation and Dose	Iodine Content, in mg.
Sodium iodide solution, 100% (w/v), 1 min.	52
Sodium iodide solution, 19.17% (w/v), 1 min.	10
Potassium iodide, 5 grs.	248
Potassium iodide solution, 100% (w/v), 1 min.	47
Potassium iodide solution, 100% (w/v), 5 min.	236
Potassium iodide solution, 21.23% (w/v), 1 min.	10
Lugol's solution, 1 min. (total iodine)	7.8
Lugol's solution, 30 min. (total iodine)	234
Lugol's solution, 1 cc. (total iodine)	126
Hydriodic Acid Syrup, U.S.P., 5 cc. (1 av. tsp.)	70
Hydriodic Acid Syrup, U.S.P., 10 min.	8.6

tion, U.S.P.), which contains 5 percent elemental iodine in a 10 percent solution of potassium iodide. Lugol's solution has no advantage as a source of iodine, and it is needlessly complex and has an extraordinarily unpleasant taste.

Not all clinicians are in agreement as to iodine dosage in syphilis; some favor "small" doses, 15 to 30 grains daily, and others favor large, 75 to 300 or more. Stokes considers 5 to 15 grains of potassium iodide daily as small dosage to be used over long periods as a stimulator of immunity and, more specifically, in cutaneous late syphilis. "Moderate" doses of 30 to 100 grains are advocated in visceral syphilis. Small to moderate doses are recommended for syphilitic cardiovascular disease. Large doses of 150 to 1,500 grains (10 to 100 Gm.) daily are advised for all cases of active neurosyphilis, including early, asymptomatic, diffuse, meningeal, meningovascular, vascular, and gummatous lesions.

Regardless of anticipated eventual dosage level, the initial dose of iodide should not exceed 5 grains (0.32 Gm.). If no side-effects occur, dosage is increased fairly rapidly. Dilution of the drug and subdivision of dosage increase tolerance. Except when enteric-coated tablets are employed, iodides should be taken with plenty of fluid; a glass of water is recommended for each 50 grains. The drug is best taken before meals. In cases of severe gastro-intestinal intolerance, it is sometimes possible to give very large doses by dissolving the total daily quantity in six quarts of water and administering it as a beverage throughout the day.

In the granulomatous systemic fungus infections, dosage varies with the disease and with the patient. In blastomycosis the largest possible doses should be given, whereas in actinomycosis very large doses sometimes appear to be less effective than moderate doses.

For the loosening of bronchial secretions in asthma, iodide is usually given in doses of 10 grains three to five times daily.

Gastro-intestinal intolerance to iodides usually takes the form of nausea or diarrhea or both. It may, however, include anorexia, vomiting, and intestinal cramps. It seems to be due to local irritation. Many patients notice the metallic, bitter taste of the iodide which is secreted in the saliva. Rarely, iodine produces aseptic parotitis.

Although the iodides are not toxic in the ordinary sense, some patients develop an idiosyncrasy to them which goes under the name of "iodism." The condition is poorly understood, even though it has been much studied. It appears, however, to be related to the quantity of iodide administered and, more importantly, to the state of the patient. The form in which the element is administered does not seem to be of influence, and the occurrence of iodism on one occasion does not necessarily indicate recurrence if iodine is given at a later time.

Table 59 outlines the observed manifestations of iodism. With small doses, coryza and acne are most common. Curiously, they may disappear when the dosage is abruptly increased to 90 grains or more daily. External application of iodine may be followed by various kinds of rashes and swellings and even exfoliative dermatitis.

The more severe forms of iodism require immediate discontinuation of the drug, following which recovery is ordinarily rapid. In a rare patient, however, the condition may persist and even prove fatal. The elimination of iodide can be hastened by administration of large quantities of fluids (4 liters daily) and sodium chloride (5 to 10 Gm. daily). However, in cases of extreme iodism, such treatment may be ineffective.

Contraindications to iodide therapy include

TABLE 59 — *Manifestations of Iodism*

Skin	acneform, maculopapular, vegetative (including frambesiform, fungating, and granulomatous), vesicular, or bullous eruptions
Mucous membranes	coryza, conjunctivitis, bronchial irritation, general swelling, and inflammation
Vascular system	edema (including angioneurotic edema), erythema, purpura, erythema multiforme (which may affect the skin and mucous membranes)
General	fever, nervous irritability

tuberculous infection (previously discussed) and adenoma of the thyroid gland. Hyperthyroidism has occasionally appeared to be induced by iodides in the presence of an otherwise benign thyroid adenoma. Mercurial preparations should not be applied to the skin of patients receiving iodine therapy; the mercuric iodide which is formed in the skin may prove to be extremely irritating.

ANTIHISTAMINIC DRUGS

In 1933, Fourneau and Bovet developed a compound which would protect guinea pigs against lethal doses of histamine. It was, however, extremely toxic of itself. As time went on, other investigators found progressively more potent and less toxic preparations, until it became possible to apply drugs of this type clinically.

Allergic reactions are believed to be mediated by histamine or substances with similar properties ("H-substances") or a combination of them. If this is true, a compound which is capable of blocking the action of histamine should prevent the manifestations of allergy. In considerable degree this has turned out to be the case, and the antihistaminic drugs have quickly become of great value in the symptomatic treatment of allergy. However, they do not constitute an entire answer to the problem of allergy: They are relatively ineffective in some persons; they do not protect against extremely powerful stimuli; they may have side-effects; and, in practice, they have not abolished the need for avoidance of contact with allergens, correction of other contributing factors, and hyposensitization with antigen extracts.

The antihistaminic drugs which have found widest clinical use in the United States are derivatives of dimethylaminoethane (see Figure 57). Many other types of substances have antihistaminic activity, however, and the search for more effective ones is active.

The mechanism of antihistaminic activity is not known. It is postulated that these drugs compete with histamine for a receptor substance or a site of action in a manner analogous to the antibacterial action of the sulfonamides. It is of interest that antihistaminic drugs have certain resemblances to local anesthetic drugs (p. 441); parts of their molecules may be related chemically (compare Figures 37 and 57, pp. 444 and 510), many antihistaminics have a slight local anesthetic effect, and some of the local anesthetics appear to have an antihistaminic effect.

Antihistaminic drugs are most effective against the following allergic manifestations:

Hay fever (p. 264)

Pruritus, acute urticaria, or angioneurotic edema due to food or drug allergy (pp. 267 and 268)

Serum sickness (p. 268)

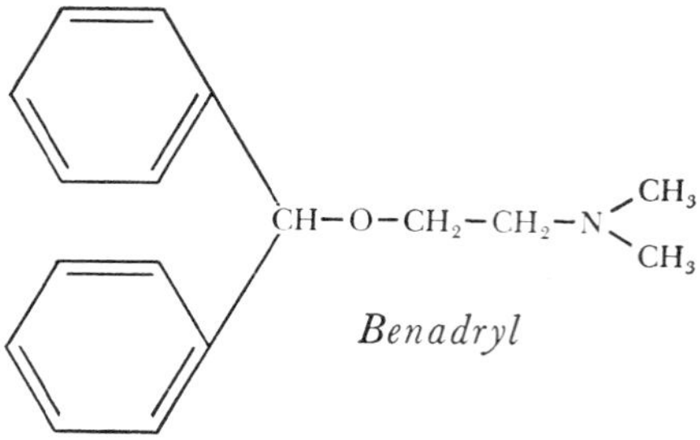

Benadryl

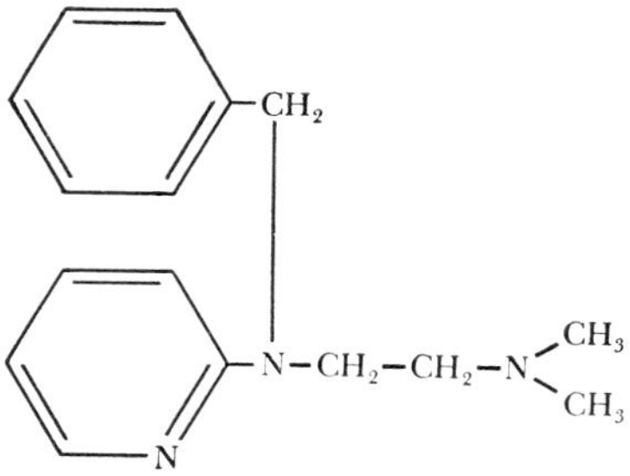

Pyribenzamine

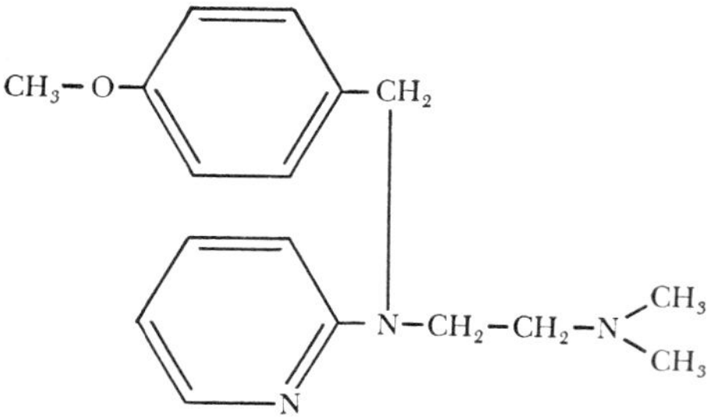

Neo-Antergan

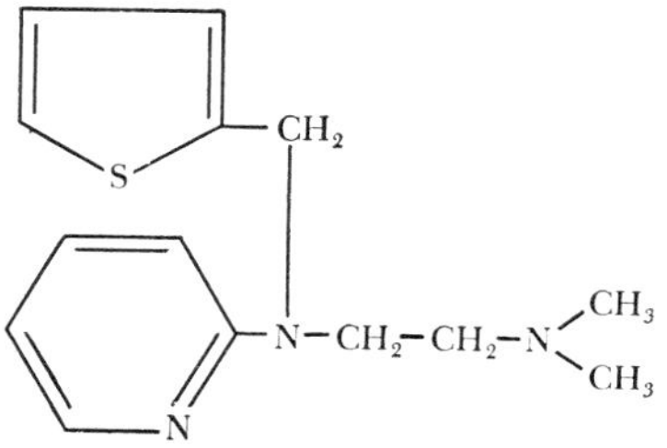

Thenylpyramine
(*'Histadyl'*)

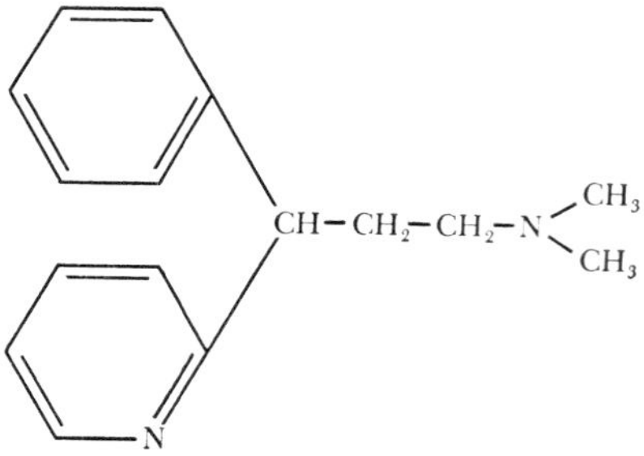

Trimeton

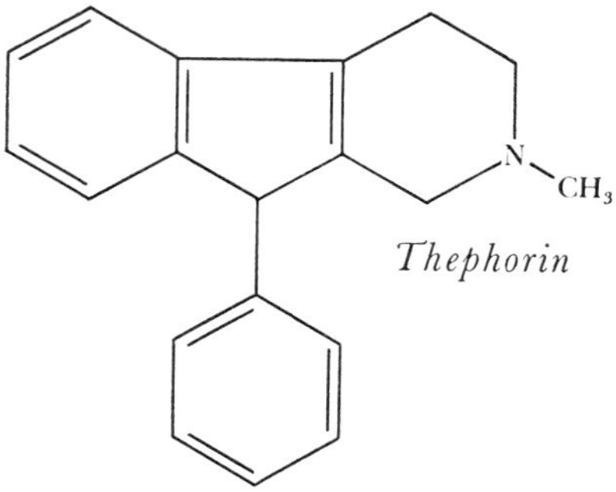

Thephorin

FIGURE 57—*Structural Formulas of Antihistaminic Drugs*

They are somewhat less effective against:
Vasomotor rhinitis
Atopic dermatitis and eczema (p. 268)
Chronic urticaria (p. 267)
Allergic cough
They are generally unsatisfactory in bronchial asthma. In headache associated with known food allergy they may give prompt relief, but in other instances headache believed to be of allergic origin has not been affected. Their value in gastro-intestinal allergy has not been adequately assessed. Recent investigations suggest that certain symptoms of infection may represent allergy to the infecting organism and may be subject to control by antihistaminic drugs. Other types of symptoms not hitherto considered to be allergic are also currently being studied.

The antihistaminic drugs are usually given by mouth for systemic effect. Some of them may be given intramuscularly or, slowly and with great caution, intravenously when a rapid and especially powerful action is needed. In allergic dermatitis they may be applied locally in lotions or ointments. Frequently they can be advantageously combined with adrenergic (such as ephedrine) and with anticholinergic drugs (such as atropine) in controlling allergic symptoms.

Different individuals vary greatly in their relative therapeutic response to the different antihistaminics; a drug that is effective in one patient may be ineffective in another. In some patients a given preparation may "wear out" and become ineffective; after a rest period its action is restored for that patient. For these reasons it is well to try a different drug if the results are or become unsatisfactory.

Side-effects are not uncommon. Usually they are mild. They include drowsiness, dizziness, visual disturbances, faintness, headache, nervousness, weakness, lassitude, dryness of the mouth, nausea and vomiting, epigastric distress, and diarrhea. Often they disappear on continued administration. Excessive doses are commonly stimulative to the central nervous system and may produce mental stimulation or convulsions.

When patients begin taking a new antihistaminic drug, they should be cautioned against driving a car or undertaking other potentially dangerous activities until they ascertain whether or not their co-ordination and skill will be temporarily affected by the drug.

Many different preparations are available for clinical use as antihistaminic drugs, and the number seems destined to increase. Six have been chosen for discussion on the basis of widespread use, outstanding effectiveness, freedom from side-effects, or unusual action.

Benadryl (diphenhydramine) is the benzhydryl ether of dimethylaminoethane (see Figure 57). It was the first antihistaminic drug to be marketed in the United States. In distinction from other antihistaminic drugs, it has an anticholinergic (atropine-like) action as well, which makes it of some value in motion sickness and Parkinsonism and may account for the side-effect of dry mouth. The usual adult dose is 50 mg. every six to eight hours, which may be doubled or halved as necessary. It may be given intramuscularly or, with caution, intravenously, the initial dose not exceeding 20 mg. Drowsiness is a common side-effect; others listed a few paragraphs above occur less frequently.

Benadryl combines chemically with 8-chlorotheophylline to form a compound called Dramamine, or dimenhydrinate, which has proved effective in preventing and relieving motion sickness.

Pyribenzamine (tripelennamine) is N,N-dimethyl-N′-benzyl-N′-α-pyridylethylenediamine (see Figure 57). It is an effective antihistaminic drug with a relatively low incidence of side-effects. The average adult dose is 50 mg. every six to eight hours by mouth.

Neo-Antergan (pyranisamine) differs chemically from Pyribenzamine in the presence of a methoxy group in the para position in the benzyl portion of the molecule. Its dosage and effects are similar to those of Pyribenzamine.

Thenylpyramine, which is marketed by Eli Lilly and Company as 'Histadyl' (other names include methapyrilene and Thenylene), differs from Pyribenzamine in having an α-thenyl group in place of the benzyl (see Figure 57). It also is an effective antihistaminic with a very low incidence of side-effects. The average oral dose is 50 to 100 mg. four or five times daily. It may be given subcutaneously or intramuscularly if necessary for rapid and powerful action, the usual dose being 20 mg. In great emergency it may be given intravenously (very slowly!); the initial dose should not exceed 10 mg.

Trimeton (prophenpyridamine), although fundamentally similar to Pyribenzamine, differs in the linkage of the phenyl and pyridyl groups and in the absence of one nitrogen atom. (Trimeton is thus not a derivative of ethylenediamine, nor does it have the ether linkage of Benadryl; see Figure 57). It is a promptly acting and powerful antihistaminic drug. The average dose is 12 to 25 mg. three or four times daily by mouth. The incidence of side-effects appears to be comparable to that with Pyribenzamine.

Thephorin (phenindamine) differs considerably in its chemical structure from the previously men-

tioned drugs; however, the pyridine ring may be looked upon as a dimethylaminoethyl group which has undergone ring closure (see Figure 57). Thephorin differs from other antihistaminics in that, in the upper therapeutic range of dosage, it may induce wakefulness and mental stimulation rather than drowsiness. The usual dosage is 25 mg. one to six times daily.

MISCELLANEOUS PREPARATIONS

THIOCYANATE

Potassium thiocyanate (sulfocyanate), KSCN, is used in the treatment of essential hypertension (p. 84). It is of most value for the relief of hypertensive headache, for which purpose it is probably the most effective agent at present available. Other symptoms such as insomnia, dizziness, emotional instability, and fatigability are affected in lesser but often satisfactory degree. In many cases, the level of blood pressure is significantly reduced. The mechanism of these effects is unknown.

The thiocyanate ion is readily absorbed from the gastro-intestinal tract and is distributed throughout the extracellular fluid. It is excreted (mainly by the kidneys) unchanged but at a variable and unpredictable rate.

Patients should be carefully selected for thiocyanate therapy. In general, greatest benefit is obtained in those who have severe symptoms and little vascular disease. Those with severe vascular degeneration or renal excretory impairment are less likely to be helped, and in them administration of thiocyanate should be cautious because the rate of excretion depends on renal function. The drug should definitely not be given if the blood nonprotein nitrogen level is elevated.

Many patients who have not improved following sympathectomy respond favorably to thiocyanate. On the other hand, the malignant form of hypertension responds poorly as a rule. The drug should be stopped during febrile periods and prior to surgical procedures because of unpredictable variations in excretion.

The effectiveness and safety of thiocyanate therapy are related to blood level of the drug rather than to dosage. For this reason, *it is essential that blood thiocyanate determinations be the guide to dosage. If close observation and frequent blood level determinations*

are not possible, the drug should not be employed. As Barker has said: "The smallest amount [of thiocyanate] that will relieve symptoms and bring clinical improvement should be used. The reduction in blood pressure is of secondary importance even though such pressure changes often parallel the clinical improvements. Perhaps the greatest abuse of thiocyanate therapy has been its casual administration with an overemphasis of the reading obtained from the blood pressure machine."

The usually effective, safe blood thiocyanate concentration is from 8 to 12 mg. per 100 cc. The Test Kit No. 1 for Blood Thiocyanate Estimation (p. 625) is available for determinations. It should be understood, however, that sometimes excellent clinical results are achieved at lower levels, and in such cases the lower levels should be maintained. Blood concentrations much higher than 12 mg. per 100 cc. predispose to toxic manifestations. The latter increase rapidly when levels exceed 20 mg. per 100 cc. and may become serious at 35 to 50 mg. per 100 cc.

Because of the variable excretion, dosage must be revised frequently in accordance with blood thiocyanate concentration. Treatment may be started with doses of 0.2 Gm. taken by mouth three times daily for the first three days and twice daily for the remainder of a week. At the end of the week, the blood level of thiocyanate is determined and inquiry is made regarding symptomatic improvement or side-effects. The dosage is decreased if the blood pressure drops sharply during the first week or two or if fatigue or depression is great enough to interfere with the patient's sense of well-being. Otherwise, the dosage is adjusted by trial in order to maintain a blood level of 8 to 12 mg. per 100 cc. Determinations are made once a week.

Clinical improvement usually begins after two to four weeks but may be delayed for several months. There may also be a fall in systolic blood pressure and, later, a drop in diastolic. Persistent symptomatic improvement may be expected in about 50 percent of patients, the figure depending partly on the choice of patients and partly on the adequacy of supervision.

During the early months of treatment, a total daily dose of 0.4 Gm. should rarely be exceeded. Later, as little as 0.3 Gm. *weekly* or as much as 1 Gm. daily may be required for maintenance. It is to be emphasized that there is no constant dosage at which either a toxic or a therapeutic effect can be expected.

Many different types of side-effects have been noted in the course of thiocyanate therapy. The drug may produce gastric irritation. For this reason and for the sake of precise dosage, potassium thiocyanate is better given as enteric-coated tablets than as a liquid preparation. Thiocyanate has a slight but definite antithyroid action (see p. 458) which can be prevented by an adequate iodine intake (use of iodized salt). In the presence of iodine deficiency, goiter and even hypothyroidism may develop, but only after long periods of thiocyanate therapy. The drug also increases calcium excretion, and an adequate calcium intake should be assured to prevent osteoporosis and the symptom of arthralgia, particularly of the arches of the feet.

Fatigue, somnolence, and mental retardation are often encountered during the first four to six weeks of thiocyanate medication. They call for reduction of dosage for a few weeks, after which they usually disappear. After several months the skin may become dry and scaly, and there may be secondary anemia. If the red cell count falls much below 4 million, thiocyanate should be discontinued until the count rises to 4.25 to 4.5 million. Toxic dermatitis may occasionally be seen in the form of a maculopapular, itching, scaling eruption which appears usually on the flexor surfaces of the wrists and forearms or on the lower third of the legs. It is ordinarily controlled by the antihistaminic drugs (p. 509) or by vitamin C (50 mg. three times daily by mouth). There may also be cracking at the corners of the mouth and eyes and falling of the hair. If these reactions are severe, the drug should be discontinued until they subside. Angina pectoris and thrombophlebitis have been noted during the course of thiocyanate therapy, but there is some question as to a causal relationship.

High blood levels of thiocyanate may lead to fever, purpura, vasomotor collapse with hypotension and weakness, anuria, delirium, convulsions, toxic psychosis, coma, and death.

A considerable early fall in blood pressure at a low blood level of thiocyanate may be a warning signal of impending toxicity. A rapid fall should also be avoided in arteriosclerotic hypertensives.

Large doses of salicylates, including acetylsalicylic acid, should be avoided during thiocyanate administration because they may give a color reaction similar to that of thiocyanate and thereby interfere with accurate colorimetric determination of blood thiocyanate level.

NEGATAN

'Negatan' (Negatol, Lilly) is a water-soluble, highly acid, colloidal compound having protein-precipitating, bactericidal, protozoacidal, fungicidal, and styptic effects. It contains polymerized disulfonic-dioxy-dimethyl-diphenyl-methane acid substances of relatively high molecular weight and is made by reacting sulfonated metacresol and formaldehyde. A 5 percent solution of 'Negatan' has a pH close to that of N/10 hydrochloric acid.

Solution 'Negatan' (about 45 percent, w/w) may be applied topically to the cervix uteri in treatment of cervicitis, erosions, and ulcerations. It is an effective styptic and is particularly useful in controlling hemorrhage from carcinoma of the cervix. For trichomonad infestation (p. 198), proper dilutions of Solution 'Negatan' may be used as vaginal douches and for instillation into the male or female urethra. Suppositories 'Negatan,' containing 0.133 to 0.147 Gm. (5 percent), are intended for vaginal use.

Solution 'Negatan' may be applied full-strength to the cervix to stimulate epithelization and promote healing two to four weeks after cautery for cervicitis. Cervical erosions may also be painted with full-strength Solution 'Negatan.' A cotton applicator saturated with the solution and placed in the external cervical os will coagulate the mucous plug and facilitate its removal. The Solution 'Negatan' may then be applied more effectively to the cervical glands. A tampon or packing, saturated with 'Negatan' in a 1:10 dilution in water or glycerin, is then inserted into the vagina. The tampon or packing is removed after twenty-four hours and may be followed by a douche of plain water or of diluted 'Negatan' (one to two teaspoonfuls of Solution 'Negatan' to a quart of water). This treatment should be repeated twice weekly until there is no longer evidence of infection.

In treating vaginitis due to *Trichomonas vaginalis*, fungi (including *Candida* [*Monilia*] *albicans*), or nonspecific cause, the following regimen may be employed. The vaginal vault is cleansed thoroughly with green soap, rinsed, and dried. All surfaces are then painted with a 1:10 dilution of 'Negatan.' (On subsequent visits, if there is no evidence of intolerance to the preparation, dilutions of 1:5 and stronger may be used.) Following the topical application, a tampon saturated with 'Negatan,' 1:10, may be inserted, with instructions that it be removed at bedtime. After removal of the tampon, a suppository of 'Negatan' should be inserted. The suppositories are used nightly for one week, and the office treatment is then repeated. A cleansing douche is used just before insertion of the suppository.

As an alternative to the above, a douche of Solution 'Negatan,' 1 1/2 tablespoonfuls to a quart, may be followed by an application of full-strength Solution 'Negatan' to the entire vaginal vault. A thick white film forms which later separates, leaving a healthy mucous membrane.

It may be advisable to paint also the urethral meatus, introitus, vulva, and anal regions, particularly if pruritus is present. Three or four office treatments are usually sufficient to eliminate the infection. Recurrence may be reduced by the use of 'Negatan' douches following active therapy, especially immediately before and after each menstrual period.

Trichomonas infection in men may be treated by urethral irrigations or instillations of diluted Solution 'Negatan,' 1 or 2 percent (2 or 4 teaspoonfuls to the quart).

'Negatan' may also be used to treat pruritus of the female perineum and labia characterized by brawny induration, diffuse dermatitis, fissures, and parchmentlike skin. 'Negatan' is destructive to inflamed epithelium but has very little effect on normal tissue. After one or two applications the pathological epithelium comes away, leaving a clean surface. Subsequent therapy consists in application of antiseptic and emollient ointments.

Very few side-effects to 'Negatan' have been reported. In clinical use, the compound seems to have little effect on intact skin. Following treatment, there may be formed in the vagina a grayish coagulum consisting of superficial layers of vaginal epithelium, precipitated protein, and the medicament itself. At times the coagulum may be discharged in the form of a cast of the vagina and cervix, but more often it comes away in fragments with the douche or is removed at the time of treatment by gentle traction with forceps. Almost invariably, the underlying mucous membrane is found to be pink and unbroken, with no evidence of inflammatory or adverse reaction of any kind.

Patients undergoing treatment with 'Negatan' should be warned to wear a perineal pad to prevent soiling of clothing, since 'Negatan,' because of its acidity, will destroy fabrics with which it comes in contact.

Some patients may complain of moderate burning when 'Negatan' is first applied. In case of persistent complaint, the use of 'Negatan' should be discontinued until the cause is determined.

DIMERCAPROL

Dimercaprol (BAL, British Anti-Lewisite) was developed during World War II for treatment of injuries due to arsenical blister gases. This drug, 2,3-dimercaptopropanol, $CH_2SH \cdot CHSH \cdot CH_2OH$, is a colorless liquid soluble in water to 6 percent. In peanut oil it dissolves to 5 percent; but if two parts of benzyl benzoate are added for each part of drug, it is soluble in all proportions.

Its therapeutic action is based on its ability to compete with the thiol groups of tissue proteins for arsenic and other heavy metals. The drug may combine with the metal before the latter combines with the tissues, or it may actually remove the metal from combination with the tissues. In either case, a soluble BAL-thio-metal compound is formed which is excreted readily by the kidneys.

Dimercaprol is effective in contact poisoning with arsenicals such as Lewisite. It is useful in the toxic manifestations of arsenotherapy, including arsenical dermatitis, hemorrhagic encephalitis, hepatitis, agranulocytosis, and "arsenical fever." Experience has shown the drug to be valuable, and in some instances remarkably so, in treating human mercury and gold poisoning. (The use of the drug to relieve toxic reactions due to gold in the treatment of arthritis has been noted by some to be followed by relapse of the disease.) In animals, the drug is an effective antidote to acute poisoning by antimony, bismuth, chromium, and nickel, but it is ineffective against lead, thallium, and selenium. The drug is not recommended for the treatment of lead poisoning in man. The compound formed by cadmium and dimercaprol appears to be toxic in itself.

Successful treatment demands that the drug be given as early as possible. In skin lesions due to contact with Lewisite or to systemic poisoning, dimercaprol may be applied locally as a 5 percent ointment. It is absorbed through damaged or intact skin.

In systemic arsenic poisoning, an effective dosage schedule is 3 mg. per Kg. intramuscularly (as a

10 percent solution in 20 percent benzyl benzoate in peanut oil) every four hours for the first two days, every six hours on the third day, and every twelve hours thereafter for ten days or until recovery. In milder cases, the dosage and duration of treatment may be reduced somewhat; a suggested schedule is 2.5 mg. per Kg. every six hours for the first two days, every twelve hours on the third day, and one injection per day for the succeeding ten days or until recovery.

In mercury poisoning an effective dosage schedule is an initial dose of 5 mg. per Kg. intramuscularly, followed in one or two hours by a dose of 2.5 mg. per Kg., with two more 2.5-mg. doses being given in the first twelve hours, two doses on the second day, and one on the third. The usual supportive therapy should not be omitted.

Toxic reactions to the drug include paresthesias (burning or tingling of the nose, eyes, mouth, and skin), perspiration and sense of warmth, generalized muscular aching, pain (limbs, jaws, abdomen, head), lacrimation, blepharospasm, salivation, nausea, vomiting, unrest, apprehension, weakness and fatigue, acceleration of heart rate, sense of constriction of the chest, and increased systolic and diastolic blood pressure. Toxic symptoms may occur after doses of 3 to 5 mg. per Kg. and are almost always seen after 8 mg. The effects of doses up to 8 mg. per Kg. are reversible and last only an hour or two. As much as 5 mg. per Kg. every four hours for four successive injections is usually without incident; however, the same quantity given at two-hour intervals may be distinctly toxic. In experimental animals the larger doses cause capillary damage.

Dimercaprol may also induce hypersensitivity, particularly on local application, with resulting erythema, edema, and papule formation in the skin following subsequent administration. Such reactions can usually be prevented by preliminary medication with ephedrine sulfate, 25 or 50 mg., or an antihistaminic drug (p. 509).

GOLD

Gold has been employed as a therapeutic agent for many centuries. In modern therapy, its use is restricted almost completely to the treatment of rheumatoid arthritis (p. 248). However, toxic effects are common, and there is some disagreement as to whether the improvement is sufficient and occurs frequently enough to outweigh the harmful potentialities.

The mechanism of action of gold is unknown.

After absorption, it is carried in the protein fraction of the blood plasma, and most of it is stored for long periods in the skin, liver, and kidneys. During its slow elimination, 70 to 80 percent is excreted in the urine and small amounts appear in the feces. Plasma levels remain fairly constant regardless of accumulation.

Gold is available as a therapeutic agent in several forms. Perhaps most commonly used is gold and sodium thiosulfate, $AuNa_3(S_2O_3)_2 \cdot 2H_2O$, which contains 37 percent gold, is water-soluble, and may be given intramuscularly or intravenously. Also available are gold sodium thiomalate (Myochrysine), $NaOOC \cdot CH_2 \cdot CHSAu \cdot COONa$, and gold thioglucose (Solganal), $C_6H_{11}O_5SAu$; these compounds contain about 50 percent gold and are water-soluble, but they are usually given intramuscularly as oil suspensions for slow absorption and to reduce the incidence of reactions. Another form is colloidal gold sulfate, which contains 87 percent gold; it disappears rapidly from the blood stream and is less toxic than the others, but it apparently has less therapeutic effect.

Various therapeutic regimens have been described, almost all calling for intravenous (gold and sodium thiosulfate) or intramuscular injections. All doses should be increased approximately one-third when the thiosulfate is used because of its lower gold content. One method consists in an initial dose of 5 mg. followed by weekly doses increasing to a maximum of 50 mg. for women and 75 mg. for men until a total of 750 to 1,000 mg. has been given in ten to fifteen weeks. Some advocate weekly doses of 12.5 to 25 mg., with a total of 500 mg. per course. Still others prefer up to 100 mg. per week, with a total dosage of 2,000 mg. All are agreed that one to three months should intervene between successive courses. It is questionable whether a second course should be undertaken if no discernible improvement has occurred with the first course. If there has been no response to 2,000 mg. of the drug, it is very doubtful whether additional doses will be successful. Maintenance doses of 50 mg. may be given every two to three weeks after completion of the courses of therapy. The drugs are contraindicated in patients with severe nephritis, hepatitis, decided hypertension, or a bleeding tendency.

Whenever gold therapy is used, great care and watchfulness must be maintained, and periodic examinations of the blood should be made. In 20 to 60 percent of cases, there are toxic manifestations varying from slight symptoms to death. Severe reactions may be expected in approximately 3 to

4 percent, and death in approximately 0.5 percent. Toxic reactions include generalized pruritus, seborrheic dermatitis, urticaria, purpura, secondary anemia, agranulocytosis, exfoliative dermatitis, stomatitis, glossitis, gastroenteritis, jaundice, and conjunctivitis. Other manifestations include peripheral neuritis, dizziness, nausea, vomiting, nephritis, nephrosis, and acute yellow atrophy of the liver. Untoward reactions demand immediate cessation of therapy and administration of dimercaprol (see p. 514). Unfortunately, dimercaprol halts the therapeutic as well as the toxic effects of gold.

SECTION *3*

Color Plates

*Plates 1 to 19**   **Anatomic Charts**

Plates 20 to 28   **Skin Lesions Commonly Misdiagnosed**

Plates 29 to 42†   **The Blood in Health and Disease**

Plate 43   **Flocculation Tests
for the Serodiagnosis of Syphilis**

Plate 44   **Pertussis Agglutination Test**

Plate 45   **Gastric Analysis**

Plate 46   **Urine Test Charts**

** The original drawings for Plates 1 to 19 inclusive were made by
Daisy Stilwell.*

*† Plates 29 to 42 inclusive were obtained through the courtesy of
Louis R. Limarzi, M.D., Associate Professor of Medicine, University of Illinois.*

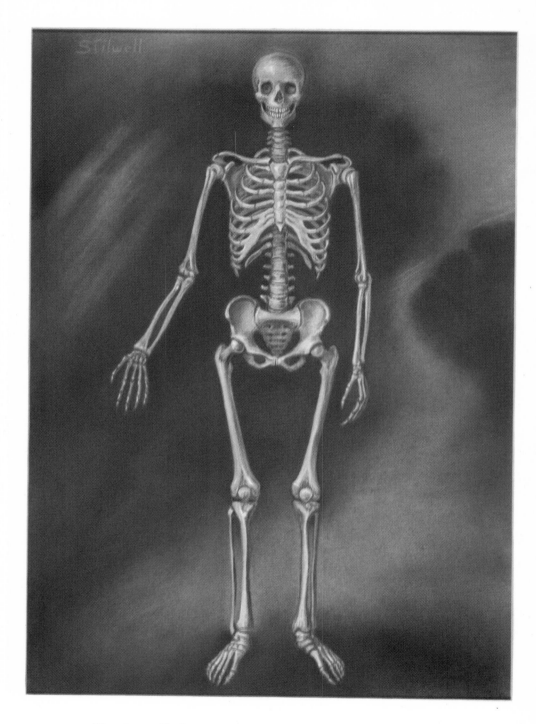

Plate 1   **Skeleton** *— anterior view*

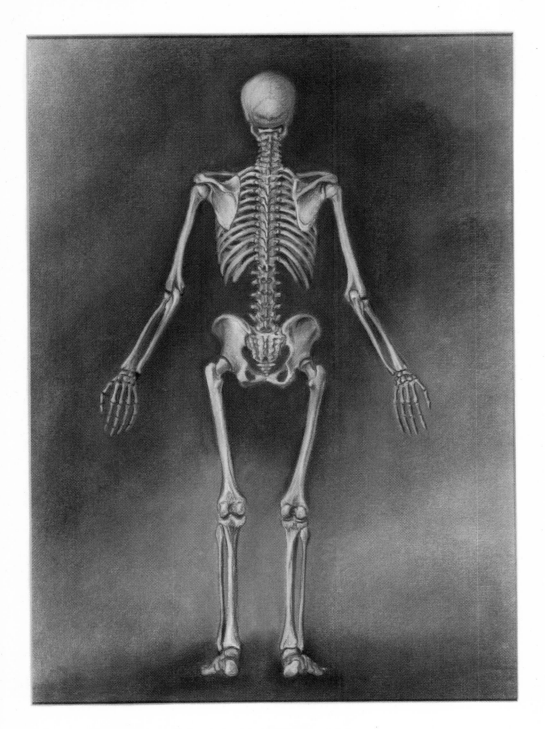

Plate 2   **Skeleton — *posterior view***

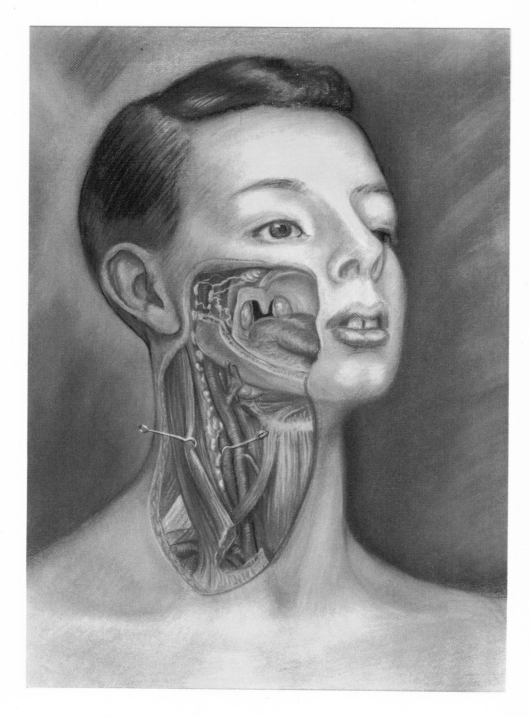

Plate 3　　Dissection of neck, including tonsils, adenoids, and their lymphatic drainage

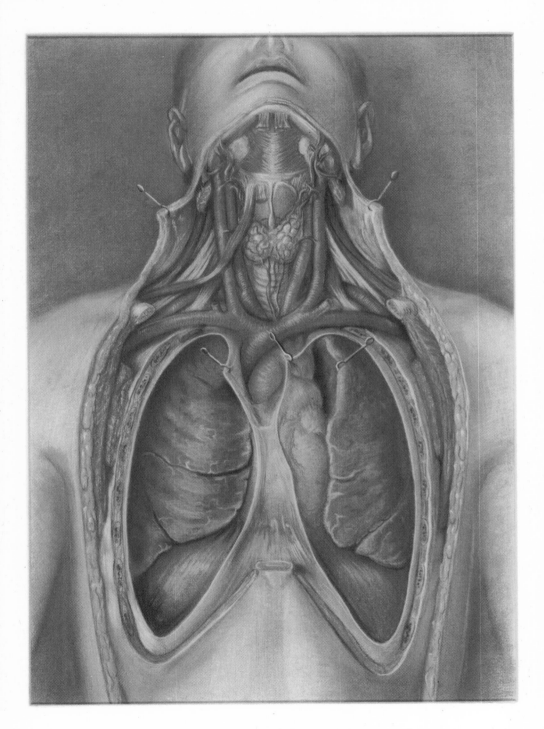

Plate 4   Chest and neck — *anterior dissection*

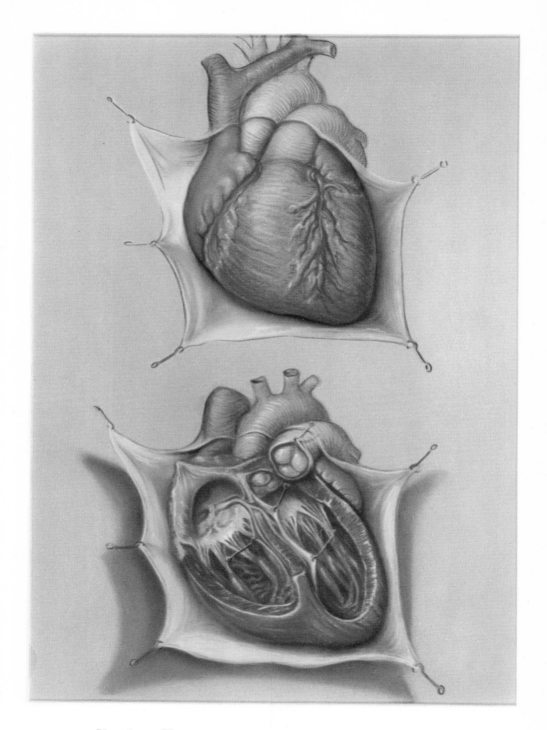

Plate 5   **Heart**

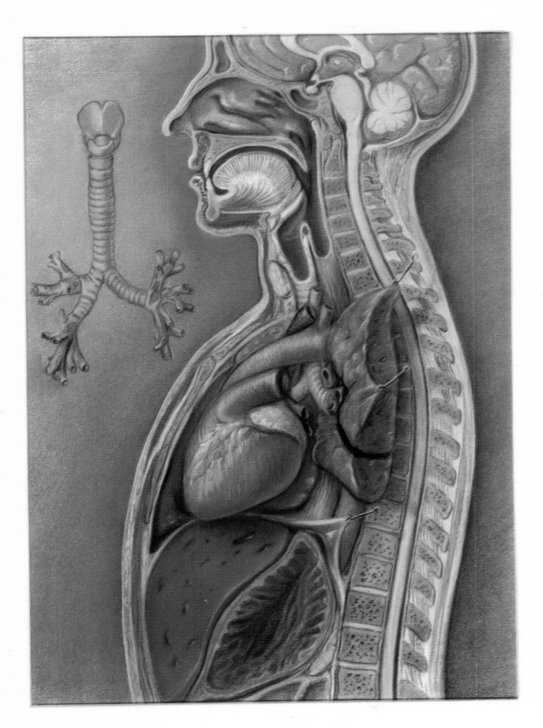

Plate 6   **Upper half of body** — *sagittal section*
Bronchial tree

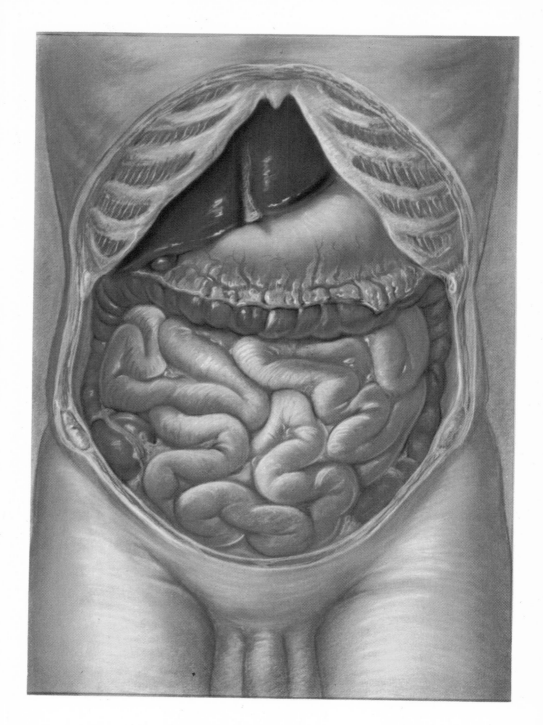

Plate 7   **Abdomen — *first view***

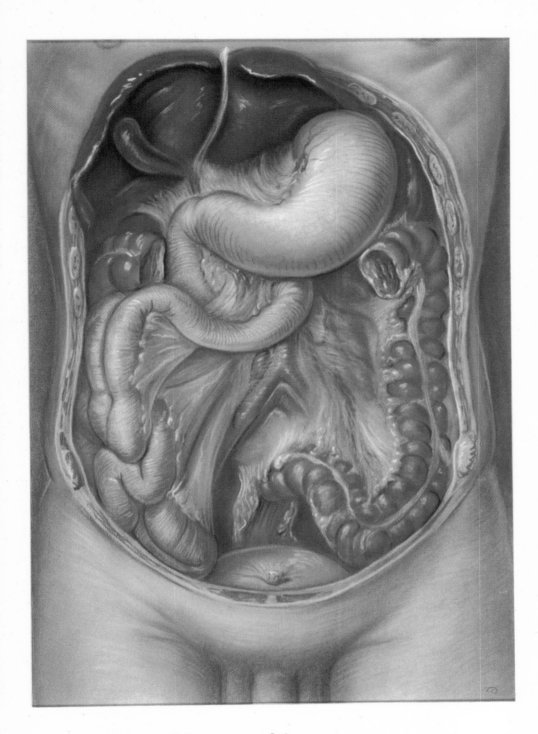

Plate 8   **Abdomen** — *second view*

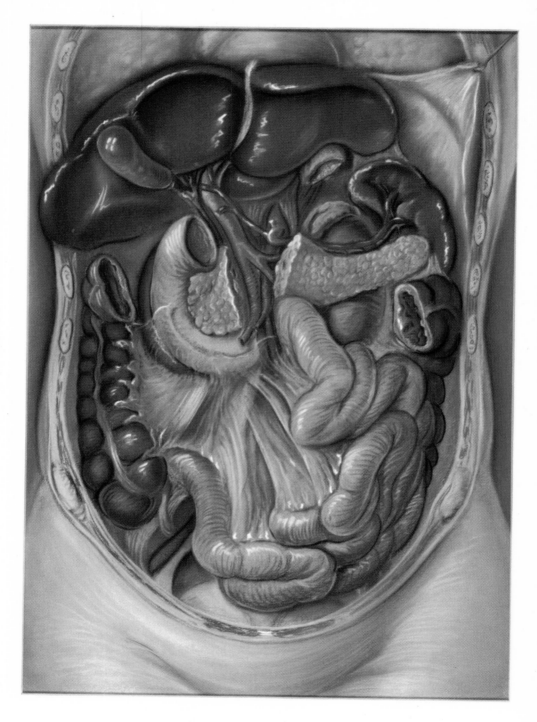

Plate 9   **Abdomen** — *third view*

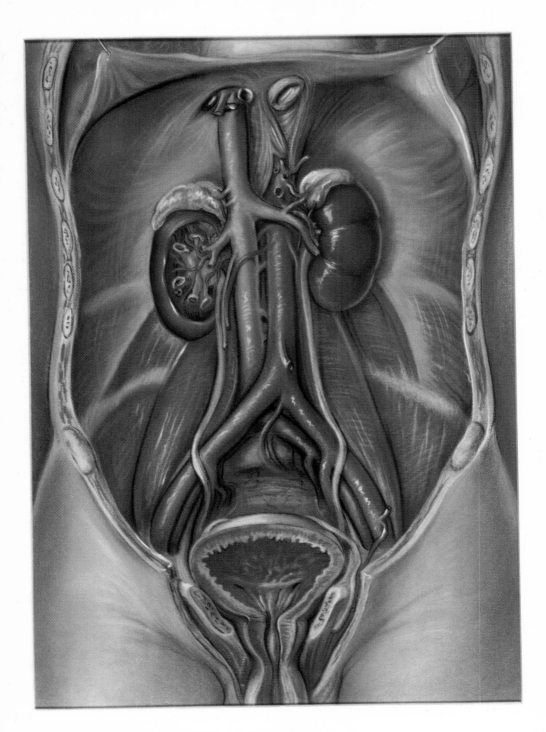

Plate 10   **Abdomen —** *fourth view*

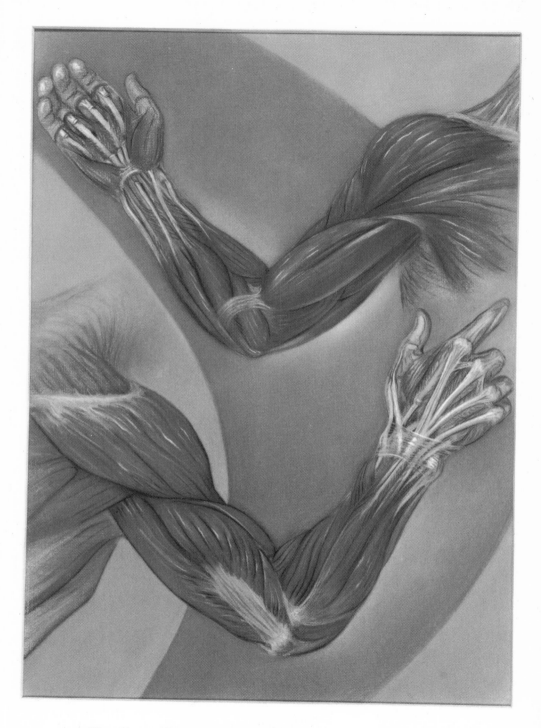

Plate 11   Upper extremity — *dissection*

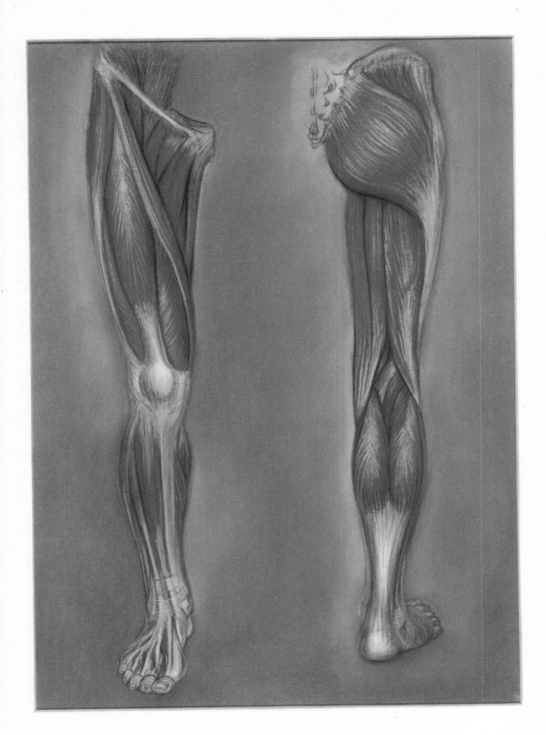

Plate 12   Lower extremity — *dissection*

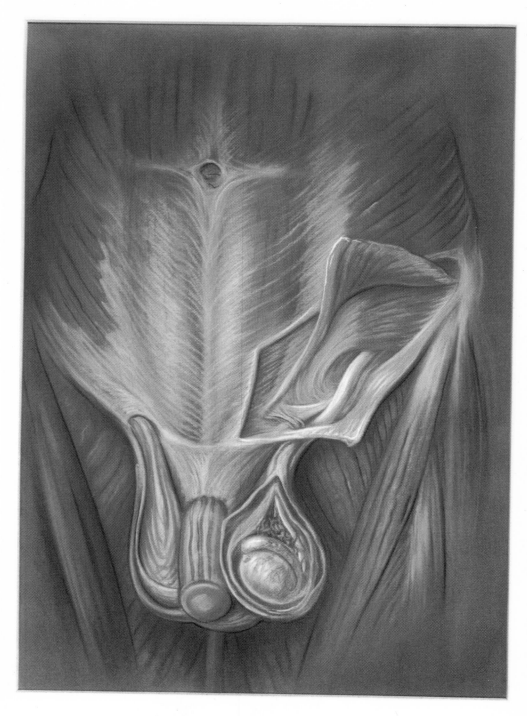

Plate 13   Abdominal wall and male genitalia

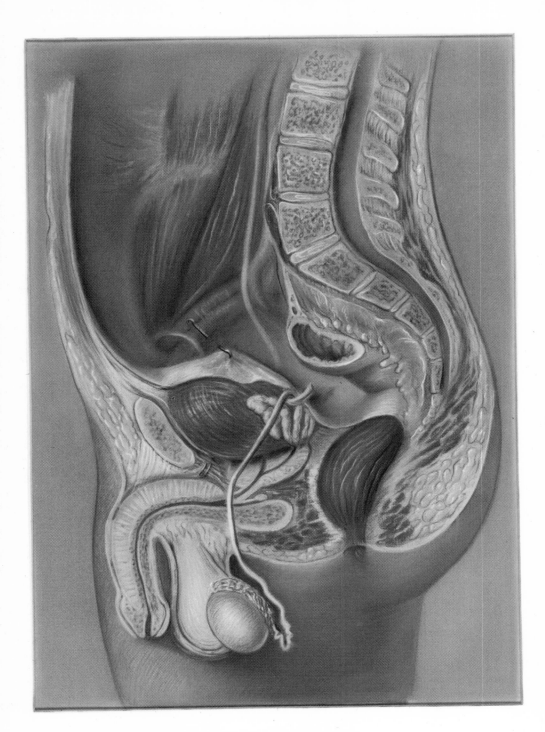

Plate 14   Male pelvis — *sagittal section*

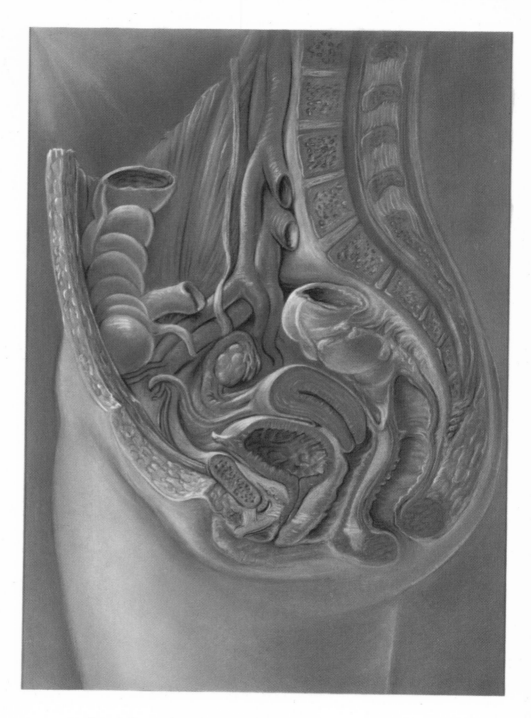

Plate 15   **Female pelvis** *— sagittal section*

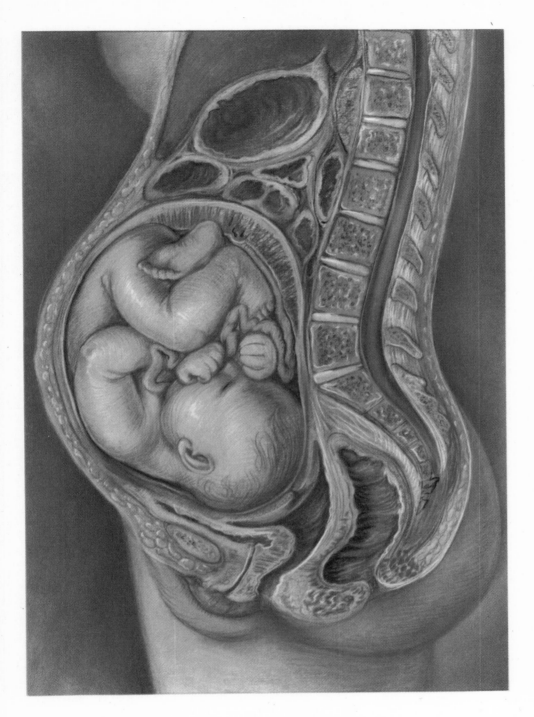

Plate 16   **Abdomen of pregnancy —** *sagittal section*

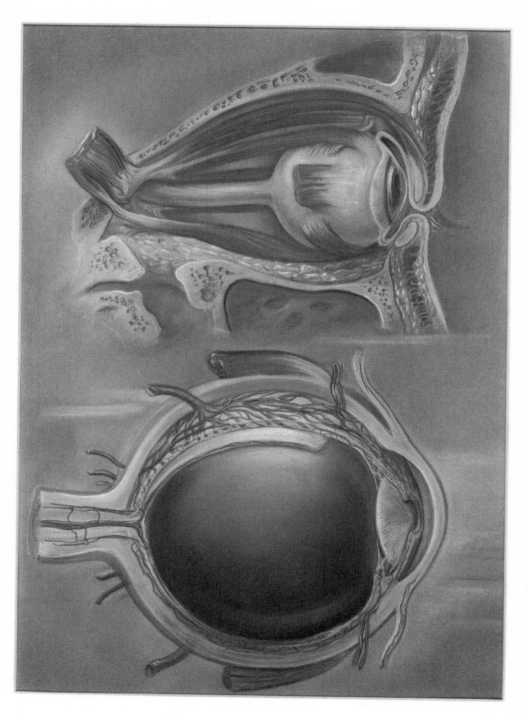

Plate 17   Eye

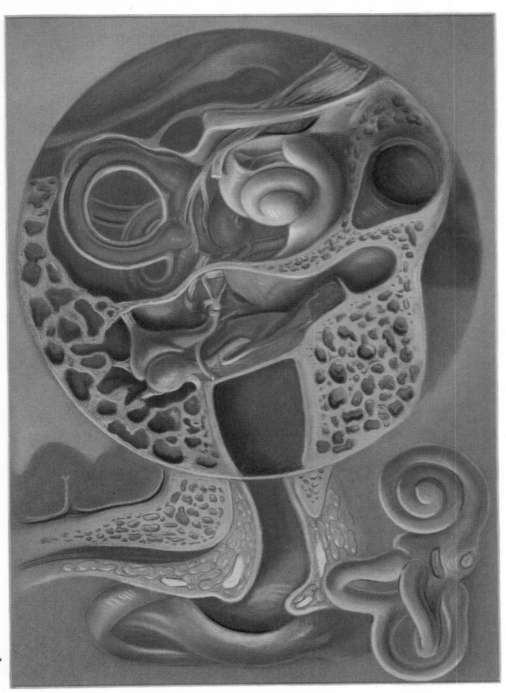

Plate 18   **Ear and inner ear** — *frontal section*

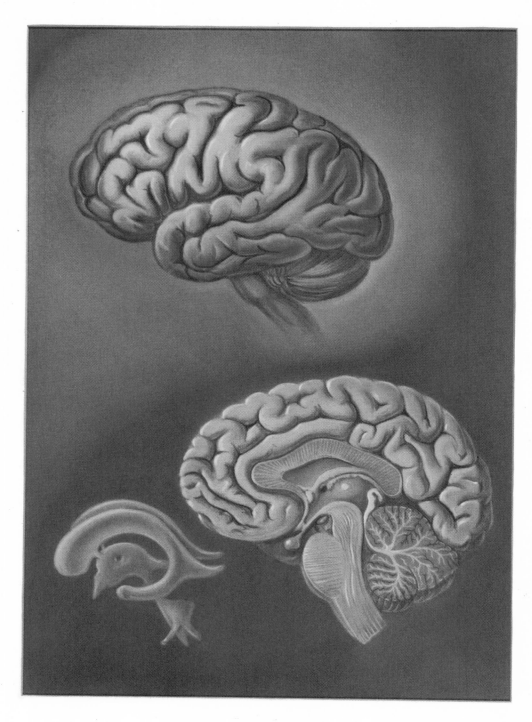

Plate 19   Brain and ventricles

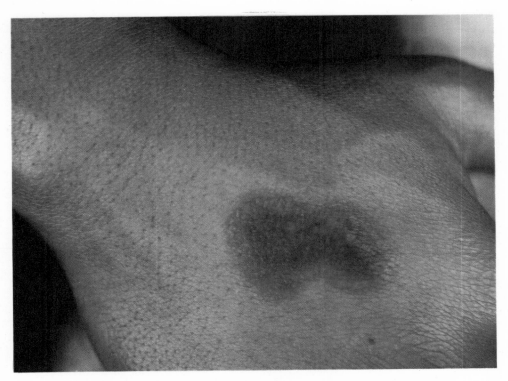

Plate 20   Fixed drug eruption on the hand of a colored man. The lesion recurs whenever he takes phenolphthalein.

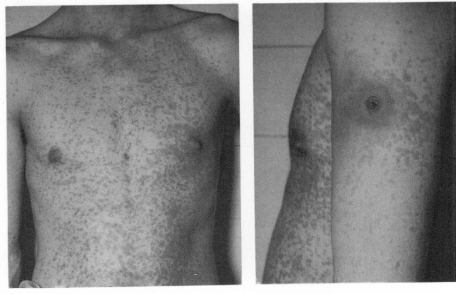

Plate 21a   *Plate 21b*

Morbilliform reaction to sulfadiazine given prophylactically, 1 Gm. daily. The eruption appeared on the tenth day. Note accentuation of the reaction about the site of a vaccinia lesion.

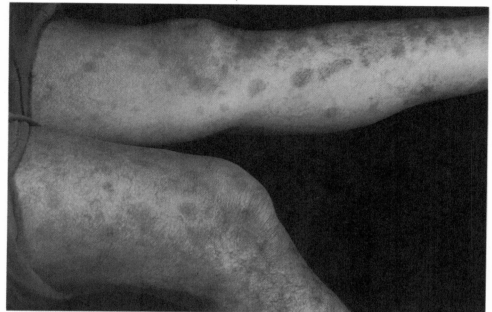

Plate 22   A toxic erythema of the multiforme type in a colored man. Drugs were ruled out in this case. There were no mucous membrane lesions. This type of eruption is not specific and may be caused by drugs, infections, or toxic states, or the cause may not be demonstrable. Note the similarity of the lesions to the phenolphthalein eruption (Plate 20).

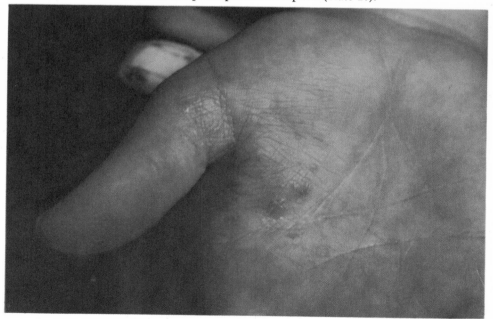

Plate 23   Contact dermatitis due, not to mechanical trauma, but to sensitivity to a metal in the scissors. This eruption resembles that seen in ivy poisoning and dermatophytosis. The distribution and history make the diagnosis.

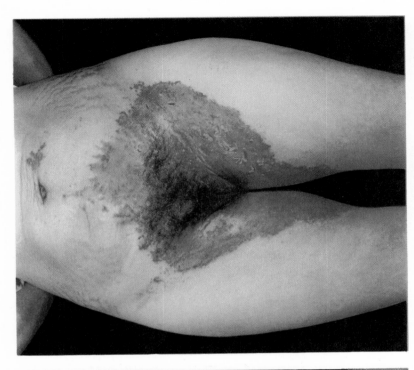

Plate 24

Chronic discoid lupus erythematosus of the face. Note the distribution and discrete nature of the lesions, loss of pigment, presence of dry scales on the nasal lesion, and alopecia in the right eyebrow.

Plate 25

Seborrheic dermatitis, showing intertriginous and other lesions. Local infection with bacteria or fungi plays an important role in such cases. The principal lesion shown is a subacute inflammatory process which began in the inguinal folds and extends around the perineum and onto the buttocks. Note the areas in and near the umbilicus. Lesions are also present on the scalp and external ears. The irregular linear marks in the lateral areas of the abdomen are lineae albicantes of pregnancy.

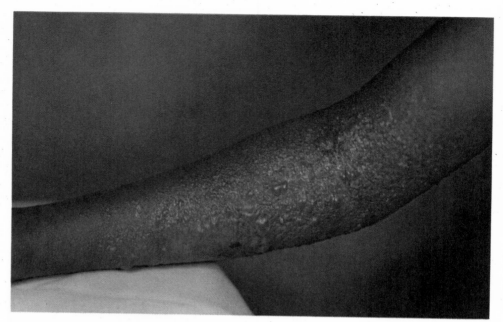

Plate 26   Contact dermatitis due to sensitization to mercury in ammoniated mercury ointment. Note resemblance to eruption of ivy poisoning.

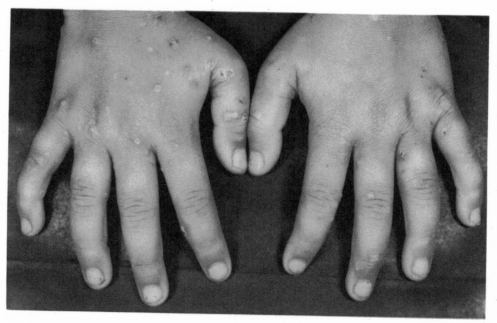

Plate 27   Scabies plus secondary infection in a child. The eruption is generalized. Note the tendency to occur on the finger webs and sides of the fingers. Note the two types of lesions, excoriated noninflammatory papules and inflammatory papules with crusts and pustulation. Scabies should always be considered in any widespread pyoderma in a child.

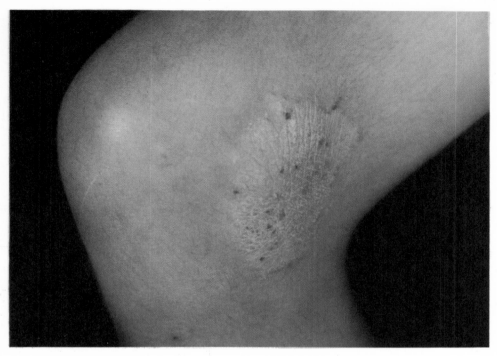

Plate 28a

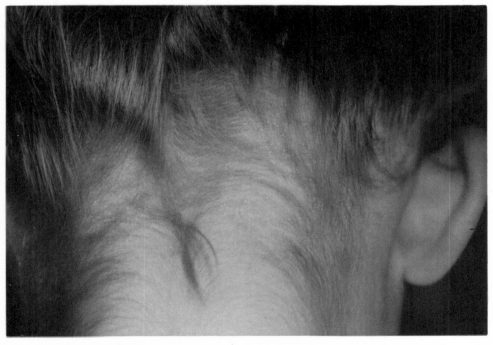

Plate 28b   Neurodermatitis, with lesions of the scalp and medial aspect of the knees
(the other knee has a lesion symmetrical to the one shown).

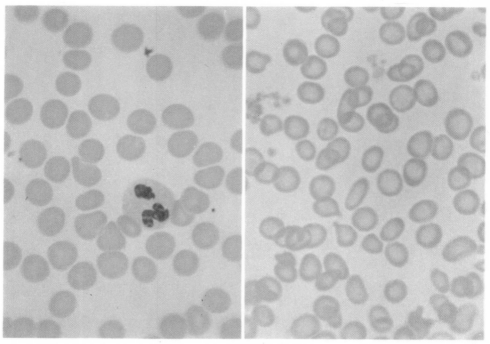

Plate 29

Normal peripheral blood

Plate 30

Iron-deficiency anemia (microcytic, hypochromic)

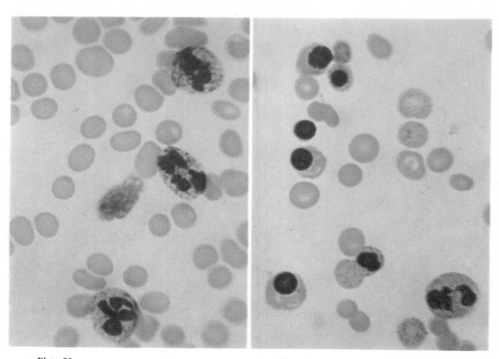

Plate 31

Toxic anemia (normocytic)

Plate 32

Erythroblastosis fetalis

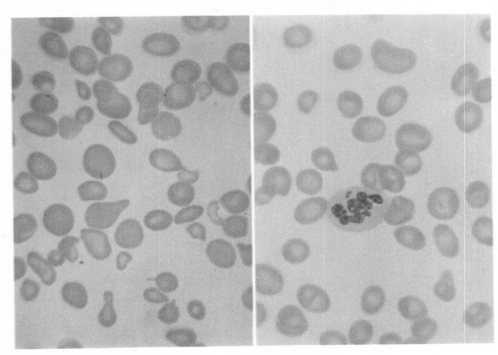

Plate 33

Pernicious anemia (Addisonian anemia)

Plate 34

Pernicious anemia of pregnancy (showing a characteristic macropolycyte [leukocyte])

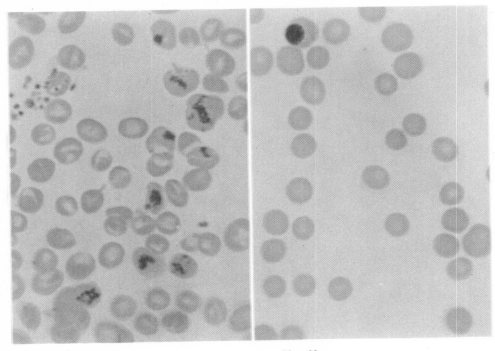

Plate 35

Reticulocytosis following liver extract therapy in pernicious anemia

Plate 36

Congenital hemolytic anemia (familial hemolytic jaundice)

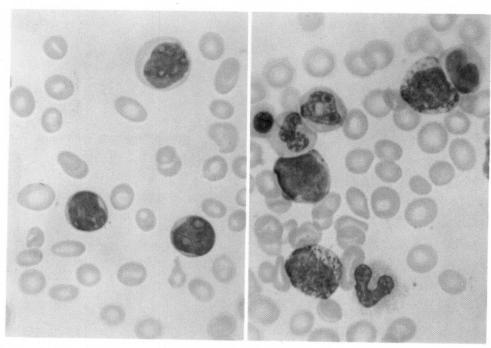

Plate 37

Acute myeloid leukemia

Plate 38

Chronic myeloid leukemia

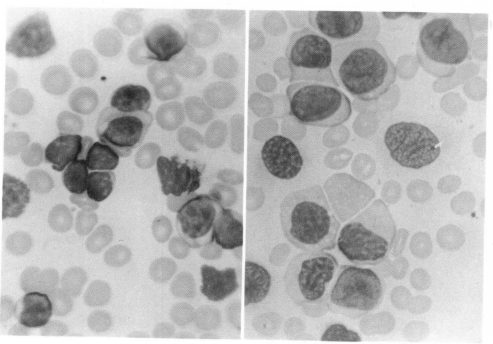

Plate 39

Chronic lymphatic leukemia

Plate 40

Monocytic leukemia

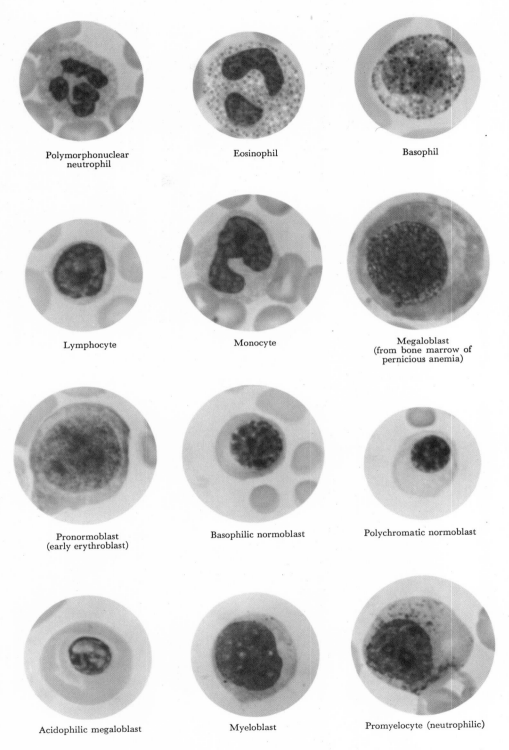

Polymorphonuclear neutrophil	Eosinophil	Basophil
Lymphocyte	Monocyte	Megaloblast (from bone marrow of pernicious anemia)
Pronormoblast (early erythroblast)	Basophilic normoblast	Polychromatic normoblast
Acidophilic megaloblast	Myeloblast	Promyelocyte (neutrophilic)

Plate 41 Individual cells from bone marrow and peripheral blood

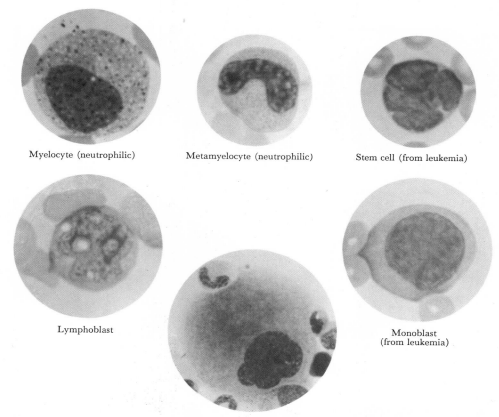

Myelocyte (neutrophilic)　　Metamyelocyte (neutrophilic)　　Stem cell (from leukemia)

Lymphoblast

Monoblast
(from leukemia)

Mature megakaryocyte (large central cell)
(somewhat reduced in relation to other cells)

Plate 42　　**Individual cells from bone marrow and peripheral blood**
(*continued*)

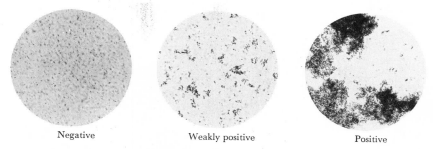

Negative　　　　Weakly positive　　　　Positive

Plate 43　　**Flocculation Tests for the Serodiagnosis of Syphilis**

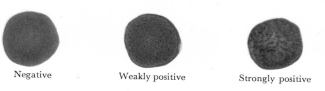

Negative　　　　Weakly positive　　　　Strongly positive

Plate 44　　**Pertussis Agglutination Test**

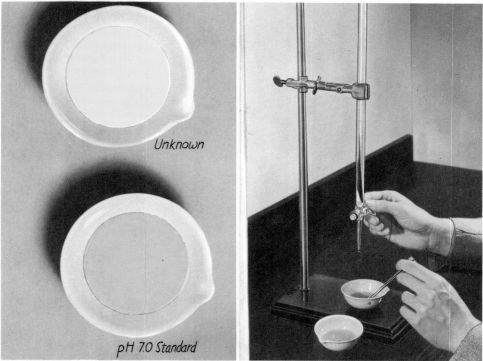

COLOR CHART A

Figure 1. Method for determination of titrable acid

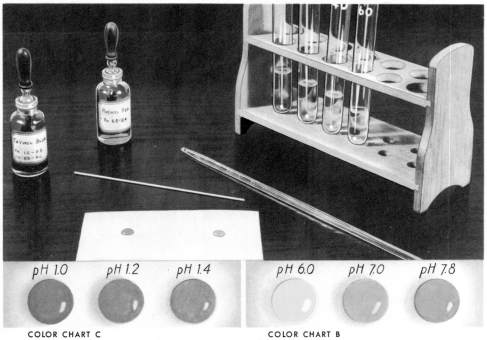

COLOR CHART C

COLOR CHART B

Figure 2. Simple method for determination of *p*H of gastric juice

Plate 45   **Gastric analysis**

BENEDICT'S TEST (SUGAR)

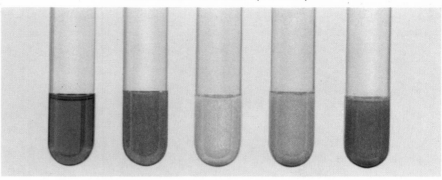

Figure 1	Figure 2	Figure 3	Figure 4	Figure 5
Negative	0.25% Sugar (+)	1% Sugar (++)	More than 1% (+++)	Over 2% (++++)

SODIUM NITROPRUSSIDE TEST (ACETONE)

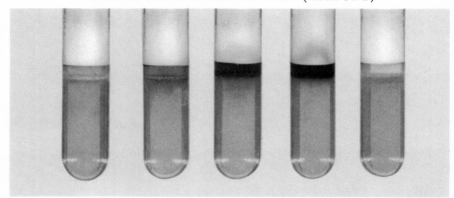

Figure 6	Figure 7	Figure 8	Figure 9	Figure 10
Negative	Trace acetone	Acetone strongly positive	Acetoacetic acid positive	Drug reaction

GERHARDT'S TEST (ACETOACETIC ACID)

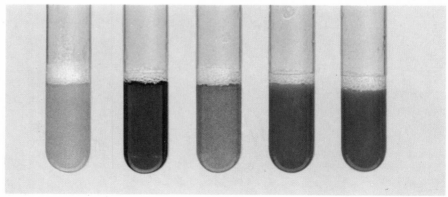

Figure 11	Figure 12	Figure 13	Figure 14	Figure 15
Negative	Positive (before boiling)	Positive (after boiling)	Drug (before boiling)	Drug (after boiling)

Plate 46   **Urine test charts**

Laboratory Tests

URINE

URINE PROTEIN, QUALITATIVE

Heat and Acetic Acid Test—Fill a test tube three-fourths full with filtered urine. Hold the lower end of the tube in the hand and boil the upper portion of the fluid. Add 2 or 3 drops of 36 percent acetic acid and boil again. A permanent white precipitate indicates protein.

Nitric Acid Test (Heller's Test)—Place 2 or 3 cc. of concentrated nitric acid in a test tube. Carefully pour an equal amount of urine down the side of the tilted tube, preferably from a pipette, so as to overlay the acid. Examine after several minutes against a dark background. If protein is present, a white ring appears at the point of contact of the two liquids.

URINE PROTEIN, QUANTITATIVE

Addis Modification of Shevky-Stafford Technic

REAGENT—Tsuchiya's Solution

phosphotungstic acid . . . . .1.5 Gm.
hydrochloric acid, concentrated, C.P. 5   cc.
ethyl alcohol, 95% . . . . .to make 100   cc.

TECHNIC—The test is usually performed in connection with the Addis count of urine sediment (p. 520). Special centrifuge tubes of 6.5-cc. capacity are used. * To such a tube add 4 cc. of urine. Dilute the urine if it contains more than a moderate cloud of protein as shown by the heat and acetic acid

test. Layer the urine with 2.5 cc. of Tsuchiya's solution. Stopper the tube, invert three times, and allow to stand for ten minutes. Centrifuge for exactly fifteen minutes at 1,800 r.p.m. Read the volume of packed precipitate. Dilute the urine and repeat the test if the volume of precipitate is greater than 1 cc.

The total twenty-four-hour excretion of protein in milligrams is the product of 7.2 times the calculated volume of urine in cubic centimeters per twenty-four hours, times the volume in cubic centimeters of protein precipitate. A twenty-four-hour excretion of 80 mg. is generally considered the upper limit of normal.

URINE SUGAR, QUALITATIVE

Benedict's Qualitative Test—To 5 cc. of Benedict's Qualitative Solution in a test tube add 8 drops of filtered urine, mix, and place in boiling water for five minutes. Allow to cool. If the urine contains no sugar, the solution remains clear. The formation of a green, yellow, or red precipitate indicates the presence of sugar in quantities ranging from traces to large amounts, in rough proportion to the color developed.

URINE SUGAR, QUANTITATIVE

Quantitative Estimation with Benedict's Qualitative Solution—Quantitatively, this test is not as

* Suitable graduated tubes may be obtained from Arthur H. Thomas Co., West Washington Square, Philadelphia, Pa.

accurate as the test in which Benedict's Quantitative Solution is used. However, it affords rough quantitative information with but little more effort than is required for the purely qualitative test.

Plate 46 shows tests that were made according to the following directions:

Drop exactly 8 drops of the urine to be tested into a test tube, and add exactly 5 cc. of Benedict's Qualitative Solution. Shake the tube. Stand the test tube in water that is already bubbling and boiling, and allow it to remain there exactly five minutes. The water in which the test tube stands should be boiling throughout the period. At the end of five minutes, remove the test tube, shake, and examine. If the contents remain blue, the urine may be considered sugar-free. If there is formation of a greenish-yellow, yellow, or reddish-brown precipitate which renders the solution opaque, an abnormal or pathological amount of sugar is present. The 8 drops should be measured with an unbroken pipette having a volume of not less than 0.4 cc. or 0.5 cc. The test tube should not be heated over an open flame, lest this impair the accuracy of the quantitative estimation.

In Figure 1 of Plate 46 the urine is sugar-free. The solution has become turbid in the process of boiling, but the color is unchanged. The faint turbidity may possibly be ascribed to precipitated urates.

Figure 2 shows the color when the urine contained less than 0.5 percent dextrose. It is filled with a finely divided precipitate. If it were allowed to stand for a number of hours, a yellow precipitate would settle to the bottom and the supernatant liquid would be a somewhat paler blue than is seen in Figure 1. A small part of the copper has been reduced, thereby lessening the blue color and causing a yellow precipitate. It is the combination of these colors that gives the greenish tinge.

Figure 3 shows the result with 8 drops of urine containing 1 percent dextrose. More copper has been reduced than in the test tube shown in Figure 2. This results in an increase in the yellow precipitate and a corresponding decrease in the blue color. Consequently, the yellow is dominant.

Figure 4 shows the color when the urine contained over 1 percent sugar. The yellow color is still dominant; however, complete reduction has not yet occurred, as would be seen if the precipitate were allowed to settle out. If this were done, the supernatant liquid would exhibit a trace of blue color.

Figure 5 shows the color when complete reduction has taken place. The muddy red color seems to depend for its appearance upon rapid and copious precipitation. With excessive heat it appears more readily. With a temperature no higher than that of boiling water, the color may be the orange-yellow of Figure 4 even with a higher sugar content. Heating the test tube over an open flame may develop the red color with lower percentages, but it is re-emphasized that the colors shown here were all obtained by standing the test tube for five minutes in boiling water.

Benedict's Quantitative Test—Transfer 25 cc. of Benedict's Quantitative Solution into a small flask with a pipette, and add to it 10 to 20 Gm. of sodium carbonate crystals (or one-half this amount of anhydrous sodium carbonate) with a bead or some talc to prevent "bumping." Heat to boiling, and add urine slowly from a burette, a drop or two at a time, until a chalk-white precipitate has formed and the blue color of the reagent begins to fade. Continue to add urine, drop by drop, until the last trace of blue color just disappears. The solution must be kept boiling vigorously, and the water lost by evaporation must be restored. Note the quantity of urine required to dissipate the blue color. This amount contains exactly 0.05 Gm. of dextrose.

For calculation:

$$\text{Percent of dextrose in urine} = \frac{5}{\text{cc. of urine required}}$$

$$\text{Total Gm. dextrose in sample} = \frac{\text{cc. in sample}}{100} \times \text{percent dextrose}$$

Sheftel Quantitative Method—This method provides a simple, accurate, and convenient means of obtaining the percentage of sugar in urine. The apparatus needed, including reagents and a source of heat, has been assembled into a small portable kit. Tests may be made almost anywhere in about five minutes, and there are no solutions to spill. Full directions for use accompany the Urine Sugar Test Case, Sheftel, which may be purchased through the drug trade.

Somogyi Rapid Quantitative Method—The basis of this method is the change of color which takes place when sugars are heated in alkaline solution.

APPARATUS—1. Test tubes of 14 mm. inside diameter.

2. Pipettes for measuring 0.5-cc. and 5-cc. portions of fluid.

REAGENTS—1. Solution of anhydrous sodium carbonate, 10 percent.

2. A series of standard dextrose solutions ranging from 0.5 to 6 percent. These solutions are best prepared from a stock 10 percent solution of dextrose in water to which is added 0.25 percent benzoic acid as a preservative. From the stock a series of 0.05, 1, 2, 3, 4, 5, and 6 percent standard solutions is prepared by dilution with water containing 0.25 percent benzoic acid. These will keep indefinitely at room temperature.

TECHNIC—Introduce into seven test tubes 0.5-cc. portions of the standard dextrose solutions and into other test tubes 0.5-cc. portions of the urines to be analyzed. Add to each test tube 5-cc. portions of the sodium carbonate reagent. Mix, place the tubes in a rack, and heat by immersing in boiling water for eight minutes. Racks accommodating one to two dozen or more tubes may be employed.

After heating, read the results without undue delay. When matching colors, view the tubes transversely, with the rack against the window or artificial source of light. If the color of the unknown lies between two of the standards, estimate the intermediate value by interpolation.

PERMANENT STANDARDS—In laboratories where urine sugars are determined throughout the day, permanent standards may be prepared from a stock 0.01 normal iodine solution in absolute alcohol by dilution with absolute alcohol according to Table 60.

TABLE 60 — *Permanent Standards for Somogyi Rapid Quantitative Method of Determining Sugar in Urine* (see text)

Normality of Iodine Solution	Corresponding Percent Dextrose Concentrations
0.0004	0.5
0.0009	1.0
0.0018	2.0
0.0028	3.0
0.0043	4.0
0.0058	5.0
0.0080	6.0

PENTOSES IN URINE

Essential pentosuria (xyloketosuria) is a rather infrequently encountered anomaly of metabolism which, although innocuous, may be confused with renal glycosuria or diabetes mellitus. It requires no treatment. When very small amounts of pentoses are suspected or when doubt exists, an increased elimination of pentose can be brought about by administration of 15 to 20 grains of aminopyrine (see p. 409) over one or two days.

The preliminary qualitative test given below yields positive results with both xyloketose and d-fructose. These two can be easily distinguished since xyloketose is not fermented by yeast, gives a positive Bial test (see below), does not form a glucosazone with phenylhydrazine, and gives a negative Seliwanoff test (see below).

Preliminary Qualitative Test (Method of Lasker and Enklewitz)—Mix 1 cc. of the urine with 5 cc. of Benedict's qualitative reagent in a test tube and place in a water bath at 55° C. Observe at the end of ten minutes. The appearance of a yellow precipitate indicates that the urine contains l-xyloketose or d-fructose.

Bial Test

REAGENT—Dissolve 1 Gm. orcinol (5-methylresorcinol) in 500 cc. of hydrochloric acid (specific gravity 1.151, or about 29.7 percent), and add 2 cc. of 10 percent ferric chloride solution. Store in a dark bottle.

TECHNIC—Boil 5 cc. of the reagent in a test tube. Remove the tube from the flame and only then add gently 5 drops of urine. A green ring at the junction is diagnostic of pentoses. Glycuronates may give a positive test also if the test tube has not been removed from the flame before the urine is added.

FRUCTOSE IN URINE

Seliwanoff Test

REAGENT—Dissolve 0.05 Gm. resorcinol in 70 cc. water and add 30 cc. of C.P. hydrochloric acid. Store in a dark bottle.

TECHNIC—Add 5 drops of urine to 2 cc. of reagent and heat in a boiling water bath for five minutes. In the presence of fructose, a deep reddish color develops which tends to remain after considerable dilution and is soluble in amyl alcohol. Dextrose in more than 2 percent concentration also gives a reddish color, but this fades rapidly on dilution. When the urine is shown to contain much sugar by the Benedict test, it should be diluted to contain less than 1.5 percent before the Seliwanoff test is performed.

ACETONE AND ACETOACETIC (DIACETIC) ACID IN URINE (KETOSIS)

The tests in common clinical use do not differentiate between acetone and acetoacetic acid, but the two substances occur under the same conditions and the former merely represents a decomposition product of acetoacetic acid. If very little acetoacetic acid is formed, it may be entirely transformed into acetone. Some clinicians advise the routine examination of the urine for acetone; others test all urines for diacetic acid first and then apply the acetone test to those which react to the Gerhardt test with a red color which does not fade on boiling. False reactions from drugs such as salicylates, aspirin, antipyrine, alkalies, acetates, phenol, and cyanates may thus be differentiated (see below).

Sodium Nitroprusside Test for Acetone

REAGENTS—1. Dry, finely powdered sodium nitroprusside, 5 Gm., mixed with 200 Gm. of ammonium sulfate is much more convenient and stable than the solutions usually employed.

2. Strong ammonia water.

TECHNIC—Add enough of the above nitroprusside mixture to saturate 2 to 3 cc. of urine in a test tube, and shake well. Overlay with a small quantity of strong ammonia water. A positive test is indicated by a color ranging from faint purplish pink to dark purple (Plate 46, Figures 6 to 10), reaching its maximum intensity within a few minutes, then fading gradually to a muddy brown. The reaction of a faint trace of acetone may be most easily determined by noting the purple track of the ammonia water through the white foam. If acetoacetic acid is present, it intensifies the test (Figure 9). Absence of color reaction may be noted in specimens which show a color reaction in the Gerhardt test due to drugs (Figure 10).

Gerhardt's Test for Acetoacetic Acid

REAGENT—10 percent aqueous solution of ferric chloride.

TECHNIC—To from 3 to 5 cc. of urine in a test tube add 10 percent ferric chloride solution, drop by drop, until no more precipitate forms. The depth of Burgundy-red color which appears indicates the presence of acetoacetic acid (Plate 46, Figures 11 to 15). Acetoacetic acid is unstable on boiling. Divide the specimen into two tubes, boil one, and then compare. If the color was due to acetoacetic acid, it will disappear on boiling (Figure 13). If due to a drug, it will remain (Figures 14 and 15). Any specimen giving a red test which does not fade on boiling should be examined in addition by the sodium nitroprusside test in order to detect acetone which is masked by "drug reaction" (Figure 10).

URINE CONCENTRATION TEST (ADDIS)

This test is used as a measure of the ability of the kidneys to perform osmotic work under the stimulus of water deprivation. Under the conditions of the test, normal kidneys can concentrate the urine to a specific gravity of not less than 1.028. A specific gravity lower than 1.026 indicates renal damage except during pregnancy, receding edema, protein undernutrition, or salt deficiency, when a lower gravity is without significance. A specific gravity

of 1.010 (that of glomerular filtrate) indicates total loss of ability to perform osmotic work.

TECHNIC—On the day before the urine is to be collected, the patient eats his usual breakfast (before 8 a.m.). Subsequently, he is to take no more fluids until after the specimen has been collected the following morning. Fluids are defined as anything liquid enough to be poured from one vessel to another. No more than the usual quantity of fruit should be taken. The patient voids during the day and again as close as possible to 8 p.m., and the urine is discarded. The exact hour at which this last voiding takes place should be recorded to the nearest minute. The patient is instructed to refrain from emptying the bladder during the night if possible. If it is necessary, however, the special bottle is used. The patient is instructed to void in the morning as close as possible to 8 a.m., using a specially prepared, clean bottle which may contain a drop or so of formaldehyde. Again the exact hour of voiding is recorded. The entire urine specimen, labeled with the patient's name and the hours of evening and morning voiding, is brought to the laboratory. There the specimen is mixed thoroughly, and the specific gravity is determined.

ADDIS COUNT OF URINE SEDIMENT

The Addis count makes possible the quantitative estimation of the daily excretion of protein and formed elements (casts, red and white blood cells, and epithelial cells) in the urine. In the diagnosis and treatment of renal disease, it plays a role similar to that of the blood count in anemia. The count is made on a specimen collected as for the urine concentration test (see above), with which it is usually combined. One difference in collection must be noted:

If an Addis count is to be made on a patient with menstrual or vaginal discharge, the patient must not void during the night, and the morning specimen is collected by catheterization.

In the laboratory, mix the specimen thoroughly and determine its volume, reaction, and specific gravity. Transfer 10 cc. to a specially graduated centrifuge tube* with a diameter so narrow toward the tip that an accurate reading of small volumes can be made. Centrifugalize the filled tube for five minutes at 1,800 r.p.m. Then discard the greater part of the supernatant urine, and remove with a pipette a part of the remainder until a volume

* Suitable graduated tubes may be obtained from Arthur H. Thomas Co., West Washington Square, Philadelphia, Pa.

remains which will vary with the amount and nature of the deposit. Allow the tube to stand for a few minutes, and then remove any additional drainage from the sides of the tube down to the exact volume desired (usually 0.3, 0.5, or 1 cc.).

Resuspend the sediment by thorough mixing, using a dry pipette, and introduce a drop of the suspension into each side of a blood counting chamber. Count the number of the various formed elements. The casts should be counted under low power over all the ruled areas. This makes a total of 18 sq. mm. of counting chamber floor for the two sides. In the urine of normal persons there are very few casts, and as many as ten drops may have to be examined before a statistically valid number are encountered. The red cells and the white and epithelial cells (omitting squamous cells) are usually counted under the high dry lens over unit areas of 1 sq. mm. or less, depending upon the number of elements encountered. For the technic of protein determination, see page 517.

In calculating the results, the output may be reduced to terms of either twelve or twenty-four hours. Most workers now prefer the latter period. If the period of urine collection is within a half hour of twelve hours, the voided volume can simply be doubled to calculate for a twenty-four-hour period. If the deviation is too great, the volume of voided urine in cubic centimeters is multiplied by twenty-four and divided by the period of urine collection in hours and fractions of an hour, the result being the equivalent twenty-four-hour volume of urine in cubic centimeters. The numbers of different formed elements may all be calculated by the same formula. The total excretion in number per twenty-four hours is the product of 1,000 times the calculated volume of urine in cubic centimeters per twenty-four hours multiplied by the volume in cubic centimeters in which the sediment was mixed, times the number of formed elements per square millimeter of counting chamber floor.*

The approximate limits of normal for twenty-four-hour excretion of formed elements are given in Table 61. It is to be noted that the hyaline matrix of casts disappears from neutral sodium chloride solutions when the salt concentration is less than 0.5 percent. On the alkaline side of neutrality, the matrix dissolves in even higher salt concentrations. A low cast count may not, therefore, be a true reflection of total cast excretion in dilute or alkaline urines.

---

* A nomograph, by which the various counts may be calculated without the need for arithmetical figuring, is available upon request.

TABLE 61—*Approximate Limits of Normal for Twenty-Four-Hour Excretion of Formed Elements in the Urine*

	Adults	Children
Casts.	20,000	80,000
Red Blood Cells.	2,000,000	2,000,000
White and Epithelial Cells	2,000,000	4,000,000 in boys 8,000,000 in girls

In normal adults, casts are 100 percent hyaline; in children, 50 percent may be granular.

URINARY *p*H ESTIMATIONS

Fairly accurate estimation of the relative acidity or alkalinity of urine may be necessary in the use of mandelic acid therapy (where a highly acid urine must be developed) and in the use of full doses of sulfadiazine, sulfathiazole, or sulfamerazine (where it is desirable that the *p*H of the urine be on the alkaline side of neutral).

The *p*H of normal urine is variable, depending chiefly upon the diet. A diet made up principally of meat, eggs, and cereals, and containing as fruits only prunes, plums, and cranberries, should produce an acid urine. A diet made up of milk, vegetables, and fruits, except the three fruits mentioned above, may give an alkaline urine. On the average American diet, normal urine is slightly acid; the average is *p*H 6, although it may vary from 5 to 7.5. Urines having *p*H values varying from 4.7 to 8 are compatible with health.

Litmus paper is often used to estimate whether the *p*H of the urine is on the acid or alkaline side of neutral. If blue litmus paper is dipped into urine and turns pink, the urine is said to be acid. If the blue litmus paper does not change color, it is necessary to place a piece of red litmus paper in the urine. If this turns blue, the urine is alkaline. If neither the red nor the blue litmus paper changes color, the urine is considered to be neutral. If it changes red litmus blue and blue litmus red, it is said to be amphoteric.

When mandelic acid therapy is being given, methyl red is the most convenient indicator. Add 5 drops of methyl red solution (0.1 percent in alcohol) to 2 cc. of urine. A red color results if the *p*H is 5.5 or less. If the color is orange or yellow, the *p*H is higher and the urine is not sufficiently acid for successful mandelic acid therapy.

The U.S.P. XIV describes a set of indicator and buffer solutions by means of which the pH of relatively colorless solutions may be accurately determined.

BLOOD PIGMENT IN URINE

Benzidine Test—To about 3 cc. of glacial acetic acid in a test tube add the amount of benzidine that can be placed on a penknife point and 1 or 2 cc. of filtered urine, and boil; add 3 cc. of fresh hydrogen peroxide (3 percent) and shake. If blood pigment is present, a blue or green color develops. A control test, using water in place of urine, may be made for comparison.

BILE IN URINE

Smith Test—Place a few cubic centimeters of urine in a test tube. With a pipette, overlay it carefully with Iodine Tincture, U.S.P. XIV, which has been diluted with twice its volume of alcohol. The presence of bile is shown by an emerald-green ring at the point of contact of the two liquids.

Harrison-Godfried Test—This test is many times more sensitive than the usual methods, since the bile is concentrated by adsorption on a precipitate. To 5 cc. of urine add an equal quantity of 10 percent solution of barium chloride. Mix and filter. Spread the filter paper on a dry piece of filter paper, and add 1 or 2 drops of Fouchet's reagent (trichloroacetic acid, 25 Gm.; 10 percent solution of ferric chloride, 10 cc.; distilled water, 100 cc.). A green or blue color indicates the presence of bilirubin.

UROBILIN IN URINE

Ehrlich's Test—To a small quantity of urine in a test tube add a few crystals of para-dimethylaminobenzaldehyde. Make acid with hydrochloric acid, and view the tube from the top over a sheet of white paper in a strong light. A cherry-red color indicates the presence of abnormal quantities of urobilin.

ASCORBIC ACID IN URINE

Method of Goldsmith and Ellenger

APPARATUS—1. Pipette, 1 cc.
2. Microburette, 5 cc.
3. Volumetric flask, 50 cc.
4. Volumetric flask, 100 cc.

REAGENTS—1. Glacial acetic acid.
2. Acetic acid, 5 percent.
3. Standard ascorbic acid solution, 0.6 mg. per cc., prepared by dissolving 60 mg. of accurately weighed ascorbic acid in 5 percent acetic acid and diluting to 100 cc. in the volumetric flask.
4. Standard 2,6-dichlorophenolindophenol solution. Extract about 0.1 Gm. of the dye twice with 25-cc. portions of boiling distilled water, pouring each extract through a small filter into a 50-cc. volumetric flask. The insoluble residue is discarded. Cool and dilute to the mark. This stock solution will keep two to three weeks. For daily use, dilute 20 cc. to 100 cc. with distilled water which has recently been boiled and cooled.

To standardize the diluted dye solution, titrate it against 2-cc. portions of the standard ascorbic acid solution which have been diluted to 50 cc. with 5 percent acetic acid. If x cc. of dye solution are required, then each cc. is equivalent to $\dfrac{1.2}{x}$ mg. ascorbic acid. The fresh ascorbic acid solution may be checked by titrating against 0.1 N iodine solution (0.114 cc. of 0.1 N iodine = 1 mg. ascorbic acid).

TECHNIC—The urine to be examined should be collected in dark, tightly stoppered bottles and should be kept on ice previous to analysis. In addition, each individual specimen should be acidified with glacial acetic acid (about 1 cc. glacial acetic acid per 100 cc. of urine). When possible, the specimens should be analyzed within two hours of the time of voiding; but if prepared as described above, a twenty-four-hour collection may be made without excessive loss of reduced ascorbic acid.

One cc. of the acidified urine specimen is diluted with 10 cc. of distilled water, and this is titrated with standardized 2,6-dichlorophenolindophenol solution from a microburette (graduated in 0.01-cc. divisions). The end point is the first faint pink color that persists thirty seconds. A distilled water blank is always run, and its value is subtracted from the final burette reading.

When the urine is highly colored, it is often necessary to dilute it with more than 10 cc. of water to obtain a satisfactory end point. If a large amount of vitamin C is present in the specimen, it may be necessary to use only one cubic centimeter of the diluted specimen for titration by the dye. In the latter case, the factor of dilution must be considered in calculating the amount of ascorbic acid in the urine.

CALCULATION—Total ascorbic acid in milligrams in the entire specimen = (cc. of dye solution required by 1 cc. of urine minus cc. of blank) × ascorbic acid equivalent of 1 cc. of dye solution × volume of urine specimen in cc.

Adults normally excrete 20 to 50 mg. ascorbic acid in the urine daily; amounts below 15 mg. are suggestive of deficiency. Children normally excrete 10 to 20 mg. daily.

SULFONAMIDES IN URINE

Method of Bratton and Marshall—The urine is tested for protein (see p. 517) and is then diluted with distilled water until it contains about 1 to 2 mg. of sulfonamide per 100 cc. If it contains protein, it is treated by the procedure for blood (p. 537). If it is protein-free, 50 cc. of the diluted urine plus 5 cc. of 4 N hydrochloric acid are further diluted to 100 cc. Ten cc. of the second dilution are treated as a blood filtrate for free sulfonamide (p. 537), and 10 cc. are heated, without further addition of acid, for total sulfonamide.

CALCULATION—Concentration of sulfonamide in

$$\text{mg. per 100 cc. urine} = \frac{\text{reading of standard}}{\text{reading of unknown}} \times$$

concentration of sulfonamide in mg. per 100 cc. of diluted standard × factor of dilution of urine.

Method of Monto—For discussion and reagents, see procedure for blood (p. 537). To make the test, 1 cc. of urine is diluted to 200 cc. with distilled water. To 10 cc. of this dilution add 1 cc. of the aldehyde reagent (Reagent No. 2 of the list on p. 537), and compare with a similarly treated standard solution as indicated in the procedure for blood. Calculation of results is the same as for the Bratton and Marshall method above.

CALCIUM IN URINE

In the treatment of hypoparathyroidism with hypercalcemic agents (p. 196) it is advisable to follow the urinary excretion of calcium. A simple rough quantitative estimate is made possible by the Sulkowitch reagent:

oxalic acid	2.5 Gm.
ammonium oxalate	2.5 Gm.
acetic acid (glacial)	5 cc.
distilled water to make	150 cc.

When equal volumes of urine and reagent are mixed, any calcium present in the urine appears as a fine precipitate of calcium oxalate. If there is no precipitate, the urine contains no calcium, and the serum calcium level is probably 5 to 7.5 mg.

per 100 cc., a very low level. A fine white cloud indicates a moderate amount of calcium and a serum calcium within normal limits. A heavy milk-white precipitate suggests the danger of hypercalcemia.

Hypoparathyroid patients are given initial dosages of hypercalcemic agents until a fine white cloud appears in the urine test. Dosage is then readjusted to maintain such a test. The serum calcium should be determined occasionally, and more frequently if the patient does not seem to be under satisfactory control.

Normal people on a low-calcium diet may show no calcium in a single specimen, and others may have an excess in the urine for a short period after drinking a glass of milk. When hypoparathyroid patients are on a high-calcium diet, they can be expected to excrete large quantities of calcium in the urine if the serum calcium is normal. The rules given above tend to maintain such patients at a slightly subnormal level of serum calcium, which is safe and harmless.

BLOOD

STAINED SMEARS

Slides and cover slips should be perfectly clean and free from grease. When new, they should be soaked in 10 percent acetic acid, rinsed in distilled water, and dried. The drop of blood, from the lobe of the ear or finger tip, should not be too large; otherwise the film will be too thick. A little practice will enable one to determine the thickness best adapted for the particular preparation required.

The two-cover-glass method is widely used. A large cover glass is touched to the top of the drop of blood, then placed, blood side down, upon another large cover glass. The blood should spread out in a very thin layer. The two cover glasses are then pulled quickly apart on a plane parallel to their surfaces.

A slide and cover slip may be used in a somewhat similar manner; or two slides may be used, one being employed as a spreader. In the latter case, place the drop of blood at the end of the spreader slide, allow the two slides to come together at an angle of 30 to 40 degrees, and push the slide across. The blood will follow. Experience will help one to regulate the thickness of the film by varying the pressure, changing the angle, and using a smaller or larger drop.

After drying, the smears are ready for staining.

Wright's Stain—The stain is best purchased in dry form, preferably in capsules each containing 0.1 Gm. To make the stock solution, the contents of one capsule are dissolved in 60 cc. of methyl alcohol especially prepared for making Wright's stain. *Ordinary methyl alcohol, even C.P., will not do.* For use, 20 cc. of the stock solution are filtered off, and 5 cc. of methyl alcohol are added to the filtrate. The bottle should be chemically clean before refilling.

Allow the blood film to be stained to dry, and then flood it with Wright's stain from a dropper, counting the drops. Leave for sixty seconds in a place where no air blows across it. Add distilled water until a greenish metallic scum appears, using approximately the same number of drops as were used of stain. Let stand two and a half to three minutes. Rinse with distilled water and dry.

NOTE: Buffer solution may be substituted with advantage for the distilled water:

monobasic potassium phosphate.............6.63 Gm.
anhydrous dibasic sodium phosphate........2.56 Gm.
chloroform................................1   cc.
distilled water.......................1,000   cc.

Giemsa's Stain—This stain is widely used for blood parasites and other protozoa and also as a routine blood stain. It is difficult to prepare and should be purchased already mixed. It consists of:

Azure II Eosin............................3   Gm.
Azure II..................................0.8 Gm.
glycerin (Merck, C.P.)....................250   cc.
methyl alcohol (reagent).................250   cc.

To stain: Fix films in methyl alcohol; then immerse for twenty minutes or longer in a freshly prepared mixture of 1 cc. of stain and 10 cc. of distilled water, placing the slides on edge in the stain. Another method is to apply 30 drops of distilled water upon the fixed film, add 3 drops of Giemsa's stain, mix, and allow to stand for fifteen to twenty minutes.

Reticulocyte Stain

OSGOOD-WILHELM METHOD—Mix in a small test tube equal parts (5 drops) of oxalated venous or capillary blood and 1 percent brilliant cresyl blue in 0.85 percent sodium chloride solution. Let stand for at least one minute, mix, and make thin smears, which are dried in air. Counterstain with Wright's stain if desired. Reticulated cells show a blue precipitate of various patterns. All red cells and reticulocytes in adjacent fields are counted, and the percentage of reticulocytes is noted.

Peroxidase Test

GOODPASTURE'S STAIN—Prepare dried films on slides or covers in the usual manner (see above). Cover with a measured amount of Goodpasture's stain for one minute. Add an equal amount of water containing 2 drops of hydrogen peroxide to each 15 cc., and let stand for three to four minutes. Rinse well in water, dry, and examine.

Nuclei are red, cytoplasm and platelets pale pink, and red corpuscles buff color. Cells giving the peroxidase reaction—the myeloid series—contain sharply defined, deep-blue granules, which distinguish them from cells of the lymphocytic series and from tissue cells.

Stain (will keep for several months):

sodium nitroprusside.....................0.05 Gm.
benzidine, C.P............................0.05 Gm.
basic fuchsin............................0.05 Gm.
alcohol................................100   cc.

TESTS ON RED CELLS

Hemoglobin Estimation

SAHLI METHOD—Fill the graduated tube to the mark 10 with N/10 hydrochloric acid. Obtain a drop of blood and draw it into the pipette to mark 20 cu. mm. Wipe off tip of pipette, transfer blood to the hydrochloric acid solution in the tube, and rinse well. Place the tube in the frame; after letting stand for one minute, dilute with water drop by drop, mixing each time, until the color of this tube exactly matches that of the standard. The percentage of hemoglobin may then be read directly off the scale. A reading of 100 percent corresponds to 17.3 Gm. hemoglobin in 100 cc. of blood. The normal therefore reads 80 to 90 percent.

OSGOOD-HASKINS METHOD—Take exactly 1 cc. of well-mixed oxalated blood (venous) in a 100-cc. volumetric flask with 40 cc. distilled water. Add 50 cc. of N/5 hydrochloric acid solution, mix well, and make up to 100 cc. Heat part of this mixture in a test tube in a water bath at 55° to 60° C. for seven minutes or longer; then cool. Place standard in colorimeter cup, set at 15 mm., and compare with the unknown, obtaining an average of three or four readings. Take temperature of standard, and refer to the table furnished with the standard for the percentage at different temperatures. One hundred percent represents 13.8 Gm. per 100 cc. when standard at 15.5° C. is set at 15 mm. and the unknown is read at 10.5 mm. (A normal blood may be kept as an acid hematin standard for about a week.)

NEWCOMER METHOD—Place the Newcomer standard disk in the colorimeter, fill this cup with water, and use as standard of comparison with the unknown, which is prepared by mixing 20 cu. mm. of blood with exactly 5 cc. of approximately N/10 hydrochloric acid solution. A table is supplied with the disk for calculating the amount of hemoglobin.

Diluting Fluid for Red Cell Count—

mercuric chloride...........................0.5 Gm.
sodium sulfate..............................5 Gm.
sodium chloride............................1 Gm.
distilled water............................200 cc.

Red Cell Volume—Place 4 cc. of well-mixed oxalated blood in a special (4.5 cc., graduated in 0.1 cc.) centrifuge tube and centrifuge at high speed for two minutes. Read total volume of blood, estimating hundredths of a cubic centimeter. Then continue to centrifuge in ten-minute periods until two successive readings show no further change in volume. Calculate the red cell volume per 100 cc. as follows:

$$\frac{\text{Cubic centimeters of packed red cells}}{\text{Cubic centimeters of blood}} \times 100$$

Red cell volume is also determined as part of the Rourke-Ernstene method for red cell sedimentation rate (p. 526).

Color Index—To calculate color index, it is necessary to have an accurate red cell count and hemoglobin determination and to know the normal standards for these in terms of the patient's sex and age. If x in the following equation represents the Gm. of hemoglobin equivalent to a 100 percent reading by the method used (17.3 Gm. for the Sahli, 13.8 Gm. for the Osgood-Haskins, and 16.92 Gm. for the Newcomer) and y represents the normal amount of hemoglobin per 100 cc. of blood (14.7 Gm. for men, 14.3 Gm. for women, and 12.0 Gm. for children), then:

$$\text{Color index} = \frac{5,000,000}{\text{red cell count}} \times$$
$$\text{hemoglobin percent} \times \frac{x}{y}$$

Red Cell Diameter—Several available methods have been described, using the eyepiece micrometer, an eriometer, or a halometer. From 200 to 1,000 cells may be directly measured by the first of these; but if one desires to make many estimations, the eriometer is much faster and probably more satisfactory on the whole.

Red Cell Fragility (Resistance to Hypotonic Salt Solution)

METHOD OF SANFORD—Make a stock preparation of exactly 0.5 percent salt solution by weighing out precisely 0.5 Gm. of freshly dried C.P. sodium

chloride in a delicate balance, dissolving it in distilled water, and making the volume up to 100 cc. in a volumetric flask.

For the test, arrange in a rack two series of twelve small test tubes, numbering them consecutively in each series from 25 down to and including 14. With a capillary pipette, place in each tube the same number of drops of the stock 0.5 percent salt solution as the number on the tube, holding the pipette always at the same angle to insure equality in size of drops. Then add to each tube, with the same pipette, distilled water in whatever number of drops is required to bring the volume in each tube to 25 drops. Mix well. The tubes now represent two identical graded series of salt solutions, the percentage strength of any of which can be found by multiplying its number by 0.02.

Venous blood is used for the test. It must be drawn into a dry syringe through a dry needle no smaller than 21 gauge. The amount required is about 1 to 1.5 cc. If possible, have the rack of prepared test tubes at the bedside so that one drop of blood can be expelled without delay into each tube of one series. If some time must elapse before the blood can be added, it may be mixed with citrated salt solution (containing 2 percent sodium citrate and 0.85 percent sodium chloride). Before use, the corpuscles are washed with 0.7 percent salt solution, and a 50 percent suspension is made.

As near as possible to the time blood is drawn from the patient, some is also drawn from a normal person and a control test is set up, using the second series of tubes containing salt solution. *The control test should not be omitted*, for it serves as a test of the correctness of the salt solutions and at the same time provides a standard for interpretation of slight deviations from average fragility.

Let both sets of tubes stand for two hours at room temperature. In that interval the corpuscles will have settled to the bottom. Hemolysis may be recognized by the color of the supernatant fluid, which will be faintly pink if hemolysis is partial ("initial hemolysis") and red, with little or no sediment, if it is complete.

With normal blood, hemolysis usually begins in the tube containing 0.44 or 0.42 percent salt solution (tube 22 or 21) and is complete in that containing 0.34 percent (tube 17). When a control is used, a variation of even 0.02 may be considered definite.

Red Cell Sedimentation Rate—An increased rate of settling of red cells in fluid blood indicates a change in the composition of the plasma which is considered to result from absorption into the blood of products of tissue destruction. The rate of red cell sedimentation therefore serves as an indirect measure of tissue breakdown without regard to etiology. Normal readings may be found in disease, but only in those conditions which do not produce inflammation or active tissue destruction. Abnormal rates do not necessarily mean disease, for in pregnancy there is almost always a moderate increase.

Gross changes in sedimentation rate occur in acute and chronic local and general infections and in severe trauma. More moderate acceleration is found in leukemia, lymphoma, malignant tumors, liver disease with jaundice, nephritis, cardiac decompensation, and thrombosis, including coronary occlusion. At the onset of a disease process, there may be a delay (amounting to a day or more) in alteration of the red cell sedimentation rate; and as recovery proceeds, the rate may be the last laboratory finding to return to normal, an abnormal rate persisting after fever and leukocytosis have disappeared. It serves, then, as a useful guide to progress in chronic or slow-healing conditions such as coronary occlusion, rheumatoid arthritis, rheumatic fever, tuberculosis, and others.

There are three phases in red cell sedimentation. The first is characterized by a progressive increase in the size of red cell clumps and rouleaux formation, with relatively slow settling. As the aggregates become larger, their rate of settling increases, and the second phase begins. This period is marked by a relatively uniform rate of sedimentation. Transition to the third phase occurs as the clumps of red cells begin to collect and pack at the bottom of the tube, gradually bringing the rate of fall to a standstill.

Major alterations in sedimentation rate are caused by variations in size of the red cell aggregates. In turn, the degree of clumping appears to vary with the concentration of certain blood constituents, particularly serum globulins and plasma fibrinogen. The exact physicochemical mechanism has not been established.

No standard method for determining red cell sedimentation rate has been adopted, and the results of different methods cannot be compared directly. Table 62 compares five methods. In general, it can be said that the internal diameter of the sedimentation tube should be no less than 2.5 mm. Narrow tubes retard settling velocity. A low red cell count increases sedimentation rate. The rate of sedimentation is also affected by the choice of anticoagulant: Potassium oxalate alone as an

anticoagulant shrinks red cells; sodium citrate retards sedimentation; a mixture of ammonium and potassium oxalate appears to have a minimal effect on settling. Three methods are described below.

WESTERGREN METHOD—This method is relatively simple and is therefore widely used. The special Westergren tube is required, with a rack that will hold it in an exactly vertical position. Exactly 0.5 cc. of 3.8 percent sodium citrate solution is used as anticoagulant. It may be placed in a test tube or in the syringe into which the blood is drawn. Exactly 4.5 cc. of blood are mixed thoroughly with the anticoagulant, and the Westergren tube is filled exactly to the zero mark and placed vertically in the rack. The level of the upper edge of the red cell mass is read at the end of exactly one hour. Normal and abnormal ranges are given in the table.

CUTLER METHOD—This method provides a graphic record and information as to the velocity during each five-minute period. The special Cutler tube is used, with a rack to hold it vertically. Exactly 0.1 cc. of 3.8 percent sodium citrate solution is placed in a 2-cc. syringe, and blood is drawn from a vein up to the 1-cc. mark. Blood and anticoagulant are thoroughly mixed, and the sedimentation tube is filled exactly to the zero mark and placed in the rack. The upper level of the red cell mass is read at intervals of five minutes, the results being recorded on the charts especially designed for this purpose. A curve is drawn connecting the points recorded. The original Cutler procedure recommended a total observation period of sixty minutes, but more recently this has been cut to thirty. Normal and abnormal ranges for the sixty-minute period are given in the table.

ROURKE-ERNSTENE METHOD—This method is the most complicated but has been chosen by many workers as the most informative. Special tubes are used, having a capacity of 1.2 to 1.25 cc. and graduated in 2-mm. divisions. Three cc. of blood are drawn from a vein without stasis into a dry syringe and transferred immediately to a tube containing 2 mg. of heparin.* The blood and heparin are thoroughly mixed, and the tube is allowed to stand for not less than fifteen minutes or more than three hours.

When the test is to be started, the blood is again mixed by inverting the tube back and forth for two to three minutes. The sedimentation tube is

---

* 150 mg. of heparin are dissolved in 1 cc. of distilled water. A capillary pipette is prepared so that it will deliver approximately 75 drops to 1 cc. One drop (2 mg. heparin) of this solution is used for 3 cc. of blood.

TABLE 62 — *Comparison of Five Sedimentation Methods*

	Linzenmeier 1920	Westergren 1920	Cutler 1926	Rourke-Ernstene 1930	Wintrobe-Landsberg 1935
Height of Blood Column	50 mm.	200 mm.	50 mm.	100 mm.	100 mm.
Internal Diameter of Tube	5.0 mm.	2.5 mm.	5.0 mm.	4.0 mm.	2.5 mm.
Anticoagulant	Sodium citrate, 5%	Sodium citrate, 3.8%	Sodium citrate, 3%	Heparin, 15%	Mixture of solid potassium and ammonium oxalate
Expression of Sedimentation Value	Minutes required to settle 18 mm.	Millimeters settled in one hour	Millimeters settled in one hour and graph of five-minute readings	Millimeters settled in fastest minute (corrected for red cell concentration)	Millimeters settled in one hour (corrected for red cell concentration)
Normal Range	200 to 600 minutes	1 to 3 mm.—men 4 to 7 mm.—women	2 to 8 mm.—men 2 to 10 mm.—women Graph approaches a horizontal line	0.08 to 0.35 mm.	0 to 9 mm.—men 0 to 20 mm.—women
Abnormal Range					9 to 15 mm.—men
Slight	100 to 200 minutes	8 to 15 mm.	Graph—diagonal line	0.35 to 0.6 mm.	20 to 25 mm.—women
Moderate	60 to 100 minutes	15 to 40 mm.	Graph—diagonal curve	0.6 to 1.0 mm.	15 to 30 mm.
Extreme	15 to 30 minutes	80 to 110 mm.	Graph—vertical curve	2.0 to 2.5 mm.	35 to 50 mm.

then filled to the mark and placed in a vertical position. The degree of settling is recorded on a graph at frequent intervals until two readings indicate a lessened rate of settling because of packing of the red cells. The sedimentation tube is then transferred to a centrifuge and spun at 3,000 r.p.m. for thirty minutes to obtain the hematocrit reading. The slope of the period of constant fall in millimeters per minute is calculated from the graph and is corrected for hematocrit value (see Red Cell Volume, p. 525) according to Figure 58 (p. 528). Normal and abnormal ranges are given in Table 62.

TESTS ON WHITE CELLS AND PLATELETS

Diluting Fluid for White Cell Count

    glacial acetic acid.............................1 cc.
    crystal violet (1 percent) ....1 cc.
    distilled water...............................100 cc.

Blood Platelet Count (Olef Method)

DILUENT

    sodium metaphosphate (Howe and French).....1 Gm.
    sodium chloride............................0.5 Gm.
    dextrose...................................0.1 Gm.
    distilled water............................100 cc.

STAIN

    sodium metaphosphate (Howe and French)....1   Gm.
    sodium chloride...........................0.4 Gm.
    dextrose..................................0.1 Gm.
    sodium bicarbonate........................0.1 Gm.
    brilliant cresyl blue.....................0.15 Gm.
    distilled water...........................100 cc.

TECHNIC—Always use a finger, prepared by immersing hand in warm water. Puncture palmar surface deeply enough to obtain free flow of blood without pressure. Discard the first drop or two; then place a drop of diluent over the puncture before the blood reaches the surface of the skin, and rapidly turn the hand over so that the palmar surface is down. The blood falls to the dependent

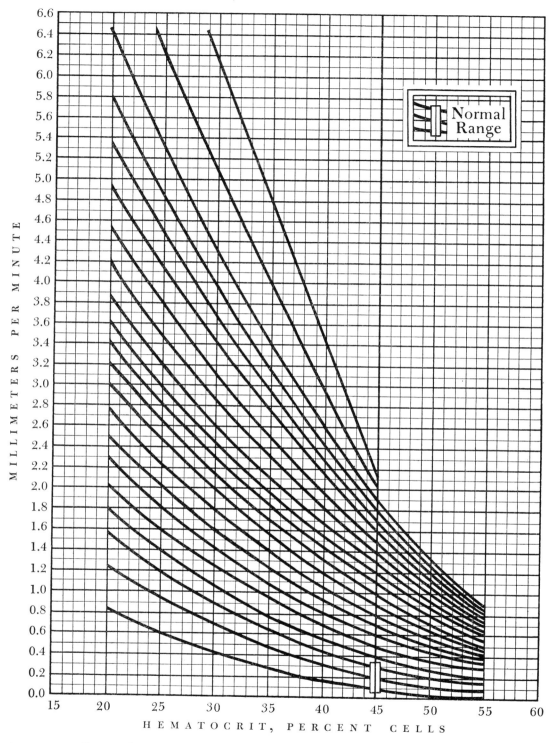

FIGURE 58 — *Chart for Correcting Blood Sedimentation Rate for Red Cell Volume According to the Rourke-Ernstene Method* (From *J. Clin. Investigation,* 8:557, 1930)

surface of the drop of diluent, and the entire mixture is then transferred to the surface of a small quantity (three or four drops) of diluting fluid in a previously prepared paraffin cup. The blood is thus diluted about 1:5. The cup is made by applying a heated glass rod to a paraffin cube about 2 cm. square.

The contents of the cup are stirred with a paraffined applicator and, after standing for a minute or two, are again stirred and transferred by the paraffined applicator to a clean glass slide. Three slides are usually obtained; after standing under cover slips for fifteen minutes, they are ready for examination. The platelets appear as clear, isolated, highly refractile bodies with numerous fine, spinelike processes projecting from the periphery. The slide may be stained if desired; both platelets and reticulocytes will be colored.

A relative platelet-red cell count is made, using the oil immersion lens. Random fields are counted until at least 1,000 cells have been seen. A red cell count is then done in the usual manner, and the absolute number of platelets per cu. mm. is calculated from these data. The average for men is 525,000; for women, 504,000.

TESTS INVOLVING BLOOD COAGULATION

Bleeding Time

DUKE'S METHOD—Make a small cut in the lobe of the ear with a blood lancet or the point of a scalpel. At one-half-minute intervals, blot off all blood with a piece of absorbent paper. The usual bleeding time is one to three minutes until the hemorrhage finally ceases.

Coagulation Time

SIMPLE METHOD—Collect several drops of blood on a clean glass slide. At one-minute intervals draw a needle through one or another drop. Coagulation has occurred when fibrin shreds cling to the needle and can be dragged along with it. The normal is seven minutes or less.

LEE AND WHITE METHOD—Obtain venous blood with a small hypodermic syringe; it is important to enter the vein quickly and without suction. Place 1 cc. of blood in a clean 8-mm. test tube which has been rinsed with physiological salt solution. Place tube in water bath at 75°F., and tilt at intervals until the tube can be inverted without displacing the clot. The normal coagulation time by this method is five to eight minutes. A larger tube prolongs the time of clotting.

Prothrombin Time

METHOD OF QUICK—Three solutions are required:

1. Sodium oxalate, 0.1 M, prepared by dissolving 1.34 Gm. anhydrous sodium oxalate, C.P., in 100 cc. of distilled water.

2. Calcium chloride, 0.025 M, made by dissolving 1.11 Gm. anhydrous calcium chloride, C.P., in 400 cc. of distilled water.

3. Thromboplastin solution. Strip the pia and all visible blood vessels from the brain of a freshly killed rabbit, and macerate the organ in a mortar under acetone (which must not be acid). Replace the acetone several times, and finally obtain a nonadhesive granular powder. Dry this on a suction filter and seal 0.3-Gm. portions in small ampoules. Before sealing, evacuate the ampoules for three minutes with an oil vacuum pump. This material will keep indefinitely in a refrigerator.

To make the thromboplastin solution, thoroughly mix the contents of one ampoule of the dry powder with 5 cc. of freshly prepared 0.9 percent sodium chloride solution, and incubate at 50°C. for fifteen minutes. Allow the coarse particles to settle out, and use the supernatant milky fluid. Centrifugation reduces activity. This fluid is stable for a few days only.

TECHNIC—To perform the test, draw 4.5 cc. of blood from a vein and mix immediately with 0.5 cc. of the 0.1 M sodium oxalate. Centrifuge to obtain plasma. Mix 0.1 cc. of plasma and 0.1 cc. of thromboplastin. On the water bath at 37.5°C., add 0.1 cc. of the 0.025 M calcium chloride and immediately click stop watch. Tip the tube each second, and record with the stop watch the time of clot formation.

Normal prothrombin time may vary from 9 to 30 seconds, depending on the activity of the thromboplastin solution. A normal standard should be established for each new solution and at intervals of forty-eight hours during the use of a given solution. This is accomplished by performing the test on the blood of two normal individuals.

KATO MODIFICATION OF THE QUICK METHOD— Kato has introduced a microtechnic for the Quick method which makes venipuncture unnecessary, although venous blood can be used. The calcium chloride solution and thromboplastin suspension of Quick are used (see above), but in place of sodium oxalate solution a 2 percent double oxalate solution is employed. This last is made by dissolving 0.75 Gm. potassium oxalate and 1.25 Gm. ammonium oxalate in 100 cc. of distilled water. A

special combination microhemopipette is used,*
and a special hanging-drop slide, with a central
depression 15 mm. in diameter and 3 mm. deep,
is recommended.

To make the test, place 20 cu. mm. of the oxalate
mixture in the hollow of the slide and allow to dry.
Make a deep puncture in the patient's heel, finger
tip, or ear lobe; and while the blood flow is free,
receive about 0.2 cc. (4 to 5 large drops) of blood
into the hollow of the slide. Mix the blood and
dry oxalate thoroughly to prevent clotting. Place
the slide in a moist chamber, such as a petri dish
containing a wet blotter or filter paper, until ready
to complete the test. Using the microhemopipette,
take exactly 10 cu. mm. each of fresh thromboplastin solution and of the calcium chloride solution (0.025 M), and mix them thoroughly in a
white porcelain spot plate or the well of a clean
hanging-drop slide. Then add exactly 10 cu. mm.
of well-mixed oxalated blood to the above mixture,
stirring thoroughly for five or six seconds with a
fine glass rod. Record with a stop watch the time
from the addition of the blood to the formation of
a clot.

The normal standard is determined in the same
way as for the original Quick method.

LINK-SHAPIRO MODIFICATION OF THE QUICK
METHOD—Four solutions are required. The first
two are the same as solutions 1 and 2 of Quick
(p. 529). The third solution is 0.85 percent sodium
chloride solution, prepared from reagent-grade salt.
The fourth is a thromboplastin-calcium chloride
mixture. The thromboplastin may be prepared
from rabbit brain (see p. 529) or from rabbit lung
(the rabbit is killed by air embolism, and the lungs
are quickly removed and dried *in vacuo*), or it may
be purchased (Maltine). Add 50 mg. of the thromboplastin to 2.5 cc. of the 0.85 percent sodium
chloride solution, stir until a uniform suspension is
obtained, place in a water bath at 54° to 56°C.,
and continue to stir for ten minutes. Remove from
the water bath, cool to 25° to 26°C., and add 2.5
cc. of the 0.025 M calcium chloride solution. Stir
this mixture for four minutes, and centrifuge for
four minutes at 1,700 to 2,000 r.p.m. Remove the
tube carefully so as not to disturb the packed sediment, and draw off the slightly turbid supernatant
fluid with a pipette. This fluid is the thromboplastin reagent. It should be stored under refrigeration.

The suggested apparatus includes the following:
1. Constant-temperature water bath (37.5°C.),
preferably made of glass.
2. Test tubes, 100 × 12 mm.
3. Copper test-tube racks.

4. Stop watch, preferably mounted on the laboratory table in such a way as to be controlled by
a foot pedal.
5. Folin-Wu micro sugar pipettes graduated to
contain 0.1 and 0.2 cc. (ml.).
6. Kahn viewer (in case the water bath is not
made of glass).

To perform the test, draw 4.5 cc. of blood from
a vein and mix it quickly with 0.5 cc. of the 0.1 M
sodium oxalate. Centrifuge for ten minutes to obtain plasma. If prothrombin time is to be determined in 12.5 percent diluted plasma, mix 0.1 cc.
whole plasma with 0.7 cc. of the sodium chloride
solution in another test tube. Mix by tapping lower
end of tube.

Transfer 0.2-cc. portions of thromboplastin-calcium chloride suspension into test tubes with a
0.2-cc. sugar pipette. Place these tubes in a rack
with the tubes containing whole and diluted plasma,
and immerse rack in the water bath for one minute.
With a sugar pipette, transfer 0.1 cc. of whole or
diluted plasma (by blowing it in quickly) to a tube
containing 0.2 cc. of thromboplastin-calcium chloride suspension. At the same time start the stop
watch. Tap the tube sharply to mix the solutions.
Introduce a small nickel-chrome wire stirrer, and
sweep it back and forth across the tube at the
rate of one cycle per second. The stirring may take
place out of the water bath and under the Kahn
viewer. The end point is that moment at which the
fibrin clot is sufficiently stable to be drawn to one
side by the stirrer, thus bringing to view a clear
area. The clot is usually turbid because of the
presence of precipitated calcium oxalate.

Normal prothrombin time by the Link-Shapiro
technic is usually 13 to 17 seconds for whole plasma
and 35 to 42 seconds for diluted plasma. However,
a normal standard should be established for each
new suspension and at intervals of forty-eight hours
during use of a given suspension.

BLOOD SUGAR

Most of the methods in common use, particularly
those depending upon copper reduction, include
in the determination a nondextrose fraction which
was formerly thought to be small and relatively
constant. More recent investigations have shown
that the nondextrose fraction may be as small as
1 mg. or as large as 78 mg. per 100 cc. of blood.
In 38 percent of one series of determinations it
was more than 30 mg. per 100 cc. The nondextrose

* Obtainable from Fisher Scientific Co., 717 Forbes Street,
Pittsburgh, Pa.

reducing substances are believed to include gluta-thione, cysteine, fructose, ergothioneine, and creat-inine.

The established normal value for the blood sugar of 80 to 120 mg. per 100 cc. includes this nondex-trose fraction. Some newer methods have been devised which record more nearly true dextrose values, and they are being adopted gradually in place of the older methods. However, since the macromethod of Folin and Wu is still the most widely employed in this country, we are describing it in detail, as well as the Folin micromethod which may be used with finger blood.

In interpreting blood-sugar values, one should bear in mind that the level is dependent upon a good many factors. For example, in the fasting state, the sugar content of capillary blood from the finger is about the same as that of venous blood, whereas in the normal person it may be 20 to 50 mg. higher than that of venous blood after a meal or after dextrose. Table 63 presents accepted levels obtained by various methods with the pa-tient in the fasting condition.

TABLE 63—*Blood Sugar: Established Normal Levels*

Method	Blood Sugar in mg. per 100 cc. of Blood
Folin-Wu	90-120
Folin-Malmros (micro)	75-105
Hagedorn-Jensen (micro)	75-105
Folin-Wu (Folin's modification) .	75-105
Folin-Wu (unlaked blood)	75-105
Benedict copper reduction	70-100
Somogyi-Shaffer-Hartman	70-100

Collection of Blood—The micromethods have the advantage of utilizing small amounts of blood which can be obtained from a finger prick with a sharp stylet. Unless the operator is skillful, how-ever, variations will occur because of the difficulty in accurately measuring 0.1 cc. of blood. The methods are of advantage in children and in in-stances when a series of observations at close inter-vals is required.

Venous specimens are still in most common use, and they are usually easily obtained from the vein in the antecubital space. Use of an ordinary hypo-dermic needle is entirely satisfactory with a little practice, and the added comfort over larger needles will be appreciated by the patient.

Dry, powdered potassium oxalate, 2 mg. to 1 cc. of blood, is quite satisfactory to prevent clotting; if the blood must stand more than an hour before it can be tested, it should be placed in the refriger-ator. If the blood must be kept several days, 10 mg. of neutral sodium fluoride should be added for each cc. of oxalated blood.

Method of Folin-Wu

PREPARATION OF PROTEIN-FREE FILTRATE (HA-DEN MODIFICATION)—To one volume of blood from a pipette, add eight volumes of N/12 sulfuric acid. Laking occurs rapidly, and the mixture becomes dark in color. Add one volume of 10 percent sodium tungstate solution, mix well, and filter. The filtrate should be water-clear, and it is suitable for other estimations besides sugar.

DETERMINATION OF DEXTROSE IN BLOOD—

REAGENTS—1. Alkaline copper tartrate solution. Dissolve 40 Gm. anhydrous sodium carbonate in 400 cc. distilled water in a liter flask. Add 7.5 Gm. of tartaric acid and, when it is dissolved, 4.5 Gm. of crystallized copper sulfate. Make volume up to one liter.

2. Molybdate-phosphate solution. Transfer 35 Gm. of molybdic acid to a beaker; add 5 Gm. of sodium tungstate, 200 cc. of 10 percent sodium hydroxide, and 200 cc. of distilled water. Boil the solution vigorously for twenty to forty minutes until the ammonia is removed. After cooling, dilute to 350 cc.; then add 125 cc. of concentrated phos-phoric acid (85 percent). Make volume up to 500 cc.

3. Standard sugar solutions.
   a. Stock solution of 1 percent dextrose in satu-rated benzoic acid solution (stable indef-initely).
   b. Standard containing 10 mg. dextrose per 100 cc. Pipette 1 cc. stock solution into a volumetric flask and dilute to mark 100 cc. with benzoic acid solution (2.5 Gm. in 1 liter). Each 2 cc. of this standard then con-tain 0.2 mg. dextrose.
   c. Standard containing 20 mg. dextrose per 100 cc. Pipette 2 cc. stock solution into 100-cc. volumetric flask and dilute to mark with benzoic acid solution.

PROCEDURE—Place 2 cc. of blood filtrate in a Folin-Wu sugar tube graduated at 25 cc., and to two other tubes add 2 cc. of the standard sugar solutions previously prepared (containing respec-tively 0.2 and 0.4 mg. of dextrose). Add 2 cc. of alkaline copper solution to each, and place in a boiling water bath for six minutes. Cool in running water; then add to each tube 2 cc. of molybdate-phosphate solution. Let stand about a minute; then dilute to 25-cc. mark with water, and mix thoroughly. Compare in a colorimeter with the standard which most nearly matches the unknown.

CALCULATION—Setting the standard at 20:

$$\frac{20}{\text{Reading of unknown}} \times 100 = \text{mg. dextrose}$$

per 100 cc. when using the standard containing 10 mg. per 100 cc. (2 cc. = 0.2 mg. dextrose).

$$\frac{20}{\text{Reading of unknown}} \times 200 = \text{mg. dextrose}$$

per 100 cc. when using the standard containing 20 mg. per 100 cc. (2 cc. = 0.4 mg. dextrose).

Folin Micromethod for Blood Sugar

REAGENTS—1. Sulfate-tungstate solution. Place 10 Gm. of C.P. anhydrous sodium sulfate and 15 cc. of 10 percent sodium tungstate solution in a 500-cc. volumetric flask, add 250 cc. distilled water, and shake until dissolved. Dilute to volume and mix.

2. Sulfuric acid. Dissolve 12 cc. of 2/3 N sulfuric acid and 2 Gm. of anhydrous sodium sulfate in a 100-cc. volumetric flask and dilute to volume.

3. Potassium ferricyanide solution. In a brown bottle place 1 Gm. of C.P. potassium ferricyanide and dilute to 250 cc. with distilled water. Keep in the dark.

4. Sodium cyanide-carbonate solution. Add 50 cc. distilled water to 8 Gm. anhydrous sodium carbonate in a 500-cc. volumetric flask and shake well. Add 150 cc. of freshly prepared 1 percent sodium cyanide solution, dilute to volume, and mix.

5. Ferric iron-gum ghatti solution. Fill a liter cylinder with cold water to the mark, and push into it a piece of wire screen to form a bowl well below the surface of the water. Place about 20 Gm. of gum ghatti in the screen, cover the flask, and let stand. After twenty-four hours, remove screen and strain through a clean laboratory towel. With the aid of heat, dissolve 5 Gm. of anhydrous ferric sulfate and 75 cc. of 85 percent phosphoric acid in 100 cc. of water in a beaker. Cool and add slowly to the gum ghatti solution. Then add 15 cc. of 1 percent potassium permanganate solution, a few cc. at a time. Keep in a warm place for several days in order to clear the turbidity of the solution.

6. Standard stock solution of dextrose. Dissolve 1 Gm. benzoic acid in 300 cc. hot distilled water. Add 980 mg. anhydrous dextrose and 400 cc. distilled water, cool to room temperature, and make up to 1 L. The working standard is prepared by diluting 1 cc. of this solution to 100 cc. with water.

PROCEDURE—Collect exactly 0.1 cc. of blood from a finger prick and add to 4 cc. sulfate-tungstate solution in a centrifuge tube. Rinse the pipette by suction a few times and stir. Allow to stand for fifteen minutes; then add 1 cc. of the sulfuric acid-sulfate solution and stir with the micropipette still in the centrifuge tube. Centrifuge for five minutes.

To a 25-cc. graduated test tube, transfer 2 cc. of the clear supernatant fluid and 2 cc. of water. Add 4 cc. of the standard working solution of dextrose to another similar tube. To both add 1 cc. (or 2 cc.) of the 0.4 percent potassium ferricyanide solution and then 1 cc. of the cyanide-carbonate solution. One cc. is accurate up to 300 mg. percent. With 2 cc., the range is from far below 100 to over 500 mg. percent, but the high values are slightly low and the low values slightly high. Heat both tubes together in a boiling water bath for eight minutes, cool, and to each add 5 cc. of the ferric iron-gum ghatti solution.

Dilute contents of each tube to 25 cc., mix, and compare in a colorimeter using a yellow light filter. Set standard at 20 mm.

CALCULATION

$$\text{Dextrose in mg. per 100 cc.} = \frac{20}{\text{reading of unknown}} \times 100.$$

Microdetermination of True Blood Dextrose—A modification has been evolved by Lauber and Mattice which is a combination of parts of well-known and established methods. Protein removal is by the technic of Somogyi, using an alkaline-zinc solution. The method is suitable for estimation by either the photoelectric colorimeter or the visual colorimeter.

REAGENTS—1. Alkaline copper tartrate solution (see p. 531).

2. Molybdate-phosphate solution (see p. 531).

3. Standard sugar solutions (see p. 531).

4. Sodium hydroxide solution, 0.25 N. Dissolve 10 Gm. sodium hydroxide in 100 cc. distilled water.

5. Zinc sulfate-sulfuric acid reagent. Dissolve 6.25 Gm. zinc sulfate ($ZnSO_4 \cdot 7H_2O$) in 200 cc. of water and transfer to a liter volumetric flask. Slowly add 62.5 cc. of 0.25 N sulfuric acid, and mix. Make up to one liter with distilled water. On titration, 25 cc. of this solution should be neutralized by 5 to 5.1 cc. of Reagent 4, phenolphthalein being used as an indicator. Freshly prepared quantities of both solutions should always be standardized in this manner before use.

PROCEDURE—Blood obtained by finger prick with a sterile needle is milked into a shallow paraffin cup. The serologic pipette calibrated for 0.1 cc. of blood is used to transfer 0.1 cc. into 1.6 cc. zinc sulfate reagent contained in a small test tube. Rinse the pipette several times with the contents of this tube. The tube is shaken, and a sample may be left corked at room temperature for several hours without danger of loss of sugar such as occurs with oxalated blood.

Add 0.3 cc. of 0.25 N sodium hydroxide and shake vigorously. Centrifuge and transfer 1 cc. of the clear, colorless supernatant fluid to a graduated 10-cc. test tube. A similar tube receives 1 cc. of the standard dextrose solution (0.005 or 0.01 percent according to the anticipated blood dextrose value).

To each tube is added 1 cc. alkaline copper tartrate reagent. The tubes are gently but thoroughly shaken, heated in a boiling water bath for exactly eight minutes, and cooled in running water for one to two minutes; then 1 cc. molybdate-phosphate reagent is added. All the cuprous oxide should react. The tubes should not be shaken at this point. If a scum of oxide persists on the surface, an additional drop of molybdate-phosphate should be allowed to fall on the film and cause its disappearance. The tubes should stand undisturbed for fifteen minutes for maximum color development.

Dilute to 6.25 cc. and invert the tube several times. After four or five minutes, match in a colorimeter fitted with a 42 filter (blue). If a visual colorimeter is used, micro cups and plunger should replace the standard equipment.

CALCULATION—For the Klett-Summerson photoelectric colorimeter:

$$\text{Dextrose in mg. per 100 cc.} = \frac{\text{reading of unknown}}{\text{reading of standard}} \times$$

(mg. dextrose in 1 cc. standard) × (factor for aliquot of filtrate analyzed) × (factor for conversion of volume of blood used to 100 cc.). When the standard 0.005 percent dextrose solution is used, when 1/2 of the filtrate is analyzed, and when 0.1 cc. of blood is used, the appropriate factors are 0.05 × 2 × 1,000, which is 100. The formula for dextrose in mg. per 100 cc. then becomes:

$$\frac{\text{Reading of unknown}}{\text{Reading of standard}} \times 100.$$

For the visual colorimeter with the same factors as above, and with the standard set at 15:

$$\text{Dextrose in mg. per 100 cc.} = \frac{15}{\text{reading of unknown}} \times 100.$$

Blood-Sugar Screening Test (Wilkerson-Heftmann Method)—For preliminary detection of diabetes mellitus, and particularly when groups are being screened, the physician needs only to know whether a patient's blood sugar has exceeded a specified level. Such information is also of value in management of diabetic patients.

A test incorporating this principle has been developed by Wilkerson and Heftmann, of the United States Public Health Service. Fixed levels have been established above which the test is positive and below which it is negative. The test is based on a method of blood-sugar analysis giving true glucose levels as devised by Hagedorn and co-workers; consequently, the levels used are lower than would be expected were other blood-sugar methods used.

On the basis of actual survey findings, 130 mg. percent true glucose was selected as the postprandial blood-sugar level which would include even borderline cases of diabetes. Obviously, a positive test at this level does not constitute a diagnosis; rather, it selects those individuals who need further diagnostic study (see p. 173).

A second level of 180 mg. percent is also included as a diagnostic level. Blood sugars above this point are in most instances indicative of diabetes mellitus.

A third level of 50 mg. percent is possible by using the kit. This hypoglycemic level may be helpful in the differential diagnosis of Insulin shock.

The kit, supplied as Test Kit No. 7, is complete, including necessary apparatus, heat source, and reagents. The reagents are all in tablet form, and the test may be completed in approximately five minutes' time. Literature containing additional information and technical details is available upon request.

Dextrose Tolerance Tests are used in the diagnosis of diabetes mellitus (p. 173) and pituitary dysfunctions. Interpretation is based on the degree and duration of the rise in blood sugar following administration of a standard quantity of dextrose.

It has been demonstrated repeatedly that the result of the dextrose tolerance test is greatly affected by the previous diet, carbohydrate restriction leading to diabetic types of response. Conn has suggested a diet of 2,800 calories, containing 80 Gm. protein, 300 Gm. carbohydrate, and 140 Gm. fat, to be given for three to seven days before the dextrose tolerance test (depending on the duration of carbohydrate restriction).

This preparatory diet seems to do no harm to the mild diabetic in whose case a dextrose tolerance test may be necessary in order to establish the diagnosis. Dextrose tolerance tests should not be performed on known diabetics.

STANDARD PROCEDURE—Before breakfast, collect a specimen of urine and one of blood to serve as controls; then administer the dextrose by mouth in 50 percent solution. The usual practice is to give 100 Gm. to the adult weighing over 100 pounds, 50 Gm. to lighter individuals, and 25 Gm. to children. Some observers prefer to give 1.5 Gm. of dextrose per kilogram of body weight. Others give the dose intravenously. Collect successive specimens of urine and blood one-half, one, two, and three hours after ingestion of the dextrose, and analyze these for sugar. A curve may then be plotted of blood-sugar level against time.

INTERPRETATION—Although there are some differences of opinion as to interpretation, most observers believe that a normal rise should not reach 170 mg. per 100 cc. when venous blood is used, or 200 mg. with capillary blood, and that the return to normal should occur within two hours. In addition to previous diet, the blood-sugar curve is influenced by age, infections, toxemia, previous administration of Insulin, hypertension, nephritis, pregnancy, hyperthyroidism or hypothyroidism, and diseases of the liver, pituitary, or adrenal cortex.

INTRAVENOUS METHOD (SOSKIN)—Because of the obvious irregularities of absorption of dextrose when given by the oral route, the intravenous tolerance test has become more popular. It is particularly valuable in distinguishing between diabetes and liver disease. It must be emphasized that the technic described by Soskin must be followed exactly if the criteria he has supplied are to be used in evaluation. The test is made in the morning before breakfast; 1/3 Gm. of dextrose per Kg. of body weight, dissolved in a 30 to 50 percent solution, is injected intravenously within three to five minutes. Blood-sugar estimations are made on capillary blood before the test and after one-half hour, one hour, and two hours by a micromethod which measures true dextrose (see p. 532).

INTERPRETATION—In the normal individual, the blood-sugar level returns to the normal value within sixty minutes. In the patient having hyperglycemia because of liver disease, the blood-sugar level does not return within sixty minutes but has returned to the normal value within one hundred twenty minutes. In the diabetic, the level has still not returned to normal at the end of one hundred twenty minutes.

ICTERUS INDEX

The icterus index is a simple and useful measure of the level of bilirubin in the blood. Its chief value is in detecting latent jaundice and in determining the progress and severity of manifest jaundice. Carotinemia gives a similar color to the serum but does not tint the sclera. Carotene can be extracted from serum by petroleum ether, in which bilirubin is not soluble.

REAGENT—Potassium dichromate solution, 0.01 percent, to which have been added 4 drops C.P. sulfuric acid per liter. The solution keeps well if stored in a dark bottle away from light.

TECHNIC—Blood is drawn with a dry needle and syringe in the fasting state, for products of digestion may produce turbidity, which disturbs the test. After the blood is clotted, the serum is withdrawn and diluted with one to four parts of water to make an approximate match to the standard. Diluted serum and standard are compared in a colorimeter.

CALCULATION

$$\text{Icterus index} = \frac{\text{reading of standard}}{\text{reading of unknown}} \times$$
$$\text{factor of dilution.}$$

Normal is 2.5 to 5.

BLOOD CHOLESTEROL

The level of total cholesterol in human serum varies widely from individual to individual, the normal ranging from about 100 to almost 400 mg. per 100 cc. Average values are 200 to 235 mg. The level increases during childhood and in a given individual is quite constant after puberty. The percentage of total cholesterol in the free form is also reasonably constant—25 to 30 percent.

The level of total cholesterol increases about 25 percent during pregnancy, returning to normal about two weeks postpartum. Typical alterations in serum cholesterol level in disease are given in Table 64.

Method of Kaye

TOTAL CHOLESTEROL—The following reagents are used:

1. Total cholesterol standard, 0.4 mg. cholesterol per cc. acetic anhydride, prepared by dissolving 100 mg. pure dry cholesterol in 250 cc. acetic anhydride.

2. Alcohol-ether solution, prepared by adding 750 cc. of 95 percent alcohol to 250 cc. ether. It is kept in a cool place in a glass-stoppered bottle.

3. Acetic anhydride-chloroform solution, prepared by mixing 1 part acetic anhydride with 2 parts chloroform. This is prepared just before use or stored in the refrigerator for a period of not more than two weeks.

4. Concentrated sulfuric acid, C.P., best kept in a dropper bottle.

5. Chloroform.

Blood is drawn from a vein and allowed to clot. Withdraw the serum and place 0.2 cc. of it in a 15-cc. test tube. To this, in a rapid stream, add 12 cc. of alcohol-ether solution. Pack the resultant precipitate by centrifugation for three minutes at 2,000 r.p.m., pour the supernatant fluid into a 25-cc. Erlenmeyer flask, and evaporate just to dryness

TABLE 64 — *Typical Alterations in Serum Cholesterol Level in Certain Diseases*

Disease	Total Cholesterol	Percent of Free Cholesterol
Impaired liver function . .	Decreased	Increased
Nephrosis or nephrotic stage of glomerulo- nephritis.	Increased	Normal
Hypothyroidism.	Increased	Normal
Hyperthyroidism.	Normal or decreased	Normal
Uncontrolled diabetes mellitus	Increased	Normal
Xanthoma tuberosum . . .	Increased	Normal

on a water bath. Because the dry residue must not be overheated, the temperature of the water bath is often reduced to 60° C. when only traces of the solvent remain. When the residue is dry and cool, add 3 cc. of the acetic anhydride-chloroform solution and then 2 drops of concentrated sulfuric acid. Mix the contents of the tube thoroughly, insert stopper, and allow to stand for ten to fifteen minutes for color development. Prepare the standard at the same time by adding 2 cc. of chloroform to 1 cc. of the total cholesterol standard. Add 2 drops of concentrated sulfuric acid, mix, stopper, and allow color to develop. During this period the two test tubes should be out of direct light. The colors are compared in a microcolorimeter.

For calculation, total cholesterol in mg.

$$\text{per 100 cc. serum} = \frac{\text{reading of standard}}{\text{reading of unknown}} \times 200.$$

FREE CHOLESTEROL—For determination of free cholesterol in serum, the following reagents are needed in addition to those used for total cholesterol:

1. Free cholesterol standard, containing 0.4 mg.

in 3 cc., made by mixing in a glass-stoppered bottle equal quantities of the total cholesterol standard, acetic anhydride, and a solution obtained by dissolving 175.6 mg. of digitonin in a small volume of glacial acetic acid at 60° C., cooling, and diluting to 100 cc. with glacial acetic acid.

2. Digitonin solution, 0.5 percent, prepared by dissolving 500 mg. digitonin in 100 cc. of 50 percent alcohol (55 cc. of 95 percent alcohol and 45 cc. of distilled water) at 60° C.

In a 30-cc. test tube, add 25 cc. of alcohol-ether solution in a rapid stream to 0.5 cc. of serum. Centrifuge at 2,000 r.p.m. for three minutes, pour the supernatant fluid into a 25-cc. Erlenmeyer flask, and evaporate to dryness on a water bath as for total cholesterol. When the residue is dry and cool, extract it with three successive 2-cc. portions of ether, transferring the extract quantitatively to a 15-cc. centrifuge tube. Evaporate the ether extract to dryness by placing the tube in a vessel of hot water. Then add 2 cc. of 95 percent alcohol, stopper the test tube, and place in a water bath at 60° C. for thirty minutes. Next, add 1 cc. of the digitonin solution, mixing thoroughly. Restopper and leave at room temperature for at least three hours; then centrifuge at 2,000 r.p.m. for ten minutes. Aspirate the supernatant liquids and suspend the precipitate in 3 cc. of ether. Centrifuge for five minutes and pour off the liquid. Suspend the precipitate once more in 3 cc. of ether, and centrifuge for five minutes before pouring off the supernatant fluid. Dry the precipitate at 60° C. and dissolve in 1 cc. of glacial acetic acid at the same temperature. Cool to room temperature and add 2 cc. of acetic anhydride and 4 drops of concentrated sulfuric acid. Mix well and set aside for twenty-seven minutes out of direct light. At the same time, prepare a standard by adding 4 drops of concentrated sulfuric acid to 3 cc. of the free cholesterol standard, and allow the mixture to stand. Compare the colors in a microcolorimeter.

For calculation, free cholesterol in mg.

$$\text{per 100 cc.} = \frac{\text{reading of standard}}{\text{reading of unknown}} \times 80.$$

CARBON-DIOXIDE COMBINING POWER OF BLOOD PLASMA (METHOD OF VAN SLYKE AND CULLEN)

For this test the special gas analysis apparatus of Van Slyke is necessary. There is also required a large separatory funnel to which is attached by glass and rubber tubing a small catch-bottle filled with glass beads. The barometric pressure must be known at the time the determination is made.

With a minimum of constriction, 6 cc. or more of blood are withdrawn from the patient's vein and with the least possible exposure to air are transferred to a centrifuge tube containing about 10 mg. dry potassium oxalate for each cubic centimeter of blood drawn. Mix gently but thoroughly, and separate the cells by centrifugation.

Transfer about 3 cc. of the plasma to the body of the separatory funnel which lies horizontal on the table. After a normal expiration, quickly blow as much air as possible from the lungs through the bottle of beads into the funnel. Insert the stopper into the funnel just before the end of the forced expiration and close the stopcock. Rotate the funnel for two minutes in such a way that the plasma is distributed as completely as possible over the inner surface. This procedure serves to saturate the plasma with carbon dioxide. Make the analysis at once.

The apparatus must be set up and tested before the analysis is made. It is set up on a ring stand and held in place by clamps, the jaws of which are covered with heavy rubber. The stopcocks should be well lubricated and held in place by heavy rubber bands. Fill the apparatus completely with mercury, making sure that both openings in the stopcocks are filled. Then, with the upper stopcock closed and the lower one open, lower the leveling bulb to a position below the lower stopcock for several seconds to produce a vacuum in the apparatus. When the bulb is returned to a position opposite the upper stopcock, a click should be heard as the rising mercury column strikes the upper stopcock. If leakage has occurred, the air forms a cushion and no click is heard. The leak must be found and eliminated.

When the apparatus has been found to be airtight and entirely filled with mercury (including all stopcock openings), rinse the cup at the top of the apparatus with distilled water, leaving 1 cc. in place. Transfer to the cup exactly 1 cc. of the plasma which has just been saturated with carbon dioxide, keeping the tip of the pipette well below the surface of the fluid. Add a small drop of caprylic alcohol. Support the bulb just below the lower stopcock, open the lower stopcock, and by carefully turning the upper stopcock allow the plasma and water to enter the main stem of the apparatus, leaving the constricted portion of the cup filled with fluid. Put 0.5 cc. of 10 percent lactic acid in the cup, and let enough of it flow into the main

stem to bring the level of the fluid exactly to the 2.5 mark. Put 1 cc. of water in the cup and then a drop of mercury. Let the mercury run into the stopcock and chamber until enough remains in the constricted portion of the cup to seal it. Remove the water from the cup.

Lower the leveling bulb to a position about 80 cm. (32 in.) below the lower stopcock; when the level of the mercury in the apparatus has fallen to the 50-cc. mark, close the lower stopcock. Then remove the apparatus from the clamp and invert it at least fifteen times to complete the carbon-dioxide extraction. Replace the apparatus and allow it to stand to drain fluid from the walls. Again lower the leveling bulb and open the lower stopcock so that the liquid drains into the trap located below the cock on the side next to the handle. Care must be used to see that all the fluid is out of the main chamber but that none of the gas follows. Raise the leveling bulb slowly and turn the lower stopcock so that mercury enters the main stem of the apparatus from the by-pass tube. Allow the mercury to rise slowly until equilibrium is reached, with the mercury in the bulb at exactly the same level as that in the graduated stem of the apparatus. Close the lower stopcock and read the gas volume present. Fill the apparatus with water when not in use.

For calculation, the following equation is sufficiently accurate if the room temperature is 65 to 70° F.:

$$\text{Volume } CO_2 \text{ in 100 cc. of plasma ("volumes percent")} = \frac{\dfrac{\text{barometric pressure in mm.}}{760}}{\text{recorded volume of gas} \times 100 - 12}$$

The normal range for adults is 53 to 75; for infants, 40 to 55. In adults, figures below 50 indicate acidosis; below 30, severe acidosis. Figures above 75 indicate alkalosis.

ASCORBIC ACID IN BLOOD

Youmans's Modification of the Method of Farmer and Abt

APPARATUS—1. Pipette, 2 cc.

2. Microburette, 5 cc.

REAGENTS—1. Standard 2,6-dichlorophenolindophenol solution, prepared as for ascorbic acid determination in urine (p. 522). For blood, however, only *10 cc.* of the stock solution, instead of 20 cc., are diluted to 100 cc. with recently boiled and cooled distilled water.

2. Metaphosphoric acid solution, 5 percent.

TECHNIC—Pipette 2 cc. of oxalated plasma into a 15-cc. centrifuge tube, and add 4 cc. of distilled water and 4 cc. of 5 percent metaphosphoric acid solution. Mix thoroughly by gentle shaking, and centrifuge. Titrate 2-cc. portions of the supernatant fluid with the diluted standard 2,6-dichlorophenol-indophenol solution, using the microburette.

The end point is the first faint pink color that persists thirty seconds. A distilled water blank is run, and its value is subtracted from the final burette reading.

Where it is possible to employ larger quantities of blood, the experimental error is correspondingly reduced; it is recommended that determinations be made on 5 cc. of blood when possible. This volume of oxalated blood would be diluted with 10 cc. of distilled water and 10 cc. of metaphosphoric acid solution, and 5-cc. portions of the supernatant fluid would be titrated. The factor of dilution in the calculation would then be 100 instead of 250.

CALCULATION—Concentration of ascorbic acid in mg. per 100 cc. plasma = (cc. of dye solution required for titration minus cc. of blank) × ascorbic acid equivalent of 1 cc. of dye solution × 250 (factor of dilution).

Standard values have not been fully established, and temporary variations in ascorbic acid intake have a great influence on blood levels. In general, normal concentrations are above 0.7 mg. per 100 cc. plasma, and 1.2 mg. or more are common in well-nourished people. From 0.4 to 0.7 mg. per 100 cc. may be considered borderline, with values of 0.4 or below strongly suggestive of scurvy.

SULFONAMIDES IN BLOOD

Method of Bratton and Marshall

REAGENTS—1. Trichloroacetic acid solution, 15 percent.

2. Sodium nitrite solution, 0.1 percent.

3. Solution of N-(1-naphthyl)ethylenediamine dihydrochloride (La Motte), 0.1 percent. This solution should be kept in a dark-colored bottle.

4. Saponin solution, 0.05 percent.

5. 4 N hydrochloric acid.

6. Ammonium sulfamate solution, 0.5 percent.

7. A stock solution of each sulfonamide for which tests are to be made. Each should contain 200 mg. per liter. They will keep for several weeks in dark bottles under refrigeration. They are diluted as needed and used as standards.

TECHNIC—Measure 2 cc. of oxalated blood into a flask and add 30 cc. of saponin solution. Mix. After one or two minutes add 8 cc. of trichloroacetic acid solution, mix again, and filter.

Free sulfonamide is determined as follows: To 10 cc. of the filtrate add 1 cc. of sodium nitrite solution. After allowing the mixture to stand for three minutes, add 1 cc. of ammonium sulfamate. Let stand for an additional two minutes, and add 1 cc. of the solution of N-(1-naphthyl)ethylenediamine dihydrochloride. Dilute a quantity of the desired standard sulfonamide solution to approximately the concentration expected to be found in the blood, and treat a 10-cc. quantity in the same way as the filtrate above. Compare unknown and standard in a colorimeter, preferably within an hour after the above treatment.

Total sulfonamide (free plus combined) is determined as follows: To 10 cc. of filtrate add 0.5 cc. of 4 N hydrochloric acid; heat in a boiling water bath for one hour, cool, adjust the volume to 10 cc. with distilled water, and proceed as for the determination of free sulfonamide.

CALCULATION—Concentration of sulfonamide in mg. per 100 cc. blood = $\dfrac{\text{reading of standard}}{\text{reading of unknown}}$ × concentration of sulfonamide in mg. per 100 cc. of diluted standard.

Method of Monto—This method is not so accurate as that of Bratton and Marshall, but it is simpler and is considered by Monto to be satisfactory for ordinary clinical purposes.

REAGENTS—1. Toluene-sulfonic acid solution, 20 percent.

2. A solution of paradimethylaminobenzaldehyde, 2 percent, in 20 percent hydrochloric acid. This solution should be kept in a dark bottle.

3. Stock solutions of the desired sulfonamides, 0.5 mg. per 100 cc.

4. 2 N sodium hydroxide solution.

TECHNIC—To 3 cc. of oxalated blood add 21 cc. of distilled water and shake until laking has occurred. Add 6 cc. of toluene-sulfonic acid solution, mix, and filter. To 10 cc. of the filtrate add 1 cc. of 2 N sodium hydroxide solution and 1 cc. of the aldehyde reagent (No. 2 above), and compare immediately in the colorimeter with a similarly treated standard solution of the given sulfonamide. Daylight or a Corning daylight lamp is the best light source.

CALCULATION is the same as for the Bratton and Marshall method given above.

FLOCCULATION TESTS FOR SYPHILIS

During the past few years, flocculation tests for the serodiagnosis of syphilis have gained favor because of their relative simplicity and economy. The "V.D.R.L. Tests" (Venereal Disease Research Laboratory), using Cardiolipin, and the Mazzini test have a high degree of specificity and sensitivity. They are quickly and easily performed, and they give clear-cut results. Cardiolipin antigen has the advantage, however, of yielding fewer false positive tests (especially in malaria), providing even higher sensitivity, and showing greater uniformity from one lot to another.

V.D.R.L. TESTS USING CARDIOLIPIN FLOCCULATION ANTIGEN

Cardiolipin is a purified phospholipid obtained from beef heart. The antigen contains:

```
Cardiolipin...............................0.03%
lecithin............................approx. 0.27%
cholesterol................................0.9 %
absolute alcohol...........................q.s.
```

Each lot is standardized serologically before release by comparison with an antigen of known reactivity. The antigen, supplied as Cardiolipin Flocculation Antigen, is dispensed in rubber-stoppered vials and should be stored at room temperature *in the dark*. Since the components of this antigen remain in solution at normal temperatures, any precipitate noted will indicate changes due to such factors as evaporation or additive materials contributed by pipettes. Antigen containing precipitate should be discarded.

A buffered saline solution (supplied with Test Kit No. 8, Cardiolipin Flocculation Antigen) is used which has the following composition:

```
sodium chloride (A.C.S.)................10    Gm.
disodium phosphate (Na₂HPO₄·12H₂O).....0.093 Gm.
potassium biphosphate (KH₂PO₄)..........0.170 Gm.
distilled water.....................1,000    cc.
   with 'Merthiolate,' 1:10,000, as a preservative.
```

This solution has a pH of 6.0 ± 0.1.

In addition, physiological salt solution (0.9 percent NaCl) is required.

Technic for V.D.R.L. Slide Flocculation Test—

To assure continued usefulness of the remaining antigen, material should be removed from the vial of antigen as supplied, in the following manner. Insert a short 27-gauge needle at an angle barely through the rubber stopper of the vial of antigen. This allows air to enter the vial during removal of material. A 22-gauge needle with hub removed (supplied with kit) is inserted perpendicularly through the rubber stopper and into the antigen solution. Place a 1-cc. pipette over the 22-gauge needle, press firmly against the rubber stopper, and withdraw antigen by suction in the usual manner. Since material allowed to dry in the needles will affect antigen subsequently withdrawn, both needles should be flushed well with 95 percent alcohol after use and dried with air. Cleaning and drying of both may be done simultaneously by placing the point of the 27-gauge needle inside the larger one and using a syringe to force the alcohol and air through them.

Clear serum, obtained by centrifuging whole clotted blood, is heated at 56°C. for thirty minutes or at 60° to 62°C. for three minutes before being tested. All serums are examined when removed from the water bath, and those found to contain particulate debris are recentrifuged. Serums to be tested more than four hours after being heated should be reheated at 56°C. for ten minutes.

Glass slides (2 x 3 in.) are used which have 12 paraffin rings with inside diameters of approximately 15 mm. as described by Kline. New slides are cleaned with Bon Ami, which is removed with a soft cloth after drying. Previously used slides are first freed of paraffin, washed with soap, and rinsed free of soap and are then treated as new slides.

While being cleaned, slides are handled by the edges so that there will be no greasy fingerprints on the testing surfaces. Serum will spread within the circles on clean slides. Failure of the serum to spread is an indication that the slide is unclean and therefore should not be used.

Paraffin rings are made by transferring heated paraffin to the slides with metal molds.*

PREPARATION OF ANTIGEN EMULSION—1. Pipette 0.4 ml. of buffered saline to the bottom of a 30-ml., round, screw-cap or glass-stoppered bottle.

2. Add 0.5 ml. of the antigen (from the lower half of a 1-ml. pipette graduated to the tip) directly to the saline while continuously but gently rotating the bottle on a flat surface. The antigen is added rapidly drop by drop so that approximately six seconds are allowed for each 0.5 ml. of antigen. The pipette tip should remain in the upper third of the bottle, and rotation should not be vigorous enough to splash saline onto the pipette.

---

* Hand or automatic-electric-type ringmakers may be obtained from Arthur H. Thomas Co., West Washington Square, Philadelphia, Pa.

3. Blow the last drop of antigen from the pipette without touching pipette to saline.

4. Continue rotation of the bottle for ten more seconds.

5. Add 4.1 ml. of buffered saline from a 5-ml. pipette.

6. Place top on bottle and shake vigorously for approximately ten seconds.

7. The antigen emulsion is then ready for use and may be used during one day. This amount (5 ml.) is sufficient for approximately 250 serum tests.

Twice this amount of antigen emulsion may be prepared at one time in a 30-ml. bottle by using doubled quantities of antigen and saline. A 10-ml. pipette should then be used for delivering the 8.2-ml. volume of saline. If larger quantities of antigen emulsion are required, more than one mixture should be prepared. These aliquots may then be pooled and tested.

Testing Antigen Emulsion Delivery Needle— The number of antigen particles per microscopic field is determined by the size of antigen emulsion drop used. For this reason the needle used each day should be checked.

Antigen emulsion is dispensed from a 22-gauge, regular-beveled or a 23-gauge, long-beveled hypodermic needle attached to a 1 or 2-ml. syringe which is allowed to stand in the antigen emulsion bottle when not in use. Sixty drops should be obtained from one milliliter of antigen emulsion. This can be accomplished by holding the syringe so that the needle bevel is down and the dropping surface is horizontal. Increasing the angle at which the syringe is held diminishes the dropping surface and consequently decreases the size of the drop. Whether this or other means of delivery are used, it is of primary importance that the proper amount (1/60 ml.) of antigen emulsion be used in each test.

Practice will allow rapid delivery of antigen emulsion, but care should be exercised to obtain drops of constant size. After it has been allowed to stand, antigen emulsion should be gently mixed before being used; this is done by rotating the bottle and filling and emptying the syringe.

Each preparation of antigen emulsion should first be examined by testing known positive and negative serums. This is accomplished by adding one drop of antigen emulsion to 0.05 ml. of each serum and completing the test as described under Qualitative Serum Test. These tests should present typically positive and negative results respectively, and the size and number of antigen particles per microscopic field in the negative serum should be optimum (see Plate 43 for typical examples).

If antigen particles in the negative serum appear too large, the fault usually will be found in the manner of preparing the antigen emulsion. An unsatisfactory antigen emulsion should not be used.

Qualitative Serum Test—1. Pipette 0.05 ml. of heated serum into one ring of a paraffin-ringed glass slide.

2. Add one drop (1/60 ml.) of antigen emulsion onto each serum.

3. Rotate slides for four minutes. (If they are rotated by hand on a flat surface, this movement should roughly circumscribe a circle two inches in diameter 120 times per minute. The Boerner type rotator* set at 180 r.p.m. also may be used for this test.)

4. Tests are read immediately after rotation. Known positive, weakly positive, and negative serum controls are always included.

Tests are read microscopically with low-power objective at 100× magnification. The antigen particles appear as short rod forms at this magnification. Aggregation of these particles into large or small clumps is interpreted as degrees of positivity (see Plate 43).

Reading	Report
No clumping or very slight roughness	Negative (N)
Small clumps	Weakly positive (WP)
Medium and large clumps	Positive (P)

Proper reading and interpretation of test results require that the technicians have had training and experience in each technic employed, but rough equivalents may be used for describing similarities between the reading of this and other slide tests. The *weakly positive* range of this test includes clumpings similar to those reported as plus-minus or one plus; and the *positive* range, those reported as 2 plus, 3 plus, or 4 plus in other slide tests. *However, it is recommended that only the terms "positive," "weakly positive," and "negative" be used for reporting the results of this test.*

Zonal reactions, due to an excess of reactive serum component, are recognized by irregular clumping and the loosely bound characteristics of the clumps. The usual positive reaction is characterized by large or small clumps of fairly uniform size, and experience will allow differentiation to be made between this type of reaction and the zonal picture wherein large or small clumps or both may be intermingled with free antigen particles.

* Obtainable from Arthur H. Thomas Co., West Washington Square, Philadelphia, Pa.

In such instances, or whenever a zonal type of reaction is suspected, the serum in question should be diluted 1:5 and 1:25 and retested. The maximum reaction produced by either of these dilutions, if greater than the reactions obtained with undiluted serum, is reported as the test finding. Dilutions may be prepared by placing 0.4 ml. of saline in each of two test tubes, adding 0.1 ml. of heated serum to tube 1, mixing well, and transferring 0.1 ml. to tube 2.

QUANTITATIVE SERUM TEST—Quantitative tests are performed on serially diluted serum in saline, each dilution of which is treated as an individual serum and tested as described under Qualitative Serum Test. Freshly prepared 0.9 percent sodium chloride solution is used for these dilutions. Serum dilutions are prepared by placing 0.5 ml. of salt solution in each of six or more tubes. Then 0.5 ml. of heated serum is added to tube 1 and mixed well, and 0.5 ml. is transferred to tube 2. This operation is continued until the sixth tube contains 1 ml. Dilutions of 1:2, 1:4, 1:8, 1:16, etc., are thus obtained.

Tests are read microscopically at 100× magnification as described for the qualitative procedure. Results are reported in terms of the greatest serum dilution that produces a positive (not weakly positive) reaction in accordance with the following example:

Serum Dilutions						Report
1:2	1:4	1:8	1:16	1:32	1:64	
P	P	P	WP	N	N	P—1:8 dilution, or 8 dils
P	WP	N	N	N	N	P—1:2 dilution, or 2 dils
WP	N	N	N	N	N	P*—undiluted only, or 1 dil

If other quantitative patterns are desired, serum dilutions of 1:5, 1:10, 1:20, etc., may be prepared, tested, and reported as above.

Under conditions of high temperature and low humidity, as are sometimes present during the summer months in certain areas, antigen emulsion may be stored in the refrigerator. To avoid surface drying under these conditions, tests should be completed and read as rapidly as possible.

Technic for V.D.R.L. Tube Flocculation Test—

Antigen and buffered saline solutions are used as in the slide flocculation test. However, the sodium chloride solution must be 1 percent strength instead of 0.9 percent. Serum is prepared as for the Slide Flocculation Test. The antigen emulsion is prepared by diluting that for the Slide Flocculation Test, using four parts of 1 percent sodium chloride solution (either buffered or unbuffered solution) to one part slide test emulsion. After thorough mixing, the diluted emulsion is allowed to stand at least five minutes (but not more than two hours) before use.

QUALITATIVE SERUM TEST—1. Pipette 0.5 ml. of heated serum into a 12 × 75-mm. (O.D.) test tube.

2. Add 0.5 ml. of diluted antigen emulsion to each serum.

3. Shake tubes on Kahn shaker for five minutes.

4. Centrifuge all tubes for ten minutes at a force equivalent to 2,000 r.p.m. in a No. 1 or to 1,700 r.p.m. in a No. 2 International Equipment Company centrifuge.

5. Return tubes to the Kahn shaking machine and shake for *exactly* one minute.

As soon as the secondary shaking period is completed, read reactions by holding tubes, at approximately eye level, close to the shade of a reading lamp having a black background. A shaded fluorescent desk lamp, or gooseneck-type lamp with a blue bulb, is a satisfactory source of light for test reading.

Record results as follows:

Positive: Visible aggregates in a clear or slightly turbid medium.

Negative: No visible clumping or aggregation of antigen particles. Appearance slightly turbid or granular. Definite silken swirl on gentle shaking. All borderline reactions, in which the observer has doubt regarding visible clumping, should be reported as negative.

Turbid or hemolyzed serums may cause completed tests to be too turbid for macroscopic reading. Fluid from these tubes may be examined microscopically. Positive reports may be rendered when large antigen-particle masses are detected microscopically if the serum tested is found to be free of particles at the same magnification.

Zonal reactions, due to excess of reactive serum component, may appear to be very weak or, in rare instances, negative. Whenever a zonal reaction is suspected, another test should be performed using 0.1 ml. of heated serum and 0.4 ml. of salt solution in place of the original 0.5 ml. of serum. If a positive result is obtained with the smaller amount of serum, a positive report should be issued.

QUANTITATIVE SERUM TEST—1. Pipette 0.5 ml. of freshly prepared 0.9 percent salt solution into each of six or more test tubes (12 × 75 mm.).

2. Add 0.5 ml. of heated serum to first tube and mix.

3. Transfer 0.5 ml. from first to second tube and mix.

---

* Positive reaction obtained with undiluted serum.

4. Continue transferring 0.5 ml. from each tube to the next and mixing until the last tube is reached.

5. Discard 0.5 ml. from last tube.

6. Add 0.5 ml. of diluted antigen emulsion to each tube and proceed as described under Qualitative Serum Test.

The greatest serum dilution producing a definitely positive reaction is reported as the reactivity end point in accordance with the following example:

Serum Dilutions						Report
1:2	1:4	1:8	1:16	1:32	1:64	
P	P	P	P	N	N	P—1:16 dilution, or 16 dils
P	P	N	N	N	N	P—1:4 dilution, or 4 dils
N	N	N	N	N	N	P*—undiluted only, or 1 dil

Technic for V.D.R.L. Spinal-Fluid Test — Each specimen of spinal fluid is centrifuged and decanted. Those which are visibly contaminated or contain gross blood are unsatisfactory for testing. Heat spinal fluid at 56°C. for fifteen minutes. Cool to room temperature before testing.

Antigen emulsion is prepared as for the Slide Flocculation Test (p. 538). To one part of the slide test emulsion, add one part 10 percent sodium chloride solution; mix well, and let stand not less than five minutes or more than two hours before use.

QUALITATIVE SPINAL-FLUID TEST—1. Pipette 1 ml. of heated spinal fluid into a 13 × 100-mm. test tube. Include positive and negative spinal-fluid controls in each test run.

2. Add 0.2 ml. of sensitized antigen emulsion to each spinal fluid. Resuspend the sensitized antigen emulsion immediately before use by inverting container several times.

3. Shake racks of tubes on Kahn shaking machine for fifteen minutes.

4. Centrifuge all tubes for five minutes at a force equivalent to 1,800 r.p.m. in a No. 1 or to 1,600 r.p.m. in a No. 2 International Equipment Company centrifuge.

5. Return tubes to Kahn shaking machine and shake for *exactly* two minutes.

Read reactions immediately after the secondary shaking period by holding tubes close to the shade of a desk lamp having a black background.

Each tube may be held motionless or shaken gently during the reading. Excessive agitation should be avoided.

Record results as follows:

Positive: Definitely visible aggregates suspended in a water-clear or turbid medium.

Negative: No aggregation; complete dispersion of particles; appearance turbid or slightly granular.

QUANTITATIVE SPINAL-FLUID TEST

1. Prepare spinal-fluid dilutions.

    a. Pipette 1 ml. of 0.9 percent sodium chloride solution into each of five or more tubes.

    b. Add 1 ml. of heated spinal fluid to tube No. 1; mix well, and transfer 1 ml. to tube No. 2.

    c. Continue mixing and transferring from one tube to the next until the last tube contains 2 ml. Discard 1 ml. from the last tube. The respective dilution ratios are 1:2, 1:4, 1:8, 1:16, 1:32, etc.

2. Test each spinal-fluid dilution as described under Qualitative Spinal-Fluid Test.

Each tube is read as described for the Qualitative Spinal-Fluid Test.

Report test results in terms of the highest dilution of spinal fluid producing a positive reaction in accordance with the following example:

Spinal-Fluid Dilutions					Report
1:2	1:4	1:8	1:16	1:32	
P	P	P	P	N	P—1:16 dilution, or 16 dils
P	P	P	N	N	P—1:8 dilution, or 8 dils
N	N	N	N	N	P†—undiluted only, or 1 dil

MAZZINI TEST

The Mazzini test requires the same glassware, pipettes, and ringed glass slides as the V.D.R.L. Slide Flocculation Test (p. 538). However, Mazzini recommends a mixture of Zubian sealing wax, 50 Gm., and paraffin, 20 Gm., for preparation of rings. The reagents are supplied as Mazzini Cholesterinized Antigen, Lilly, and consist of a 4-cc. bottle of antigen and a 30-cc. bottle of buffered saline solution for dilution of the antigen; a 22-gauge needle with hub removed is included in each package.

Clear serum, obtained by centrifuging whole clotted blood, is heated at 56°C. for thirty minutes before testing. In emergency before transfusion, the serum may be inactivated at 60°C. for ten minutes. If it is necessary to retest a weakly positive serum which was heated several hours before, a fresh portion should be drawn from the clot and heated.

Qualitative Test—1. Put 3 cc. of buffered saline solution directly into the bottom of a 20-cc. to 30-cc. bottle.

2. Remove exactly 0.4 cc. of the antigen from its container, using the technic described for Car-

---

* Positive reaction obtained with undiluted serum.

† Positive reaction obtained with undiluted spinal fluid in the Qualitative Test.

diolipin Antigen (p. 539) (and observe the same precautions in cleaning the needles). Quickly take the bottle containing the 3 cc. of saline in the left hand and impart a rapid rotating motion to it, at the same time discharging the antigen directly into the saline solution from the pipette in the right hand. The volume of 3.4 cc. is sufficient for about 300 tests.

The bottle is corked and shaken for ten seconds, then allowed to stand at room temperature for three hours, at which time the suspension reaches its optimum sensitivity. If room temperature exceeds 25°C. (77°F.), the bottle of suspension should be kept in a water bath at 23° to 25°C.

In emergencies, the newly prepared antigen suspension may be placed in the refrigerator at 6° to 8°C. for fifteen minutes to accelerate the ripening process. However, at this stage of ripening, it will not possess the degree of sensitivity that it does when the suspension has stood at room temperature for three hours. Any specimen showing the slightest flocculation with the fifteen-minute-refrigerated antigen must be retested after the suspension has reached its maximum sensitivity.

The suspension kept at room temperature is satisfactory for use for twenty-four hours; after this time it loses its potency and must be discarded.

3. After the required ripening period either at room or icebox temperature, the suspension is shaken gently from the bottom to cork and back ten times and transferred to a 5-cc. glass syringe fitted with a 25-gauge needle. It is then ready for immediate use.

4. Place one-, two-, or three-ringed glass slides on a slide holder, depending on the number of specimens to be tested. Pipette 0.05 cc. of each patient's properly prepared serum into one of the chambers of the glass slide. Discharge one drop of the ripened antigen suspension into each of the serums in the chambers. Known negative and positive serums should be included at the beginning of the day's tests as controls on the antigen suspension.

5. Rotate the slide holder with a circular, slightly "jerky" motion for four minutes at 120 rotations per minute.

It is important that the number of rotations be as indicated and that the proper motion be given to the slide to insure that the antigen particles become well dispersed throughout the area of the ring.

6. First examine every one of the rings macroscopically to make certain that no serum has "jumped" the ring and contaminated another. Then examine them microscopically under the low-power objective with subdued light. Inspection of the periphery of the rings for clumps should be made routinely, for occasionally the clumps are very compact and have a tendency to locate in the outer portion of the ring.

7. Record results as follows:

No clumping—negative; very small to small clumps—doubtful; medium to large clumps—positive. Representative examples are shown in Plate 43.

In reading weakly positive reactions, care should be taken to differentiate red blood cells, oil globules, or debris—which may be contained in the serum, on the slide, or in the antigen suspension—from the true flocculate of a positive reaction. This caution obviously applies only in weakly positive reactions, since in strongly positive ones debris or blood cells are masked by the large clumps of the reaction. Although no experience is needed to read strongly positive reactions, time and observation alone will lead to correct interpretation of the weakly positive reactions.

When tested undiluted (as above), very strongly positive serums sometimes give reactions of doubtful character. It is recommended that the addition of a second drop of antigen be made a routine practice whenever weakly positive reactions are obtained. Preparation of serial dilutions, as in the quantitative test, avoids all of these so-called "zone reactions."

Quantitative Test—The procedure for the quantitative test is exactly the same as for the routine test except that each serum is tested in serial dilutions.

Qualitative Test with Spinal Fluid—Spinal fluid should be tested as soon as possible after it is drawn. A grossly contaminated fluid is not dependable; it should not contain blood in appreciable quantity. The heating of spinal fluid is neither necessary nor desirable.

Rapid Test—1. Centrifuge the fresh fluid at 2,000 r.p.m. for five minutes; pour off the clear supernatant into a clean tube.

2. With a 0.2-cc. pipette graduated in hundredths, place exactly 0.01 cc. of 6 percent acetic acid in one side of as many chambers of a glass slide as there are fluids to be tested. Accurate preparation of the acid solution and precise measurement of the volume delivered to each chamber are obviously necessary, for stronger concentrations or larger amounts will flocculate the suspension even in the absence of antibody.

3. With a 1-cc. pipette, deliver 0.1 cc. of spinal fluid into the side of the chamber opposite to that in which the acid was placed. Mix acid and fluid evenly over the surface of the chamber with a wood applicator.

4. Rotate slide holder with a circular motion for one minute. Thorough mixing is essential.

5. Add one drop of the same antigen suspension that is used for testing serum to each chamber containing spinal fluid.

6. Rotate slide holder for ten minutes at 120 rotations per minute. The results are examined and recorded in the same manner as for the test with blood serum.

CONCENTRATION TEST — Weakly positive fluids and negative fluids are subjected to the concentration test. The fluid (1.5 cc.) is evaporated to a volume of 0.2 cc. or 0.3 cc. by a hot-air blower (accomplished in about six to eight minutes); and the technic for the rapid test is used.

Quantitative Test with Spinal Fluid — Serial dilutions are prepared and tested by the acid test.

LIVER FUNCTION

Hippuric Acid Excretion Test of Liver Function (Quick) — The test is based on the principle that, in the normal liver, benzoic acid is combined with aminoacetic acid to form hippuric acid, which is excreted in the urine. In the presence of liver damage this function is impaired, and the degree of impairment is presumed to be measured by the diminution of hippuric acid excretion following the ingestion of a standard quantity of benzoic acid. Its reliability obviously depends on normal absorption of the ingested material and on prompt and quantitative excretion of the hippuric acid by the kidneys.

The test is usually performed in the morning, one hour after the patient has had a light breakfast of toast or cereal with tea, coffee, or milk. He must have taken no drugs during the preceding two days. Immediately before the test, have the patient empty the bladder; then have him drink 6 Gm. sodium benzoate dissolved in 30 cc. of water flavored with oil of peppermint, followed by a half glass of water. Subsequently, have him empty the bladder every hour for four hours.

Measure the volume of each specimen and add solid ammonium sulfate in the proportion of 5 Gm. for every 10 cc. When the salt is dissolved, filter or centrifuge the urine and acidify with hydrochloric acid. The urine must be distinctly acid to Congo red or thymol blue. A slight excess of acid is desirable. Usually 1 cc. of concentrated acid is adequate. Stir the mixture vigorously and allow to stand for thirty minutes, during which time hippuric acid crystallizes out. Filter off the crystals, and dry and weigh them on the filter paper, using another filter paper as counterweight.

If the hourly urine output exceeds 150 cc., it is advisable to concentrate the urine on a water bath to about 50 cc. before adding the ammonium sulfate. Since the urine must not at any time become alkaline, it should be made acid with acetic acid before being concentrated.

In calculating the result, add 0.1 Gm. hippuric acid for every 100 cc. of final urine filtrate to allow for that remaining in solution. The total weight of hippuric acid obtained is multiplied by 22.7, and the resulting figure is the percentage of normal excretion.

An excretion of over 90 percent is considered nonpathological. Excretion of less than 90 percent, in the presence of normal absorption of the sodium benzoate and normal excretion of the hippuric acid, is indicative of impaired hepatic function. The meaning of an excretion of over 120 percent is not known at present.

GASTRIC ANALYSIS

Histamine Test — The subcutaneous administration of histamine affords a maximal stimulation to gastric secretion, at the same time avoiding dilution of the juice with ingested material.

APPARATUS — 1. A stomach tube, preferably a Levine tube, since it is of uniform size and not too stiff. It should be marked 40 cm., 56 cm., and 70 cm. from the lower end.

2. A syringe, such as a 50-cc. Luer.

3. A pan of ice for cooling the tube.

4. Glycerin (50 percent) or mineral oil to lubricate tube.

5. Five to seven clean 8-oz. bottles, numbered.

6. A kidney basin or other vessel.

7. A sterile hypodermic syringe and needle.

8. A sterile solution of histamine (see p. 366).

PROCEDURE — The test is performed after at least eight hours of fasting. Passage of the tube is facilitated by having it ice-cold and the tip lubricated. The patient should be in a comfortable sitting position. Instruct the patient to swallow it rapidly, to grip the sides of the chair or bed firmly with his hands, and to breathe rapidly with mouth open if he feels nauseated or choked. In some patients, passage through the nose (with a tube not larger than 15F) is more convenient than through the mouth. Have the patient continue to swallow the tube until the teeth are halfway between the 40-cm. and 56-cm. marks. Caution the patient to expectorate saliva instead of swallowing it.

After the tube is in place, the fasting contents are withdrawn and placed in bottle No. 1. The time is noted, and the histamine is injected hypodermically. Leaving about 25 cc. of air in the stomach, continuously aspirate the contents by passing the air in and out of the stomach. The secretion obtained during each ten-minute period following histamine injection is collected in a separate bottle. Aspiration is continued until the volume of secretion passes its maximum, usually within forty to sixty minutes after histamine.

DOSAGE OF HISTAMINE—Cheney and Bloomfield and Polland use 0.1 mg. histamine per 10 Kg. of body weight. Johansen uses 0.4 to 0.5 mg., adjusting the dose to the age, weight, and general condition of the patient (histamine is supplied as histamine acid phosphate; for dosage calculation, see p. 367). Pulse and blood pressure readings should be recorded; a slight drop in blood pressure and increase in pulse rate are usually observed. Flushing of the skin and feelings of fullness and pounding in the head are brief and normal sequelae of injection.

DETERMINATION OF TITRABLE ACID (see Plate 45, Figure 1)—Gastric secretion contains mucus, salts, and protein which, acting as buffers, combine with some of the acid. It is considered that "free" acid is present only when the pH is less than 3. The total quantity of acid and the question of the presence of free acid are considered of importance.

Dimethylamino-azobenzene (Töpfer's reagent) changes color at a pH of approximately 3 and is commonly used for the determination of free acid. On the alkaline side of pH 3, it is yellow; on the acid side, red. Thus, a specimen showing a red color when the indicator is added contains free acid, whereas a yellow specimen shows absence of free acid. A specimen containing no free acid may still contain combined acid.

In the complete absence of acid, the pH of the secretion will approximate 7; phenol red is used for the test. This indicator is yellow on the acid side of pH 7 and red on the alkaline.

To make the test, pipette 1 cc. of filtered or centrifuged gastric juice into a 60-cc. porcelain evaporating dish (or a flask held against a white background) and dilute with 20 cc. of distilled water. Add 2 drops of 0.1 percent phenol red indicator* and titrate with N/100 sodium hydroxide solution until the color of the sample (un-

known) matches the standard color chart for pH 7 (see Plate 45, Figure 1, Color Chart A), or compare with a control buffered solution in another evaporating dish made up to a pH of 7. The results are expressed in "clinical units" by multiplying by 10 the number of cubic centimeters of N/100 sodium hydroxide solution required to bring the sample of gastric juice to neutrality. A "clinical unit" is defined as the amount of N/10 sodium hydroxide needed to bring 100 cc. of gastric juice to neutrality.

This procedure is carried out in turn for each sample, including the fasting juice.

DETERMINATION OF pH—Adequate information for clinical purposes can be obtained by the use of one or two simple tests. Spread a thin coat of petrolatum on a piece of white paper or a filing card. Place a drop of gastric juice on the greased surface of the card (see Plate 45, Figure 2) and add a drop of phenol red indicator,* mixing with a glass rod, toothpick, or applicator. At once compare the color of the resulting mixture with the standard (Color Chart B).

If the drop has turned deep red, the pH is greater than 8, anacidity is definitely present, and no further test of the secretion is needed. If the drop has turned yellow, acid is present, and it is desirable to determine whether the acidity falls within normal limits. For this purpose, place a second drop of gastric juice on the greased paper and add a drop of thymol blue indicator†; mix well, and compare with the standard (Color Chart C). The development of any of the three shades of red shown in the chart indicates that the gastric acidity is within normal limits. The presence of an orange or yellow color indicates that the pH of the specimen is greater than 1.6; hypoacidity is present, but not anacidity. These tests are carried out on each sample of gastric juice.

STAINS FOR VAGINAL SMEARS

Stains are of particular value in the detection of estrogenic effects, which include cornification and an increase in glycogen content of the epithelial cells.

---

* Phenol Red Stock Solution. A 0.1 percent stock solution is made by dissolving 0.1 Gm. of the solid dye with the aid of 28.2 cc. of N/100 sodium hydroxide, and diluting with distilled water to make 100 cc.

† Thymol Blue. A 0.1 percent stock solution is made by dissolving 0.1 Gm. of the solid dye with the aid of 21.5 cc. of N/100 sodium hydroxide, and diluting to 100 cc. with distilled water. For use in determination of the pH of the gastric juice, 40 cc. of the stock solution are diluted to 200 cc. with distilled water.

The specimen of vaginal fluid for staining is obtained either with a medicine dropper or pipette or by inserting a cotton applicator into the vagina and twirling it lightly (one complete rotation) against the vaginal wall. The material is spread on a slide (by rolling rather than rubbing in the case of the applicator).

Iodine Vapor Technic (Mack)—After it is dry, the slide is placed, face down, over a shallow (petri) dish containing Lugol's solution (iodine, 5 Gm.; potassium iodide, 10 Gm.; distilled water to make 100 cc.). Glycogen-containing cells will be stained brown by iodine vapor in two to three minutes, when the slide is ready to be examined under the microscope. The stain fades in one or two days, but the slide can be restained repeatedly. Cells not containing glycogen stain light yellow; those containing glycogen stain dark brown.

Shorr Stain—Fix the slide while wet in a mixture of equal parts of ether and 95 percent alcohol. Carry it through graded dilutions of alcohol to water (70 percent, 50 percent, and 25 percent will do). Greater differentiation of cell morphology can be obtained by staining for one minute with Harris hematoxylin and washing in running water for five minutes, but this step can be omitted if desired. Stain for one minute in a solution containing 1 percent Biebrich Scarlet, water soluble,* and 0.4 percent Orange G in 1 percent acetic acid. Rinse in water. Mordant for one minute in a mixture of equal parts of 5 percent solutions of phosphomolybdic and phosphotungstic acids. Rinse. Stain for two minutes in a solution of 0.5 percent Fast Green FCF* in 0.3 percent acetic acid. Do not rinse, but differentiate in 1 percent acetic acid for one minute, carry through alcohols to xylol, and mount.

With this stain, the cells of an atrophic smear usually appear lavender or pale blue. In less atrophic smears the prevailing tint is a pale greenish-blue. After estrogenic activity, the cells become progressively greener in addition to undergoing morphological changes. With cornification, the cells change abruptly to a brilliant orange red.

BACTERIOLOGICAL METHODS
Direct Tests on Material from Patients

MALARIA PARASITES IN BLOOD

Thick-smear technic is generally preferred by those experienced in searching for malaria parasites in blood. For the relatively inexperienced, the thin smear may be preferable, even though it is much more time-consuming because of the greater area which must be examined.

Thick Smear (Field's Method)

REAGENTS

Solution A—

methylene blue	0.8 Gm.
Azure I	0.5 Gm.
disodium hydrogen phosphate (anhydrous)	5 Gm.
potassium dihydrogen phosphate (anhydrous)	6.25 Gm.
distilled water	500 cc.

Solution B—

eosin	1 Gm.
disodium hydrogen phosphate (anhydrous)	5 Gm.
potassium dihydrogen phosphate (anhydrous)	6.25 Gm.
distilled water	500 cc.

The phosphate salts are first dissolved, and then the stain is added. Solution of the granular Azure I is aided by grinding in a mortar with a small quantity of the phosphate solvent. The solutions of stain should be set aside for twenty-four hours and then filtered, after which they are ready for use. Should a scum later appear on the surface, or a dye precipitate on the stained films, subsequent filtration is necessary. The same solution may be used continuously for many weeks without apparent deterioration, but the eosin solution should be renewed when it becomes greenish from the slight carry-over of the methylene blue. The stains are kept in covered jars of such a size that the depth of solution is about three inches, the level being maintained by the addition of fresh stain as necessary.

PREPARATION OF BLOOD FILMS—Blood films should be thick, but not too thick—about ten to fifteen times the thickness of those used for differential blood counts. The dried film should not be so thick that the hands of a watch cannot be seen through it. It may be made by any of the conventional methods (p. 523) and is ready to stain as soon as it ceases to be obviously moist. Fixation is unnecessary, and freshly prepared films stain better than those which have been kept for a day or two.

TECHNIC—Dip the film for one second in Solution A. Immediately rinse by moving it gently in clean water for a few seconds, until stain ceases to flow from the film and the glass of the slide is free from stain. Dip for one second in Solution B. Rinse by moving gently for two or three seconds in clean water. Place vertically against a rack to drain and dry.

The concentration of the stain is adjusted for a

---

* Obtainable from National Aniline Division, Allied Chemical & Dye Corp., 40 Rector Street, New York, N.Y.

staining time of one second with an immediate wash of five seconds, but the relative times may need slight adjustment to suit different batches of stain. Varying periods of from one to five seconds should be tried until the results are optimal for the particular stains and washing water in use.

Staining is optimal at the lower edge of the film toward which the hemoglobin has drained. In this area the color differentiation under the oil immersion lens is as follows:

The general ground is creamy-yellow in color, sometimes uniform, sometimes mottled with pale blue. In the leukocytes the nuclei are deep blue and sharply defined; the eosinophilic granules are large, dull red, and well defined; and the neutrophilic granules are small, pale, purple, and vague.

In the malaria parasites, the cytoplasm is blue; the chromatin, dark purplish-red; the pigment, unstained yellow of varying shades depending on the depth of the cytoplasm in which it lies.

Thin Smear — Thin blood films prepared as for counting blood cells may be stained with Wright's or Giemsa's stain and examined under oil immersion. This method facilitates positive identification of the malaria species but is far less accurate for establishing the diagnosis of malaria.

DIRECT CULTURE FOR PERTUSSIS

Although the cough-plate technic has been extensively used in obtaining direct cultures for *H. pertussis*, the nasopharyngeal swab technic is now believed to be more accurate. A sterile-cotton-tipped metal applicator is bent into a suitable curve and is swabbed over the posterior surface of the nasopharynx above and behind the soft palate. It is then streaked over a culture plate containing special glycerin-potato-blood agar and incubated for two days. Diagnosis is facilitated if there is added to the medium a suitable concentration of penicillin, which inhibits the growth of most of the common bacterial inhabitants of the nose and throat without interfering with the reproduction of *H. pertussis*.

Pertussis colonies appear as minute, glistening, mercury-like droplets (amid larger saprophytic colonies if no penicillin has been added). They usually double in size by the third or fourth day and are then about one millimeter in diameter, translucent, raised, and definitely circular. When viewed against strong transmitted light, the colony and the surrounding zone appear lighter than the rest of the medium (because of hemolysis). The following are other aids to identification:

1. On the third or fourth day of incubation, gentle scraping of the colony with a pointed platinum wire will remove most of the soft, slightly sticky growth.

2. Colonies do not slide from their original position on the medium when touched with a platinum loop.

3. A colony on the loop diffuses evenly in a droplet of water on a clean slide without much mixing.

4. An unstained capsule is often seen in thin gram-stained smears (counterstained with double-strength carbolfuchsin). Stained by Gram's method (negative), the smears consist of small, delicately staining, ovoid bacilli, some of which show bipolar staining. After frequent transfers they appear more coccoid.

5. Cultures should give a positive Dold test before (and after) intensive vaccine cultivation.

PNEUMOCOCCUS TYPING OF SPUTUM (NEUFELD QUELLUNG TEST)

A loopful of sputum is mixed separately with an equal amount of each of the available specific-type serums (rabbit) and an equal quantity of Loeffler's alkaline methylene blue (p. 547). Examination is made with the oil immersion lens, with light dimmed. When a positive reaction occurs, which is usually in a few minutes, there is a decided swelling of the capsule of the pneumococcus that is present. In the preparation in which there is no reaction, the capsule of the pneumococcus appears as a halo of refracted light.

When organisms are too few in a specimen of sputum to permit the use of the Neufeld method, the mouse inoculation method will often yield a positive result.

EXAMINATION FOR TRICHOMONAS VAGINALIS

The patient should be instructed to report without previous douches or vaginal treatment. Insert a speculum into the vagina, and secure a large drop of purulent secretion. Place a loopful in a hanging drop of warm physiological salt solution. The protozoa can be seen moving about freely. Dark-field illumination will show the flagella and undulating membrane.

Occasionally, if the organisms are few or their motility is suspended, a contrast stain is of assistance in making the diagnosis. A drop of 0.1 percent safranine can be added to the pus as a diluent. The nuclear material and protoplasm of the accompanying leukocytes take the stain, but the trichomonad remains unstained and conspicuous against a pale-pink background. The stain appears to stimulate the motility of the organism.

EXAMINATION FOR INTESTINAL PARASITES

For Vegetative Endamoeba Histolytica—The best method of obtaining this organism is through the proctoscope. Ulcers are swabbed or bits of mucus or pus are obtained, and the material is smeared on a warm slide holding a drop of warm physiological salt solution. After a cover glass is applied, the slide is examined under the microscope.

Less success attends the examination of material passed at stool. If this method is used, the feces should be passed into a warm vessel and examined as soon as possible. It may be advisable, in carriers or chronic cases, to administer a saline cathartic. The first liquid stool should be examined. Grayish or blood-streaked particles of mucus are most likely to contain the organism. They are prepared on a slide as described above.

The most important characteristics of *E. histolytica* in its vegetative stage are its active motility in fresh specimens of stool and the presence of ingested red blood cells. It is grayish or colorless, granular, and varies in size from 20 to 40 microns in diameter. There is no contractile vacuole, and the nucleus is small, round, and indistinct. The presence of red blood cells in the digestive vacuole is of diagnostic importance. The parasites may be rendered more conspicuous by vital staining. A loopful of feces is mixed with a drop of 1:10,000 solution of neutral red in physiological salt solution. The dye is taken up by the amebae.

Zinc-Flotation Method for Cysts of Endamoeba Histolytica—Prepare the flotation solution by dissolving 331 Gm. of granular Zinc Sulfate, U.S.P., ($ZnSO_4 \cdot 7H_2O$) in one liter of distilled water. The specific gravity at room temperature should be 1.180.

Place a stool sample the size of a pea in 2 or 3 cc. of lukewarm tap water in a test tube measuring 13 by 100 mm., and break up thoroughly by means of a glass rod. Add water to 1/2 inch from the top, stir thoroughly, and centrifuge at 1,200 to 1,800 r.p.m. for forty-five seconds. Decant the supernatant fluid, fill again with water, stir, and centrifuge. If the supernatant fluid is cloudy, again decant, refill, and centrifuge. When the supernatant remains clear, decant it and fill the tube one-fourth full with the zinc sulfate solution. Stir thoroughly and then fill to 1/4 inch from the top with zinc sulfate solution. Centrifuge at 2,500 r.p.m. for forty-five to sixty seconds, being sure that the centrifuge stops smoothly. By means of a 3/16-inch platinum loop, transfer the surface film onto a glass slide containing a drop of 0.5 percent iodine solution (Lugol's solution diluted 1:10). Apply a cover glass and examine under the microscope.

An alternative technic makes use of a cup or 50-cc. beaker instead of a test tube. The stool sample is broken up thoroughly and then mixed with the zinc sulfate solution, more being added until the cup is full to the brim. After it has stood for twenty minutes, a slide is gently placed in contact with the surface and lifted away. The adhering drop is covered with a cover glass after addition of a drop of the dilute iodine solution.

The method provides a means of concentrating cysts of *E. histolytica* and also ova of many of the common intestinal parasites. Cysts of *E. histolytica* may be seen with the 16-mm. objective. They are colorless, refractile, spherical bodies, 7 to 15 microns in diameter, looking not unlike oil globules. After full development, the cysts contain four small nuclei which lie at different levels. These can best be found by reducing the light and focusing carefully with the 4-mm. objective. Young cysts have only one or two nuclei and contain refractile, colorless chromatin bodies and a small amount of glycogen.

Bacterial Stains

Loeffler's Alkaline Methylene Blue is an excellent stain for studying morphology of organisms. To prepare it, dissolve 0.3 Gm. methylene blue in 30 cc. of 95 percent ethyl alcohol and filter. Dissolve 0.01 Gm. potassium hydroxide in 100 cc. of distilled water (or, more conveniently, dilute 17.8 cc. of N/100 potassium hydroxide solution to 100 cc.). Mix the two solutions. The resultant preparation keeps indefinitely.

To use, fix the smear with heat, cover with stain, allow to remain thirty seconds (for diphtheria or Vincent's organisms, five minutes are required), wash in water, and allow to dry.

Gram's Method is extremely useful as an aid in differentiating bacteria. It is based on the observation that when bacteria are treated successively with certain dyes (gentian violet, methyl violet, or crystal violet) and iodine, some types tend to retain the stain when subsequently treated with acetone or alcohol, whereas others lose it quickly. The former are termed *gram-positive;* the latter, *gram-negative.* The staining characteristics of the more common organisms are given in Table 65.

TABLE 65—*Common Pathogenic Micro-Organisms and Their Staining Characteristics*

Organism	Stain
Staphylococcus (aureus, albus) . . .	Gram-positive
Streptococcus (beta-hemolytic, viridans, indifferent)	Gram-positive
Pneumococcus (*Diplococcus pneumoniae*)	Gram-positive
Gonococcus (*Neisseria gonorrhoeae*)	Gram-negative
Meningococcus (*Neisseria intracellularis*)	Gram-negative
Micrococcus catarrhalis (*Neisseria catarrhalis*)	Gram-negative
Bacillus anthracis	Gram-positive
Clostridium perfringens (*C. welchii*)	Gram-positive
Clostridium septicum (*Vibrion septique*)	Gram-positive
Clostridium botulinum (*B. botulinus*)	Gram-positive
Clostridium tetani (*B. tetani*)	Gram-positive
Corynebacterium diphtheriae (Klebs-Loeffler bacillus)	Gram-positive
Eberthella typhosa (*B. typhosus*)	Gram-negative
Salmonella paratyphi (*B. paratyphosus A*)	Gram-negative
Salmonella schottmülleri (*B. paratyphosus B*)	Gram-negative
Salmonella enteritidis (Gärtner's bacillus)	Gram-negative
Shigella dysenteriae (*B. dysenteriae*)	Gram-negative
Proteus vulgaris (*B. proteus*)	Gram-negative
Pseudomonas aeruginosa (*B. pyocyaneus*)	Gram-negative
Klebsiella pneumoniae (Friedländer's bacillus)	Gram-negative
Hemophilus influenzae (Pfeiffer's bacillus)	Gram-negative
Mycobacterium tuberculosis (Koch's bacillus)	Acid-fast
Mycobacterium leprae	Acid-fast

Burke's modification of Gram's method gives sharp differentiation and has the advantage of simplicity.

BURKE'S REAGENTS—1. Crystal violet (85 percent dye content), 1 percent in distilled water.

2. Sodium bicarbonate solution, 5 percent.

3. Iodine solution containing 1 percent iodine and 2 percent potassium iodide. This solution may be prepared by diluting 20 cc. of Lugol's solution to 100 cc. with distilled water.

4. Acetone.

5. Safranin O, 2 percent aqueous solution.

TECHNIC—Dry a thin smear in air and fix with the minimum effective amount of heat. Flood the smear with the crystal violet solution, and mix 3 to 8 drops of the sodium bicarbonate solution with the dye on the slide. Allow to stand two to three minutes. Some prefer to steam the slide. Flush off the dye with iodine solution, cover with fresh iodine solution, and let stand one minute or longer. Wash with water for as brief a period as possible (excess washing has an adverse effect on differentiation), and blot film until almost but not quite dry. Apply acetone decolorizer, allow to stand for a few seconds, and drain off. Then allow fresh decolorizer to flow over slide until it drops off clear (not more than ten seconds). Dry the slide completely (this is essential). Counterstain for five to ten seconds or longer with the safranin O solution, wash briefly with water, and dry.

Ziehl-Neelsen Stain for Acid-Fast Bacilli—Czaplewski's carbolfuchsin may be used; to make it, add 5 cc. of warm, liquefied phenol and 50 cc. of glycerin to 1 Gm. basic fuchsin (90 percent dye), stirring constantly, and then add 50 cc. of water. Filter. The solution keeps indefinitely.

Only clean, unscratched slides should be used. The smear is fixed and immersed for thirty minutes or longer in the carbolfuchsin at room temperature. Wash the slide in water and decolorize in acid alcohol (5 cc. of C.P. hydrochloric acid in 100 cc. of 95 percent ethyl alcohol) until the stain has been removed from all but the thick parts of the slide. Wash in water and counterstain lightly with Loeffler's alkaline methylene blue (p. 547). Wash again in water and allow to dry.

When the smear and stain are correctly made, everything in the slide will appear light blue except acid-fast bacilli (tubercle, smegma, and lepra bacilli), which are bright red.

It is essential that suitable portions of sputum be chosen for smears. The more purulent parts are best. Pieces of necrotic tissue are good, but they must be differentiated from bits of food. Better selection can be made from fresh sputum than from that which has liquefied on standing.

If acid-fast bacilli are not found on direct smears, the sputum may be concentrated. The Haynes trypsin-digestion method is rapid and satisfactory. The trypsin solution is prepared by adding 0.5 Gm.

powdered trypsin (1:250, Difco) to 100 cc. freshly distilled water, mixing by shaking, and adding 0.7 cc. normal sodium hydroxide solution. This solution is kept in the refrigerator. Since acid-fast organisms often grow in it as contaminants, it is necessary to run controls (using only reagents) each time the trypsin solution is used. If acid-fast organisms are found in the control smears, the trypsin solution is put through a Seitz filter.

To concentrate the specimen, add to it an equal quantity of trypsin solution, or more if the specimen is very thick, in a bottle or large test tube. Mix thoroughly with an applicator stick or glass rod. Incubate at 37°C. for thirty minutes or until the mucus is thoroughly digested, stirring at intervals. After digestion is complete, centrifuge at 3,000 r.p.m. for five minutes or at 1,500 r.p.m. for ten minutes. If the sediment obtained by centrifugation is large, decant the supernatant fluid, add an equal volume of 4 percent sodium hydroxide solution, incubate for an additional half hour, dilute to 50 cc. with distilled water, and centrifuge again. Prepare slides from the sediment, fix, and stain as with unconcentrated material (see above).

Poisons and Antidotes

IMMEDIATE EMERGENCY MEASURES

If the nature of the poisoning is immediately apparent, appropriate specific treatment should be undertaken. Whether the poison is known or not, certain general measures are applicable. If the poison was taken by mouth, the stomach should be emptied. If the patient is conscious, vomiting can be induced by one or more of the following:

EMETICS

1. Strong suds of laundry soap in warm water.
2. Table salt in warm water, two tablespoonfuls in 8 ounces.
3. Mustard and warm water, 1 tablespoonful to 8 ounces.
4. Zinc sulfate, 15 grains (1 Gm.), in 8 ounces of warm water.
5. Apomorphine hydrochloride, 1/10 grain (6.5 mg.), hypodermically.

In the unconscious patient, and in the conscious patient who will co-operate, the stomach may be emptied by the passage of a tube. With corrosive poisons and in patients in convulsions or deep coma, passage of a stomach tube may be dangerous.

After evacuation of the stomach, the following may be given repeatedly:

UNIVERSAL ANTIDOTE

```
pulverized charcoal (or
    powdered burnt toast)....................2 parts
tannic acid (or strong tea) ..................1 part
magnesium oxide (or milk of magnesia)........1 part
```

If all ingredients are dry, a teaspoonful of the mixture is given in water. One gram of charcoal will absorb 40 mg. of phenol and over 500 mg. of strychnine. Tannic acid precipitates alkaloids, certain glucosides, and many metals, and the magnesia serves to neutralize acids. Vomiting should be induced, or the stomach washed out, after each dose. Vomiting is dangerous in unconscious patients because of the possibility of the aspiration of vomitus into the trachea.

The patient's body should be kept warm, since shock occurs in severe poisoning. For treatment of shock, see page 90. For respiratory depression, use oxygen plus caffeine and nikethamide. If respiratory paralysis is imminent, place patient in Drinker respirator if possible; otherwise use artificial respiration. Use atropine for excessive secretions and in mushroom poisoning. Do not exhaust patient by too active treatment.

Information should be obtained, if possible, from the patient's friends or relatives and the poison identified as soon as possible in order that specific measures may be instituted promptly. Save any bottle or container for later evidence or analysis.

CHEMICAL BURNS

Acid burns or acid in the eye should be treated immediately by washing with water and with sodium bicarbonate solution (1/2 percent). Alkali burns should be washed with water, followed by 1 percent acetic acid solution (vinegar contains about 4 percent acetic acid).

POISON KIT*

Cases of poisoning almost always occur as unexpected emergencies; thus the physician may save a life by keeping a kit prepared against such an exigency. A small box will serve the purpose. It may contain the following:

  1 50-cc. sterile syringe and needle
  1 10-cc. sterile syringe and needle
  1 Ampoule 'Amytal Sodium,' 1 Gm. (15 1/2 grains)
  2 Ampoules Sodium Thiosulfate, 1 Gm. (15 1/2 grains), 10 cc.
  2 Ampoules Ephedrine and Caffeine, 2 cc. (Ephedrine Sulfate, 3/8 grain, and Caffeine and Sodium Benzoate, 7 1/2 grains)
  Hypodermic Tablets Strychnine Sulfate, 1/60 grain (0.0011 Gm.)
  2 ampoules of nikethamide, 25 percent
  12 Aspirols Amyl Nitrite, 5 min. (0.3 cc.)
  12 Aspirols Ammonia Aromatic, 0.4 cc.

*Adapted from emergency kit, Indianapolis General Hospital.

  1 ampoule of sodium nitrite, 0.3 Gm., 10 cc.
  1 ampoule of sodium thiosulfate, 12.5 Gm., 50 cc.
  1 ampoule of sodium formaldehyde sulfoxylate, 10 Gm.
  1 package of tannic acid powder
  1 package of copper sulfate
  1 pound of sodium bicarbonate
  2 Ampoules Picrotoxin, 0.003 Gm. (1/20 grain)
  2 Ampoules Dimercaprol (BAL), 10 percent, in oil, 4.5 cc.

The physician's regular case in daily use should provide a supply of the more usual hypodermic tablets and ampoules, such as:

  Pilocarpine Hydrochloride, 1/4 grain (16 mg.)
  Apomorphine Hydrochloride, 1/10 grain (6.5 mg.)
  Atropine Sulfate, 1/100 grain (0.65 mg.)
  Morphine Sulfate, 1/4 grain (16 mg.)
  Codeine Sulfate, 1/2 grain (32.5 mg.)
  Caffeine and Sodium Benzoate, 0.5 Gm. (7 1/2 grains)

TREATMENT OF POISONING

Poison	Smallest Fatal Dose	Immediate Treatment	Supportive Treatment
Acetanilid Acetone Aniline Antipyrine	5–10 grains 6 oz. 6 dr. 15–30 grains	Gastric lavage or emetic. Artificial respiration or respirator if necessary, and oxygen. Methylene blue solution (1%) intravenously for methemoglobinemia.	Recumbent position, external heat to body, cold to head. Stimulation with caffeine and ammonia. Atropine if secretions become excessive. Blood transfusion.
☐ ACIDS Hydrochloric Nitric Sulfuric Acetic Phosphoric	1–4 dr. 2 dr. 1 dr. * *	Avoid stomach tube and also emetics if corrosion of tissues has occurred. Give alkalies (magnesia, lime water, sodium bicarbonate solution, soap, chalk) and demulcents (white of egg, milk).	Recumbent position, general stimulants, external heat. Morphine and atropine usually necessary.
Oxalic	1/2–2 dr.	Never use stomach pump. Induce vomiting immediately, and give any form of lime (plaster from wall if necessary) at once. Avoid salts of sodium and potassium on account of injurious soluble oxalate formation. Calcium chloride by vein.	Recumbent position, external heat. Ammonia, caffeine, atropine if necessary. Morphine for pain.

* Not determined

Poison	Smallest Fatal Dose	Immediate Treatment	Supportive Treatment
□ ACIDS — (*contd.*) Carbolic (Phenol) Cresol (Lysol) Creosote Guaiacol	1–4 dr. 1 dr. * *	Death may occur rapidly. Use stomach tube cautiously; give sodium or magnesium sulfate, lime water, soap, and milk, egg white, or other demulcents. Avoid oil, alcohol, and glycerin.	Recumbent position, external heat to body, cold to head. Artificial respiration and oxygen if necessary, with stimulation by caffeine, ammonia, and atropine. Morphine if needed for pain.
Carbonic	*	Respirator if necessary. Artificial respiration.	Oxygen, fresh air, friction and heat to extremities. Stimulation if necessary.
Hydrocyanic (Prussic)		*See* Cyanides	
Aconite Aconitine	4 grains 1/10 grain	Tannic acid (10–30 grains in water), charcoal (1 tablespoonful in water). Stomach lavage, tea, strong coffee. Respirator and oxygen if necessary. Avoid emetics.	Horizontal position, with head covered; external heat to body; friction of back with hot towels. Stimulation with aromatic ammonia, caffeine, and atropine.
□ ALCOHOL, ETHYL Acute	3 1/2–7 oz.	Wash out stomach. Respirator, and oxygen and carbon dioxide if necessary. Give slowly by vein 50 cc. of 50% dextrose solution containing 15 units of Insulin, 50 mg. of thiamin chloride, and 50 mg. of nicotinamide.	Keep warm; cold to head; caffeine and sodium benzoate, 7 1/2–15 grains; ephedrine sulfate, 1/2 grain p.r.n.; paraldehyde, 4–15 cc., or barbiturates if patient is violent.
Chronic		*See* page 159	
□ ALCOHOL, METHYL	1–2 oz.	Empty stomach by emesis or tube, and wash repeatedly with sodium bicarbonate solution; give large volumes of fluid; pilocarpine, potassium iodide, and purgatives aid in relieving eye symptoms.	Recumbent posture. Morphine for pain; caffeine for stimulation; artificial respiration if necessary; venesection if edema of lungs. Combat acidosis with fluids, alkalies, and sodium lactate (*see* p. 59).
□ ALDEHYDES Formaldehyde (Formalin)	1 oz.	Wash out stomach; give dilute ammonia (0.1 percent) and ammonium acetate.	Recumbent posture. Cardiac stimulants, atropine if excessive secretions, morphine for pain, artificial respiration and oxygen if necessary.

* Not determined

Poison	Smallest Fatal Dose	Immediate Treatment	Supportive Treatment
☐ **ALKALIES** Lye Caustic Soda Potash Ammonia Lime	1/2–4 dr. * * * *	Avoid stomach tube; neutralize with large volume of weak acid, vinegar, lemon juice, or grapefruit juice; boric acid for use in eye; give milk, egg white, or other demulcents.	Recumbent posture. Morphine, stimulants, caffeine. Ammonia, cold air.
☐ **ALKALOIDS** (Specific measures given under name of alkaloid)		Precipitate with tannic acid solution; adsorb with charcoal. Evacuate stomach by emetic or lavage.	Maintain circulation and respiration; artificial respiration if necessary.
☐ **ANESTHETICS** Chloroform Ether		Maintain free airway. If drug was swallowed, evacuate stomach; give sodium bicarbonate solution and demulcents. Oxygen and carbon dioxide, and respirator if necessary.	Head low, recumbent posture; external heat; caffeine, atropine, strychnine, ouabain intravenously.
Antimony	3/4– 1 1/2 grains	Gastric lavage with warm tannic acid solution or tea, repeated several times. Demulcents (milk, egg white) or magnesium oxide. Give dimercaprol as in arsenic poisoning (below).	Caffeine, atropine, morphine. External heat.
☐ **ARSENIC** Arsenious Acid Fowler's Solution Paris Green "Rough on Rats"	1 1/2 grains * * *	Prompt gastric lavage with large quantities of warm water. Saline laxatives, followed by castor oil. Give dimercaprol (BAL, British Anti-Lewisite) in doses of 3 mg. per Kg. of body weight by intramuscular injection every four hours for two days; for subsequent therapy, *see* page 514.	Recumbent posture. Large quantities of fluids. Watch for collapse; keep warm; give atropine, caffeine, if necessary.
Atropine Belladonna Hyoscyamus Stramonium	1 grain ± * * *	Tannic acid solution orally if taken by mouth; gastric lavage or emetic. Give 'Amytal Sodium' and physostigmine, muscarine, or pilocarpine to antagonize.	Recumbent posture. Alternate hot and cold applications. Morphine if needed. Artificial respiration or respirator if required.

*Not determined

Poison	Smallest Fatal Dose	Immediate Treatment	Supportive Treatment
Barbiturates	15 grains	Prompt evacuation and lavage of stomach; give large volumes of fluid, magnesium sulfate purge, and diuretics. Ephedrine in 3/4-grain doses and strychnine, 1/12 grain, every two hours are useful. In severe poisoning, give 10 mg. of picrotoxin intramuscularly or intravenously at intervals of one to thirty minutes until signs of stimulation occur or there is evidence of returning corneal sensitivity. Avoid overdosage.	Recumbent posture. Watch for bronchopneumonia, and give atropine if pulmonary edema occurs. Third day is critical. Stimulate with ammonia, and provide external heat. Respirator if necessary. (*See also* p. 395)
Barium (Soluble Salts)	15 grains	Evacuate stomach by tube or emetic; lavage with magnesium or sodium sulfate solution; follow with milk or other demulcents.	Treat pain with morphine and atropine. Give artificial respiration and oxygen if needed.
Belladonna		*See* Atropine	
Benzene Benzol		*See* Solvents	
Botulism		*See* Food Poisoning, page 557	
Bromides	*	Discontinue drug; give sodium chloride by mouth, 4–10 Gm. daily, to hasten excretion of bromide. Give fluids, at least 4,000 cc. daily. Do not confine to bed unless necessary.	Keep warm; stimulate with caffeine, or calm with paraldehyde, 4–16 cc. by mouth or 12–24 cc. by rectum, or 'Seconal Sodium,' 1 1/2–3 grains (0.1–0.2 Gm.), as indicated.
Bromine Chlorine	* *	By INHALATION: Infusions of normal saline solution during initial period of blood concentration; venesection when blood is diluted.	Symptomatic stimulation.
		By MOUTH: Gastric lavage with diluted egg white or boiled starch solution.	Symptomatic stimulation. Treat also for bromide poisoning.
Brucine		*See* Strychnine	
Cannabis American Hemp Indian Hemp Marijuana	* * * *	Evacuate stomach by tube or emetic; precipitate drug with tannic acid solution. Respirator if necessary.	External heat to body, cold to head. Stimulate with ammonia, caffeine, atropine, and oxygen if needed.

* Not determined

Poison	Smallest Fatal Dose	Immediate Treatment	Supportive Treatment
Carbon Monoxide		*See* Gas	
Carbon Tetrachloride		*See* Solvents	
Chloral Hydrate Chloralformamide	20 grains *	Evacuate stomach, and wash out with tea or coffee. Intravenous administration of 10–20 mg. of picrotoxin may save life.	External heat, ammonia, caffeine, artificial respiration.
Chlorine		*See* Bromine	
Chloroform		*See* Anesthetics	
Cocaine and Its Substitutes	1/2–15 grains	If drug was taken by mouth and if patient is seen early, give tannic acid solution and remove by stomach tube. Emetics have no effect. If convulsions occur, give 'Amytal Sodium' intravenously to control.	Keep horizontal, in fresh air. Use artificial respiration and oxygen inhalations if needed. (*See also* p. 442)
Conium Coniine Poison Hemlock	* 2 grains ± *	Evacuate stomach by tube or emetic; use tannic acid to precipitate the alkaloid, and follow with demulcents.	Recumbent position. Watch for respiratory failure; stimulate with ammonia and nikethamide. Maintain body temperature; apply artificial respiration and oxygen if needed.
☐ COPPER Sulfate (Blue Vitriol) Subacetate (Verdigris) Acetoarsenite (Paris Green)	5 dr.	Give potassium ferrocyanide or sodium thiosulfate; empty stomach and wash out thoroughly. Follow with demulcents and magnesia.	External heat; stimulants if indicated; morphine if necessary for pain.
Corrosive Sublimate		*See* Mercury	
Creosote		*See* Acids, Carbolic	
Croton Oil	20 gtt.	Evacuate stomach, wash with warm water, and follow with demulcents.	External heat; circulatory and respiratory stimulation with ammonia, nikethamide, caffeine. Morphine for pain.

* Not determined

Poison	Smallest Fatal Dose	Immediate Treatment	Supportive Treatment
□ CYANIDES Hydrocyanic Acid (Prussic Acid) (Fumigating Gas) Bitter Almonds Chokeberries	1–2 grains * *	Rapid work is essential, and a team of three individuals should carry out the following steps: 1. Physician in charge loads 10-cc. syringe with 10 cc. (0.3 Gm.) of sodium nitrite while assistant No. 1 washes out stomach and assistant No. 2 gives amyl nitrite by inhalation (one aspirol every three minutes). 2. Physician injects sodium nitrite intravenously, assistant No. 1 finishes washing stomach, and assistant No. 2 withdraws amyl nitrite and loads 50-cc. syringe with sodium thiosulfate (12.5 Gm. in 50-cc. ampoule). 3. The physician injects the 50 cc. of thiosulfate solution intravenously while more amyl nitrite is given if needed.	Support respiration. Give artificial respiration as long as heart beats. Watch patient for twenty-four to forty-eight hours. If relapse occurs, repeat treatment, using one-half these amounts. The value of methylene blue has been questioned.
Digitalis	40 grains	Give tannic acid solution, evacuate stomach by tube, and lavage with tannic acid solution or strong tea. Empty bowel with magnesium sulfate.	Maintain horizontal position' for arising may be fatal. Stimulate with ammonia, caffeine; give atropine in 1/65-grain doses as needed to combat bradycardia; and morphine, 1/4 grain, may reduce excessive irritability.
Ergot and Derivatives	12 grains	Repeated gastric lavage; purgation with magnesium sulfate. Vasodilators, such as papaverine and nitrites.	Caffeine and strychnine stimulation.
Eserine		*See* Physostigmine	
□ FOOD POISONING (Ptomaines) Botulism		Produce emesis, and lavage stomach; give magnesium sulfate or castor oil, and colonic irrigations. Strychnine may be used freely for stimulation, accompanied by pilocarpine and digitalis as indicated. Barbiturates and morphine delay acute symptoms in animals and should be tried. Specific antitoxin, 20–50 cc., must be given early to be of value.	Recumbent position. Fluids by rectum and under skin. Watch for evidence of paralysis of muscles of swallowing. Be ready with artificial respiration and carbon dioxide. (*See also* p. 271)

* Not determined

Poison	Smallest Fatal Dose	Immediate Treatment	Supportive Treatment
□ FOOD POISONING —(contd.) Salmonella Group		Gastric lavage, and purgation with magnesium sulfate and castor oil.	Symptomatic stimulation. (See also p. 271)
Staphylococcus Group		Gastric lavage, purgation with magnesium sulfate and castor oil, colonic irrigations.	Symptomatic measures. (See also p. 271)
Formaldehyde		See Aldehydes	
□ GAS Carbon Monoxide Illuminating Gas Automobile Exhaust Gas	*	Remove at once to fresh air; give oxygen and carbon dioxide if possible. Use artificial respiration or respirator (call police or fire department or local gas company). Blood transfusion has been effective if carried out within an hour. Stimulate with ammonia inhalations. Value of methylene blue has been questioned.	Hypodermic medication is of little value. Keep the patient breathing fresh air and oxygen.
Gelsemium	1 dr.	Give tannic acid solution; empty and lavage stomach; follow with castor oil.	Maintain external heat; give atropine, nikethamide, and caffeine. Artificial respiration if needed.
Hydrocyanic Acid		See Cyanides	
Hyoscyamus		See Atropine	
Iodine	1 dr.	Starch or flour with water; evacuate stomach; then give demulcents.	Give stimulants if needed, keep warm, and use morphine if necessary for pain.
Jaborandi		See Pilocarpine	
□ LEAD SALTS Acetate White Lead	300 grains	Give 4 or 5 Gm. of sodium citrate dissolved in 30 cc. of water, three or four times daily by mouth, until lead excretion falls to normal. For severe colic, give 50 cc. of 2.5% sodium citrate solution by vein. In acute poisoning by ingestion, evacuate stomach, give a cathartic, and follow with demulcents.	

*Not determined

Poison	Smallest Fatal Dose	Immediate Treatment	Supportive Treatment
Lobelia	*	Tannic acid solution; evacuate stomach; follow with castor oil.	Stimulants, artificial heat, morphine.
□ MERCURY Bichloride (Corrosive Sublimate)	3–5 grains	1. Administer 1 raw egg white in milk for every 4 grains of bichloride of mercury taken. 2. Evacuate stomach and wash out thoroughly with 5% solution of sodium formaldehyde sulfoxylate. Allow 6 or 7 oz. to remain in stomach (or use 1 Gm. sodium hypophosphite, 10 cc. water, and 5 cc. hydrogen peroxide for each estimated 1 1/2 grains of mercury bichloride taken). Lavage with diluted solution should follow this treatment. 3. Give dimercaprol (BAL) intramuscularly, 5 mg. per Kg. of body weight at once, and follow in one or two hours with 2.5 mg. per Kg. For subsequent doses, *see* page 514.	Give morphine for pain, and stimulate with caffeine, nikethamide, and atropine if indicated. Maintain body fluids, give dextrose intravenously, and begin the Lambert and Patterson treatment: 1. Every two hours give 8 oz. of the following mixture: potassium bitartrate . . 1 dr. sugar . . . . 1 dr. lactose . . . . 1/2 oz. lemon juice . . . . 1 oz. water . . . . 16 oz. 2. Give 8 oz. of milk on the alternate two hours. 3. Rectal irrigation with potassium acetate, 1 dr. to pint, given by continuous-drip method. 4. Wash out stomach twice daily.
Morphine		*See* Opium	
Mushroom Muscarine	* *	Tannic acid and charcoal in suspension; evacuate stomach; wash out with sodium or magnesium sulfate. Atropine repeatedly hypodermically, or even intravenously for muscarine.	Treat shock (*see* p. 90). 'Amytal,' 3–6 grains, every few hours if excitement. Maintain body temperature with artificial heat. Alternate intravenous 10% dextrose solutions with hypertonic saline solution.
Nicotine Black Leaf 40	1–4 min. *	Tannic acid solution; emetic or gastric lavage.	Symptomatic stimulation.
□ NITRITES Amyl Nitrite Nitroglycerin Spirit of Nitre	*	Gastric lavage and purgation by magnesium sulfate. Methylene blue, 6 cc. of 1 percent solution intramuscularly followed by 1 or 2 grains daily by mouth, for methemoglobinemia. Blood transfusion if necessary.	Horizontal position, cold packs to head; stimulate with caffeine, ephedrine. Oxygen inhalation.
Nux Vomica		*See* Strychnine	

* Not determined

Poison	Smallest Fatal Dose	Immediate Treatment	Supportive Treatment
□ OPIUM Codeine Heroin Laudanum Morphine Paregoric	3–4 grains * * * 1–2 grains *	Evacuate stomach in all cases and lavage with potassium permanganate (1:1,000 solution). Give subsequent doses of 2 grains dissolved in 4 oz. of water. Keep warm and awake; stimulate with strychnine and caffeine. Most important is O_2 and 5% or 10% CO_2 by inhalation.	Artificial respiration or respirator; coffee, atropine (not more than 1/40 grain). Empty bowel with salines after few hours. Continue artificial respiration as long as any sign of life is present.
Paris Green		*See* Arsenic	
□ PETROLEUM Kerosene Gasoline Benzene	*	Gastric lavage or emetic.	Symptomatic stimulation, oxygen, external heat, artificial respiration.
□ PHOSPHORUS Rat and Roach Paste Matches	1–3 grains * *	Copper sulfate, 1/2% solution, potassium permanganate, 1:1,000, or dilute hydrogen peroxide will oxidize phosphorus to phosphoric acid. Old oil of turpentine forms an insoluble compound with phosphorus; use 1 teaspoonful to a pint of water. Repeat lavage frequently, and give mucilaginous drinks and magnesium sulfate.	Intravenous dextrose and calcium salts will aid in protecting the liver from damage following absorption. Glycine has been recommended. Morphine and symptomatic stimulation with caffeine may be required; give oxygen inhalations if necessary.

□ PHYSOSTIG-
  MINE (Eserine)
Calabar Bean
  (Ordeal Bean)
	
	2–3 grains
	
	6 beans
		Lavage stomach, and give as antagonist 1/40–1/60 grain of atropine. Magnesium sulfate intramuscularly has been recommended.	Keep body warm; treat shock (*see* p. 90); give oxygen if needed.

□ PICROTOXIN Cocculus Indicus	*	Evacuate stomach and wash out freely. In animals, fifty times the fatal dose may be combated by barbiturates. Control convulsions by slow intravenous injections of 'Amytal Sodium' or pentobarbital sodium.	Symptomatic stimulation and artificial respiration with O_2 and CO_2 if necessary.
□ PILOCARPINE Jaborandi	2 grains *	Combat effects with atropine, the physiological antagonist. Treat collapse by stimulation; prepare to carry on artificial respiration.	Morphine, ammonia, oxygen.

*Not determined

Poison	Smallest Fatal Dose	Immediate Treatment	Supportive Treatment
Ptomaines		*See* Food Poisoning	
□ **SILVER SALTS** Lunar Caustic Silver Nitrate	30 grains	Large quantities of common salt and water, given as lavage or emetic. Follow with eggs and milk for demulcent effect.	Morphine; stimulants if necessary.
□ **SOLVENTS** Benzene Benzol Toluol Xylol	*	Remove patient to fresh air, and change clothing if it contains the poison. If ingested, wash out stomach with warm water. Artificial respiration and O_2 and CO_2.	Place in recumbent posture, give caffeine, and combat asphyxia. Later, blood transfusions and liver extract parenterally to combat anemia. Watch blood count. Pentnucleotide may be of value.
Carbon Tetrachloride	1 dr.	Remove patient from contact with the vapor; or, if ingested, wash out stomach with warm water. Respirator, with O_2 and CO_2, may be necessary.	Stimulate symptomatically, maintain free catharsis, force fluids, and give high-carbohydrate diet. Dextrose and calcium salts intravenously may aid in treatment of resulting liver necrosis. Blood transfusions have been recommended.
Stramonium		*See* Atropine	
Strophanthus Ouabain	*	Tannic acid solution, gastric lavage, and magnesium sulfate. Use respirator, and give 'Amytal Sodium' intravenously to control convulsions.	Horizontal position. May give alcohol, ammonia, chloral, or bromide. Be ready with artificial respiration and O_2.
□ **STRYCHNINE** Nux Vomica	1/4–1 grain 0.75 Gm.	If time allows, give 1 pint of warm potassium permanganate (1:1,000), iodine (15 drops of tincture in 1/2 glass of water), or tannic acid solution (1 teaspoonful in 1/2 glass of hot water). Remove immediately from stomach by tube. When convulsions are present, give slowly by vein just enough 'Amytal Sodium' to control the convulsions. This may be repeated at intervals as indicated. Ether, chloroform, or other barbiturates may be employed if at hand.	Give artificial respiration if indicated, and continue to control seizures with 'Amytal Sodium.' Intravenous dextrose may aid in combating collapse.

* Not determined

Poison	Smallest Fatal Dose	Immediate Treatment	Supportive Treatment
Sulfonal Trional	30 grains 30 grains	Treatment as given under Barbiturates.	
Tobacco		*See* Nicotine	
Turpentine	2 oz.	Empty and wash out stomach; follow with demulcents.	Morphine if large dose was taken. Symptomatic stimulation.
□ VERATRUM Veratrine V. viride	1 dr. (fl. ext.)	Give tannic acid solution, wash out stomach, and purge with magnesium sulfate.	Horizontal position; apply external heat, and keep in fresh air. Use caffeine, ammonia, and digitalis for stimulation. Apply artificial respiration if necessary.
□ ZINC SALTS Chloride Sulfate	90 grains 4 dr. ±	Give tannic acid solution, evacuate stomach, and wash out with sodium bicarbonate solution. Follow with lime water, soap, mucilaginous drinks, or milk.	Recumbent position, with application of external heat. Give morphine for pain, treat shock, and stimulate with atropine and caffeine.

Useful Tables

LATIN WORDS AND ABBREVIATIONS

Abbreviation	Latin	Meaning	Abbreviation	Latin	Meaning
aā	ana	of each	. . . .	idem	the same
ad	ad	to, up to	m. dict.	more dicto	in the manner directed
ad lib.	ad libitum	at pleasure			
agit.	agita	shake or stir	non rep.	non repetatur	do not repeat
. . . .	alternis horis	every other hour	omn. hor.	omni hora	every hour
a. c.	ante cibum	before meals	omn. bih.	omni bihorio	every two hours
aq. bull.	aqua bulliens	boiling water	omn. quadr.	omni quadrante	every quarter of
aq. dest.	aqua destillata	distilled water	hor.	horae	an hour
aq. ferv.	aqua fervens	hot water	omn. man.	omni mane	every morning
bib.	bibe	drink	omn. noct.	omni nocte	every night
b. i. d.	bis in die	twice a day	p. ae.	partes aequales	equal parts
cap.	capiat	let him (or her) take	p. c.	post cibum	after eating
chart.	charta	paper	p. r. n.	pro re nata	as needed
c.	cum	with	q. s.	quantum sufficiat	a sufficient quantity
e. m. p.	ex modo prescripto	after the manner prescribed, as directed	ss.	semis	half
			Sig.	signa	let it be marked
			s.	sine	without
f., ft.	fac, fiat, fiant	make, let it be made, let them be made	si op. sit	si opus sit	if necessary
			stat.	statim	immediately
gtt.	gutta	a drop	t. i. d.	ter in die	three times a day
h. s.	hora somni	at bedtime	ut dict.	ut dictum	as directed

WEIGHTS AND MEASURES

The official standard for length, area, and cubic measure in the United States is the International Prototype Meter; other units are derived from this. Similarly, the International Prototype Kilogram is the standard for mass; the liter is a derived unit of capacity or volume, being defined as the volume of one kilogram of water at standard atmospheric pressure and at the temperature of its maximum density (about 4°C.). The meter and the kilogram are by definition independent of each other. Actually, a liter (based on the kilogram) is equal to 1,000.027 cubic centimeters (based on the meter). For practical purposes, however, a milliliter (ml.) can be taken as equal to a cubic centi-

meter (cc.), and a gram of water at room temperature can be regarded, somewhat less accurately, as occupying 1 cc.

Although the metric system is official in the United States Pharmacopoeia and National Formulary and is constantly gaining in usage, the English systems are still employed. Under them, when weight is the basis of calculation, the pharmacist buys and sells all goods, other than those dispensed on prescription, by the avoirdupois system; in dispensing prescriptions, the apothecaries system is used. The U. S. apothecaries (or wine) measure is employed for all statements of volume or capacity under the English systems.

563

METRIC MEASURES OF LENGTH

1 decimeter	(dm.)	= 0.1	meter (M.)
1 centimeter	(cm.)	= 0.01	M.
1 millimeter	(mm.)	= 0.001	M.
1 micron	(μ)	= 0.001	mm.
1 millimicron	(mμ)	= 0.001	μ
1 micromicron	($\mu\mu$)	= 0.001	mμ

METRIC WEIGHTS

1 kilogram	(Kg.)	= 1,000	grams (Gm.)
1 milligram	(mg.)	=	0.001 Gm.
1 microgram (gamma)	(μg; γ)	=	0.001 mg.

METRIC MEASURES OF VOLUME

1 liter	(L.)	= 1,000 milliliters (ml.)
		= 1,000 cubic centimeters (cc.)

AVOIRDUPOIS WEIGHT

1 ounce	(oz.)	= 437.5 grains (grs.)
1 pound	(lb.)	= 16 oz.
		= 7,000 grs.

APOTHECARIES WEIGHT

1 scruple	(Ɔ)	=	20 grains (grs.)
1 drachm	(ʒ)	=	60 grs.
1 ounce	(ʒ)	=	8 ʒ
		=	480 grs.
1 pound	(lb. apoth.)	=	12 ʒ
		=	5,760 grs.

APOTHECARIES (WINE) MEASURE (U.S.)

1 fluidrachm	(fʒ)	=	60 minims (min.) (♏)
1 fluidounce	(fʒ)	=	8 fʒ
		=	480 ♏
1 pint	(pt.) (O.)	=	16 fʒ
		=	7,680 ♏
1 gallon	(Cong.)	=	8 O.

RELATIVE VALUES OF VARIOUS WEIGHTS AND MEASURES

1 gr. (apoth.)	=	1	gr. (avoir.)
	=	0.0648	Gm.
15.43 grs.	=	1	Gm.
16.23 minims (♏)	=	1	cc.
1 fluidrachm (fʒ)	=	3.70	cc.
1 oz. (avoir.)	=	28.35	Gm.
1 ʒ (apoth.)	=	31.10	Gm.
1 fluidounce (fʒ)	=	29.57	cc.
1 lb. (apoth.)	=	373.24	Gm.
1 lb. (avoir.)	=	453.59	Gm.
1 pint	=	473.17	cc.
33.815 fluidounces	=	1	L.
2.11 pts.	=	1	L.
2.205 lb. (avoir.)	=	1	Kg.
1 inch (in.)	=	2.54	cm.
1 foot (ft.)	=	30.48	cm.
0.62 mile	=	1	kilometer (Km.)
1 mile	=	1.61	Km.

Approximate Equivalents

The *approximate* dose equivalents given below represent the quantities which would probably be prescribed under similar conditions by physicians trained respectively in the metric or in the apothecaries system of weights and measures. As such, they have been adopted by the U.S.P. and N.F. *They are not suitable for conversion (1) of specific quantities in a prescription which requires compounding, or (2) of a pharmaceutical formula from one system to another.* For such purposes the *exact* equivalents must be used.

1 quart	1,000	cc.
1 pint	500	cc.
3 fluidounces	100	cc.
1 3/4 fluidounces	50	cc.
1 fluidounce	30	cc.
2 1/2 fluidrachms	10	cc.
1 fluidrachm	4	cc.
15 minims	1	cc.
5 minims	0.3	cc.
3 minims	0.2	cc.
1 minim	0.06	cc.
3/4 minim	0.05	cc.
1 ounce apoth.	30	Gm.
2 1/2 drachms apoth.	10	Gm.
2 drachms apoth.	7.5	Gm.
1 drachm (60 grains)	4	Gm.
15 grains	1	Gm.
12 grains	0.75	Gm.
10 grains	0.6	Gm.
7 1/2 grains	0.5	Gm.
6 grains	0.4	Gm.
4 grains	0.25	Gm.
1 1/2 grains	0.1	Gm.
1 grain	60	mg.
3/4 grain	50	mg.
1/8 grain	8	mg.
1/50 grain	1.2	mg.
1/60 grain	1	mg.

UNOFFICIAL APPROXIMATE EQUIVALENTS

1 glass	250	cc.
1 tablespoonful	15	cc.
1 teaspoonful	5	cc.

NOTE: One drop does not equal one minim. The size of a drop varies with the size and shape of the orifice and of the wall of the tube from which it is dropped, the angle at which the tube is held, the viscosity of the liquid, and possibly other factors.

Molar and Ionic Equivalents

A *mole* (M) is the weight of a substance in grams which is numerically equal to the molecular weight; a mole of any substance must, therefore, contain the same number of molecules, which is estimated to be 6.02×10^{23}. A *millimole* (mM) is one one-thousandth of a mole. A *molar solution* contains one mole (or gram molecular weight) of solute per liter of solution.

An *equivalent weight* is the weight of an atom, radical (group of atoms reacting chemically as a unit), or molecule divided by its valence. The amounts of substances which take part in chemical reactions are always proportional to their equivalent weights. A *milliequivalent* (mEq) is one one-thousandth of an equivalent weight. The values of milliequivalents of various ions per liter in terms of milligrams per 100 cc. are as follows:

	mEq/L.	mg./100 cc.
Hydrogen [H^+]	1	0.1
Sodium [Na^+]	1	2.30
Potassium [K^+]	1	3.91
Calcium [Ca^{++}]	1	2.00
Magnesium [Mg^{++}]	1	1.22
Chloride [Cl^-]	1	3.55
Bicarbonate [HCO_3^-]	1	6.10
Biphosphate [$H_2PO_4^-$]	1	9.70
Phosphate [HPO_4^{--}]	1	4.80
Bisulfate [HSO_4^-]	1	9.71
Sulfate [SO_4^{--}]	1	4.80

Thus, 1 mEq of sodium combines with 1 mEq of chloride to form 1 mM (millimole) of sodium chloride, which will contain 2.30 plus 3.55 or 5.85 mg. sodium chloride per 100 cc. A solution supplying 154 mEq/L. each of sodium and of chloride will contain 154 (2.30 + 3.55) or 900 mg./100 cc., or 0.9 percent sodium chloride.

Percentage Solutions

Percentage concentrations of solutions are expressed as follows:

Percent weight in volume (w/v) expresses the number of grams of an active constituent in 100 cubic centimeters of solution and is used in prescription practice regardless of whether water or some other liquid is the solvent.

Percent volume in volume (v/v) expresses the number of cubic centimeters of an active constituent in 100 cubic centimeters of solution.

Percent weight in weight (w/w) expresses the number of grams of an active constituent in 100 grams of solution.

The U.S.P. XIV specifies: "When per cent is used in prescriptions without qualification, it means: for solutions of solids in liquids, per cent weight in volume; for solutions of liquids in liquids, per cent volume in volume; and for solutions of gases in liquids, per cent weight in volume."

"In dispensing prescriptions, slight changes in volume owing to variations in room temperatures may be disregarded."

COMMON INCOMPATIBILITIES

Physical Incompatibilities most commonly result from either (1) incorporation of immiscible liquids in the same prescription or (2) precipitation of a substance from solution by addition of a liquid in which it is not soluble. Some of these difficulties are discussed below.

1. Mixtures containing oil and water can often be dispensed in the form of a smooth, homogeneous preparation by the use of a gum as an emulsifying agent (see p. 481).

2. Phenol may be made water-soluble by using an amount of glycerin equal to its own volume.

3. When metallic salts are dissolved in medicated waters, an oily separation sometimes develops because of the selective action of the solvent. In some cases it is advisable to remove the oil globules by filtration. In others it may be more desirable to reduce the "salting out" tendency by using more of the solvent and increasing the dose accordingly.

4. Gums, mucilages, and albuminous materials are generally incompatible with strongly alcoholic liquids. Their precipitation can usually be avoided by diluting the alcoholic liquid with water.

5. Precipitation frequently takes place in mixtures containing fluidextracts or tinctures which have widely different alcoholic content. This may involve the separation of active principles that are desirable in the mixture. The proper procedure would obviously be to dispense the entire mixture with a "shake" label. The addition of a small amount of honey or of syrup of acacia often prevents resinous matter from adhering to the sides of the bottle and aids in forming a homogeneous mixture.

6. Liquefaction is likely to occur when certain organic compounds such as camphor, thymol, menthol, or salol are mixed or rubbed together. When

Centigrade and Fahrenheit Equivalents

°C.	°F.	°C.	°F.	°C.	°F.
−25	−13.0	17	62.6	59	138.2
−24	−11.2	18	64.4	60	140.0
−23	− 9.4	19	66.2	61	141.8
−22	− 7.6	20	68.0	62	143.6
−21	− 5.8	21	69.8	63	145.4
−20	− 4.0	22	71.6	64	147.2
−19	− 2.2	23	73.4	65	149.0
−18	− 0.4	24	75.2	66	150.8
−17	+ 1.4	25	77.0	67	152.6
−16	3.2	26	78.8	68	154.4
−15	5.0	27	80.6	69	156.2
−14	6.8	28	82.4	70	158.0
−13	8.6	29	84.2	71	159.8
−12	10.4	30	86.0	72	161.6
−11	12.2	31	87.8	73	163.4
−10	14.0	32	89.6	74	165.2
− 9	15.8	33	91.4	75	167.0
− 8	17.6	34	93.2	76	168.8
− 7	19.4	35	95.0	77	170.6
− 6	21.2	36	96.8	78	172.4
− 5	23.0	37	98.6	79	174.2
− 4	24.8	38	100.4	80	176.0
− 3	26.6	39	102.2	81	177.8
− 2	28.4	40	104.0	82	179.6
− 1	30.2	41	105.8	83	181.4
0	32.0	42	107.6	84	183.2
+ 1	33.8	43	109.4	85	185.0
2	35.6	44	111.2	86	186.8
3	37.4	45	113.0	87	188.6
4	39.2	46	114.8	88	190.4
5	41.0	47	116.6	89	192.2
6	42.8	48	118.4	90	194.0
7	44.6	49	120.2	91	195.8
8	46.4	50	122.0	92	197.6
9	48.2	51	123.8	93	199.4
10	50.0	52	125.6	94	201.2
11	51.8	53	127.4	95	203.0
12	53.6	54	129.2	96	204.8
13	55.4	55	131.0	97	206.6
14	57.2	56	132.8	98	208.4
15	59.0	57	134.6	99	210.2
16	60.8	58	136.4	100	212.0

two or more of these ingredients are used in a mixture which is intended to be in the form of a dry powder, it may be desirable to employ an absorbent powder, such as althea.

7. 'Amytal' dissolves freely in alcohol but is only very sparingly soluble in water. When 'Amytal' is prescribed in a liquid preparation, for example, its solution can be effected only when the proportion of alcohol present is relatively high. The addition of aqueous liquids tends to precipitate the 'Amytal.' For this reason, it is always more desirable to administer 'Amytal' in the form of tablets or in capsules.

8. Physical incompatibilities can very often be avoided by using care in the order of mixing the ingredients. It is always easier to prevent an incompatibility than it is to remedy one that has already taken place. The pharmacist is frequently able to make a presentable mixture containing two or more ingredients that are known to be incompatible by mixing the offending agents with other ingredients in the mixture with which they may be compatible. For example, by bringing the incompatible ingredients together in the form of separate dilutions, advantage may be taken of a certain amount of protective or buffering action which serves to retard their precipitation.

Chemical Incompatibilities always involve some change in the chemical nature of the ingredients. As a general rule, these changes bring about the formation of a precipitate, the evolution of a gas, or a change in the color of the mixture. Some of them are discussed below.

1. Alkaloids generally are precipitated from solutions of their salts by the action of alkalies or by the usual alkaloidal precipitating agents, such as tannic acid, mercuric chloride, or a solution of iodine with potassium iodide. It is good policy to place a "shake well" label on the bottle of a mixture when there is the slightest suspicion that such precipitation may occur, even though the liquid may be perfectly clear at the time it is dispensed.

2. Free acids may cause the separation of sparingly soluble organic acids from solutions of their soluble salts. Sometimes there is sufficient alcohol present to redissolve this precipitate.

3. Free acids also can be expected to liberate gases from solutions containing carbonates, bicarbonates, sulfites, bisulfites, thiosulfates, nitrites, and sulfides.

4. Sodium barbital, sodium phenobarbital, and **'Amytal Sodium'** generally form precipitates in their water solutions upon the addition of an excess of free acid. This is due to the decomposition of the sodium salts and to the separation of free barbital, phenobarbital, or 'Amytal,' all three of which are insoluble in water but soluble in alcohol.

5. Most local anesthetics, such as procaine hydrochloride and 'Metycaine Hydrochloride,' behave like alkaloidal salts and are consequently incompatible with soluble alkalies and with the usual alkaloidal precipitating agents.

6. Aminopyrine frequently gives difficulty in that it forms a sticky mass with acetylsalicylic acid and also with citric, tartaric, and salicylic acids. In solution, aminopyrine often gives pronounced colors, particularly with many oxidizing agents and with acacia.

7. Colloidal silver solutions are made turbid by precipitation when an electrolyte, such as an acid, a base, or a salt, is added to the mixture. For this reason it is advisable not to use other ingredients in aqueous solutions of the various silver proteinates.

8. Ephedrine alkaloid differs from most free alkaloids by being appreciably soluble in water and in the immiscible solvents. For this reason, ephedrine base is not so likely to be precipitated in aqueous solutions by the action of the usual alkaloidal precipitating agents; however, caution should be exercised with complex mixtures and a "shake well" label should be placed on the bottle.

9. Thiamin chloride is extremely soluble in water (1:1) but only slightly in alcohol (1:100). If it is dispensed in liquids, they should be slightly acid; thiamin decomposes rapidly in an alkaline medium.

10. Solution 'Merthiolate' is a carefully adjusted preparation containing mercury in organic combination. Solution 'Merthiolate' is particularly incompatible with acids, salts of the heavy metals, and oxidizing agents in general. Because of its delicate nature, this solution should be prescribed alone rather than with other ingredients.

11. When chloral hydrate is dispensed with soluble salts in a hydroalcoholic solution such as an elixir, an oily layer may separate, consisting of alcohol, chloral, chloral alcoholate, and perhaps some of the dissolved salt, depending on the nature and concentration of the mixture. It is best to direct that such a mixture be well shaken before use, even though no separation may be noted when the mixture is dispensed.

12. Ferric chloride usually gives pronounced color changes with phenol, resorcinol, salicylates, tannic acid, and tannin-containing drugs.

NORMAL HEIGHT—WEIGHT, ½ TO 21 YEARS*

AGE	BOYS		GIRLS		AGE	BOYS		GIRLS	
Years	Height Inches	Weight Pounds	Height Inches	Weight Pounds	Years	Height Inches	Weight Pounds	Height Inches	Weight Pounds
½	26	17	26	16	11	55	75	55	74
1	29	21	29	20	12	57	81	57	82
2	33	26	33	25	13	59	90	60	94
3	36	31	36	30	14	62	103	62	105
4	39	35	39	34	15	64	112	63	112
5	42	38	41	37	16	66	126	64	117
6	45	43	44	43	17	67	133	64	122
7	47	50	47	47	18	68	138	65	124
8	49	55	49	54	19	69	138	65	126
9	51	61	51	60	20	69	139	65	126
10	53	67	53	67					

"IDEAL" WEIGHTS FOR MEN—
AGES 25 AND OVER

"IDEAL" WEIGHTS FOR WOMEN—
AGES 25 AND OVER

(from Metropolitan Life Insurance Co.)

Height (with shoes)		Weight in Pounds (as ordinarily dressed)			Height (with shoes)		Weight in Pounds (as ordinarily dressed)		
		Small Frame	Medium Frame	Large Frame			Small Frame	Medium Frame	Large Frame
Feet	Inches				Feet	Inches			
5	2	116-125	124-133	131-142	4	11	104-111	110-118	117-127
5	3	119-128	127-136	133-144	5	0	105-113	112-120	119-129
5	4	122-132	130-140	137-149	5	1	107-115	114-122	121-131
5	5	126-136	134-144	141-153	5	2	110-118	117-125	124-135
5	6	129-139	137-147	145-157	5	3	113-121	120-128	127-138
5	7	133-143	141-151	149-162	5	4	116-125	124-132	131-142
5	8	136-147	145-156	153-166	5	5	119-128	127-135	133-145
5	9	140-151	149-160	157-170	5	6	123-132	130-140	138-150
5	10	144-155	153-164	161-175	5	7	126-136	134-144	142-154
5	11	148-159	157-168	165-180	5	8	129-139	137-147	145-158
6	0	152-164	161-173	169-185	5	9	133-143	141-151	149-162
6	1	157-169	166-178	174-190	5	10	136-147	145-155	152-166
6	2	163-175	171-184	179-196	5	11	139-150	148-158	155-169
6	3	168-180	176-189	184-202	6	0	141-153	151-163	160-174

GROWTH CHART—BOYS*

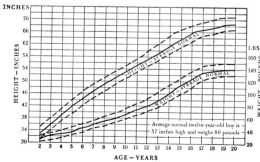

Solid lines indicate average normals; broken lines, 10 percent above or below ideal normals.

GROWTH CHART—GIRLS*

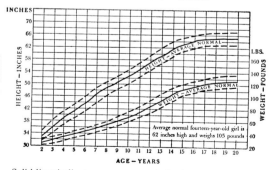

Solid lines indicate average normals; broken lines, 10 percent above or below ideal normals.

* (Reproduced by courtesy of J. H. BARACH, M.D.—Director, Falk Clinic, University of Pittsburgh)

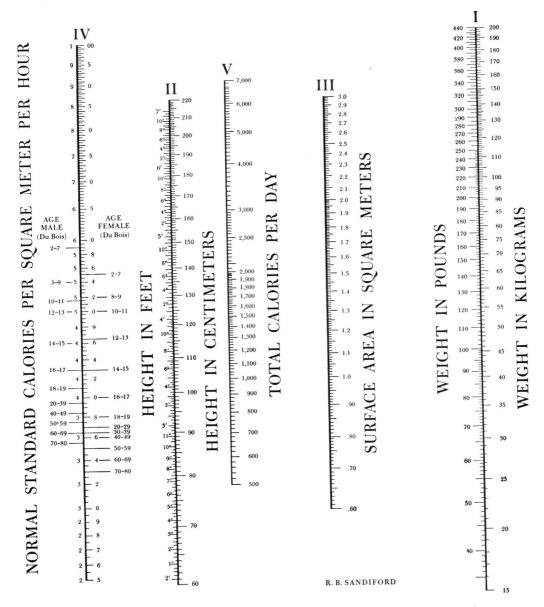

Chart for Determination of Basal Caloric Requirement
(Reprinted by Permission of the Mayo Clinic)

Lay the chart flat. Use only a ruler with a true straight edge. Do not draw lines on the chart, but merely indicate their positions by the straight edge of the ruler. Locate the various points by means of needles (pin stuck through the eraser of a lead pencil). Locate the patient's normal weight on Scale I and his height on Scale II. The ruler joining these two points intersects Scale III at the patient's surface area. Locate the age and sex of the patient on Scale IV. A ruler joining this point with the patient's surface area on Scale III crosses Scale V at the *basal* caloric requirement. For the *maintenance* requirement, 10 to 50 percent of the figure thus obtained is added to that figure.

LIST OF FOODS

Grouped According to Approximate Percentage Composition of Carbohydrate, Protein, and Fat

(Based on Tables of U. S. Department of Agriculture*)

Average Values for Calculation of Carbohydrate, Protein, and Fat of Fruits and Vegetables in the Several Groups (Fresh or Water-Packed)

GROUP	FRUITS				VEGETABLES		
Number	Carbohydrate	Protein	Fat	Cal.	Protein	Fat	Cal.
	%	%	%		%	%	
I	3	1	0.3	12	2	0.3	20
II	6	1	0.3	28	2	0.3	32
III	9	1	0.3	40	3	0.3	50
IV	12	1	0.3	52	4	0.3	64
V	15	1	0.3	64	3	0.3	75
VI	18	1	0.3	76	3	0.3	85

Fresh, canned, and dried fruits and vegetables are included in these lists. A serving is to be considered as the solid portion with its share of liquor from the can. Of the canned fruits, only the water-packed and the juice-packed products come in the six classified groups. Fruits canned in syrup are high in carbohydrate and are therefore placed in the miscellaneous group, where they are listed collectively.

Dried fruits, as such, also come in this miscellaneous group. They average about 67 percent of carbohydrate, but when they are stewed for serving, dilution lowers this figure. If the fruit is cooked without the addition of sugar and with enough water so that the finished product weighs about *four times* as much as the dried fruit used, then the dilution will be such that the cooked fruit may be classified in the 18 percent group.

Dried vegetables, represented by dry legumes and dried corn, fall in the miscellaneous high-carbohydrate group. Even fresh green corn and fresh peas may be placed in this group if they are not sufficiently young. Only *very young* green corn and only *young* or medium peas are low enough in carbohydrate to be included in the classified lists.

Mushrooms and algae are not included in these lists since their content of available carbohydrate is negligible. Avocados, though not high in carbohydrate, are not listed because their fat content is extremely variable and is likely to be very high.

---

* NOTE: If the composition of foods not listed in these tables is desired, please refer to Circular No. 549, U. S. Department of Agriculture. For sale by the Superintendent of Documents, Washington, D. C.—Price, 15 cents.

Vegetables

Group I (Approximately 3% Carbohydrate)

	100 Grams	*Approximate Household Measures*
A 100-Gm. portion contains approximately C 3, P 2, F 0 = 20 Cal.	Asparagus, fr.	10 to 12 stalks—5″ long
	Asparagus, cn.	½ c. tips, drained, or 8 tips
	Bamboo shoots, fr.	¾ c.
	Beans, green or wax, cn.	¾ c.—1″ pieces
	Beet greens, fr.	½ c., ck.
	Broccoli, fr.	3 stalks—5″ long
	Cabbage, fr., raw	1 c., shredded
	Cabbage, fr.	⅔ c., ck.

Vegetables—*continued*

Group I—*continued*

100 Grams	Approximate Household Measures
Cabbage, Chinese, fr., raw	¾ c., sliced
Cauliflower, fr. or cn.	3 sm. clusters or ⅓ sm. head
Celery, fr., raw	2 lg. hearts or 4 stalks
Celery, ck.	⅔ c.
Chard, fr.	⅔ c.
Chicory leaves, fr.	10 to 14 sm. inner leaves
Corn salad, fr.	2 c.
Cress, garden, fr.	2 c.
Cucumber	12 med. slices
Dock, fr.	2 c., raw, or ½ c., ck.
Endive, fr.	2 stalks—5¾″ long
Escarole, fr.	⅔—3″ d.
Fennel, fr.	⅔—3″ d.
Lettuce, fr.	¼—4″ head
Mung bean sprouts, fr.	1 c., scant
Mustard greens, fr.	½ c., ck.
Pokeberry or poke shoots	½ c., ck.
Radishes, fr.	10—1″ d.
Rhubarb, fr. or cn., w.p.	⅔ c.
Sauerkraut, fr. or cn.	¾ c.
Sea kale, fr.	1 c., ck.
Sorrel, fr.	2 c.
Spinach, fr.	½ c., ck.
Spinach, cn.	½ c.
Squash, summer, fr.	½ c., diced, ck.
Tomato, fr., raw	1 med.
Tomatoes, cn.	½ c.
Tomato jc., fr. or cn.	½ gl. or 3⅓ oz.
Turnip tops, fr.	½ c., ck.
Vegetable marrow, fr.	½ to ⅔ c.
Water cress, fr.	1 bunch—3″ long, 3″ d.

Group II (Approximately 6% Carbohydrate)

A 100-Gm. portion contains approximately C 6, P 2, F 0 = 32 Cal.

100 Grams	Approximate Household Measures
Beans, snap, fr., green or wax, fr.	¾ c.—1″ pieces
Carrots, cn.	⅔ c., cubed
Celery root or celeriac, fr.	¾ c., sliced
Chives, fr.	1 c., chopped
Collards, fr.	½ c., ck.
Dandelion greens, fr.	½ c., ck.
Eggplant, fr.	1 c., diced; or 1 slice—4½″ x ½″
Kale, fr.	⅔ c., ck.
Kohlrabi, fr.	½ to ⅔ c., diced
Lamb's-quarters, fr.	½ c., ck.
Leeks, fr.	1 c.—½″ pieces
Okra, fr.	½ c., sliced, or 5 pods
Parsley, fr.	100 av. sprigs
Pepper, green or red, fr.	1 med.
Pumpkin, fr.	½ c., diced
Pumpkin and squash, cn.	½ c., diced
Soybeans, green, shelled, fr.	½ c.
Soybean sprouts, fr.	⅔ c.
Squash, cushaw, fr.	⅘ c., diced
Squash, winter, fr.	⅔ c., ck.
Turnips, fr.	½ c., diced

ABBREVIATIONS: av.—average. C—carbohydrate. c.—cup. ck.—cooked. cn.—canned. d.—diameter. dr.—dried. e.p.—edible portion. F—fat. fr.—fresh. gl.—glass. Gm.—gram. jc.—juice. j.p.—juice-packed. lg.—large. med.—medium. oz.—ounces. P—protein. sm.—small. T.—tablespoon. t.—teaspoon. tk.—thick. tom.—tomato. uns.—unsweetened. veg.—vegetable. w.p.—water-packed.

VEGETABLES—*continued*

Group III (Approximately 9% Carbohydrate)

	100 Grams	*Approximate Household Measures*
A 100-Gm. portion contains approximately C 9, P 3, F 0 = 50 Cal.	Artichoke, globe or French, fr.	1 med.
	Asparagus beans, pods, fr.	1 c.
	Beets, fr. or cn.	½ c., diced
	Brussels sprouts, fr.	6—about 1½″ d.
	Carrots, fr.	⅔ c., sliced
	Onions, fr.	2 to 3 sm. or 1 lg.
	Peas, fr. (very young)	¾ c.
	Peas, cn.	½ c.
	Rutabagas, fr.	½ c., ck.

Group IV (Approximately 12% Carbohydrate)

	100 Grams	*Approximate Household Measures*
A 100-Gm. portion contains approximately C 12, P 4, F 0 = 64 Cal.	Beans, Lima, green, cn.	½ c.

Group V (Approximately 15% Carbohydrate)

	100 Grams	*Approximate Household Measures*
A 100-Gm. portion contains approximately C 15, P 3, F 0 = 75 Cal.	Beans, broad, green, shelled	⅔ c.
	Beans, red kidney, cn.	½ c.
	Corn, fr. (very young)	½ c., ck.
	Jerusalem artichoke, tuber, fr.	1 lg. tuber
	Onions, top, fr.	15 to 20 sm.
	Parsnip, fr.	1 med., or ⅔ c., sliced
	Peas, fr. (med. mature)	⅔ c.
	Salsify, fr.	2—6″ long
	Shallot, fr.	32 sm. bulbs

Group VI (Approximately 18% Carbohydrate)

	100 Grams	*Approximate Household Measures*
A 100-Gm. portion contains approximately C 18, P 3, F 0 = 85 Cal.	Beans, baked, cn.	½ c.
	Corn, sweet, cn.	⅜ c.
	Garlic, fr.	3—1½″ bulbs
	Horse-radish, fr.	20 t.
	Potato, fr.	1 med.—2½″ d.

Fruits

Group I (Approximately 3% Carbohydrate) — None

Group II (Approximately 6% Carbohydrate)

	100 Grams	*Approximate Household Measures*
A 100-Gm. portion contains approximately C 6, P 1, F 0 = 28 Cal.	Blackberries, cn., w.p.	¾ c.
	Cantaloupe	⅓—4½″ d. melon
	Chayote, fruit, fr.	¾ c.
	Gooseberries, cn., w.p.	½ c.
	Honeydew melon	1″ wedge from 7″ d. melon
	Spanish melon	⅓—4½″ d. melon
	Muskmelon	⅓—4½″ d. melon
	Peaches, cn., w.p.	2 med. halves—2½″ d.
	Plums (excluding prunes), cn., w.p.	3 med.
	Strawberries, fr.	⅔ c.
	Strawberries, cn., w.p. or j.p.	½ c.
	Strawberry juice, fr.	½ gl. or 3⅓ oz.
	Watermelon, fr.	e.p.—2½″ x 2½″ x 1″

Fʀᴜɪᴛs — *continued*

Group III (Approximately 9% Carbohydrate)

	100 Grams	*Approximate Household Measures*
A 100-Gm. portion contains approximately C 9, P 1, F 0 = 40 Cal.	Applesauce, cn., uns.	⅜ c.
	Apricots, cn., w.p.	3 med.
	Blackberries, fr.	¾ c.
	Blackberries, cn., j.p.	¾ c.
	Blackberry juice, fr.	½ gl. or 3⅓ oz.
	Blueberries, cn., w.p.	⅔ c.
	Blueberries, cn., j.p.	½ c.
	Cherries, red or white, cn., w.p.	⅔ c.
	Cranberries, fr.	1 c., raw
	Currants, fr.	½ c.
	Currant juice, fr.	½ gl. or 3⅓ oz.
	Gooseberries, fr.	⅔ to 1 c.
	Grapefruit, fr.	½—4″ d.; or ½ c. sections
	Grapefruit, cn., w.p.	½ c. sections
	Grapefruit, cn., j.p.	½ c. sections
	Grapefruit juice, fr.	½ gl. or 3⅓ oz.
	Lemons, fr.	2—2¾″ long (e.p.)
	Lemon juice, fr. or cn.	½ gl. or 3⅓ oz.
	Limes, fr.	3 med. (e.p.)
	Lime juice, fr.	½ gl. or 3⅓ oz.
	Loganberries, cn., w.p.	⅔ c.
	Loganberry juice, fr.	½ gl. or 3⅓ oz.
	Papaya, fr.	¼—5″ d.
	Peaches, cn., j.p.	2 med. halves—2½″ d.
	Pears, cn., w.p.	2 med. halves
	Prunes, cn., w.p.	4 med.
	Quince juice, fr.	½ gl. or 3⅓ oz.
	Raspberries, cn., w.p.	¾ c.
	Tangerines, fr.	2—2″ d.
	Tangerine juice, fr.	½ gl. or 3⅓ oz.

Group IV (Approximately 12% Carbohydrate)

	100 Grams	*Approximate Household Measures*
A 100-Gm. portion contains approximately C 12, P 1, F 0 = 52 Cal.	Apple juice, fr.	½ gl. or 3⅓ oz.
	Applesauce, cn., j.p.	½ c.
	Apricots, fr.	2—1⅝″ d.
	Apricots, cn., j.p.	2—1⅝″ d.
	Apricots, cn., sieved, uns.	½ c.
	Cherries, sour, fr.	⅔ c.
	Cherries, red or white, cn., j.p.	½ c.
	Crab apple juice, fr.	½ gl. or 3⅓ oz.
	Figs, cn., w.p.	4 sm.
	Grapefruit juice, cn., uns.	½ gl. or 3⅓ oz.
	Grapes, cn., w.p.	1 sm. bunch or ⅔ c.
	Guavas, fr.	¾ c. or 10 med.
	Kumquats, fr.	5 med.
	Loganberries, fr.	¾ to 1 c.
	Loganberries, cn., j.p.	½ c.
	Mulberries, fr.	⅔ c.
	Orange, fr.	1 med.—2½″ d.
	Orange juice, fr. or cn.	½ gl. or 3⅓ oz.
	Peach, fr.	1 med.—2½″ d.
	Peach juice, fr.	½ gl. or 3⅓ oz.
	Pears, cn., j.p.	1 med.
	Pineapple, fr. or cn., w.p.	2½ slices—¼″ tk., 3″ d.

ABBREVIATIONS: av.—average. C—carbohydrate. c.—cup. ck.—cooked. cn.—canned. d.—diameter. dr.—dried. e.p.—edible portion. F—fat. fr.—fresh. gl.—glass. Gm.—gram. jc.—juice. j.p.—juice-packed. lg.—large. med.—medium. oz.—ounces. P—protein. sm.—small. T.—tablespoon. t.—teaspoon. tk.—thick. tom.—tomato. uns.—unsweetened. veg.—vegetable. w.p.—water-packed.

FRUITS — *continued*

Group IV— *continued*

100 Grams	*Approximate Household Measures*
Pineapple juice, fr. or cn.	½ gl. or 3⅓ oz.
Plums, fr. (excluding prunes)	3—1½″ d.
Quince, fr.	⅓—3″x2½″
Raspberries, fr.	¾ c.
Raspberries, cn., j.p.	½ c.
Raspberry juice, fr.	½ gl. or 3⅓ oz.

Group V (Approximately 15% Carbohydrate)

A 100-Gm. portion contains approximately C 15, P 1, F 0 = 64 Cal.

100 Grams	*Approximate Household Measures*
Apple, fr.	1—2½″ d.
Blueberries, fr.	⅔ c.
Blueberry juice, fr.	½ gl. or 3⅓ oz.
Cherries, black, cn., w.p.	⅓ c. or 10 lg., pitted
Grapes, fr.	1 av. bunch or 24 grapes
Huckleberries, fr.	⅔ c.
Huckleberry juice, fr.	½ gl. or 3⅓ oz.
Mango, fr.	1 sm.
Nectarines, fr.	2 med.
Papaws, fr.	2—4″ long
Pear, fr.	1 med.
Pineapple, cn., j.p.	2 slices—¼″ tk., 3″ d.

Group VI (Approximately 18% Carbohydrate)

A 100-Gm. portion contains approximately C 18, P 1, F 0 = 76 Cal.

100 Grams	*Approximate Household Measures*
Cherries, sweet, fr.	⅔ c. or 15 cherries
Cherries, black, cn., j.p.	⅓ c. with 1 T. jc.
Crab apples, fr.	2 sm.
Figs, fr.	2 med.—1½″ d.
Grape juice, fr. or bottled	½ gl. or 3⅓ oz.
Persimmon, Japanese	1 lg.
Pomegranate, fr.	⅓—6½″ d.
Prunes, cn., j.p.	3 med. with 1 T. jc.
Prune juice, cn.	½ gl. or 3⅓ oz.

Miscellaneous Group (High Carbohydrate)

100 Grams	*Approximate Household Measures*	C	P	F
Apples, dr.	½ c. packed or 14 sm. halves	73	1	1
Apricots, dr.	½ c. packed or 16 sm. halves	67	5	0
Banana, fr.	1 med.—6″ long (e.p.)	23	1	0
Banana, dr.	10 T.	70	4	0
Beans, broad, dr.	½ c., shelled	58	25	2
Beans, Lima, fr.	⅔ c., shelled	23	7	1
Beans, Lima, dr.	⅔ c.	62	22	1
Beans, soy, dr. seeds	½ c.	12	35	18
Black-eyed peas, dr.	½ c.	62	23	1
Cherries, maraschino, cn.	½ c.	52	0	0
Corn, fr. (med. mature and old)	½ c. or 1 med. 8″ ear	25	4	1
Corn, dr., sweet or field	½ c.	71	11	3
Cowpeas, fr., green, shelled	⅔ c.	23	9	1
Cowpeas, dr.	½ c.	62	23	1
Currants, dr.	½ c.	71	2	0
Dates, fr.	20 med.	66	2	0
Dates, dr.	15 med.	66	2	0
Figs, dr.	6 med.	68	4	1
Lentils, dr., whole or split	½ c.	60	24	1

MISCELLANEOUS GROUP — *continued*

100 Grams	Approximate Household Measures	C	P	F
Peaches, dr.	6—1¾″ d.	69	3	1
Pears, dr.	5 med.	72	2	0
Peas, fr. (mature)	⅔ c., shelled	25	8	0
Peas, dr., whole or split	½ c.	60	24	1
Persimmons, native, fr.	2 sm.	28	1	0
Plantain, or baking banana, fr.	1 sm. (e.p.)	33	1	0
Prunes, fr.	4 med.	20	1	0
Prunes, dr.	12 med.	60	2	1
Raisins, dr.	⅔ c.	71	2	0
Sweet potato, fr.	½ med.	28	2	1
Sweet potato, cn.	1 sm.	31	1	0
Tomato catchup	7 T.	24	2	0
Yam, winged, fr.	1—4½″x1½″	24	2	0

Meat and Poultry, Cooked

This approximate classification includes *cooked* beef, veal, lamb, chicken, turkey, rabbit, pork, and ham.

	Amount in Grams	Approximate Household Measures	C	P	F
Meat and poultry, lean, med. done	60	2 slices—3½″x2½″x¼″	0	18	4
Meat and poultry, med. fat, med. done	60	2 slices—3½″x2½″x¼″	0	16	11
Meat and poultry, fat, med. done	60	2 slices—3½″x2½″x¼″	0	13	18

MISCELLANEOUS MEATS

	Amount in Grams	Approximate Household Measures	C	P	F
Bacon, crisp	15	3 strips—3¼″ long	0	4	8
Beef, dr. and smoked	20	½ c. diced, or 1 av. serving	0	7	1
Bologna, all meat	60	2 slices—4½″ d., ⅛″ tk.	0	8.6	10.7
Bologna, with added cereal	60	2 slices—4½″ d., ⅛″ tk.	2.2	8.9	9.5
Braunschweiger	30	1 slice—3″ d., ¼″ tk.	0	4.6	7.1
Frankfurter, all meat	60	1 av.	0	8.5	12.5
Frankfurter, with added cereal	60	1 av.	2	9.1	8.5
Lamb chop, rib, lean, e.p.	60	1 sm. thin chop	0	10.6	9.4
Liver, raw	100	1 slice—3″x6″x½″	4	19	5
Luncheon meat	30	1 slice—¼″ tk.	0	4.8	7.1
Pork chop, lean, e.p.	60	1 sm. chop, med. fat	0	20	15
Pork sausage, raw	60	1 patty—2″ d., ½″ tk.	0	6.5	27
Salami	60	2 slices—3¼″ d., ¼″ tk.	0	14.3	22
Summer sausage, all types	60	2 slices—3¾″ d., ¼″ tk.	0	14.1	20.9
Veal chop, med. fat, e.p.	90	1 thin chop	0	17.3	9.9
Wieners, all meat	60	2 av.	0	8.5	12.5
Wieners, with added cereal	60	2 av.	2	9.1	8.5

Fish and Sea Foods

	Amount in Grams	Approximate Household Measures	C	P	F
Fish, cooked, broiled, or steamed, lean or med. fat	100	1 piece—4″x2″x½″	0	21	2
fatter fish only	100	1 piece—4″x2″x½″	0	21	11
Oysters, fr.	100	⅓ c., standard	6	10	2
Shrimp, cn.	100	½ c.	1	18	1

ABBREVIATIONS: av.—average. C—carbohydrate. c.—cup. ck.—cooked. cn.—canned. d.—diameter. dr.—dried. e.p.—edible portion. F—fat. fr.—fresh. gl.—glass. Gm.—gram. jc.—juice. j.p.—juice-packed. lg.—large. med.—medium. oz.—ounces. P—protein. sm.—small. T.—tablespoon. t.—teaspoon. tk.—thick. tom.—tomato. uns.—unsweetened. veg.—vegetable. w.p.—water-packed.

Soybeans

	Amount in Grams	Approximate Household Measures	C	P	F
*Soybeans, fr., edible varieties, e.p.	100	⅔ c.	6	12.5	6.5
*Soybeans, dr., edible varieties	100	½ c.	12	34.9	18.1
*Soybeans, dr., edible varieties, ck.	100	½ c.	4	11.6	6.1

* Soybeans as marketed at present are really by-products of the oil production process and contain only 5 to 6 percent of the original 20 percent (*J. Am. Dietet. A., 19*:36, 1943).

Oils and Fats

	Amount in Grams	Approximate Household Measures	C	P	F
Butter	10	1 pat or 2 t.	0	0	8
Cooking fats	14	1 T.	0	0	14
Mayonnaise	10	2 t.	0	0	8
Oleomargarine	10	1 pat or 2 t.	0	0	8
Salad oils, pure	10	2 t.	0	0	10

Cereals and Cereal Products

	Amount in Grams	Approximate Household Measures	C	P	F
Bread, av.	100	3⅓ av. slices	50	8.9	2.4
Bread, av.	30	1 av. slice	15	3	1
Cereal, av., dry	100	13⅓ T., dry measure	75.9	10.7	2.3
i.e., oatmeal	20	2⅔ T. dry, or scant ½ c. ck.	15	2	0
Cereal, prepared:					
Bran flakes	15	1 c.	10	1	0
Corn flakes	15	1 c.	11	2	0
Puffed rice	15	¾ c.	12.5	1	0.4
Puffed wheat	15	¾ c.	11.3	2	0.3
Rice Krispies	20	⅔ c.	17.7	1.2	0
Shredded wheat	30	1 biscuit	24.5	2.3	0.3
Crackers, graham	10	1 cracker	7.4	0.8	0.2
Crackers, saltines	8	1 double saltine	5.7	0.7	0.9
Crackers, soda	3	1—2″ square	2.2	0.3	0.3
Hominy, ck.	100	½ c.	14.9	1.8	0.2
Macaroni, ck.	100	½ c.	19.4	3.7	0.4
Noodles, ck.	100	½ c.	19.4	3.7	0.4
Rice, ck.	100	½ c.	23.2	2.2	0.1
†Ry-Krisp	6	1 wafer	4.8	0.8	0.1
Spaghetti, ck.	100	½ c.	19.4	3.7	0.4
Zwieback	8	1—3¼″x1¼″x½″	5.9	0.9	0.7

† Analysis made by the manufacturer.

Dairy Products

	Amount in Grams	Approximate Household Measures	C	P	F
Buttermilk, genuine	200	1 gl.	9.2	7	1
Buttermilk, artificial culture	200	1 gl.	10	7	0.4
Cheese, American Cheddar	30	1 slice—3½″x2½″x⅛″	0.5	7.2	9.7
Cheese, cottage, skim	30	2 T.	1.3	5.7	0.2
Cheese, Philadelphia cream	30	⅓ package	0.3	3.4	11.3
Cheese, Swiss-processed	30	1 slice—3″x3″x⅛″	0.5	7.1	7.8
Cream, coffee, 20% fat	30	1 oz. or 2 T.	1.2	0.9	6
Cream, whipping, 35% fat	30	1 oz. or 2 T.	1	0.7	11
Egg, white, e.p.	34	1 av.	0.3	3.7	0
Egg, whole, e.p.	50	1 av.	0.3	6.4	5.7
Egg, yolk, e.p.	16	1 av.	0.1	2.6	5.1
Milk, evaporated	100	½ gl.	10	7	8
Milk, malted, powder	100	10 T.	71	15	8
Milk, skim	200	1 gl.	10	7	0.4
Milk, whole	200	1 gl.	10	7	8

Nuts

	Amount in Grams	Approximate Household Measures	C	P	F
Almonds	10	9 to 10 nuts (e.p.)	2	1.9	5.4
Brazil nuts	30	4 to 5 nuts (e.p.)	3.3	4.3	19.8
Cashews	15	10 nuts (e.p.)	4	3	7
Chestnuts	35	7 to 8 nuts (e.p.)	14.5	0.4	0.2
Coconut, fr.	35	1 slice—2"x2"x½" (e.p.)	4.9	1.1	12.1
Coconut, dr.	20	2 T. or ¼ c. (e.p.)	10.6	0.7	7.8
Peanuts	30	25 nuts (e.p.)	7	8	13.3
Peanut butter	15	1 T.	3	4	7.2
Pecans	15	4 to 5 nuts (e.p.)	2	1.4	11
Pistachios	15	15 nuts (e.p.)	2.8	2.9	8
Walnuts, California, soft-shell	15	9 halves (e.p.)	2.3	2.2	9.6
Walnuts, California, black	15	9 halves (e.p.)	2.8	2.7	8.7

Miscellaneous

	Amount in Grams	Approximate Household Measures	C	P	F
*Beef juice	30	1 oz. or 2 T.	0	1.5	0
Beer, 4% alcohol	240	1 c. or 8 oz.	10	0	0
Bouillon cube	4	1	0	0.2	0.1
Catchup	25	1 T.	6.6	0.5	0
Chili sauce	25	1 T.	5.9	0.7	0
Chocolate, sweet	30	1 square	18	0.6	8.9
Chocolate, uns.	30	1 square	5.4	1.6	15.9
Cocoa, dry, uns.	8	1 T.	2.5	0.7	1.5
Coca-Cola	180	1 bottle	14.4	0	0
Corn syrup	30	2 T.	22.2	0	0
Dextrose or glucose	30	2 T.	29.9	0	0
Gelatin, granulated, dry	3	1 t.	0	3	0
Ginger ale	200	1 gl.	18	0	0
Honey, strained	30	1⅓ T.	23.8	0	0
Jello, dry	5	1 t.	4.4	0.5	0
Jelly	30	1⅔ T.	19.5	0	0
Lactose	30	3 T.	29.9	0	0
Mustard, prepared	15	1 T.	0.5	0.6	1
Olives, green	30	5 to 6	1.2	0.4	4
Olives, ripe	30	5 to 6	0.9	0.5	6
Pickles, sour	40	1 T., sliced	0.8	0.2	0
Popcorn, popped	25	1½ c.	19.4	2.8	1.3
Sugar, cane or beet	30	2 T.	29.9	0	0
Vinegar	15	1 T.	0.7	0	0
Yeast, compressed	15	1 cake	2	2	0
*Yeast, Fleischmann's	15	1 cake	1.2	2.1	0.1

* Bridges, M. A.: *Dietetics for the Clinician*, Ed. 3. Philadelphia: Lea & Febiger, 1937.

ABBREVIATIONS: av.—average. C—carbohydrate. c.—cup. ck.—cooked. cn.—canned. d.—diameter. dr.—dried. e.p.—edible portion. F—fat. fr.—fresh. gl.—glass. Gm.—gram. jc.—juice. j.p.—juice-packed. lg.—large. med.—medium. oz.—ounces. P—protein. sm.—small. T.—tablespoon. t.—teaspoon. tk.—thick. tom.—tomato. uns.—unsweetened. veg.—vegetable. w.p.—water-packed.

EQUIVALENTS AND SUBSTITUTES

Substitution of certain foods is necessary because of (1) inability to obtain the food listed in the menu; (2) dislike for that kind of food; (3) idiosyncrasy to the item listed; (4) a desire to prevent monotony.

The following lists of foods or combinations of foods are approximately equivalent in carbohydrate, protein, and fat content to some article that appears frequently in the menus.

These equivalents are selected for their equality in carbohydrates, proteins, fats, and calories but not necessarily for equality in bulk or in vitamin and mineral content. In making substitutions, therefore, care should be exercised that the diet does not become too low in vitamin and mineral content, or too concentrated in bulk. In general, bulky foods, that

is, foods with low percentages of C, P, and F, can be measured with greater accuracy than more concentrated foods. A given error in weighing a food containing 50 percent carbohydrate will be ten times as serious as the same error made in weighing a food containing 5 percent carbohydrate.

APPROXIMATE MEASURE EQUIVALENTS FRUITS AND VEGETABLES

100 Gm. 3% (see Approximate Household Measures) = 1/2 approximate measure of 100 Gm. 6% = 1/3 approximate measure of 100 Gm. 9% = 1/4 approximate measure of 100 Gm. 12% = 1/5 approximate measure of 100 Gm. 15% = 1/6 approximate measure of 100 Gm. 18%.

APPROXIMATE EQUIVALENTS OF FRUITS AND VEGETABLES*

100 Gm.	GROUP I 3%	GROUP II 6%	GROUP III 9%	GROUP IV 12%	GROUP V 15%	GROUP VI 18%
Group I, 3%		50	34	25	20	18
Group II, 6%	200		70	50	40	35
Group III, 9%	300	150		75	60	50
Group IV, 12%	400	200	130		80	70
Group V, 15%	500	250	170	125		85
Group VI, 18%	600	300	200	150	120	
Household measure specified	See approximate equivalents	½	⅓	¼	⅕	⅙

* See lists of vegetables and fruits for approximate household measures.

Food Equivalent Tables

Cereals—Approximate Equivalents of 10 Gm. Cereal
C 8, P 1, F 1

	Amount in Grams	Approximate Household Measures
Cream of wheat	10	1 T. uncooked, or ¼ c. ck.
Farina	10	1 T. uncooked, or ¼ c. ck.
Ralston	10	1 T. uncooked, or ¼ c. ck.
Rice	10	⅔ T. uncooked, or ¼ c. ck.
Oatmeal	10	1⅓ T. uncooked, or ¼ c. ck.
Corn flakes	10	½ c.
Puffed wheat	10	⅔ c.
Puffed rice	10	1 c.
Shredded wheat	10	⅓ lg. biscuit
Rice Krispies	10	⅓ c.
40% Bran Flakes	10	¼ c.
Bread	10	½ slice
6% Fruit	130	See Group II list of fruits
9% Fruit	90	See Group III list of fruits
12% Fruit	70	See Group IV list of fruits
15% Fruit	55	See Group V list of fruits

Approximate Equivalents of 30 Gm. Bread
C 15, P 3, F 1

	Amount in Grams	Approximate Household Measures
Cereal.........................	20	2 times the amount of any of the cereals (see cereal list, 10-Gm. portions)
18% vegetable or 18% fruit...........	80	See Group VI vegetable or fruit list for equivalent measure
15% vegetable or 15% fruit...........	100	See Group V vegetable or fruit list for equivalent measure
12% vegetable or 12% fruit...........	125	See Group IV vegetable or fruit list for equivalent measure
9% vegetable or 9% fruit.............	170	See Group III vegetable or fruit list for equivalent measure
6% vegetable or 6% fruit.............	250	See Group II vegetable or fruit list for equivalent measure
Apricots, dr........................	25	4 sm. halves
Banana.............................	65	½ med.
Dates, dr...........................	20	2
Figs, fr.............................	75	2½
Figs, dr.............................	20	1½
Figs, cn., w.p.......................	100	3
Peaches, dr.........................	21	3 halves
Pears, dr...........................	21	1¼ halves
Prunes, dr..........................	25	2 med.
Prunes, fr...........................	70	2¾ med. (e.p.)
Raisins, seeded or seedless...........	21	1 scant T.
Beans, dr. (navy, kidney, pinto, Lima, dr. peas, and others)................	25	⅙ c. dr., or ½ scant c. ck.
Lima beans, fr.......................	60	⅓ c. or 2½ T.
Lentils, dr., whole and split...........	25	⅛ scant c. dr., or ½ scant c. ck.
Sweet potato........................	55	1½ full T., or ½ sm. (e.p.)
Tomato catchup.....................	60	3 T.
Crackers, soda......................	20	6⅔
Saltines............................	20	2½—4″x2″
Ry-Krisp...........................	19	3 wafers
Crackers, Ritz......................	25	7
Rice, ck............................	70	½ c.
Macaroni, ck., or plain noodles........	80	⅓ c.
Potato chips........................	30	20 lg. pieces, *minus* 12 Gm. (2½ t.) butter or fat
Milk...............................	100	½ gl. or 3⅓ oz., *plus* 100 Gm. 9% fruit, *minus* 1 scant t. butter

Approximate Equivalents of One Egg
C 0, P 6, F 6

	Amount in Grams	Approximate Household Measures
Cheese, American...................	20	1 slice—3¼″x2½″x⅛″
Cheese, Philadelphia cream...........	60	⅔ pkg., *minus* 19 Gm. (4 t.) butter or fat
Cheese, Swiss.......................	30	1½ slices—3¼″x2½″x⅛″, *minus* 3 Gm. (½ t.) butter or fat
Cheese, cottage, creamed.............	30	2 T., *plus* 5 Gm. (1 t.) butter or fat
Milk	180	1 gl. (6 oz.), *minus* 75 Gm. 12% fruit (see Group IV list of fruits)
Meat, lean.........................	20	⅔ oz., *plus* 5 Gm. (1 t.) butter (see list of meats)
Fish, fr., baked or broiled..........	30	1 slice—2″x2″x½″, or 1 oz., *plus* 3 Gm. (½ t.) butter or fat
Fish, boiled or steamed..............	30	1 slice—2″x2″x½″, or 1 oz., lean or med. fat, *plus* 6 Gm. (1 full t.) butter or fat
Fish, boiled or steamed.............	30	1 slice—2″x2″x½″, or 1 oz., fatter fish only, *plus* 3 Gm. (½ t.) butter or fat
Tuna fish, cn., with or without added oil.	30	⅙ c. flaked, or 1 piece—1″x1″x1″, or 1 oz., *plus* 4 Gm. (1 scant t.) butter or fat
Salmon, cn..........................	30	¼ scant c. flaked, or 1 oz., *plus* 4 Gm. (1 scant t.) butter or fat
Sardines, cn. in oil..................	20	2, each 3″ long, *plus* 5 Gm. (1 t.) butter or fat

ABBREVIATIONS: av.—average. C—carbohydrate. c.—cup. ck.—cooked. cn.—canned. d.—diameter. dr.—dried. e.p.—edible portion. F—fat. fr.—fresh. gl.—glass. Gm.—gram. jc.—juice. j.p.—juice-packed. lg.—large. med.—medium. oz.—ounces. P—protein. sm.—small. T.—tablespoon. t.—teaspoon. tk.—thick. tom.—tomato. uns.—unsweetened. veg.—vegetable. w.p.—water-packed.

Approximate Equivalents of One Egg — *continued*
C 0, P 6, F 6

	Amount in Grams	*Approximate Household Measure*
Oysters...........................	60	3 med., *plus* 6 Gm. (1 full t.) butter or fat
Crab meat........................	40	¼ scant c. flaked, *plus* 5 Gm. (1 t.) butter or fat
Shrimp, cn. or cooked...............	40	3 to 5, or ½ c., *plus* 8 Gm. (1½ t.) butter or fat
Bacon, crisp......................	25	5 strips—3¼″ long, *minus* 30 Gm. (2 T.) butter or fat
Peanuts, roasted...................	22	22 to 23, no skins, *minus* 5 Gm. (1 t.) butter or fat and *minus* 45 Gm. 12% fruit (see Group IV list of fruits)
Peanut butter.....................	23	1½ T., *minus* 6 Gm. (1 full t.) butter or fat and *minus* 40 Gm. 12% fruit (see Group IV list of fruits)
Walnuts, black.......	33	18 halves, *minus* 16 Gm. (1 full T.) butter or fat and *minus* 50 Gm. 12% fruit (see Group IV list of fruits)
Walnuts, English....................	40	24 halves, or 3⅓ T. chopped, *minus* 25 Gm. (1⅔ T.) butter or fat and *minus* 50 Gm. 12% fruit (see Group IV list of fruits)
Cashews..........................	30	16 to 20 med., *minus* 17 Gm. (3½ t.) butter or fat and *minus* 65 Gm. 12% fruit (see Group IV list of fruits)

Approximate Equivalents of 30 Gm. Cooked Lean Meat
C 0, P 9, F 2

	Amount in Grams	*Approximate Household Measures*
Beef, veal, or lamb, lean, ck............	30	1 thin slice—3½″x2½″x¼″
Lamb chop, lean.....................	60	1 thin, *minus* 8 Gm. (1½ t.) butter
Pork chop, lean.....................	30	½ sm., *minus* 5 Gm. (1 t.) butter
Veal chop, lean.....................	30	1 sm.
Pork, fr., or smoked ham, lean........	30	1 thin slice—2½″x1½″x¼″
Chicken, turkey, rabbit, fowl (roast, lean)	30	1 slice—3½″x2½″x¼″
Sausage, fat cooked out..............	30	1½—each 3″ long x ¾″ d.
Bologna...........................	30	2 slices—2⅛″ d., ⅓″ tk., *minus* 10 Gm. (2 t.) butter
Wieners	60	2
Frankfurter........................	60	1, *minus* 10 Gm. (2 t.) butter
Liver, raw.........................	50	1 slice—3″x3″x½″
Heart.............................	30	1 slice—2″x1″x½″
Sweetbreads.......................	30	1 piece—2½″x1″x¾″, or ¼ c.
Bacon, crisp.......................	36	7 strips—3¼″ long, *minus* 22 Gm. (1½ T.) butter or fat
Beef, dr..........................	27	5 slices—3½″x7½″, or ⅔ c. diced
Beef, corned, cn., med. fat............	36	1 slice—3½″x3″x¼″, or 1¼ oz., *minus* 3 Gm. (½ t.) butter or fat
Beef, corned, fr., lean...............	50	1⅔ slices—3½″x3″x½″, *minus* 5 Gm. (1 t.) butter or fat
Eggs.............................	75	1½, *minus* 9 Gm. (2 scant t.) butter or fat
Cheese, American...................	40	2 slices—3¼″x2½″x⅛″, *minus* 12 Gm. (2½ t.) butter or fat
Cheese, Philadelphia cream...........	90	1 pkg., 3 oz., *minus* 38 Gm. (2 T. and 1½ t.) butter or fat
Cheese, cottage, creamed.............	45	3 level T.
Cheese, Swiss......................	40	1 slice—3¼″x3¼″x¼″, *minus* 10 Gm. (2 t.) butter or fat
Milk, whole.......................	255	8½ oz., *minus* 12 Gm. (2½ t.) butter or fat, *minus* 100 Gm. 12% fruit (see Group IV list of fruits)
Fish, fr., baked or broiled............	40	1 slice—2″x3″x½″, *minus* 4 Gm. (1 scant t.) butter or fat
Fish, steamed or boiled, lean or med. fat.	40	1 slice—2″x3″x½″
Fish, boiled or steamed, fatter fish only..	40	1 slice—2″x3″x½″, *minus* 4 Gm. (1 scant t.) butter or fat
Tuna fish, cn., with or without added oil..	40	⅓ c. flaked, *minus* 6 Gm. (1 full t.) butter or fat
Salmon, cn.........................	45	⅓ c. flaked, or 1½ oz., *minus* 3 Gm. (½ t.) butter or fat
Sardines, cn. in oil..................	35	3½, each 3″ long, *minus* 3 Gm. (½ t.) butter or fat
Oysters...........................	90	4 to 5 med.
Crab meat.........................	55	⅓ c. flaked
Shrimp, ck. or cn....................	50	4 to 7, *plus* 3 Gm. (½ t.) butter or fat
Peanuts, roasted....................	33	33 to 34, no skins, *minus* 15 Gm. (1 T.) butter or fat, *minus* 75 Gm. 12% fruit (see Group IV list of fruits)
Peanut butter......................	34	2¼ T., *minus* 17 Gm. (3½ t.) butter or fat, *minus* 60 Gm. 12% fruit (see Group IV list of fruits)

Approximate Equivalents of 20 Gm. American Cheese
C 0, P 5, F 6

Equal approximately one egg or any of the equivalents of one egg.

Approximate Equivalents of 30 Gm. American Cheese
C 0, P 7, F 10

	Amount in Grams	Approximate Household Measures
Egg..........................	50	1, *plus* 5 Gm. (1 t.) butter or fat
Cheese, Philadelphia cream...........	30	⅓ pkg., *plus* 1 egg (9 Gm.) or 2 scant t. butter
Cheese, Swiss......................	30	1½ slices—3¼"x2½"x⅛", *plus* 3 Gm. (½ t.) butter or fat
Cheese, cottage, creamed.............	35	2⅓ T., *plus* 10 Gm. (2 t.) butter or fat
Milk..........................	200	6⅔ oz., *plus* 3 Gm. (½ t.) butter or fat, *minus* 85 Gm. 12% fruit (see Group IV list of fruits)
Meat, lean........................	25	⅚ oz., *plus* 10 Gm. (2 t.) butter or fat
Fish, baked or broiled...............	30	1 slice—2"x2"x½", or 1 oz., *plus* 8 Gm. (1½ t.) butter or fat
Fish, boiled or steamed, lean or med. fat..	30	1 slice—2"x2"x½", or 1 oz., *plus* 11 Gm. (2 full t.) butter or fat
Fish, boiled or steamed, fatter fish only..	30	1 slice—2"x2"x½", or 1 oz., *plus* 9 Gm. (2 scant t.) butter or fat
Fish, tuna, cn., with or without added oil.	30	⅙ scant c. flaked, or 1 piece—1"x1"x1", or 1 oz., *plus* 9 Gm. (2 scant t.) butter or fat
Salmon, cn........................	35	¼ c. flaked, or 1⅙ oz., *plus* 9 Gm. (2 scant t.) butter or fat
Sardines, cn. in oil..................	30	3, each 3" long, *plus* 9 Gm. (2 scant t.) butter or fat
Oysters...........................	70	3½ med., *plus* 11 Gm. (2 full t.) butter or fat
Crab meat........................	45	¼ c. flaked, *plus* 11 Gm. (2 full t.) butter or fat
Shrimp, ck. or cn....................	40	3 to 5, or ½ c., *plus* 12 Gm. (2½ t.) butter or fat
Bacon, crisp.......................	30	6 strips—3¼" long, *minus* 7 Gm. (1½ t.) butter or fat
Peanuts, roasted....................	35	37 to 38 nuts, no skins, *minus* 6 Gm. (1 full t.) butter or fat
Peanut butter......................	28	2 scant T., *minus* 5 Gm. (1 t.) butter or fat
Walnuts, black.....................	40	21 halves, *minus* 16 Gm. (1 full T.) butter or fat
Walnuts, English...................	45	24 to 30 halves, or 3¾ T. chopped, *minus* 23 Gm. (4½ t.) butter or fat
Nuts, cashew......................	35	18 to 20 med., *minus* 8 Gm. (1½ t.) butter or fat

Approximate Equivalents of 40 Gm. American Cheese
C 0, P 9, F 12

	Amount in Grams	Approximate Household Measures
Meat, lean........................	30	1 oz., *plus* 12 Gm. (2½ t.) butter or fat; or equivalents of 30 Gm. of meat
Eggs..........................	75	1½, *minus* 4 Gm. (1 scant t.) butter or fat; or 1½ times the equivalents of 1 egg

Approximate Equivalents of 200 Gm. Milk
C 10, P 7, F 8

	Amount in Grams	Approximate Household Measures
Egg..........................	50	1, *plus* 85 Gm. 12% fruit (see Group IV list of fruits), *plus* 3 Gm. (½ t.) butter or fat
Milk, skim.........................	200	6⅔ oz., *plus* 10 Gm. (2 t.) butter or fat
Bacon, crisp.......................	28	5½ strips—3¼" long, *minus* 9 Gm. (2 scant t.) butter or fat, *plus* 85 Gm. 12% fruit (see Group IV list of fruits)
Cheese, American..................	30	1½ slices—3¼"x2½"x⅛", *minus* 3 Gm. (½ t.) butter or fat, *plus* 85 Gm. 12% fruit (see Group IV list of fruits)
Cheese, cottage, creamed.............	36	2¼ T., *plus* 10 Gm. (2 t.) butter or fat, *plus* 85 Gm. 12% fruit (see Group IV list of fruits)

ABBREVIATIONS: av.—average. C—carbohydrate. c.—cup. ck.—cooked. cn.—canned. d.—diameter. dr.—dried. e.p.—edible portion. F—fat. fr.—fresh. gl.—glass. Gm.—gram. jc.—juice. j.p.—juice-packed. lg.—large. med.—medium. oz.—ounces. P—protein. sm.—small. T.—tablespoon. t.—teaspoon. tk.—thick. tom.—tomato. uns.—unsweetened. veg.—vegetable. w.p.—water-packed.

Approximate Equivalents of 10 Gm. Bacon
C 0, P 2, F 5

	Amount in Grams	Approximate Household Measures
Egg	20	⅓, plus 4 Gm. (1 scant t.) butter or fat
Cream, coffee	30	2 t.
Cheese, American	10	1 slice—3¼"x1"x⅛", plus 3 Gm. (½ t.) butter or fat

One-third of any of the equivalents of one egg.

Approximate Equivalents of 30 Gm. Coffee Cream
C 1, P 1, F 16

	Amount in Grams	Approximate Household Measures
Milk	30	2 T., plus 6 Gm. (1 full t.) butter or fat
Bacon, crisp	5	1 strip—3¼" long, plus 4 Gm. (1 scant t.) butter or fat

Approximate Equivalents of 50 Gm. Coffee Cream
C 2, P 1, F 10

	Amount in Grams	Approximate Household Measures
Milk	50	1⅔ oz., or 3⅓ T., plus 10 Gm. (2 t.) butter or fat
Bacon	5	1 strip—3¼" long, plus one soda cracker, plus 10 Gm. (2 t.) butter or fat

DIETS

Daily Protein Intake for Normal Adult (154 lb., 70 Kg.)

	Protein Content, in Gm.
16 oz. whole cow's milk* (or 8 oz. condensed milk or 5 T. dried skim milk)	15
3 oz. meat, poultry, or fish (or 1 1/2 oz. soybean flour or 5 oz. [3/4 c.] cooked soybeans)	18
1 egg (or 1 oz. American or cottage cheese)	6
3 oz. (1/2 c.) cooked peas, navy beans, or Lima beans (or 2/3 oz. [1 1/2 T.] peanut butter or 1/4 c. cooked soybeans)	6
3 oz. (1/2 c.) potato	2
3 servings vegetables (including one green leafy or yellow)	3
2 servings fruit (including one citrus or tomato)	2
6 slices enriched or whole-grain bread†	18
	70

The above foods provide the basic requirement of 70 Gm. protein. They are to be divided appropriately among the three daily meals.

* 1 serving (4 oz.) milk pudding or ice cream equals 3 oz. fluid milk.

† 1 slice of bread is equivalent in protein content to 1 oz. cereal (dry weight), 1/2 c. cooked spaghetti or noodles, 6 soda crackers, 1 sm. piece cake, a 2-in. cube of corn bread, or 3 graham crackers.

Low-Calorie Diet

The low-calorie diet is intended to yield less energy than the individual dissipates, so that body fat will be oxidized to make up the difference. Such a diet should be low in fat and concentrated carbohydrate and rather high in protein (1 Gm. per kilo-gram of "ideal" weight—not actual weight). In order to fill the stomach and induce a feeling of satiety, ample quantities of leafy vegetables and the less sweet fruits are allowed. A sample day's menu follows; it can be modified as desired.

Meals	Gm.	Household Measures	C	P	F
Breakfast					
Orange or equivalent..............	100	1 med.—2½″ d..........	12	1	0
Cereal (see table, p. 578)..........	10		8	1	1
Skim milk.......................	180	¾ c.....................	9	6	0
Egg............................	50	1 med..................	0	6	6
Cream (20%)....................	15	1 T.....................	0	1	3
Coffee or tea (uns.)................		1 c.....................	0	0	0
			29	15	10
Luncheon					
Vegetable soup*..................	200	1 c.....................	3	1	0
Cottage cheese...................	30	2 T.....................	1	6	0
Group I vegetable................	100	(see p. 570).............	3	2	0
Lean meat.......................	60	2 slices—3½″x2½″x¼″....	0	18	4
Group II fruit....................	150	(see p. 572).............	9	1	0
Tea or coffee (uns.)...............			0	0	0
			16	28	4
Dinner					
Broth (fat-free)..................	100	½ c.....................	0	2	0
Lean meat.......................	60	2 slices—3½″x2½″x¼″....	0	18	4
Group I vegetable................	100	(see p. 570).............	3	2	0
Salad—					
Group I vegetable..............	100		3	2	0
Group II vegetable or equivalent...	50	(see p. 571).............	3	1	0
Vinegar dressing..................			0	0	0
Bread or equivalent (see table, p. 579).	30	1 slice..................	15	3	1
Group II fruit....................	100	(see p. 572).............	6	1	0
Tea or coffee (uns.)..............			0	0	0
			30	29	5
Total for the day, Gm.............			75	72	19
Calories.........................			300	288	171
Total calories....................					759

* Made by cooking Group I vegetables in fat-free broth.

ABBREVIATIONS: av.—average. C—carbohydrate. c.—cup. ck.—cooked. cn.—canned. d.—diameter. dr.—dried. e.p.—edible portion. F—fat. fr.—fresh. gl.—glass. Gm.—gram. jc.—juice. j.p.—juice-packed. lg.—large. med.—medium. oz.—ounces. P—protein. sm.—small. T.—tablespoon. t.—teaspoon. tk.—thick. tom.—tomato. uns.—unsweetened. veg.—vegetable. w.p.—water-packed.

High-Calorie Diet

The purpose of the high-calorie diet is to provide a high caloric intake in a relatively small bulk.

The emphasis is therefore on fat and concentrated carbohydrate. A sample day's menu follows.

Meals	Gm.	Household Measures	C	P	F
Breakfast					
Banana or equivalent (see p. 579).....		1 med.—6″ long (e.p.).....	23	1	0
Cereal (see table, p. 578)............	20		16	2	2
Sugar.............................	20	4 t......................	20	0	0
Cream (20%).....................	60	4 T......................	2	2	12
Bacon, crisp.......................	15	3 strips—3¼″ long........	0	4	8
Eggs..............................	100	2 med....................	0	13	11
Toast.............................	30	1 slice...................	15	3	1
Butter............................	20	2 pats or 4 t.............	0	0	16
Jelly..............................	12	1 T.....................	8	0	0
Coffee or tea......................			0	0	0
			84	25	50
Midmorning Lunch					
Orange juice......................	200	1 c......................	24	2	0
Sugar............................	10	2 t......................	10	0	0
			34	2	0
Noon Lunch					
Salad					
Cheese, Philadelphia cream........	30	2 T......................	0	3	11
Pineapple......................	80	2 slices—¼″ tk., 3″ d......	10	1	0
Mayonnaise....................	15	3 t......................	0	0	12
Lettuce.......................	50	⅛ head..................	1	0	0
Bread....	30	1 slice...................	15	3	1
Butter............................	20	2 pats or 4 t.............	0	0	16
Egg or protein equivalent (see p. 579).	50	1 med....................	0	6	6
Group V vegetable................	100	(see p. 572)..............	15	3	0
Group VI fruit...................	150	(see p. 574)..............	27	2	0
Milk.............................	200	1 c......................	10	7	8
Cream (20%).....................	60	4 T......................	2	2	12
			80	27	66
Midafternoon Lunch					
Orange juice.....................	200	1 c......................	24	2	0
Sugar............................	10	2 t......................	10	0	0
			34	2	0
Dinner					
Meat, med. fat....................	120	4 slices—3½″x2½″x¼″....	0	32	22
Potato............................	100	1 med.—2½″ d...........	18	3	0
Salad.............................	50		2	0	0
Mayonnaise.......................	10	2 t......................	0	0	8
Bread............................	30	1 slice...................	15	3	1
Butter............................	20	2 pats or 4 t.............	0	0	16
Ice cream.........................	85	¼ pint..................	22	5	12
Cake.............................	60	2″x2″x3″................	35	4	9
			92	47	68
Bedtime Lunch					
Milk.............................	200	1 c......................	10	7	8
Graham crackers..................	20	2........................	15	1	0
			25	8	8
Total for the day, Gm.............			349	111	192
Calories...........................			1,396	444	1,728
Total calories......................					3,568

Low-Residue Diet

The low-residue diet is most commonly employed as a temporary measure to minimize peristalsis and to reduce the bulk of the intestinal contents in intestinal disease or in connection with operations on the intestines. Any desired degree of reduction can be achieved by suitable restriction of the kind and quantity of food. Supplements of vitamins and minerals may be indicated in diets of extremely low residue.

Foods of little residue are listed below, beginning with those producing least residue:

> Lean meat (but avoid connective tissue which cannot be chewed up)
> Gelatin
> Concentrated broth
> Rice (polished)
> Hard-cooked egg
> Sugars (except lactose)
> Fruit and vegetable juices, tea, coffee (small amounts)
> Cottage cheese
> Refined cereal

Cellulose, fats, and calcium salts produce a large residue. The following foods are to be taken sparingly because of their high residue:

> Fruits
> Potato
> Bread
> Butter
> Lard
> Swiss cheese
> Soft-cooked egg
> Raw egg white
> Milk
> Lactose
> Any food containing obvious roughage

Low-Sodium Diet

A diet low in sodium may be indicated in generalized edema from any cause, for localized edema such as is thought to occur in Ménière's syndrome, and in some cases of cardiovascular disease without edema. Suggested below are menu plans which will provide daily sodium intakes of not more than 0.5, 1, and 1.5 Gm. respectively.

Certain **general rules** should be explained to patients:

1. Because no food is completely free of sodium, quantitative limits are placed on most allowed foods, and the patient must take no food, beverage, or medication not authorized by the physician.

2. The following are absolutely forbidden. They are not to be taken by themselves, added to food, or used in cooking:

> Ordinary table salt (sodium chloride)
> Baking soda (sodium bicarbonate)
> Saline laxatives
> Effervescent powders
> Symptomatic remedies for colds, headache, rheumatism, and the like, unless known to be free of sodium

3. If the patient's drinking water contains more than 0.1 Gm. of sodium per liter (10 mg. per 100 cc.), he should drink only distilled or deionized water. (Information on the sodium content of public water supplies can usually be obtained from the local health department.) If these precautions are followed, the patient can take water, tea, and coffee as desired.

4. Vegetables should be fresh or frozen, not canned. They may be served raw or cooked without salt. A pressure cooker helps to preserve natural flavor and make salt-free vegetables more palatable.

5. Meat (from the diet list only!) should be baked, roasted, broiled, or boiled without salt.

6. In place of ordinary salt, the patient may, at the discretion of the physician, add to his food at the table potassium chloride, ammonium chloride, or Neo-Curtasal.

7. Sugar, clear jellies, and salt-free butter may be used as desired and are consequently not listed under menu plans. The physician may wish to add clear, hard sugar candies and soft drinks such as Coca-Cola and ginger ale (but not prepared or alkaline waters for mixed drinks).

Foods Allowed

FRUITS

> *Group I*—100-Gm. portions containing 1 mg. sodium or less
> Apple, 1 sm. (without skin)
> Apricots, 2 (without skin)
> Banana, 1 med.
> Blackberries, ½ c.
> Blueberries, ½ c.
> Dates, 3
> Grapefruit, ½ med. or ½ c. sections
> Grapefruit juice, ½ c.
> Lemon, 1 med.
> Orange, 1 med. or ½ c. sections
> Orange juice, ½ c.
> Peaches, 2 halves

ABBREVIATIONS: av.—average. C—carbohydrate. c.—cup. ck.—cooked. cn.—canned. d.—diameter. dr.—dried. e.p.—edible portion. F—fat. fr.—fresh. gl.—glass. Gm.—gram. jc.—juice. j.p.—juice-packed. lg.—large. med.—medium. oz.—ounces. P—protein. sm.—small. T.—tablespoon. t.—teaspoon. tk.—thick. tom.—tomato. uns.—unsweetened. veg.—vegetable. w.p.—water-packed.

Pineapple, 1¾ slices or ½ c.
Plums, 2 (without skin)
Raspberries, ½ c.
Rhubarb, 1 c.
Strawberries, ¾ c.

Group II—100-Gm. portions containing 5 mg.
  sodium or less
Grapes, 16
Pear, 1 (without skin)
Prunes, 3
Tangerine, 1 med.

VEGETABLES

Group I—100-Gm. portions containing 1 mg.
  sodium or less
Beans, great northern, green, or Lima, ½ c.
Corn, ½ c. or 1 med. ear
Cucumber, 12 slices
Eggplant, ½ c.
Okra, ½ c.
Onions, 2 med.
Peas, ½ c.
Pepper, green, fr., 1 med.
Potato, white, 1 med. or ½ c. (without skin)
Pumpkin, ½ c.
Squash, ½ c.

Group II—100-Gm. portions containing 3 mg.
  sodium or less
Cabbage, 1 c.
Mushrooms, ½ c.
Parsnips, ½ c.
Potato, sweet, 1 med. or ½ c.
Tomato, fr., 1 med. or ½ c.

Group III—100-Gm. portions containing 12 to
  35 mg. sodium
Broccoli, ⅔ c.
Brussels sprouts, ⅔ c.
Carrots, ½ c.
Cauliflower, ⅔ c.
Lettuce, ¼ head

MEATS—Each portion containing about 65 mg.
  sodium
Roast beef, 4 slices—3½″ × 2½″ × ¼″
Beefsteak, 3″ × 2″ × 1″
Lamb chop, 1 sm. thin chop
Roast lamb, 2 slices—3½″ × 2½″ × ¼″
Veal cutlet, 1 med.
Roast veal, 4 slices—3½″ × 2½″ × ¼″
Beef patties, 2 sm.
Chicken, white meat, 3 slices—
  3½″ × 2½″ × ¼″
Turkey, white meat, 3 slices—4″ × 3″ × ⅓″

CEREALS—Each portion containing about 1 mg.
  sodium
Cream of wheat, ½ c.
Wheatena, ½ c.
Farina (not enriched), ½ c.
Oatmeal, ½ c.
Macaroni or spaghetti, ½ c.
Noodles, ½ c.
Rice, ½ c.

MISCELLANEOUS
Egg, 1—70 mg. sodium
Bread, salt-free, 1 slice—10 mg. sodium
Bread, whole wheat, 1 slice—130 mg. sodium
Cream, 4 T. or ¼ c.—25 mg. sodium
Milk, 1 gl.—105 mg. sodium

Menu Plan to contain not more than 0.5 Gm. sodium
  per day

BREAKFAST
Fruit, Group I, 1 portion
Cereal, 1 portion
Salt-free bread, 1 slice*
Egg, 1
Cream, ½ c.
Coffee or tea

LUNCH
Meat, 1 portion
Macaroni, rice, or noodles, 1 portion
Vegetable, Group I, 1 portion
Vegetable, Group II, 1 portion
Salt-free bread, 1 slice*
Fruit, Group II, 1 portion (or 2 portions from
  Group I)
Coffee or tea

DINNER
Meat, 1 portion
Potato, white, 1 portion
Vegetable, Group I, 1 portion
Vegetable, Group II, 1 portion
Salt-free bread, 1 slice*
Fruit, Group I, 1 portion
Milk, 1 gl.

If desired, 1 portion of Group I fruit may be
  taken in the afternoon and at bedtime.

---

* Salt-free bread can be made in the home by using a yeast
roll recipe, substituting vegetable shortening for lard, and
water or dialyzed milk (Lonalac) for ordinary milk. Salt
is omitted. One average-sized roll is equivalent to one
slice of bread.